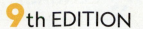
9th EDITION

SIMMERS
DHO
CAREER EXPLORATION AND SKILL DEVELOPMENT
Health Science

Louise Simmers, BSN, MEd, RN

Karen Simmers-Nartker, BSN, RN

Sharon Simmers-Kobelak, BBA

Janet Fuller

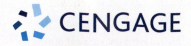

Australia • Brazil • Canada • Mexico • Singapore • United Kingdom • United States

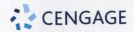

Acknowledgments

Grateful acknowledgment is given to the authors, artists, photographers, museums, publishers, and agents for permission to reprint copyrighted material. Every effort has been made to secure the appropriate permission. If any omissions have been made or if corrections are required, please contact the Publisher.

Photographic Credits

Cover: SCIEPRO/SCIENCE PHOTO LIBRARY/Getty Images.

For product information and technology assistance, contact us at Customer & Sales Support, 888-915-3276

For permission to use material from this text or product, submit all requests online at
www.cengage.com/permissions

Further permissions questions can be emailed to
permissionrequest@cengage.com

National Geographic Learning | Cengage
200 Pier 4 Blvd., Suite 400
Boston, MA 02210

National Geographic Learning, a Cengage company, is a provider of quality core and supplemental educational materials for the PreK–12, adult education, and ELT markets. Cengage is a leading provider of customized learning solutions with employees residing in nearly 40 different countries and sales in more than 125 countries around the world. Find your local representative at **NGL.Cengage.com/RepFinder**

Visit National Geographic Learning online at **NGL.Cengage.com**

ISBN: 978-0-357-41999-1

Printed in the United States of America
Print Number: 03   Print Year: 2022

CONTENTS

PART 1 — BASIC HEALTH CARE CONCEPTS AND SKILLS — 1

CHAPTER 1 — HISTORY AND TRENDS OF HEALTH CARE — 2

CHAPTER 2 — HEALTH CARE SYSTEMS — 26

CHAPTER 3 — CAREERS IN HEALTH CARE — 42

PREFACE

DHO Health Science, ninth edition, was written to provide the beginning student in health science education (HSE) with the basic entry-level knowledge and skills required for a variety of health care careers. Although each specific health care career requires specialized knowledge and skills, some knowledge and skills are applicable to many different health careers. In short, this book was developed to provide the core knowledge and skills that can be used in many different fields.

Health care is in a state of constant change. The scientific foundation presented in this textbook is required in over 200 different health care careers. *DHO Health Science,* together with *Body Structures and Functions and Medical Terminology,* provides a thorough introduction to the health sciences.

ORGANIZATION OF TEXT

DHO Health Science, ninth edition, is divided into two main parts. **Part 1** provides the student with the basic knowledge and skills required for many different health care careers. **Part 2** introduces the student to basic entry-level skills required for some specific health care careers. Each part is subdivided into chapters.

Chapter Organization

Each chapter has a list of learning objectives and a list of key terms (with pronunciations for more difficult words). For each skill included in the text, both the knowledge necessary for the skill and the procedure to perform the skill are provided. By understanding the principles and the procedure, the student will develop a deeper understanding of why certain things are done and will be able to perform more competently. Procedures may vary slightly depending on the type of agency and on the kind of equipment and supplies used. By understanding the underlying principles, however, the student can adapt the procedure as necessary and still observe correct technique.

Information Sections (Textbook): The initial numbered sections for each topic in this text are information sections that provide the basic knowledge the student must acquire. These sections explain why the knowledge is important, the basic facts regarding the particular topic, and how this information is applied in various health care careers. Most information sections refer the student to the assignment sheets found in the student workbook.

Assignment Sheets (Workbook or MindTap): After students have read the information in the initial section of a topic, they are instructed to go to the corresponding assignment sheet. The assignment sheets allow them to test their comprehension and to return to the information section to check their answers. This enables them to reinforce their understanding of the information presented prior to moving on to another information section.

Procedure Sections (Textbook) The procedure sections provide step-by-step instructions on how to perform specific procedures. The student follows the steps while practicing the procedures. Each procedure begins with a list of the necessary equipment and supplies. The terms *Note, Caution,* and *Checkpoint* may appear within the procedure. **Note** urges careful reading of the comments that follow. These comments usually stress points of knowledge or explain why certain techniques are used. **Caution** indicates that a safety factor is involved and that students should proceed carefully while doing the step in order to avoid injuring themselves or a patient. **Checkpoints** at the end of each section alert teachers to check in with how students are processing the information. **Final Evaluations** alert students to ask the instructor to check their work at that point in the procedure. Each procedure section refers the student to a specific evaluation sheet in the workbook.

Evaluation Sheets (Workbook or MindTap): Each evaluation sheet contains a list of criteria on which the student's performance will be tested after they have mastered a particular procedure. When a student feels they mastered a particular procedure, they sign the evaluation sheet and give it to the instructor. The instructor can grade the student's performance by using the listed criteria and checking each step against actual performance.

Because regulations vary from state to state regulating which procedures can be performed by a student in health science education, it is important to check the specific regulations for your state. A health care worker should never perform any procedure without checking legal responsibilities. In addition, a student should not perform a procedure unless the student has been properly taught the procedure and has been authorized to perform it.

Special Features

- The text material covers the *National Health Care Foundation Standards*, helping instructors implement the curriculum elements of this important document. An appendix provides a table showing the correlation of chapters in the book to the *National Health Care Foundation Standards*.

- Mandates of the Health Insurance Portability and Accountability Act (HIPAA) have been incorporated throughout the textbook to emphasize the student's responsibilities in regard to this act.

- Learning objectives, included in every chapter, help focus the student on content discussed in the chapter.

- Review questions and activities are at the end of each chapter to enable the student to test their knowledge of information provided in the chapter.

- Career information has been updated and is stressed throughout the textbook to provide current information on a wide variety of health care careers. Careers have been organized according to the National Health Science Career Clusters. Several new careers have been added.

- Additional emphasis has been placed on cultural diversity, technological advances, legal responsibilities, new federal legislation pertaining to health care providers, infection control standards, and safety.

- Various icons have been included throughout the textbook. These icons denote the integration of academics, such as math, science, and communication; occupational safety issues, such as standard precautions; federal requirements such as HIPAA, electronic health records (EHRs), and OBRA; and workplace readiness issues such as career, legal, and technology information. The icons and their meaning are as follows:

 Observe Standard Precautions

 Instructor's Check—Call Instructor at This Point

 Safety—Proceed with Caution

 OBRA Requirement—Based on Federal Law for Nurse Assistants

 Math Skill

 Legal Responsibility

 Science Skill

 Career Information

 Communications Skill

 Technology

 Health Insurance Portability and Accountability Act

 Electronic Health Records

Enhanced Content New to the Ninth Edition

- Case Study Investigations and Case Study Investigation Conclusions offer a real-life scenario of a patient's medical case and are located at the beginning and end of each chapter. Students instantly connect skills they will learn throughout the chapter to real patients and review new concepts to re-analyze the case after the chapter reading.

- Issues in Health Care have been added to discuss timely topics from our modern-day culture. Topics such as telemedicine present an insight into the ever-changing world of health care.

- Critical Thinking questions have been added to the end of each chapter to give students an opportunity to further investigate the content and topics taught within the chapter.

- Activities give students the opportunity to use active learning and work in small groups to practice skills featured in the chapter from preparing a classroom debate and conducting research to lively competitions as students solve real-world problems and synthesize key terms.

- 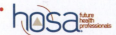 The HOSA Connection highlights HOSA competitive events that correspond with chapter content. This textbook is listed as the recommended resource for nine competitions including Health Science Events, Knowledge Tests, Health Professions Events, Emergency Preparedness Events and HOSA Bowl.

EXTENSIVE TEACHING AND LEARNING PACKAGE

DHO Health Science, ninth edition, has a complete and specially designed supplement package to enhance student learning and workplace preparation. It is also designed to assist instructors in planning and implementing their instructional programs for the most efficient use of time and resources. The package contains the following instructor and student support materials.

DHO Health Science, Ninth Edition, Instructor's Manual

The online *Instructor's Manual* provides easy-to-find answers to questions found in the *Student Workbook*. New to this edition are answers to the end-of-chapter review questions found in the textbook.

DHO Health Science, Ninth Edition, Student Workbook

ISBN-13: 9780357646434
This workbook, updated to reflect the *DHO Health Science* ninth edition text, contains perforated, performance-based assignment and evaluation sheets. The assignment sheets help students review what they have learned. The evaluation sheets provide criteria or standards for judging student performance for each procedure in the text.

Instructor Companion Website to Accompany *DHO Health Science*, Ninth Edition

Everything you need for your course in one place! This collection of product-specific lecture and class tools is available online via the instructor resource center. You will be able to access and download materials such as PowerPoint® presentations, lesson plans, solution files, Precision Exams Correlations, and more.

Components include:

- Teacher's Resource Kit offers a complete guide to implementing a *DHO Health Science* course. The kit explains how to apply content to applied academics and the *National Health Care Foundation Standards*.
- *Cognero®, Customizable Test Bank Generator* is a flexible, online system that allows you to import, edit, and manipulate content from the text's test bank or elsewhere, including your own favorite test questions; create multiple test versions in an instant; and deliver tests from your Learning Management System, your classroom, or wherever you want.

- Teacher support slides created in PowerPoint® supporting the text for use in classroom lectures
- Online Instructor's Manual in PDF format
- Multimedia animations narrating difficult-to-visualize anatomical and physiological processes, including "The Anatomy of a Cell," "The Process of Hearing," "Blood Flow Through the Heart," and much more
- A comprehensive guide maps the textbook content to the *National Consortium for Health Science Education's National Healthcare Foundation Standards and Accountability Criteria*

Download your resources at companion-sites.cengage.com.

Don't have an account? Request access from your Sales Consultant, ngl.cengage.com/repfinder.

Visit us at ngl.cengage.com/cte.

MindTap to accompany *DHO Health Science*, Ninth Edition ✦ MINDTAP

ISBN-13: 9780357646458
MindTap for *DHO Health Science*, ninth edition is the online learning solution for career and technical education courses that helps teachers engage and transform today's students into critical thinkers. Through paths of dynamic assignments and applications that you can personalize, real-time course analytics, and an interactive eBook, MindTap helps teachers organize and engage students. Every MindTap course includes data analytics with engagement tracking as well as student tools, such as flashcards, practice quizzes, auto-graded homework, and tests.

Whether you teach this course in the classroom or in hybrid/e-learning models, MindTap for *DHO Health Science*, ninth edition enhances the course experience with *Learning Lab Simulations* for career exploration, health careers, critical thinking, and foundational skills like infection control, anatomy & physiology, medical terminology, and more. Gain insight into student knowledge and skill competency before you get hands-on in the lab as students work through video-based, real-world scenarios in clinics and make decisions using E.H.R. resources, talking to colleagues, and gain feedback from their clinic administrator.

The *Career Exploration Learning Lab for DHO Health Science* introduces health science students to the variety of health care career paths available to them. Using video simulations that follow a young, seriously injured patient from an accident scene through all aspects of required health care to home care, the student is exposed to 31 primary careers and various additional related careers. From the patient's point of view, the student watches video segments of each primary professional that offer a glimpse of the health care professional's role in the care of the young patient. Students are introduced to career paths that require various levels of education and training and offer a variety of salary ranges—careers that range from phlebotomist to occupational therapist to psychiatrist. Accompanying career profile screens offer interview videos for each primary career and provide basic information such as duties and responsibilities, career attributes, and educational and certification requirements.

Teachers and students who have adopted MindTap can access their courses at nglsync.cengage.com. Request access from your Sales Consultant, ngl.cengage.com/repfinder.

Additional Student Resources

Audio podcasts of medical terminology and animations are available for download at companion-sites.cengage.com. Search by author last name, book title, or 13-digit ISBN to access these bonus resources available with the textbook. Look for the Free Materials tab.

This edition of *DHO Health Science* is aligned to Precision Exams' *Health Sciences* Career Cluster exams listed below, and with the *National Health Science Certificate* sponsored by NCHSE (National Consortium for Health Educators). Precision Exams' standards are validated by industry, allowing students to earn a certification that connects skills taught in the classroom to a future profession, creating a successful transition

from high school to college and/or career. Working together, Precision Exams and National Geographic Learning, a part of Cengage, focus on preparing students for the workforce, with exams and content that are kept up to date and relevant to today's jobs.

PRECISION EXAMS
by youscience

DHO Health Science correlates to the following Precision Exams:

- Medical Assistant: Medical Office Management;

- Medical Assistant: Clinical and Laboratory Procedures;

- Medical Assistant: Anatomy & Physiology;

- Medical Anatomy: Anatomy & Physiology;

- Dental Assistant: Dental Science I & II;

- Health Science Fundamentals;

- Medical Terminology; and

- Medical Assistant: Medical Terminology,

To access the corresponding correlation guides, visit the accompanying Online Instructor Companion Website for this title in NGLsync or at companion-sites.cengage.com. For more information on how to administer the *DHO Health Science* exam or to gain access to any of the 180+ Precision Exams, contact your local NGL/Cengage Sales Consultant. You can find your rep at ngl.cengage.com/repfinder.

HOW TO USE
THIS TEXTBOOK

LEARNING OBJECTIVES

Review these goals before you begin reading a chapter to help you focus your study. Then, when you have completed the chapter, go back and review these goals to see if you have grasped the key points of the chapter.

▪ LEARNING OBJECTIVES

After completing this chapter, you should be able to:

- Describe at least eight types of private health care facilities.
- Analyze at least three government health services agencies and the services offered by each.
- Describe at least three services offered by voluntary or nonprofit agencies.
- Explain the purpose of organizational structures in health care facilities.

ICONS

Icons are used throughout the text to highlight specific pieces of information. An icon key is presented at the beginning of each part to reinforce the meaning of the icons.

 Precaution   Science Check   Safety OBRA HIPAA

 Math Legal   Career 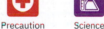 Comm   Technology   EHR

KEY TERMS

Key terms highlight the critical vocabulary words you will need to learn. Pronunciations are also included for the harder-to-pronounce words. These terms are highlighted within the text where they are defined. You will also find most of these terms listed in the Glossary section. Use this listing as part of your study and review of critical terms.

▪ KEY TERMS

Agency for Healthcare Research and Quality (AHRQ)
assisted living facilities
Centers for Disease Control and Prevention (CDC)
clinics
concierge medicine
dental offices
emergency care services
fee-for-service compensation
Food and Drug Administration (FDA)
genetic counseling centers

health departments
health insurance plans
Health Insurance Portability and Accountability Act (HIPAA)
health maintenance organizations (HMOs)
home health care
hospice
hospitals
independent living facilities
industrial health care centers
laboratories

long-term care facilities (LTCs or LTCFs)
managed care
Medicaid
medical offices
Medicare
Medigap policy
mental health facilities
National Institutes of Health (NIH)
nonprofit agencies
Occupational Safety and Health Administration (OSHA)

TODAY'S RESEARCH: TOMORROW'S HEALTH CARE AND ISSUES IN HEALTH CARE

Today's Research: Tomorrow's Health Care and *Issues in Health Care* boxes are located in each chapter. These commentaries help you learn about the many different types of research occurring today. If the research is successful, it may lead to possible cures and/ or better methods of treatment in the future for a wide range of diseases and disorders. These boxes of information also highlight the fact that health care changes constantly because of new ideas and technology.

Today's Research | **Tomorrow's** Health Care

Nature as a Pharmacy?

Throughout history, many medicines have been derived from natural resources. Examples include aspirin, which comes from willow bark; penicillin, which comes from fungus; and the cancer drug Taxol, which comes from the Pacific yew tree. Recognizing this, many scientists believe that nature is a pharmaceutical gold mine and are exploring the vast supply of materials present in the oceans and on the earth.

The National Cancer Institute (NCI) has more than 50,000 samples of plants and 10,000 samples of marine organisms stored in Frederick, Maryland. Every sample is crushed into a powder and made into extracts that can be tested against human cancer cells. More than 110,000 extracts of these samples are available to other scientists who evaluate their effectiveness against conditions such as viral diseases and infections. To date, more than 4,000 extracts have shown promise and are being used in more advanced studies. One compound, Halichondrin B, labeled "yellow slimy" by researchers, is an extract taken from a deep-sea sponge found in New Zealand. Scientists created a synthetic version of the active component in Halichondrin B, called E7389. After extensive testing, the drug Eribulin, which was created from this compound, was approved by the FDA in 2010 as a treatment for metastatic breast cancer. Bristol-Myers received FDA approval for another drug, Ixabepilone, that is extracted from garden soil bacteria and is also used to treat metastatic breast cancer. Wyeth's drug Rapamune was isolated from soil on Easter Island and approved for preventing kidney rejection after transplants. Another novel drug involves photodynamic activity. A substance called psoralen is obtained from a Nile-dwelling weed called ammi. Psoralen is inactive until it is exposed to light. When it is activated, it attaches to the DNA of cancer cells and kills them. Research led to the approval of a psoralen-like drug that is exposed to certain wavelengths of light and used to treat some forms of lymphoma, a cancer of white blood cells. By creating synthetic versions of the compounds, scientists are preserving natural resources while also benefiting from them.

RELATED HEALTH CAREERS

Related Health Careers appear in Chapter 7, *Anatomy and Physiology*, and in other chapters that contain information related to specific careers. By reviewing the information presented in these boxes, you will relate specific health careers to specific body systems or chapter content.

Related Health Careers

- Activity director
- Assisted living administrator
- Biogerontologists
- Geriatric aide
- Geriatric case manager
- Geriatric counselor

CAREER HIGHLIGHTS

Career Highlights appear in the Special Health Care Skills chapters. By reading and understanding the material presented in these boxes, you will learn the educational requirements of each profession, potential places of employment, and additional tasks you may have to perform that are not specifically discussed within the chapter.

Career Highlights

Dental assistants work under the supervision of doctors called dentists, and they are important members of the dental health care team. Educational requirements vary from state to state, but can include on-the-job training, one- or two-year health science education programs, and/or an associate's degree.

 Legal Certification is available through the Dental Assisting National Board (DANB) after an individual has graduated from a Commission on Dental Accreditation (CODA)–accredited program of dental assisting or has met the requirements established in their state for completing a specific number of hours of work experience in a period of two years of full-time or four years of part-time employment as a dental assistant. The duties of dental assistants vary depending on the size and type of practice, and on the dental practice laws of the state in which they work. Each state has a dental practice act that governs which duties dental assistants can perform under the scope of practice. It is the responsibility of the dental assistant to know and follow the state regulations. In addition to the knowledge and skills presented in this chapter, dental assistants must also learn and master skills such as:

- Presenting a professional appearance and attitude
- Obtaining knowledge regarding health care delivery systems, organizational structure, and teamwork
- Meeting all legal responsibilities
- Communicating effectively

- Being sensitive to and respecting cultural diversity
- Comprehending human anatomy, physiology, and pathophysiology with an emphasis on oral anatomy and physiology
- Observing all safety precautions

FULL-COLOR PHOTOS AND ILLUSTRATIONS

Illustrations are presented in full color and demonstrate important health care concepts, including the inner workings of the body. Use these illustrations for review while studying.

Full-color photos are used throughout the text to illustrate important techniques you will be required to know and demonstrate when working within a health care field.

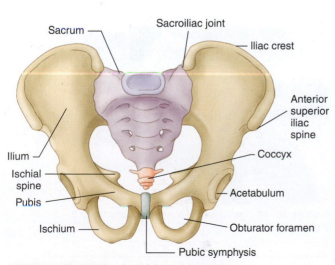

FIGURE 7–22 Anterior view of the pelvic girdle.

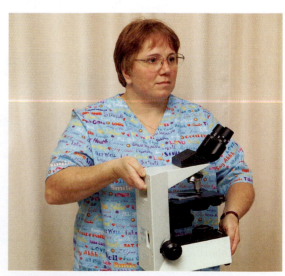

FIGURE 20–3 To carry a microscope, place one hand firmly on the arm and the other hand under the base.

PROCEDURE SECTIONS

Procedure sections provide step-by-step instructions on how to perform the procedure outlined in the initial information section at the start of each topic. Practice these procedures until you perform them correctly and proficiently.

Procedure 20:1

Operating the Microscope

Equipment and Supplies

Microscope; lens paper; slide and coverslip; hair, paper, or other small object; drop of water; immersion oil; gloves for a biological specimen

Procedure

1. Assemble equipment.

2. Wash hands. Put on gloves if needed.

    CAUTION: Wear gloves and observe standard precautions while handling any specimen contaminated by blood or body fluids, or while examining pathogenic organisms. If splashing of the specimen is possible, wear a gown, mask or face shield, and eye protection.

3. Use a prepared slide or get a clean slide. Place a human hair, shred of paper, or other small object on the slide. Add a drop of water or normal saline. Cover with a clean coverslip by holding the coverslip at an angle and allowing it to drop on the specimen.

   NOTE: Make sure there are no air bubbles between the slide and coverslip. If air bubbles are present, remove the coverslip and position it again.

4. Use lens paper to clean the eyepiece (ocular viewpiece) and the objectives (**Figure 20–4A**).

    CAUTION: Do not use any other material to clean these surfaces. Towels, rags, and tissues can scratch these surfaces.

5. Turn on the illuminating light. Open the iris diaphragm so that the largest hole is located directly under the hole in the stage platform.

6. Turn the revolving nosepiece until the low-power objective clicks into place.

7. Place the slide on the stage. Fasten it with the slide clips (**Figure 20–4B**).

   NOTE: Avoid getting fingerprints or smudges on the slide.

8. Watch the stage and slide. Turn the coarse adjustment so that the objective moves down close to the slide.

    CAUTION: Do not look into the eyepiece while moving the objective down. The objective could crack the slide and/or be damaged.

9. Now, look through the eyepiece. Slowly turn the body tube upward until the object comes into focus.

10. Change to the fine adjustment. Turn the knob slowly until the object comes into its sharpest focus (**Figure 20–4C**).

11. Do the following while still using low power:

    a. Move the slide to the right while looking through the eyepiece. In which direction does the image move?

    b. Move the slide to the left. In which direction does the image move?

    c. Open and close the iris diaphragm. How does this affect the image?

12. Without moving the body tube, turn the revolving nosepiece until the high-power objective is in place. Focus with the fine adjustment only.

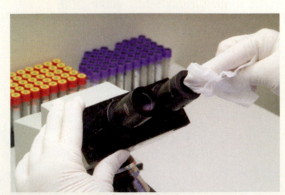

FIGURE 20–4A Use lens paper to clean the eyepiece and objectives.

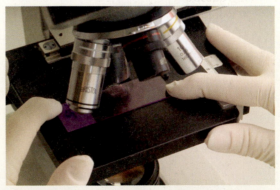

FIGURE 20–4B Place the slide on the stage and fasten it in place with the slide clips.

HOSA CONNECTION

HOSA Connections are included to offer you an insight as to how the content will prepare you for HOSA competitive events.

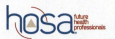 | CONNECTION

Pathophysiology

Purpose: To encourage HOSA members to improve their ability to identify, spell, define and apply the prefixes, suffixes, roots, anatomy and physiology of human diseases impacting the health community.

Description: This event shall be a written test requiring competitors to apply, analyze, synthesize, and evaluate information related to pathophysiology. Competitors will recognize, identify, define, interpret, and apply terms related to human diseases and conditions in a 100-item multiple choice test plus one tiebreaker essay question. Written test will measure knowledge and understanding at the recall, and application.

Details of this competitive event may be found at www.hosa.org/guidelines

REVIEW QUESTIONS

Review Questions enhance your comprehension of chapter content. After you have completed the chapter reading, try to answer the review questions at the end of the chapter. If you find yourself unable to answer the questions, go back and review the chapter again.

■ REVIEW QUESTIONS

1. Differentiate between antisepsis, disinfection, and sterilization.

2. List the five (5) essential times for handwashing as identified by the World health Organization (WHO).

3. Name the different types of personal protective equipment (PPE) and state when each type must be worn to meet the requirements of standard precautions.

4. What level of infection control is achieved by an ultrasonic cleaner? Chemicals? An autoclave?

CRITICAL THINKING

Critical Thinking questions offer you the ability to build upon the content learned throughout the chapter. You will form greater knowledge by investigating complementary topics.

■ CRITICAL THINKING

1. Josh Merkowski is a pharmacist that has been found guilty of falsifying drug records at the pharmacy. He has also revealed that he is addicted to Vicodin. Investigate industry standards for substance abuse related to health care providers. Based on these facts, write a report predicting Dr. Merkowski's remediation.

2. Analisa Gallegos is admitted to a hospital to give birth to her premature baby. Identify at least 10 health care team members who may be on the team that provides her care. Review the different careers in Chapter 3 to prepare your list. Why do you think teamwork is important in this scenario? How do healthy professional relationships promote a healthy community?

3. After a building explodes, EMS delivers 22 critically injured patients to a hospital emergency room. Which type of leader do you think would be most effective in directing the group of emergency room personnel? Why?

ACTIVITIES

Activities give you the chance to work with fellow classmates. Using real-life medical scenarios, you will have the opportunity to apply what you learned in a creative and challenging way.

■ ACTIVITIES

1. With a partner, stand back to back. The shorter person should draw a figure. The taller partner will then draw a figure that the shorter partner describes. After 2 minutes, compare original figure with what the taller partner drew. Why is listening important? Is accurate recording important? What are four (4) factors that may be a barrier in communicating the desired figure?

2. In a small group, create a medical scene involving communication between two (2) different age groups or two (2) different cultures. Exchange your scenario with another group. Using consensus-building techniques, plan how to role play the new scene using effective communication techniques for five (5) minutes. Present to the class.

SUPPLEMENTS AT A GLANCE

Supplement	Where to Find It	What's In It
Online Teacher's Resource Kit	Available on the Instructor Companion Website via NGLsync.cengage.com. if you have purchased a MindTap online course, or at companion-sites.cengage.com.	Classroom Management Activities Lesson Plans Ready-to-Use Tests and Quizzes Classroom Activities Internet Activities Leadership Development Activities Applied Academics Clinical Rotations Resources
Online Instructor's Manual	Available on the Instructor Companion Website via NGLsync.cengage.com. if you have purchased a MindTap online course, or at companion-sites.cengage.com.	Answers to Student Workbook Assignment Sheets Answers to end-of-chapter review questions
Workbook ISBN-13: 9780357646434	Print product	Assignment Sheets for student review Evaluation Sheets for judging student performance for each procedure in the textbook
Instructor Companion Website	Accessed via NGLsync.cengage.com. if you have purchased a MindTap online course, or at companion-sites.cengage.com.	Computerized test banks powered by Cognero® software Slide presentations in PowerPoint® Image Library Animations Standards mapping grid Online Instructor's Manual Online Teacher's Resource Kit
MindTap to Accompany *DHO Health Science* ISBN-13: 9780357646441	Accessed via NGLsync.cengage.com.	Flexible learning path to meet diverse classroom needs and learning styles Chapter-level simulations to apply knowledge and elevate learning Adaptable Table of Contents and customizable Learning Path
Student Online Companion	Additional online student resources; web access via NGLsync.cengage.com with purchase of a MindTap online course.	Audio podcasts of medical terminology Animations of anatomical and physiological processes

*Online Teacher and Student resources require a Cengage Account at NGLsync or for our Companion sites. Don't have an account? Request access from your Sales Consultant, ngl.cengage.com/repfinder.

ABOUT THE AUTHORS

Louise Simmers received a Bachelor of Science degree in nursing from the University of Maryland and an MEd from Kent State University. She has worked as a public health nurse, medical-surgical nurse, charge nurse in a coronary intensive care unit, instructor of practical nursing, health science education teacher, and school-to-work coordinator at the Madison Comprehensive High School in Mansfield, Ohio. She is a member of the University of Maryland Nursing Alumni Association, Sigma Theta Tau, Phi Kappa Phi, National Education Association, and Association for Career and Technical Education (ACTE), and she is a volunteer worker for the Red Cross. Mrs. Simmers received the Vocational Educator of the Year Award for Health Occupations in the State of Ohio and the Diversified Health Occupations Instructor of the Year Award in the State of Ohio. Mrs. Simmers is retired and lives with her husband in Venice, Florida. The author is pleased that her twin daughters are now assisting with the revisions of this textbook.

Karen Simmers-Nartker graduated from Kent State University, Ohio, with a Bachelor of Science degree in nursing. She has been employed as a telemetry step-down, medical intensive care, surgical intensive care, and neurological intensive care nurse. She is currently employed as a charge nurse in an open-heart intensive care unit. She has obtained certification from the Emergency Nurses Association for the Trauma Nursing Core Course (TNCC) and from the American Heart Association for Advanced Cardiac Life Support (ACLS). In her current position as charge nurse in her ICU, she coordinates patient care and staff assignments; manages interpersonal conflicts among staff and/or patients and family members; is responsible for ensuring quality care to meet the diverse needs of patients and/or family; actively participates in in-services to evaluate new equipment, medications, hospital services, and supplies; and teaches and mentors newly employed nurses.

Sharon Simmers-Kobelak graduated from Miami University, Ohio, with a Bachelor of Business Administration degree. She is currently employed in the educational publishing industry as an Integrated Solutions Specialist. In this position, she assists instructors at private career schools to find appropriate print and digital materials for classroom instruction. Sharon also provides in-service training for instructors on how to utilize digital assets and instructor and student resources in the most productive manner. She achieved President's Club status for 2 years, number one representative status 1 year, and has repeatedly achieved quota in her 20 years in the educational publishing market.

Janet Fuller graduated from Bellevue University, Nebraska, with a Bachelor of Science degree in Health Care Administration. She obtained a Texas LVN nursing license from St. Philip's College and a Texas teaching certification from Region 13 in San Antonio. She has worked as a medical-surgical nurse, a clinic lead nurse, a surgical clinic nurse, and a home health nurse. She developed, owned, and instructed certified nursing assistants with South Texas School of Nurse Aides, LLC.

Ms. Fuller has taught medical terminology courses for Texas Lutheran College and San Antonio College. She is currently a health science education instructor at New Braunfels High School in New Braunfels, Texas. She is a sponsor and member of Future Health Professionals (HOSA), a member of the Career and Technology Association of Texas (CTAT), and a board member of Texas Health Occupations Association (THOA). Ms. Fuller has been in charge of coordinating health science conference speakers for both THOA and CTAT state events.

ACKNOWLEDGMENTS

This ninth edition of *DHO Health Science* is dedicated to my daughters, Karen Simmers-Nartker and Sharon Simmers-Kobelak, who have worked so hard the past two years as we revised both this textbook and *Practical Problems in Mathematics for Health Science Careers*. Even though they are parents of young children and work full time, they devoted many hours to working on these projects.

The author would like to thank everyone who participated in the development of this text, including:

Nancy L. Raynor, former Chief Consultant, Health Occupations Education, State of North Carolina, who served as a consultant and major mentor in the initial development of this textbook

Dr. Charles Nichols, Department Head, and Ray Jacobs, Teacher Educator, Kent State University, who provided the encouragement I needed when I wrote the first edition of this textbook

My best friend and colleague, the late Nancy Webber, RN, who taught health science education with me for over 20 years and critiqued many chapters of this textbook

Carolynn Townsend, Lisa Shearer Cooper, Donna Story, Dorothy Fishman, Dakota Mitchell, and Lee Haroun who contributed chapter information

The author and Cengage Learning would like to thank those individuals who reviewed the manuscript and offered suggestions, feedback, and assistance. The text has been improved as a result of the reviewers' helpful, insightful, and creative suggestions. Their work is greatly appreciated.

Nancy H. Allen
Health Science Education Associate
South Carolina Department of Education
Office of Career and Technology Education
Columbia, South Carolina

Michelle Baker, MEd, DC
Health Science Teacher
Texas HOSA Board of Directors
Deer Park, TX

Bethanne Reichard Bean, MLS, CLSup, BSMT (ASCP)
Medical Science Academy Coordinator/Instructor,
Grades 6–12
State of Florida Licensed Clinical Laboratory
Supervisor of Microbiology, Hematology, Clinical
Chemistry, Molecular Pathology, Serology, and
Immunohematology
School District of Palm Beach County, Florida

Kimberly Davidson, RN, BSN, MEd
Level 1 Tech Prep Health Occupations Instructor
Madison Comprehensive High School
Mansfield, Ohio

Laura C. Fink, RN, Ed. S
Academy of Health Science
Coral Reef High School
Miami, FL

Staci Gramling Gardner, RRT
Health Science Instructor
Gadsden City High School
Gadsden, Alabama

Alice Graham, RN
Coordinator and Instructor
Chiefland High School Academy of Health Related Professions
Chiefland, Florida

Beth Hardee
Director, Fire and EMS Academy at the Professional
Academies Magnet
Loften High School
Gainesville, Florida

Katrina L. Haynes, RN, BSN MIT
Health Science Educators Association

Robin Hill
Health Careers Instructor
Four County Career Center
Archbold, OH

Mrs. Randi Hunewill, NDOE, NREMT-I
Nevada Department of Education Health Science
Consultant

Grant Iannelli, DC
Professor of Chiropractic Medicine
National University of Health Sciences
Lombard, Illinois

Kathleen Iannucci, LAc, PTA, LMT
Adjunct Professor, Palm Beach State College
Boca Raton, Florida

Thalea J. Longhurst
Health Science Specialist
Career, Technical, and Adult Education
Utah State Office of Education
Salt Lake City, Utah

Clarice K.W. Morris, PhD
Coordinator, Academy of Medical Professions,
Charles E. Gorton High School
Yonkers, New York

Amy Parker-Ferguson, MEd, BS, RN, LP, NREMT-P
Chief Nursing Officer for Dallas Medical Center
Adjunct Faculty, Dallas Community College
Dallas, Texas

Anne B. Regier, RDH, BS
Health Science Coordinator
J. Frank Dobie High School
Pasadena I.S.D.
Houston, Texas

Linda Roberts
Teacher, Nampa School District Health Professions
Academy
Nampa, Idaho

Christa G. Ruber, EdD
Department Head, Allied Health
Pensacola State College
Pensacola, Florida

Debra A. Sawhill, RN, BAEd, CMA-AAMA OEA-NEOEA,
AAMA, SkillsUSA Advisor, American Red Cross Instructor
Program Coordinator for Portage Lakes Career Center
NATCEP, Program Instructor for Portage Lakes Career
Center
Health Care Academy
Uniontown, Ohio

Lara Skaggs
State Program Manager, Health Careers Education
Oklahoma Department of Career and Technology
Education
Stillwater, Oklahoma

Elisabeth A. Smith, RN, EdS
National Academy Foundation (NAF) Academy of Health
Science
CNA Program Coordinator and Instructor
William R. Boone High School
Orlando, Florida

Karen Ruble Smith, RN, BSN
Health Science Consultant/Biomedical Science State Leader
High Schools That Work Coordinator
Kentucky Department of Education
College & Career Readiness
Frankfort, Kentucky

Kathy B. Turner, RN, BSN
Assistant Chief, Health Care Personnel Registry
Division of Health Service Regulation
Raleigh, North Carolina

Jackie Uselton, RDH, CPhT, MEd
Health Science Instructor
TEKS Trainer, HOSA Advisor
THOA Inc. Board of Directors
Austin, Texas

The author also wishes to thank the following companies,
associations, and individuals for information and/ or
illustrations:

Air Techniques, Inc.

American Cancer Society

Atago, USA

Becton Dickinson

Timothy Berger, MD

Bigstock

Bruce Black, MD

Brevis Corporation

Briggs Corporation

Marcia Butterfield

Carestream Health

Care Trak International, Inc.

Carson's Scholar Fund

Centers for Disease Control and Prevention

Chart Industries, Inc.

Sandy Clark

The Clorox Company

Control-o-fax Office Systems

Covidien

DMG America

Dynarex

Empire Blue Cross/Blue Shield

Food and Drug Administration (FDA)

Deborah Funk, MD

Steve Greg, DDS

Hager Worldwide

HOSA: Future Health Professionals

HemoCue®

Hu-Friedy Manufacturing Company

Integra Miltex

Invacare

Iris Sample Processing Company

i-Stock

J.T. Posey Company

Kardex Systems

Kerr Corporation

McKesson Automation Solutions

Medical Indicators, Inc.

Medline Industries

Midmark Corporation

Miltex Instrument Company

National Archives, Brady Collection

National Cancer Institute

National Consortium for Health Science Education

National Eye Institute

National Hospice and Palliative Care Organization

National Institutes of Health

National Library of Medicine

National Multiple Sclerosis Society

National Pressure Ulcer Advisory Panel

National Uniform Claim Committee

NexTemp

Nonin Medical, Inc.

NPS Corporation Omron Healthcare

Pfizer

Physicians' Record Company

Polara Studios

Poly-Medco

Practicon

Quinton Cardiology, Inc.

Sage Products, Inc.

Salk Institute

Science Photo Library, David Martin, MD

Shutterstock

Robert A. Silverman, MD

SkillsUSA

Smead Manufacturing

Spacelabs Medical, Inc.

SPS Medical

Statlab Medical Products

STERIS Corporation

Ron Stram, MD

Sunrise Medical

Larry Torrey

Unico

UPI/Newscom

U.S. Administration on Aging

U.S. Army

U.S. Department of Agriculture

U.S. Postal Systems

Vertex-42

Victorian Adult Burns Service, Melbourne, Australia

W. A. Baum Company, Inc.

Wake Forest Institute for Regenerative Medicine, Dr. Atala

Winco

Zuma Press/Newscom

BASIC HEALTH CARE CONCEPTS AND SKILLS

Welcome to the world of health science education!

You have chosen a career in a field that offers endless opportunities. If you learn and master the knowledge and skills required, you can find employment in any number of rewarding careers.

What would you do?

Annalisa is a 19-year-old college student who has recently started to experience headaches, fainting, and heart flutters. Her boyfriend, Joe, rushes her to the ER when she faints three times in one day while they are at the park.

What could be wrong?

Annalisa was brought into your freestanding ER because of her fainting and general disorientation. What lab tests would you order? Is a cardiac or neuro workup in order? Should she have some radiology testing?

What is the answer?

Annalisa is experiencing some troubling changes in her health status. After being cleared to go home, the ER doctor recommends that Annalisa's family take her to be further evaluated by her doctor.

Let's get started using this book to lay the foundation and learn the principles of health science you will need to help this patient.

HISTORY AND TRENDS OF HEALTH CARE

Case Study Investigation

Mrs. Anita Perez is a 66 year-old Hispanic female that has been battling high blood pressure for 3 years. Mrs. Perez is taking care of her terminally ill mother and is still working full time, resulting in elevated stress levels. She has been on high blood pressure medication for 6 months and has added an anti-anxiety medication this month. Mrs. Perez complains about headaches, an upset stomach and nervousness. She has experienced an 8 pound weight loss over the last 2 months and developed mouth ulcers. She has complained of increasing fatigue and muscle aches as well. Mr. Perez is worried about Anita and is looking for ways to help his wife manage these symptoms. What alternative or complimentary therapies might you recommend to the Perez family? Would any of those therapies conflict with her traditional medications or medical treatments?

LEARNING OBJECTIVES

After completing this chapter, you should be able to:

- Differentiate between early and current beliefs about the causes of disease and treatment.

- Name at least six historic individuals that impacted medicine and explain how each one helped to improve health care.

- Create a timeline showing what you believe are the most important discoveries in health care and explain why you believe they are important.

- Identify at least five current trends or changes in health care.

- Explain how discoveries in health care have led to the advancement of this field.

- Define, pronounce, and spell all key terms.

KEY TERMS

alternative therapies

biotechnology

complementary therapies

cost containment

diagnostic related groups (DRGs)

energy conservation

geriatric care

holistic health care

home health care

integrative (integrated) health care

Omnibus Budget Reconciliation
  Act (OBRA)

outpatient services

pandemic

telemedicine

wellness

NOTE: *To further emphasize the key terms, they appear in color within the chapter. You will notice beginning in Chapter 3 on page 42 that pronunciations have been provided for the more difficult key terms. The single accent mark, _"_, shows where the main stress is placed when saying the word. The double accent, _"_, shows secondary stress (if present in the word).*

1:1 HISTORY OF HEALTH CARE

Why is it important to understand the historical significance of health care? Would you believe that some of the treatment methods in use today were also used in ancient times? In the days before drug stores, people used many herbs and plants as both food and medicine. Many of these herbs remain in use today. A common example is a medication called *morphine*. Morphine is made from the poppy plant and is used to manage pain. As you review each period of history, think about how the discoveries made in that period have helped to improve the health care you receive today.

ANCIENT TIMES

Table 1–1 lists many of the historical events of health care in ancient times. In primitive times, the common belief was that disease and illness were caused by evil spirits and demons. Treatment was directed toward eliminating the evil spirits. As civilizations developed, people began to study the human body and make observations about how it functions.

Religion played an important role in health care. It was commonly believed that illness and disease were punishments from the gods. Religious ceremonies were frequently used to eliminate evil spirits and restore health. Exploring the structure of the human body was limited because most religions did not allow dissection, or cutting the body apart. For this reason, animals were frequently dissected to learn about different body parts.

The ancient Egyptians were the first people to keep health records. It is important to remember that many people could not read; therefore, knowledge was limited to an educated few. Most of the records were inscribed on stone and were created by priests, who also acted as physicians.

The ancient Chinese strongly believed in the need to cure the spirit and nourish the entire body. This form of treatment remains important today, when holistic health methods stress treating the entire patient—mind, body, and soul. Chinese herbal medicine, acupuncture, and massage (Tui na) are still commonly used.

Hippocrates (ca. 460–377 BC), called the "Father of Medicine," was one of the most important physicians in ancient Greece (see the Biography box for more information about Hippocrates). The records that he and other physicians created helped establish that disease is caused by natural causes, not by supernatural spirits and demons. The ancient Greeks were also among the first to stress that a good diet and cleanliness help to prevent disease.

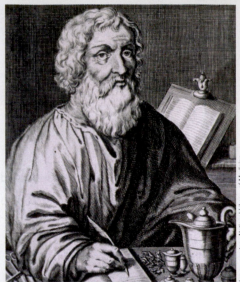
The Rod of Asclepius (**Figure 1–1A**), the Greek symbol associated with medicine and healing, originated in ancient Greece. The caduceus symbol (**Figure 1–1B**) is often mistaken as the medical symbol, but it is actually the symbol for commerce. Different variations of both of these symbols are in use today. All contain the staff, but many have wings and either one or two serpents.

TABLE 1–1 History of Health Care in Ancient Times

Historical Events of Health Care in Ancient Times	
4000 BC–3000 BC Primitive Times	People believed that illness and disease were caused by supernatural spirits and demons Tribal witch doctors treated illness with ceremonies to drive out evil spirits Herbs and plants were used as medicines, and some are still used today Average life span was 20 years
3000 BC–300 BC Ancient Egyptians	Earliest people known to maintain accurate health records Called on the gods to heal them when disease occurred Physicians were priests who studied medicine and surgery in temple medical schools Used magic and medicinal plants to treat disease Average life span was 20 to 30 years
1700 BC–220 AD Ancient Chinese	Religious prohibitions against dissection resulted in inadequate knowledge of body structure Monitored the pulse to determine the condition of the body Believed in the need to treat the whole body by curing the spirit and nourishing the body Recorded a pharmacopoeia (an official drug directory) of medications based mainly on the use of herbs Used acupuncture to relieve pain and congestion Began the search for medical reasons for illness Average life span was 20 to 30 years
1200 BC–200 BC Ancient Greeks	Began modern medical science by observing the human body and effects of disease Hippocrates (460–377 BC), called the Father of Medicine: • Developed an organized method to observe the human body • Recorded signs and symptoms of many diseases • Created a high standard of ethics, the Oath of Hippocrates, used by physicians today Believed illness is a result of natural causes Stressed diet and cleanliness as ways to prevent disease Average life span was 25 to 35 years
753 BC–410 AD Ancient Romans	First to organize medical care by providing care for injured soldiers Early hospitals developed when physicians cared for ill people in rooms in their homes Began public health and sanitation systems: • Created aqueducts to carry clean water to the cities • Built sewers to carry waste materials away from the cities • Drained marshes to reduce the incidence of malaria Claudius Galen (129–199? AD), a physician, described the symptoms of inflammation and studied infectious diseases in addition to dissecting animals and determining the functions of muscles, the kidney, and the bladder Average life span was 25 to 35 years

FIGURE 1–1 Symbols of medicine include (A) the Rod or Staff of Asclepius and (B) a caduceus. © Maximus256//Shutterstock.com

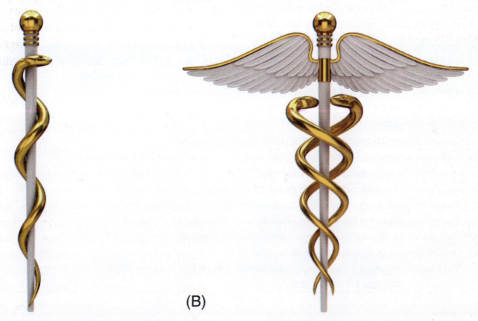

(A)

(B)

With knowledge obtained from the Greeks, the Romans realized that some diseases were connected to filth, contaminated water, and poor sanitation. They began to develop sanitary systems by building sewers to carry away waste and aqueducts (waterways) to deliver clean water. They drained swamps and marshes to reduce the incidence of malaria. They created laws to keep streets clean and eliminate garbage. The first hospitals were also established in ancient Rome when physicians began caring for injured soldiers or ill people in their homes.

Although many changes occurred in health care during ancient times, treatment was still limited. The average person had poor personal hygiene, drank contaminated water, and had unsanitary living conditions. Diseases such as typhoid, cholera, malaria, dysentery, leprosy, and smallpox infected many individuals. Because the causes of these diseases had not been discovered, the diseases were usually fatal. The average life span was 20 to 35 years. Today, individuals who die at this age are considered to be young people.

THE DARK AGES AND MIDDLE AGES

Table 1–2 lists many of the historical events of health care during the Dark Ages and the Middle Ages. During the Dark Ages, after the fall of the Roman Empire, the study of medicine stopped. Individuals again lived in unsanitary conditions with little or no personal hygiene. Epidemics of smallpox, dysentery, typhus, and the plague were rampant. Monks and priests stressed prayer to treat illness and disease.

The Middle Ages brought a renewed interest in the medical practices of the Romans and Greeks. Monks obtained and translated the writings of the Greek and Roman physicians and recorded the knowledge in handwritten books. Medical universities were created in the 9th century to train physicians how to use this knowledge to treat illness. Later, the Arabs began requiring that physicians pass examinations and obtain licenses.

In the 1300s, a major epidemic of bubonic plague killed almost 75 percent of the population of Europe and Asia. Other diseases such as smallpox, diphtheria, tuberculosis, typhoid, and malaria killed many others. The average life span of 20 to 35 years was often reduced even further by the presence of these diseases. Many infants died shortly after birth. Many children did not live into adulthood. Today, most of these diseases are almost nonexistent because they are prevented by vaccines or treated by medications.

THE RENAISSANCE

Table 1–3 lists many of the historical events of health care that occurred between 1350 and 1650 AD, a period known as the Renaissance. This period is often referred to as the "rebirth of the science of medicine." New information about the human body was discovered as a result of human dissection becoming accepted and allowed. Physicians could now view body organs and see the connections between different systems in the body. Artists, such as Michelangelo and Leonardo da Vinci, were able to draw the body accurately. In addition, the development of the printing press resulted in the publication of medical books that were used by students at medical universities. Knowledge spread more rapidly. Physicians became more educated.

The life span increased to an average age of 30 to 40 years during the Renaissance, but common infections still claimed many lives. At this point in time, the actual causes of disease were still a mystery.

TABLE 1–2 History of Health Care in the Dark Ages and the Middle Ages

Historical Events of Health Care in the Dark Ages and the Middle Ages	
400–800 AD Dark Ages	Emphasis was placed on saving the soul, and the study of medicine was prohibited Prayer and divine intervention were used to treat illness and disease Monks and priests provided custodial care for sick people Average life span was 20 to 30 years
800–1400 AD Middle Ages	Renewed interest in the medical practice of Greeks and Romans Physicians began to obtain knowledge at medical universities in the 9th century A pandemic (worldwide epidemic) of the bubonic plague (black death) killed three-quarters of the population of Europe and Asia Major diseases were smallpox, diphtheria, tuberculosis, typhoid, the plague, and malaria Rhazes (al-Razi), an Arab physician, became known as the Arab Hippocrates: • Based diagnoses on observations of the signs and symptoms of disease • Suggested blood was the cause of many infectious diseases • Began the use of animal gut as suture material Arabs began requiring that physicians pass examinations and obtain licenses Average life span was 20 to 35 years

TABLE 1–3 History of Health Care in the Renaissance

Historical Events of Health Care in the Renaissance	
1350–1650 AD Renaissance	Rebirth of the science of medicine
	Dissection of the body began to allow a better understanding of anatomy and physiology
	Artists Michelangelo (1475–1564) and Leonardo da Vinci (1452–1519) used dissection to draw the human body more realistically
	Development of the printing press allowed knowledge to be more easily spread to others
	First anatomy book was published by Andreas Vesalius (1514–1564)
	Michael Servetus (1511–1553):
	• Described the circulatory system in the lungs
	• Explained how digestion is a source of heat for the body
	Roger Bacon (1214?–1292?) researched optics and refraction (bending of light rays)
	Average life span was 30 to 40 years

THE 16TH, 17TH, AND 18TH CENTURIES

Table 1–4 lists many of the historical events of health care that occurred during the 16th, 17th, and 18th centuries. During this period, physicians gained an increased knowledge of the human body. William Harvey described the circulation of blood. Gabriel Fallopius described the tympanic membrane in the ear and the fallopian tubes in the female reproductive system. Bartolomeo Eustachio identified the tube between the ear and throat. These discoveries allowed other physicians to see how the body functioned.

A major development occurred after Anton van Leeuwenhoek built a microscope that increased magnification ability and produced clear and bright images (see the Biography box for more information about Anton van Leeuwenhoek). This instrument allowed physicians to see organisms that are too small to be seen by the human eye. Even though they were not aware of it at the time, physicians were looking at many of the pathogenic organisms (germs) that cause disease. The microscope continues to be a major diagnostic tool.

This period also saw the start of drug stores, or pharmacies. Apothecaries (early pharmacists) made, prescribed, and sold medications. Many of these medications were made from plants and herbs similar to those used in ancient times. At the end of the 18th century, Edward Jenner developed a vaccine to prevent smallpox, a deadly disease.

During this time, the average life span increased to 40 to 50 years. However, the causes of many diseases were still unknown, and medical care remained limited.

TABLE 1–4 History of Health Care in the 16th, 17th, and 18th Centuries

Historical Events of Health Care in the 16th, 17th, and 18th Centuries	
16th and 17th Centuries	Causes of disease were still not known, and many people still died from infections and puerperal (childbirth) fever
	Ambroise Paré (1510–1590), a French surgeon, known as the Father of Modern Surgery:
	• Established the use of ligatures to bind (use of thread or suture to tie off) arteries and stop bleeding
	• Promoted use of artificial limbs
	Gabriel Fallopius (1523–1562):
	• Identified the fallopian tubes in the female reproductive system
	• Described the tympanic membrane in the ear
	William Harvey (1578–1657) described the circulation of blood to and from the heart in 1628
	Anton van Leeuwenhoek (1632–1723) built a microscope with increased magnification in 1666
	First successful blood transfusion was performed on animals in England in 1667
	Bartolomeo Eustachio identified the eustachian tube leading from the ear to the throat
	Apothecaries (early pharmacists) made, prescribed, and sold medications
	Average life span was 35 to 45 years
18th Century	Gabriel Fahrenheit (1686–1736) created the first mercury thermometer in 1714
	John Hunter (1728–1793), an English surgeon:
	• Established scientific surgical procedures
	• Introduced tube feeding in 1778
	Benjamin Franklin (1706–1790) invented bifocals for eyeglasses
	Dr. Jesse Bennett performed the first successful Cesarean section operation to deliver an infant in 1794
	James Lind prescribed lime juice containing vitamin C to prevent scurvy in 1795
	Edward Jenner (1749–1823) developed a vaccination for smallpox in 1796
	Average life span was 40 to 50 years

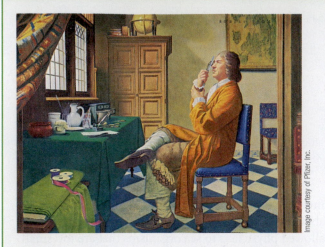

Image courtesy of Pfizer, Inc.

In 1668, he visited London and saw a copy of Robert Hooke's *Micrographia*, a book depicting Hooke's own observations with the microscope. This stimulated van Leeuwenhoek's interest, and he began to build microscopes that magnified more than 200 times, with clearer and brighter images than were available at the time. Using the improved microscope, van Leeuwenhoek began to observe bees, bugs, water, and other similar substances. He noticed tiny single-celled organisms that he called *animalcules*, now known as microorganisms. When van Leeuwenhoek reported his observations to the Royal Society of London, he was met with skepticism. However, other scientists researched his findings, and eventually his ideas were proved and accepted.

Anton van Leeuwenhoek (1632–1723) is one of several individuals who are called the "Father of Microbiology" because of his discovery of bacteria and other microscopic organisms. He was born in Delft, Holland, and worked as a tradesman and apprentice to a textile merchant. He learned to grind lenses and make simple microscopes to use while examining the thread densities of materials.

Anton van Leeuwenhoek was the first individual to record microscopic observations on muscle fibers, blood vessels, and spermatozoa. He laid the foundations of plant anatomy and animal reproduction. He developed a method for grinding powerful lenses and made more than 400 different types of microscopes. Anton van Leeuwenhoek's discoveries are the basis for microbiology today.

THE 19TH CENTURY

Table 1–5 lists many of the historical events of health care that occurred during the 19th century, a period also known as the Industrial Revolution. Major progress in medical science occurred because of the development of machines and the wide availability of books.

Early in the century, René Laënnec invented the stethoscope (see the Biography box for more information about René Laënnec). This invention allowed physicians to listen to internal body sounds, which increased their knowledge of the human body.

Formal training for nurses began during this century. After training at a program in Germany, Florence Nightingale established sanitary nursing care units for injured soldiers during the Crimean War. She is known as the founder of modern nursing (see the Biography box for more information about Florence Nightingale).

TABLE 1–5 History of Health Care in the 19th Century

Historical Events of Health Care in the 19th Century	
19th Century	Royal College of Surgeons (medical school) founded in London in 1800
	French barbers acted as surgeons by extracting teeth, using leeches for treatment, and giving enemas
	René Laënnec (1781–1826) invented the stethoscope in 1816
	In 1818, James Blundell performed the first successful blood transfusion on humans
	Dr. Philippe Pinel (1755–1826) began humane treatment for mental illness
	Cholera pandemic in 1832
	Theodor Fliedner started one of the first training programs for nurses in Germany in 1836, which provided Florence Nightingale with her formal training
	In the 1840s, Ignaz Semmelweis (1818–1865) encouraged physicians to wash their hands with lime after performing autopsies and before delivering babies to prevent puerperal (childbirth) fever
	Dr. William Morton (1819–1868), an American dentist, began using ether as an anesthetic in 1846
	American Medical Association was formed in Philadelphia in 1847
	Elizabeth Blackwell (1821–1910) became the first female physician in the United States in 1849; she started the first Women's Medical College in New York in 1868

(continues)

TABLE 1–5 History of Health Care in the 19th Century *(continued)*

Historical Events of Health Care in the 19th Century

Florence Nightingale (1820–1910), the founder of modern nursing:
- Established efficient and sanitary nursing units during Crimean War in 1854
- Began the professional education of nurses

Dorothea Dix (1802–1887) was appointed Superintendent of Female Nurses of the Army in 1861

International Red Cross was founded in 1863

Joseph Lister (1827–1912) started using disinfectants and antiseptics during surgery to prevent infection in 1865

Elizabeth Garrett Anderson (1836–1917) became the first female physician in Britain in 1870 and the first woman member of the British Medical Association in 1873

Paul Ehrlich (1854–1915), a German bacteriologist, developed methods to detect and differentiate between various diseases, developed the foundation for modern theories of immunity, and used chemicals to eliminate microorganisms

Clara Barton (1821–1912) founded the American Red Cross in 1881

Robert Koch (1843–1910), another individual who is also called the "Father of Microbiology," developed the culture plate method to identify pathogens and in 1882 isolated the bacteria that causes tuberculosis

Louis Pasteur (1822–1895) contributed many discoveries to the practice of medicine, including:
- Proving that microorganisms cause disease
- Pasteurizing milk to kill bacteria
- Creating a vaccine for rabies in 1885

Gregory Mendel (1822–1884) established the principles of heredity and dominant/recessive patterns

Wilhelm Roentgen (1845–1923) discovered roentgenograms (X-rays) in 1895

Bayer introduced aspirin in powdered form in 1899

Average life span was 40 to 60 years

Biography René Laënnec

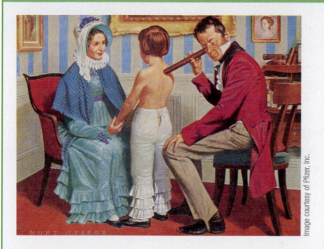

Image courtesy of Pfizer, Inc.

René-Théophile-Hyacinthe Laënnec (1781–1826) was a French physician who is frequently called the "Father of Pulmonary Diseases." In 1816, he invented the stethoscope, which began as a piece of rolled paper and evolved into a wooden tube that physicians inserted into their ears.

Laënnec used his stethoscope to listen to the various sounds made by the heart and lungs. For years, he studied chest sounds and correlated them with diseases found on autopsy. In 1819, he published a book on his findings, *De l'auscultation mediate*, also known as *On Mediate Auscultation*. Laënnec's use of auscultation (listening to internal body sounds) and percussion (tapping body parts to listen to sounds) formed the basis of the diagnostic techniques used in medicine today.

Laënnec studied and diagnosed many medical conditions such as bronchiectasis, melanoma, cirrhosis, and tuberculosis. Cirrhosis of the liver is still called *Laënnec's cirrhosis* because Laënnec was the first physician to recognize this condition as a disease entity. Laënnec also conducted extensive studies on tuberculosis, but unfortunately he was not aware of the contagiousness of the disease, and he contracted tuberculosis himself. He died of tuberculosis at the age of 45, leaving a legacy of knowledge that is still used by physicians today.

Infection control was another major development. Physicians began to associate the tiny microorganisms seen under the microscope with diseases. Methods to stop the spread of these organisms were developed by Theodor Fliedner, Joseph Lister, and Louis Pasteur (see the Biography box for more information about Louis Pasteur).

Women became active participants in medical care in the 19th century. Elizabeth Blackwell was the first female physician in the United States. Dorothea Dix was appointed superintendent of female nurses in the U.S. Army. Clara Barton founded the American Red Cross (see the Biography box for more information about Clara Barton).

Biography Florence Nightingale

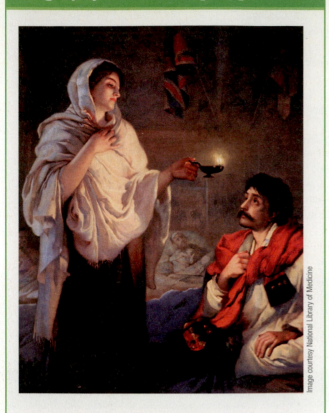

Image courtesy National Library of Medicine

Florence Nightingale (1820–1910) is known as the founder of modern nursing. In 1854, Nightingale led 38 nurses to serve in the Crimean War. During the war, the medical services of the British army were horrifying and inadequate. Hundreds of soldiers died because of poor hygiene and unsanitary conditions. Nightingale fought for the reform of the military hospitals and for improved medical care.

Nightingale encouraged efficiency and cleanliness in the hospitals. Her efforts decreased the patient death rate by two-thirds. She used statistics to prove that the number of deaths decreased with improved sanitary conditions. Because of her statistics, sanitation reforms occurred and medical practice improved.

One of Nightingale's greatest accomplishments was starting the Nightingale Training School for nurses at St. Thomas' Hospital in London. Nurses attending her school received a year's training, which included lectures and practical ward work. Trained nurses were then sent to work in British hospitals and abroad. These trained nurses also established other nursing schools using Nightingale's model. Nightingale published more than 200 books, pamphlets, and reports. Her writings on hospital organization had a lasting effect in England and throughout the world. Many of her principles are still used in health care today.

Biography Louis Pasteur

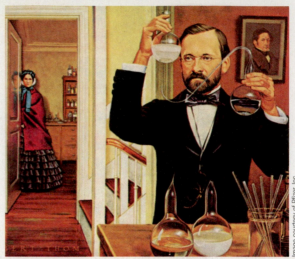

Image courtesy of Pfizer, Inc.

Louis Pasteur (1822–1895) was a French chemist and biologist. He is also called the "Father of Microbiological Sciences and Immunology" because of his work with the microorganisms that cause disease. Pasteur developed the germ theory and discovered the processes of pasteurization, vaccination, and fermentation. His germ theory proved that microorganisms cause most infectious diseases. In addition, he proved that heat can be used to destroy harmful germs in perishable food, a process now known as *pasteurization*. Pasteur also discovered that weaker microorganisms could be used to immunize against more dangerous forms of a microorganism. He developed vaccines against anthrax, chicken cholera, rabies, and swine erysipelas. Through his studies of fermentation, he proved that each disease is caused by a specific microscopic organism.

Pasteur's principles for sanitation helped control the spread of disease and provided ideas about how to prevent disease. These discoveries reformed the fields of surgery and obstetrics. Pasteur is responsible for saving the lives of millions of people through vaccination and pasteurization. His accomplishments are the foundation of bacteriology, immunology, microbiology, molecular biology, and virology in today's health care.

The average life span during this period increased to 40 to 65 years. Treatment for disease was more specific after the causes for diseases were identified. Many vaccines and medications were developed.

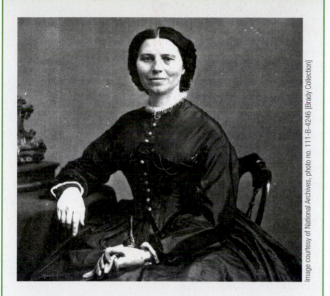

Image courtesy of National Archives, photo no. 111-B-4246 [Brady Collection]

Clara Barton (1821–1912) was the founder of the American Red Cross. During the American Civil War, she volunteered to provide aid to wounded soldiers. She appealed to the public to provide supplies and, after collecting the supplies, personally delivered them to soldiers of both the North and the South.

In 1869, Barton went to Geneva, Switzerland, to rest and improve her health. During her visit, she learned about the Treaty of Geneva, which provided relief for sick and wounded soldiers. A dozen nations had signed the treaty, but the United States had refused. She also learned about the International Red Cross, which provided disaster relief during peacetime and war.

When Barton returned to the United States, she campaigned for the Treaty of Geneva until it was ratified. In 1881, the American Red Cross was formed, and Barton served as its first president. She represented the American Red Cross by traveling all over the United States and the world to assist victims of natural disasters and war.

THE 20TH CENTURY

Table 1–6 lists many of the historical events of health care that occurred during the 20th century. This period showed the most rapid growth in advancements in health care. Physicians were able to use new machines such as X-rays to view the body. Medicines—including insulin for diabetes, antibiotics to fight infections, and vaccines to prevent diseases—were developed. The causes for many diseases were identified. Physicians were now able to treat the cause of a disease to cure the patient.

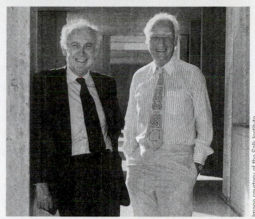

Image courtesy of the Salk Institute

Francis Crick and **James Watson** shared the Nobel Prize in 1962 with Maurice Wilkins for discovering the structure of deoxyribonucleic acid (DNA). Crick was a biophysicist and chemist; Watson studied zoology; Wilkins was a physicist and molecular biologist who worked with Rosalind Franklin, a chemist whose contribution to the discovery is not well known. They all shared a desire to solve the mystery of the structure of DNA.

Crick and Watson built a three-dimensional model of the molecules of DNA to assist them in discovering its structure. In 1953, they discovered that the structure of DNA is a double helix, similar to a gently twisted ladder. It consists of pairs of bases: adenine and thymine, and guanine and cytosine. The order in which these bases appear on the double helix determines the identity of the organism. That is, DNA carries life's hereditary information. Wilkins and Franklin studied DNA using X-ray diffraction. Franklin's X-ray crystallographic technique allowed her to be the first to obtain an X-ray image of DNA that clearly established DNA was a helical structure. When this image was shown to Crick and Watson by Wilkins, it provided the final clue and allowed them to combine this information with their research to create the three-dimensional model of DNA. Franklin died of cancer several years later and her contribution was not recognized for many years.

Crick and Watson's model of the DNA double helix provided motivation for research in molecular genetics and biochemistry. Their work showed that understanding how a structure is arranged is critical to understanding how it functions. This discovery is the foundation for most of the genetic research that is being conducted today.

TABLE 1–6 History of Health Care in the 20th Century

Historical Events of Health Care in the 20th Century	
20th Century	Carl Landsteiner classified the ABO blood groups in 1901
	Female Army Nurse Corps was established as a permanent organization in 1901
	Marie Curie (1867–1934) isolated radium in 1910
	Sigmund Freud's (1856–1939) studies formed the basis for psychology and psychiatry
	Influenza (Spanish flu) pandemic killed more than 40 million people in 1918
	Frederick Banting and Charles Best discovered and used insulin to treat diabetes in 1922
	Health insurance plans and social reforms were developed in the 1920s
	Sir Alexander Fleming (1881–1955) discovered penicillin in 1928
	Buddy, a German shepherd, became the first guide dog for the blind in 1928
	The Ransdell Act reorganized the Laboratory of Hygiene into the National Institutes of Health (NIH) in 1930
	Dr. Robert Smith (Dr. Bob) and William Wilson founded Alcoholics Anonymous in 1935
	Gerhard Domagk (1895–1964) developed sulfa drugs to fight infections
	Dr. George Papanicolaou developed the Pap test to detect cervical cancer in women in 1941
	The first kidney dialysis machine was developed in 1944
	Jonas Salk (1914–1995) developed the polio vaccine using dead polio virus in 1952
	In 1953, Francis Crick and James Watson described the structure of DNA and how it carries genetic information
	The first heart–lung machine was used for open-heart surgery in 1953
	Joseph Murray performed the first successful kidney transplant in humans in 1954
	Albert Sabin (1906–1993) developed an oral live-virus polio vaccine in the mid-1950s
	Birth control pills were approved by the U.S. Food and Drug Administration (FDA) in 1960
	An arm severed at the shoulder was successfully reattached to the body in 1962
	The Medicare and Medicaid 1965 Amendment to the Social Security Act marked the entry of the federal government into the health care arena as a major purchaser of health services
	Christian Barnard performed the first successful heart transplant in 1967
	The first hospice was founded in England in 1967
	The U.S. Congress created the Occupational Safety and Health Administration (OSHA) in 1970
	The Health Maintenance Organization Act of 1973 established standards for HMOs and provided an alternative to private health insurance
	Physicians used amniocentesis to diagnose inherited diseases before birth in 1975
	Computerized axial tomography (CAT) scan was developed in 1975
	In 1975, the New Jersey Supreme Court ruled that the parents of Karen Ann Quinlan, a comatose woman, had the power to remove her life support systems
	The first "test tube" baby, Louise Brown, was born in England in 1978
	Acquired immune deficiency syndrome (AIDS) was identified as a disease in 1981
	In 1982, Dr. William DeVries implanted the first artificial heart, the Jarvik-7, in a patient
	Cyclosporine, a drug to suppress the immune system after organ transplants, was approved in 1983
	In 1984, the human immunodeficiency virus (HIV), which causes AIDS, was identified
	The Omnibus Budget Reconciliation Act (OBRA) of 1987 established regulations for the education and certification of nursing assistants
	The Clinical Laboratory Improvement Act (CLIA) was passed in 1988 to establish standards and regulations for performing laboratory tests
	The first gene therapy to treat disease occurred in 1990
	President George H.W. Bush signed the Americans with Disabilities Act in 1990
	The Patient Self-Determination Act was passed in 1990 to require health care providers to inform patients of their rights in regard to making decisions about their medical care and to provide information and assistance in preparing advance directives
	OSHA's Bloodborne Pathogens Standards became effective in 1991
	A vaccine for hepatitis A became available in 1994
	A vaccine for chicken pox (varicella) was approved in 1995
	President Clinton signed the Health Insurance Portability and Accountability Act (HIPAA) of 1996 to protect patient privacy and to make it easier to obtain and keep health insurance
	Identification of genes that caused diseases increased rapidly in the 1990s
	Oregon enacted the Death with Dignity Act in 1997 to allow terminally ill individuals to end their lives
	A sheep was cloned in 1997
	An international team of scientists sequenced the first human chromosome in 1999
	Average life span was 60 to 80 years

A major development in understanding the human body occurred in the 1950s when Francis Crick and James Watson described the structure of DNA and how it carries genetic information (See the Biography box for more information about Francis Crick and James Watson. See also **Figure 1–2**.). Their studies began the search for gene therapies to cure inherited diseases. This research continues today.

Health care plans that help pay the costs of care also started in the 20th century. At the same time, standards were created to make sure that every individual had access to quality health care. This remains a major concern of health care in the United States today.

The first open-heart surgery, which took place in the 1950s, has progressed to the heart transplants that occur today. Surgical techniques have provided cures for what were once fatal conditions. Also, infection control has helped decrease surgical infections that previously killed many patients.

The contribution of computer technology to medical science has helped medicine progress faster in the 20th century than in all previous periods combined. Today, computers and technology are used in every aspect of health care. Their use will increase even more in the 21st century.

All of these developments have helped increase the average life span to 60 to 80 years. In fact, it is not unusual for people to live to be 100. With current pioneers such as Ben Carson (see the Biography box for more information about Ben Carson), as well as many other medical scientists and physicians, there is no limit to what future health care will bring.

THE 21ST CENTURY

The potential for major advances in health care in the 21st century is unlimited. Early in this century, the completion of the Human Genome Project by the U.S. Department of Energy and the National Institutes of Health (NIH) provided the basis for much of the current research on genetics. Clustered Regularly Interspaced Short Palindromic Repeats (CRISPR) technology has built on that information, and this new technology allows advanced genetic editing. Research with embryonic stem cells and the development of cloned cells could lead to treatments that will cure many diseases.

Some major threats to health care exist in this century. Bioterrorism, the use of microorganisms or biologic agents as weapons to infect humans, is a real and present threat. New viruses, such as the H1N1, or swine flu virus, and the COVID-19 or coronavirus, can mutate and cause disease in humans. Pandemics, or worldwide epidemics, could occur quickly in our global society because people can travel easily from one country to another.

Organizations such as the World Health Organization (WHO), an international agency sponsored by the United Nations, are constantly monitoring health problems throughout the world and taking steps to prevent pandemics. Health care has become a global concern and countries are working together to promote good health in all individuals. Technology is allowing

FIGURE 1–2 The discovery of the structure of DNA and how it carries genetic (inherited) information was the beginning of research on how to cure inherited diseases by gene therapy.

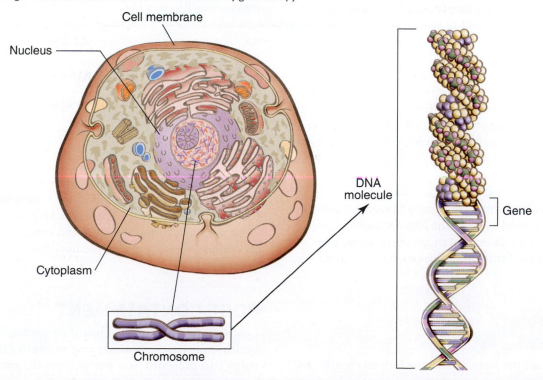

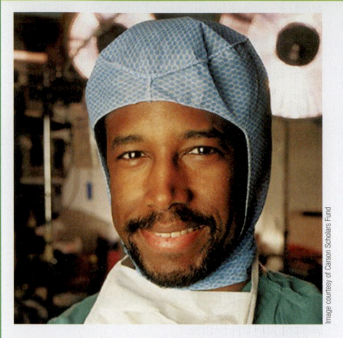

Image courtesy of Carson Scholars Fund

Benjamin Carson, MD, has become famous for his landmark surgeries to separate conjoined twins. Dr. Carson is one of the most skilled and accomplished neurosurgeons today.

In 1987, he was the primary surgeon of a 70-member surgical team that separated conjoined twins born in West Germany. The 7-month-old boys were joined at the back of the head, sharing the major cerebral blood drainage system. After the operation, both boys were able to survive independently. This was the first surgery to separate occipital craniopagus twins, meaning they were joined at the head near the occipital bone. In 1997, Dr. Carson was the lead surgeon in South Africa in another successful operation to separate 11-month-old boys who were vertical craniopagus twins, meaning they were joined at the top of the head looking in opposite directions.

Dr. Carson continues to perform landmark surgeries and conduct research for new techniques and procedures. He has refined hemispherectomy, a revolutionary surgical procedure performed on the brain to stop seizures that are difficult to treat or cure. He also works with craniofacial (head or facial disfigurement) reconstructive surgery. Dr. Carson has developed an important craniofacial program that combines neurosurgery and plastic surgery for children with congenital (at birth) deformities. He is also known for his work in pediatric neuro-oncology (brain tumors).

Dr. Carson is the author of three best-selling books: *Gifted Hands*, the story of his life; *Think Big*, a story inspiring others to use their intelligence; and *The Big Picture*, a closeup look at the life of a professional surgeon. Dr. Carson is also cofounder and president of the Carson Scholars Fund, which was established to recognize young people for superior academic performance and humanitarian achievement.

In 2017, the U.S. Senate confirmed Dr. Carson to become the U.S. Secretary of Housing and Urban Development.

---

scientists to remotely monitor patient health status. Robots assist and enhance surgery all across the globe. 3-D printers are revolutionizing the cost and availability of implants and joints to match individual measurements precisely. Nanotechnology is pushing medical devices to become smaller and more efficient. Implanted insulin pumps can now measure glucose levels and respond seamlessly.

Table 1–7 lists some of the events of health care that have occurred so far in the 21st century and some possible advances that might occur soon. The potential for the future of health care has unlimited possibilities.

check**point**

1. Who was responsible for keeping health records?
2. When was the Human Genome Project completed?

1:2 TRENDS IN HEALTH CARE

Health care has seen many changes during the past several decades, and many additional changes will occur in the years to come. Robotics and technology have increased the pace of new innovations in the medical field.

An awareness of such changes and trends is important for any health care provider. Medical professionals are lifelong learners.

COST CONTAINMENT

Cost containment, a term heard frequently in health care circles, means trying to control the rising cost of health care and achieve the maximum

TABLE 1–7 History of Health Care in the 21st Century

Historical Events of Health Care in the 21st Century	
21st Century	Adult stem cells were used in the treatment of disease early in the 2000s
	The FDA approved Da Vinci, the first robotic surgical system, which allows for smaller surgical incisions, less pain, and faster recovery in 2000
	President George W. Bush approved federal funding for research using only existing lines of embryonic stem cells in 2001
	The first totally implantable artificial heart was placed in a patient in Louisville, Kentucky, in 2001
	In 2002, smallpox vaccinations were given to military personnel and first responders to limit the effects of a potential bioterrorist attack
	The Netherlands became the first country in the world to legalize euthanasia in 2002
	The Human Genome Project to identify all of the approximately 20,000 to 25,000 genes in human DNA was completed in 2003
	The Standards for Privacy of Individually Identifiable Health Information, required under the Health Insurance Portability and Accountability Act (HIPAA) of 1996, went into effect in 2003
	The virus that causes severe acute respiratory syndrome (SARS) was identified in 2003 as a new coronavirus, never before seen in humans
	National Institutes of Health (NIH) researchers discovered that primary teeth can be a source of stem cells in 2003
	In 2005, the first face transplant was performed in France on a woman whose lower face was destroyed by a dog attack
	Stem cell researchers at the University of Minnesota coaxed embryonic stem cells to produce cancer-killing cells in 2005
	The National Cancer Institute (NCI) and the National Human Genome Research Institute started a project in 2006 to map genes associated with cancer so mutations that occur with specific cancers can be identified
	Researchers proposed a new method to generate embryonic stem cells from a blastocyst without destroying embryos in 2006
	Gardasil, a vaccine to prevent cervical cancer, was approved by the FDA in 2006
	Zostavax, a vaccine to prevent herpes zoster (shingles), was approved by the FDA in 2006
	The CDC issued Transmission-Based Precautions for preventing the spread of infectious diseases in 2007
	The FDA approved the first molecular test to detect metastatic breast cancer in 2007
	Scarless surgery using the body's own openings was first performed in 2008
	In 2008, a genetic screen for cancer was developed, allowing physicians to determine who would best respond to Herceptin, a breast cancer drug
	In 2009, the funding ban on stem cell research was lifted, leading to advancements that used adult skin stem cells to create the first stem cell mice and to regenerate fully functioning teeth in rodents
	A new set of three genes linked to Alzheimer's disease was discovered in 2009
	By November of 2009, 71% of the U.S. population was banned from smoking in bars, restaurants, and the workplace
	WHO declared a pandemic of the H1N1 virus, commonly called swine flu, in 2009
	In 2010, Dr. Craig Venter, co-mapper of the human genome, synthesized an entire genome of a bacterium that was then able to reproduce
	In 2010, the first artificial ovary was created, a major advancement in infertility research
	The Patient Protection and Affordable Care Act was signed into law in March 2010
	An experimental vaccine for glioblastoma, a deadly brain tumor, was developed in 2011
	In 2011, the FDA approved an implant that is inserted in the brain through blood vessels—without brain surgery—to treat brain aneurysms
	In 2013, the FDA approved a bionic eye to treat retinitis pigmentosa, a leading cause of blindness
	Sofosbuvir, the first oral pill to treat hepatitis C, was approved by the FDA in 2013
	In 2013, the FDA approved Neuropace, a responsive neurostimulator that is surgically implanted into the brain, as a treatment for intractable epilepsy
	A woman in Sweden with a transplanted uterus gave birth to a baby boy in 2014
	A major epidemic of Ebola occurred in West African countries in 2014
	In September 2014, the CDC declared the first case of Ebola in the United States and issued transmission-based guidelines for the Ebola virus disease (EVD)
	In 2014, surgeons in the Netherlands used a 3-D printer to create a custom-made skull that was used in a complete skull transplant
	Shringrex, a more effective vaccine to prevent herpes zoster (shingles), was approved by the FDA in 2017
	In 2019, an outbreak of coronavirus spurred the World Health Organization (WHO) to declare a pandemic
	Average life span is 75 to 85 years
Potential for the 21st Century	Cures for AIDS, cancer, and heart disease are found
	Genetic manipulation to prevent inherited diseases is a common practice
	Development of methods to slow the aging process or stop aging are created
	Nerves in the brain and spinal cord are regenerated to eliminate paralysis
	Transplants of every organ in the body, including the brain, are possible
	Antibiotics are developed that do not allow pathogens to develop resistance
	Enhanced biology using prosthetics
	Average life span is increased to 90 to 100 years and beyond

benefit for every dollar spent. Some reasons for high health care costs include:

- **Technological advances**: Highly technical procedures such as heart, lung, liver, or kidney transplants can cost hundreds of thousands of dollars. Even so, many of these procedures are performed daily throughout the United States. Artificial hearts are another new technology being used. Computers and technology that can examine internal body parts are valuable diagnostic tools, but these devices can cost millions of dollars. Advanced technology does allow people to survive illnesses that used to be fatal, but these individuals may require expensive and lifelong care.

- **The aging population**: Older individuals use more pharmaceutical products (medications), have more chronic diseases, and often need more frequent health care services.

Lawsuits force health care providers to obtain expensive malpractice insurance, order diagnostic tests even though they might not be necessary, and make every effort to avoid lawsuits. Because these expenses must be paid, a major concern is that health care costs could rise to levels that could prohibit providing services to all individuals. Health services can have a detrimental effect on the economy. Health care is a growing expense for businesses and individuals. Health care is a driver of U.S. debt at the federal level. National health spending—which includes government spending, the private sector, and individual spending—has risen by trillions from 1960 to the present and continues to rise. It is projected to be 19.9 percent in 2025, as opposed to 17.9 percent in 2016. The average health insurance premium has risen 19 percent over the past 5 years. Thus, all aspects of health care focus on cost containment. Although there is no absolute answer to how to control health costs, most agencies that deliver health care are trying to provide quality care at the lowest possible price. Some methods of cost containment include:

- **Diagnostic related groups (DRGs)**: This is one way Congress is trying to control costs for government insurance plans such as Medicare and Medicaid. Under this plan, patients with certain diagnoses who are admitted to hospitals are classified in one payment group. A limit is placed on the cost of care, and the agency providing care receives this set amount. This encourages the agency to make every effort to provide care within the expense limit allowed.

- **Replace fee-for-service compensation with value-based compensation or bundled payments**: Fee-for-service compensation pays health care providers for each service rendered, so there is little incentive to consider the cost or necessity of services provided. Replacing this payment type with value-based or bundled payments, in which providers are paid a certain amount for each diagnosis or disease, makes health care providers consider the necessity of various services or treatments.

- **Combination of services**: This is done to eliminate duplication of services. Clinics, laboratories shared by different agencies, health maintenance organizations (HMOs), preferred provider organizations (PPOs), and other similar agencies all represent attempts to control the rising cost of health care. When health care agencies join together or share specific services, care can be provided to a larger number of people at a decreased cost per person. For example, a large medical laboratory with expensive computerized equipment performing thousands of tests per day can provide quality service at a much lower price than smaller laboratories with less expensive equipment capable of performing only a limited number of tests per day.

- **Outpatient services**: Patients who use these services receive care without being admitted to hospitals or other care facilities. Hospital care is expensive. Reducing the length of hospital stays or decreasing the need for hospital admissions lowers the cost of health care. For example, patients who had open-heart surgery used to spend several weeks in a hospital. Today, the average length of stay is 4 to 7 days. Less expensive home care or transfer to a skilled-care facility can be used for individuals who require additional assistance.

- **Mass or bulk purchasing**: This means buying equipment and supplies in larger quantities at reduced prices. This can be done by combining the purchases of different departments in a single agency or by combining the purchases of several different agencies. A major health care system purchasing medical supplies for hundreds or thousands of health care agencies can obtain much lower prices than an individual agency. Computerized inventory can be used to determine when supplies are needed and to prevent overstocking and waste.

- **Early intervention and preventive services**: Providing care before acute or chronic disease occurs is crucial. Preventing illness is always more cost-effective than treating illness. Methods used to prevent illness include patient education, immunizations, regular physical examinations to detect problems early, incentives for individuals to participate in preventive activities, and easy access for all individuals to preventive health care services. Studies have shown that individuals with limited access to health services and restricted finances use expensive emergency rooms and acute care facilities much more frequently.

- **Environmental Protection**: A major expense is the correct disposal of the toxic waste that health care produces. All hazardous medical waste must be collected by a licensed medical waste collector/hauler.

  - **Categories of waste**: There are three categories of hazardous medical waste that must be treated differently than general waste. *Infectious Medical Waste* can transmit infection and includes bloody bandages, sharps, body parts, and lab cultures. *Radioactive Medical Waste* contains radioactive material such as nuclear medicine for cancer treatment and diagnostic test material. *Hazardous Medical Waste* is dangerous but not necessarily infectious such as chemotherapy agents and unused sharps.

  - **Management of waste**: Ways to improve management of these potential environmental hazards include building systems for long-term improvements, reducing volume, autoclave or steam on-site, providing easy-to-use waste disposal, proper air venting, and protecting water from facility containments.

- **Energy conservation**: This means monitoring the use of energy to control costs and conserve resources. Some of the major expenses for every health care industry/agency are electricity, water, and/or gas. Most large health care facilities perform energy audits to determine how resources are being used and to calculate ways to conserve energy. Methods that can be used for energy conservation include designing new energy-efficient facilities, maintaining heating/cooling systems, using insulation and thermopane windows to prevent hot/cool air loss, repairing plumbing fixtures immediately to stop water loss, replacing energy-consuming lightbulbs with energy-efficient bulbs, installing infrared sensors to turn water faucets on and off, and using alternative forms of energy such as solar power. Recycling is also a form of energy conservation, and most health care facilities recycle many different materials.

The preceding are just a few examples of cost containment. Many other methods will undoubtedly be applied in the years ahead. It is important to note that the quality of health care should not be lowered simply to control costs. The Agency for Healthcare Research and Quality (AHRQ) researches the quality of health care services to make health care safer; more accessible, equitable, and affordable; and of higher quality. In addition, every health care worker must make every effort to provide quality care while doing everything possible to avoid waste and keep expenditures down. Health care consumers must assume more responsibility for their own care, become better informed of all options for health care services, and follow preventive measures to avoid or limit illness and disease. Everyone working together can help control the rising cost of health care.

HOME HEALTH CARE

Career

Home health care is a rapidly growing field. Diagnostic-related groups and shorter hospital stays have created a need for care in the home. Years ago, home care was the usual method of treatment. Doctors made house calls, private duty nurses cared for patients in the patients' homes, babies were delivered at home, and patients died at home. Current trends show a return to some of these practices. Home care is also another form of cost containment because it is usually less expensive to provide this type of care. All aspects of health care can be involved. Nursing care, physical and occupational therapy, respiratory therapy, social services, nutritional and food services, and other types of care can be provided in the home environment.

GERIATRIC CARE

Career

Geriatric care, or care for the elderly, is another field that will continue to experience rapid growth in the future (**Figure 1–3**). This is caused in part by the large number of individuals who are experiencing longer life spans because of advances in health care. Many people now enjoy life spans of 80 years or more. Years ago, very few people lived to be 100 years old, but this experience is becoming more and more common. Also, the "baby boom" generation—the large number of people born after World War II—is now reaching the geriatric age. Projections from the U.S. Census Bureau indicate that the rate of population growth during the next 50 years will be slower for all age groups, but the number of people in older age groups will continue to grow more than twice as rapidly as the total population. Many different facilities will be involved in providing care and resources for this age group. Adult day care centers, retirement communities, assisted/independent living facilities, long-term care facilities, and other organizations will all see increased demand for their services.

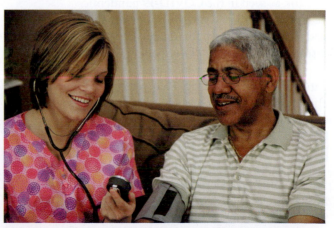

FIGURE 1–3 Home health care and geriatric care are fields that will continue to experience rapid growth. © iStock.com/Brad Killer

OBRA, the **Omnibus Budget Reconciliation Act** of 1987, has led to the development of many regulations regarding long-term care and home health care. This act requires states to establish training and competency evaluation programs for nursing and geriatric assistants. Each assistant working in a long-term care facility or home health care is now required under federal law to complete a state-approved training program and pass a written and competency examination to obtain certification. OBRA also requires continuing education, periodic evaluation of performance, and retraining and testing if a nursing assistant does not work in a health care facility for more than 2 years. Each state then maintains a registry of qualified individuals.

The minimum skills required are specified in the National Nurse Aide Assessment Program (NNAAP), the largest nurse aide certification examination in the United States, developed by the National Council of State Boards of Nursing (NCSBN). Programs that prepare nursing and geriatric assistants use NNAAP as a guideline to ensure that the minimum requirements of OBRA are met. OBRA also requires compliance with patients'/residents' rights and forces states to establish guidelines to ensure that such rights are observed and enforced.

TELEMEDICINE

Telemedicine involves the use of video, audio, and computer systems to provide medical and/or health care services. New technology now allows interactive services between health care providers even though they may be in different locations. For example, emergency medical technicians (EMTs) at the scene of an accident or illness can use technology to transmit medical data such as an electrocardiogram to an emergency department physician. The physician can then monitor the data and direct the care of the patient. This fills an especially critical need when personal exposure and limited travel is a factor, as seen in the COVID-19 pandemic. Telemedicine allows medical professionals to diagnose and treat patients without unnecessary exposure to disease for either provider or patient. Practitioners can also disseminate information and take care of noncritical patients in a home setting. That type of treatment helps eliminate pressure on hospital systems and resources that are already stressed.

Electronic health records (EHRs), also called electronic medical records (EMRs), facilitate rapid transmission of patient information. When physician offices, hospitals, and other health care providers have access, a doctor or authorized individual can obtain hospital laboratory results, radiology reports, and EHRs at any location. Patients can also access their EHRs to obtain information about their medical care.

The use of satellite and video technology also enhances medical care. Surgeons using a computer can guide a remote-controlled robotic arm to perform surgery on a patient many miles away. In other instances, one surgeon can direct the work of another surgeon by watching the procedure on video beamed by a satellite system.

Telephone apps are already allowing individuals with chronic illnesses or disabilities to receive care in the comfort of their own homes. This decreases the need for trips to medical care facilities. Patients can test their own blood sugar levels, oxygen levels, blood pressure measurements, and other vital signs as well and send the results to a health care provider. They can also monitor pacemakers, use online courses to learn how to manage their condition(s), schedule an appointment to talk with a health care provider "face-to-face" through phone apps, receive electronic reminders to take medications or perform diagnostic tests, and receive answers to specific health questions. In rural areas, where specialty care is often limited, telemedicine can provide a patient with access to specialists thousands of miles away. Telemedicine is an important way to deliver health care.

WELLNESS

Wellness—or the state of being in optimum health with a balanced relationship between physical, mental, and social health—is another major trend in health care. People are more aware of the need to maintain health and prevent disease because disease prevention improves their quality of life and saves costs. More individuals are recognizing the importance of exercise, good nutrition, weight control, and healthy living habits (**Figure 1–4**). This trend has led to the establishment of wellness centers, weight-control facilities, health food stores, nutrition services, stress reduction counseling, and habit cessation management.

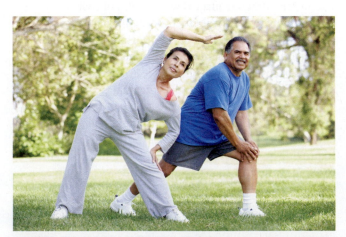

FIGURE 1–4 Individuals are recognizing the importance of exercise and healthy living habits. © iStock.com/Catherine Yeulet

Wellness is determined by the lifestyle choices made by an individual and involves many factors. Some of the factors and ways to promote wellness include:

- **Physical wellness**: promoted by a well-balanced diet; regular exercise; routine physical examinations and immunizations; regular dental and vision examinations; and avoidance of alcohol, tobacco, caffeine, drugs, environmental contaminants, and risky sexual behavior

- **Emotional wellness**: promoted by understanding personal feelings and expressing them appropriately, accepting one's limitations, adjusting to change, coping with stress, enjoying life, and maintaining an optimistic outlook

- **Social wellness**: promoted by showing concern, fairness, affection, tolerance, and respect for others; communicating and interacting well with others; sharing ideas and thoughts; and practicing honesty and loyalty

- **Mental and intellectual wellness**: promoted by being creative, logical, curious, and open-minded; using common sense; continually learning; questioning and evaluating information and situations; learning from life experiences; and using flexibility and creativity to solve problems

- **Spiritual wellness**: promoted by using values, ethics, and morals to find meaning, direction, and purpose in life; often includes believing in a higher authority and observing religious practices

The trend toward wellness has led to **holistic health care**, or care that promotes physical, emotional, social, intellectual, and spiritual well-being by treating the whole body, mind, and spirit. Each patient is recognized as a unique person with different needs. Holistic health care uses many methods of diagnosis and treatment in addition to traditional Western medical practice. Treatment is directed toward protection and restoration. It is based on the body's natural healing powers, the various ways different tissues and systems in the body influence each other, and the effect of the external environment. It is essential to remember that the patient is responsible for choosing his or her own care. Health care workers must respect the patient's choices and provide care that promotes the well-being of the whole person.

COMPLEMENTARY AND ALTERNATIVE METHODS OF HEALTH CARE

The most common health care system in the United States is the biomedical or "Western" system. It is based on evaluating the physical signs and symptoms of a patient, determining the cause of disease, and treating the cause. A major trend, however, is an increase in the use of complementary and alternative (CAM)

health care therapies. **Complementary therapies** are methods of treatment that are used in conjunction with conventional medical therapies. **Alternative therapies** are methods of treatment that are used in place of biomedical therapies. Even though the two terms are different, the term *alternative* is usually applied whether or not the therapy is used in place of, or in conjunction with, conventional medical therapies.

Many health care facilities now offer **integrative (integrated) health care**, which uses both mainstream medical treatments and CAM therapies to treat patients. For example, chronic pain is treated with both medications and CAM therapies that encourage stress reduction and relaxation. Integrative health care is based on the principle that individuals have the ability to bring greater wellness and healing into their own lives and that the mind affects the healing process. In addition, integrative care recognizes that each person is unique and may require different medical treatments and a variety of CAM therapies. For this reason, an integrative treatment plan must be individualized to meet the patient's own special needs and circumstances.

The interest in holistic health care has increased the use of CAM therapies. Common threads in these therapies are that they consider the whole individual and recognize that the health of each part has an effect on the person's total health status; that each person has a life force or special type of energy that can be used in the healing process; and that skilled practitioners, rituals, and specialized practices are a part of the therapy. Many of these therapies are based on cultural values and beliefs. A few examples of CAM practitioners include the following:

- **Ayurvedic practitioners**: use an ancient philosophy, ayurveda, which was developed in India, to determine a person's predominant *dosha* (body type) and prescribe diet, herbal treatment, exercise, yoga, massage, minerals, and living practices to restore and maintain harmony in the body.

- **Chinese medicine practitioners**: use an ancient holistic-based healing practice based on the belief that a life energy (Chi) flows through every living person in an invisible system of meridians (pathways), linking the organs together and connecting them to the external environment or universe; they use acupuncture (**Figure 1–5**), acupressure, tai chi, and herbal remedies to maintain the proper flow of energy and promote health.

- **Chiropractors**: believe that the brain sends vital energy to all body parts through nerves in the spinal cord, and, when there is a misalignment of the vertebrae (bones), pressure is placed on spinal nerves that results in disease and pain; they use spinal manipulation, massage, and exercise to adjust the position of the vertebrae and restore the flow of energy.

- **Homeopaths**: believe in the ability of the body to heal itself through the actions of the immune system; they use minute diluted doses of drugs made from plant, animal, and mineral substances to cause symptoms similar to the disease and activate the immune system.

- **Hypnotists**: help an individual obtain a trancelike state with the belief that the person will be receptive to verbal suggestions and make a desired behavior change.

- **Naturopaths**: use only natural therapies such as fasting, special diets, lifestyle changes, and supportive approaches to promote healing; they avoid the use of surgery or medicinal agents to treat disease.

Many different therapies are used in CAM medicine. Some of these therapies are discussed in **Table 1–8**. Most of the therapies are noninvasive and holistic. In many instances, they are less expensive than other traditional treatments: An excellent example is pet therapy (**Figure 1–6**). Many insurance programs now cover a wide variety of CAM therapies.

 Legal

Because of the increased use of CAM therapies, the federal government established the National Center for Complementary and Alternative Medicine (NCCAM) at the National Institutes of Health in 1992. Its purpose is to research the various therapies and determine standards of quality care. In addition, many states have passed laws to govern the use of various therapies. Some states have established standards for some therapies, forbidden the use of others, labeled specific therapies experimental, and require a

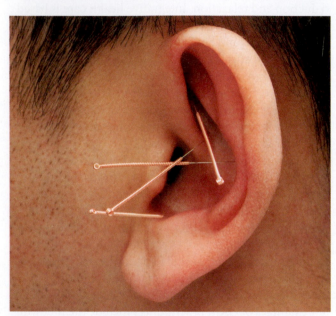

FIGURE 1–5 Acupuncture therapists insert very thin needles into specific points along the meridians (pathways) in the body to stimulate and balance the flow of energy. © iStock.com/Eliza Snow

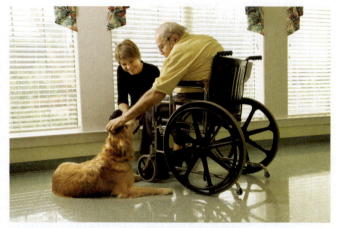

FIGURE 1–6 Pet therapy helps individuals overcome physical limitations, socialize, increase self-esteem, and lower stress levels and blood pressure. © iofoto/Shutterstock.com

TABLE 1–8 Complementary and Alternative Therapies

Therapy	Basic Description
Acupressure (*Shiatsu*)	Pressure is applied with fingers, palms, thumbs, or elbows to specific pressure points of the body to stimulate and regulate the flow of energy; based on the belief that Chi (life energy) flows through meridians (pathways) in the body, and illness and pain occur when the flow is blocked; used to treat muscular–joint pain, depression, digestive problems, and respiratory disorders; *Shiatsu* is the Japanese form of acupressure
Acupuncture	Ancient Chinese therapy that involves the insertion of very thin needles into specific points along the meridians (pathways) in the body to stimulate and balance the flow of energy; at times, heat (moxibustion) or electrical stimulation is applied to the needles; based on the belief that Chi (life energy) flows through the meridians, and illness and pain occur when the flow is blocked; used to relieve pain (especially headache and back pain), reduce stress-related illnesses, and treat drug dependency and obesity
Antioxidants (Free Radicals)	Nutritional therapy that encourages the use of substances called *antioxidants* to prevent or inhibit oxidation (a chemical process in which a substance is joined to oxygen) and neutralize free radicals (molecules that can damage body cells by altering the genetic code); examples of antioxidants are vitamins A, C, and E, and selenium; antioxidants may prevent heart disease, cataracts, and some types of cancer
Aromatherapy	Therapeutic use of selected fragrances (concentrated essences or essential oils that have been extracted from roots, bark, plants, and/or flowers) to alter mood and restore the body, mind, and spirit; fragrances may be diluted in oils for massages or placed in warm water or candles for inhalation; used to relieve tense muscles and tension headaches or backaches, lower blood pressure, and create a stimulating, uplifting, relaxing, or soothing effect
Biofeedback	Relaxation therapy that uses monitoring devices to provide a patient with information about his/her reaction to stress by showing the effect of stress on heart rate, respirations, blood pressure, muscle tension, and skin temperature; patient is then taught relaxation methods to gain voluntary control over these physical responses; used to treat hypertension (high blood pressure), migraine headaches, and stress-related illnesses, and to enhance relaxation

(continues)

TABLE 1–8 Complementary and Alternative Therapies *(continued)*

Therapy	Basic Description
Healing Touch (*Reiki*)	Ancient Japanese/Tibetan healing art based on the idea that disease causes an imbalance in the body's energy field; begins with centering (inward focus of total serenity) before gentle hand pressure is applied to the body's chakras (energy centers) to harness and balance the life energy force, help clear blockages, and stimulate healing; at times, hands are positioned slightly above the energy centers; used to promote relaxation, reduce pain, and promote wound healing
Herbal or Botanical Medicine	Herbal medicine treatments that have been used in almost all cultures since primitive times; based on the belief that herbs and plant extracts from roots, stems, seeds, flowers, and leaves contain compounds that alter blood chemistry, remove impurities, strengthen the immune system, and protect against disease
Homeopathy	Treatment based on using very minute, dilute doses of drugs made from natural substances to produce symptoms of the disease being treated; based on the belief that these substances stimulate the immune system to remove toxins and heal the body; very controversial form of treatment
Hydrotherapy	Type of treatment that uses water in any form, internally and externally, for healing purposes; common external examples include water aerobics and exercises, massage in or under water, soaking in hot springs or tubs, and steam vapors; a common internal example is a diet that encourages drinking large amounts of water to help cleanse the body and stimulate the digestive tract
Hypnotherapy (Hypnosis)	Technique used to induce a trancelike state so a person is more receptive to suggestion; enhances a person's ability to form images; used to encourage desired behavior changes such as losing weight, stopping smoking, reducing stress, and relieving pain
Imagery	Technique of using the imagination and as many senses as possible to visualize a pleasant and soothing image; used to decrease tension, anxiety, and adverse effects of chemotherapy
Ionization Therapy	Special machines called *air ionizers* are used to produce negatively charged air particles or ions; used to treat common respiratory disorders
Macrobiotic Diet	Macrobiotic (meaning "long life") is a nutrition therapy based on the Taoist concept of the balance between yin (cold, death, and darkness) and yang (heat, life, and light) and the belief that different foods represent yin (sweet foods) and yang (meat and eggs); the diet encourages balanced foods such as brown rice, whole grains, nuts, vegetables, fruits, and fish; discourages overindulgence in yin or yang foods; emphasizes that processed and treated foods, red meat, sugar, dairy products, eggs, and caffeine should be avoided; similar to the American Dietary Association's low-fat, low-cholesterol, and high-fiber diet
Meditation	Therapy that teaches breathing and muscle relaxation techniques to quiet the mind by focusing attention on obtaining a sense of oneness within oneself; used to reduce stress and pain, slow heart rate, lower blood pressure, and stimulate relaxation
Pet Therapy	Therapy that uses pets, such as dogs, cats, and birds, to enhance health and stimulate an interest in life; helps individuals overcome physical limitations, decrease depression, increase self-esteem, socialize, and lower stress levels and blood pressure
Phytochemicals	Nutritional therapy that recommends foods containing phytochemicals (nonnutritive plant chemicals that store nutrients and provide aroma and color in plants) with the belief that the chemicals help prevent disease; phytochemicals are found mainly in a wide variety of fruits and vegetables, so these are recommended for daily consumption; used to prevent heart disease, stroke, cancer, and cataracts
Play Therapy	Therapy that uses toys to allow children to learn about situations, share experiences, and express their emotions; important aspect of psychotherapy for children with limited language ability
Positive Thought	Therapy that involves developing self-awareness, self-esteem, and love for oneself to allow the body to heal itself and eliminate disease; based on the belief that disease is a negative process that can be reversed by an individual's mental processes
Reflexology	Ancient healing art based on the concept that the body is divided into ten equal zones that run from the head to the toes; illness or disease of a body part causes deposits of calcium or acids in the corresponding part of the foot; therapy involves applying pressure on specific points on the foot so energy movement is directed toward the affected body part; used to promote healing and relaxation, reduce stress, improve circulation, and treat asthma, sinus infections, irritable bowel syndrome, kidney stones, and constipation
Spiritual Therapies	Therapies based on the belief that a state of wholeness or health depends not only on physical health but also the spiritual aspects of an individual; uses prayer, meditation, self-evaluation, and spiritual guidance to allow an individual to use the powers within to increase the sense of well-being and promote healing
Tai Chi	Therapies based on the ancient theory that health is harmony with nature and the universe and a balanced state of yin (cold) and yang (heat); uses a series of sequential, slow, graceful, and precise body movements combined with breathing techniques to improve energy flow (Chi) within the body; improves stamina, balance, and coordination and leads to a sense of well-being; used to treat digestive disorders, stress, depression, and arthritis
Therapeutic (Swedish) Massage	Treatment that uses kneading, gliding, friction, tapping, and vibration motions of the hands to increase circulation of the blood and lymph, relieve musculoskeletal stiffness, pain, and spasm, increase range of motion, and induce relaxation
Therapeutic Touch	Therapy based on an ancient healing practice with the belief that illness is an imbalance in an individual's energy field; the practitioner assesses alterations or changes in a patient's energy fields, places his/her hands on or slightly above the patient's body, and balances the energy flow to stimulate self-healing; used to encourage relaxation, stimulate wound healing, increase the energy level, and decrease anxiety
Yoga	Hindu discipline that uses concentration, specific positions, and ancient ritual movements to maintain the balance and flow of life energy; encourages the use of both the body and mind to achieve a state of perfect spiritual insight and tranquility; used to increase spiritual enlightenment and well-being, develop an awareness of the body to improve coordination, relieve stress and anxiety, and increase muscle tone

license or certain educational requirements before a practitioner can administer a particular therapy. It is essential for health care providers to learn their states' legal requirements regarding the different CAM therapies. Health care providers must also remember that patients have the right to choose their own type of care. Thus, a nonjudgmental attitude is essential.

PANDEMIC

A **pandemic** exists when the outbreak of a disease occurs over a wide geographic area and affects a high proportion of the population. A major concern today is that worldwide pandemics will become more and more frequent as individuals can travel rapidly throughout the world.

The World Health Organization (WHO) is concerned about influenza pandemics occurring in the near future. Throughout history, influenza pandemics have killed large numbers of people. For example, the 1918 Spanish flu pandemic killed approximately 2.6 percent of individuals who contracted it, or more than 40 million people. Researchers recently identified the virus that caused this epidemic as an avian (bird) flu virus, or H5N1, that was transmitted directly to humans. The *H5N1* viruses present today devastate bird flocks but the spread from one person to another has been reported only rarely. In 2009 a new virus, H1N1, was discovered. The respiratory infection caused by this virus is commonly called the swine flu. Swine flu is an influenza in pigs, and it can occasionally be transmitted to humans. H1N1 spreads quickly and easily between humans when infected people cough or sneeze and others breathe in the virus or come in contact with a contaminated surface. H1N1 spread to almost all parts of the world, and the WHO declared it to be a global pandemic in 2009.

In 2014, a widespread epidemic of Ebola virus disease (EVD) occurred in West African countries, primarily in Guinea, Liberia, and Sierra Leone. Conservative estimates from WHO show that more than 23,000 people were infected and more than 70 percent of these people died from the disease. Ebola is a filovirus that was first discovered in 1976. It spreads to humans after close contact with the blood or body fluids of animals such as fruit bats, monkeys, chimpanzees, and gorillas who are infected with the disease. The disease starts by causing flu-like symptoms. As the disease becomes more severe, external and internal hemorrhaging occurs, and major organs such as the heart, kidney, and liver fail, causing death.

In September 2014, the first case of Ebola in the United States occurred when an infected person traveled from Liberia to Texas. Even with intensive treatment, the individual died from the disease. Two nurses who provided care for the patient were diagnosed with Ebola. Both nurses survived, but fear developed that a pandemic would occur. Many other cases developed in health care

personnel who provided care in West Africa. Some were transported to their home countries for treatment and care. As a result, Ebola cases were present not only in the United States but also in other countries—including Spain, Britain, France, Germany, Norway, Switzerland, Italy, and the Netherlands. To prevent a pandemic, WHO began coordinating the construction and staffing of treatment centers in the highly infected areas and providing education about the disease. In the United States, the Centers for Disease Control and Prevention issued very strict transmission-based guidelines that must be followed when providing care to infected individuals.

The major concern is that flu viruses can mutate quickly and may create a new, even more lethal virus. In addition to H5N1, H1N1, and Ebola, WHO is concerned about many other viruses. Examples include the hantavirus spread by rodents, severe acute respiratory syndrome (SARS), monkeypox, and the Marburg virus, which is a filovirus similar to Ebola. In 2018, for the first time in history, the United States had flu outbreaks in 49 states at the same time.

In 2019, COVID-19, or coronavirus, spread from China to the rest of the world. WHO declared an international public health emergency and eventually a pandemic. China quarantined 15 cities, and international travel with China was restricted. The United States declared a national emergency. The rapid global spread of this disease caused further international travel restrictions, and cities issued "shelter in place" orders that closed schools and nonessential businesses and restricted how many people could gather. States had phased reopenings. When out in public, the recommended physical distance between people was 6 feet apart, and this was called social distancing. The use of masks by the general population was encouraged, especially indoors. Personal protective equipment like N95 masks, face shields, and gowns for health care providers were sometimes in short supply. Hospitals filled and a shortage of ventilators was a concern and occurred in some parts of the world.

As the number of coronavirus cases and deaths increased, major research was directed toward finding effective methods of treatment and developing a vaccine.

Many governments are creating pandemic influenza plans to protect their populations. Components of most plans include the following:

- **Education**: Information about the pandemic and ways to avoid its spread must be given to the entire population.

- **Vaccine production**: In 2018, newly developed vaccines were freeze-dried for ease of transportation to remote areas. Patients can now choose to take their vaccine by not just an injection but also intranasal, oral, or patch.

- **Antiviral drugs**: Drugs that are currently available must be stockpiled so they will be ready for immediate use.

- **Development of protective public health measures**: Influenza and other viruses like COVID-19 must be diagnosed rapidly and accurately, strict infection control methods must be implemented to limit the spread of the virus, first responders and health care personnel must be immunized so they will be able to care for infected individuals, and quarantine measures must be used if necessary to control the spread of the disease.

- **International cooperation**: Countries must be willing to work with each other to create an international plan that will limit the spread of lethal viruses and decrease the severity of a pandemic.

Of growing concern are the drug-resistant bacteria, or superbugs. Infections such as MRSA (methicillin-resistant Staphylococcus aureus), VRE (vancomycin-resistant Enterococcus), CRA (carbapenem-resistant Enterobacteriaceae), and MRAB (multidrug-resistant Acinetobacter baumannii) are believed to be caused by decades of unnecessary antibiotic use. This overuse caused genetic mutations in bacteria that made them resistant to commonly used antibiotics.

In the near future, much effort will be directed toward identifying and limiting the effect of any organism that could lead to a pandemic. Health care providers must stay informed and be prepared to deal with the consequences of a pandemic. Cooperation to prevent pandemics must be a global effort. WHO and the governments of all countries must constantly be alert to the dangers that pandemics can present and be ready to act when one occurs.

BIOTECHNOLOGIES

Science

Biotechnology is the use of the genetic and biochemical processes of living systems and organisms to develop or modify useful products or, as defined by the UN Convention on Biological Diversity, "any technological application that uses biological systems, living organisms, or derivatives thereof, to make or modify products or processes for specific use." Engineers have made equipment smaller and more implantable. 3-D printing has provided cost-effective and individualized choices. Some recent examples are sleep apnea implants and combination glucose monitor and insulin pumps. Even though biotechnology has been used for thousands of years in agriculture, food production, energy, medicine, and other fields, it has expanded to include new and diverse sciences. Some of these include genomics, pharmacogenomics, proteomics, stem cell research, and nanotechnology.

Genomics is the study of all the genes in the human genome, or the complete set of DNA within a single cell of an organism. It analyzes the structure and function of genes, what they express, how they are regulated, how they interact with the environment, and ways they mutate or change. Research is directed at basing treatments on an individual's genetic makeup and identifying inherited genetic conditions. In 2019, scientists, using Clustered Regularly Interspaced Short Palindromic Repeats (CRISPR), were able to pinpoint defective or malfunctioning genes and provide advanced gene editing to treat disease.

Genomic (genetic) testing is the use of specific tests to check for the presence of inherited genes known to cause disease. These tests allow preventive methods and/or early diagnosis to eliminate or decrease the effects of the disease. Approved genetic tests are available for cancers such as breast, ovarian, colorectal, gastric, lung, leukemia, lymphoma, and melanoma and for diseases such as osteoporosis and AIDS. In addition, prenatal screening tests can be performed for diseases such as cystic fibrosis, sickle cell anemia, and Tay-Sachs. As research continues, many more genetic tests will become available to diagnose disease.

Pharmacogenomics is defined by the National Human Genome Research Institute as using a person's genetic makeup to choose the drugs and drug doses that are likely to work best for that individual. It is based on recognizing that individuals respond differently to medications according to their genetic makeup. The hope is to provide *personalized medicine* in which medications and dosages are optimized for each individual. Personalized medicine can lead to more accurate and effective treatments for many cancers and other diseases. The targeted drugs would decrease adverse reactions or side effects, provide accurate dosages based on how the individual's body metabolizes the drug, and treat the diseased area while limiting damage to nearby healthy cells.

Proteomics studies the structure and function of proteins. Proteins are substances in the protoplasm of cells that cause biochemical reactions, act as messengers, influence growth and development of tissues, transport oxygen in the blood, defend the body against disease, regulate cell reproduction, and perform many other vital functions. Research is directed toward mapping a proteome, or the entire set of proteins produced or modified by an organism, similar to the way genomics maps the human genome. When researchers identify defective proteins that cause specific diseases, new drugs can be developed that correct a defective protein or replace a missing one. Other research on finding biomarkers that identify unique patterns of protein to diagnose diseases, such as the prostate specific antigen (PSA) test used for prostate cancer, will lead to better diagnostic tests.

Stem cell research studies stem cells, or cells that are capable of becoming any of the specialized cells in the body such as skin, muscle, or nerve cells. The two main types include embryonic stem cells from a developing fetus and somatic or adult stem cells. Stem cells can be used to replace defective cells and treat diseases such as cancer, diabetes, and heart disease. Research is directed toward determining how the stem cells can be delivered to a specialized organ/cell and continue with specific function.

Nanotechnology uses a wide range of techniques to manipulate atoms and molecules to create new materials and devices. *Nanomedicine* is the use of nanotechnology

The Food and Drug Administration Regulating Maggots and Leeches as Medical Devices?

Throughout the history of health care, maggots and leeches have been used to treat infection and encourage blood flow. Maggots clean festering, gangrenous wounds that fail to heal. They eat the dead tissue and discharges to clean the wound and promote the growth of new tissue. Leeches drain excess blood from tissue and encourage new circulation.

Microsurgeons—physicians who specialize in reattaching fingers, hands, and other body appendages—have come to rely on the assistance of leeches. When microsurgeons reattach or transplant a body part, they can usually connect arteries that bring blood to the appendage. They find it more difficult to attach veins, which carry blood away from the appendage, because veins are smaller and more fragile. Without a good venous supply, blood tends to collect in the new attachment, clot, and in some cases, kill the tissue. To allow time for the body to create its own veins to the new appendage, physicians apply leeches. The leeches naturally inject the area with a chemical that includes an anticoagulant (a substance that prevents clotting), an anesthetic, an antibiotic, and a vasodilator (a substance that dilates or enlarges blood vessels). This chemical encourages the blood to flow quickly. The leeches drain this blood to reduce pressure and allow veins to form.

Now, researchers are evaluating the use of maggots to treat burns and skin cancer. Surgeons are determining if maggots can decrease the risk of infection after surgery, especially as so many infectious agents are antibiotic resistant. German scientists are evaluating the use of leech therapy to lessen pain and decrease the inflammation associated with osteoarthritis and other inflammatory diseases. Many other alternative uses of this biotherapy (including using living animals to aid in diagnosis or treatment) are possible in the future.

Even though many individuals are squeamish about the use of maggots and leeches, they have proved to be an effective method of treatment for chronic infections and microsurgery. The FDA has classified maggots and leeches as medical devices and regulates how maggots and leeches are grown, transported, sold, and disposed of after use. This regulation provides a safe source for this unique method of treatment and encourages future research on the use of maggots and leeches as methods of treatment.

---

for medical applications. A nanometer (nm) is a very small structure, 1 one-billionth of a meter. To visualize this size, think of a nanometer as a marble; a meter would be the size of the Earth. Research using these small particles has led to the development of nanodevices that can deliver drugs in precise amounts to targeted body cells, such as the delivery of cancer drugs directly to a brain tumor. This decreases the side effects of drugs and damage to other body cells. *Tissue engineering* is attempting to use nanotechnology to build structures that repair or reproduce damaged tissue. This has the potential to replace organ transplants or artificial implants. *Neuro-electronic* research is directed at using nanodevices to link computers to the nervous system to treat paralysis and nerve damage. Research has also led to the development of diagnostic devices, contrast agents for imaging, energy-based treatments using heat and radiation, and biosensors that measure very minute amounts of substances in biological fluids. The potential for this science is almost unlimited.

Cloning describes a number of different lab processes that can be used to produce genetically identical copies of a biological entity. Researchers have cloned tissues, genes, and cells. They have also cloned a sheep. Human cloning is still fiction. It is much more difficult to clone primates than other mammals. In 2004, Woo-Suk Hwang of Seoul National University in South Korea published a paper in the journal *Science* claiming to have cloned a human embryo. Independent scientists could not verify these results, and in January 2006, Hwang's paper was retracted.

Biotechnologies will have a major impact on the future of medicine. The opportunities in this field are unlimited, and many new health care careers will develop as research continues. However, it is important to mention that biotechnology research has also created bioethical concerns. For example, should a human being be cloned using biotechnology? Solving bioethical issues is a major concern as science advances.

checkpoint

1. Identify five current trends in health care and what medical advances made each possible.

PRACTICE: Go to the workbook and complete the assignment sheet for Chapter 1, History and Trends of Health Care.

Case Study Investigation Conclusion

What specific alternative treatments might help Mrs. Perez with her symptoms? Would anything in the treatment interfere with or block the effectiveness of her regular medications?

CHAPTER 1 SUMMARY

- Even in ancient times, people thought disease was caused by supernatural spirits, and plants and herbs were used to treat disease.

- New discoveries throughout the centuries developed our modern view of disease and treatments.

- Modern technology has caused major changes in health care in the past century. Computers have accelerated the rate of these changes.

- Cost containment, home health care, geriatric care, telemedicine, wellness to prevent disease, complementary and alternative methods (CAM) of health care, pandemic preparation, and biotechnologies are some current changes and trends in health care. An awareness of of such changes and trends is important for any health care provider.

REVIEW QUESTIONS

1. Name the person responsible for each of the following events in the history of health care. Briefly state how their accomplishments contributed to the current state of health care.
    a. The ancient Greek who is known as the Father of Medicine
    b. An artist who drew the human body during the Renaissance
    c. The individual who built a microscope that led to the discovery of microorganisms
    d. The individual who discovered roentgenograms (X-rays)
    e. The person who discovered penicillin
    f. The 19th-century individual that encouraged washing hands in lime before delivering babies
    g. The person that started using disinfectants and antiseptics during surgery

2. List six (6) specific ways to control the rising cost of health care.

3. You are employed in a medical office with four physicians. Identify and sketch or construct a model of four (4) specific ways to conserve energy and protect the health care environment in the office.

4. Review all the CAM therapies shown in Table 1–8. Identify two (2) therapies that you believe would be beneficial and explain why you think the therapies might be effective.

5. What is a pandemic? List four (4) pandemics and the cause of each.

6. Choose one (1) of the biotechnological sciences and identify what you feel might be a bioethical concern. How do you think this issue should be resolved?

CRITICAL THINKING

1. Write a brief essay describing how you maintain physical, emotional, social, mental, and spiritual wellness. Be sure to include specific examples for each type of wellness.

2. You and your team of three are in charge of pandemic disease plans for your country. Using news medias and research identify four (4) main ways your government agency team can help prevent the spread of disease in your country during a pandemic.

ACTIVITIES

1. Assemble in teams. After reading professional journals and watching news media about health care, use index cards and create a timeline for the history of health care, showing the twenty (20) events your team believes had the most impact on modern-day care. Record why your team believes these events are the most important. When complete, exchange cards with rival teams, and have a timeline assembly race.

2. Research and synthesize information found using news media and trade magazines to create a paper on the figure you believe is the most important in medical history. Include how this person's work or discoveries led to the advancement of health care. Be ready to defend your choice in a debate.

Case Study Investigation

A homeless man, John, arrives at a county shelter and is found to be a drug addict and in need of medical care. John does have a primary care provider, Dr. Brinthall, and he is sent there for medical care. Dr. Brinthall refers John to a drug treatment clinic for his addiction under a county program. The addiction center must report treatment information back to the county for program reimbursement and back to the shelter to verify that John is in treatment. Someone claiming to be a relation of John requests information from the shelter on all the health services John has received. The staff at the homeless shelter is working to connect the homeless man with his relative. At the end of the chapter, you will be asked to identify two private facilities where John was treated, one government agency that would be involved, and how HIPAA laws would impact the amount of information the facilities and the relative would be able to obtain about John's condition.

▮ LEARNING OBJECTIVES

After completing this chapter, you should be able to:

- Describe at least eight types of private health care facilities.
- Analyze at least three government health services agencies and the services offered by each.
- Describe at least three services offered by voluntary or nonprofit agencies.
- Explain the purpose of organizational structures in health care facilities.
- Compare the basic principles of at least four different health insurance plans.
- Define, pronounce, and spell all key terms.

KEY TERMS

Agency for Healthcare Research and Quality (AHRQ)

assisted living facilities

Centers for Disease Control and Prevention (CDC)

clinics

concierge medicine

dental offices

emergency care services

fee-for-service compensation

Food and Drug Administration (FDA)

genetic counseling centers

health departments

health insurance plans

Health Insurance Portability and Accountability Act (HIPAA)

health maintenance organizations (HMOs)

home health care

hospice

hospitals

independent living facilities

industrial health care centers

laboratories

long-term care facilities (LTCs or LTCFs)

managed care

Medicaid

medical offices

Medicare

Medigap policy

mental health facilities

National Institutes of Health (NIH)

nonprofit agencies

Occupational Safety and Health Administration (OSHA)

Office of the National Coordinator for Health Information Technology (ONC)

optical centers

organizational structure

Patient Protection and Affordable Care Act (PPACA)

pharmaceutical services

preferred provider organization (PPO)

rehabilitation facilities

school health services

technology

The Joint Commission

TRICARE

U.S. Department of Health and Human Services (USDHHS)

value-based compensation

Veteran's Administration

voluntary agencies

workers' compensation

World Health Organization (WHO)

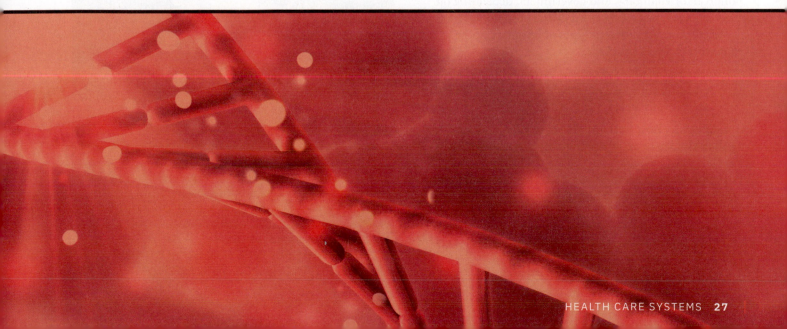

2:1 PRIVATE HEALTH CARE FACILITIES

Today, health care systems include the many agencies, facilities, and personnel involved in the delivery of health care. According to U.S. government statistics, health care is one of the largest and fastest-growing industries in the United States. This industry employs more than 17 million workers in more than 200 different health care careers. It attracts people with a wide range of educational backgrounds because it offers multiple career options. By the year 2026, health care employment is expected to increase by 11.6 million jobs to more than 28.1 million workers. Health care spending in the United States is projected to increase from more than $3.8 trillion in 2020 or 17.8 percent of the GDP to 19.9 percent of the GDP in 2025.

Many different health care facilities provide services that are a part of the industry called *health care* (**Figure 2–1**). Most private health care facilities require a fee for services. In some cases, grants and contributions provide some financial support for these facilities. A basic description of the various facilities will help provide an understanding of the many different types of services included under the umbrella of the health care industry.

HOSPITALS

Hospitals are one of the major types of health care facilities. They vary in size and types of services provided. Some hospitals are small and serve the basic needs of a community; others are large, complex centers offering a wide range of services including diagnosis, treatment, education, and research. Hospitals are also classified as private or proprietary (operated for profit), religious, nonprofit or voluntary, and government, depending on the sources of income received by the hospital.

There are many different types of hospitals. Some of the more common ones include:

- **General hospitals**: treat a wide range of conditions and age groups; usually provide diagnostic, medical, surgical, and emergency care services for acute care

- **Specialty hospitals**: provide care for special conditions or age groups; examples include burn hospitals, oncology (cancer) hospitals, pediatric (children's) hospitals, psychiatric hospitals (dealing with mental diseases and disorders), orthopedic hospitals (dealing with bone, joint, or muscle diseases), cosmetic surgery, and rehabilitative hospitals (offering services such as physical and occupational therapy)

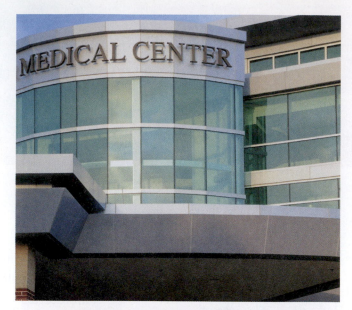

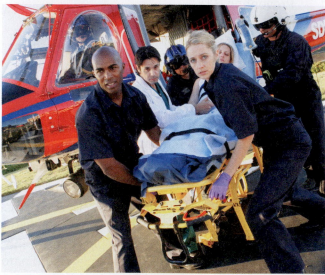

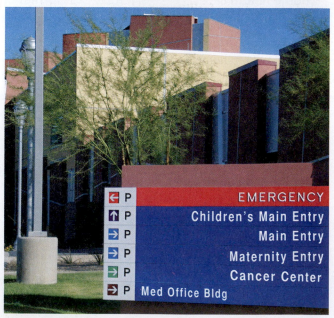

FIGURE 2–1 Different health care facilities. Top image, © iStock.com/ Steve Shepard; middle Image, © iStock.com/Catherine Yeulet; and bottom image, © iStock.com/Paul Hill

- **Government hospitals**: operated by federal, state, and local government agencies; include the many facilities located throughout the world that provide care for government service personnel and their dependents; examples are Veterans Administration hospitals (which provide care for veterans), state psychiatric hospitals, and state rehabilitation centers

- **University or college medical centers**: provide hospital services as well as research and education; can be funded by private and/or governmental sources

In many instances, the classifications and types of hospitals can overlap. For example, a hospital in a major city can be a for-profit hospital but still receive government funding. A hospital can also be a general hospital but offer specialty services such as oncology and pediatrics.

LONG-TERM CARE FACILITIES

Long-term care facilities (LTCs or LTCFs) mainly provide assistance and care for elderly patients, usually called *residents*. However, they also provide care for individuals with disabilities or handicaps and individuals with chronic or long-term illnesses.

There are many different types of long-term care facilities. Some of the more common ones include:

- **Residential care facilities (nursing homes or geriatric homes)**: designed to provide basic physical and emotional care for individuals who can no longer care for themselves; help individuals with activities of daily living (ADLs), provide a safe and secure environment, and promote opportunities for social interactions

- **Extended care facilities or skilled care facilities**: designed to provide skilled nursing care and rehabilitative care to prepare patients* or residents for return to home environments or other long-term care facilities; some have *subacute units* designed to provide services to patients who need rehabilitation to recover from a major illness or surgery, treatment for cancer, or treatments such as kidney dialysis or heart monitoring

- **Independent living facilities** and **assisted living facilities**: allow individuals who can care for themselves to rent or purchase an apartment in the facility; provide services such as meals, housekeeping, laundry, transportation, social events, and basic medical care (such as assisting with medications)

Most assisted or independent living facilities are associated with nursing homes, extended care facilities,

and/or skilled care facilities. This arrangement allows an individual to move readily from one level of care to the next when health needs change. Many long-term care facilities also offer special services such as the delivery of meals to the homes of older adults, the chronically ill, or people with disabilities. Some facilities offer senior citizen or adult day care centers, which provide social activities and other services for older people. The need for long-term care facilities has increased dramatically because of the large increase in the number of older people. Many health care career opportunities are available in these facilities, and there is a shortage of nurses and other trained personnel.

MEDICAL OFFICES

Medical offices vary from offices that are privately owned by one physician to large complexes that operate as corporations and employ many physicians and other health care professionals. Medical services obtained in these facilities can include diagnosis (determining the nature of an illness), treatment, examination, basic laboratory testing, minor surgery, and other similar care. Some physicians treat a wide variety of illnesses and age groups, but others specialize in and handle only certain age groups or conditions. Examples of specialties include pediatrics (infants and children), cardiology (diseases and disorders of the heart), obstetrics (care during pregnancy), and pulmonology (respiratory diseases).

CONCIERGE MEDICINE

Concierge medicine, or *retainer medicine*, is a type of personalized health care. In exchange for an annual or monthly fee, an enhanced level of care is provided by a primary care physician. The physician is able to care for fewer patients while having more availability. The rates and services vary among providers.

DENTAL OFFICES

Dental offices vary in size from offices that are privately owned by one or more dentists to dental clinics that employ a group of dentists. In some areas, major retail or department stores operate dental clinics. Dental services can include general care provided to all age groups or specialized care offered to certain age groups or for certain dental conditions like orthodontics (straighten teeth).

CLINICS OR SATELLITE CENTERS

Clinics, also called *satellite clinics* or *ambulatory centers*, are health care facilities found in many types of health care. Some clinics are composed of a group of medical or

---

*In some health care facilities, patients are referred to as *clients*. For the purposes of this text, *patient* will be used.

dental doctors and other personnel who share a facility. Other clinics are operated by private groups who provide special care. Examples include:

- **Surgical clinics or surgicenters**: perform minor surgical procedures and some cosmetic surgeries; frequently called "one-day" surgical centers because patients are sent home immediately after they recover from their operations
- **Urgent, walk-in, or emergency care clinics**: provide first aid or emergency care to acutely ill or injured patients
- **Rehabilitation clinics**: offer physical, occupational, speech, and other similar therapies
- **Substance abuse clinics**: provide rehabilitation for drug and alcohol abuse
- **Specialty clinics**: provide care for specific diseases; examples include diabetic clinics, kidney dialysis centers, and oncology (cancer) clinics
- **Outpatient or ambulatory clinics**: usually operated by hospitals or large medical groups; provide care for outpatients (patients who are not admitted to the hospital)
- **Health department clinics**: may offer clinics for pediatric health care, treatment of sexually transmitted diseases, treatment of respiratory disease, immunizations, and other special services
- **Medical center clinics**: usually located in colleges or universities; offer clinics for various health conditions; offer care and treatment and provide learning experiences for medical students

OPTICAL CENTERS

Optical centers can be individually owned by an ophthalmologist or optometrist, or they can be part of a large chain of stores. They provide vision examinations, prescribe eyeglasses or contact lenses, and check for the presence of eye diseases.

EMERGENCY CARE SERVICES

Emergency care services provide special care for victims of accidents or sudden (acute) illness. Facilities providing these services include ambulance services, both private and governmental; rescue squads, frequently operated by fire departments; emergency care clinics and centers; emergency departments operated by hospitals; and helicopter or airplane emergency services that rapidly transport patients to medical facilities for special care.

LABORATORIES

Laboratories are often a part of other facilities but can operate as separate health care services. Medical laboratories can perform special diagnostic tests such as blood or urine tests. Dental laboratories can prepare dentures (false teeth) and many other devices used to repair or replace teeth. Medical and dental offices, small hospitals, clinics, and many other health care facilities frequently use the services provided by laboratories.

HOME HEALTH CARE

Home health care agencies are designed to provide care in a patient's home (**Figure 2–2**). Older adults and people with disabilities frequently use the services of these agencies. Examples of such services include nursing care, personal care, therapy (physical, occupational, speech, respiratory), and homemaking (food preparation, cleaning, and other household tasks). Health departments, hospitals, private agencies, government agencies, and nonprofit or volunteer groups can offer home care services.

HOSPICE

Hospice agencies provide care for people who are terminally ill and who usually have life expectancies of 6 months or less. Care can be provided in a person's home or in a hospice facility. Hospice offers palliative care, or care that provides support and comfort and is directed toward allowing the person to die with dignity. Psychological, social, spiritual, and financial counseling are provided for both the patient and the family. Hospice also provides support to the family following a patient's death.

MENTAL HEALTH FACILITIES

Mental health facilities treat patients who have mental disorders and diseases. Examples of these facilities include guidance and counseling centers, psychiatric clinics and hospitals, chemical abuse treatment centers (dealing with alcohol and drug abuse), and physical abuse treatment centers (dealing with child abuse, spousal abuse, and geriatric [elder] abuse).

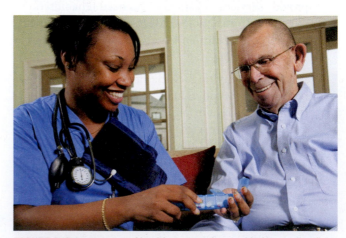

FIGURE 2–2 Many types of health care can be provided in a patient's home. © iStock.com/Steve Debenport

GENETIC COUNSELING CENTERS

Genetic counseling centers can be independent facilities or can be located in another facility such as a hospital, clinic, or physician's office. Genetic counselors work with couples or individuals who are pregnant or considering a pregnancy. They perform prenatal (before birth) screening tests, check for genetic abnormalities and birth defects, explain the results of the tests, identify medical options when a birth defect is present, and help the individuals cope with the psychological issues caused by a genetic disorder. Examples of genetic disorders include Down syndrome and cystic fibrosis. Counselors frequently consult with couples before a pregnancy if the pregnancy occurs in the late childbearing years, there is a family history of genetic disease, or it involves a specific race or nationality with a high risk for genetic disease.

REHABILITATION FACILITIES

Rehabilitation facilities are located in hospitals, clinics, and/or private centers. They provide care to help patients who have physical or mental disabilities obtain the maximum self-care and function. Services may include physical, occupational, recreational, speech, and hearing therapy.

HEALTH MAINTENANCE ORGANIZATIONS

Health maintenance organizations (HMOs) are both health care delivery systems and a type of health insurance. They provide total health care services that are primarily directed toward preventive health care for a fee that is usually fixed and prepaid. Services include examinations, basic medical services, health education, and hospitalization or rehabilitation services, as needed. Some HMOs are operated by large industries or corporations; others are operated by private agencies. They often use the services of other health care facilities including medical and dental offices, hospitals, rehabilitative centers, home health care agencies, clinics, and laboratories.

INDUSTRIAL HEALTH CARE CENTERS

Industrial health care centers or *occupational health clinics* are found in large companies or industries. Such centers provide health care for employees of the industry or business by performing basic examinations, teaching accident prevention and safety, and providing emergency care. Major resort industries, such as Disney, may also provide emergency health care to visitors.

SCHOOL HEALTH SERVICES

School health services are found in schools and colleges. These services provide emergency care for victims of accidents and sudden illness; perform tests to check for health conditions such as speech, vision, and hearing problems; promote health education; and maintain a safe and sanitary school environment. Many school health services also provide counseling.

PHARMACEUTICAL SERVICES

Pharmaceutical services, also called pharmacies, chemists, or drug stores, link health science with chemical science. A pharmacist prepares and dispenses medications and provides expertise on drug therapy. Pharmacists also ensure patient safety through education. Pharmaceutical services can be found in many settings—including hospitals, community stores, clinics, nursing homes, and even online. In addition to prescription drugs, many pharmaceutical services also offer over-the-counter drugs (for conditions such as pain, colds, and allergies), vitamins, and herbal remedies.

check**point**

1. Describe eight (8) types of private health care facilities.

2:2 GOVERNMENT HEALTH AGENCIES

In addition to the government health care facilities mentioned previously, other health services are offered at the international, national, state, and local levels. Government services are tax supported. State and local health departments serve critical roles in promoting the health of residents in their jurisdictions. Examples of government agencies include:

- **World Health Organization (WHO):** an international agency sponsored by the United Nations; compiles statistics and information on disease, publishes health information, and investigates and addresses serious health problems throughout the world; the main objective of the WHO, per its constitution, "is the attainment by all people of the highest possible level of health care"; Internet address: *www.who.int*

- **U.S. Department of Health and Human Services (USDHHS):** a national agency that deals with the health problems in the United States; its goal is to protect the health of all Americans, especially those people who are in need; provides more grant money than any other federal agency; Internet address: *www.hhs.gov*

- **National Institutes of Health (NIH)**: a division of the USDHHS; involved in researching disease and conducting scientific studies; Internet address: *www.nih.gov*

- **Centers for Disease Control and Prevention (CDC)**: another division of the USDHHS; concerned with the causes, spread, and control of diseases in populations (**Figure 2–3**); Internet address: *www.cdc.gov*

- **Food and Drug Administration (FDA)**: a federal agency responsible for regulating food and drug products sold to the public; also protects the public by regulating things such as medical devices, cosmetics, and cell phones; Internet address: *www.fda.gov*

- **Agency for Healthcare Research and Quality (AHRQ)**: a federal agency established to improve the quality, safety, efficiency, and effectiveness of health care for Americans; Internet address: *www.ahrq.gov*

- **Occupational Safety and Health Administration (OSHA)**: establishes and enforces standards that protect workers from job-related injuries and illnesses; issues standards on things such as limits on chemical and radiation exposure and use of personal protective equipment; Internet address: *www.osha.gov*

- **Office of the National Coordinator for Health Information Technology (ONC)**: leads national efforts to build a private and secure nationwide health information exchange; its goal is to improve health care by allowing health information to be exchanged quickly among providers. Internet address: *www.healthit.gov*

- **Public Health Systems/Health departments**: provide health services as directed by the U.S. Department of Health and Human Services (USDHHS); the public health system in the United States is a complex network of people and organizations in both public and private sectors that collaborate in various ways at national, state and local levels to promote and protect public health. When facing global pandemics or health threats, these agencies can recommend mandates like "shelter in place" and self-quarantine requirements to protect the public. They also provide specific services needed by the state or local community; examples of services include testing and immunization for disease control, inspections for environmental health and sanitation, collection of statistics and records related to health, health education, clinics for health care and prevention, and other services needed in a community; local health care services provide information on home care, recreation activities, meal and food assistance programs, transport, and other resources that will support people's well-being; Internet address: *www.hhs.gov*; use the search box to locate the web address of a specific state or local health department

- **Veteran's Administration**: a federal agency that provides health care for veterans and their families; also is America's largest integrated health care system, providing care at hospitals, medical centers and outpatient sites serving 9 million enrolled veterans each year; Internet address: *https://www.va.gov*

check**point**

1. Name three (3) ways that national government agencies provide services to the health care community.
2. Name three (3) ways that the health department provides services for both state and local health care.

2:3 VOLUNTARY OR NONPROFIT AGENCIES

Voluntary agencies, frequently called **nonprofit agencies**, are supported by donations, membership fees, fundraisers, and federal or state grants. They provide health services at the national, state, and local levels.

The Joint Commission is a nonprofit, U.S.-based organization that was created to ensure that patients receive the safest, highest quality care in any health care setting. Meeting the standards of The Joint Commission is recognized as a symbol of quality. In many states, a Joint Commission accreditation is required to receive Medicaid reimbursement. Its Internet address is *www.jointcommission.org*.

Other examples of nonprofit agencies include the American Cancer Society, American Heart Association, American Respiratory Disease Association, American Diabetes Association, National Mental Health Association, Alzheimer's Association, National Kidney Foundation,

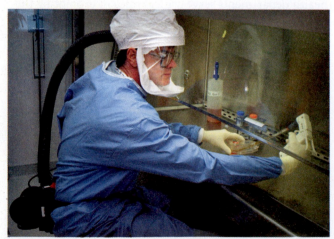

FIGURE 2–3 The Centers for Disease Control and Prevention (CDC) deals with the causes, spread, and control of diseases in populations.
CDC/James Gathany

Leukemia and Lymphoma Society, March of Dimes Foundation, American Red Cross, and Autism Speaks. Many of these organizations have national offices as well as branch offices in states and/or local communities.

As indicated by their names, many such organizations focus on one specific disease or group of diseases. Each organization typically studies the disease, provides funding to encourage research directed at curing or treating the disease, and promotes public education regarding the information obtained through research. These organizations also provide special services to victims of disease, such as purchasing medical equipment and supplies, providing treatment centers, and supplying information regarding other community agencies that offer assistance.

Nonprofit agencies employ many health care workers in addition to using volunteers to provide services.

checkpoint

| **1.** What is The Joint Commission?

2:4 ORGANIZATIONAL STRUCTURE

All health care facilities must have some type of **organizational structure**. The structure may be complex, as in larger facilities, or simple, as in smaller facilities. Organizational structure always, however, encompasses a line of authority or chain of command. The organizational structure should indicate areas of responsibility and lead to the most efficient operation of the facility.

A sample organizational chart for a large general hospital is shown in **Figure 2–4**. This chart shows organization by department. Each department, in turn, can have an organizational chart similar to the one shown for the nursing department in Figure 2–4. A sample organizational chart for a small medical office is shown in **Figure 2–5**. The organizational structure will vary with the size of the office and the number of people employed.

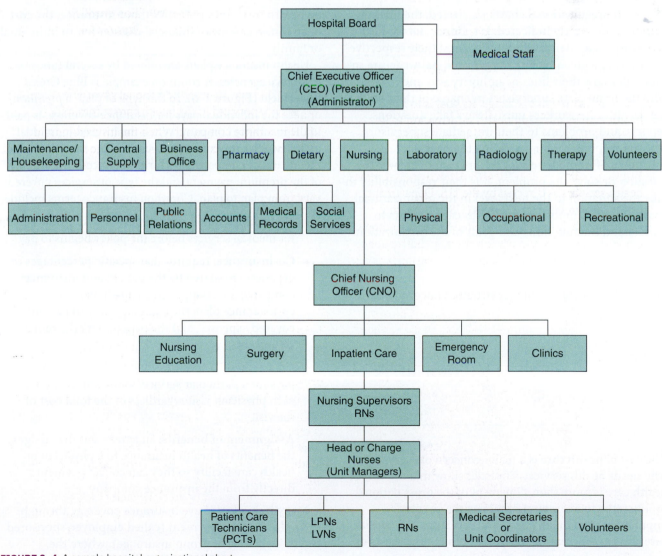

FIGURE 2–4 A sample hospital organizational chart.

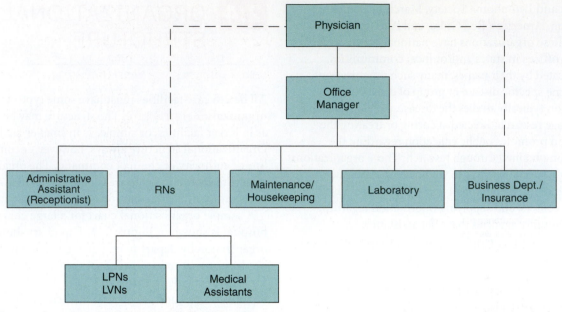

FIGURE 2–5 A sample medical office organizational chart.

In both organizational charts illustrated, the lines of authority are clearly indicated. It is important for health care workers to identify and understand their respective positions in a given facility's organizational structure so they will know their lines of authority and understand who the immediate supervisors in charge of their work are. Health care workers must always take questions, reports, and problems to their immediate supervisors, who are responsible for providing the necessary assistance. If immediate supervisors cannot answer the question or solve the problem, it is their responsibility to take the situation to the next level in the organizational chart. It is also important for health care workers to understand the functions and goals of the organization.

checkpoint

1. What does organizational structure encompass?

2:5 HEALTH INSURANCE PLANS

The cost of health care is a major concern of everyone who needs health services. Statistics show that the cost of health care is more than 17 percent of the gross national product (the total amount of money the country's population spent on all goods and services). Also, health care costs are increasing much faster than other costs of living. To pay for the costs of health care, most people rely on **health insurance plans**. Without insurance, the cost of an illness can mean financial disaster for an individual or family.

Health insurance plans are offered by several thousand insurance agencies. A common example is Blue Cross/Blue Shield (**Figure 2–6**). In this type of plan, a *premium*, or a fee the individual pays for insurance coverage, is paid to the insurance company. When the insured individual incurs health care expenses covered by the insurance plan, the insurance company pays for the services. The amount of the premium payment and the type of services covered vary from plan to plan. Common insurance terms include:

- **Deductibles**: amounts that must be paid by the patient for medical services before the policy begins to pay

- **Co-insurance**: requires that specific percentages of expenses are shared by the patient and insurance company; for example, in an 80–20 percent co-insurance plan, the company pays 80 percent of covered expenses, and the patient pays the remaining 20 percent

- **Co-payment**: a specific amount of money a patient pays for a particular service, for example, $20 for each physician visit regardless of the total cost of the visit

- **Assignment of benefits**: an agreement that assigns the benefits of health insurance to a physician or health care facility so they can collect payment directly from the insurance company

Many individuals have insurance coverage through their places of employment (called employer-sponsored health insurance or group insurance), where the premiums are paid by the employer. In most cases,

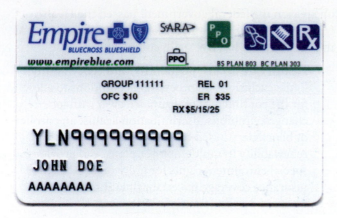

FIGURE 2–6 Health insurance plans help pay for the costs of health care. *Courtesy of Empire Blue Cross and Blue Shield*

the individual also pays a percentage of the premium. Private policies are also available for purchase by individuals.

A health maintenance organization (HMO) is another type of health insurance plan that provides a managed care plan for the delivery of health care services. A monthly fee or premium is paid for membership, and the fee stays the same regardless of the amount of health care used. The premium can be paid by an employer and/or an individual. The care provided is directed toward preventive-type health care. Therefore, an individual insured under this type of plan has ready access to health examinations and early treatment and detection of disease. Because most other types of insurance plans do not cover routine examinations and preventive care, an individual insured by an HMO can therefore theoretically maintain a better state of health. The disadvantage of an HMO is that the insured is required to use only HMO-affiliated health care providers (doctors, laboratories, hospitals) for health care. If a nonaffiliated health care provider is used instead, the insured usually must pay for the care.

A **preferred provider organization (PPO)** is another type of managed care health insurance plan usually provided by large industries or companies to their employees. The PPO forms a contract with certain health care agencies, such as a large hospital and specific doctors and dentists, to provide certain types of health care at reduced rates. Employees are restricted to using the specific hospital and doctors, but the industry or company using the PPO can provide health care at lower rates. PPOs usually require a deductible and a co-payment. If an enrollee uses a nonaffiliated provider, the PPO may require co-payments of 40–60 percent.

The government also provides health insurance plans for certain groups of people. Two of the main plans are Medicare and Medicaid.

Medicare is a federal government program that provides health care for almost all individuals age 65 and older, for any person with a disability who has received Social Security benefits for at least 2 years, and for any person with end-stage renal (kidney) disease. Medicare consists of three kinds of coverage: type A for hospital insurance, type B for medical insurance, and type D for pharmaceutical (medication) expenses. Type A covers hospital services, care provided by an extended care facility or home health care agency after hospitalization, and hospice care for people who have terminal illnesses. Type B offers additional coverage for doctors' services, outpatient treatments, therapy, clinical laboratory services, and other health care. The individual does pay a premium for type B coverage and also must pay an initial deductible for services. In addition, Medicare pays for only 80 percent of these medical services; the individual must either pay the balance or have another insurance policy to cover the expenses.

A **Medigap policy** is a health insurance plan that helps pay medical expenses not covered by Medicare. These policies are offered by private insurance companies and require the enrollee to pay a premium. Medigap policies must meet specific federal guidelines. They provide options that allow enrollees to choose how much coverage they want to purchase.

Medicaid is a medical assistance program that is jointly funded by the federal government and state governments but operated by individual states. Benefits and individuals covered under this program vary slightly from state to state because each state has the right to establish its own eligibility standards, determine the type and scope of services, set the rate of payment for services, and administer its own program. In most states, Medicaid pays for the health care of individuals with low incomes, children who qualify for public assistance, and individuals who are physically disabled or blind. Generally, all state Medicaid programs provide hospital services, physician's care, long-term care services, and some therapies. In some states, Medicaid offers dental care, eye care, and other specialized services.

The Children's Health Insurance Program (CHIP) was established in 1997 to provide health care to uninsured children of working families who earn too little to afford private insurance but too much to be eligible for Medicaid. It provides inpatient and outpatient hospital services, physician's surgical and medical care, laboratory and X-ray tests, and well-baby and well-child care, including immunizations.

Workers' compensation is a health insurance plan providing treatment for workers injured on the job. It is administered by the state, and payments are made by employers and the state. In addition to providing payment for needed health care, this plan also reimburses the worker for wages lost because of an on-the-job injury.

TRICARE is a U.S. government health insurance plan for all military personnel. It provides care for all active duty members and their families, survivors of military personnel, and retired members of the Armed Forces. The Veterans Administration provides care for military veterans.

Managed care is an approach that has developed in response to rising health care costs. Employers, as well as insurance companies who pay large medical bills, want to ensure that such money is spent efficiently rather than wastefully. The principle behind managed care is that all health care provided to a patient must have a purpose. A second opinion or verification of need is frequently required before care can be provided. Every effort is made to provide preventive care and early diagnosis of disease to avoid the high cost of treating disease. For example, routine physical examinations, well-baby care, immunizations, and wellness education to promote good nutrition, exercise, weight control, and healthy living practices are usually provided under managed care. Employers and insurance companies create a network of doctors, specialists, therapists, and health care facilities that provide care at the most reasonable cost. HMOs and PPOs are the main providers of managed care, but many private insurance companies are establishing health care networks to provide care to their subscribers. As these health care networks compete for the consumer dollar, they are required to provide quality care at the lowest possible cost. The health care consumer who is enrolled in a managed care plan receives quality care at the most reasonable cost but the choice of health care providers is restricted.

Fee-for-service compensation is a health payment plan in which doctors or providers are paid for each service they render. They are paid a set amount for each office visit, test, and procedure. With this form of compensation, there is little incentive to consider the cost or necessity of services provided.

Value-based compensation, or bundled payments, is a health payment plan in which doctors are paid for their performance. This form of compensation takes into account quality, cost, patient satisfaction, and patient outcomes. Doctors and providers are paid a certain amount for each diagnosis or disease. This type of plan has been met with resistance because the uniqueness of each patient and each disease complicates the idea of placing a measurable value on each case.

Health insurance plans do not solve all the problems of health care costs, but they do help many people by paying for all or part of the cost of health services. However, as the cost of insurance increases, many employers are less willing to offer health care insurance. Individuals with chronic illnesses often find they cannot obtain insurance coverage if their place of employment changes. This is

HIPAA

one reason the federal government passed the **Health Insurance Portability and Accountability Act (HIPAA)** in 1996. This act has five main components:

- **Health care access, portability, and renewability**: limits exclusions on preexisting conditions to allow for the continuance of insurance even with job changes, prohibits discrimination against an enrollee or beneficiary based on health status, guarantees renewability in multiemployer plans, and provides special enrollment rights for individuals who lose insurance coverage in certain situations such as divorce or termination of employment

- **Preventing health care fraud and abuse; administrative simplification and medical liability reform**: establishes methods for preventing fraud and abuse and imposes sanctions or penalties if fraud or abuse does occur, reduces the costs and administration of health care by adopting a single set of electronic standards to replace the wide variety of formats used in health care, provides strict guidelines for maintaining the confidentiality of health care information and the security of health care records, and recommends limits for medical liability. The confidentiality requirement is discussed in more detail in Section 5:1 under Privacy Act.

- **Tax-related health provisions**: promotes the use of medical savings accounts (MSAs) by allowing tax deductions for monies placed in the accounts, establishes standards for long-term care insurance, allows for the creation of state insurance pools, and provides tax benefits for some health care expenses

- **Application and enforcement of group health plan requirements**: establishes standards that require group health care plans to offer portability, access, and renewability to all members of the group

- **Revenue offsets**: provides changes to the Internal Revenue Code for HIPAA expenses

Compliance with all HIPAA regulations was required by April 2004 for all health care agencies. These regulations have not solved all of the problems of health care insurance, but they have provided consumers with more access to insurance and greater confidentiality in regard to medical records. In addition, standardization of electronic health care records, reductions in administrative costs, increased tax benefits, and decreased fraud and abuse in health care have reduced health care costs for everyone.

Major changes to health care insurance have been provided by the **Patient Protection and Affordable Care Act (PPACA)**, also called the *Affordable Care Act (ACA)*. This act was signed into law in March 2010, and by 2014 most of the provisions of the act were in place. The primary provisions of this law are:

- Guaranteed issue that requires all insurers to charge the same premium to all applicants of the same gender, age, and geographic location, regardless of preexisting conditions

- Prohibits insurance companies from rescinding coverage to any individual as long as premiums are paid

- Expands Medicaid eligibility to include families and individuals with incomes up to 133 percent of the poverty level unless a particular state opts out of this requirement

- Creates affordable insurance exchanges in every state that provide a more organized and competitive market for insurance, offers a choice of plans to individuals or small businesses, and establishes common rules regarding the offering and pricing of insurance

- Provides subsidies for low-income families, individuals, or very small businesses, on a sliding income scale of between 100 percent and 400 percent of the poverty level, to purchase insurance through a health insurance exchange

- Allows a young adult to be covered under a parent's policy up to age 26

- Provides increased enrollment for Medicaid and CHIP

- Improves benefits for Medicare and prescription drug coverage

- Allows a restructuring of Medicare reimbursement from fee-for-service to bundled payments; for example, a specific amount is paid to a group of physicians for treating a patient with a specific diagnosis instead of individual payments for each treatment provided

- Gives a small business tax credit to qualified small businesses and nonprofit organizations that provide health insurance for employees

- Establishes a national voluntary insurance program that allows individuals to purchase community living assistance services and support for long-term care

- Establishes a Prevention and Public Health Fund to create programs that promote good health and prevent disease

- Provides additional support for medical research and the National Institutes of Health

- Requires minimum health insurance standards and removes annual and lifetime coverage caps

- Eliminates co-payments for insurance benefits that have been mandated as essential coverage benefits such as those for specified preventive care services

- Requires insurance companies to spend at least 80 to 85 percent of premiums collected on medical costs or to refund excess money to the insured individuals

- Mandates that insurance companies provide coverage for individuals participating in clinical trials

Consumer responsibility for health care costs continues to increase as both consumers and health care plans struggle to control cost. It is essential for individuals to take an active role and become responsible consumers of health care. Some ways consumers can meet this responsibility include:

- **Take an active role in maintaining good health**: Maintain a healthy lifestyle by eating a healthy diet, exercising regularly, getting adequate rest, avoiding tobacco and drugs, getting immunizations to prevent disease, practicing wellness, and obtaining screening tests for early detection of disease.

- **Evaluate different health care plans**: Compare different plans based on cost, benefits, and quality of care and choose the plan that will provide quality care at the most reasonable cost.

- **Research quality of care:** Use resources available on the Internet and media to see which health care providers are rated high for quality care, and try to use these providers whenever possible; seek recommendations from friends and family and check credentials for any health care provider.

- **Make informed decisions regarding health care**: Ask questions regarding different treatments and choose care based on their own values and beliefs; choose health care providers who make every effort to provide information about choices available and the risks and benefits of each choice.

- **Use health care plan benefits wisely**: Be informed about what co-insurance, deductibles, and other costs are with any plan and try to minimize these costs; for example, a visit to an urgent care is usually much cheaper than a visit to an emergency room for many acute illnesses.

- **Make every effort to save money on health care costs**: Use in-network physicians and facilities whenever possible; price medications to see if a generic equivalent- or lower-priced mail-order is available; check medical bills carefully for accuracy, and question any charges that do not seem appropriate.

- **Help prevent medical errors**: Question any care that does not seem appropriate; keep track of test results, and ask for explanations about abnormal results; check medications to ascertain they are correct.

Nature as a Pharmacy?

Throughout history, many medicines have been derived from natural resources. Examples include aspirin, which comes from willow bark; penicillin, which comes from fungus; and the cancer drug Taxol, which comes from the Pacific yew tree. Recognizing this, many scientists believe that nature is a pharmaceutical gold mine and are exploring the vast supply of materials present in the oceans and on the earth.

The National Cancer Institute (NCI) has more than 50,000 samples of plants and 10,000 samples of marine organisms stored in Frederick, Maryland. Every sample is crushed into a powder and made into extracts that can be tested against human cancer cells. More than 110,000 extracts of these samples are available to other scientists who evaluate their effectiveness against conditions such as viral diseases and infections. To date, more than 4,000 extracts have shown promise and are being used in more advanced studies. One compound, Halichondrin B, labeled "yellow slimy" by researchers, is an extract taken from a deep-sea sponge found in New Zealand. Scientists created a synthetic version of the active component in Halichondrin B, called E7389. After extensive testing, the drug Eribulin, which was created from this compound, was approved by the FDA in 2010 as a treatment for metastatic breast cancer. Bristol-Myers received FDA approval for another drug, Ixabepilone, that is extracted from garden soil bacteria and is also used to treat metastatic breast cancer. Wyeth's drug Rapamune was isolated from soil on Easter Island and approved for preventing kidney rejection after transplants. Another novel drug involves photodynamic activity. A substance called psoralen is obtained from a Nile-dwelling weed called ammi. Psoralen is inactive until it is exposed to light. When it is activated, it attaches to the DNA of cancer cells and kills them. Research led to the approval of a psoralen-like drug that is exposed to certain wavelengths of light and used to treat some forms of lymphoma, a cancer of white blood cells. By creating synthetic versions of the compounds, scientists are preserving natural resources while also benefiting from them.

Other natural products are now being tested and modified. Clinical trials are being conducted on ecteinascidin, which is a substance obtained from a sea creature called a tunicate (a marine organism that spends most of its life attached to docks or rocks). Lab tests show it is safe for humans and that it may be an effective treatment for soft-tissue sarcomas (tumors of the muscles, tendons, and supportive tissues). In 2015, the FDA did give limited approval to trabectedin (Yondelis), a medication derived from ecteinascidin, for liposarcomas and leiomyosarcomas that cannot be removed or that have metastasized. Further clinical trials are being conducted.

Other unique studies involve cone snails found in the reefs surrounding Australia, Indonesia, and the Philippines. These animals produce a unique venom containing nerve toxins. Some of these venoms are being studied as pain relievers because they block pain signals from reaching the brain. Researchers in Oslo, Norway, are studying and testing plant extracts from the sweet wormwood plant and the bark of the cinchona tree to determine if an effective drug can be created to destroy both the malaria parasite and the mosquitoes that carry the parasite. An intriguing bioluminescent bacterium named *Vibrio fischeri* has researchers trying to develop antibiotics that prevent bacterial resistance. This special bacterium emits light when it senses that there are enough bacteria to draw prey that can be used as sources of nourishment, a phenomenon called "quorum sensing," similar to the "safety in numbers" concept. When there are enough of these bacteria, they signal each other and produce an enzyme that creates light. Disease-producing bacteria also use quorum sensing, and when a quorum is reached, they form slimy, sticky biofilms and produce toxins that make people sick. If researchers can develop a class of antibiotics that disrupt the signals bacteria use to sense a quorum or destroy the biofilms that are formed, they can destroy the action of the bacteria and render them harmless. Because the drugs do not kill the bacteria, the bacteria would be less likely to develop resistance. As scientists continue to explore all that nature has to offer, it is possible they will find cures for many cancers, diseases, and infections.

It is essential to remember that all health care consumers have the right and responsibility to fully participate in all decisions related to their health care, and if they are unable to participate, they have the right to be represented by parents, family members, or guardians.

check**point**

1. What does the term *deductible* mean?
2. What group of people does Medicare insurance cover?

2:6 IMPACT OF EMERGING ISSUES ON DELIVERY SYSTEMS

Technology, applying scientific knowledge for practical purposes to find answers and fix problems, has brought about a massive and welcome change to the health care industry. Patients now have access to some of the best diagnostic tools and new cutting-edge treatments. The digitalization of health records has made for quick, secure, and accessible information to remote providers. Mobile app technology allows patients to easily obtain accurate information and track their own health status over time. Another example of technology in health care is 3-D printing, which is used to create prosthetics, hearing aids, and more. Virtual reality devices help depression and isolation in older patients. Developments in technology are constantly streamlining and improving how patients interact with their health care providers.

Addictions and substance use disorders are medical conditions and their treatment has impacts on and is impacted by other mental and physical health conditions. Individuals with substance use disorders often access the health care system for reasons other than their substance use disorder.

Effective integration of prevention, treatment, and recovery services across health care systems is key to addressing substance misuse and its consequences. It represents the most promising way to improve access to and quality of treatment. Recent health care reform laws are facilitating greater integration to better serve individual and public health, reduce health disparities, and reduce costs to society.

Epidemiology is the study of disease in populations. Epidemiological methods are used for disease surveillance to identify which hazards are the most important. They also identify risk factors that may represent critical control points in health and food/drug production systems. Fast and effective management of resources to maintain and promote the health of populations helps control costs. The use of epidemiological concepts and tools to improve decisions about the management of health services helps pinpoint specific areas of concentration to efficiently improve the health of a population.

Bioethics comes into play as medical technology advances at a rapid pace, and health care providers are tasked with examining the resulting ethical dilemmas. Applying the principles of ethics to the field of medicine, bioethics aims to investigate and study how health care decisions are made. It is a core component of ensuring that medical practices and procedures benefit society as a whole. Deciding who gets what is a main task for medical ethics. Should scarce health care resources be divided according to need, ability to pay, potential for economic productivity, or some other criteria? Should doctors at the bedside be the gatekeepers, or should financial managers or others make the rules from a distance? Should people get health care whether or not they "deserve" it—for example, should criminals or heavy smokers receive transplants that are currently in shortage? Should cosmetic surgery be publicly funded? Should health care be a right for all, and if so, does it mean that taxes ought to pay for it all? Should people be forced to purchase health insurance, and if so, at what income level? These ethical questions involve a myriad of complexities. The answers to these pressing questions directly impact health care delivery system risk, efficiency, and, ultimately, cost.

Socioeconomic status (SES) affects individuals' health outcomes and the health care they receive. Low-socioeconomic patients receive fewer diagnostic tests and medications for many chronic diseases and have limited access to health care due to cost and coverage. Patients find it difficult to find providers who are able and/or willing to care for them. The limited number of physicians and hospitals treating patients of low SES create distance and time barriers, which discourage them even further from seeking care. Patients at times drive for more than an hour to find hospitals that will treat them, and some wait several months to get an appointment with a doctor. These problems make it especially difficult for those who cannot afford to pay for gas, lack reliable transportation, or require emergency treatment. Many patients delay or avoid seeking care because of cost, which typically only results in the worsening of their condition and an even more expensive hospital visit. Health care delivery systems continue to grapple with the best way to provide affordable accessible health care to the growing number of low SES patients.

check**point**

1. What is epidemiology?
2. Identify at least two (2) ways to provide more efficient care for low SES patients.

PRACTICE: Go to the workbook and complete the assignment sheet for Chapter 2, Health Care Systems.

Case Study Investigation Conclusion

What can you conclude about John's care for his medical conditions? Did the agencies involved address his issues adequately? What would explain the sudden appearance of a relative? Does this relative have the right to know John's medical information? Based on what you know about HIPAA law, formulate your theory about the correct flow of information between the agencies and medical facilities involved.

CHAPTER 2 SUMMARY

- Health care, one of the largest and fastest-growing industries in the United States, encompasses many different types of facilities. These include hospitals, long-term care facilities, medical and dental offices, clinics, laboratories, industrial health care centers, school health services, and many others.

- Government, nonprofit, and voluntary agencies also provide health care services. All health care facilities require different health care providers at all levels of training.

- Organizational structure is important in all health care facilities. The structure can be complex or simple, but it should show a line of authority and indicate areas of responsibility.

- Many types of health insurance plans are available to help pay the costs of health care. It is important for consumers to be aware of the types of coverage provided by their respective insurance plans.

- Emerging issues such as technology, addictive and substance disorders, epidemiology, bioethics, and socioeconomic class also have an impact on health care delivery systems.

REVIEW QUESTIONS

1. Differentiate between private, nonprofit, and government types of hospitals.

2. Name each of the following government agencies and briefly describe the services offered by each:
   a. CDC
   b. FDA
   c. NIH
   d. OSHA
   e. USDHHS
   f. WHO
   g. ONC

3. Why is it important for every health care provider to know the organizational structure for their place of employment?

4. What does the term *deductible* mean in regard to health insurance policies? *Co-insurance*? *Co-payment*? *Premium*? *Assignment of benefits*?

5. Describe three (3) services offered by voluntary or nonprofit agencies.

6. Describe the impact of local and state government on the health science industry.

CRITICAL THINKING

1. Mr. and Mrs. Moreno brought their daughter Mia into the emergency room after she fell off the swing in the backyard. They were not worried because they had insurance. They found that their policy stated that they have a co-payment of 80–20 percent and a deductible of $500. If Mia's emergency department bill is $10,660.00, what amount will the Morenos have to pay?

2. What are the five (5) components of HIPAA? Using what you know, give three (3) examples of how a health care facility or a health care worker could be in violation of HIPAA regulations.

3. Create a chart to compare the basic principles of four (4) different health insurance plans.

ACTIVITIES

1. In a group of three, create a medium-sized rehabilitation clinic. Determine a mission statement. Based on what you have learned, create an organizational chart that will reflect the function and goals of your rehab clinic.

2. Does the Patient Protection and Affordable Care Act provide health care insurance to every individual living in the United States? Why or why not?

   Take a position on this topic and write a response.

3. With a partner, compare and contrast the U.S. health care delivery system with those of two other countries that have high efficiency scores in health care as rated by agencies like the World Health Organization. Create a chart along with a report for your team presentation.

CAREERS IN HEALTH CARE

Career

Case Study Investigation

A 6-year-old boy, Luke, was riding his bike on ramps in his backyard while his 4-year-old sister, Hazel, played with the family dog, Rex, nearby. Luke lost control of his bike and crashed into the fence. Before the fence stopped him, he ran over Rex, and the dog pushed Hazel to the ground. The two children were taken by ambulance to the local hospital ER. Luke has a 6-inch laceration, disfigured right arm and is complaining of pain. Hazel was knocked out and is now dizzy and throwing up and has a 2 cm swollen area superior to her right eye. Rex was found under a bush with a swollen abdomen and a crooked leg. He was taken to the Pet Emergency Clinic. At the end of the chapter, you will be asked to identify the health careers that might be involved in the care of Luke, Hazel, and Rex.

■ LEARNING OBJECTIVES

After completing this chapter, you should be able to:

- Compare the educational requirements for associate's, bachelor's, master's, and doctorate degrees.
- Contrast certification, registration, and licensure.
- Describe at least five different health care careers by including a definition of the career, three duties, the educational requirements, and employment opportunities.
- Investigate at least one health care career by contacting online sources to request additional information about the career.
- Interpret at least 10 abbreviations used to identify health care team members.
- Define, pronounce, and spell all key terms.

■ KEY TERMS

admitting officers/clerks

associate's degree

athletic trainers certified (ATCs)

audiologists

bachelor's degree

biological (medical) scientists

biomedical/clinical engineers

biomedical equipment technicians (BETs) (CBETs certified)

cardiovascular technologist

central/sterile service/supply technicians

certification

clinical account managers

clinical account technicians (CATs)

clinical laboratory scientists (CLSs)

clinical laboratory technicians (CLTs)

continuing education units (CEUs)

dental assistants (DAs)

dental hygienists (DHs) *(den'-tall hi-gen'-ists)*

dental laboratory technicians (DLTs)

dentists (DMDs or DDSs)

dialysis technicians *(die-ahl'- ihsis tek-nish'-ins)*

dietetic assistants

KEY TERMS *(continued)*

dietetic technicians (DTs)

dietitians (RDs)

Doctor of Chiropractic (DC) *(Ky-row-prak'-tik)*

Doctor of Medicine (MD)

Doctor of Osteopathic Medicine (DO) *(Oss-tee-oh-path'-ik)*

Doctor of Podiatric Medicine (DPM) *(Poh"-dee'-ah-trik)*

doctorate/doctoral degree

electrocardiograph (ECG) technicians *(ee-lek"-trow-car'-dee-oh-graf tek-nish'-ins)*

electroencephalographic (EEG) technologist *(ee-lek"-trohen-sef-ahl-oh-graf'-ik tek-nahl'-oh-jist)*

electroneurodiagnostic technologist (END) *(ee-lek"-troh-new-roh-die-ag-nah'-stik)*

embalmers *(em-bahl'-mers)*

emergency medical responder (EMR)

emergency medical technician (EMT)

endodontics *(en"-doe-don'-tiks)*

entrepreneur *(on-trah-preh-nor')*

environmental services facilities managers

epidemiologists

ethicists

forensic science technicians

funeral directors

genetic counselors

geneticists

geriatric aides/assistants *(jerry-at-rik)*

health care administrators

health care risk managers

health educators

health information (medical records) administrators (HIAs)

health information (medical records) technicians (HITs)

health science education (HSE)

home health care assistants

housekeeping workers/sanitary managers

industrial hygienists

licensed practical/vocational nurses (LPNs/LVNs)

licensure *(ly'-sehn-shur)*

massage therapists

master's degree

medical administrative assistants

medical assistants (MAs)

medical coders

medical illustrators

medical interpreters/translators

medical (clinical) laboratory assistants

medical laboratory technicians (MLTs)

medical laboratory technologists (MTs)

medical librarians

medical secretaries/health unit coordinators

medical transcriptionists

medication aides/assistants

mortuary assistants

multicompetent/multiskilled health care provider

nurse assistants

occupational therapists (OTs)

occupational therapy assistants (OTAs)

ophthalmic assistants (OAs)

ophthalmic laboratory technicians

ophthalmic medical technologists (OMTs)

ophthalmic technicians (OTs)

ophthalmologists (MD)

opticians *(ahp-tish'-ins)*

optometrists (ODs) *(ahp"-tom'-eh-trists)*

oral surgery

orthodontics *(or"-thow-don'-tiks)*

paramedic (EMT-P)

patient care technicians (PCTs)

pedodontics *(peh"-doe-don'-tiks)*

perfusionists *(purr-few'-shun-ists)*

periodontics *(pehr"-ee-oh-don'-tiks)*

pharmaceutical/clinical project managers

pharmacists (PharmDs) *(far'-mah-sists)*

pharmacologists

pharmacy technicians

phlebotomists

physical therapist assistants (PTAs)

physical therapists (PTs)

physician assistants (PAs)

physicians

process technicians

prosthodontics *(pross"-thow-don'-tiks)*

psychiatric/mental health technicians

psychiatrists

psychologists *(sy-koll'-oh-jists)*

quality control technicians

radiologic technologists (RTs) *(ray'-dee-oh-loge'-ik tek-nahl'-oh-jists)*

recreational therapists (TRs)

recreational therapy assistants

registered nurses (RNs)

registration

respiratory therapists (RTs)

respiratory therapy technicians (RTTs)

scope of practice

social workers (SWs)

speech-language pathologists

surgical technologists/technicians (STs)

toxicologists

transport technicians

veterinarians (DVMs or VMDs) *(vet"-eh-ran-air'-e-ans)*

veterinary assistants

veterinary technologists/technicians (VTs)

3:1 INTRODUCTION TO HEALTH CARE CAREERS

There are more than 250 different health care careers, so it would be impossible to discuss all of them in this chapter. A broad overview of a variety of careers is presented, however.

Math Science

Educational requirements for health care careers depend on many factors and can vary from state to state. Basic preparation begins in high school (secondary education) and should include the sciences, social studies, English, and mathematics. Computer applications and accounting skills are also used in most health care careers. Secondary **health science education (HSE)** programs can prepare a student for immediate employment in many health care careers or for additional education after graduation. Postsecondary education (after high school) can include training in a career/technical school, community college, university, or an accredited online program. Some careers require an **associate's degree**, which is awarded by a career/technical school or a community college after completion of a prescribed two-year course of study. Other careers require a **bachelor's degree**, which is awarded by a college or university after a prescribed course of study that usually lasts for four or more years. In some cases, a **master's degree** is required. This degree is awarded by a college or university after completion of one or more years of work beyond a bachelor's degree. Other careers require a **doctorate** or **doctoral degree**, which is awarded by a college or university after completion of two or more years of work beyond a bachelor's or master's degree. Some doctorates can require four to six years of additional study.

A health science career cluster has been developed by the National Consortium for Health Science Education (NCHSE) (**Figure 3–1**). This cluster allows a student to see how early career awareness and exploration

HEALTH SCIENCE CAREER CLUSTER

Employment in Career Specialties

POST SECONDARY

CAREER PREPARATION PATHWAY STANDARDS

- Diagnostic
- Therapeutic
- Biotechnology Research and Development
- Health Informatics
- Support Services

WORK PLACE

PLACES OF LEARNING

HIGH SCHOOL

CAREER ORIENTATION/PREPARATION CLUSTER FOUNDATION STANDARDS

- Academic Foundation
- Communications
- Systems
- Employability Skills
- Legal Responsibilities
- Ethics
- Safety Practices
- Teamwork
- Health Maintenance Practices
- Technical Skills
- Information Technology Applications

MIDDLE

PLACES OF LEARNING WORK PLACE

ELEMENTARY

CAREER EXPLORATION/ORIENTATION

CAREER AWARENESS

FIGURE 3–1 This cluster shows how early career awareness and exploration can provide a foundation for making informed choices to prepare for a career in health care. Courtesy National Consortium for Health Science Education (NCHSE)

provide the foundation for making informed choices to prepare for a career in health care. Students who take the required courses in middle school and high school have the foundation for success at the postsecondary level. Detailed information and guidance on specific careers can be found on the states' Career Cluster Internet Site, *www.careertech.org*. Additional information can be found at *www.healthscienceconsortium.org*.

CERTIFICATION, REGISTRATION, AND LICENSURE

Three other terms associated with health care careers are *certification*, *registration*, and *licensure*. These are methods used to ensure the skill and competency of health care personnel and to protect the consumer or patient.

Certification means that a person has fulfilled the requirements of education and performance and meets the standards and qualifications established by the professional association or government agency that regulates a particular career. A certificate or statement is issued to the qualified person by the appropriate association. Examples of certified positions include certified dental assistant, certified laboratory technician, and certified medical assistant.

Registration is required in some health care careers. This testing is performed by a regulatory body (professional association or state board) that administers examinations and maintains a current list ("registry") of qualified personnel in a given health care area. Examples of registered positions include registered dietitian, registered respiratory therapist, and registered radiologic technologist.

Licensure is a process whereby a government agency authorizes individuals to work in a given occupation. The license clearly defines the **scope of practice** or the procedures, processes, and actions that health care providers are legally permitted to perform in keeping within the terms of their professional license. Health care careers requiring licensure can vary from state to state. Obtaining and retaining licensure usually requires that a person complete an approved educational program, pass a state board test, and maintain certain standards. Examples of licensed positions include physician, dentist, physical therapist, registered nurse, and licensed practical/vocational nurse.

ACCREDITATION

For most health care careers, graduation from an accredited program is required before certification, registration, and/or licensure will be granted. Accreditation ensures that the program of study meets the established quality competency standards and prepares students for employment in the health care career. It is important for a student to make sure that a technical school, college, or university offers accredited programs of study before enrolling. Two major accrediting agencies for health care programs are the Commission on Accreditation of Allied Health Education Programs (CAAHEP) at *www.caahep.org* and the Accrediting Bureau of Health Education Schools

(ABHES) at *www.abhes.org*. A student can contact these agencies to determine whether an HSE program at a specific school is accredited.

CONTINUING EDUCATION UNITS

Legal

Continuing education units (CEUs) are required to renew licenses or maintain certification or registration in many states (**Figure 3–2**). An individual must obtain additional hours of education in the specific health care career area during a specified period. For example, many states require registered nurses to obtain 24 to 48 CEUs every 1 to 2 years to renew licenses. Health care team members should be aware of the state requirements regarding CEUs for their given careers.

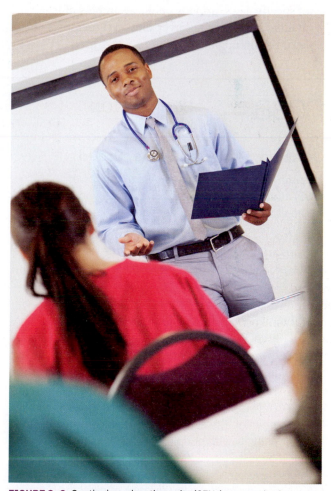

FIGURE 3–2 Continuing education units (CEUs) are required to renew licenses or maintain certification or registration in many states. © iStock. com/Steve Debenport

PROFESSIONAL ORGANIZATIONS

Professional organizations are an important component of many health care careers. A list of professional organizations associated with specific health care careers is provided in this chapter at the end of each career cluster. Individuals benefit greatly by becoming members and being in close contact with other individuals in the same profession. Even though the purposes of the organizations may vary, most provide the following benefits:

- **Professional development**: provide publications, seminars, conferences, and CEUs to keep members current with accurate information relating to the career

- **Career information**: promote the health care career by providing information about the career, encouraging networking among members, and educating the public about the career

- **Influence legislation**: monitor legislative and regulatory actions, advocate for laws that affect the health care career, inform legislators of the impact of specific laws, provide public awareness of legal matters affecting the career, and alert members about legal requirements

- **Assistance with certification, registration, or licensure**: offer certification or registration examinations, assist with testing and assessment of individuals in the career, and help define and endorse the standards of practice for the career

- **Financial support**: provide grants for research, education, scholarships, and other specific causes

- **Code of ethics**: establish a standard of conduct or code of behavior for the profession

HOSA - Future Health Professionals is a student-led professional organization for future health care team members. It allows like-minded individuals to learn, experience, and expand their knowledge of the health care field. Competition at the regional, state, and international level is available to increase knowledge base and master skills that you practice through health science courses and the HOSA club membership. More details regarding HOSA may be found at *HOSA.org* (see **Figure 3–3**).

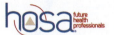 | CONNECTION

Mission, Purpose, Goals, Creed

Mission: The mission of HOSA is to empower HOSA-Future Health Professionals to become leaders in the global health community through education, collaboration, and experience.

Purpose: The purpose of HOSA-Future Health Professionals is to develop leadership and technical HOSA skill competencies through a program of motivation, awareness and recognition, which is an integral part of the Health Science Education instructional program.

Goals: The goals that HOSA believes are vital to each member are:

- To promote physical, mental and social well-being.
- To develop effective leadership qualities and skills.
- To develop the ability to communicate more effectively with people.
- To develop character.
- To develop responsible citizenship traits.
- To understand the importance of pleasing oneself as well as being of service to others.
- To build self-confidence and pride in one's work.
- To make realistic career choices and seek successful employment in the health care field.
- To develop an understanding of the importance in interacting and cooperating with other students and organizations.

- To encourage individual and group achievement.
- To develop an understanding of current health care issues, environmental concerns, and survival needs of the community, the nation and the world.
- To encourage involvement in local, state and national health care and education projects.
- To support Health Science Education instructional objectives.
- To promote career opportunities in health care.

Creed:

I recognize the universal need for quality, compassionate health care.

I understand the importance of academic excellence, skills training, and leadership development in my career pathway.

I believe through service to my community and to the world, I will make the best use of my knowledge and talents.

I accept the responsibility of a health professional and seek to find my place on a team equally committed to the well-being of others.

Therefore, I will dedicate myself to promoting health and advancing health care as a student, a leader, an educator, and a member of HOSA-Future Health Professionals.

FIGURE 3–3

EDUCATION LEVELS, TRENDS, AND OPPORTUNITIES

Generally speaking, training for most health care careers can be categorized into four levels: professional, technologist or therapist, technician, and aide or assistant, as shown in **Table 3–1**.

A common trend in health care is the **multicompetent** or **multiskilled health care provider**. Because of high health care costs, smaller facilities and rural areas often cannot afford to hire a specialist for every aspect of care. Therefore, health care providers who can perform a variety of health care tasks are hired. For example, a health care provider may be hired to perform the tasks of both an electrocardiograph (ECG) technician (who records electrical activity of the heart) and an electroencephalographic (EEG) technologist (who records electrical activity of the brain). Another example might involve combining the basic skills of radiology, medical (clinical) laboratory, and respiratory therapy. At times, health care providers trained in one field or occupation receive additional education to work in a second and even third occupation. In other cases, educational programs have been established to prepare multicompetent health care providers.

Another opportunity available in many health care careers is that of entrepreneur. An **entrepreneur** is an individual who organizes and manages a business and assumes its risks. Some health care careers allow an individual to work as an independent entrepreneur, while others encourage the use of groups of cooperating individuals. Many entrepreneurs must work under the direction or guidance of physicians or dentists. Because the opportunity to be self-employed and to be involved in the business area of health care exists, educational programs are including business skills with career objectives. A common example is combining a bachelor's degree in a specific health care career with a master's degree in business. Some health care providers who may be entrepreneurs include dental laboratory technicians, dental hygienists, nurse practitioners, physical therapists, physician assistants, respiratory therapists, recreational therapists, physicians, dentists, chiropractors, and optometrists. Although entrepreneurship involves many risks and requires a certain level of education and ability, it can be an extremely satisfying choice for the individual who is well motivated, self-confident, responsible, creative, and independent.

NATIONAL HEALTHCARE STANDARDS

The National Healthcare Standards were developed to indicate the knowledge and skills that are expected of health care team members. These standards answer the question, "What does a team member need to know and be able to do to contribute to the delivery of safe and effective health care?" The standards allow students to set goals for future education and employment, educators to design quality curriculums that meet the expectations of health care agencies, and consumers to receive high-quality health care from well-educated providers. The groups of standards include:

- **Healthcare Foundation Standards**: specify the knowledge and skills that most health care team members should have; discuss the academic foundation, communication skills, employability skills, legal responsibilities, ethics, safety practices, teamwork, information technology applications, technical skills, health maintenance practices, and knowledge about the systems in the health care environment

- **Therapeutic Services Standards**: specify the knowledge and skills required of team members in health care careers that are involved in changing the health status of the patient over time; include interacting with patients, communicating with other team members, collecting information, planning treatment, implementing procedures, monitoring patient status, and evaluating patient response to treatment

TABLE 3–1 Education and Levels of Training

Career Level	Educational Requirement	Examples
Professional	4 or more years of college with a bachelor's, master's, or doctoral degree	Medical doctor Dentist Pharmacist Physical therapist
Technologist or Therapist	3–4 years of college plus work experience, usually a bachelor's degree and, at times, a master's degree	Medical laboratory technologist (MT) Speech therapist Respiratory therapist
Technician	2-year associate's degree, special health science education (HSE), or 3–4 years of on-the-job training	Dental laboratory technician Medical laboratory technician (MLT) Surgical technician
Aide or Assistant	1–2 years in HSE program, associate's degree, or 2–4 years of on-the-job training	Dental assistant Medical assistant Nurse assistant

- **Diagnostic Services Standards**: specify the knowledge and skills required of team members in health care careers that are involved in creating a picture of the health status of the patient at a single point in time; include communicating oral and written information, assessing patient's health status, moving and positioning patients safely and efficiently, explaining procedures and goals, preparing for procedures, performing diagnostic procedures, evaluating test results, and reporting required information

- **Health Informatics Standards**: specify the knowledge and skills required of team members in health care careers that are involved with the documentation of patient care; include communicating information accurately within legal boundaries; analyzing information, abstracting and coding medical records and documents, designing and/or implementing effective information systems, documenting information, and understanding operations to enter, retrieve, and maintain information

- **Support Services Standards**: specify the knowledge and skills required of team members in health care careers that are involved with creating a therapeutic environment to provide direct or indirect patient care; include developing and implementing the administration, quality control, and compliance regulations of a health care facility; include maintaining a clean and safe environment through aseptic techniques, managing resources, and maintaining an aesthetically appealing environment

- **Biotechnology Research and Development Standards**: specify the knowledge and skills required of team members in health care careers that are involved in bioscience research and development; include comprehending how biotechnology contributes to health and the quality of life, developing a strong foundation in math and science principles, performing biotechnology techniques, understanding and following laboratory protocols and principles, working with product design and development, and complying with bioethical policies

Examples of some of the health care careers included in each of the classifications are shown in **Table 3–2**. Many of the careers listed are discussed in detail in this chapter.

INTRODUCTION TO HEALTH CARE CAREERS

In the following discussion of health care careers, a basic description of the job duties for each career is provided. The various levels in each health care career are also given. In addition, tables for each career group show educational requirements, job outlook, and average yearly earnings.

To simplify the information presented in these tables, the highest level of education for each career group is listed. The designations used are:

- **On-the-job**: training while working at a job
- **HSE program**: health science education program
- **Associate's degree**: two-year associate's degree
- **Bachelor's degree**: four-year bachelor's degree
- **Master's degree**: one or more years beyond a bachelor's degree to obtain a master's degree
- **Doctoral degree**: doctorate with four or more years beyond a bachelor's degree

It is important to note that, although many health care careers begin with HSE programs, obtaining additional education after graduation from HSE programs allows health care providers to progress in career level to higher-paying positions.

The job outlook or expected job growth is stated in the tables as "below average," "average," or "above average."

Average yearly earnings are presented as ranges of income because earnings will vary according to geographical location, specialty area, level of education, and work experience.

Legal

All career information presented includes a basic introduction. *Because requirements for various health care careers can vary from state to state, it is important for students to obtain information pertinent to their respective states.* More detailed information about any discussed career can be obtained from the sources listed for that occupation's career cluster. Another excellent resource for current information about health care careers is the *Occupational Outlook Handbook*. It is published by the Bureau of Labor Statistics of the U.S. Department of Labor and can be found online at *www.bls.gov/ooh*. Additional information can be found at *www.explorehealthcareers.org*.

checkpoint

1. With a partner, create a chart that compares the educational requirements for associate's, bachelor's, master's and doctorate degrees.
2. Compare and contrast certification, registration, and licensure.

3:2 THERAPEUTIC SERVICES CAREERS

Therapeutic services careers in health care are directed toward changing the health status of the patient over time.

Providers in the therapeutic services use a variety of treatments to help patients who are injured, physically or mentally disabled, or emotionally disturbed.

TABLE 3-2 Health Science Pathways and Sample Career Specialties

Pathways

Therapeutic Services	Diagnostic Services	Health Informatics	Support Services	Biotechnology Research and Development
Acupuncturist	Audiologist	Admitting Clerk	Behavioral Disorder Counselors	Biochemist
Advanced Practice Registered Nurse (APRN)	Blood Bank Technician	Applied Researcher	Biomedical/Clinical Engineer	Bioinformatics Associate
Anesthesiologist Assistant	Cardiovascular Technologist	Cancer Registrar	Biomedical/Clinical Technician	Bioinformatics Scientist
Art/Music/Dance Therapist(s)	Clinical Laboratory Technician	Certified Compliance Technician	Clinical Simulator Technician	Bioinformatics Specialist
Athletic Trainer	Computer Tomography (CT) Technologist	Clinical Account Manager	Central Service Manager	Biomedical Chemist
Audiologist	Cytogenetic Technologist	Clinical Account Technician	Central Service Technician	Biomedical/Clinical Engineer
Certified Nursing Assistant	Cytotechnologists	Clinical Coder	Community Health Worker	Biomedical/Clinical Technician
Certified Registered Nurse Anesthetist (CRNA)	Diagnostic Medical Sonographers	Clinical Data Miner	Dietary Manager	Biostatistician
Chiropractor	Electrocardiographic (ECG) Technician	Clinical Data Management Specialist	Dietary Aide	Cell Biologist
Dental Assistant	Exercise Physiologist	Clinical Data Specialist	Environmental Services Facilities Manager	Clinical Data Management Associate/Consultant
Dental Hygienist	Genetic Counselor	Community Services Specialist	Healthcare Administrator	Clinical Pharmacologist
Dental Lab Technician	Histotechnician	Data Quality Manager	Healthcare Economist	Clinical Trials Monitor
Dentist	Histotechnologist	Decision Support Analyst	Maintenance Engineer	Clinical Trials Research Associate
Dialysis Technician	Magnetic Resonance (MR) Technologist	Epidemiologist	Industrial Hygienist	Clinical Trials Research Coordinator
Dietitian/Nutritionist	Mammographer	Ethicist	Interpreter	Geneticist
Dietetic Technician	Medical Technologist/Clinical Laboratory Scientist	Health Educator	Materials Manager	Laboratory Assistant-Genetics
Dosimetrist	Neurodiagnostic Technologist	Health Information Administrator	Patient Navigator	Laboratory Technician
Emergency Medical Technician	Nuclear Medicine Technologist	Health Information Technician	Substance Abuse Counselors	Medical Editor/Writer
Home Health Aide	Nutritionist/Dietitian	Health Information Services	Transport Technician	Microbiologist
Kinesiotherapist	Occupational Therapist	Healthcare Administrator		Molecular Biologist
Licensed Practical Nurse	Ophthalmic Technician/Technologist	Healthcare Finance Professional		Pharmaceutical/Clinical Project Manager
Massage Therapist	Ophthalmic Dispensing Optician	Information Privacy Officer		Pharmaceutical Sales Representative
Medical Assistant	Optometrist	Information Security Officer		Pharmaceutical Scientist
Mortician	Phlebotomist	Managed Care Contract Analyst		Pharmacologist
Occupational Therapist	Physical Therapist	Medical Assistant		Product Safety Associate/ Scientist
Occupational Therapy Assistant	Polysomnographic Technologist	Medical Illustrator		Process Development Associate/ Scientist
Ophthalmic Technician		Medical Information Technologist		Processing Technician
Orientation & Mobility Specialist		Medical Librarian		
Orthotist/Prosthetist		Medical Records Technician		
		Patient Account Manager		

(continues)

TABLE 3–2 Health Science Pathways and Sample Career Specialties (continued)

Pathways			
Therapeutic Services	**Diagnostic Services**	**Health Informatics**	**Support Services**	**Biotechnology Research and Development**
Paramedic	Positron Emission Tomography (PET) Technologist	Patient Account Technician		Quality Assurance Technician
Pedorthist	Radiologic Technician	Patient Advocate		Quality Control Technician
Personal Care Aide	Respiratory Therapist	Patient Information Coordinator		Regulatory Affairs Specialist
Pharmacist		Project Manager		Research Assistant
Pharmacy Technician		Quality Management Specialist		Research Scientist
Physical Therapist		Quality Data Analyst		Toxicologist
Physical Therapy Assistant		Reimbursement Specialist		
Physician (MD/DO)		Risk Manager		
Physician Assistant		Transcriptionist		
Podiatrist		Unit Coordinator		
Psychiatrist		Utilization Manager		
Psychologist		Utilization Review Manager		
Radiation Therapist				
Recreational Therapist				
Registered Nurse				
Rehabilitation Counselor				
Respiratory Therapist				
Social Worker				
Speech Language Pathologist				
Surgeon				
Surgical Technologist				
Veterinarian				
Veterinarian Technician				
Wellness Coach				

Courtesy National Consortium for Health Science Education (NCHSE)

All treatment is directed toward allowing patients to function at their maximum capacity.

Places of employment include rehabilitation facilities, hospitals, clinics, mental health facilities, day care facilities, long-term care facilities, home health care agencies, schools, and government agencies.

There are many health care careers in the therapeutic services cluster. Some of these careers are discussed in the following sections.

3:2A DENTAL CAREERS

Dental providers focus on the health of the teeth and the soft tissues of the mouth. Care is directed toward preventing dental disease, repairing or replacing diseased or damaged teeth, and treating the gingiva (gums) and other supporting structures of the teeth.

Places of employment include private dental offices, laboratories, and clinics as well as dental departments in hospitals, schools, health departments, and government agencies.

Most dental professionals work in general dentistry practices where all types of dental conditions are treated in people of all ages. Some, however, work in specialty areas such as the following:

- **Endodontics**: treatment of diseases of the pulp, nerves, blood vessels, and roots of the teeth; often called root canal treatment
- **Orthodontics**: alignment or straightening of the teeth
- **Oral Surgery**: surgery on the teeth, mouth, jaw, and facial bones; often called *maxillofacial surgery*

- **Pedodontics**: dental treatment of children and adolescents
- **Periodontics**: treatment and prevention of diseases of the gums, bone, and structures supporting the teeth
- **Prosthodontics**: replacement of natural teeth with artificial teeth or dentures

Levels of providers in dentistry include dentist, dental hygienist, dental laboratory technician, and dental assistant (see **Table 3–3**).

Dentists (DMDs or DDSs) are doctors who examine teeth and mouth tissues to diagnose and treat disease and abnormalities; perform corrective surgery on the teeth, gums, tissues, and supporting bones; and work to prevent dental disease. They also supervise the work of other dental providers. Most are entrepreneurs.

Dental hygienists (DHs) work under the supervision of dentists. They perform preliminary examinations of the teeth and mouth, remove stains and deposits from teeth, expose and develop radiographs, apply cavity-preventing agents such as fluorides or pit and fissure sealants to the teeth, and perform other preventive or therapeutic (treatment) services to help the patient develop and maintain good dental health (**Figure 3–4**). In some states, dental hygienists are authorized to place and carve restorative materials, polish restorations, remove sutures, and/or administer anesthesia. Dental hygienists can be entrepreneurs.

Dental laboratory technicians (DLTs) make and repair a variety of dental prostheses (artificial devices) such as dentures, crowns, bridges, and orthodontic appliances according to the specifications of dentists. Specialties include dental ceramist and orthodontic technician. Some dental laboratory technicians are entrepreneurs.

TABLE 3–3 Dental Careers

Occupation	Education Required	Job Outlook	Average Yearly Earnings
Dentist (DMD or DDS)	• Doctor of Dental Medicine (DMD) or Doctor of Dental Surgery (DDS) • 2 or more years additional education for specialization • Licensure in state of practice	Above average growth	$80,500–$210,000
Dental Hygienist (DH) Licensed Dental Hygienist (LDH)	• Associate's, bachelor's, or master's degree • Licensure in state of practice	Above average growth	$61,300–$98,200
Dental Laboratory Technician (DLT), Certified Dental Laboratory Technician (CDLT)	• 3–4 years on the job or 1–2 years HSE program or associate's or bachelor's degree • Certification can be obtained from National Board for Certification in Dental Laboratory Technology	Below average growth	$30,000–$70,300
Dental Assistant (DA), Certified Dental Assistant (CDA)	• 2–4 years on the job or 1–2 years in HSE program or associate's degree • Licensure or registration required in most states • Certification can be obtained from Dental Assisting National Board after graduating from a Commission on Dental Accreditation (CODA)—approved program or 2 years full-time or 4 years part-time employment as a dental assistant	Above average growth	$27,950–$52,800

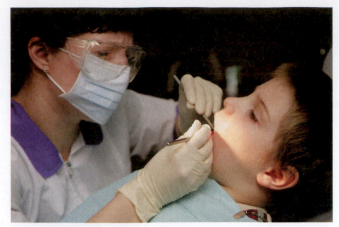

FIGURE 3–4 Dental hygienists perform preliminary examinations of the teeth and mouth, and remove stains and deposits from teeth.
© Vasiliy Koval/Shutterstock.com

Dental assistants (DAs), working under the supervision of dentists, prepare patients for examinations, pass instruments, prepare dental materials for impressions and restorations, take and develop radiographs, teach preventive dental care, sterilize instruments, and/or perform dental receptionist duties such as scheduling appointments and handling accounts. Their duties may be limited by the dental practice laws of the state in which they work.

RESEARCH HEALTH CAREERS

- American Dental Assistants Association
  www.adaausa.org

- American Dental Association
  www.ada.org

- American Dental Education Association
  www.adea.org

- American Dental Hygienists' Association
  www.adha.org

- Dental Assisting National Board, Inc.
  www.danb.org

- National Association of Advisors for the Health Professions, Inc.
  www.naahp.org

- National Association of Dental Laboratories
  www.nadl.org

- For information about the specific tasks of a dental assistant, see the Guidelines for Clinical Rotations in the *Teacher's Resource Kit* online. Additional career information is provided in the Career Highlight Section of Chapter 19 in this text and on the Companion Site.

3:2B EMERGENCY MEDICAL SERVICES CAREERS

Emergency medical services personnel (**Figure 3–5**) provide emergency, prehospital care to victims of accidents, injuries, or sudden illnesses. Although sometimes individuals with only basic training in first aid work in this field, **emergency medical technician (EMT)** training is required for most jobs. Formal EMT training is available in all states and is offered by fire, police, and health departments; hospitals; career/technical schools; and as a nondegree course in technical/community colleges and universities.

Places of employment include fire and police departments, rescue squads, ambulance services, hospital or private emergency rooms, urgent care centers, industry, emergency helicopter services, and the military. Some EMTs are entrepreneurs. Emergency medical technicians sometimes serve as volunteers in fire and rescue departments.

Levels of EMT include EMT, advanced EMT, and paramedic (see **Table 3–4**). Another emergency medical person is an emergency medical responder.

An **emergency medical responder (EMR)** is the first person to arrive at the scene of an illness or injury. Common examples include police officers, security guards, and fire department personnel. The EMR interviews and examines the victim to identify the illness or cause of injury, calls for emergency medical assistance as needed, maintains

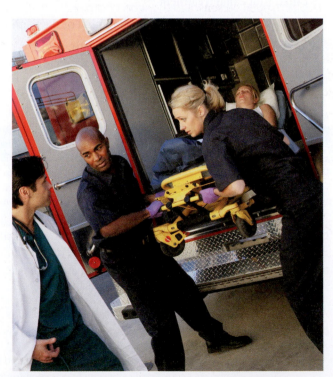

FIGURE 3–5 Emergency medical technicians (EMTs) provide emergency, prehospital care to victims of accidents, injuries, or sudden illness. © iStock.com/Catherine Yeulet

TABLE 3–4 Emergency Medical Services Careers

Occupation	Education Required	Job Outlook	Average Yearly Earnings
Paramedic	• Advanced EMT—plus an additional 6–9 months to 2 years (approximately 1,200 to 1,800 hours) approved paramedic training or associate's degree • 6 months experience as paramedic • Licensure required in all states • Certification can be obtained from the National Registry of EMTs (NREMT)	Above average growth	$36,400–$68,200
Advanced Emergency Medical Technician (AEMT)	• EMT plus additional approved training of approximately 1,000 hours with clinical experience • Licensure required in all states • Certification can be obtained from the NREMT	Above average growth	$28,900–$51,700
Emergency Medical Technician (EMT)	• Usually minimum of 110 hours approved EMT program with 10 hours of internship in an emergency department • Licensure required in all states • Certification can be obtained from the NREMT	Above average growth	$23,700–$41,200
Emergency Medical Responder (EMR)	• Minimum of 40 hours of approved training program • Certification can be obtained from the NREMT	Average growth	Salary depends on individual's regular job

safety and infection control at the scene, and provides basic emergency medical care. A certified emergency medical responder course prepares individuals by teaching airway management, oxygen administration, bleeding control, and cardiopulmonary resuscitation (CPR).

Emergency medical technicians (EMTs) provide care for a wide range of illnesses and injuries including medical emergencies, bleeding, fractures, airway obstruction, basic life support (BLS), oxygen administration, emergency childbirth, rescue of trapped persons, and transport of victims.

Advanced emergency medical technicians (AEMT) perform the same tasks as EMTs as well as assessing patients, interpreting electrocardiograms (ECGs), administering defibrillation as needed, managing shock, using intravenous equipment, and inserting esophageal airways.

Paramedics (EMT-P) perform all the basic EMT duties plus in-depth patient assessment, provision of advanced cardiac life support (ACLS), ECG interpretation, endotracheal intubation, drug administration, and operation of complex equipment.

RESEARCH HEALTH CAREERS

- National Association of Emergency Medical Technicians
  www.naemt.org
- National Highway Transportation Safety Administration (NHTSA)
  www.nhtsa.dot.gov
- National Registry of Emergency Medical Technicians
  www.nremt.org
- Office of Emergency Medical Services
  www.ems.gov

3:2C MEDICAL CAREERS

Medical careers is a broad category encompassing physicians and other individuals who work in any of the varied careers under the supervision of physicians. All such careers focus on diagnosing, treating, or preventing diseases and disorders of the human body.

Places of employment include private practices, clinics, hospitals, public health agencies, research facilities, health maintenance organizations (HMOs), government agencies, and colleges or universities.

Levels include physician, physician assistant, and medical assistant (see **Table 3–5**).

Physicians examine patients, obtain medical histories, order tests, make diagnoses, perform surgery, treat diseases/disorders, and teach preventive health. Several classifications are:

- **Doctor of Medicine (MD)**: diagnoses, treats, and prevents diseases or disorders; may specialize, as noted in **Table 3–6**

- **Doctor of Osteopathic Medicine (DO)**: treats diseases/disorders, placing special emphasis on the nervous, muscular, and skeletal systems, and the relationship between the body, mind, and emotions; may also specialize, as noted in **Table 3–6**

- **Doctor of Podiatric Medicine (DPM)**: examines, diagnoses, and treats diseases/disorders of the feet or of the leg below the knee

- **Doctor of Chiropractic (DC)**: focuses on ensuring proper alignment of the spine and optimal operation of the nervous and muscular systems to maintain health

TABLE 3–5 Medical Careers

Occupation	Education Required	Job Outlook	Average Yearly Earnings
Physician	• Doctoral degree • 3–8 years additional postgraduate training of internship and residency depending on specialty selected • State licensure • Board certification in specialty area	Above average growth	$144,400–$459,300
Physician Assistant (PA), PAC (certified)	• 2 or more years of college and usually a bachelor's or master's degree • 2 or more years accredited physician assistant program with certificate, associate's, bachelor's, or master's degree • Licensure required in all states • Certification can be obtained from National Commission on Certification of Physician Assistants • Specialization option	Above average growth	$80,100–$150,800
Medical Assistant (MA), CMA (certified), RMA (registered)	• 1–2-year HSE program or associate's degree • Certification can be obtained from American Association of Medical Assistants (AAMA) after graduation from CAAHEP- or ABHES-accredited medical assistant program • Registered credentials can be obtained from American Medical Technologists (AMT) • Certification for clinical medical assistants can be obtained from the National Healthcareer Association (NHA)	Above average growth	$27,900–$54,700

TABLE 3–6 Medical Specialties

Physician's Title	Specialty
Anesthesiologist	Administration of medications to cause loss of sensation or feeling during surgery or treatments
Cardiologist	Diseases of the heart and blood vessels
Dermatologist	Diseases of the skin
Emergency Physician	Acute illness or injury
Endocrinologist	Diseases of the endocrine glands
Family Physician/Practice	Promote wellness, treat illness or injury in all age groups
Gastroenterologist	Diseases and disorders of the stomach and intestine
Gerontologist	Diseases of older individuals
Gynecologist	Diseases of the female reproductive organs
Hospitalist	Provides care to patients who are in a hospital
Infectious Disease Physician	Diseases and conditions caused by a pathogenic agent such as a bacteria or virus
Internist	Diseases of the internal organs (lungs, heart, glands, intestines, kidneys)
Nephrologist	Diseases of the kidneys
Neurologist	Disorders of the brain and nervous system
Obstetrician	Pregnancy and childbirth
Oncologist	Diagnosis and treatment of tumors (cancer)
Ophthalmologist	Diseases and disorders of the eye
Orthopedist	Diseases and disorders of muscles and bones
Otolaryngologist	Diseases of the ears, nose, and throat
Pathologist	Diagnosis of diseases by studying changes in organs, tissues, and cells
Pediatrician	Diseases and disorders of children
Physiatrist	Physical medicine and rehabilitation
Plastic Surgeon	Corrective surgery to repair injured or malformed body parts
Proctologist	Diseases of the lower part of the large intestine
Psychiatrist	Diseases and disorders of the mind
Pulmonologist	Diseases and disorders of the lungs
Radiologist	Use of X-rays and radiation to diagnose and treat disease
Sports Medicine	Prevention and treatment of injuries sustained in athletic events
Surgeon	Surgery to correct deformities or treat injuries or disease
Thoracic Surgeon	Surgery of the lungs, heart, or chest cavity
Urologist	Diseases of the kidney, bladder, or urinary system

Physician assistants (PAs), working under the supervision of physicians, take medical histories; perform routine physical examinations and basic diagnostic tests; make preliminary diagnoses; treat minor injuries; and prescribe and administer appropriate treatments. *Pathology assistants*, working under the supervision of pathologists, perform both gross and microscopic autopsy examinations.

Medical assistants (MAs), working under the supervision of physicians, prepare patients for examinations, take vital signs and medical histories, assist with procedures and treatments, perform basic laboratory tests, prepare and maintain equipment and supplies, and/or perform secretarial-receptionist duties (**Figure 3–6**). The type of facility and physician determines the kinds of duties. The range of duties is also determined by state law. Assistants working for physicians who specialize are called *specialty assistants*. For example, an assistant working for a pediatrician is called a *pediatric assistant*.

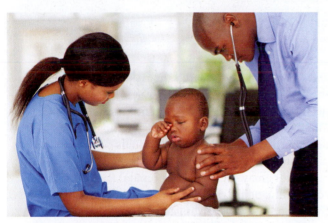

FIGURE 3–6 Medical assistants prepare patients for examinations and assist with the examinations. © michaeljung/Shutterstock.com.

RESEARCH HEALTH CAREERS

- American Academy of Physician Assistants
  www.aapa.org
- American Association of Medical Assistants
  www.aama-ntl.org
- American Chiropractic Association
  www.acatoday.org
- American Medical Association
  Internet address: *www.ama-assn.org*
- American Medical Technologists Association
  www.americanmedtech.org
- American Osteopathic Association
  www.osteopathic.org
- American Podiatric Medical Association
  www.apma.org

- American Society of Podiatric Medical Assistants
  www.aspma.org
- For information about the specific tasks of a medical assistant, see the Guidelines for Clinical Rotations in the *Teacher's Resource Kit* online. Additional career information is provided in the Career Highlight Section of Chapter 21 in this text.

3:2D MENTAL HEALTH SERVICES AND SOCIAL SERVICES CAREERS

Mental health services professionals focus on helping people who have mental or emotional disorders or those who are developmentally delayed or mentally impaired. Social workers help people deal with illnesses, employment, or community problems. Professionals in both fields try to help individuals function to their maximum capacities.

Places of employment include hospitals, psychiatric hospitals or clinics, home health care agencies, public health departments, government agencies, crisis or counseling centers, drug and alcohol treatment facilities, prisons, educational institutions, and long-term care facilities.

Levels of employment range from psychiatrist (a physician), who diagnoses and treats mental illness, to psychologist and psychiatric technician. There are also various levels (including assistant) employed in the field of social work (see **Table 3–7**).

Psychiatrists are physicians who specialize in diagnosing and treating mental illness. Some specialties include child or adolescent psychiatry, geriatric psychiatry, and drug/chemical abuse.

Psychologists study human behavior and use this knowledge to help individuals deal with problems of everyday living. Many specialize in specific aspects of psychology, which include child psychology, adolescent psychology, geriatric psychology, behavior modification, drug/chemical abuse, and physical/sexual abuse.

Psychiatric/mental health technicians, working under the supervision of psychiatrists or psychologists, help patients and their families follow treatment and rehabilitation plans. They provide understanding and encouragement, assist with physical care, observe and report behavior, and help teach patients constructive social behavior. Assistants or aides who have completed one or more years in an HSE program are also employed in this field.

TABLE 3-7 Mental Health Services and Social Services Careers

Occupation	Education Required	Job Outlook	Average Yearly Earnings
Psychiatrist	• Doctoral degree • 2–7 years postgraduate specialty training • State licensure • Certification in psychiatry	Above average growth	$121,800–$297,100
Psychologist, PsyD (Doctor of Psychology)	• Master's or doctoral degree • Doctor of psychology required for many positions • Licensure or certification required in all states • Certification for specialty areas available from American Board of Professional Psychology	Above Average growth	$58,300–$129,500
Psychiatric/Mental Health Technicians	• Associate's degree • Licensure required in some states • A few states require a nursing degree • Certification can be obtained from American Association of Psychiatric Technicians	Above average growth	$25,300–$63,200
Social Workers	• Bachelor's or master's degree or Doctorate in Social Work (DSW) • Licensure, certification, or registration required in all states • Credentials available from National Association of Social Workers	Above average growth	$35,500–$83,400
Genetic Counselor (GC)	• Master's degree • Certification can be obtained from the American Board of Genetic Counseling (ABGC)	Above average growth	$65,300–$92,910

Social workers (SWs), also called case managers, or counselors (**Figure 3–7**), aid people who have difficulty coping with various problems by helping them make adjustments in their lives and/or by referring them to community resources for assistance. Specialties include child welfare, geriatrics, family, correctional (jail), and occupational social work. Many areas employ assistants or technicians who have completed one or more years of an HSE program.

Genetic counselors provide information about genetic diseases or inherited conditions to individuals and families. They research the risk for occurrence of the disease or birth defect, analyze inheritance patterns, perform screening tests for potential genetic defects, identify medical options when a genetic disease or birth defect is present, and help individuals cope with the psychological issues caused by genetic diseases. Genetic counselors may specialize in prenatal (before birth) counseling, pediatric (child) counseling, neurogenetics (brain and nerves), cardiogenetics (heart and blood vessels), or genetic influences on cancer.

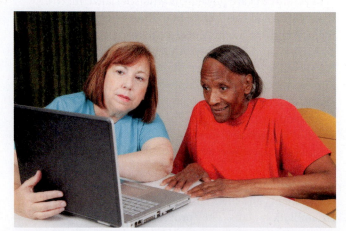

FIGURE 3–7 Social workers help people make life adjustments and refer patients to community resources for assistance. © iStock.com/Alina Solovyova-Vincent

RESEARCH HEALTH CAREERS

- American Association of Psychiatric Technicians
  www.psychtechs.org
- American Board of Genetic Counseling
  www.abgc.net
- American Psychiatric Association
  www.psych.org
- American Psychological Association
  www.apa.org
- American Sociological Association
  www.asanet.org
- Mental Health America
  www.nmha.org
- National Association of Social Workers
  www.socialworkers.org

- National Institute of Mental Health
  www.nimh.nih.gov
- National Society of Genetic Counselors
  www.nsgc.org

3:2E MORTUARY CAREERS

Team members employed in mortuary careers provide a service that is needed by everyone. Even though funeral practices and rites vary because of cultural diversity and religion, most services involve preparation of the body, performance of a ceremony that honors the deceased and meets the spiritual needs of the living, and cremation or burial of the remains.

Places of employment are funeral homes or mortuaries, crematoriums, or cemetery associations.

Levels include funeral director, embalmer, and mortuary assistant (see **Table 3–8**).

Funeral directors, also called *morticians* or *undertakers*, provide support to the survivors, interview the family of the deceased to establish details of the funeral ceremonies or review arrangements the deceased person requested before death, prepare the body following legal requirements, secure information for legal documents, file death certificates, arrange and direct all the details of the wake and services, make arrangements for burial or cremation, and direct all business activities of the funeral home. Frequently, funeral directors help surviving individuals adapt to the death by providing post-death counseling and support group activities. Most funeral directors are also licensed embalmers.

Embalmers prepare the body for interment by washing the body with germicidal soap, replacing the blood with embalming fluid to preserve the body, reshaping and restructuring disfigured bodies, applying cosmetics to create a natural appearance, dressing the body, and placing it in a casket. They are also responsible for maintaining embalming reports and itemized lists of clothing or valuables.

Mortuary assistants work under the supervision of the funeral director and/or embalmer. They may assist with preparation of the body, drive the hearse to pick up the body after death or take it to the burial site, arrange flowers for the viewing, assist with preparations for the funeral service, help with filing and maintaining records, clean the funeral home, and other similar duties.

RESEARCH HEALTH CAREERS

- American Board of Funeral Service Education
  www.abfse.org
- Cremation Association of North America
  www.cremationassociation.org
- International Cemetery, Cremation, and Funeral Association
  www.iccfa.com
- International Conference of Funeral Service Examining Boards
  www.theconferenceonline.org
- National Funeral Directors Association
  www.nfda.org

3:2F NURSING CAREERS

Those in the nursing careers provide care for patients as directed by physicians. Care focuses on the mental, emotional, and physical needs of the patient.

Hospitals are the major places of employment, but people in nursing careers are also employed in long-term care facilities, rehabilitation centers, physicians' offices, clinics, public health agencies, home health care agencies, health maintenance organizations (HMOs), schools, government agencies, and industry.

Levels include registered nurse, licensed practical/vocational nurse, and nurse assistant/technician (see **Table 3–9**).

TABLE 3–8 Mortuary Careers

Occupation	Education Required	Job Outlook	Average Yearly Earnings
Funeral Director (Mortician)	• 2–4 years in a mortuary science college or associate's or bachelor's degree • Licensure required in all states except Colorado	Average growth	$36,800–$156,700
Embalmer	• 2–4 years in a mortuary science college or associate's or bachelor's degree • Licensure required in all states except Colorado	Average growth	$35,300–$68,500
Mortuary Assistant	• 1–2 years on-the-job training or 1-year HSE program	Average growth	$18,300–$38,800

TABLE 3–9 Nursing Careers

Occupation	Education Required	Job Outlook	Average Yearly Earnings
Registered Nurse (RN)	• Bachelor's degree, associate's degree, or 2–3-year diploma program in a hospital or school of nursing • Master's or doctorate for some administrative/educational positions and for advanced practice nursing positions (doctorate may be required for advanced practice nurses after 2015) • Licensure in state of practice	Above average growth	$52,600–$99,900 $64,300–$138,900 with advanced specialties
Licensed Practical/Vocational Nurse (LPN/LVN)	• 1–2-year state-approved HSE practical/vocational nurse program • Licensure in state of practice	Above average growth	$36,700–$68,400
Nurse Assistant, Geriatric Aide, Home Health Care Assistant, Medication Aide, Certified Nurse Technician, Patient Care Technician (PCT)	• HSE program • Certification or registration required in all states for long-term care facilities—obtained by completing 75–120-hour state-approved program	Above average growth, especially in geriatric or home care	$20,100–$44,200

Registered nurses (RNs) (**Figure 3–8**) work under the direction of physicians and provide total care to patients. The RN observes patients, assesses patients' needs, reports to other health care personnel, administers prescribed medications and treatments, teaches health care, and supervises other nursing personnel. The type of facility determines specific job duties. Registered nurses with an advanced education can specialize. Examples of advanced practice nurses include:

- **Nurse practitioners (CRNPs):** take health histories, perform basic physical examinations, order laboratory tests and other procedures, refer patients to physicians, help establish treatment plans, treat common illnesses such as colds or sore throats, and teach and promote optimal health

- **Nurse midwives (CNMs):** provide total care for normal pregnancies, examine the pregnant woman at regular intervals, perform routine tests, teach childbirth and childcare classes, monitor the infant and mother during childbirth, deliver the infant, and refer any problems to a physician

- **Nurse educators:** teach in HSE programs, schools of nursing, colleges and universities, wellness centers, and health care facilities

- **Nurse anesthetists (CRNAs):** administer anesthesia, monitor patients during surgery, and assist anesthesiologists (who are physicians)

- **Clinical nurse specialists (CNSs):** use advanced degrees to specialize in specific nursing areas such as intensive care, trauma or emergency care, psychiatry, pediatrics (infants and children), neonatology (premature infants), and gerontology (older individuals)

Licensed practical/vocational nurses (LPNs/LVNs), working under the supervision of physicians or RNs, provide patient care requiring technical knowledge but

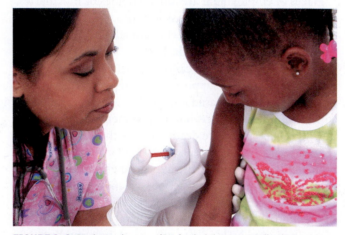

FIGURE 3–8 Registered nurses (RNs) administer prescribed medications to patients. © iStock.com/Jaimie Duplass

not the level of education required of RNs. The type of care is determined by the work environment, which can include the home, hospital, long-term care facility, adult day care center, physician's office, clinic, wellness center, and health maintenance organization. The care provided by LPNs/LVNs is also determined by state laws regulating the extent of their duties.

Nurse assistants—also called nurse aides, nurse technicians, **patient care technicians (PCTs),** or orderlies—work under the supervision of RNs or LPNs/LVNs. They provide patient care such as baths, bed making, and feeding; assist in transfer and ambulation; and administer basic treatments. **Geriatric aides/assistants** acquire additional education to provide care for older patients in environments such as extended care facilities, nursing homes, retirement centers, adult day care facilities, and other similar agencies. **Home health care assistants** are trained to work in the patient's home and may perform additional duties such as meal preparation or cleaning. **Medication aides/assistants** receive special training such as a 40-hour or more state-approved medication aide course to administer medications to patients or residents in long-term care facilities or patients receiving home health care. Most states that have the medication aide program require that the aide be on the state-approved list for nurse or geriatric assistants before taking the medication aide course. In addition, many states require a competency test.

OBRA Each nursing assistant working in a long-term care facility or in home health care is now required under federal law to complete a mandatory, state-approved training program and pass a written and/or competency examination to obtain certification or registration. Health care providers in these environments should check the requirements of their respective states.

RESEARCH HEALTH CAREERS

- All Nursing Schools
  www.allnursingschools.com
- American Association of Nurse Practitioners
  www.aanp.org
- American Health Care Association
  www.ahcancal.org
- American Nurses' Association
  www.nursingworld.org
- National Association for Home Care and Hospice
  www.nahc.org
- National Association for Practical Nurse Education and Service
  www.napnes.org
- National Association of Health Care Assistants
  www.nahcacares.org
- National Council of State Boards of Nursing
  www.ncsbn.org
- National Federation of Licensed Practical Nurses
  www.nflpn.org

- National League for Nursing
  www.nln.org
- National Network of Career Nursing Assistants
  www.cna-network.org
- Registered Nurse, RN
  www.registerednursern.com
- For information about the specific tasks of a geriatric assistant/technician or nursing assistant/technician, see the Guidelines for Clinical Rotations in the *Teacher's Resource Kit* online. Additional career information is provided in the Career Highlight Section of Chapter 22 in this text and on the Companion Site.

3:2G NUTRITION AND DIETARY SERVICES CAREERS

Health, nutrition, and physical fitness have become a way of life. Individuals employed in the nutrition and dietary services recognize the importance of proper nutrition to good health. Using knowledge of nutrition, they promote wellness and optimum health by providing dietary guidelines used to treat various diseases, teaching proper nutrition, and preparing foods for health care facilities.

Places of employment include hospitals, long-term care facilities, child and adult day care facilities, wellness centers, schools, home health care agencies, public health agencies, clinics, industry, and offices.

Levels include dietitian, dietetic technician, and dietetic assistant (see **Table 3–10**).

Dietitians (RDs), or *nutritionists*, manage food service systems, assess patients'/residents' nutritional needs, plan menus, teach others proper nutrition and special diets, research nutrition needs and develop

TABLE 3–10 Nutrition and Dietary Services Careers

Occupation	Education Required Job	Outlook	Average Yearly Earnings
Dietitian, RD (registered)	• Bachelor's or master's degree • Registration can be obtained from the Commission on Dietetic Registration of the Academy of Nutrition and Dietetics • Licensure, certification, or registration required in most states	Above average growth	$47,100–$93,200
Dietetic Technician, DTR (registered)	• Associate's or bachelor's degree • Licensure, certification, or registration required in most states • Registration can be obtained from the Commission on Dietetic Registration of the Academy of Nutrition and Dietetics	Average growth	$25,400–$59,600
Dietetic Assistant	• On-the-job training • One or more years of HSE or food service career/technical program	Average growth	$16,600–$29,900

recommendations based on the research, purchase food and equipment, enforce sanitary and safety rules, and supervise and train other personnel. Some dietitians specialize in the care of pediatric (child), renal (kidney), or diabetic patients, or in weight management.

Dietetic technicians (DTs), working under the supervision of dietitians, plan menus, order foods, standardize and test recipes, assist with food preparation, provide basic dietary instruction, and teach classes on proper nutrition.

Dietetic assistants, also called *food service workers*, work under the supervision of dietitians and assist with food preparation and service, help patients select menus, clean work areas, and assist other dietary team members.

RESEARCH HEALTH CAREERS

- Academy of Nutrition and Dietetics *www.eatright.org*

- Association of Nutrition and Foodservice Professionals *www.anfponline.org*

- Institute of Food Technologists *www.ift.org*

- For information about the specific tasks of a dietetic assistant/food service provider, see the Guidelines for Clinical Rotations in the *Teacher's Resource Kit* online.

3:2H VETERINARY CAREERS

Veterinary careers focus on providing care to all types of animals—from house pets to livestock to wildlife.

Places of employment include animal hospitals, veterinarian offices, laboratories, zoos, farms, animal shelters, aquariums, drug or animal food companies, and fish and wildlife services.

Levels of employment include veterinarian, animal health technician, and assistant (see **Table 3–11**).

Veterinarians (DVMs or VMDs) (**Figure 3–9**) work to prevent, diagnose, and treat diseases and injuries in animals. Specialties include surgery, small-animal care, livestock, fish and wildlife, and research.

Veterinary technologists/technicians (VTs), also called *animal health technicians*, working under the supervision of veterinarians, assist with the handling and care of animals, collect specimens, assist with surgery, perform laboratory tests, take and develop radiographs, administer prescribed treatments, and maintain records.

Veterinary assistants, also called *animal caretakers*, feed, bathe, and groom animals; exercise animals; prepare animals for treatment; assist with examinations; clean and sanitize cages, examination tables, and surgical areas; and maintain records.

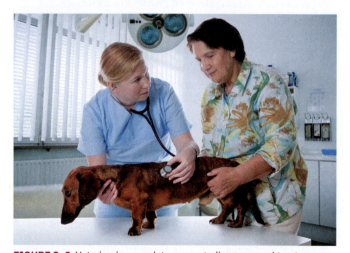

FIGURE 3–9 Veterinarians work to prevent, diagnose, and treat diseases and injuries in animals. © Alexander Raths/Shutterstock.com

TABLE 3–11 Veterinary Careers

Occupation	Education Required	Job Outlook	Average Yearly Earnings
Veterinarian (DVM or VMD)	• 3–4 years pre-veterinary college • 4 years veterinary college and Doctor of Veterinary Medicine degree • State licensure required in all states • Certification for specialties can be obtained from the American Veterinary Medical Association	Above average growth	$59,300–$171,500
Veterinary (Animal Health) Technologist/ Technician, VTR (registered)	• Associate's degree for veterinary technician • Bachelor's degree for veterinary technologist • Registration, certification, or licensure required in all states • Certification for technologists/technicians employed in animal laboratory research facilities can be obtained from the American Association for Laboratory Animal Science (AALAS)	Above average growth	$26,300–$63,800
Veterinary Assistant (Animal Caretakers)	• 1–2 years on the job or a 1–2-year HSE program	Average growth	$22,400–$47,700

RESEARCH HEALTH CAREERS

- American Association for Laboratory Animal Science
www.aalas.org

- American Veterinary Medical Association
www.avma.org

- Animal Caretakers Information, The Humane Society of the United States
www.humanesociety.org

- Association of American Veterinary Medical Colleges
www.aavmc.org

- National Association of Veterinary Technicians in America (NAVTA)
www.navta.net

- National Dog Groomers Association of America
www.nationaldoggroomers.com

- For information about the specific tasks of a veterinary assistant, see the Guidelines for Clinical Rotations in the *Teacher's Resource Kit* online.

3:2I OTHER THERAPEUTIC SERVICES CAREERS

There are many other therapeutic service careers. Some are discussed in this section. Most therapeutic occupations include levels of therapist, technician, and assistant/aide (see **Table 3–12**).

Occupational therapists (OTs) (**Figure 3–10**) often work under the direction of a physiatrist, a physician specializing in physical medicine and rehabilitation. OTs help people who have physical, developmental, mental, or emotional disabilities overcome, correct, or adjust to their particular problems. The occupational therapist uses various activities to assist the patient in learning skills or activities of daily living (ADL), adapting job skills, or preparing for return to work. Treatment is directed toward helping patients acquire independence, regain lost functions, adapt to disabilities, and lead productive and satisfying lives.

TABLE 3–12 Other Therapeutic Services Careers

Occupation	Education Required	Job Outlook	Average Yearly Earnings
Occupational Therapist (OT), OTR (registered)	• Master's degree and internship and some doctoral degrees • Licensure required in all states • Certification can be obtained from the National Board for Certification in Occupational Therapy	Above average growth	$67,900–$120,300
Occupational Therapy Assistant, COTA (certified)	• Associate's degree or certificate and internship • Licensure or certification required by most states • Certification can be obtained from the National Board for Certification in Occupational Therapy	Above average growth	$48,200–$79,300
Pharmacist (PharmD)	• 5–6-year college program with Doctor of Pharmacy degree plus internship • Licensure required in all states	Above average growth	$110,800–$162,400
Pharmacy Technician	• 1 year on the job or 1 year HSE program • Certification required in many states • Certification can be obtained from the Pharmacy Technician Certification Board and the National Healthcareer Association	Above average growth	$25,900–$48,100
Physical Therapist (PT)	• Doctoral degree • Licensure required in all states	Above average growth	$71,500–$130,200
Physical Therapist Assistant (PTA)	• Associate's degree plus internship • Licensure required in most states except Hawaii	Above average growth	$28,500–$75,000
Massage Therapist	• 3-month–1-year accredited Massage Therapy Program • Certification, registration, or licensure required in most states • Certification can be obtained from the National Certification Board for Therapeutic Massage and Bodywork (NCBTMB)	Above average growth	$45,8000–$68,500
Recreational Therapist (TR), Certified Therapeutic Recreation Specialist (CTRS)	• Possibly associate's but usually bachelor's degree plus internship • Licensure or certification required in some states • Certification can be obtained from the National Council for Therapeutic Recreation Certification (NCTRC)	Average growth	$29,500–$77,100
Recreational Therapist Assistant (Activity Director or Therapeutic Recreation Assistant)	• Associate's degree • Certification can be obtained from the NCTRC	Average growth	$17,100–$46,300

(continues)

TABLE 3–12 Other Therapeutic Services Careers (continued)

Occupation	Education Required	Job Outlook	Average Yearly Earnings
Respiratory Therapist, RRT (registered), CRT (certified)	• Associate's, bachelor's, or master's degree • Licensure required in all states except Alaska • Registration and certification can be obtained from the National Board for Respiratory Care	Above average growth	$50,800–$88,300
Respiratory Therapy Technician (RTT), CRTT (certified)	• Associate's degree or postsecondary certificate from an accredited school • Licensure or certification required in most states • Certification can be obtained from the National Board for Respiratory Care	Average growth	$36,500–$78,500
Speech-Language Therapist/ Pathologist and/or Audiologist	• Master's degree and 9 months postgraduate clinical experience • Licensure required in most states • Clinical doctoral degree for audiologists • Audiologists may obtain certification from the American Board of Audiology • Certificate of Clinical Competence in Speech-Language Pathology (CCC-SLP) or Audiology (CCC-A) can be obtained from the American Speech-Language-Hearing Association (ASHA) • Specialty certifications for audiology can be obtained from the American Board of Audiology	Above average growth	$60,800–$159,200
Surgical Technician/ Technologist, CST (certified)	• 1–2-year HSE program • Certificate, diploma, or associate's degree • Certification can be obtained from the National Board of Surgical Technology and Surgical Assisting or the National Center for Competency Testing (NCCT)	Above average growth	$38,400–$66,800
Art, Music, Dance Therapist	• Bachelor's or master's degree • Certification for art therapist can be obtained from the American Art Therapy Association • Certification for music therapist can be obtained from the American Music Therapy Association • Registration for dance/movement therapist (RDMT) can be obtained from the American Dance Therapy Association • Registration for art therapist (ATR) can be obtained from the Art Therapy Credentials Board	Average growth	$35,600–$126,500
Athletic Trainer, ATC (certified)	• Bachelor's, master's, or doctoral degree • Licensure or registration required in most states • Nearly all states require certification • Certification can be obtained from the Board of Certification (BOC) for the Athletic Trainer	Above average growth	$44,900–$89,300
Dialysis Technician (Nephrology Technician)	• Varies with states • Some states require RN or LPN/LVN license and state-approved dialysis training • Other states require 1–2-year HSE state-approved dialysis program or associate's degree • Certification can be obtained from the National Association of Nephrology Technicians/Technologists	Above average growth	$24,800–$59,700
Perfusionist/Certified Clinical Perfusionist (CCP)/ Extracorporeal Circulation Technologist	• Bachelor's or master's degree • Specialized extracorporeal circulation training and supervised clinical experience • Licensure required in most states • Certification can be obtained from the American Board of Cardiovascular Perfusion	Above average growth	$88,300–$166,200

Occupational therapy assistants (OTAs), or *certified occupational therapy assistants* (COTAs), working under the guidance of occupational therapists, help patients carry out programs of prescribed treatment. They direct patients in arts and crafts projects, recreation, and social events; teach and help patients carry out rehabilitation activities and exercises; use games to develop balance and coordination; assist patients to master the activities of daily living; and inform therapists of patients' responses and progress.

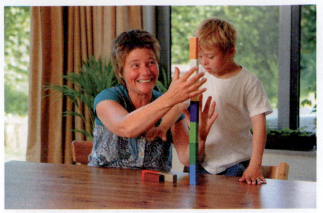

FIGURE 3–10 Occupational therapists (OTs) help patients who have disabilities overcome, correct, or adjust to the disabilities.
© iStock.com/Ema Vader

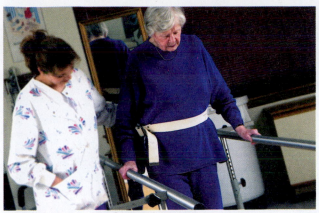

FIGURE 3–12 Physical therapists (PTs) provide treatment to improve mobility of patients who have disabling injuries or diseases.
© CWImages/Shutterstock.com

Pharmacists (PharmDs) (**Figure 3–11**) dispense medications per written orders from physicians, dentists, and other health care professionals authorized to prescribe medications. They provide information about drugs and the correct ways to use them; order and dispense other health care items such as surgical and sickroom supplies; recommend nonprescription items to customers/patients; ensure drug compatibility; maintain records on medications dispensed; and assess, plan, and monitor drug usage. Pharmacists can also be entrepreneurs or work for one of the many drug manufacturers involved in researching, manufacturing, and selling drugs.

Pharmacy technicians, working under the supervision of pharmacists, help prepare medications for dispensing to patients, label medications, perform inventories and order supplies, prepare intravenous solutions, help maintain records, and perform other duties as directed by pharmacists.

Physical therapists (PTs) (**Figure 3–12**) often work under the direction of a physiatrist, a physician specializing in physical medicine and rehabilitation. PTs provide treatment to improve mobility and prevent or limit

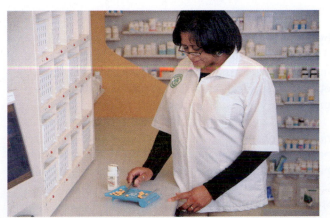

FIGURE 3–11 Pharmacists dispense medications and provide information about drugs.

permanent disability of patients who have disabling joint, bone, muscle, and/or nerve injuries or diseases. Treatment may include exercise, massage, and/or applications of heat, cold, water, light, electricity, or ultrasound. Therapists assess the functional abilities of patients and use this information to plan treatment programs. They also promote health and prevent injuries by developing proper exercise programs and teaching patients correct use of muscles. Some physical therapists are entrepreneurs.

Physical therapist assistants (PTAs), working under the supervision of physical therapists, help carry out prescribed plans of treatment. They perform exercises and massages; administer applications of heat, cold, and/or water; assist patients to ambulate with canes, crutches, or braces; provide ultrasound or electrical stimulation treatments; inform therapists of patients' responses and progress; and perform other duties, as directed by therapists.

Massage therapists usually work under the supervision of physicians or physical therapists. They use many variations of massage, bodywork (manipulation or application of pressure to the muscular or skeletal structure of the body), and therapeutic touch to muscles to provide pain relief for chronic conditions (such as back pain) or inflammatory diseases, improve lymphatic circulation to decrease edema (swelling), and relieve stress and tension (**Figure 3–13**). Some massage therapists are entrepreneurs.

Recreational therapists (TRs), or *therapeutic recreation specialists*, use recreational and leisure activities as forms of treatment to minimize patients' symptoms and improve physical, emotional, and mental well-being. Activities might include organized athletic events, dances, arts and crafts, musical activities, drama, field trips to shopping centers or other places of interest, movies, or poetry or book readings. All activities are directed toward allowing the patient to gain independence, build self-confidence, and relieve anxiety. Some recreational therapists are entrepreneurs.

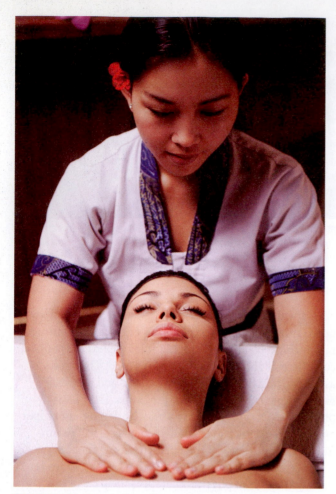

FIGURE 3–13 Massage therapists use massage, bodywork, and therapeutic touch to provide pain relief, improve circulation, and relieve stress and tension. © g-stockstudio/Shutterstock.com

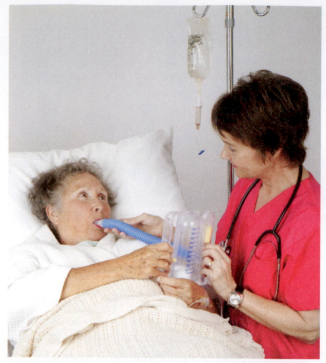

FIGURE 3–14 Respiratory therapists (RTs) provide treatments to patients with heart and lung diseases. © Lisa F. Young/Shutterstock.com

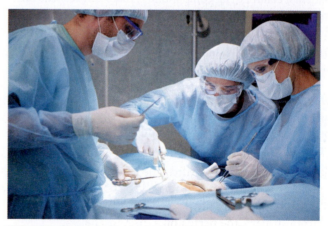

FIGURE 3–15 Surgical technologists assist by passing instruments and supplies to the surgeon. © iStock.com/Anastasia Pelikh

Recreational therapy assistants, also called *activity directors* or *therapeutic recreation assistants*, work under the supervision of recreational therapists or other health care professionals. They assist in carrying out the activities planned by therapists and, at times, arrange activities or events. They note and inform therapists of patients' responses and progress.

Respiratory therapists (RTs), under physicians' orders, treat patients with heart and lung diseases by administering oxygen, gases, or medications; using exercise to improve breathing; monitoring ventilators; and performing diagnostic respiratory function tests (**Figure 3–14**). Some respiratory therapists are entrepreneurs.

Respiratory therapy technicians (RTTs) work under the supervision of respiratory therapists and administer respiratory treatments, perform basic diagnostic tests, clean and maintain equipment, and note and inform therapists of patients' responses and progress.

Surgical technologists/technicians (STs), also called *operating room technicians* (**Figure 3–15**), working under the supervision of RNs or physicians, prepare patients for surgery; set up instruments, equipment, and sterile supplies in the operating room; and assist during surgery by passing instruments and supplies to the surgeon. Although most surgical technologists/technicians work in hospital operating rooms, some are employed in outpatient surgical centers, emergency departments, urgent care centers, physicians' offices, and other facilities.

Speech-language pathologists, also called *speech therapists* or *speech scientists*, identify, evaluate, and treat patients with speech and language disorders. They help patients communicate as effectively as possible and also teach patients to cope with the problems created by speech impairments.

Audiologists provide care to individuals who have hearing impairments. They test hearing, diagnose problems, and prescribe treatment, which may include hearing aids, auditory training, or instruction in speech or lip reading. They also test noise levels in workplaces and develop hearing protection programs.

Art, music, and dance therapists use the arts to help patients deal with social, physical, or emotional problems. Therapists usually work with individuals who are emotionally disturbed, mentally disabled, or physically disabled, but they may also work with adults and children who have no disabilities in an effort to promote physical and mental wellness.

Athletic trainers certified (ATCs) prevent and treat athletic injuries and provide rehabilitative services to athletes. The athletic trainer frequently works with a physician who specializes in sports medicine. Athletic trainers teach proper nutrition, assess the physical condition of athletes, give advice regarding physical conditioning programs to increase strength and flexibility or correct weaknesses, put tape or padding on players to protect body parts, treat minor injuries, administer first aid for serious injuries, and help carry out any rehabilitation treatment prescribed by sports medicine physicians or other therapists (**Figure 3–16**).

Dialysis technicians,—also called *renal dialysis technicians*, *hemodialysis technicians*, or *nephrology technicians*—operate the kidney hemodialysis machines used to treat patients with limited or no kidney function. Careful patient monitoring is critical during the dialysis process. The dialysis technician must also provide emotional support for the patient and teach proper nutrition (because many patients must follow restricted diets).

Perfusionists, also called *extracorporeal circulation technologists*, are members of open-heart surgical teams and operate the heart–lung machines used in coronary bypass surgery (surgery on the coronary arteries in the heart). This field is expanding to include new advances such as artificial hearts. Monitoring and operating a heart–lung machine correctly is critical because the patient's life depends on the machine. During surgery, the perfusionist monitors blood gases and vital signs; administers blood products,

anesthetic agents, and/or drugs as needed; and induces hypothermia (low body temperature) to decrease the body's need for oxygen. After the surgery, the perfusionist must restore normal body circulation when the heart starts beating and wean the patient from the extracorporeal machine.

RESEARCH HEALTH CAREERS

- American Academy of Audiology
  www.audiology.org
- American Art Therapy Association
  www.arttherapy.org
- American Association for Respiratory Care
  www.aarc.org
- American Association of Colleges of Pharmacy
  www.aacp.org
- American Association of Pharmacy Technicians
  www.pharmacytechnician.com
- American Board of Audiology
  www.americanboardofaudiology.org
- American Dance Therapy Association
  www.adta.org
- American Massage Therapy Association
  www.amtamassage.org
- American Music Therapy Association
  www.musictherapy.org
- American Occupational Therapy Association
  www.aota.org
- American Pharmacists Association
  www.pharmacist.com
- American Physical Therapy Association
  www.apta.org
- American Society of Extracorporeal Technologists
  www.amsect.org
- American Speech-Language-Hearing Association
  www.asha.org
- American Therapeutic Recreation Association
  www.atra-online.com
- Associated Bodywork and Massage Professionals
  www.abmp.com
- Association of Surgical Technologists
  www.ast.org
- Massage and Bodywork Resource Center
  www.massageresource.com
- National Association of Nephrology Technicians/ Technologists
  www.dialysistech.net

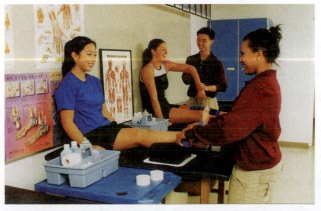

FIGURE 3–16 Athletic trainers (ATCs) apply tape or padding to players to protect body parts or treat minor injuries.

- National Athletic Trainers Association
  www.nata.org

- National Council for Therapeutic Recreation Certification
  www.nctrc.org

- National Pharmacy Technician Association
  www.pharmacytechnician.org

- National Surgical Assistant Association
  www.nsaa.net

- Pharmacy Technician Certification Board
  www.ptcb.org

- Society of Health and Physical Educators
  www.shapeamerica.org

- For information about the specific tasks of a pharmacy technician/assistant, physical therapist assistant/technician, or respiratory therapy assistant/ technician, see the Guidelines for Clinical Rotations in the *Teacher's Resource Kit* online. Additional career information for physical therapy is provided in the Career Highlight Section of Chapter 23 in this text and on the Companion Site.

checkpoint

1. Name five (5) career opportunities in Therapeutic Services and what education is required.

Individuals employed in diagnostic services are involved with creating a picture of the health status of a patient at a single point in time. They perform tests or evaluations that aid in the detection, diagnosis, and treatment of disease, injury, or other physical conditions.

Many team members are employed in hospital laboratories, but others work in private laboratories, outpatient centers, physicians' offices, clinics, public health agencies, pharmaceutical (drug) firms, and research or government agencies. In some careers, individuals are entrepreneurs, owning and operating their own businesses.

Many careers fall under the designation of diagnostic services; some of the more common ones are discussed in this chapter. There are various levels of education required in most fields (**Table 3–13**).

Electrocardiograph (ECG) technicians operate electrocardiograph machines, which record electrical impulses that originate in the heart. Physicians (especially cardiologists) use the electrocardiogram (ECG) to help diagnose heart disease and to note changes in the condition of a patient's heart. *ECG or cardiographic technicians (CT)* with more advanced training perform stress tests (which record the action

TABLE 3–13 Diagnostic Services Careers

Occupation	Education Required	Job Outlook	Average Yearly Earnings
Cardiovascular Technologist, Registered Vascular Technologist (RVT)	• Associate's or bachelor's degree • Certification or registration can be obtained from Cardiovascular Credentialing International • Registration can be obtained from the American Registry for Diagnostic Medical Sonography	Above average growth	$39,600–$94,500
Electrocardiograph (ECG) Technician, Certified Cardiographic Technician (CCT)	• 1–12 months on the job or 6–12-month HSE program • Certification can be obtained from Cardiovascular Credentialing International and the National Healthcareer Association	Average growth	$20,400–$42,600
Electroencephalographic (EEG) Technologist, R-EEG (registered)	• A few have 1–2 years of on-the-job training • Most have 1–2-year HSE certification program or associate's degree • Registration can be obtained from the American Board of Registration of Electroencephalographic and Evoked Potential Technologists	Average growth	$24,500–$52,600
Electroneurodiagnostic Technologist, (END) Neurodiagnostic Technologist	• 1–2-year program usually leading to associate's degree • Registration can be obtained from the American Board of Electroencephalographic and Evoked Potential Technologists • Polysomnographic technologists can obtain registration from the Association of Polysomnographic Technologists	Above average growth	$39,800–$69,900
Clinical Laboratory Scientist (CLS), Medical Laboratory Technologist (MT)	• Bachelor's or master's degree • Licensure, registration, or certification required in some states • Certification can be obtained from the Board of Certification of the American Society for Clinical Pathology, the American Medical Technologists (AMT), and the National Credentialing Agency for Laboratory Personnel	Above average growth	$46,800–$88,900

(continues)

TABLE 3–13 Diagnostic Services Careers (continued)

Occupation	Education Required	Job Outlook	Average Yearly Earnings
Medical Laboratory Technician (MLT), Clinical Laboratory Technician (CLT)	• 2-year HSE certification program or associate's degree • Licensure or registration required in some states • Certification can be obtained from the Board of Certification of the American Society for Clinical Pathology, the AMT, and the National Credentialing Agency for Laboratory Personnel	Above average growth	$29,400–$68,300
Medical (Clinical) Laboratory Assistant	• 1–2-year HSE program or on-the-job training • Certification can be obtained from the AMT and the National Credentialing Agency for Laboratory Personnel	Above average growth	$22,600–$43,600
Phlebotomist	• 1–2 years on the job or HSE program or 100–300-hour certification program • Certification can be obtained from the National Credentialing Agency for Laboratory Personnel and the American Society of Phlebotomy Technicians • Registration (RPT) can be obtained from the American Medical Technologists	Above average growth	$24,500–$44,400
Ophthalmologist (MD)	• Doctoral degree • 2–8 years postgraduate specialty training • State licensure • Certification in ophthalmology	Above average growth	$112,000–$324,800
Optometrist (OD)	• 3–4 years pre-optometric college • 4 years at college of optometry for Doctor of Optometry degree • State licensure	Above average growth	$110,300–$190,600
Ophthalmic Medical Technologist, COMT (certified)	• Associate's degree • Certification can be obtained from the Joint Commission on Allied Health Personnel in Ophthalmology (JCAHPO)	Above average growth	$32,200–$74,600
Ophthalmic Technician, COT (certified)	• 1-year certificate program or associate's degree • Certification can be obtained from JCAHPO	Average growth	$31,500–$69,700
Ophthalmic Assistant, COA (certified)	• Some on-the-job training • 1-month–1-year HSE program • Certification can be obtained from the JCAHPO	Average growth	$29,100–$44,900
Optician	• 2–4 years on the job or 2–4-year apprenticeship or HSE program or associate's degree • Licensure or certification required in some states • Certification can be obtained from American Board of Opticianry and National Contact Lens Examiners	Above average growth	$28,100–$64,700
Ophthalmic Laboratory Technician	• 2–3 years on the job or 1-year HSE certificate program • Licensure or certification required in some states	Below average growth	$24,300–$68,500
Radiologic Technologist, ARRT (Registered)	• Associate's or bachelor's degree • Licensure or certification required in most states • Registration that can lead to state licensure can be obtained from the American Registry of Radiologic Technologists (ARRT)	Above average growth	$50,200–$94,800

of the heart during physical activity; see **Figure 3–17**), Holter monitor tests (ECGs lasting 24–48 hours), thallium scans (a nuclear scan after thallium is injected), and other specialized cardiac tests that frequently involve the use of computers. An associate's or bachelor's degree leads to a position as a **cardiovascular technologist**. These individuals assist with cardiac catheterization procedures and angioplasty (a procedure to remove blockages in blood vessels), monitor patients during open-heart surgery and the implantation of pacemakers, and perform tests to check circulation in blood vessels. Some specialize in using ultrasound (high-frequency sound waves) to

assess heart function and diagnose heart conditions and are called *echocardiographers* or *cardiac sonographers*. Others use ultrasound to diagnose disorders of blood vessels by checking blood pressure, oxygen saturation, and circulation of blood throughout the body. They are called *vascular technologists* or *vascular sonographers*.

An **electroencephalographic (EEG) technologist** operates an instrument called an *electroencephalograph*, which records the electrical activity of the brain. The record produced, called an *electroencephalogram*, is used by a variety of physicians, especially neurologists (physicians specializing in nerve and brain diseases), to

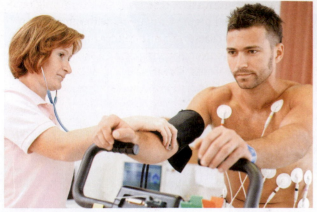

FIGURE 3–17 Cardiographic technicians perform stress tests to aid in the diagnosis of heart disease. © iStock.com/Zsolt Nyulaszi

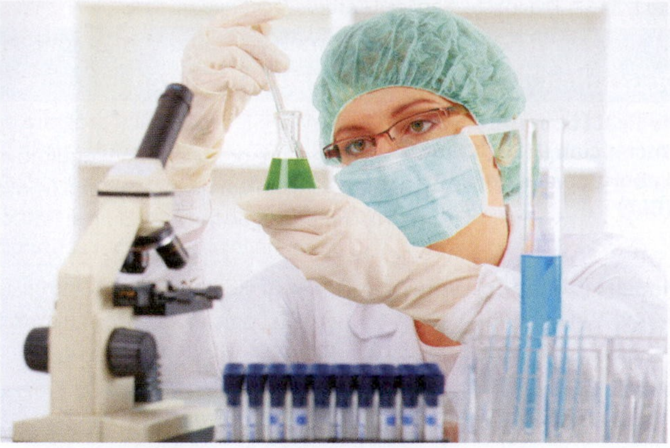

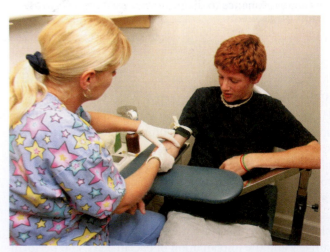

FIGURE 3–18 Medical laboratory technologists perform tests to help determine the presence and/or cause of disease. © Monika Wisnieswka/Shutterstock.com

diagnose and evaluate diseases and disorders of the brain such as brain tumors, strokes, toxic/metabolic disorders, epilepsy, and sleep disorders. Advanced training leads to a position as an **electroneurodiagnostic technologist (END)**, also called *neurodiagnostic technologist*. In addition to performing EEGs, these individuals perform nerve conduction tests, measure sensory and physical responses to specific stimuli, perform evoked potential (EP) tests that measure brain response when specific nerves are stimulated, and operate other monitoring devices. Technologists who specialize in administering sleep disorder evaluations are called *polysomnographic technologists*.

Medical laboratory technologists (MTs), also called **clinical laboratory scientists (CLSs)**, work under the supervision of physicians called *pathologists*. They study the tissues, fluids, and cells of the human body to help determine the presence and/or cause of disease. They perform complicated chemical, microscopic, and automated analyzer/computer tests (**Figure 3–18**). In small laboratories, technologists perform many types of tests. In larger laboratories, they may specialize. Examples of specialization include:

- **Biochemistry or clinical chemistry**: chemical analysis of body fluids
- **Blood bank technology**: collection and preparation of blood and blood products for transfusions
- **Cytotechnology**: study of human body cells and cellular abnormalities
- **Hematology**: study of blood cells
- **Histology**: study of human body tissue
- **Molecular biology**: complex protein and nucleic acid testing on cell samples
- **Microbiology**: study of bacteria and other microorganisms

Medical laboratory technicians (MLTs), also called **clinical laboratory technicians (CLTs)**, work under the supervision of medical technologists or pathologists and

perform many of the routine tests (Figure 3–18) that do not require the advanced knowledge held by a medical technologist. Like the technologist, the technician can specialize in a particular field or perform a variety of tests.

Medical (clinical) laboratory assistants—working under the supervision of medical technologists, technicians, or pathologists—perform basic laboratory tests, prepare specimens for examination or testing, and perform other laboratory duties such as cleaning and helping to maintain equipment.

Phlebotomists (**Figure 3–19**), or *venipuncture technicians*, collect blood and prepare it for testing. In some states, they perform blood tests under the supervision of medical technologists or pathologists.

Ophthalmologists are medical doctors specializing in diseases, disorders, and injuries of the eyes. They diagnose and treat disease, perform surgery, and correct vision problems or defects.

Optometrists (ODs), doctors of optometry, examine eyes for vision problems and defects, prescribe corrective lenses or eye exercises, and, in some states, use drugs for

FIGURE 3–19 Phlebotomists collect blood and prepare it for testing.
© iStock.com/Joseph Abbott

diagnosis and/or treatment. If eye disease is present or if eye surgery is needed, the optometrist refers the patient to an ophthalmologist.

Ophthalmic medical technologists (OMTs), working under the supervision of ophthalmologists, obtain patient histories, perform routine eye tests and measurements, fit patients for contacts, administer prescribed treatments, assist with eye surgery, perform advanced diagnostic tests such as ocular motility and biocular function tests, administer prescribed medications, and perform advanced microbiological procedures. In addition, they may perform any tasks that ophthalmic technicians or assistants perform.

Ophthalmic technicians (OTs) (**Figure 3–20**) work under the supervision of ophthalmologists and optometrists. Technicians prepare patients for examinations, obtain medical histories, take ocular measurements, administer basic vision tests, maintain ophthalmic and surgical instruments, adjust glasses, teach eye exercises, measure for contacts, instruct patients on the care and use of contacts, and perform receptionist duties.

Ophthalmic assistants (OAs) work under the supervision of ophthalmologists, optometrists, and/or ophthalmic medical technologists or technicians. Assistants prepare patients for examinations, measure visual acuity, perform receptionist duties, help patients with frame selections and fittings, order lenses, perform minor adjustments and repairs of glasses, and teach proper care and use of contact lenses.

Opticians make and fit the eyeglasses or lenses prescribed by ophthalmologists and optometrists. Some specialize in contact lenses.

Ophthalmic laboratory technicians cut, grind, finish, polish, and mount the lenses used in eyeglasses, contact lenses, and other optical instruments such as telescopes and binoculars.

Radiologic technologists (RTs), working under the supervision of physicians called radiologists, use X-rays, radiation, nuclear medicine, ultrasound, and magnetic resonance to diagnose and treat disease. Most

techniques are noninvasive, which means examining or treating the internal organs of patients without entering the body. In many cases, recent advances in this field have eliminated the need for surgery and, therefore, offer less risk to patients. Radiologic technologists use different types of scanners to produce images of body parts. Examples include X-ray machines, fluoroscopes, ultrasonic scanners, computerized tomography (CT) scanners (formerly known as computerized axial tomography [CAT] scanners), magnetic resonance imagers (MRI), and positron emission tomography (PET) scanners. Many radiologic technologists also provide radiation treatment. Specific job titles exist for technologists who specialize:

- **Radiographers**: take X-rays of the body for diagnostic purposes.

- **Radiation therapists**: administer prescribed doses of radiation to treat disease (usually cancer).

- **Nuclear medicine technologists**: prepare radioactive substances for administration to patients. Once administered, these professionals use films, images on a screen, or body specimens such as blood or urine to determine how the radioactive substances pass through or localize in different parts of the body. This information is used by physicians to detect abnormalities or diagnose disease.

- **Ultrasound technologists or diagnostic medical sonographers**: use equipment that sends high-frequency sound waves into the body. As the sound waves bounce back from the part being examined, an image of the part is viewed on a screen. This can be recorded on a printout strip or be photographed. Ultrasound is frequently used to examine the fetus (developing infant) in a pregnant woman and can reveal the sex of the unborn child. Ultrasound is also used for neurosonography (the brain), vascular (blood vessels and blood flow), and echocardiography (the heart) examinations.

- **Mammographer**: uses a special mammography machine to produce images of the breast. The mammograms are used to assist in the early detection and treatment of breast cancer.

- **Computer tomography technologists**: use a computerized axial tomography (CT or CAT) scanner to obtain cross-sectional images of body tissues, bones, and organs (**Figure 3–21**). CT scans help locate tumors and other abnormalities.

- **Magnetic resonance imaging (MRI) technologists**: use superconductive magnets and radio waves to produce detailed images of internal anatomy. The information is processed by a computer and displayed on a video screen. Examples of MRI uses include identifying multiple sclerosis and detecting hemorrhaging (bleeding) in the brain.

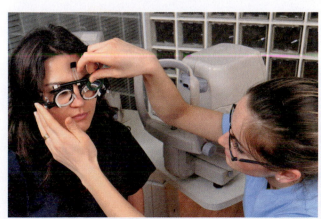

FIGURE 3–20 Ophthalmic technicians perform basic vision tests, adjust glasses, and measure for contacts. © Levent Konuk/Shutterstock.com

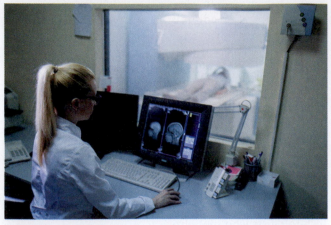

FIGURE 3–21 Radiologic technologists may use a computerized axial tomography (CT) scanner to obtain cross-sectional images of body tissues, bones, and organs. © Shutterstock/Drazen Zigic

- **Positron emission tomography (PET) technologists**: inject a slightly radioactive substance into the patient and then operate the PET scanner, which uses electrons to create a three-dimensional image of body parts and to scan the body for disease processes. This allows physicians to see an organ or bone from all sides, similar to a three-dimensional model.

RESEARCH HEALTH CAREERS

- Alliance of Cardiovascular Professionals
  www.acp-online.org
- American Association of Bioanalysts
  www.aab.org
- American Board of Opticianry National Contact Lens Examiners
  www.abo-ncle.org
- American College of Radiology
  www.acr.org
- American Medical Technologists
  www.americanmedtech.org
- American Optometric Association
  www.aoa.org
- American Registry for Diagnostic Medical Sonography
  www.ardms.org
- American Registry of Radiologic Technologists
  www.arrt.org
- American Society for Clinical Laboratory Science
  www.ascls.org
- American Society of Radiologic Technologists
  www.asrt.org
- ASET—The Neurodiagnostic Society
  www.aset.org
- Association of Schools and Colleges of Optometry
  www.opted.org

- Association of Schools of Allied Health Professions
  www.asahp.org
- Cardiovascular Credentialing International (CCI)
  www.cci-online.org
- Clinical Laboratory Management Association
  www.clma.org
- Commission on Opticianry Accreditation
  www.coaccreditation.com
- Joint Commission on Allied Health Personnel in Ophthalmology
  www.jcahpo.org
- National Accrediting Agency for Clinical Laboratory Sciences
  www.naacls.org
- National Credentialing Agency for Laboratory Personnel
  www.phlebotomycertificationzone.com/national-credentialing-agency-for-laboratory-personnel.html
- National Federation of Opticianry Schools
  www.nfos.org
- National Healthcareer Association
  www.nhanow.com
- Opticians Association of America
  www.oaa.org
- Society for Vascular Ultrasound
  www.svunet.org
- Society of Diagnostic Medical Sonography
  www.sdms.org
- The Vision Council Optical Lab Division
  www.thevisioncouncil.org
- For information about the specific tasks of a medical laboratory assistant/technician or a radiology assistant/technician, see the Guidelines for Clinical Rotations in the *Teacher's Resource Kit* online. Additional career information for medical laboratory assistants/technicians is provided in the Career Highlight Section of Chapter 20 in this text and on the Companion Site.

checkpoint

1. How do Diagnostic and Therapeutic Services work together for positive patient outcomes?

3:4 HEALTH INFORMATICS CAREERS

Health informatics providers are involved with documentation of patient records and health information. Because of the increase in the use of electronic health records (EHRs), also called electronic medical records

(EMRs), the job responsibilities of these providers have increased. Maintaining security, using EHR software programs, analyzing information, and creating networks for health information are critical components of health informatics careers. There are many different types of health informatics providers at all levels. Some examples of careers in health informatics include health information administrators or technicians, health educators, medical transcriptionists, admitting office personnel, epidemiologists, medical illustrators, photographers, writers, and librarians (see **Table 3–14**). Computer technology is used in all these careers.

TABLE 3–14 Health Informatics Careers

Occupation	Education Required	Job Outlook	Average Yearly Earnings
Health Information (Medical Records) Administrator, RHIA (registered)	• Bachelor's or master's degree • Registration can be obtained from the American Health Information Management Association (AHIMA)	Above average growth	$63,500–$156,100
Health Information (Medical Records) Technician, RHIT (registered)	• Associate's degree • Certification can be obtained from the AHIMA after passing a written examination	Above average growth	$36,800–$74,500
Medical Coder/Certified Coding Specialist (CCS)	• On-the-job training (usually a minimum of 2 years), HSE program, or accredited medical coding program • Certification can be obtained from the AHIMA for coding associate (CCA) or coding specialist (CCS) • Certification can be obtained from the American Academy of Professional Coders (AAPC) for professional coder (CPC)	Above average growth	$28,900–$66,700
Medical Transcriptionist, CMT (certified), RMT (registered)	• 1 or more years career or technical education program, on-the-job training, or associate's degree • Certification can be obtained from the Association for Healthcare Documentation Integrity (AHDI)	Average growth	$28,900–$57,300
Clinical Account Manager	• Bachelor's degree or Registered Nurse	Above average growth	$51,083–$99,730
Clinical Account Technician, CCAT (certified)	• On-the-job training Certification may be obtained from American Association of Healthcare Administrative Management (AAHAM)	Above average growth	$28,000–$34,760
Admitting Officer or Clerk	• 1–2 year HSE or business/office career/technical education • Admitting manager may require bachelor's degree • Few have on-the-job training	Below average growth	$20,600–$39,700
Medical Administrative Assistant, CMAA (certified)	• 1–2 years HSE program or associate's degree • Certification can be obtained from National Healthcareer Association	Above average growth	$23,200–$52,800
Medical Secretary/ Health Unit Coordinator/ Medical Records Clerk	• 1 or more years career or technical education program • Some have on-the-job training	Average growth	$28,100–$51,500
Health Educator, CHES (certified specialist)	• Bachelor's or master's degree • Certification can be obtained from the National Commission for Health Education Credentialing	Above average growth	$40,200–$98,500
Health Care Risk Manager	• Bachelor's or master's degree • Certification can be obtained from the Professional Association of Health Care Office Management (PAHCOM) or the American College of Health Care Administrators (ACHCA)	Above average growth	$60,500–$182,600
Ethicist	• Master's or doctoral degree • Certification can be obtained from the American Society for Bioethics and Humanities (ASBH)	Average growth	$78,400–$164,500
Epidemiologist	• Master's or doctoral degree in environmental health, public health, or health management sciences	Average growth	$56,200–$129,300
Medical Illustrator	• Bachelor's or master's degree • Certification can be obtained from the Association of Medical Illustrators	Average growth	$45,600–$146,900
Medical Librarian	• Master's degree in library science • Certification or licensure required in most states	Below average growth	$43,800–$144,600

Places of employment include hospitals, clinics, research centers, health departments, long-term care facilities, colleges, law firms, health maintenance organizations (HMOs), and insurance companies.

Health information (medical records) administrators (HIAs) develop and manage the systems for storing and obtaining information from records, prepare information for legal actions and insurance claims, compile statistics for organizations and government agencies, manage medical records departments, ensure the confidentiality of patient information, and supervise and train other personnel. Because computers are used in almost all aspects of the job, it is essential for the medical records administrator to be able to operate and use a variety of computer programs.

Health information (medical records) technicians (HITs) (Figure 3–22) organize and code patient records, gather statistical or research data, record information on patient records, monitor electronic and paper-based information to ensure confidentiality, and calculate bills using health care data. Computers have simplified many of these duties and are used to organize records, compile and report statistical data, and perform similar tasks. Computer operation is an essential part of the education program for health information technicians. Medical records departments also employ clerks who organize records. Clerks typically complete a 1- or 2-year career/technical program, or they are trained on the job.

Medical coders, or *coding specialists*, identify diagnoses, procedures, and services shown in a patient's health care record and assign specific codes to each. The two main coding systems used are the *International Classification of Diseases* or ICD codes for diagnoses, and the *Current Procedural Terminology* or CPT codes for procedures and services. The codes allow the health care provider to obtain reimbursement or payment for services, provide information for research on health care services, verify compliance with medical standards, and allow for an audit of the health care provided. Some medical coders specialize in a specific field, such as coding the diagnosis and treatment of cardiovascular disease or cancerous tumors. Other coders specialize in coding for specific health care agencies such as hospitals or medical offices.

Medical transcriptionists use a computer and word-processing software to enter data that has been dictated on a recorder by physicians or other health care professionals. Examples of data include physical examination reports, surgical reports, consultation findings, progress notes, and radiology reports.

Clinical account managers promote, sell, and educate clients, sales associates, and the public about health care products and services. They are responsible for making appointments with both customers and sales staff, scheduling educational programs, and account interactions. They coordinate personnel and support needs in their territory and promote a firm's health care services and products in order to build new business.

Clinical account technicians (CATs) assist patients that have questions about their bill or need help to make payment arrangements. The duties of a CAT would include sending bills, collecting payments, and communicating with insurance companies and patients. Clinical account technicians must understand all aspects of the bill in order to identify possible errors and be able to articulate this to the patient. They have access to confidential information and must understand and comply with HIPAA standards and protect their patients' privacy.

Admitting officers/clerks work in the admissions department of a health care facility. They are responsible for obtaining all necessary information when a patient is admitted to the facility, assigning rooms, maintaining records, and processing information when the patient is discharged. An *admitting manager* is a higher level of provider in this field, usually having an associate's or bachelor's degree. The admitting manager is responsible for supervising staff, developing and implementing policies and procedures for the department, monitoring performance standards, and coordinating the operation of the department with other departments in the health care facility.

Medical administrative assistants perform general administrative duties as well as tasks that are specific to the health care industry. Duties may include answering the phone, scheduling appointments, maintaining patient records, processing insurance forms, and scheduling medical procedures or lab services.

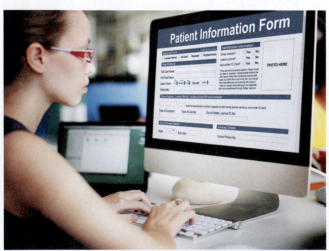

FIGURE 3–22 Health information (medical records) technicians organize and code patients' records. © Shutterstock/Rawpixel.com

Medical secretaries, or **health unit coordinators**, are employed in hospitals, extended-care facilities, clinics, and other health facilities to record information in records, schedule procedures or tests, answer telephones, order supplies, and work with computers to record or obtain information.

Health educators teach people the behaviors that promote wellness. They collect data and speak with populations about their health concerns. They evaluate, design, present, recommend, and disseminate culturally appropriate health education information and materials. They may hold workshops to present information effectively to diverse audiences.

Health care risk managers assess risks in order to minimize them to staff, patients, and the public. They manage legal and insurance claims and communicate with internal and external legal counsel. They prepare reports and analyze risk data. They also provide training to key staff and frontline supervisors. They employ preemptive techniques to reduce potential safety, financial, and patient problems.

Ethicists for health care recognize that modern technology has created many ethical problems for the delivery of health care. They study and review the history, philosophy, theology, medical research, and sociology of health care to make judgments about treatment options and the effectiveness of these options as they relate to ethical standards regarding patient rights, quality of life, privacy, death, and how health care funds and resources should be allocated. They discuss their findings with patients, families, medical professionals, health care providers, health care facilities, and ethic committees and review boards. They act as consultants to provide information that allows medical personnel, patients, and their families to work together in a constructive way to identify, analyze, and resolve many of the ethical problems that arise in clinical medicine to determine the best course of action to provide treatment to the patient. Ethicists may also help develop policy, do research, and provide education about ethical standards for health care facilities.

Epidemiologists identify and track diseases as they occur in a group of people. They determine risk factors that make a disease more likely to occur, evaluate situations that may cause occupational exposure to toxic substances, develop methods to prevent or control the spread of new diseases, and evaluate statistics and data to help governments, health agencies, and communities deal with epidemics and other health issues. Some may specialize in areas such as cancer, cardiovascular (heart and blood vessels) diseases, occupational diseases, infectious or communicable (spread rapidly from person to person) diseases, and health care research.

Medical illustrators use their artistic and creative talents to produce illustrations, charts, graphs, and diagrams for health textbooks, journals, magazines, and exhibits. Another related field is a *medical photographer*, who photographs or videotapes surgical procedures, health education information, documentation of patient conditions before and after reconstructive surgery, and legal information such as injuries received in an accident.

Medical librarians, also called *health sciences librarians*, organize books, journals, and other print materials to provide health information to other health care professionals. They use computer technology to create information centers for large health care facilities or to supply information to health care providers. Some librarians specialize in researching information for large pharmaceutical companies, insurance agencies, lawyers, industry, or government agencies.

RESEARCH HEALTH CAREERS

- American Academy of Professional Coders
  www.aapc.com
- American Health Information Management Association
  www.ahima.org
- American Association of Healthcare Administrative Management
  www.aaham.org
- Association for Healthcare Documentation Integrity
  www.ahdionline.org
- American Society for Bioethics and Humanities
  www.asbh.org
- Association for Professionals in Infection Control and Epidemiology
  www.apic.org
- Association of Medical Illustrators
  www.ami.org
- Council of State and Territorial Epidemiologists
  www.cste.org
- Medical Library Association
  www.mlanet.org
- National Commission for Health Education Credentialing
  www.nchec.org
- Professional Association of Healthcare Coding Specialists
  www.pahcs.org

checkpoint

1. How are health informatics and cybersecurity interrelated?

3:5 SUPPORT SERVICES CAREERS

Support services providers are involved with creating a therapeutic environment to provide direct or indirect patient care. Any hospital or health care facility requires personnel to operate the support departments such as administration, the business office, the admissions office, central/sterile supply, plant operations, equipment maintenance, and housekeeping. Each department has providers at all levels and with varying levels of education (see Table 3–15).

Places of employment include hospitals, clinics, long-term care facilities, HMOs, and public health or governmental agencies.

Health care administrators, also called *health care executives* or *health services managers*, plan, direct, coordinate, and supervise delivery of health care and manage the operation of health care

TABLE 3–15 Support Services Careers

Occupation	Education Required	Job Outlook	Average Yearly Earnings
Health Care Administrator/ Health Services Manager	• Usually a master's or doctoral degree • Licensure required for long-term care facilities in all states • Certification can be obtained from the American College of Health Care Executives	Above average growth	$54,300–$181,000
Biomedical/Clinical Engineer	• Bachelor's or master's degree • Licensure required in some states • Certification available from the International Certification Commission for Clinical Engineering and Biomedical Technology of the Association for the Advancement of Medical Instrumentation	Above average growth	$63,900–$144,300
Biomedical Equipment Technician, BET or CBET (certified)	• Associate's or bachelor's degree • Certification can be obtained from the International Certification Commission for Clinical Engineering and Biomedical Technology of the Association for the Advancement of Medical Instrumentation	Above average growth	$33,100–$81,700
Medical Interpreter/ Translator	• Associate's, bachelor's, or master's degree • Certification can be obtained from the American Translators Association • Certification for sign language interpreters can be obtained from the National Association of the Deaf and the Registry of Interpreters for the Deaf • Certification for associate health care interpreter (AHI) and certified health care interpreter (CHI) can be obtained from the Certification Commission for Healthcare Interpreters	Above average growth	$34,900–$96,600
Industrial Hygienist, CIH (certified)	• Bachelor's or master's degree • Certification can be obtained from the American Board of Industrial Hygiene	Average growth	$42,800–$102,900
Environmental Services Facility Manager, CFM (certified)	• Bachelor's or master's degree • Certification can be obtained from the International Facility Management Association • Certification for a Certified Healthcare Environmental Services Professional (CHESP) can be obtained from the American Hospital Association Certification Center	Average growth	$48,500–$136,400
Central/Sterile Service/ Supply Technician	• On-the-job training or 1–2-year HSE program • Certification for a sterile processing technician can be obtained from the Certification Board for Sterile Processing and Distribution (CBSPD)	Average growth	$24,400–$42,500
Housekeeping Worker/ Sanitary Manager	• On-the-job training or 1-year career/technical program	Average growth	$19,900–$39,600
Transport Technician	• On-the-job training or HSE program • Certification can be obtained from the National Association of Transport Management	Average growth	$20,100–$38,500

facilities. One type of health care administrator is a called a chief executive officer (CEO). A health care administrator may be responsible for personnel, supervise department heads, determine budget and finance, establish policies and procedures, perform public relations duties, and coordinate all activities in the facility. Duties depend on the size of the facility.

Biomedical/clinical engineers combine knowledge of engineering with knowledge of biology and biomechanical principles to assist in the operation of health care facilities. They design and build sensor systems that can be used for diagnostic tests, such as the computers used to analyze blood; develop computer systems that can be used to monitor patients; design and produce monitors, imaging machines, surgical instruments, lasers, and other similar medical equipment; design clinical laboratories and other units in a health care facility that uses advanced technology; and monitor and maintain the operation of the technologic systems. They frequently work with other health team members such as physicians or nurses to adapt instrumentation or computer technology to meet the specific needs of the patients and health care teams.

Biomedical equipment technicians (BETs) (CBETs certified) work with the many different machines used to diagnose, treat, and monitor patients (**Figure 3–23**). They install, test, service, and repair equipment such as patient monitors, kidney hemodialysis units, diagnostic imaging scanners, incubators, electrocardiographs, X-ray units, pacemakers, sterilizers, blood-gas analyzers, heart–lung machines, respirators, and other similar devices. Lives depend on the accuracy and proper operation of many of these machines, so constant maintenance and testing

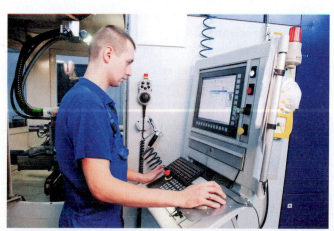

FIGURE 3–23 Biomedical equipment technicians (BETs) work with the many different machines used to diagnose, treat, and monitor patients.
© Dmitry Kalinovsky/Shutterstock.com

for defects is critical. Some biomedical equipment technicians also teach other staff members how to use biomedical equipment.

Medical interpreters/translators assist cross-cultural communication processes by converting one language to another. Interpreters convert the spoken word while translators convert written material. Medical interpreters/translators must be proficient at translating words, relaying concepts and ideas between languages, practicing cultural sensitivity, editing written language, and determining that the communication has been comprehended. *Sign language interpreters* facilitate communication for individuals who are deaf or hard of hearing

Industrial hygienists identify and analyze workplace hazards. They measure the level of exposure that can cause sickness or impair the health of providers when they are exposed to biological, chemical, physical, or ergonomic stressors. They develop programs, policies, and procedures to create a safe and healthy environment. They are responsible for clean water, safe air, efficient waste disposal, and even protecting food from contaminants.

Environmental services facilities managers oversee buildings, grounds, equipment, and supplies. Their responsibilities include making sure that the building meets the needs of the people that work there. They identify environmental hazards and evaluate ways to eliminate them. They are in charge of security, parking, maintenance and repair, and cleaning to make sure the facility meets environmental, health, and security standards and complies with government regulations.

Central/sterile service/supply technicians, also called *sterile processing technicians*, are involved in ordering, maintaining, and supplying all the equipment and supplies used by other departments in a health care facility. They sterilize instruments or supplies, maintain equipment, inventory materials, and fill requisitions from other departments.

Housekeeping workers/sanitary managers, also called *environmental service workers*, help maintain the cleanliness of the health care facility to provide a pleasant, sanitary environment. They observe all principles of infection control to prevent the spread of disease.

Transport technicians transport patients by assisting them to move in and out of vehicles, ambulances and helicopters. They are trained to lift patients on and off beds, wheelchairs, stretchers, and mechanical lifts and then move them to different areas such as special treatment rooms, operating rooms, and testing areas.

RESEARCH HEALTH CAREERS

- American Board of Industrial Hygiene
  www.abih.org
- American College of Health Care Administrators
  www.achca.org
- American College of Healthcare Executives
  www.ache.org
- American Health Care Association
  www.ahcancal.org
- American Hospital Association
  www.aha.org
- American Industrial Hygiene Association
  www.aiha.org
- American Translators Association
  www.atanet.org
- Association for the Advancement of Medical Instrumentation
  www.aami.org
- Biomedical Engineering Society
  www.bmes.org
- Certification Board for Sterile Processing and Distribution (CBSPD)
  www.sterileprocessing.org
- Certification Commission for Health Care Interpreters
  www.cchicertification.org
- IEEE Engineering in Medicine and Biology Society
  www.embs.org
- International Facility Management Association
  www.ifma.org
- Medical Group Management Association
  www.mgma.com
- National Association of Healthcare Transport Management
  www.nahtm.org
- National Board of Certification for Medical Interpreters
  www.certifiedmedicalinterpreters.org
- Registry of Interpreters for the Deaf
  www.rid.org

checkpoint

1. List at least one (1) example of how support services impacts every other career area.

3:6 BIOTECHNOLOGY RESEARCH AND DEVELOPMENT CAREERS

Biotechnology career providers are involved with using living cells and their molecules to make useful products. They work with cells and cell products from humans, animals, plants, and microorganisms. Through research and development, they help produce new diagnostic tests, forms of treatment, medications, vaccines to prevent disease, methods to detect and clean up environmental contamination, and food products. The potential uses of biotechnology are unlimited.

Places of employment include pharmaceutical companies, chemical companies, agricultural facilities, research laboratories, colleges or universities, government facilities, forensic laboratories, hospitals, and industry. There are many career opportunities at all levels (**Table 3–16**).

Biological (medical) scientists study living organisms such as viruses, bacteria, protozoa, and other infectious substances. They assist in the development of vaccines, medicines, and treatments for diseases; evaluate the relationships between organisms and the environment; and administer programs for testing food and drugs. Some work on isolating and identifying genes associated with specific diseases or inherited traits, and perform research to correct genetic defects. Some specialties include:

- **Biochemists**: study the chemical composition of living things
- **Cell Biologist**: study the function, systems, structure of cells and their interaction with living organisms
- **Microbiologists**: investigate the growth and characteristics of microscopic organisms
- **Physiologists**: study the life functions of plants and animals
- **Forensic scientists**: study cells, fibers, and other evidence to obtain information about a crime
- **Biophysicists**: study the response and interrelationship of living cells and organisms to the principles of physics, such as electrical or mechanical energy

Most biological (medical) scientists use research associates and assistants. These associates or assistants must have high-level math and science skills, computer technology proficiency, effective written and oral communication skills, knowledge of aseptic techniques, and laboratory skills.

Biomedical/clinical engineers use engineering knowledge to develop solutions to complex medical problems. They develop devices such as cardiac pacemakers, blood oxygenators, and defibrillators that aid in the diagnosis and treatment of disease; research various metals and other biomaterials to determine which

TABLE 3–16 Biotechnology Research and Development Careers

Occupation	Education Required	Job Outlook	Average Yearly Earnings
Biological (Medical) Scientists	• Master's or doctoral degree • Licensure required in some states	Average growth	$54,500–$162,100
Biomedical/Clinical Engineers	• Bachelor's but usually Master's degree • Licensure required in some states • Certification available from the International Certification Commission for Clinical Engineering and Biomedical Technology of the Association for the Advancement of Medical Instrumentation	Above average growth	$63,900–$144,300
Biomedical/Clinical Technicians	• Bachelor's degree • Certification can be obtained from the National Credentialing Agency for Laboratory Personnel	Average growth	$34,800–$74,800
Process Technician/ Chemical Technicians	• Associate's degree • Some have bachelor's degree	Average growth	$34,800–$76,500
Quality Control Technician	• On-the job training or associate's degree • Certification from the American Society for Quality (ASQ)	Average growth	$31,000–$64,250
Forensic Science Technicians	• Bachelor's or master's degree • Most states do not have licensing or certification requirements • Must meet proficiency levels established by national accreditation associations for criminal laboratories • Certification can be obtained from the American Society for Clinical Pathology	Below average growth	$42,300–$98,700
Pharmaceutical/clinical project manager	• Bachelor's or master's degree in Business	Above average growth	$71,335–$142,339
Geneticist	• Bachelor's degree • Master's and doctoral degrees for advancement	Average growth	$43,500–$147,000
Pharmacologist	• Doctoral degree in pharmacy (PharmD) or in related medical field • Licensure required in all states	Above average growth	$86,700–$160,520
Toxicologist	• Bachelor's, master's, or doctoral degree • Licensure required in some states • Certification can be obtained from the American Board of Toxicology	Above average growth	$51,900–$109,000 and higher with doctoral

can be used as implants in the human body; design and construct artificial organs such as hip replacements, kidneys, heart valves, and artificial hearts; and research the biomechanics of injury and wound healing.

Biomedical/clinical technicians, working under the supervision of biological scientists or biotechnological engineers, assist in the study of living organisms. They perform many of the laboratory experiments used in medical research on diseases such as cancer and acquired immune deficiency syndrome (AIDS). They also assist in the development, testing, and manufacturing of pharmaceuticals or medications (**Figure 3–24**). Biomedical technicians must be proficient in the use of clinical laboratory equipment and computers. They must also be adept at compiling statistics and preparing research reports to document experiments.

Process technicians, also called *chemical technicians*, working under the supervision of biological scientists or research physicians, operate and monitor the machinery that is used to produce biotechnology products. They may install new equipment, monitor the operating processes of the equipment, assess quality control of

the finished product, and enforce environmental and safety regulations. For example, a process technician manufacturing drugs for a pharmaceutical company may prepare and measure raw materials, load the raw materials into the machinery, set the controls, operate the machinery, take test samples for quality control, and record required information. Process technicians must use aseptic techniques and follow all safety and environmental regulations during the manufacturing process.

Quality control technicians test materials and products before, during, and after production to make sure the characteristics of the material or product are correct and to ensure they conform to specifications. Quality control technicians must be meticulous in their work. They must know about measurements and be able to test equipment

Forensic science technicians, also called *criminalists*, investigate crimes by collecting physical evidence. Examples of physical evidence include weapons, clothing, shoes, fibers, hair, body tissues, blood, body fluids, fingerprints, chemicals, and even vapors in the air. After the physical evidence is analyzed and preserved, the

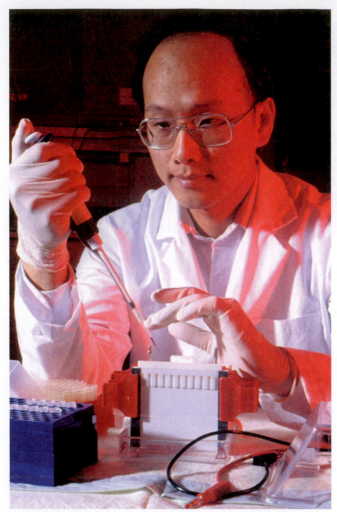

FIGURE 3–24 Biomedical technicians perform many of the laboratory experiments used for medical research. Courtesy CDC/James Gathany

clinical trial team in order to make sure everyone is up to date on any relevant issues that may arise.

Geneticists study genes and how they are inherited, mutated, and activated, or inactivated. They supervise other geneticists, biologists, and technicians that are working on genetic research projects. They maintain lab notebooks or electronic data records that record procedures, research methods, analyses of lab tests, and results of the research.

Pharmacologists are medical researchers that work with patients and doctors to test and evaluate effectiveness as well as safety of new drugs. They design and carry out experiments, analyze and interpret data, manage lab staff and equipment, prepare research grants, and publish findings. They are employed in a variety of settings like government, industry, and academia.

Toxicologists design, plan, and conduct experiments and trials to study the safety and biological effects of chemical agents, drugs, and other substances on the body. They develop hypotheses and test them. They use appropriate techniques to identify and quantify toxins. They analyze and interpret data. Toxicologists must have patience and focus. They must be able to follow procedures to obtain reliable results.

RESEARCH HEALTH CAREERS

- American Academy of Forensic Sciences
  www.aafs.org

- American Board of Toxicology
  www.abtox.org

- American Institute of Biological Sciences
  www.aibs.org

- American Society for Biochemistry and Molecular Biology (ASBMB)
  www.asbmb.org

- American Society for Clinical Pathology
  www.ascp.org

- American Society for Quality
  www.asq.org

- Biotechnology Industry Organization
  www.bio.org

- Biotechnology Institute
  www.biotechinstitute.org

- Federation of American Societies for Experimental Biology
  www.faseb.org

- Genetics Society of America
  www.genetics-gsa.org

- Pharmaceutical Research and Manufacturers of America
  www.phrma.org

forensic science technician works with other investigative officers such as police detectives to reconstruct a crime scene and find the individual who committed the crime. Forensic science technicians must be proficient in the use of laboratory equipment and computers. They must also be adept at preparing reports, compiling statistics, and testifying in trials or hearings.

Pharmaceutical/clinical project managers plan and manage all aspects of scientific research studies. Pharmaceutical project managers direct drug clinical trials while clinical project managers direct trials to obtain information to help prevent, screen, diagnose, and/or treat disease or medical conditions. They must make sure that the research project stays on task and complies with all aspects of regulation. They must evaluate the safety and effectiveness of the pharmaceutical or clinical research in order to submit it for regulation, obtain FDA approval, write scientific studies, or prepare marketing/ad claims. These managers must also supervise staff and manage the project budget. They spend a lot of time communicating with other professionals and the

Memories Restored by Flipping a Switch?

Do you wish that you could forget the time you dropped a plate of spaghetti in your lap at a restaurant or that you could always remember the names of people you have met before? Wouldn't it be nice to be able to turn memories on and off with the flip of a switch? You could eliminate all of your bad memories and improve your good ones. Someday this may be possible.

Theodore Berger, a biomedical engineer at the University of Southern California, has figured out how to manipulate brain cells in rats so that they can be activated or suppressed. The study involved an area of the brain called the hippocampus, a region crucial for memory formation. The team inserted electrical probes in the hippocampus. They then taught rats to learn which of several levers had to be pressed to receive a reward. During the learning process, the researchers recorded changes in the brain activity of the rats between two major internal divisions of the hippocampus, subregions known as CA3 and CA1. Through research, they learned these subregions interact to convert short-term memory into long-term memory. They were also able to pinpoint the pattern of nerve-cell activity involved in creating a solid memory. The scientists then used the electrical probes to stimulate the nerves in the same pattern and found that the rats' performance improved, and the rats could remember the correct lever for a longer period of time. In order to evaluate if memory could be suppressed, the researchers gave the rats a drug that blocked the nerve-cell activity and caused the rats to forget the task. A prosthetics (artificial devices) team then created an artificial system that duplicated the pattern of interaction between CA3 and CA1 in the hippocampus. When this system was inserted into the animals and the brain cells were stimulated with the correct pattern, long-term memory returned. A final discovery was that when the prosthetic hippocampus with its electrodes was implanted in animals with normal function, the device strengthened the memory being created. In 2018, Dr. Berger worked with a team of doctors to implant the hippocampal prosthetic in patients as part of a medical diagnostic procedure for epilepsy. While the electrodes were in place, memory tests were performed, and the team was able to demonstrate up to 37 percent improvement in memory function. Additional research is now being conducted to customize the implants and test memory codes to see if memories can be retained over a period of time.

If research is successful, it might be possible to create a prosthetic that can be permanently implanted in humans. This could help victims of Alzheimer's disease, stroke, or brain injury recover memory that has been lost and could improve mental function. In addition, if the prosthetic can be used to suppress memories, the device might be a method for treating individuals with posttraumatic stress disorder or other psychiatric conditions such as fears caused by a previous memory. Even though this research will require many more years of study due to the complex nature of memory in humans, if it is successful, it will be a major breakthrough for many individuals.

checkpoint

1. List three (3) characteristics needed by professionals in the biotechnology research and development field.

PRACTICE: Go to the workbook and complete the assignment sheet for Chapter 3, Careers in Health Care.

Case Study Investigation Conclusion

What careers can you identify that might be involved in the transport, assessment, diagnosis, and treatment of Luke, Hazel, and Rex? It may seem obvious that they need to see a physician, but who performs the field assessment and safe transport to the ER? What support staff provide a clean welcoming environment? What careers are involved in the diagnosis and treatment? Rex went to a different facility, and professionals with different careers took care of him. With a partner, formulate a probable list of medical providers that were involved in the care of these individuals.

CHAPTER 3 SUMMARY

More than 250 different careers in health care provide individuals with opportunities to find occupations they enjoy.

This chapter describes:

- Major health care careers
- Basic job duties
- Educational requirements
- Anticipated need for health care providers
- Average yearly salaries

REVIEW QUESTIONS

1. Explain the differences and similarities between secondary and postsecondary health care education.

2. For each of the postsecondary degrees listed, state how many years of education are required to obtain the degree. For each degree, give three (3) examples of specific health care careers that require the degree for entry-level providers.
   a. Associate's degree
   b. Bachelor's degree
   c. Master's degree
   d. Doctorate

3. What are CEUs? Why are they required in many health care careers?

4. Name at least four (4) specific careers within each cluster of the National Health Care Standards.

5. What is an entrepreneur? Identify five (5) examples of health care careers that may be an entrepreneur.

6. Choose one (1) health care career in which you have an interest. Use references or search the Internet to identify three (3) different schools that offer accredited programs in the career.

7. Match the abbreviations used to identify each health care provider.

_____ Dentist

_____ Certified Athletic Trainer

_____ Doctor of Medicine

_____ Social Worker

_____ Veterinarian

_____ Optometrist

_____ Registered Respiratory Therapist

_____ Electrocardiograph Technician

_____ Registered Health Information Administrator

_____ Certified Biomedical Equipment Technician

a.	CBET	f.	SW
b.	DDS	g.	OD
c.	ECG	h.	DVM
d.	RRT	i.	CAT
e.	MD	j.	RHIA

CRITICAL THINKING

1. Prepare a paper for one (1) occupation in each of the health science career pathways. Use and document at least two (2) online resources. Each career paper must include:
   - Job description with roles and responsibilities
   - The knowledge and skills needed for the career
   - Track the pathway of education or study from high school through postsecondary; include employment opportunities
   - Traits required to excel in the career
   - Licensure or credentialing requirements
   - Non-educational requirements, i.e., age, physical fitness testing
   - Include between one (1) to three (3) photographs to illustrate this career

2. Write a brief report comparing each of the five (5) careers you investigated and conclude which would be for you.

■ ACTIVITIES

1. With a partner, conduct an interview with a health care provider in one (1) of the health science career pathways. Create a video. The video should include information about how this individual became employed in this field and the pros and cons of working in this field.

2. With a partner, investigate a career in the medical field. Use the criteria for the HOSA competitive event, "Health Career Display." Prepare your display and present it to your class. Go to *www.hosa.org/guidelines* for more information.

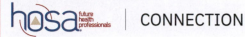 | CONNECTION

Health Career Display

Event Summary: Health Career Display provides members with the opportunity to research a career of interest, create a display board of associated career materials, and improve their presentation skills as they communicate the career information to others. This competitive event consists of 2 rounds, and each team consists of 2 people. Round One is the judging of the Health Display Board. The top scoring teams will advance to Round Two for the presentation. This event aims to inspire members to become future health professionals by exciting them about a career of their choosing.

Details of this competitive event may be found at www.hosa.org/guidelines

CHAPTER 4

PERSONAL AND PROFESSIONAL QUALITIES OF A HEALTH CARE TEAM MEMBER 💼
Career

Case Study Investigation

Gregg, a 50-year-old CEO of a large restaurant chain with a family history of high cholesterol, has come to your hospital for cardiac bypass surgery. He has been married to Lynn for 25 years, and they have two college-aged children, Jake and Josh. The surgeon and anesthesiologist are both members of different multi-specialty physician groups.

The hospital has recently purchased a new piece of equipment for blood administration during a surgical procedure. The anesthesiologist is the only one that has been trained on this and has used it successfully in five surgical cases. Two units of blood have been administered during the case using this equipment. As the anesthesiologist administers the last unit of blood,

the patient suddenly goes into cardiac arrest. CPR was undertaken with successful results. Over the next few days, it is clear Gregg has suffered brain injury due to lack of oxygen and is discharged to a skilled nursing facility with little prospects of returning to work.

The root cause analysis suggests that there were several causes but identifies a breakdown in communication between the anesthesiologist, perfusionist, and surgeon, along with a lack of familiarity with the new equipment. At the end of this chapter, you will be asked to identify barriers to communication, how health care teamwork is beneficial, and the characteristics of an effective team.

■ LEARNING OBJECTIVES

After completing this chapter, you should be able to:

- Explain how diet, rest, exercise, good posture, preventive screenings, and avoiding use of tobacco, alcohol, and drugs contribute to good health.
- Demonstrate the standards of a professional appearance as they apply to uniforms, shoes, nails, hair, jewelry, and makeup.
- Create a characteristic profile of a health care team member that includes at least eight personal/professional traits or attitudes.
- Identify four factors that interfere with communication.
- Explain the importance of listening, nonverbal behavior, reporting, and recording in the communication process.

LEARNING OBJECTIVES *(continued)*

- Differentiate between the positive and negative effects of relationships on emotional, physical, and mental health.
- Identify why teamwork is beneficial.
- Identify six basic characteristics of leaders.
- Differentiate among democratic, laissez-faire, and autocratic leaders.
- Conduct a meeting following the basic principles of parliamentary procedure.
- Differentiate between positive and negative stressors by identifying the emotional response.
- List six ways to eliminate or decrease stress.
- Explain how time management, problem solving, and goal setting reduce stress.
- Define, pronounce, and spell all key terms.

KEY TERMS

acceptance of criticism
autocratic leader
communication
competence (*kom'-peh-tense*)
cultural diversity
democratic leader
dependability
discretion
empathy (*em"-pa-thee'*)
enthusiasm
feedback

goal
honesty
initiative
laissez-faire leader
leader
leadership
listening
nonverbal communication
parliamentary procedure
patience
personal hygiene

professionalism
responsibility
self-motivation
stress
tact
team player
teamwork
time management
willingness to learn

INTRODUCTION

Although health care team members are employed in many different career areas and in a variety of facilities, certain personal/professional characteristics, attitudes, and rules of appearance apply to all health care providers. This chapter discusses these basic requirements.

4:1 PERSONAL APPEARANCE

As a team member in any health care career, it is important to present an appearance that inspires confidence and a positive self-image. Research has shown that within the first 7 seconds, people form an impression about another person based mainly on appearance. Although the rules of suitable appearance may vary, certain professional standards apply to most health care careers and should be observed to create a positive impression.

GOOD HEALTH

Health care involves promoting health and preventing disease. Therefore, health care team members should present a healthy appearance. Six factors contribute to good health:

- **Diet**: Eating well-balanced meals and nutritious foods provides the body with the materials needed for optimum health. Foods from each of the five major food groups should be eaten daily. *MyPlate*, discussed in Section11:4, identifies the major food groups.

- **Rest**: Adequate rest and sleep provide energy and the ability to deal with stress. The amount of sleep required varies for each individual.

- **Exercise**: Exercise maintains circulation, improves muscle tone, enhances mental attitude, aids in weight control, and contributes to more restful sleep. In addition, regular physical activity reduces risk for coronary heart disease, diabetes, colon cancer, hypertension (high blood pressure), and osteoporosis. Individuals should choose the form of exercise best suited to their own needs, but they should exercise daily.

- **Good posture**: Good posture helps prevent fatigue and puts less stress on muscles. Basic principles include standing straight with stomach muscles pulled in, shoulders relaxed, and weight balanced equally on each foot.

- **Avoid use of tobacco, alcohol, and drugs**: The use of tobacco, alcohol, and drugs can seriously affect good health. Tobacco affects the function of the heart, circulatory system, lungs, and digestive system. In addition, the odor of smoke is offensive to many individuals, and secondhand smoke (smoke people inhale when someone is smoking around them) has proven to be harmful to their health. Health care facilities are "smoke-free" environments, and some of them will not hire any health care professionals who smoke, even if it is outside of the health care facility. These facilities require a potential employee to pass a nicotine test before that person is hired. The use of alcohol and drugs impairs mental function, decreases the ability to make decisions, and adversely affects many body systems. The use of alcohol or drugs can also result in job loss. Avoiding tobacco, alcohol, and drugs helps prevent damage to the body systems and contributes to good health.

- **Preventative screenings**: The health care team member should schedule routine medical exams and dental screenings in order to promote good health and prevent disease. Immunizations and stress management are just two things that may be addressed at regularly scheduled checkups.

PROFESSIONAL APPEARANCE

When you obtain a position in a health care field, it is important to learn the rules or standards of dress and personal appearance that have been established by your place of employment. Abide by the rules and make every effort to maintain a neat, clean, and professional appearance.

Uniform

Many health care careers require personnel to wear uniforms, usually called scrubs. A uniform should always be neat, well fitting, clean, and wrinkle-free (**Figure 4–1**). Some agencies require a white uniform, but most use differently colored scrubs to identify the different groups of personnel in the facility. It is important that the health care team member learn what type and color uniform is required or permitted and follow the standards established by the place of employment.

Clothing

If regular clothing is worn in place of a uniform, the clothing must be clean, neat, and in good condition (**Figure 4–2**). The style should allow for freedom of body movement and should be appropriate for the job. For example, while clean, neat jeans might be appropriate at times for a recreational therapist, they are not proper

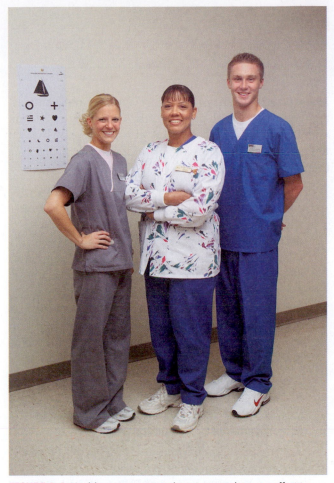

FIGURE 4–1 Health care team members must make every effort to maintain a neat, clean, and professional appearance.

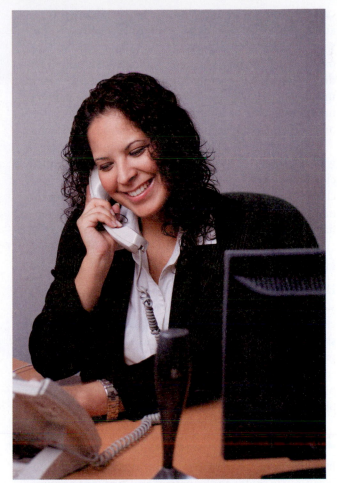

FIGURE 4–2 If regular clothing is worn in place of a uniform, the clothing should reflect a professional appearance. © iStock.com/Aldo Murillo

attire for most other health professionals. Washable fabrics are usually best because frequent laundering is necessary.

Name Badge or Identification Tag

Most health care facilities require personnel to wear name badges or photo identification tags (ID tags) at all times. The badge or tag usually states the name, title, and department of the health care team member. Most also contain a photo of the individual. In some health care settings, such as long-term care facilities, team members are required by law to wear identification badges or tags. In addition, a health care facility's security regulations may require photo ID tags to gain access into the building or into certain areas inside the facility.

Shoes

Although white shoes made of a nonabsorbent material such as leather are frequently required, many health care careers allow other types of shoes. Any shoes should fit well and provide good support to prevent fatigue. Low heels are usually best because they help prevent fatigue and accidents. Avoid wearing sandals, open-toe shoes,

or Crocs™ unless they are standard dress for a particular career. Shoes should be cleaned daily. If shoelaces are part of the shoes, these must also be cleaned or replaced frequently.

Personal Hygiene

Good **personal hygiene** is essential. Because health care team members typically work in close contact with others, body odor must be controlled. A daily bath or shower, use of deodorant or antiperspirant, good oral hygiene, and clean undergarments all help prevent body odor. Strong odors caused by tobacco, perfumes, scented hairsprays, and aftershave lotions can be offensive. In addition, certain scents can cause allergic reactions in some individuals. The use of these products should be avoided when working with patients and team members.

Nails

Nails should be kept short, clean, and natural. Many health care facilities prohibit the use of artificial nails. If fingernails are long and/or pointed, they can injure patients. They can also transmit germs because dirt can collect under long nails and artificial nails. In addition, health care personnel are now required to wear gloves for most procedures. Long nails can tear or puncture gloves. The use of colored nail polish is discouraged because the color can conceal any dirt that may collect under the nails. Further, because frequent handwashing causes polish to chip, germs can collect on the surfaces of nails.

Finally, the flash of bright colors may bother a person who does not feel well. If nail polish is worn, it should be clear or colorless, and the nails must be kept thoroughly clean. Hand cream or lotion should be used to keep the hands from becoming chapped and dry from frequent handwashing.

Hair

Hair should be kept clean and neat. It should be neatly styled and easy to care for. Fancy or extreme hairstyles, excessive hair accessories, and/or unnatural hair colors should be avoided. If the job requires close contact with patients, long hair must be pinned back and kept off the shoulders. This prevents the hair from touching the patient/resident, falling on a tray or on equipment, or blocking necessary vision during procedures.

Jewelry

Jewelry is usually not permitted with a uniform because it can cause injury to the patient and transmit germs or pathogens. Exceptions sometimes include a watch, wedding ring, and small, pierced earrings. Also, medical alert bracelets such as diabetic or heart disease bracelets are permitted in all situations. Earrings with hoops or dangling earrings should be avoided. Body jewelry—such as nose, eyebrow, or tongue piercings—detracts from a professional appearance and is prohibited in many health care facilities. When a uniform is not required, jewelry should still be limited. Excessive jewelry can interfere with patient care and detracts from the professional appearance of the health care team member.

Makeup and Tattoos

Excessive and unnatural makeup should be avoided. The purpose of makeup is to create a natural appearance and add to the attractiveness of a person.

Tattoos that are visible detract from a professional appearance and are prohibited in many health care facilities. Some health care facilities require that any tattoo be covered by clothing at all times. An exception to the rule is medical alert tattoos, which are permitted in all situations. Follow the policies established by your place of employment.

checkpoint

| **1.** What six (6) main factors contribute to good health?

Many personal/professional characteristics and attitudes are required in health care careers. As a health care team member, you should make every effort to develop the following characteristics and attitudes and to incorporate them into your personality:

- **Empathy**: Empathy means being able to identify with and understand another person's feelings, situation, and motives. As a health care team member, you may care for persons of all ages—from the newborn infant to the elderly adult. To be successful, you must be sincerely interested in working with people. You must care about others and be able to communicate and work with them (**Figure 4–3**). Understanding the needs of people and learning effective communication techniques is one way to develop empathy. This topic is covered in greater detail in Section 4:3 of this text.

- **Honesty**: Truthfulness and integrity are important in any health care field. Others must be able to trust you at all times. You must be willing to admit mistakes so they can be corrected.

- **Dependability**: Employers and patients rely on you, so you must accept the responsibility required by your position. You must be prompt in reporting to work, and you must maintain a good attendance record. You must perform assigned tasks on time and accurately.

- **Willingness to learn**: You must be willing to learn and to adapt to changes. The field of health care changes constantly because of research, new inventions, and technological advances. Change often requires learning new techniques or procedures. At times, additional education may be required to remain competent in a particular field. Be prepared for lifelong learning to maintain a competent level of knowledge and skills.

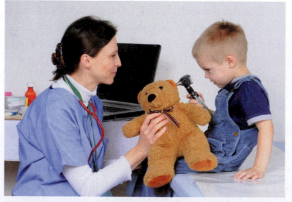

FIGURE 4–3 An empathetic health care provider tries to help a child who is frightened about a medical procedure. © iStock.com/Yarinca

- **Patience**: You must be tolerant and understanding. You must learn to control your temper and "count to 10" in difficult situations. Learning to deal with frustration and overcome obstacles is important.

- **Acceptance of criticism**: Patients, families, employers, team members, doctors, and others may criticize you. Some criticism will be constructive and will allow you to improve your work. Remember that everyone has some areas where performance can be improved. Instead of becoming resentful, you must be willing to accept criticism and learn from it.

- **Enthusiasm**: You must enjoy your work and display a positive attitude. Enthusiasm is contagious; it helps you do your best and encourages others to do the same. If you do not like some aspects of your job, concentrating on the positive points can help diminish the importance of the negative points.

- **Self-motivation**: Self-motivation, or **initiative**, is the ability to begin or to follow through with a task. You should be able to determine things that need to be done and do them without constant direction. You must set goals for yourself and work to reach those goals.

- **Tact**: Being tactful means having the ability to say or do the kindest or most fitting thing in a difficult situation. It requires constant practice. Tactfulness implies a consideration for the feelings of others. It is important to remember that all individuals have a right to their respective feelings and that these feelings should not be judged as right or wrong.

- **Competence**: Being competent means that you are qualified and capable of performing a task. You follow instructions, use approved procedures, and strive for accuracy in all you do. You know your limits and ask for help or guidance if you do not know how to perform a procedure.

- **Responsibility**: Responsibility implies being willing to be held accountable for your actions. Others can rely on you and know that you will meet your obligations. Responsibility means that you do what you are supposed to do.

- **Discretion**: You must always use good judgment in what you say and do. In any health care career, you will have access to confidential information. This information should not be told to anyone without proper authorization. A patient is entitled to confidential care; you must be discreet and ensure that the patient's rights are not violated.

- **Professionalism**: This involves a blending of many different personal qualities to meet the standards expected in a health care career. Displaying good judgment, proper behavior, courtesy, good communication skills, honesty, politeness, responsibility, integrity, competence, and a proper appearance are all components of professionalism. It is important to note that if you are employed in health care, you should show professionalism on social media sites. Negative comments about your employer or a display of unprofessional photographs can be seen by your employer and result in the loss of your job. Remaining on task, following the rules and regulations of the facility, and avoiding distractions are other traits of a professional. Using a cell phone to talk, text, or play games while you are working is not professional. Wait until you have your break before using these devices.

- **Team player**: In any health care field, you will become part of a team. It is essential that you become a team player and learn to work well with others. Each member of a health care team will have different responsibilities, but each member must do his or her part to provide the patient with quality care. By working together, a team can accomplish goals much faster than an individual can.

Each of the preceding characteristics and attitudes must be practiced and learned. Some take more time to develop than others. By being aware of these characteristics and striving constantly to improve, you will provide good patient/resident care and be a valuable asset to your employer and other members of the health care team.

check**point**

1. What are ten (10) characteristics of a health care team member?

4:3 EFFECTIVE COMMUNICATIONS

Communicating effectively with others is an important part of any health care profession. The health care team member must be able to relate to patients and their families, to fellow team members, and to other professionals. An understanding of communication skills will assist the health care team member who is trying to relate effectively.

Communication is the exchange of information, thoughts, ideas, and feelings. It can occur through *verbal* means (spoken words), written communications, and *nonverbal* behavior such as facial expressions, body language, and touch. While all types of communication are important, research has shown that a large percentage of the communication we do is nonverbal, so it is very important to remember that your facial expressions, body language, and use of touch have a large impact on the communication process.

COMMUNICATION PROCESS

The communication process involves three essential elements:

- **Sender**: an individual who creates a message to convey information or an idea to another person
- **Message**: the information, ideas, or thoughts
- **Receiver**: an individual who receives the message from the sender

Without a sender, message, and receiver, communication cannot occur.

Feedback is a method that can be used to determine whether a communication was successful. This occurs when the receiver responds to the message. Feedback allows the original sender to evaluate how the message was interpreted and to make any necessary adjustments or clarification. Feedback can be verbal or nonverbal.

Even though the communication process seems simple, many factors can interfere with the process. Important elements of effective communication include:

- **The message must be clear.** The message must be in terms that both the sender and receiver understand. Health care team members learn and use terminology that is frequently not understood by those people who are not employed in health care. Even though these terms are familiar to the health care team member, they must be modified, defined, or substituted with other words when messages are conveyed to people not employed in health care. For example, if a health care team member needs a urine specimen, some patients can be told to urinate in a container. Others, such as very small children or individuals with limited education, may have to be told to "pee" or "do number one." Even a term such as *apical pulse* is not understood by many individuals. Instead of telling a patient, "I am going to take your apical pulse," say, "I am going to listen to your heart." Keep in mind that while it is important to use terms the receiver can understand, it is also important not to use obscene or offensive terms. It requires experience and constant practice to learn to create a message that can be clearly understood.

- **The sender must deliver the message in a clear and concise manner.** Correct pronunciation and the use of good grammar are essential. The use of slang words or words with double meanings should be avoided. Meaningless phrases or terms such as "you know," "all that stuff," "um," and "OK" distract from the message and also must be avoided. In verbal communications, the tone and pitch of voice is important. A moderate level, neither too soft nor too loud, and good inflection to avoid speaking in a monotone, are essential. Think of the many different ways the sentence "I really like this job" can be said and the different meanings that can be inferred

depending on the tone and pitch of the voice. The proper rate, or speed, of delivering a message is also important. If a message is delivered too quickly, the receiver may not have enough time to hear all parts of the message. In written communications, the message should be spelled correctly, contain correct grammar and punctuation, and be concise but thorough.

- **The receiver must be able to hear and receive the message.** Patients who are heavily medicated or are weak may nod their heads as if messages are heard, when, in reality, the patients are not receiving the information. They may hear it, but it is not being interpreted and understood because of their physical states. Patients with hearing or visual impairments or patients with limited English-speaking abilities are other examples of individuals who may not be able to easily receive messages (**Figure 4–4**). Repeating the message, changing the form of the message, and getting others to interpret or clarify the message are some ways to help the receiver receive and respond to the message.

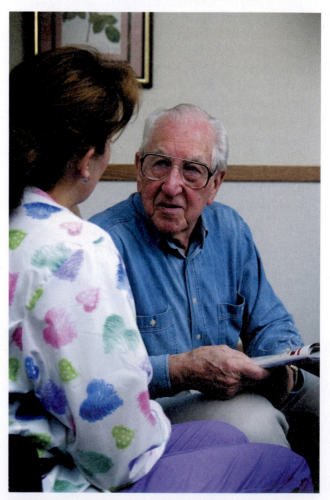

FIGURE 4–4 In communicating with a person who has a hearing impairment, face the individual and speak slowly and distinctly.
© GWImages/Shutterstock.com

- **The receiver must be able to understand the message.** Using unfamiliar terminology can cause a breakdown in communication. Many people do not want to admit that they do not understand terms because they think others will think they are stupid. The health care team member should ask questions or repeat information in different terms if it appears that the patient does not understand the information. The receiver's attitude and prejudices can also interfere with understanding. If a patient feels that health care team members do not know what they are talking about, the patient will not accept the information presented. Receivers must have some confidence and belief in the sender before they will accept and understand a message. It is important that health care team members be willing to say, "I don't know, but I will try to find out that information for you," when they are asked a question about which they do not have the correct knowledge. It is also important for health care team members to be aware of their own prejudices and attitudes when they receive messages from patients. If health care team members feel that certain patients are lazy, ignorant, or uncooperative, they will not respond correctly to messages sent by these patients. Health care team members must be aware of these feelings and work to overcome them so they can accept patients as they are.

- **Interruptions or distractions must be avoided.** Interruptions or distractions can interfere with any communication. Trying to talk with others while answering the phone, responding to a text, reading an e-mail, or writing a message can decrease the effectiveness of spoken and/or written communication. Loud noises or distractions in the form of bright lights or uncomfortable temperatures can interrupt communication. When two people are talking outside in freezing temperatures, for example, the conversation will be limited because of their discomfort from the cold. A small child jumping around or climbing up and down off a mother's lap will distract the mother as she is getting instructions from a health care team member. A loud television or radio interferes with verbal messages because receivers may pay more attention to the radio or television than to the person speaking to them. It is important to eliminate or at least limit distractions if meaningful communication is to take place.

LISTENING

Listening is another essential part of effective communication. Listening means paying attention to and making an effort to hear what the other person is saying.

Good listening skills require constant practice. Techniques that can be used to learn good listening skills include:

- Show interest and concern for what the speaker is saying
- Be alert and maintain eye contact with the speaker
- Avoid interrupting the speaker
- Pay attention to what the speaker is saying
- Avoid thinking about how you are going to respond
- Try to eliminate your own prejudices and see the other person's point of view
- Eliminate distractions by moving to a quiet area for the conversation
- Watch the speaker closely to observe actions that may contradict what the person is saying
- Reflect statements back to the speaker to let the speaker know that statements are being heard
- Ask for clarification if you do not understand part of a message
- Keep your temper under control and maintain a positive attitude

Good listening skills will allow you to receive the entire message a person is trying to convey to you. For example, if a patient says, "I'm not worried about this surgery," but is very restless and seems nervous, the patient's body movements may indicate fear that she or he is denying in words. The health care team member could reflect the patient's statement by saying, "You're not at all worried about this surgery?" The patient may respond by saying, "Well, not really. It's just that I worry about my family if something should happen to me." Good listening allowed the patient to express fears and opened the way to more effective communication. In this same case, the entire pattern of communication could have been blocked if the health care team member had instead responded, "That's good."

NONVERBAL COMMUNICATION

Nonverbal communication involves the use of facial expressions, body language, gestures, eye contact, and touch to convey messages or ideas (**Figure 4–5**).

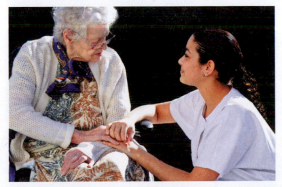

FIGURE 4–5 What aspects of listening and nonverbal behavior can you see in this picture? © Gilles Lougassi/Shutterstock.com

If a person is smiling and sitting in a very relaxed position while saying, "I am very angry about this entire situation," two different messages are being conveyed. A smile, a frown, a wink, a shrug of the shoulders, a bored expression, a tapping of fingers or feet, and other similar gestures or actions all convey messages to the receiver. It is important for health care team members to be aware of both their own and patients' nonverbal behaviors because these are an important part of any communication process. A touch of the hand, a pat on the back, a firm handshake, and a hug can convey more interest and caring than words ever could. When verbal and nonverbal messages agree, the receiver is more likely to understand the message being sent.

BARRIERS TO COMMUNICATION

A communication barrier is something that gets in the way of clear communication. Three common barriers are physical disabilities, psychological attitudes and prejudices, and cultural diversity.

Physical and Sensory Disabilities

- **Deafness or hearing loss**: People who are deaf or hearing impaired have difficulty receiving messages. To improve communication, it is essential to use body language such as gestures and signs, speak clearly in short sentences, face the individual to improve the potential for lip reading, write messages if necessary, and make sure that any hearing aids have good batteries and are inserted correctly (**Figure 4–6**). At times, it may be necessary to obtain the assistance of a sign language interpreter to communicate with an individual who is deaf.

- **Blindness or impaired vision**: People who are blind or visually impaired may be able to hear what is being said, but they will not see body language, gestures, or facial expressions. To improve communication, use a soft tone of voice, describe events that are occurring, announce your presence as you enter a room, explain sounds or noises, and use touch when appropriate.

- **Aphasia or speech impairments**: Aphasia is the loss or impairment of the power to use or comprehend words, usually as a result of injury or damage to the brain. Individuals with aphasia or speech impairments can have difficulty with not only the spoken word but also written communications. They may know what they want to say but have difficulty remembering the correct words, may not be able to pronounce certain words, or may have slurred and distorted speech. Patience is essential while working with these individuals. Allow them to try to speak, encourage them to take their time, ask questions that require only short responses, speak slowly and clearly, pause between sentences to allow them to comprehend what has been said, repeat messages to be sure they are correct, encourage them to use gestures or point to objects, provide writing materials if they can write messages, or use pictures with key messages to communicate (**Figure 4–7**).

- **Cognitive impairments**: Cognitive impairments occur when an individual has problems with memory, learning, making decisions, solving problems, confusion, and ability to think. Simple things like pain and medications can cause confusion and disorientation. Conditions such as dementia, autism, Down syndrome, and traumatic brain injuries can also be causes. Again, patience is essential while communicating with these individuals. Speak slowly, provide time for the patient to respond, use feedback to determine if information is understood, provide written directions if possible, and work with the patient's family or guardian to make sure instructions are understood.

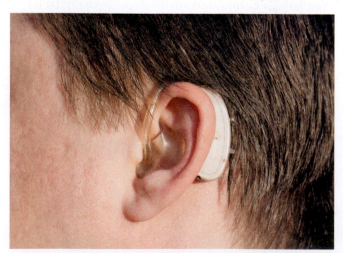

FIGURE 4–6 To be effective, hearing aids must be inserted correctly and have good batteries. © andras_csontos/Shutterstock.com

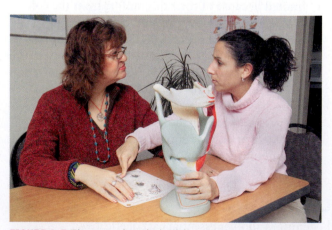

FIGURE 4–7 Picture cards make it easier to communicate with a patient who has aphasia or a speech impairment.

Psychological Barriers

Psychological barriers to communication are often caused by bias, prejudice, stereotyping, attitudes, and personality. Examples include closed-mindedness, judging, preaching, moralizing, lecturing, overreacting, arguing, advising, and prejudging. Our judgments of others are too often based on appearance, lifestyle, and social or economic status. Accepting stereotypes such as "dumb blonde," "lazy bum," or "fat slob" causes us to make snap judgments about an individual and affects the communication process. More information on bias, prejudice, and stereotyping may be found in Section 10:2.

Health care team members must learn to put prejudice aside and show respect to all individuals. A homeless person deserves the same quality of health care as the president of the United States. It is important to respect each person as an individual and to remember that each person has the right to good care and considerate treatment. At times, this can be extremely difficult, and patience and practice are essential. When individuals have negative attitudes or constantly complain or criticize your work, it can be difficult to show them respect. The health care team member must learn to see beyond the surface attitude to the human being underneath.

Frequently, fear is the cause of anger or a negative attitude. Allow patients to express their fears or anger, encourage them to talk about their feelings, avoid arguing, remain calm, talk in a soft and nonthreatening tone of voice, and provide quality care. If other health care team members seem to be able to communicate more effectively with patients, watch these team members to learn how they handle difficult or angry patients. This is often the most effective means of learning good communication skills.

Cultural Diversity

Cultural diversity, discussed in detail in Chapter 10, is another possible communication barrier. Culture consists of the values, beliefs, attitudes, and customs shared by a group of people and passed from one generation to the next. It is often defined as a set of rules because culture allows an individual to interpret the environment and actions of others and behave appropriately. The main barriers created by cultural diversity include:

- **Beliefs and practices regarding health and illness**: Individuals from different cultures may have their own beliefs about the cause of an illness and the type of treatment required (refer to **Table 10-1**). It is important to remember that they have the right to determine their treatment plans and even to refuse traditional treatments. At times, these individuals may accept traditional health care but add their own cultural remedies to the treatment plan.

- **Language differences**: Language differences can create major barriers. In the United States, English is the primary language used in health care. If a person has difficulty communicating in English and a health care team member is not fluent in another language, a barrier exists. When providing care to people who have limited English-speaking abilities, speak slowly, use simple words, use gestures or pictures to clarify the meaning of words, and use nonverbal communication in the form of a smile or gentle touch. Avoid the tendency to speak louder because this does not improve comprehension. Whenever possible, try to find an interpreter who speaks the patient's language. Frequently, another health care team member, a consultant, or a family member may be able to assist in the communication process. In addition, many health care facilities provide written instructions or explanations in several different languages to facilitate the communication process (**Figure 4–8**).

- **Eye contact**: In some cultures, direct eye-to-eye contact while communicating is not acceptable. These cultures believe that looking down shows proper respect for another individual. A health care team member who feels that eye contact is important must learn to accept and respect this cultural difference and a person's inability to engage in eye contact while communicating.

- **Ways of dealing with terminal illness and/or severe disability**: In the United States, a traditional health care belief is that the patient should be told the truth about his or her diagnosis and should be informed about the expected outcome. Some cultural groups believe that a person should not be told of a fatal diagnosis or be burdened with making decisions about treatment. In these cultures, the family, the mother or father, or another designated individual is expected to make decisions about care,

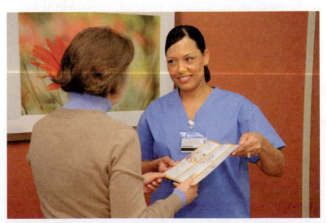

FIGURE 4–8 Many health care facilities provide written instructions or explanations in several different languages to facilitate communication with individuals who have limited English-speaking abilities.

treatment, and information given to the patient. In such instances, it is important for health care team members to recognize and respect this practice and to involve these individuals in the patient's care. At times, it may be necessary for a patient to use legal means, such as a power of attorney for health care, to transfer responsibility for his or her care to another person.

- **Touch**: In some cultures, it is inappropriate to touch someone on the head. Other cultures have clearly defined areas of the body that should not be touched. Even a simple handshake can be regarded as showing a lack of respect. In some cultures, only family members provide personal care. For this reason, health care team members should always get permission from the patient before providing care and should avoid any use of touch that seems to be inappropriate for the individual.

Respect for and acceptance of cultural diversity is essential for any health care team member. When beliefs, ideas, concepts, and ways of life are different, communication barriers can result. By making every attempt to learn about cultural differences and by showing respect for an individual's right to cultural beliefs, a health care team member can provide *transcultural health care*, or care based on the cultural beliefs, emotional needs, spiritual feelings, and physical needs of a person.

RECORDING AND REPORTING

In health care, an important part of effective communication is reporting or recording all observations while providing care. To do this, it is important not only to listen to what the patient is saying but also to make observations about the patient. Urgent abnormal observations should be both orally reported to the immediate supervisor and recorded in the chart. Most senses are used to make observations:

- **Sense of sight**: notes the color of skin, swelling or edema, the presence of a rash or sore, the color of urine or stool, the amount of food eaten, and other similar factors
- **Sense of smell**: alerts a health care team member to body odor or unusual odors of breath, wounds, urine, or stool
- **Sense of touch**: used to feel the pulse, dryness or temperature of the skin, perspiration, and swelling
- **Sense of hearing**: used while listening to respirations, abnormal body sounds, coughs, and speech

By using all senses, the health care team member can learn a great deal about a patient's condition and be able to report observations accurately.

Abnormal observations should verbally be reported promptly to an immediate supervisor. There are two types of observations:

- **Subjective observations**: These cannot be seen or felt, and are commonly called *symptoms*. They are usually statements or complaints made by the patient. They should be reported in the exact words the patient used.
- **Objective observations**: These can be seen or measured, and are commonly called *signs*. A bruise, cut, rash, or swelling can be seen. Blood pressure and temperature are measurable. For example, the health care team member should not state, "I think Mr. B. has a fever." The report should state, "Mr. B. is complaining of feeling hot. His skin is red and flushed, and his temperature is 102°."

WRITTEN COMMUNICATION

EHR

In most health care facilities, observations are recorded in a patient's health care record using a computer to access the patient's electronic health record (EHR), also called an electronic medical record (EMR). Effective communication requires these written observations to be precise, accurate, concise, and complete (**Figure 4–9**). Spelling and grammar should be correct, and objective observations should be noted. Subjective observations that the health care team member feels or thinks should be avoided. If a patient's statement is recorded, the statement should be written in the patient's own words and enclosed in quotation marks. All information should be signed with the name and title of the person recording the information. Errors should be crossed out neatly with a straight line, have the word "error" recorded by them, and show the initials of the person fixing the error. Incorrect data on an EHR should be corrected by

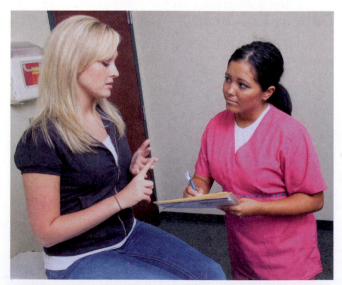

FIGURE 4–9 Information recorded on health care records must be accurate, concise, and complete.

following the directions for making corrections in the particular software being used. In this way, recorded communication will be effective communication. When using portable electronic communication, keep the screen view secure and make sure you have signed out when your documentation is complete.

Incident reports are an important part of written communications. An incident is any unplanned or unintended event or situation that could have resulted in or did result in harm to a patient or any situation that affects the health, safety, and welfare of others. For example, if a patient falls while being transferred to a wheelchair, the health care team member should immediately complete an incident report. Facilities have a specific form to fill out and document these occurrences or dangers. Most forms require information such as the time and date, where the incident happened, a concise but thorough description of the incident, information about any injury or damage caused, names and contact information for all involved individuals and any witnesses, and in some cases, photographs of the damage. If a situation exists that could endanger team members and/or patients, it also should be reported and documented immediately. An example might be a health care team member noticing that dangerous chemicals are being stored incorrectly in a closet. Effective incident remediation requires prompt reporting of any occurrence.

There are also different types of writing used in health care. The main form used is *technical writing*, which is a more formal type of writing that is used to provide pertinent information. This differs from *creative writing* that is used to entertain and to describe personal feelings and thoughts. For example, information entered into a patient's record should be clear and concise and report objective observations. It should not contain feelings or unsupported facts. Technical writing can be used to write reports, research papers, manuals, instructions, information about a medical condition or medication, and other similar documents. Health care team members may also be required to give reports or summaries. Reports can be described as an oral or written presentation of information or activities that have been observed, performed, and/or investigated. At times, a summary is presented that basically describes the main points of a report. Research papers are a more formal type of report that describe the result or conclusion the author has obtained after performing independent research on a topic, product, or concept. For all types of documents, the health care team member should always prepare a draft, revise the draft as necessary, and then edit the material to make sure all information is correct and there are no errors in spelling, punctuation, or grammar.

 The Health Insurance Portability and Accountability Act (HIPAA) established strict standards for maintaining confidentiality of health care records. Under this act, patients have total control of how information in their medical records is used. Patients must be able to see and obtain copies of their records. They can set limits on who can obtain this information; they can even prevent other family members from seeing the information. If any health care provider allows information to be released from a medical record without the patient's permission, the patient can file a complaint that the privacy act has been violated. This act is discussed in more detail in Section 5:1. It is important for every health care provider to be aware of all parts of this act and to make every effort to protect the privacy and confidentiality of the patient's health care records.

Good communication skills allow health care team members to develop good interpersonal relationships. Patients feel accepted, they feel that others have an interest and concern for them, they feel free to express their ideas and fears, they develop confidence in the health care team members, and they feel they are receiving quality health care. In addition, the health care team member will relate more effectively with team members and other individuals.

checkpoint

1. List four (4) barriers to communication.
2. Define objective and subjective observations. List two (2) examples for each type of observation.

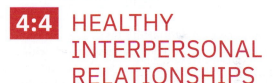

4:4 HEALTHY INTERPERSONAL RELATIONSHIPS

Interpersonal relationships are relationships between people. Healthy interpersonal relationships are a major factor in any individual's life and even influence career goals. Every day, an individual is likely to have interactions with many different groups of people such as family, friends, individuals at school or work, neighbors, members of the community, and new acquaintances. Some of the interactions may be positive, but some may be negative. However, every interaction can have an effect on the physical, mental, and emotional health of the individual.

Humans are basically social and tend to enjoy spending time with others. Healthy interpersonal relationships can provide the following benefits:

- Provide a sense of belonging and self-worth
- Allow an individual to learn to trust and respect others and receive trust and respect in return
- Encourage participation in new ideas or activities
- Encourage personal growth

- Support ambitious career goals
- Increase self-confidence
- Offer safety and security
- Improve physical health by decreasing stress
- Provide support during tough times
- Share celebrations of good times
- Make life more enjoyable

At the same time, poor or negative relationships can have adverse effects including:

- Contributing to low self-esteem
- Contributing to feelings of being powerless or worthless
- Creating suspicion about the sincerity of other relationships
- Feeling isolated from others and hesitant to participate in social activities
- Creating stress
- Weakening or interfering with your career goals
- Distracting your attention from workplace duties
- Developing depression and withdrawing from others
- Causing physical illnesses such as headaches, chronic pain, digestive disorders, hypertension (high blood pressure), insomnia and sleep problems, and a weak immune system

Healthy interpersonal relationships take time and effort to develop and require a willingness to work with others. Effectively communicating needs, wants, and emotions can be a learned skill. Strategies to build healthy relationships and techniques to convey needs, wants, and emotions include:

- Maintain a positive attitude and learn to laugh at yourself
- Be friendly and cooperate with others
- Assist others when you see that they need help
- Listen carefully when another person is sharing ideas or beliefs
- Respect the opinions of others even though you may not agree with them
- Be open-minded and willing to compromise
- Avoid criticizing others
- Learn good communication skills so you can share ideas, concepts, and knowledge
- Support and encourage others
- Perform your duties to the best of your ability

It is also important for everyone to evaluate the relationships that they have. Because you do not have control over what other people say or do, you have to think about things you can say or do to protect and care for yourself. Try to maximize positive relationships, especially among other health care providers. Good relationships between health care community team members result in better health care for everyone. A trusting relationship promotes seamless care for patients. Effective communication is a supporting element of a healthy professional relationship. Research has shown that individuals who have a network of positive relationships are healthier, have lower blood pressure, experience less anxiety, manage stress and conflict more appropriately, heal faster, have less pain or better control of pain, are less likely to be depressed or abuse substances such as drugs and alcohol, and tend to live longer, happier lives.

checkpoint

1. List three (3) benefits of good interpersonal relationships.

4:5 TEAMWORK

In almost any health care career, you will be a part of an interdisciplinary health care team. The team concept was created to provide quality holistic health care to every patient. Teamwork consists of many professionals—with different levels of education, ideas, backgrounds, and interests—working together for the benefit of the patient. For example, a surgical team might include the following people:

- **Admitting clerk**: collects admission information
- **Insurance representative**: obtains approval for the surgery
- **Nurses or patient care technicians**: prepare the patient for surgery
- **Surgeons**: perform the operation
- **Anesthesiologist**: administers anesthetics, medications that decrease pain and/or consciousness
- **Operating room nurses**: assist the surgeon
- **Surgical technicians**: prepare and pass instruments
- **Housekeepers**: clean and sanitize the area
- **Sterile supply personnel**: sterilize the instruments
- **Recovery room personnel**: care for the patient after surgery

After the surgery is complete, a dietitian, social worker, physical therapist, occupational therapist, home health care personnel, and other team members might be needed to assist the patient as he or she recuperates. Each team member has an important job to do. When the team members cooperate, the patient receives quality care.

Comm

Teamwork improves communication and continuity of care. When a team is assigned to a particular patient, the patient knows her or his caregivers and support staff. All the team members can help to identify the needs of the patient, offer opinions about the best type of care, participate in decisions about care options, and suggest additional professionals who might be able to assist with specific needs. This allows a patient to become more educated about health care options and to make informed decisions regarding treatment and care.

For a team to function properly, every person on the team must understand the role of each team member. Effective teams have the following attributes: active participation, commitment, common goals, cultural sensitivity, flexibility, open to feedback, positive attitude, reliability, trust, and a respect for individual contributions. Most teams have frequent patient care conferences, where the patient is an active participant (**Figure 4–10**). Opinions are shared, options are discussed, decisions are made, and goals are established. During the conference, each team member must listen, be honest, express his or her own opinion, and be willing to try different solutions.

A leader is an important part of any team. The leader is responsible for establishing an effective team by organizing and coordinating the team's activities, encouraging everyone to share ideas and give opinions, motivating all team members to work toward established goals, assisting with problems, monitoring the progress of the team, and providing reports and feedback to all team members on the effectiveness of the team. A good team leader will also allow others to assume the leadership role when circumstances indicate that another person can handle a particular situation more effectively. Creating effective *mentorships,* where a more experienced or knowledgeable team member provides guidance and support to a less experienced or knowledgeable member, is also an important role for a team leader. Leadership is discussed in more detail in Section 4:6.

Healthy interpersonal relationships are also essential. Poor interpersonal relationships among team members can harm the quality of care and prevent the team from meeting its goals. In the same way, good interpersonal relationships can improve the quality of care. Members of a team will have different cultural and ethnic backgrounds, sexes, ages, socioeconomic statuses, lifestyle preferences, beliefs, and levels of education. Each team member must understand that these differences affect the way a person thinks and acts. Each person must be sensitive to the hopes, feelings, and needs of other team members. The Golden Rule of "treat others as you would want to be treated" should be the main rule of teamwork.

Conflict among individuals with different personalities is a problem that can occur when a group of people are working as a team. Using the strategies for communicating needs, wants, and emotions found in Section 4:4 will promote team conflict resolution. When conflict occurs, it is essential for each person to deal with the conflict in a positive way. The people involved in the conflict should meet, talk with each other to identify the problem, listen to the other person's point of view, avoid accusations and hostility, try to determine a way to resolve the problem in a cooperative manner, and put the agreed-on solution into action. If two people do not feel comfortable talking privately with each other, a mediator may be able to assist with finding a solution to the problem. Some health care facilities have grievance committees to assist with conflicts that may occur. During this negotiation, the committee will gather facts to determine the details of the tension and set clear expectations for a resolution. Assertive communication is the ability to express your ideas in a clear and unafraid way. This type of communication is essential in dispute resolution. If a team is to meet its goals, conflict must be resolved.

Legal

Legal responsibilities are another important aspect of teamwork. Each member of a team must be aware of the legal limitations on duties that can be performed. All members must function within legal boundaries. No team member should ever attempt to solve a problem or perform a duty that is beyond the range of duties legally permitted.

Effective teams are the result of hard work, patience, commitment, and practice. When each individual participates fully in the team and creates healthy relationships, the team achieves success.

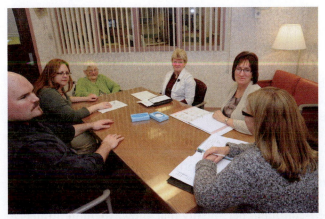

FIGURE 4–10 Most health care teams have frequent patient care conferences to establish team goals.

Checkpoint

| **1.** List two (2) results of forming an effective team.

4:6 PROFESSIONAL LEADERSHIP

Leadership is an important concept in health care careers. **Leadership** is defined by Haroun and Mitchell (2012) in *Introduction to Health Care* as "the skill or ability to encourage people to work together and do their best to achieve common goals" (p. 303). A **leader** is frequently defined as an individual who leads or guides others, or who is in charge or in command of others. A myth exists that leaders are born. In fact, leaders develop by their own efforts. Leaders define clear goals, share the goals with others in the group, help provide the information and knowledge the group needs to work toward the goals, adapt or revise the goals based on the input of others, and allow the group to achieve the goals. Anyone can learn to be a leader by making an effort to understand the principles of leadership. In a group, every member who makes a contribution to an idea can be considered a leader. The leadership in the group passes from person to person as each individual contributes to the achievement of the group's goals.

Many different characteristics are assigned to a leader. All the characteristics can be learned. In this way, leadership becomes a skill or function that can be learned, rather than an inherited set of characteristics.

Some common leadership characteristics may include:

- Respects the rights, dignity, opinions, and abilities of others
- Understands the principles of democracy
- Works with a group and guides the group toward a goal
- Inspires and motivates others
- Participates in continuing education and professional development and understands the concept of lifelong learning
- Understands own strengths and weaknesses
- Displays self-confidence and willingness to take a stand
- Communicates effectively and verbalizes ideas clearly
- Thinks creatively and asks "What if?"
- Shows initiative, a willingness to work, and completes tasks
- Shows optimism, is open-minded, and can compromise
- Praises others and gives credit to others

Leaders can often be classified into broad categories. Some of the categories include religious, political, club or organizational, business, community, expertise in a particular area, and even informal or peer group. Leaders in these categories often develop based on their involvement with the particular category. An individual who joins a club or organization may become a leader when the group elects the individual to an office or position of leadership within the group.

Leaders are frequently classified as one of three types based on how they perform their leadership skills. The three main types of leader are *democratic, laissez-faire,* and *autocratic*.

- **Democratic leader**: encourages the participation of all individuals in decisions that have to be made or problems that have to be solved. This leader listens to the opinions of others and then bases decisions on what is best for the group as a whole. By guiding the individual group members to a solution, the leader allows the group to take responsibility for the decision.

- **Laissez-faire leader**: more of an informal type of leader. This leader believes in noninterference in the affairs of others. A laissez-faire leader will strive for only minimal rules or regulations and allow the individuals in a group to function in an independent manner with little or no direction. This leader almost has a "hands-off" policy and usually avoids making decisions until forced by circumstances to do so. The term *laissez-faire* comes from a French idiom meaning "to let alone" and can be translated to mean "allow to act"; therefore, it is an appropriate term for this type of leader.

- **Autocratic leader**: often called a "dictator." This individual maintains total rule, makes all of the decisions, and has difficulty delegating or sharing duties. This type of leader seldom asks for the opinions of others, emphasizes discipline, and expects others to follow directions at all times. Individuals usually follow this type of leader because of a fear of punishment or because of an extreme loyalty. In certain situations, such as an emergency, autocratic leaders are very beneficial.

There are also different theories about leadership that correlate with the types of leaders. One theory compares *charismatic* leaders to *noncharismatic* leaders. Charismatic leaders have a vision of a course of action, are opposed to the status quo, and attempt to change it. They have the ability to build confidence and inspire others, and they are willing to use unconventional methods to achieve the desired change. Most charismatic leaders have a very strong, self-confident personality that allows them to influence others and convince them that the leader's vision is the best solution to the situation. Noncharismatic leaders are satisfied with the status quo and resist change. They discourage the opinions of others and stress why the current situation is the best solution. Other theories of leadership identify leaders as transformational, transactional, or stewardship. Here are basic descriptions of these types of leaders.

- **Transformational leaders**: want to change the current situation so they stress what is wrong and provide a vision of what a new plan of action could do; visionaries who see themselves as agents of change; often described as inspirational, influential, articulate, and charismatic; can readily state goals that must be obtained; encourage others to shift their focus from self-interests to collective interests; believe in people and show sensitivity to their needs; encourage teamwork and commitment to shared goals to create significant change while also encouraging each person to fulfill his or her own potential

- **Transactional leaders**: prefer to maintain stability in an organization by catering to the interests of others; are often described as task oriented; focus on defining roles and requirements; want others to obey the commands of the leader and accept the status quo; motivate others by rewards and punishments based on their performance; reward others if they are successful in assigned tasks; reprimand or punish others if they fail assigned tasks; tend to discourage creativity, so followers may be prevented from achieving their full potential

- **Stewardship leaders**: concentrate on serving the needs of others rather than the self-interest of obtaining power and control over others; empower others to make decisions and grow personally and professionally; emphasize respect, honesty, patience, kindness, and commitment to encourage others to share the responsibility for achieving a goal; listen carefully to opinions of others and work with them to formulate goals and strategies to solve a problem or find the best course of action; serve as a negotiator or support agent rather than a commander or authority agent

All types of leadership have advantages and disadvantages. In some situations, an autocratic or even transactional leader may be beneficial. However, the democratic or transformational leader is the model frequently presented as most effective for group interactions. By allowing a group to share in deciding what, when, and how something is to be done, members of the group will usually do what has to be done because they want to do it. Respecting the rights and opinions of others becomes the most important guide for the leader.

checkpoint

1. List six (6) characteristics of an effective leader.

2. Identify the three (3) types of leaders and describe their style of leadership.

NOTE: To obtain more detailed information about leadership, see the worksheets provided in the Leadership Section of the *Teacher's Resource Kit* online.

4:7 PARLIAMENTARY PROCEDURE

When health care team members join one of the many professional health care organizations, they will be participating in meetings. A working knowledge of parliamentary procedure is essential. **Parliamentary procedure** can be defined as a set of rules or guidelines that determine the conduct and order followed during a meeting. It is based on three basic principles:

- Right of the majority to rule
- Right of the minority to be heard
- Right of the individual to be heard and represented

Although organizations develop their own bylaws, most follow the principles of parliamentary procedure established by *Robert's Rules of Order*. When these principles are followed effectively, the business being conducted in the meeting proceeds in an orderly manner, with only one issue being considered at a time. All members have the opportunity to participate. Order is maintained, and business is conducted in a uniform and efficient manner.

Meetings conducted with parliamentary procedure usually follow an *agenda*, or a fixed order of business. A standard agenda usually consists of the following:

- **Call to order**: the chairperson (person running the meeting) announces that the meeting is starting; alerts members that they must be quiet and orderly

- **Roll taken by the secretary**: done to have an official record of members present; in many cases, a quorum, or minimum number of members to conduct business, must be present; roll call can be taken by reading names aloud or having members sign in on a list

- **Minutes of previous meeting**: the secretary reads the minutes aloud or written copies are given to the members to remind the members about topics that were covered in the last meeting and issues still pending; the chairperson asks for any corrections to the minutes; if there are no corrections, the minutes are approved as read

- **Treasurer's report**: the treasurer informs the members about disbursements (money spent) and receipts (money received) since the last meeting; the chairperson may ask if there are any questions; the report is then filed for audit

- **Report of officers**: some of the officers may give a report or update; during this time, any correspondence that has been received is usually read

- **Standing committee reports**: reports are given by representatives of any standing committees, or committees that usually remain the same every year; examples include a membership committee or a fundraising committee

- **Special committee reports**: reports are given by representatives of any special committees or committees that were established for a specific purpose or activity; examples include a field trip committee or a special party committee

- **Unfinished business**: this includes any issues that were brought before the members at a previous meeting that could not be resolved at that time; these issues are presented one at a time in an orderly fashion

- **New business**: new actions or business that must be considered by the members; can be introduced by the chairperson or any member present; brought up in the form of a motion and then discussed following the correct procedure for motions

- **Program and/or announcements**: optional parts of a meeting; announcements may be made at this time or a special program such as entertainment or a mini-workshop may be presented

- **Adjournment**: occurs after all business is completed or there is no more time available for the meeting to continue; the chairperson can call for the meeting to end or a member may make a motion that the meeting end

Meetings that follow parliamentary procedure use different types of motions to conduct business. A motion allows an order of business to be introduced in an official manner. A member makes a motion to present an idea or proposal. Another member seconds the motion to express support for discussion of the idea. After the motion is seconded, the idea is discussed, and every individual in the meeting has the right to express his or her opinion about the topic. After discussion is complete, the members vote on the motion to decide if it passes or fails. There are four basic types of motions:

- **Main motion**: This introduces a topic to the membership for their consideration; it cannot be made when any other motion is on the floor for consideration.

- **Subsidiary motion**: The purpose of this type of motion is to change or affect how the main motion is handled; it may change or modify the main motion

or may dispose of the motion (postpone or table it); it must be seconded and adopted before voting can occur on the main motion.

- **Privileged motion**: The purpose of this motion is to bring up items that are urgent or important matters unrelated to the pending motion; an example is a motion to recess the meeting to secure additional information.

- **Incidental motion**: This motion allows a member to question the procedure concerning other motions; it must be considered before voting on the main motion; an example is a point of order calling on the chairperson for enforcement of the rules.

Some of the more common motions that may be used in a meeting are discussed in **Table 4–1**. Each type of motion has a specific purpose and leads to an efficiently conducted meeting.

The type of vote that is made on any motion depends on the situation and the bylaws of the organization. Some common methods of voting on motions include:

- **Voice vote**: the chairperson asks those in favor of the motion to say "aye" or "yes" and those opposed to say "nay" or "no"; provides an approximate count of votes

- **Roll call**: each member says "yes" or "no" as his or her name is called; provides for an accurate count of the votes

- **General consent**: used by a chairperson when a motion is not likely to be opposed; chairperson says, "If there are no objections. . . the motion will pass"; members show agreement by silence; if anyone objects, the motion must be put to a vote

- **Division**: vote similar to a voice vote but members stand or raise their hands so an accurate count can be obtained

- **Ballot**: members write their vote on a slip of paper or enter into a computer program; permits secrecy in voting; usually used to elect officers or for other sensitive motions

Proper conduct by the members of an organization is also an important part of parliamentary procedure. If all members act appropriately during a meeting, the business of the meeting can be handled much more efficiently while allowing all individuals to voice their own opinions. Some basic guidelines that should be followed by all members include:

- Wait until the last speaker has finished.

- Wait until the chairperson recognizes you before speaking out loud.

- Speak in a clear and concise manner to present your opinion.

- Stay on the motion or topic being discussed.

TABLE 4–1 Types of Motions

Types of Motion	Purpose of Motion
Refer to committee	Asks that a motion be referred to a committee to provide time for a smaller group to study the motion and report back to the members; allows time to obtain more information, organize details, and secure a recommendation from a smaller group of people who have time to research the motion; this motion must have a second, allows for discussion or debate, can be amended, and requires a majority vote to pass
Postpone definitely	Delays an action or motion until a specific date or meeting; allows individuals more time to think about the motion or to obtain additional information before a vote is taken; this motion must have a second, allows for discussion or debate, can be amended, and requires a majority vote to pass
Postpone indefinitely	Delays voting on a motion with no set time to reconsider the motion; if it passes, the only way the members will vote on the motion is if it is presented as a new motion at another meeting; this motion must have a second, allows for discussion or debate, cannot be amended, and requires a majority vote to pass
Call for previous question	Calls for an end to debate or discussion and calls for an immediate vote; if the motion is unqualified, the question applies only to the question immediately pending, for example, an amendment to a motion; if the motion is qualified, it applies to everything being discussed and requires an immediate vote on any amendments and the motion without further discussion; this motion must have a second, allows for discussion or debate, cannot be amended, and requires a two-thirds vote to pass
Lay on the table	Temporarily postpones a discussion or vote on a motion; allows members to obtain more information, permits consideration of more urgent business, and delays action until the motion is taken from the table; this motion must have a second, does not allow for discussion or debate, cannot be amended, and requires a majority vote to pass
Take from table	Allows a motion that was previously tabled to be brought back for discussion; must be taken from the table during the meeting in which it was tabled or at the next regular meeting; this motion must have a second, does not allow for discussion or debate, cannot be amended, and requires a majority vote to pass
Raise a question of privilege	Used to make a request during a debate or discussion; permits a member to secure immediate action regarding someone's rights or comfort; may be made at any time during the meeting; usually used to request an adjustment of sound, room temperature, lack of chairs, or similar items; this motion does not require a second, does not allow for discussion, cannot be amended, and is decided by the chairperson
Take a recess	Provides a break during a meeting or dismisses the meeting for a specific period; this motion requires a second, does not allow for discussion, can be amended, and requires a majority vote to pass
Division of the assembly or house	Provides for a more accurate verification of a vote that was taken by voice or a show of hands; automatically requires a standing vote or ballot; this motion does not require a second, does not allow for discussion, cannot be amended, and does not require a vote; when this motion is made, the chairperson must immediately ask members for a standing vote or ballot so an exact count can be taken
Point of order	Used to call attention to a violation of the rules or a mistake in parliamentary procedure; this motion does not require a second, does not allow for discussion, cannot be amended, and is decided by the chairperson; the chairperson can obtain information from the parliamentarian or *Robert's Rules of Order* before making a decision
Adjourn	Ends or dismisses the meeting; can be made by any member when the business is complete; this motion requires a second, does not allow for discussion, cannot be amended, and requires a majority vote to pass

- Avoid personal attacks on the opinions of others.
- Direct your comments to the chairperson and general membership, not to another individual in the group.
- Respect and follow the time limit that has been established for each speaker.
- Obey the rules of debate.
- Respect the right of others to have opposing opinions.

Learning and following the rules of parliamentary procedure will allow a health care team member to effectively participate in meetings and to express an opinion for others to discuss. It is the most democratic manner for all individuals to express their ideas and then allow the majority to rule.

checkpoint

1. What are the three (3) basic principles of parliamentary procedure?
2. What are a few common motions used during a meeting?

NOTE: To obtain more detailed information about parliamentary procedure, see the worksheets provided in the Leadership Section of the *Teacher's Resource Kit* online.

4:8 STRESS

Stress can be defined as the body's reaction to any stimulus that requires a person to adjust to a changing environment. Change always initiates stress. The stimuli to change, alter behavior, or adapt to a situation are called *stressors*. Stressors can be situations, events, or concepts. Stressors can also be external or internal forces. For example, a heart attack is an internal stressor, and a new job is an external stressor.

No matter what the cause, a stressor will cause the body to go into an alarm or warning mode. This mode is frequently called the "fight or flight" reaction because of the physical changes that occur in the body. When a warning is received from a stressor, the sympathetic nervous system prepares the body for action, and the following changes occur:

- Adrenaline, a hormone from the adrenal glands, is released into the bloodstream.
- Blood vessels to the heart and brain dilate to increase blood circulation to these areas.
- Blood vessels to the skin and other internal organs constrict, resulting in cool skin, decreased movement in the digestive tract, and decreased production of urine.
- The pupils in the eyes dilate to improve vision.
- Saliva production decreases and the mouth becomes dry.
- The heart beats more rapidly.
- Blood pressure rises.
- The respiratory rate increases.

These actions by the sympathetic nervous system provide the body with a burst of energy and the stamina needed to respond to the stressor.

After the individual responds to the stressor and adapts or changes as needed, the parasympathetic system slowly causes opposite reactions in the body. This results in fatigue or exhaustion while the body returns to normal and recuperates. If the body is subjected to continual stress with constant "up and down" nervous system reactions, the normal functions of the body will be disrupted. This can result in a serious illness or disease. Many diseases have stress-related origins. Examples include migraine headaches, anxiety reactions, depression, allergies, asthma, digestive disorders, hypertension (high blood pressure), insomnia (inability to sleep), and heart disease.

PTSD or posttraumatic stress disorder is a psychiatric disorder that can occur in people who have experienced a traumatic event like a natural disaster, a terrorist act, a violent personal assault, a serious accident, or war/combat. Long after the initial trauma has ended, people with PTSD have intense upsetting feelings and thoughts related to that event. They may have flashbacks or nightmares and feel sad, fearful, angry, or detached from people. The people suffering from PTSD may avoid situations that remind them of what happened and may have strong reactions to ordinary loud noises or accidental touch. These simple events can set off a stress reaction that is out of proportion to reality. Some people's symptoms subside over time, but others require mental health care professionals to recover.

Everyone experiences a certain degree of stress on a daily basis. The amount of stress felt usually depends on the individual's reaction to and perception of the situation causing stress. For example, a blood test can be a routine event for some individuals, such as a diabetic who performs three or four blood tests on a daily basis. Another individual who is terrified of needles might feel extreme stress when a blood test is necessary. Many different things can cause stress. Examples include:

- Relationships with family, friends, and team members
- Job or school demands
- Foods such as caffeine, excessive sweets, and salt
- Illness or disability
- Lifestyle
- Financial problems
- Family events such as birth, death, marriage, or divorce
- Overwork or excessive activities
- Boredom and negative feelings
- Time limitations (too much to do and not enough time to do it)
- Failure to achieve goals

Not all stress is harmful. In fact, a small amount of stress is essential to an individual's well-being because it makes a person more alert and raises his or her energy level. The individual is able to make quick judgments and decisions, becomes more organized, and is motivated to accomplish tasks and achieve goals. The way in which an individual responds to or copes with stressors determines whether the situation is helpful or harmful. If stress causes positive feelings such as excitement, anticipation, self-confidence, and a sense of achievement, it is helpful. If stress causes negative feelings such as boredom, frustration, irritability, anger, depression, distrust of others, self-criticism, emotional and physical exhaustion, and emotional outbursts, it is harmful. Negative stress can also lead to substance abuse. An individual may smoke more, drink large amounts of alcohol, take drugs, or eat excessively to find comfort and escape from negative feelings. Prolonged periods of harmful stress can lead to burnout or mental breakdown. For this reason, an individual must become aware of the stressors in his or her life and learn methods to control them.

The first step in learning how to control stress is to identify stressors. Recognizing the symptoms of "fight or flight" can lead to an awareness of the factors that cause these symptoms. By keeping a list or diary of stressors, an individual can begin to evaluate ways to deal with the stressors and ways to eliminate them. When stressful events occur, note what the event was, why you feel stress, how much stress you experience, and how you deal with the stress. Do you tackle the cause of the stress or the symptom? This type of information allows you to understand the level of stress you are comfortable with, the type of stress that motivates you effectively, and the type of stress that is unpleasant for you. If a chronic daily stressor is heavy traffic on the road to work, it may be time to evaluate the possibility of finding a new way to work, leaving earlier or later to avoid traffic, or finding a way to relax while stuck in traffic.

Stressors are problems that must be solved or eliminated. One way to do this is to use the *problem-solving method*. It consists of the following steps:

- **Gather information or data**: Assess the situation to obtain all facts and opinions.

- **Identify the problem**: Try to identify the real stressor and why it is causing a reaction.

- **List possible solutions**: Look at all ways to eliminate or adapt to the stressor. Include both good and bad ideas. Evaluate each of the ideas and try to determine how effective it will be.

- **Make a plan**: After evaluating the solutions, choose the one that you think will have the best outcome.

- **Act on your solution**: Use the solution to your problem to see if it has the expected outcome. Does it allow you to eliminate or adapt to the stressor?

- **Evaluate the results**: Determine whether the action was effective. Did it work, or is another solution better?

- **Change the solution**: If necessary, use a different solution that might be more effective.

Learning to manage a stress reaction is another important way to deal with stressors. When you become aware that a stressor is causing a physical reaction in your body, use the following four-step plan to gain control:

- **Stop**: Immediately stop what you are doing to break out of the stress response.

- **Breathe**: Take a slow deep breath to relieve the physical tension you are feeling.

- **Reflect**: Think about the problem at hand and the cause of the stress.

- **Choose**: Determine how you want to deal with the stress.

The brief pause that the four-step method requires allows an individual to become more aware of the stressor, the physical reaction to the stressor, and the actual cause of the stress. This awareness can then be used to determine whether a problem exists. If a problem does exist, a solution to the problem must be found.

Many other stress-reducing techniques can be used to manage stress. Some of the more common techniques include:

- **Live a healthy life**: Eat balanced meals, get sufficient amounts of rest and sleep, and exercise on a regular basis (**Figure 4–11**).

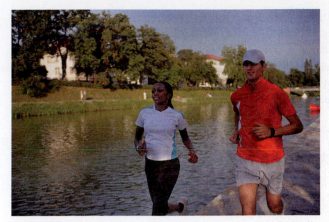

FIGURE 4–11 Exercising on a regular basis is one way to reduce stress.
© iStock.com/technotr

- **Take a break from stressors**: Sit in a comfortable chair with your feet up.

- **Relax**: Take a warm bath.

- **Escape**: Listen to quiet, soothing music.

- **Relieve tension**: Shut your eyes, take slow deep breaths, and concentrate on relaxing each tense muscle.

- **Rely on others**: Talk with a friend and reach out to your support system.

- **Meditate**: Think about your values or beliefs in a higher power.

- **Use imagery**: Close your eyes and use all your senses to place yourself in a scene where you are at peace and relaxed.

- **Enjoy yourself**: Find an enjoyable leisure activity or hobby to provide "time-outs."

- **Renew yourself**: Learn new skills, take part in a professional organization, participate in community activities, and make every effort to continue growing as an individual.

- **Think positively**: Reflect on your accomplishments and be proud of yourself.

- **Develop outside interests**: Provide time for yourself; do not allow a job to dominate your life.

- **Seek assistance or delegate tasks**: Ask others for help or delegate some tasks to others. Remember that no one can do everything all of the time.

- **Avoid too many commitments**: Learn to say "no."

It is important to remember that stress is a constant presence in every individual's life and cannot be avoided. However, by being aware of the causes of stress, by learning how to respond when a stress reaction occurs, by solving problems effectively to eliminate stress, and by practicing techniques to reduce the effect of stress, an individual can deal with the daily stressors in his or her life and even benefit from them. It is also important for every health care team member to remember that patients also experience stress, especially when they are dealing with an illness and/or disability. The same techniques can be used by the health care team member to help patients learn to deal with stress.

checkpoint

1. List six (6) stress-reducing techniques that can be beneficial. State why they help reduce stress.

4:9 TIME MANAGEMENT

One way to help prevent stress is to use time management. **Time management** is a system of practical skills that allows an individual to use time in the most effective and productive way possible. Time management helps prevent or reduce stress by putting the individual in charge, keeping things in perspective when events are overwhelming, increasing productivity, using time more effectively, improving enjoyment of activities, and providing time for relaxing and enjoying life.

The first step of time management is to keep an activity record for several days. This allows an individual to determine how he or she actually uses the time available. Most mobile devices offer applications that can be used to record and prioritize activities, and they can be used to help manage time more effectively. By listing activities as they are performed, noting the amount of time each activity takes, and evaluating how effective the activity was, an individual can see patterns emerge. Certain periods of the day will show higher energy levels and an improved quantity of work. Other periods may indicate that accomplishments are limited because of fatigue. Wasted time will also become apparent. Time spent listening to music, talking on the telephone, texting, playing video games, watching TV, and doing things that are not worthwhile is time that can be put to more constructive use. After this information has been obtained, an individual can begin to organize his or her time. Important projects can be scheduled during the periods of the day when energy levels are high. Rest or relaxation periods can be scheduled when energy levels are low.

SETTING GOALS

Goal setting is another important factor of time management. A **goal** can be defined as a desired result or purpose toward which one is working. Goals can be compared with maps that help you find your direction and reach your destination. An old saying states, "If you don't know where you are going, you will never get there." Goals allow you to know where you are going and provide direction to your life.

Everyone should have both short- and long-term goals. *Long-term goals* are achievements that may take years or even a lifetime to accomplish. *Short-term goals* usually take days, weeks, or months to accomplish. They are the smaller steps that are taken to reach the long-term goal. For example, a long-term goal might be to graduate from college with a health care degree.

If the person with this goal is starting high school, short-term goals might include:

- Research and learn about the wide variety of health care careers.

- Job-shadow health care professions that seem most interesting.

- Talk with people in different health care professions to find out about the professions.

- Complete job interest surveys to determine how your own skills and interests match requirements for different health care professions.

- Discuss career opportunities with a guidance or career counselor.

- Attend job fairs or career planning days to obtain information about specific health care professions.

- Use a computer to research health care professions on the Internet.

- Narrow your career choices to the health care professions that you like best.

- Investigate which high school courses you should take to meet college entry requirements for these health care professions.

- Take the required courses in English, math, science, computer technology, and other specific academic areas.

- Explore the career and technology programs offered by your high school.

- Enroll in a health science education (HSE) program if one is available.

- Join a student organization such as HOSA, which allows HSE students to network with other people who have similar interests.

- Obtain a job or work as a volunteer in different health care areas to determine which career you like best.

- Research and visit different colleges or technical schools to learn about course offerings, financial aid, entry requirements, and other similar information.

When this person is in the junior or senior year of high school, short-term goals might include:

- Complete all required high school courses and maintain a high grade point average.
- Confer with guidance or career counselors to obtain information about scholarships, financial help, career planning, college life, and other similar topics.
- Apply to several colleges or technical schools that have accredited programs in the chosen health field.
- Arrange for financial assistance and obtain a part-time job to save money for college.
- Check living arrangements at the college campuses if living away from home will be necessary.
- After being accepted by colleges or technical schools, evaluate each individually to choose the school you will attend.
- Notify the school you have selected before the established deadline for enrollment.

These short-term goals are basic suggestions. Each individual has to establish her or his own goals. It is important to remember that short-term goals will change constantly as one set is completed and a new set is established. The completion of a goal, however, will lead to a sense of satisfaction and accomplishment and provide motivation to attempt other goals. To set goals effectively, you must observe certain points, including:

- **State goals in a positive manner**: Use words such as "accomplish" rather than "avoid."
- **Define goals clearly and precisely**: If possible, set a time limit to accomplish the goal.
- **Prioritize multiple goals**: Determine which goals are the most important, and complete them first.
- **Write goals down**: This makes the goal seem real and attainable.
- **Make sure each goal is at the right level**: Goals should present a challenge but not be too difficult or impossible to complete.

After goals have been established, concentrate on ways to accomplish them. Review necessary skills, information that must be obtained, resources you can use, problems that may occur, and which goal should be completed first. Basically, this is just organizing the steps that will lead to achieving the goal. After the goal has been achieved, enjoy your sense of accomplishment and satisfaction for a job well done. If you fail to obtain the goal, evaluate the situation and determine why you failed. Was the goal unrealistic? Did you lack the skills or knowledge to obtain the goal? Is there another way to achieve the goal? Remember that failure can be a positive learning experience.

TIME MANAGEMENT PLAN

Time management is used to ensure success in meeting established goals. A daily planner, calendar, or computerized calendar and schedule are essential tools. These tools allow an individual to record all activities and obligations, organize all information, become aware of conflicts (two things to do at the same time), and provide an organized schedule to follow. An effective time management plan involves the following seven steps:

- **Analyze and prioritize**: review and list established goals; determine what tasks must be completed to achieve goals; list tasks in order, from the most important to the least important; decide if any tasks can be delegated to another person to complete and delegate whenever possible; eliminate unnecessary tasks
- **Identify habits and preferences**: know when you have the most energy to complete work and when it is best to schedule rest, exercise, or social activities
- **Schedule tasks**: use the daily planner and calendar to record all events; be sure to include time for rest, exercise, meals, hobbies, and social activities; if a conflict arises with two things scheduled at the same time, prioritize and reschedule
- **Make a daily "to do" list**: record all tasks required on a daily basis; as you complete each one, delete it from the list; enjoy the sense of satisfaction that occurs as you complete each job; if some things on the list are not completed at the end of the day, determine if they should be added to the next day's list or if they can be eliminated
- **Plan your work**: work at a comfortable pace; try to do the hardest tasks first; do one thing at a time whenever possible so you can complete it and delete it from the list; make sure you have everything you need to complete the task before you begin; ask for assistance when needed; work smarter, not harder
- **Avoid distractions**: make every effort to avoid interruptions; use caller ID to screen calls; avoid procrastination; learn to say "no" when asked to interrupt your work for something that is not essential
- **Take credit for a job well done**: when a job is complete, recognize your achievement; delete the completed work from the list; if the task was a particularly hard one, reward yourself with a short break or other positive thing before going on to the next job on the list

These steps of time management provide for an organized and efficient use of time. However, even with

There are few subjects that can stir up stronger emotions among doctors, scientists, researchers, policy makers, and the public than medical marijuana. What conditions is it useful for? Should it be legal? Decriminalized? Has its effectiveness been proven? This is an effort to present facts vs. fiction.

The term medical marijuana refers to using the whole, unprocessed marijuana plant or its basic extracts to treat symptoms of illness and other conditions. The U.S. Food and Drug Administration (FDA) has not recognized or approved the marijuana plant as medicine. Scientific study of the chemicals in marijuana, called cannabinoids, has led to FDA-approved medications that contain cannabinoid chemicals.

The two main cannabinoids from the marijuana plant that are of medical interest are THC and CBD. THC can increase appetite and reduce nausea. THC may also decrease pain, inflammation (swelling and redness), and muscle-control problems. Unlike THC, CBD is a cannabinoid that doesn't make people "high." These drugs aren't popular for recreational use because they aren't intoxicating. It may be useful in reducing pain and inflammation, controlling epileptic seizures, and possibly even treating mental illness and addictions.

According to the National Institute of Health (NIH), drugs containing cannabinoids may be helpful in treating certain rare forms of epilepsy, nausea and vomiting associated with cancer chemotherapy, and loss of appetite and weight loss associated with HIV/AIDS. In addition, some evidence suggests modest benefits of cannabis or cannabinoids for chronic pain and multiple sclerosis symptoms. Studies on cannabis or cannabinoids for other conditions are in early stages.

Research is in progress on cannabis or cannabinoids for these specific health conditions:

- Anxiety
- Epilepsy
- Glaucoma
- HIV/AIDS symptoms
- Posttraumatic stress disorder (PTSD)
- Sleep problems
- Inflammatory bowel disease
- Irritable bowel syndrome
- Movement disorders due to Tourette syndrome
- Multiple sclerosis
- Pain
- Opioid use
- Nausea and vomiting related to cancer chemotherapy

Research may lead to more medications. Since the marijuana plant contains chemicals that may help treat a range of illnesses and symptoms, many people argue that it should be legal for medical purposes. In fact, a growing number of states have legalized marijuana for medical use. U.S. federal law prohibits the use of whole plant *Cannabis sativa* or its derivatives for any purpose. CBD derived from the hemp plant (<0.3 percent THC) is legal under federal law to consume.

Many states allow THC use for medical purposes. Federal law regulating marijuana supersedes state laws. Because of this, people may still be arrested and charged with possession in states where marijuana for medical use is legal.

---

careful planning, things do not always get done according to plan. Unexpected emergencies, a new assignment, a complication, and overscheduling are common events in the life of a health care team member. When a time management plan does not work, try to determine the reasons for failure. Reevaluate goals and revise the plan. Patience, practice, and an honest effort will eventually produce a plan that provides self-satisfaction for achieving goals, less stress, quality time for rest and relaxation, a sense of being in control, a healthier lifestyle, and increased productivity.

check**point**

1. Differentiate between short-term and long-term goals.

PRACTICE: Go to the workbook and complete the assignment sheet for Chapter 4, Personal and Professional Qualities of a Health Care Team Member.

Case Study Investigation Conclusion

What fundamentally went wrong in this case? Was lack of leadership at fault? What communication improvement might best have contributed to this critical situation? What professional characteristics may have improved Gregg's outcome from this surgery? With a partner, list three policies or procedures that might be implemented to avoid this type of outcome for future patients.

CHAPTER 4 SUMMARY

- Certain personal characteristics, attitudes, and rules of appearance apply to health care team members in all health care careers.

- A professional appearance helps inspire confidence and a positive self-image. Good health is an important part of appearance. Eating correctly, obtaining adequate rest, exercising daily, avoiding the use of tobacco, alcohol, and drugs, and obtaining preventative screenings are actions a team member can take to strive to maintain good health.

- Wearing the appropriate uniform or clothing and shoes is essential to projecting a professional image. Proper hair and nail care, good personal hygiene, and limited makeup also help create a professional appearance.

- Personal characteristics such as empathy, honesty, dependability, willingness to learn, patience, acceptance of criticism, enthusiasm, self-motivation or initiative, tact, responsibility, discretion, professionalism, and competence are essential.

- Effective communication is an important aspect of helping individuals through stages of growth and development and in meeting their emotions, wants, and needs. A health care team member must have an understanding of the communication process, factors that interfere with communication, the importance of listening, and verbal and nonverbal communication. The proper reporting or recording of all observations noted while providing care is essential.

- Communication barriers such as physical and sensory disabilities, psychological barriers, and cultural diversity can interfere with the communication process. Special consideration must be given to these barriers to improve communication. Some cultural groups have beliefs and practices that may relate to health and illness. Because individuals will respond to health care according to their cultural beliefs, a health care team member must be aware of and show respect for different cultural values in order to provide optimal patient care.

- Developing good interpersonal relationships is important for the physical, mental, and emotional health of an individual. It is important to evaluate relationships to try to maximize positive relationships and minimize negative ones as much as possible.

- Teamwork is important in any health care career. For a team to function effectively, it needs a qualified leader, good interpersonal relationships, ways to avoid or deal with conflict, positive attitudes, and respect for legal responsibilities. Effective teams are the result of hard work, patience, commitment, and practice.

- Leadership is a skill that can be learned by mastering the characteristics of a leader. Of the three types of leaders—democratic, laissez-faire, and autocratic—the democratic leader is the most effective for group interaction. Other theories of leadership that correlate with the types of leaders include charismatic, noncharismatic, transformational, transactional, and stewardship.

- Parliamentary procedure can be defined as a set of rules or guidelines that determines the conduct and order followed during a meeting. Health care team members must be familiar with parliamentary procedure because they will be participating in meetings as members of health care organizations.

- Stress is a component of every individual's life. Stress can be good or bad, depending on the person's perception of and reaction to the stress. By being aware of the causes of stress and learning how to respond when a stress reaction occurs, an individual can deal with stress and even benefit from it.

- Time management is a system of practical skills that allows an individual to use time in the most effective and productive way possible. An effective time management plan will reduce stress, help an individual attain goals, increase self-confidence, and lead to a healthier lifestyle.

REVIEW QUESTIONS

1. Three-year-old Lucy fell off the swing. She is crying, rubbing her head, and holding her abdomen. What are the nonverbal and verbal cues Lucy is displaying. What message is being conveyed? Why is it important to observe both verbal and nonverbal communication?

2. Decide on a topic for discussion. After identifying the motions, conduct a meeting following the basic principles of parliamentary procedure to discuss the topic based on these motions.

   Identify each of the following types of motions:
   a. Introduces a topic to the membership for their consideration
   b. Temporarily postpones a discussion or vote on a motion
   c. Allows a member to ask that the chairperson speak louder so he or she can be heard
   d. Calls for an immediate, more accurate verification of a vote that was taken by voice or a show of hands
   e. Calls for an end to debate or discussion and an immediate vote
   f. Informs the chairperson that a vote cannot be made on the main motion until the amendment to the motion has been voted on
   g. Ends or dismisses the meeting

3. Identify at least one (1) major stressor in your life. List the steps of the problem-solving method, and then apply each of these steps to the stressor you have chosen. Identify at least three (3) courses of action that you can take.

4. What are the main goals of time management? Using what you have learned, why does time management result in less stress?

CRITICAL THINKING

1. Josh Merkowski is a pharmacist that has been found guilty of falsifying drug records at the pharmacy. He has also revealed that he is addicted to Vicodin. Investigate industry standards for substance abuse related to health care providers. Based on these facts, write a report predicting Dr. Merkowski's remediation.

2. Analisa Gallegos is admitted to a hospital to give birth to her premature baby. Identify at least 10 health care team members who may be on the team that provides her care. Review the different careers in Chapter 3 to prepare your list. Why do you think teamwork is important in this scenario? How do healthy professional relationships promote a healthy community?

3. After a building explodes, EMS delivers 22 critically injured patients to a hospital emergency room. Which type of leader do you think would be most effective in directing the group of emergency room personnel? Why?

4. Based on the information in question 3, with a partner, identify four (4) barriers to communication that may arise during this disaster response and how you would use therapeutic communication to overcome them.

5. Your family moved to a wonderful new house last month. This is a stressful event. Identify emotional responses to this event by listing two (2) positive and two (2) negative stressors of this new home.

ACTIVITIES

1. With a partner, stand back to back. The shorter person should draw a figure. The taller partner will then draw a figure that the shorter partner describes. After 2 minutes, compare original figure with what the taller partner drew. Why is listening important? Is accurate recording important? What are four (4) factors that may be a barrier in communicating the desired figure?

2. In a small group, create a medical scene involving communication between two (2) different age groups or two (2) different cultures. Exchange your scenario with another group. Using consensus-building techniques, plan how to role play the new scene using effective communication techniques for five (5) minutes. Present to the class.

3. Think of a person that has impacted your life in a positive way. Write a letter to them expressing how their influence has impacted your emotional, physical, and mental health as well as your career goals. In a separate report, predict what the effect on each area of your life would be if you did NOT have a positive relationship with someone.

4. With a partner, create a drawing depicting a person that has negative relationships. Label an effect of negativity on each body system.

CHAPTER
5 LEGAL AND ETHICAL RESPONSIBILITIES

Legal

Case Study Investigation

Jennifer is a new registered nurse on the surgical floor of her medium-sized community hospital. Her patient, Mr. Eddie Cruz, is a 34-year-old male that has end-stage AIDS. He has not told his family or his current girlfriend Brianna. The family is demanding to know why this young man is not getting better since being admitted to the hospital. Mr. Cruz dies without disclosing his health status to anyone. Brianna and

Eddie's family are demanding a meeting with Jennifer and the rest of the staff regarding their loved one's care. "What did he die from? Why didn't the hospital make him better—he was young!" Jennifer must decide how to respond to their inquiries. At the end of this chapter, you will be asked what information and to whom Jennifer can disclose Mr. Eddie Cruz's medical status.

■ LEARNING OBJECTIVES

After completing this chapter, you should be able to:

- Provide one example of a situation that might result in legal action for each of the following: malpractice, negligence, assault and battery, invasion of privacy, false imprisonment, abuse, and defamation.

- Describe how contract/consent laws affect health care.

- Define *privileged communications* and explain how electronic health care records impact confidentiality.

- State the legal regulations that apply to health care records.

- Define HIPAA and explain how it provides confidentiality for health care information.

- List at least six basic rules of ethics for health care providers.

- List at least six rights of the patient who is receiving health care.

- Justify at least six professional standards by explaining how they help meet legal/ethical requirements.

- Define, pronounce, and spell all key terms.

■ KEY TERMS

abuse

advance directives

agent

assault and battery

civil law

confidentiality *(con"-fih-den-chee"-ahl'-ih-tee)*

Consumer Bill of Rights and Responsibilities

contract

criminal law

defamation *(deff'-ah-may'-shun)*

Designation of Health Care Surrogate

Durable Power of Attorney (POA)

ethics *(eth'-iks)*

expressed consents

false imprisonment

health care records

Health Insurance Portability and Accountability Act (HIPAA)

implied consents

informed consent

invasion of privacy

legal

legal disability

libel *(ly'-bull)*

living wills

malpractice

negligence *(neg'-lih-gents)*

Omnibus Budget Reconciliation Act (OBRA) of 1987

Patient Protection and Affordable Care Act (PPACA)

Patient Self-Determination Act (PSDA)

patients' rights

privileged communications

Resident's Bill of Rights

scope of practice

slander

tort

INTRODUCTION

In every aspect of life, there are certain laws and legal responsibilities formulated to protect you and society. An excellent example is the need to obey traffic laws when driving a motor vehicle. An employee in any health care career also has certain responsibilities. Being aware of and following legal regulations is important for your own protection, the protection of your employer, and the safety and well-being of the patient.

Legal responsibilities are those that are authorized or based on law. A law is a rule that must be followed. Laws are created and enforced by the federal, state, or local governments. Health care providers must follow any laws that affect health care. In addition, *health care professionals/providers are also required to know and follow the state laws that regulate their respective licenses or registrations or set standards for their respective professions.* Failure to meet your legal responsibilities can result in legal action against you, your employer, and loss of your health care license or certification.

Two main types of laws affect health care providers: criminal laws and civil laws.

- **Criminal law**: focuses on behavior known as crime; deals with the wrongs against a person, property, or society; examples include practicing in a health profession without having the required license, illegal possession of drugs, misuse of narcotics, theft, sexual assault, and murder. The penalty for criminal crimes is usually incarceration.

- **Civil law**: focuses on the legal relationships between people and the protection of a person's rights; in health care, civil law usually involves torts and contracts. The penalty for civil violations is usually fines, but sometimes incarceration.

TORTS

A **tort** is a wrongful act that does not involve a contract. It is called a civil wrong instead of a crime. A tort occurs when a person is harmed or injured because a health care provider does not meet the established or expected standards of care. Many different types of torts can lead to legal action. These offenses may be quite complex and may be open to different legal interpretations. Some of the more common torts include the following:

- **Malpractice**: Malpractice can be interpreted as "bad practice" and is commonly called "professional negligence." It can be defined as the failure of a professional to use the degree of skill and learning commonly expected in that individual's profession, resulting in injury, loss, or damage to the person receiving care. Examples might include a physician not administering a tetanus injection when a patient has a puncture wound, or a nurse performing minor surgery without having any training.

- **Negligence**: Negligence can be described as failure to give care that is normally expected of a person in a particular position, resulting in injury to another person (**Figure 5–1**). Examples include falls and injuries that occur when side rails are left down, using or not reporting defective equipment, infections caused by the use of nonsterile instruments and/or supplies, and burns caused by improper heat or radiation treatments.

- **Assault and battery**: Assault includes a threat or attempt to injure, and battery includes the unlawful touching of another person without consent. They are closely related and often used together. Examples of assault and battery include performing a procedure after a patient has refused to give permission, threatening a patient, and improper handling or rough treatment of a patient while providing care.

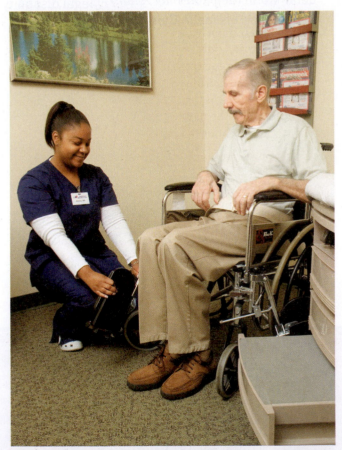

FIGURE 5–1 A medical assistant could be charged with negligence if a patient is injured because the foot rests on a wheelchair are not moved up and out of the way before the patient is transferred out of the chair.

It is important to remember that patients must give consent for any care and that they have the right to refuse care. Some procedures or practices require written consent from the patient. Examples include surgery, certain diagnostic tests, experimental procedures, treatment of minors (individuals younger than legal age, which varies from state to state) without parental consent, and even simple things such as side rail releases for a patient who wants side rails left down when other factors indicate that the side rails should be up to protect the patient. Verbal consent is permitted in other cases, but the law states that this must be "informed consent." **Informed consent** is permission granted voluntarily by a person who is of sound mind and who has been instructed, in terms the person can understand, about all the risks involved. It is important to remember that a person has the right to withdraw consent at any time. Therefore, all procedures must be explained to the patient, and no procedure should be performed if the patient does not give consent.

- 🔒 **HIPAA** **Invasion of privacy**: There are two kinds of invasion of privacy, physical and informational. Physical invasion of privacy includes unnecessarily exposing an individual, while informational invasion of privacy refers to revealing personal information about an individual without that person's consent. Examples include improperly draping or covering a patient during a procedure so that other patients or personnel can see the patient exposed, sending information regarding a patient to an insurance company without the patient's written permission, or informing the news media of a patient's condition without the patient's permission.

- **False imprisonment**: False imprisonment refers to restraining an individual or restricting an individual's freedom without authorization. Examples include keeping patients hospitalized against their will or applying physical restraints without proper authorization or with no justification.

It is important to remember that patients have the right to leave a hospital or health care facility without a physician's permission. If this situation occurs, the patient is usually asked to sign an AMA (Against Medical Advice) form. If the patient refuses to sign the form, this refusal must be documented in the patient's record and the physician must be notified.

Physical restraints, devices used to limit a patient's movements, are discussed in detail in Section 22:11. They should be used *only* to protect patients from harming themselves or others and when all other measures to control the situation have failed. A physician's order must be obtained before they are used, and strict guidelines must be observed while they are in use.

- **Abuse**: Abuse includes any care that results in physical harm, pain, or mental anguish. Examples of types of abuse include:
  - **Physical abuse**: hitting, forcing people against their will, restraining movement, depriving people of food or water, and not providing physical care
  - **Verbal abuse**: speaking harshly, swearing or shouting, using inappropriate words to describe a person's race or nationality, and writing threats or abusive statements
  - **Psychological abuse**: threatening harm; denying rights; belittling, intimidating, or ridiculing the person; and threatening to reveal information about the person
  - **Sexual abuse**: any sexual touching or act, using sexual gestures, and suggesting sexual behavior, even if the patient is willing or tries to initiate it

Patients may experience abuse before entering a health care facility. *Domestic abuse* occurs when an intimate partner uses threats, manipulation, aggression, or violent behavior to maintain power and control over another person. If abuse is directed toward a child, it is *child abuse*. If it is directed toward an older person, it is *elder abuse*. Health care providers must be alert to the signs and symptoms that may indicate patients in their care are victims of abuse. These may include:

- Unexplained bruises, fractures, burns, or injuries
- Signs of neglect such as poor personal hygiene
- Irrational fears or a change in personality
- Aggressive or withdrawn behavior
- Patient statements that indicate abuse or neglect

Many of the other torts can lead to charges of abuse, or a charge of abuse can occur alone. Laws in all states require that any form of abuse be reported to the proper authorities. Even though the signs and symptoms do not always mean a person is being abused, their presence indicates a need for further investigation. Health care providers are required to report any signs or symptoms of abuse to their immediate supervisor or to the individual in the health care facility responsible for reporting suspicions to the proper authorities.

- **Defamation**: Defamation occurs when false statements either cause a person to be ridiculed or damage the person's reputation. Incorrect information given out in error can result in defamation. If the information is spoken, it is **slander**; if it is written, it is **libel**. Examples include reporting that a patient has an infectious disease to a government agency when laboratory results are inaccurate, telling others that a person has a drug problem when actually another medical condition exists, or saying that a fellow team member is incompetent.

CONTRACTS OR CONSENTS

In addition to tort laws, contract laws also affect health care. A **contract** is an agreement between two or more parties. Most contracts have three parts:

- **Offer**: a health care facility or provider has a treatment or services they can offer to a patient; a competent individual offers to be a patient
- **Acceptance**: a patient makes an appointment with the health care facility or provider and accepts the treatment or services offered; the health care facility or provider accepts the individual as a patient
- **Consideration**: the patient receives treatment or services; the health care facility or provider receives payment from the patient

Contracts or consents in health care are implied or expressed. **Implied consents** are those obligations that are understood without verbally expressed terms. For example, when a qualified health care provider prepares a medication and a patient takes the medication, it is implied that the patient accepts this treatment. **Expressed consents** are stated in distinct and clear language, either orally or in writing. An example is a surgery consent. Promises of care must be kept. Therefore, all risks associated with treatment must be explained completely to the patient (**Figure 5–2**).

All parties entering into a contract must be free of **legal disability**. A person who has a legal disability does not have the legal capacity to form a contract. Examples of people who have legal disabilities are minors (individuals under legal age), mentally incompetent persons, individuals under the influence of drugs that alter the mental state, and semiconscious or unconscious people. In such cases, parents, guardians, or others permitted by law must form the contract for the individual.

A contract requires that certain standards of care be provided by competent, qualified individuals. If the contract is not performed according to the agreement, the contract is breached. Failure to provide care and/or giving improper

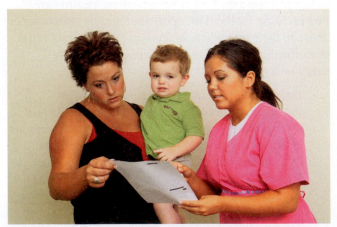

FIGURE 5–2 All risks of treatment must be explained to a patient before asking the patient for permission to administer treatment.

care on the part of the health provider, or failure on the part of the patient to pay according to the consideration, can be considered a breach of contract and cause for legal action.

Comm

To comply with legal mandates, an interpreter/translator must be used when a contract is explained to an individual who does not speak English. In addition, many states require the use of interpreter services for individuals who are deaf or hard of hearing. Most health care agencies have a list of interpreters who can be used in these situations.

A final important consideration in contract law is the role of the **agent**. When a person works under the direction or control of another person, the employer is called the *principal*, and the person working under the employer is called the *agent*. The principal may be held *vicariously liable* or responsible for the actions of the agent and can be required to pay or otherwise compensate people who have been injured by the agent. For example, if a dental assistant tells a patient "your dentures will look better than your real teeth," the dentist, because of vicarious liability, may have to compensate the patient financially should this statement prove false. Health care team members should therefore be aware of their role as agents of their employers and work to protect the interests of their employers.

PRIVILEGED COMMUNICATIONS

Comm

Privileged communications are another important aspect of legal responsibility. Privileged communications comprise all information given to health care personnel by a patient. By law, this information must be kept confidential and shared only with other members of the patient's health care team. It cannot be told to anyone else without the written consent of the patient. The consent should state what information is to be released, to whom the information should be given, and any applicable time limits. Certain information is exempt by law and must be reported in accordance with facility policy. Examples of exempt information are births and deaths; injuries caused by violence (such as assault and battery, abuse, or stabbings) that may require police involvement; drug abuse; communicable diseases; and sexually transmitted diseases.

Health care records are also considered privileged communications. Such records contain information about the care provided to the patient. Although the records belong to the health care provider (for example, the physician, dentist, hospital, or long-term care facility), the patient has a right to obtain a copy of any information in the record. Health care records can be used as legal records in a court of law. Erasures are therefore not allowed on such records. Errors should be crossed out with a single line so the material is still readable. Correct information should then be inserted, initialed, and dated. If necessary, an explanation for the correction should also be provided. Incorrect data on an electronic health record

(EHR) should be corrected by following the directions for making corrections in the particular software being used or by following agency policy. All health care records must be properly maintained, kept confidential, and retained for the amount of time required by state law. When records are disposed of after the legal time for retention, they should be burned or shredded to maintain confidentiality.

 The growing use of electronic health records (EHRs) has created a dilemma in maintaining confidentiality (**Figure 5–3**). In a large health care facility such as a hospital, many different individuals may have access to a patient's records. For this reason, health care providers are creating safeguards to maintain computer confidentiality. Some examples include limiting the personnel who have access to such records, requiring the use of iris scans or fingerprints to access records, using codes to prevent access to certain information, requiring passwords to access specific information on records, and constantly monitoring and evaluating computer use.

In 2009, under the American Recovery and Reinvestment Act (ARRA), the Health Information Technology for Economic and Clinical Health Act (HITECH) was enacted. Its purpose was to promote the adoption and meaningful use of health information technology. As a result of this act, the Office of the National Coordinator for Health Information (ONC) was authorized to establish programs to improve health care quality, safety, and efficiency through the use and transfer of electronic health records (EHRs) in a secure network exchange. The ONC established a national electronic health record exchange called a *health information exchange (HIE)* that is being developed with the help of government funding. The HIE allows all medical facilities to electronically transfer and receive patient electronic health records. The HIE provides many benefits to patients and facilities, including:

- A greater degree of patient safety with quick access to medical history and lab tests

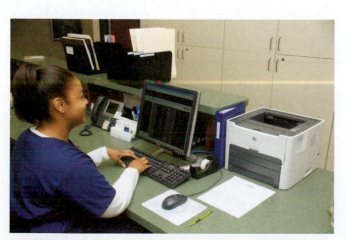

FIGURE 5–3 The growing use of electronic health records (EHRs) has created the need to limit access to computers to maintain confidentiality.

- Better-coordinated care across different health care facilities and across different levels of specialization within those facilities
- Patient access to the EHR
- Information for research and public health monitoring
- Reduction in health care costs due to eliminating repetition of the same tests in different facilities

One problem of the HIE is coordinating the system so that all facilities use compatible software that can interpret the information. Policies and standards are being developed to solve this communication problem. However, the biggest challenge for the HIE is keeping the transferred information secure. If the networks for all transferring facilities are not completely secure, then the security of the health care records can be compromised. This is a major issue that will need to be monitored continually with use of the HIE.

PRIVACY ACT

The federal government is concerned about protecting privileged communications and maintaining confidentiality of health care records. In the **Health Insurance Portability and Accountability Act (HIPAA)** of 1996, Congress required the U.S. Department of Health and Human Services (USDHHS) to establish standards to protect health information. The USDHHS published the *Standards for Privacy of Individually Identifiable Health Information* (commonly called the Privacy Rule), which went into effect in 2003. These standards provide federal protection for privacy of health information in all states. These mandates for privacy were strengthened by the passage of the Health Information Technology for Economic and Clinical Health Act (HITECH) of 2009, which increased the civil and criminal enforcement of the HIPAA codes.

HIPAA regulations in the Privacy Rule require every health care provider to inform patients about how their health information is used. Patients must sign a consent form (**Figure 5–4**) acknowledging that they have received the information before any health care provider can use the health information for diagnosis, treatment, billing, insurance claims, or quality of care assessments.

In addition, before a health care provider can release information to anyone else—such as another health care provider, attorney, insurance company, federal or state agency, or even other members of the patient's family—a patient must sign an authorization form for the release of this information (**Figure 5–5**). This authorization form must identify the purpose or need for the information, the extent of the information that may be released, any limits on the release of information, the date of authorization, and the signature of the person authorized to give consent. These requirements are used to ensure the privacy and confidentiality of a patient's health care information. The only exception to these regulations is for the release of information about diseases or injuries that must be reported by law to protect the safety and welfare of the public. Examples of exempt information include births, deaths, injuries caused by violence that require police involvement, victims of abuse or neglect, communicable diseases, and sexually transmitted infections.

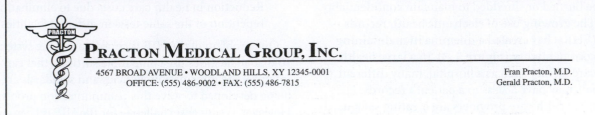

CONSENT TO THE USE AND DISCLOSURE OF HEALTH INFORMATION

I understand that this organization originates and maintains health records which describe my health history, symptoms, examination, test results, diagnoses, treatment, and any plans for future care or treatment. I understand that this information is used to:

- ◆ plan my care and treatment
- ◆ communicate among health professionals who contribute to my care
- ◆ apply my diagnosis and services, procedures, and surgical information to my bill
- ◆ verify services billed by third-party payers
- ◆ assess quality of care and review the competence of health care professionals in routine health care operations

I further understand that:

- ◆ a complete description of information uses and disclosures is included in a *Notice of Information Practices* which has been provided to me
- ◆ I have a right to review the notice prior to signing this consent
- ◆ the organization reserves the right to change their notice and practices
- ◆ any revised notice will be mailed to the address I have provided prior to implementation
- ◆ I have the right to object to the use of my health information for directory purposes
- ◆ I have the right to request restrictions as to how my health information may be used or disclosed to carry out treatment, payment, or health care operations
- ◆ the organization is not required to agree to the restrictions requested
- ◆ I may revoke this consent in writing, except to the extent that the organization has already taken action in reliance thereon.

☐ I request the following restrictions to the use or disclosure of my health information.

June 29, 20XX
Date

June 29, 20XX
Notice Effective Date

Consuelo Hernandez
Signature of Patient or Legal Representative

Witness

Signature

Title

_____ Accepted _____ Rejected

Date

FIGURE 5–4 Example of a Health Insurance Portability and Accountability Act (HIPAA) required form granting consent for the use and disclosure of health information.

AUTHORIZATION FOR RELEASE OF INFORMATION

Section A: Must be completed for all authorizations.

I hereby authorize the use or disclosure of my individually identifiable health information as described below.

I understand that this authorization is voluntary. I understand that if the organization authorized to receive the information is not a health plan or health care provider, the released information may no longer be protected by federal privacy regulations.

Patient name: _Hilda F. Goodman_   ID Number: _4309_

Identity of person/organization disclosing protected health information →

Persons/organizations providing information:
Practon Medical Group, Inc.
4567 Broad Avenue
Woodland Hills, XY 12345-4700

Persons/organizations receiving information:
Jennifer P. Lee, MD
400 North M Street
Anytown, XY 54098-1235

← *Identity of those authorized to use protected health information*

Specific description of information [including from and to date(s)]:
Complete medical records from 4-22-XX to 9-15-XX

← *Specific description of information to be used or disclosed with dates*

Section B: Must be completed only if a health plan or a health care provider has requested the authorization.

Purpose for disclosure →

1. The health plan or health care provider must complete the following:
   a. What is the purpose of the use or disclosure? _Patient relocating to another city_

   b. Will the health plan or health care provider requesting the authorization receive financial or in-kind compensation in exchange for using or disclosing the health information described above? Yes___ No _X_

2. The patient or the patient's representative must read and initial the following statements:
   a. I understand that my health care and the payment for my health care will not be affected if I do not sign this form.

   Initials: _hfg_

   b. I understand that I may see and copy the information described on this form if I ask for it, and that I get a copy of this form after I sign it.

   Initials: _hfg_

Section C: Must be completed for all authorizations.

The patient or the patient's representative must read and initial the following statements:

Expiration date →

1. I understand that this authorization will expire on _12_ / _31_ / _20XX_ (DD/MM/YR).

   Initials: _hfg_

Individual's right to revoke this authorization in writing →

2. I understand that I may revoke this authorization at any time by notifying the providing organization in writing, but if I do it will not have any effect on any actions they took before they received the revocation.

   Initials: _hfg_

Redisclosure conditions →

3. I understand that any disclosure of information carries with it the potential for an unauthorized redisclosure and the information may not be protected by federal confidentiality rules.

   Initials: _hfg_

Individual's signature →

Hilda F. Goodman   _September 15, 20XX_ ← *Date of signature*

Signature of patient or patient's representative   **Date**
(Form MUST be completed before signing)

Printed name of patient's representative:_____

Relationship to the patient:_____

FIGURE 5–5 Example of an authorization form to release health information.

Another requirement of the privacy standards is that patients must be able to see and obtain copies of their medical records. Many health care agencies provide a *patient portal* or an Internet site patients can use to access their electronic health records (EHRs). If an error is found in the EHR, it should be flagged, and a comment indicating that an error has been made and is being corrected should be added to the amended report, not overwritten, which would obscure the original entry. In addition, every patient must be provided with information on how to file a complaint against a health care provider who violates the privacy act. Health care providers must be aware of these standards and make every effort to protect the privacy and confidentiality of a patient's health care information.

If a health care team member has violated information confidentiality, an investigation must be started. If the breech was found to be unintentional, internal policies will determine if retraining may address this issue. The facility may elect to suspend with a warning or terminate the employee. If the level of violation is reportable, criminal penalties can range up to $250,000 and 10 years in prison.

REGULATION OF HEALTH CARE PROVIDERS

All states have laws, regulations, and licensing boards that govern health care providers. The regulations usually determine the **scope of practice**—or the procedures, processes, and actions that health care providers are legally permitted to perform in keeping with the terms of their professional license or registration. Each medical practitioner must understand the scope of practice that his or her license, certification, or registration falls under. Failure to abide by the regulations can result in the suspension or loss of a license, certification, or registration.

The federal government has established national standards that regulate health care. Some of the regulations are mandated by federal laws. A few examples of these laws include:

- Health Insurance Portability and Accountability Act (HIPAA)

- Health Information Technology for Economic and Clinical Health Act (HITECH)

- Americans with Disabilities Act (ADA)

- Patient Self-Determination Act (PSDA)

- Genetic Information Non-Discrimination Act (GINA)

- Mental Health Parity Act (MHPA)

- Newborns' and Mothers' Health Protection Act (NMHPA)

- Omnibus Budget Reconciliation Act (OBRA) of 1987

- Patient Protection and Affordable Care Act (PPACA)

Health care providers are responsible for knowing and following the provisions of these laws. In addition, federal agencies such as the Centers for Disease Control and Prevention (CDC), the Occupational Safety and Health Administration (OSHA), the Centers for Medicare and Medicaid Services (CMS), the Food and Drug Administration (FDA), the National Highway Traffic Safety Administration (NHTSA), and the U.S. Department of Health and Human Services (USDHHS) issue standards and regulations. For example, OSHA established *Bloodborne Pathogen Standards* that must be followed by all health care facilities and health care providers. The NHTSA Office of EMS established the educational standards for emergency medical services. The CDC developed *Standard Precautions* and *Transmission Based Precautions*.

Professional organizations in all of the health care careers assist in the establishment of educational requirements for the career, professional standards that should be observed, certification and/or registration requirements that must be met, and a code of ethics or conduct that must be followed. The organizations strive to establish standards that are followed by every individual working in the career field. In addition, they monitor legislative and regulatory actions and advocate for laws

that affect the health care career. Again, every health care provider in the specific career field must be aware of and follow these professional guidelines and standards.

In addition, most health care agencies have specific rules, regulations, and standards that determine the activities performed by individuals employed in different positions. These standards are usually in the facility's policy or procedure manual. Every health care team member should read and follow the guidelines presented in the manual.

 Standards and regulations can vary from state to state and even from agency to agency. It is important to remember that you are liable, or legally responsible, for your own actions regardless of what anyone tells you or what position you hold. Therefore, when you undertake a particular position of employment in a health care agency, *it is your responsibility to learn exactly what you are legally permitted to do and to familiarize yourself with your exact responsibilities.*

check**point**

1. List four (4) legal disabilities that would prevent a person from signing a consent form or contract.
2. Define the term *tort*.
3. Define *privileged communications* and explain how they apply to health care.

5:2 ETHICS

Medical legal responsibilities are determined by medical laws. Medical providers are liable for their own actions under the law. **Ethics** are a set of principles relating to what is morally right or wrong. Ethics provide a standard of conduct or code of behavior. This allows a health care provider to analyze information and make decisions based on what he or she believes is right and good conduct. Modern health care advances, however, have created many medical ethical dilemmas for health care providers. Some of these dilemmas include:

- Should a person have the right to euthanasia (assisted death) if he or she is terminally ill and in excruciating pain?

- Should a patient be told that a health care provider has AIDS?

- When should life support be discontinued?

- Do parents have a religious right to refuse a lifesaving blood transfusion for their child?

- Can a health care facility refuse to provide expensive treatment such as a bone marrow transplant if a patient cannot pay for the treatment?

- Who decides whether a 75-year-old patient or a 56-year-old patient gets a single kidney available for transplant?

- Should people be allowed to sell organs for use in transplants?

- If a person can benefit from marijuana, should a physician be allowed to prescribe it as a treatment?

- Should animals be used in medical research even if it results in the death of the animal?

- Should genetic researchers be allowed to transplant specific genes to create the "perfect" human being?

- Should human beings be cloned?

- Should aborted embryos be used to obtain stem cells for research, especially as scientists may be able to use the stem cells to cure diseases such as diabetes, osteoporosis, and Parkinson's?

As medical technology advances, the implications on ethical decisions become more complex. For example, digital medicine combines information technology, artificial intelligence, and big data with pharmaceutical, biotechnology, and medical device companies. An example of this is the digital pill. It combines sensor technology with a drug that is used to treat a range of serious mental illnesses. A psychiatrist who prescribes it to a patient with schizophrenia might be better positioned to help that patient by being certain he or she is taking the medicine as prescribed. On the other hand, there is the potential for a negative effect on the doctor–patient relationship with regard to mutual trust. Another consideration is whether patients fully understand how their health information may be collected, used, stored, and shared. Ethics must keep up with the rapid pace of technology and the challenges of managing a large amount of patients' behavioral, medical, and personal information.

Although there are no easy answers to any of these questions, some guidelines are provided by an ethical code. Most of the national organizations affiliated with the different health care professions have established ethical codes for personnel in their respective occupations. Although such codes differ slightly, most contain the same basic principles:

- Put the saving of life and the promotion of health above all else.

- Make every effort to keep the patient as comfortable as possible and to preserve life whenever possible.

- Respect the patient's choice to die peacefully and with dignity when all options have been discussed with the patient and family and/or predetermined by advance directives.

- Treat all patients equally, regardless of race, religion, social or economic status, gender, age, or nationality. Bias, prejudice, and discrimination have no place in health care.

- Provide care for *all* individuals to the best of your ability.

- Maintain a competent level of skill consistent with your particular health care career.

- Stay informed and up to date, and pursue continuing education as necessary.

- Maintain **confidentiality**. Confidentiality means that information about the patient must remain private and can be shared *only* with other members of the patient's health care team. A legal violation can occur if a patient suffers personal or financial damage when confidential information is shared with others, including family members. Information obtained from patients should not be repeated or used for personal gain. Gossiping about patients is ethically wrong.

- Refrain from immoral, unethical, and illegal practices. If you observe others taking part in illegal actions, report such actions to the proper authorities. Failure to report these actions may result in legal actions taken against you.

- Show loyalty to patients, team members, and employers. Avoid negative or derogatory statements, and always express a positive attitude.

- Be sincere, honest, and caring. Treat others as you want to be treated. Show respect and concern for the feelings, dignity, and rights of others.

When you enter a health care career, learn the code of ethics for that career. Make every effort to abide by the code and to become a competent and ethical health care provider. In doing so, you will earn the respect and confidence of patients, team members, and employers.

checkpoint

1. What does the term *confidentiality* mean?

5:3 PATIENTS' RIGHTS

Federal and state legislation requires health care agencies to have written policies concerning **patients' rights**, or the factors of care that patients can expect to receive. Agencies expect all personnel to respect and honor these rights.

The Department of Health and Human Services implemented a **Consumer Bill of Rights and Responsibilities** in 1998 that must be recognized and honored by health care providers. This bill of rights states, in part, that patients have the right to:

- Receive accurate, easily understood information and assistance in making informed health care decisions about their health care plans, professionals, and facilities

- A choice of health care providers that is sufficient to ensure access to appropriate high-quality health care

- Access emergency health services when and where the need arises

- Fully participate in all decisions related to their health care (**Figure 5–6**)

- Be represented by parents, guardians, family members, or other conservators if they are unable to fully participate in treatment decisions

- Considerate and respectful care

- Not be discriminated against in the delivery of health care services based on race, ethnicity, national origin, religion, gender, age, mental or physical disability, sexual orientation, genetic information, or source of payment

- Communicate with health care providers in confidence and have the confidentiality of their individually identifiable health care information protected

- Review and copy their own medical records and request amendments to their records

- A fair and efficient process for resolving differences with their health care plans, health care providers, and the institutions that serve them, including a rigorous system of internal review and an independent system of external review

Residents in long-term care facilities are guaranteed certain rights under the **Omnibus Budget Reconciliation Act (OBRA) of 1987**. Every long-term care facility must inform residents or their guardians of these rights, and a copy must be posted in each facility. This is often called a **Resident's Bill of Rights**, and it states, in part, that a resident has the right to:

- Free choice regarding physician, treatment, care, and participation in research

- Freedom from abuse and chemical or physical restraints

- Privacy and confidentiality of personal and clinical records

- Accommodation of needs and choice regarding activities, schedules, and health care

- Voice grievances without fear of retaliation or discrimination

- Organize and participate in family/resident groups and in social, religious, and community activities

- Information about medical benefits, medical records, survey results, deficiencies of the facility, and advocacy groups, including the ombudsman program (state representative who checks on resident care and violations of rights)

- Manage personal funds and use personal possessions

- Unlimited access to immediate family or relatives and to share a room with his or her spouse if both are residents (**Figure 5–7**)

- Remain in the facility and not be transferred or discharged except for medical reasons, the welfare of the resident or others, failure to pay, or if the facility either cannot meet the resident's needs or ceases to operate

The **Patient Protection and Affordable Care Act (PPACA)**, commonly called the *Affordable Care Act (ACA)*, also guarantees certain rights pertaining to health insurance coverage. Some of the main provisions of this act state, in part, that consumers have the right to:

- An easy-to-understand summary of insurance benefits and coverage

- Coverage for essential health benefits such as emergency care, hospitalization, prescription drugs, maternity care, and newborn care

- Preventive care for specific procedures at no cost to the consumer

- Coverage even if a pre-existing illness or condition exists

- Coverage to age 26 under a parent's health care plan if eligible

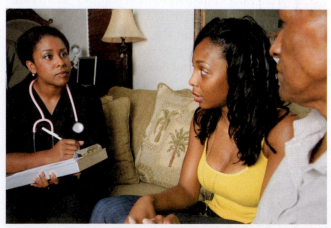

FIGURE 5–6 Patients have the right to fully participate in all decisions related to their health care. © iStock.com/Steve Debenport

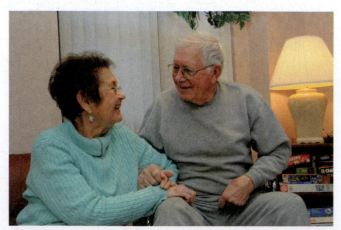

FIGURE 5–7 A married couple in a long-term care facility has the legal right to share a room if both members of the couple are residents in the facility.

- Choose any available participating primary care provider as their doctor
- Receive care for emergency medical conditions at any emergency care facility without pre-authorization and without higher co-payments for out-of-network services
- No annual or lifetime limits on health care benefits
- No arbitrary withdrawal or cancellation of insurance coverage (exceptions include no payment of premiums, lying on an application form, or the company ceases to offer insurance in the region)
- Appeal any health care plan decision if the health insurance company denies payment for a medical treatment or service
- A review by an independent organization (outside review) if a health insurance company denies payment for a claim or terminates insurance coverage
- A refund of a percentage of their premiums if an insurance company does not spend at least 80–85 percent of premiums paid on health care versus administrative costs such as salaries and marketing

All states have adopted these rights, and some have added additional rights. It is important to check state law and obtain a list of the rights established in your state.

Health care providers can face job loss, fines, and even imprisonment if they do not follow and grant established patients' or residents' rights. By observing these rights, the health care provider helps ensure the patient's safety, privacy, and well-being and provides quality care at all times.

checkpoint

1. Which of the components of the Affordable Care Act will impact you the most as you move from high school student to independent adult?

5:4 ADVANCE DIRECTIVES FOR HEALTH CARE

Advance directives for health care, also known as *legal directives*, are legal documents that allow individuals to state what medical treatment they want or do not want in the event that they become incapacitated and are unable to express their wishes regarding medical care. The two main directives are a living will and a Designation of Health Care Surrogate or a Durable Power of Attorney (POA) for Health Care (**Figure 5–8**).

FLORIDA ADVANCE DIRECTIVE – PAGE 1 OF 5

INSTRUCTIONS

PRINT YOUR NAME

Part One. Designation of Health Care Surrogate

Name: _____

(Last)   (First)   (Middle Initial)

In the event that I have been determined to be incapacitated to provide informed consent for medical treatment and surgical and diagnostic procedures, I wish to designate as my surrogate for health care decisions:

PRINT THE NAME, HOME ADDRESS AND TELEPHONE NUMBER OF YOUR SURROGATE

Name: _____

Address: _____

_____ Zip Code: _____

Phone: _____

If my surrogate is unwilling or unable to perform his or her duties, I wish to designate as my alternate surrogate:

PRINT THE NAME, HOME ADDRESS AND TELEPHONE NUMBER OF YOUR ALTERNATE SURROGATE

Name: _____

Address: _____

_____ Zip Code: _____

Phone: _____

I fully understand that this designation will permit my designee to make health care decisions and to provide, withhold, or withdraw consent on my behalf; to apply for public benefits to defray the cost of health care; and to authorize my admission to or transfer from a health care facility.

When making health care decisions for me, my health care surrogate should think about what action would be consistent with past conversations we have had, my treatment preferences as expressed in Part Two (if I have filled out Part Two), my religious and other beliefs and values, and how I have handled medical and other important issues in the past. If what I would decide is still unclear, then my health care surrogate should make decisions for me that my health care surrogate believes are in my best interest, considering the benefits, burdens, and risks of my current circumstances and treatment options.

© 2005 National Hospice and Palliative Care Organization. 2011 Revised.

FLORIDA ADVANCE DIRECTIVE - PAGE 2 OF 5

ADD OTHER INSTRUCTIONS, IF ANY, REGARDING YOUR ADVANCE CARE PLANS

THESE INSTRUCTIONS CAN FURTHER ADDRESS YOUR HEALTH CARE PLANS, SUCH AS YOUR WISHES REGARDING HOSPICE TREATMENT, BUT CAN ALSO ADDRESS OTHER ADVANCE PLANNING ISSUES, SUCH AS YOUR BURIAL WISHES

ATTACH ADDITIONAL PAGES IF NEEDED

Additional instructions (optional):

_____

© 2005 National Hospice and Palliative Care Organization. 2011 Revised.

FIGURE 5–8 Advance directives include a living will that allows an individual to state what measures should or should not be taken to prolong life, and a designation of a health care surrogate that allows an individual to appoint another person to make health care decisions if the individual is unable to make his or her own decisions. © 2005 National Hospice and Palliative Care Organization 2011 Revised. All rights reserved. Reproduction and distribution by an organization or organized group without the written permission of the National Hospice and Palliative Care Organization is expressly forbidden. Visit caringinfo.org for more information.

(continues)

Part Two. Declaration

INSTRUCTIONS

PRINT THE DATE

Declaration made this _____ day of _____, _____,
(day)   (month)   (year)

PRINT YOUR NAME

I, _____,
willfully and voluntarily make known my desire that my dying not be
artificially prolonged under the circumstances set forth below, and I do
hereby declare that:

If at any time I am incapacitated and

(initial all that apply)

INITIAL EACH THAT
APPLIES

_____ I have a terminal condition, or

_____ I have an end-stage condition, or

_____ I am in a persistent vegetative state

and if my attending or treating physician and another consulting physician
have determined that there is no reasonable medical probability of my
recovery from such condition, I direct that life-prolonging procedures be
withheld or withdrawn when the application of such procedures would
serve only to prolong artificially the process of dying, and that I be
permitted to die naturally with only the administration of medication or
the performance of any medical procedure deemed necessary to provide
me with comfort care or to alleviate pain.

It is my intention that this declaration be honored by my family and
physician as the final expression of my legal right to refuse medical or
surgical treatment and to accept the consequences for such refusal.

© 2005 National
Hospice and
Palliative Care
Organization.
2011 Revised.

ORGAN DONATION
(OPTIONAL)

ORGAN DONATION (OPTIONAL)
I hereby make this anatomical gift, if medically acceptable, to take effect
on death. The words and marks below indicate my desires:

I give (initial one choice below):

_____ any needed organs, tissues, or eyes for the purpose of
transplantation, therapy, medical research, or education;

_____ only the following organs, tissues, or eyes for the purpose of
transplantation, therapy, medical research, or education:
_____
_____
_____

INITIAL ONLY ONE
OF THE FOUR
OPTIONS

_____ my body for anatomical study if needed. Limitations or special
wishes, if any:
_____
_____
_____

IF YOU HAVE
ALREADY
ARRANGED TO
DONATE YOUR
ORGANS TO A
SPECIFIC DONEE,
INITIAL THIS
OPTION, AND
INDICATE THE
DETAILS OF YOUR
ARRANGEMENT
HERE

_____ I have already arranged to donate
_____ Any needed organs, tissues, or eyes,
_____ The following organs, tissues, or eyes:
_____
_____
_____

to the following donee:_____

Phone:_____

Address:_____

_____ Zip Code:_____

© 2005 National
Hospice and
Palliative Care
Organization.
2011 Revised.

Part Three. Execution

PRINT YOUR NAME

I, _____
understand the full impact of this declaration, and I am emotionally and
mentally competent to make this declaration. I further affirm that this
designation is not being made as a condition of treatment or admission
to a health care facility.

SIGN AND DATE
THE DOCUMENT

Signed: _____

Date: _____

Witness 1:

Signed: _____

Address: _____
_____

TWO WITNESSES
MUST SIGN AND
PRINT THEIR
ADDRESSES

Witness 2:

Signed: _____

Address: _____
_____

(Optional) I will notify and send a copy of this document to the following
persons other than my surrogate, so they may know who my surrogate
is:

OPTIONAL

Name: _____

PRINT THE NAMES
AND ADDRESSES OF
THOSE WHO YOU
WANT TO KEEP
COPIES OF THIS
DOCUMENT

Address:_____

_____

Name: _____

Address:_____

_____

Courtesy of Caring Connections
1731 King St., Suite 100, Alexandria, VA 22314
www.caringinfo.org, 800/658-8898

© 2005 National
Hospice and
Palliative Care
Organization.
2011 Revised.

FIGURE 5–8 *(continued)* © 2005 National Hospice and Palliative Care Organization 2011 Revised. All rights reserved. Reproduction and distribution by an organization or organized group without the written permission of the National Hospice and Palliative Care Organization is expressly forbidden. Visit caringinfo.org for more information.

Living wills are documents that allow individuals to state what measures should or should not be taken to prolong life when their conditions are terminal (death is expected). The document must be signed when the individual is competent and witnessed by two adults who cannot benefit from the death. Most states now have laws that honor living wills and allow life-sustaining procedures to be withheld. A living will frequently results in a Do Not Resuscitate (DNR) order for a terminally ill individual. The DNR order means that cardiopulmonary resuscitation is not performed when the patient stops breathing. The patient is allowed to die with peace and dignity. At times, this is extremely difficult for health care team members to honor. It is important to remember that many individuals believe that the quality of life is important and a life on support systems has no meaning or purpose for them.

A **Designation of Health Care Surrogate**, also called a **Durable Power of Attorney (POA)** for Health Care, is a document that permits an individual (known as a principal) to appoint another person (known as an agent) to make any decisions regarding health care if the principal should become unable to make decisions. This includes providing or withholding specific medical or surgical procedures, hiring or dismissing health care providers, spending or withholding funds for health care, and having access to medical records. Although they are most frequently given to spouses or adult children, POAs can be given to any qualified adult. To meet legal requirements, the POA must be signed by the principal, agent, and one or two adult witnesses.

A federal law called the **Patient Self-Determination Act (PSDA)** of 1990 mandates that all health care facilities receiving any type of federal aid comply with the following requirements:

- Inform every adult, both orally and in writing, of his or her right under state law to make decisions concerning medical care, including the right to refuse treatment and right-to-die options
- Provide information and assistance in preparing advance directives
- Document any advance directives on the patient's record
- Provide written statements to implement the patient's rights in the decision-making process
- Affirm that there will be no discrimination or effect on care because of advance directives
- Educate the staff on the medical and legal issues of advance directives

The PSDA ensures that patients are informed of their rights and have the opportunity to determine the care they will receive.

All health care providers must be aware of and honor advance or legal directives. In addition, health care team members should give serious consideration to preparing their own advance directives.

checkpoint

1. What is a living will? How does it differ from a Designation of Health Care Surrogate?

5:5 PROFESSIONAL STANDARDS

Legal responsibilities, ethics, patients' rights, and advance directives all help determine the type of care provided by health care providers. By following certain standards at all times, you can protect yourself, your employer, and the patient. Some of the basic standards are:

- **Perform only those procedures for which you have been trained and you are legally permitted to do**. Never perform any procedure unless you are qualified. The necessary training may be obtained from an educational facility, from your employer, or in special classes provided by an agency. If you are asked to perform any procedure for which you are not qualified, it is your responsibility to state that you have not been trained and to refuse to do it until you receive the required instruction. If you are not legally permitted to either perform a procedure or to sign documents, it is your responsibility to refuse to do so because of legal limitations.

- **Use approved, correct methods while performing any procedure**. Follow specific methods taught by qualified instructors in educational facilities, or observe and learn procedures from your employer or authorized personnel. Most health care facilities have an approved procedure manual that explains the step-by-step methods for performing tasks. Use this manual or read the manufacturer's instructions for specific equipment or supplies.

- **Obtain proper authorization before performing any procedure**. In some health care careers, you will obtain authorization directly from the doctor, therapist, or individual in charge of a

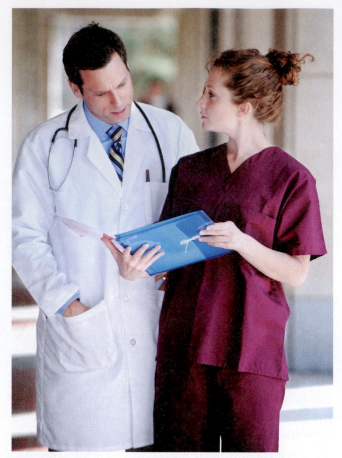

FIGURE 5–9 Obtain proper authorization before performing any procedure on a patient. © iStock.com/Eric Hood

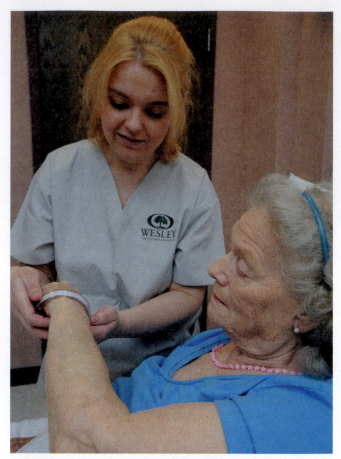

FIGURE 5–10 If a name band is present, use it to identify the patient.

patient's care (**Figure 5–9**). In other careers, you will obtain authorization by checking written orders. In careers where you have neither access to patients' records nor direct contact with the individuals in charge of care, an immediate supervisor will interpret orders and then direct you to perform procedures.

- **Identify the patient**. In some health care facilities, patients wear identification bands. If this is the case, check this name band (**Figure 5–10**). In addition, state the patient's name clearly, repeating it if necessary. For example, say "Miss Jones?" followed by "Miss Sandra Jones?" to be sure you have the correct patient. Some health care facilities now use bar codes on patient identification bands. A scanner is used to check the bar code and verify the identity of the patient. Some long-term care facilities use photo IDs for patients because sometimes the patients are disoriented and are not able to state their name.

- **Obtain the patient's consent before performing any procedure**. Always explain a procedure briefly or state what you are going to do, and obtain the patient's consent. It is best to avoid

statements such as "May I take your blood pressure?" because the patient can say "No." By stating, "The doctor would like me to check your blood pressure," you are identifying the procedure and obtaining consent by the patient's acceptance or lack of objection. If a patient refuses to allow you to perform a procedure, check with your immediate supervisor. Some procedures require written consent from the patient. Follow the agency policy with regard to such procedures. Never sign your name as a witness to any written consent or document unless you are authorized to do so.

- Safety **Observe all safety precautions**. Handle equipment carefully. Be alert to all aspects of safety to protect the patient. Know and follow safety rules and regulations. Be alert to safety hazards in any area and make every effort to correct or eliminate such hazards as quickly as possible.

- HIPAA **Keep all information confidential**. This includes oral and written information. Ensure that you do not place patient records in any area where they can be seen

Frozen Stem Cells That Cure Major Diseases?

Stem cells are a major area of research today. Stem cells are important because they can become any of the specialized cell types needed in the human body. They can turn into muscle cells in the heart, nerve cells in the brain, or cells that secrete the insulin needed by a patient with diabetes. The major sources of stem cells are a developing embryo (infant); adult tissues such as bone marrow, brain, muscle, skin, and liver; and blood from the umbilical cord of a newborn infant. Currently, parents have the option of preserving the umbilical cord blood for its stem cells. When their baby is born, blood from the umbilical cord can be collected and stored in liquid nitrogen. If the child later develops a disease such as cancer and needs stem cells, the cells can be recovered and used for the transplant. The cost of this procedure still limits its widespread use.

Scientists the world over are finding ways to grow stem cells and force them to generate special cells that can be used to treat injury or disease. Early research has proved it is easier to work with embryonic cells, but this has created ethical dilemmas because it means embryos are destroyed. However, if adult cells can be harvested and grown, it would be easier to use an adult's own cells because they would not be rejected by the body.

Many scientists believe that, eventually, the study of stem cells will help explain how cells grow and develop. Conditions such as cancer and birth defects are caused by abnormal cell division. If scientists can learn how the abnormal development occurs, they could find ways to treat and even prevent the conditions. Major research is directed toward learning what makes the cells specialize to become a specific type of cell in the body.

Some of the latest research on stem cells involves treatment for heart disease. If the muscle of the heart is deprived of oxygen because of a blocked artery, the muscle cells die. Researchers are using embryonic cells, cardiac stem cells that naturally reside within the heart, myoblasts (muscle stem cells), and umbilical cord blood cells to try to repair damaged heart tissue. Most of their work has been performed on rats or larger animals such as pigs. However, some experiments have been performed on humans undergoing open-heart surgery. Initial studies showed that stem cells injected directly into the injured heart tissue appeared to improve cardiac function. However, much more research is needed to determine the safety and effectiveness of this treatment. Another major area of research is directed toward patients with Type 1 or insulin-dependent diabetes, a condition in which the cells of the pancreas do not produce sufficient insulin. New studies are showing some success in directing embryonic stem cells in a cell culture to form insulin-producing cells. A recent study by a group of scientists at ViaCyte has developed a method for turning embryotic stem cells into pancreatic progenitor cells that can mature into fully functioning insulin-producing beta cells. The team is currently implanting a device about the size of a credit card into patients with Type 1 or insulin-dependent diabetes. This device contains the pancreatic progenitor cells, and the scientists hope that they will mature into beta cells and produce insulin. Again, years of intensive research will be required before this is an effective treatment for diabetes, but stem cells do offer exciting promise for future therapies.

by unauthorized individuals. Do not reveal any information contained in the records without proper authorization and patient consent. If you are reporting specific information about a patient to your immediate supervisor, ensure that your conversation cannot be heard by others. Avoid discussing patients with others at home, in social situations, in public places, or anywhere outside the agency.

- **Think before you speak and carefully consider everything you say.** Do not reveal information to the patient unless you are specifically permitted to do so.

- **Treat all patients equally regardless of race, religion, social or economic status, gender, age, or nationality.** Provide care for *all* individuals to the best of your ability.

- **Accept no tips or bribes for the care you provide.** You receive a salary for your services, and the care you provide should not be influenced by the amount of money a patient can afford to pay. A polite refusal, such as "I'm sorry, I am not allowed to accept tips," is usually the best way to handle this situation. An exception to this rule is if a patient or family member brings the entire floor/unit a thank-you gift such as cookies or candy.

- **If any error occurs or you make a mistake, report it immediately to your supervisor**. Never try to hide or ignore an error. Make every effort to correct the situation as soon as possible, and take responsibility for your actions.

- **Behave professionally in dress, language, manners, and actions**. Take pride in your profession and in the work you do. Promote a positive attitude at all times.

Even when standards are followed, errors leading to legal action sometimes still occur. Liability insurance constitutes an additional form of protection in such cases. Many insurance companies offer policies at reasonable cost for health care providers and students. Some companies will even issue liability protection under a homeowner's policy or through a liability policy that protects the person against all liabilities, not just those related to their profession.

Legal

Again, remember that it is your responsibility to understand the legal and ethical implications of your particular health care career. Never hesitate to ask specific questions or to request written policies from your employer. Contact your state board of health or state board of education to obtain information regarding the regulations and guidelines for your health care field. By obtaining this information and by following the basic standards listed, you will protect yourself, your employer, and the patient to whom you provide health care.

checkpoint

1. Choose three (3) professional standards and explain how they protect yourself, your employer, and the patient.

PRACTICE: Go to the workbook and complete the assignment sheet for Chapter 5, Legal and Ethical Responsibilities.

Case Study Investigation Conclusion

Mr. Eddie Cruz died of the highly infectious disease AIDS without consenting to let anyone except his direct caregivers know that information. What can you conclude about Mr. Cruz's patient rights? What is Jennifer able to disclose to his girlfriend Brianna? His family? What about Eddie's mom? Support what you think Jennifer's decision should be based on evidence in this chapter. What might be the reaction from Mr. Cruz's family to Jennifer's response to their questions? How can Jennifer help this grieving family?

CHAPTER 5 SUMMARY

- All health care professionals have legal and ethical responsibilities that exist to protect the health care team member, employer, and patient.

- Legal responsibilities in health care involve torts and contracts. Torts are wrongful acts that do not involve contracts. Contracts are agreements between two or more parties that create obligations that must be met.

- Understanding privileged communications is another important aspect of legal responsibilities. Health care records are privileged communications and can be used as legal records in a court of law.

- Health care providers must know and follow all of the regulations that determine which procedures, processes, and actions they can legally perform. They are responsible for determining their scope of practice.

- Ethical responsibilities are based on right or wrong. Most health care careers have established codes of ethics that provide standards of conduct.

- Health care providers must respect patients' rights. Health care facilities have written policies concerning these rights.

- Advance directives for health care are legal documents that allow individuals to state what medical treatment they want or do not want in the event that they become incapacitated. Two main examples are a living will and Durable Power of Attorney for Health Care.

- Professional standards of care provide guidelines for meeting legal responsibilities, ethics, and patients' rights. All health care providers should know and follow the laws that regulate their respective careers.

REVIEW QUESTIONS

1. What is the difference between an implied consent and an expressed consent? Write a paragraph explaining the importance of these contracts in health care.

2. Differentiate between medical law and medical ethics.

3. You are employed as a geriatric assistant. A resident tells you that he is saving sleeping pills so he can commit suicide. He has terminal cancer and is in a great deal of pain. What should you do? Why is reporting an incident important?

4. What is HIPAA? Identify three (3) specific ways that HIPAA protects the privacy and confidentiality of health care information.

5. What are two (2) legal regulations that apply to health care records?

6. Obtain codes of ethics and state standards for two (2) different health professions by contacting professional organizations or searching the Internet. Compare these codes of ethics and describe the scope of practice for each profession.

7. Mr. Gonzales is a healthy 55-year-old man with a living will that contains a DNR (Do Not Resuscitate) order for terminal conditions. He goes into cardiac arrest as a result of an allergic reaction to an injection of dye for a laboratory test. Should cardiopulmonary resuscitation (CPR) be started? Why or why not?

8. List six (6) different patient or resident rights.

9. Identify six (6) professional standards and explain how they meet legal responsibilities, ethics, or patient's rights. Why are they important?

CRITICAL THINKING

1. Laura is an area finalist in cross country but can't quite make it past state to national competition. She suffered a major car accident in her junior year that left her with a knee injury, a mangled left ankle, and traumatic amputation of the distal end of her foot. After consulting with her physician and surgeon, Laura has decided to replace her entire left leg with a prosthetic that would allow her to run without fatigue and navigate anything blocking her running path more smoothly and efficiently. In a small group, predict what would happen if she competes with her team after this mechanical enhancement. Come to a consensus and decide if this is fair. What ideas or technology supports your group's decision?

2. With a partner, research and describe advance directives generally; then focus on an explanation of two (2) specific advance directive documents and what issues they address. Provide an example of each document.

3. In an essay, define privileged communications and explain how electronic health care records can sometimes complicate keeping the medical record confidential.

4. Assemble a health care think tank. Here is your dilemma:

    There is a major shortage of kidneys available for transplant. Should an individual be allowed to sell a kidney to a facility or an individual in renal failure who needs the kidney in order to live and is willing to pay for the kidney? Why or why not? What six (6) basic ethical rules would be involved in this decision?

ACTIVITES

1. With a small group, create a terms chart that defines each term listed below and a brief description of how each might be demonstrated in a health care setting.

    TERMS: abuse, slander, assault and battery, libel, false imprisonment, malpractice, invasion of privacy, negligence, defamation of character

2. In a small group, using the information in the terms chart, research a legal case for each term. Lead the class in a discussion regarding these cases in which you would include the legal responsibilities and implications of all involved.

3. With a small group, in five (5) minutes, write down as many patient basic rights as you can. Summarize the class findings on the board.

4. In a small group, research the PPACA. How does it influence health care insurance plans and health care delivery? Is this influence positive or negative for our country? Be prepared to defend your team's view in a class debate.

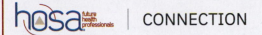
Medical Law & Ethics

Event Summary: Medical Law & Ethics provides members with the opportunity to gain knowledge and skills regarding medical law, ethics, and bioethics. This competitive event consists of a written test with a tie-breaker essay question. This event aims to inspire members to learn about ethical and legal terms as well as how to analyze, synthesize, and evaluate information related to this field.

Details on this competitive event may be found at

www.hosa.org/guidelines

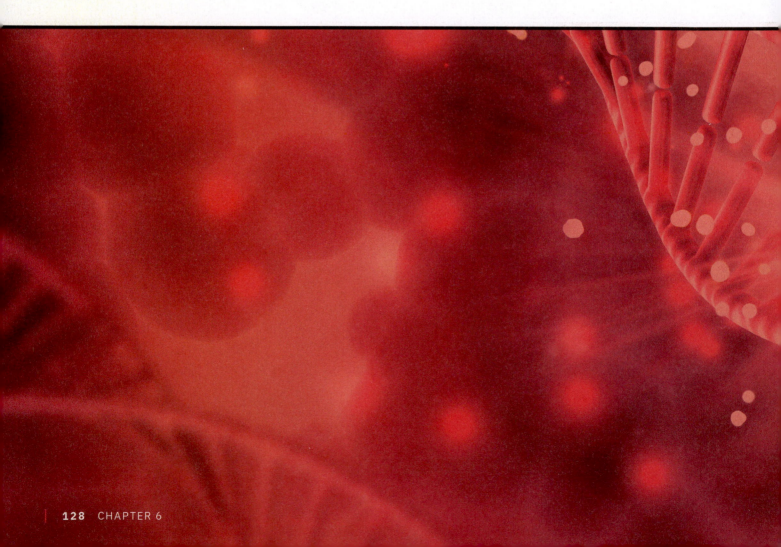

CHAPTER 6

MEDICAL TERMINOLOGY

Comm

Case Study Investigation

Loni Keller went to the ER with her mother and brother when her brother fell out of a tree and broke his arm. While waiting for discharge papers, they were given a copy of chart notes to take to their regular doctor. Mrs. Keller took one look and could not understand the note at all! Luckily, Loni had taken medical terminology and could interpret the information for her mother.

Here is what it said: "Ray Keller a 12 yo male presents c/o Rt arm pain and HA. Lateral X-ray show Colles Fx of the Rt distal radius. BP 120/80, P 100, R 22, afebrile. Casted Rt arm, RICE recommended, ASA for HA and Vicodin I tab q 4h prn pain. Pt activity ad lib. See GP in 3 days." At the end of this chapter, you will be asked to transcribe and communicate what is written.

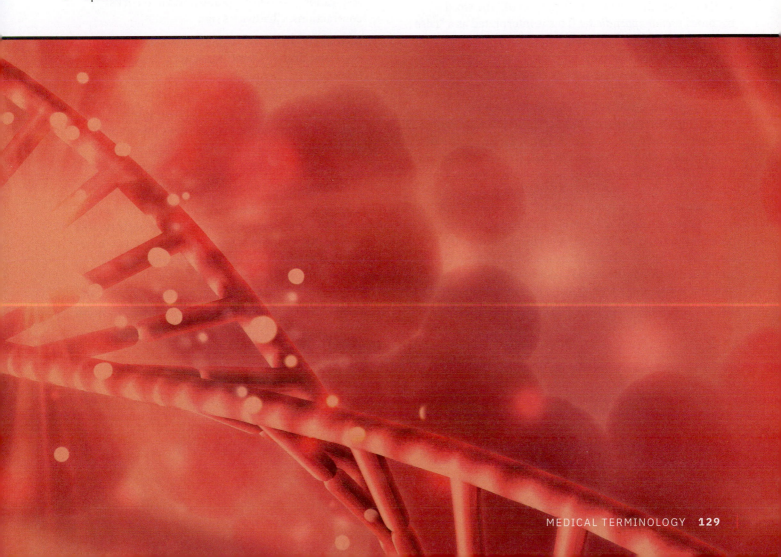

LEARNING OBJECTIVES

After completing this chapter, you should be able to:

- Define prefixes, suffixes, and word roots selected from a list of words.
- Identify basic medical abbreviations selected from a standard list.
- Transcribe and communicate medical terms correctly.
- Define, pronounce, and spell all key terms.

KEY TERMS

abbreviations	prefix	transcribe
eponyms	suffix	word roots
opioids		

Medical dictionaries have been written to include the many words used in health care careers. It would be impossible to memorize all such words. By breaking the words into parts, however, it is sometimes possible to figure out their meanings.

A word is often a combination of different parts. The parts include prefixes, suffixes, and word roots (see **Figure 6–1**).

A **prefix** can be defined as a syllable or word placed at the beginning of a word. A **suffix** can be defined as a syllable or word placed at the end of the word.

The meanings of prefixes and suffixes are set. For example, the suffix *itis* means "inflammation of." *Tonsillitis* means "an inflammation of the tonsils," and *appendicitis* means "an inflammation of the appendix." Note that the meaning of the suffix is usually placed first when the word is defined.

Word roots can be defined as main words or parts to which prefixes and suffixes can be added. In the example *appendicitis*, the word root is *appendix*. By adding the prefix *pseudo-*, which means "false," and the suffix *itis*, which means "inflammation of," the word becomes *pseudoappendicitis*. This is interpreted as a "false inflammation of the appendix."

The prefix usually serves to further define the word root. The suffix usually describes what is happening to the word root.

When prefixes, suffixes, and/or word roots are joined together, vowels are frequently added. Common examples include *a, e, i, ia, io, o,* and *u*. These are listed in parentheses in the lists that follow. The vowels are not used if the word root or suffix begins with a vowel. For example, *encephal (o)* means brain. When it is combined with *itis*, meaning "inflammation of," the vowel is not used for *encephalitis*. When it is combined with *gram*, meaning "tracing" or "record," the vowel *o* is added for *encephalogram*. *Hepat (o)* means liver. When it is combined with *itis*, the vowel is not used for *hepatitis*. When it is combined with *megaly*, meaning "enlarged," the vowel *o* is added for *hepatomegaly*.

Eponyms are terms used in medicine that are named after people, places, or things. They are usually used to identify the individual who identified or discovered a substance, disease, or structure. An eponymous individual is someone who uses his or her name to describe something. Common uses for eponyms in medicine include naming:

- **Anatomical parts**: Achilles tendon, Adam's apple, Eustachian tube, Langerhans cells, Bartholin's gland, Cowper's gland, circle of Willis, Golgi apparatus

- **Diagnostic tests**: Coombs test, Papanicolaou (Pap) test, Ishihara plates, Wright's stain, Gram's stain, Mantoux test, Hirschberg test

- **Diseases**: Alzheimer's disease, Down syndrome, Parkinson's disease, Legionnaire's disease, Lou Gehrig's disease, Kaposi's sarcoma, Hodgkin's disease, Bell's palsy, Munchausen syndrome

- **Fractures**: Colles' fracture, Hill-Sachs fracture, hang-man's fracture

- **Instruments or medical devices**: Adson forceps, Auvard speculum, Allis clamp, Holter monitor, Leur lock, Glenn shunt, Milwaukee brace, St. Jude valve

- **Medical signs**: Babinski sign, Cheyne-Stokes respiration, Korotkoff sounds, Braxton-Hicks contractions, Chadwick's sign

- **Medical treatments**: Heimlich maneuver, Kegel exercises, Brandt-Daroff maneuver, Pasteur's treatment

- **Microorganisms**: Listeria, Escherichia coli, Norwalk virus, Klebsiella pneumonia, Weichselbaum's cocci, Friedlander's pneumonia, Epstein-Barr virus

- **Surgeries**: Trendelenburg operation, Whipple's procedure, Syme's amputation

By learning basic prefixes, suffixes, and word roots and being aware of eponyms, you will frequently be able to interpret the meaning of a word even when you have never before encountered the word. You must also be able to **transcribe** or put the word and/or its meaning in written form. A list of common prefixes, suffixes, and word roots follows. An example of a medical term using

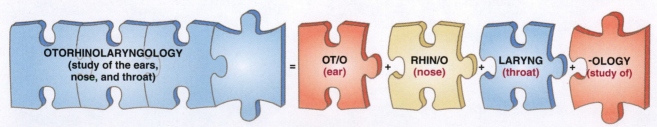

FIGURE 6–1 Prefixes, suffixes, and word roots can be used to interpret the meaning of a word.

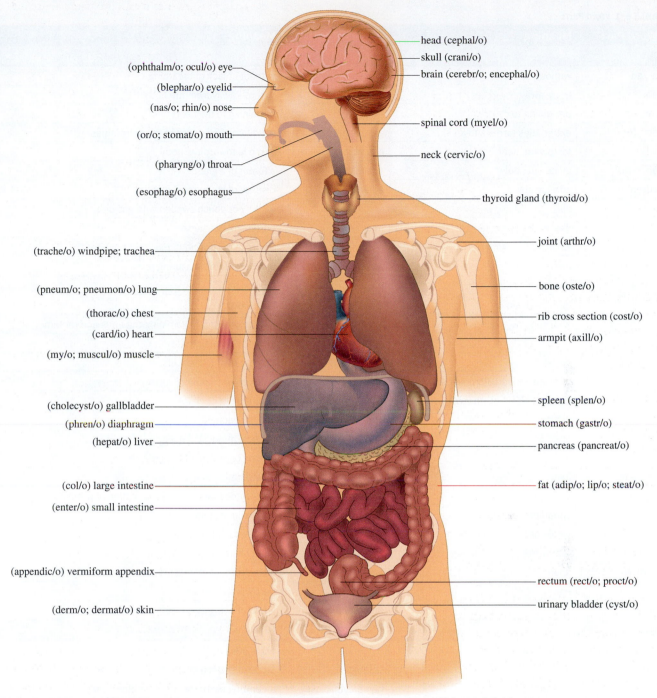

FIGURE 6–2 The prefixes, suffixes, and word roots for parts of the human body.

the word part and the meaning of the medical term is also provided. In addition, the prefixes, suffixes, and word roots for parts of the human body are shown in **Figure 6–2**.

Learn the prefixes, suffixes, and word roots in the following way:

- Use a set of index cards to make flashcards of the word parts found on the prefix, suffix, and word root list (see **Table 6-1**). Place one prefix, suffix, or word root on each card. Put the word part on the front of the card and the meaning of the word part on the back of the card. Ensure that each is spelled correctly.

- Use the flashcards to learn the meanings of the word parts. A realistic goal is to learn one letter per week. For example, learn all word parts starting with the letter *A* the first week, all of those starting with *B* the second week, all of those starting with *C* the third week, and so on until all are learned. Practice correct spelling of all of the word parts.

- Follow the instructor's guidelines for tests on the word parts. Many instructors give weekly tests. The tests may be cumulative. They may cover the letter of the week plus any letters learned in previous weeks. Words may be presented that use the various word parts.

TABLE 6-1 Word Parts

Word Part	Meaning	Medical Term	Meaning
A			
a-, an-	without, lack of	a/pnea	without or lack of breathing
ab-	from, away	ab/duct	to move away from the body
-ac, -ic	pertaining to	cardi/ac	pertaining to the heart
acr- (o)	extremities (arms and legs)	acro/cyan/osis	condition of blueness of the extremities
ad-	to, toward, near	ad/duct	to move toward the body
aden- (o)	gland, glandular	adeno/cele	a tumor of a gland
adren- (o)	adrenal gland	adreno/pathy	disease of the adrenal gland
aer- (o)	air	aero/cele	a cavity or pouch swollen with gas or air
-al	like, similar, pertaining to	neur/al	pertaining to a nerve
alba-, albi-	white	albi/no	an organism deficient in pigment, white
alges- (i, ia)	pain	algesi/meter	instrument for measuring pain
-algia	pain	my/algia	muscle pain
ambi-	both, both sides	ambi/lateral	both sides
an- (o, us)	anus (opening to rectum)	ano/scope	an instrument for examining the anus and rectum
andr- (o)	man, male	andr/ology	study of male diseases
angi- (o)	vessel	angio/pathy	disease of blood vessels
ankyl-	crooked, looped, immovable, fixed	ankyl/osis	stiffness or fixation of a joint
ante- (ro)	before, in front of, ahead of	ante/partum	before labor or childbirth
anti-	against	anti/bacterial	against bacteria
append- (i, o)	appendix	append/ectomy	surgical removal of the appendix
arter- (io)	artery	aterio/gram	tracing or picture of the arteries
arthr- (o)	joint	arthr/itis	inflammation of a joint
-ase	enzyme	peptid/ase	an enzyme that aids in the digestion of proteins
-asis	condition of	chole/lithi/asis	condition of stones in the gallbladder
-asthenia	weakness, lack of strength	my/asthenia	weakness in a muscle
ather- (o)	fatty, lipid	athero/sclerosis	a fatty hardening
audi- (o)	sound, hearing	audio/meter	an instrument to measure sound or hearing
aur-	ear	aur/al	pertaining to the ear
auto-	self	auto/phobia	a fear of being by oneself or alone
B			
bi- (s)	twice, double, both	bi/lateral	two sides
bio-	life	bio/logy	study of science of life
-blast	germ/embryonic cell	hemo/cyto/blast	an embryonic or stem cell for blood cells
blephar- (o)	eyelid	blepharo/plasty	plastic surgery on an eyelid
brachi-	arm	brachi/algia	arm pain
brachy-	short	brachy/dactyl/ic	condition of having short fingers
brady-	slow	brady/cardia	slow heart
bronch- (i, o)	air tubes in lungs	bronch/itis	inflammation of the air tubes in the lungs
bucc- (a, o)	Cheek	bucco/lingu/al	pertaining to the cheek and tongue
C			
calc- (i)	calcium	calc/emia	calcium in the blood
calc- (u, ulus)	stone	calcul/osis	condition of having a stone
carcin- (o)	cancer, malignancy	carcin/oma	cancerous tumor
cardi- (a, o)	pertaining to heart	cardi/ologist	physician who studies and treats heart disease
carp- (o)	wrist	carp/itis	inflammation of the wrist
-cele, -coele	swelling, tumor, cavity, hernia	meningo/cele	swelling or tumor of the membranes of the brain and spinal cord

(continues)

TABLE 6-1 Word Parts *(continued)*

Word Part	Meaning	Medical Term	Meaning
cent- (i)	one hundred	centi/meter	a hundredth part of a meter (unit of measurement)
-centesis	surgical puncture to remove fluid	thora/centesis	surgical puncture to remove fluid from the chest
cephal- (o)	head, pertaining to head	cephal/algia	pain in the head, headache
cerebro-	brain	cerebro/spin/al	pertaining to the brain and spinal cord
cervic- (o)	neck	cervico/facial	relating to the neck and face
cheil- (o)	lip	cheilo/plasty	plastic surgery to repair lip defects
chem- (o)	drug, chemical	chemo/therapy	treatment with drugs or chemicals
chlor- (o)	green	chlor/opsia	a visual defect in which all objects appear green
chol- (e, o)	bile, gallbladder	chole/cyst/ic	pertaining to the gallbladder or bag
chond- (i, r, ri)	cartilage	chondr/itis	inflammation of cartilage
chrom- (a, at, o)	color	chromato/meter	an instrument for measuring color perception
-cide	causing death	germi/cide	causing death to germs
circum-	around, about	circum/duction	movement in a circular motion
-cise	cut	ex/cise	cut out
co- (n)	with, together	co/chromato/graphy	identifying a substance by comparing color hues with a known substance
-coccus	round	diplo/coccus	two round circles
col- (in, o)	colon, bowel, large intestine	col/ostomy	creating an opening into the colon or large intestine
colp- (i, o)	vagina	colp/orrhaphy	surgical repair of the vaginal wall
contra-	against, counter	contra/stimulant	against a stimulant
cost- (a, i, o)	rib	cost/ectomy	surgical removal of a rib
crani- (o)	pertaining to the skull	crani/otomy	cutting into the skull
-crine	secrete	exo/crine	secrete outside of
cryo-	cold	cryo/therapy	treatment with cold
crypt- (o)	hidden, obscure	crypto/genic	obscure or unknown origin
cut- (an)	skin	cutane/ous	pertaining to the skin
cyan- (o)	blue	cyan/osis	condition of blueness
cyst- (i, o)	bladder, bag, sac	cyst/itis	inflammation of the bladder
cyt- (e, o)	cell	cyt/ology	study of cells
D			
dacry- (o)	tear duct, tear	dacryo/cyst/itis	inflammation of the lacrimal (tear duct) sac
dactyl- (o)	finger, toe	dactyl/oscopy	the scientific study of fingerprints
dec- (a, i)	ten	deci/meter	a tenth part of a meter (unit of measurement)
dent- (i, o)	tooth	dent/al	pertaining to teeth
derm- (a, at, o)	pertaining to skin	dermat/itis	inflammation of the skin
-desis	surgical union or fixation	arthro/desis	surgical immobilization of a joint to allow the bones to grow together
dextr- (i, o)	to the right	dextro/ocular	right eye
di- (plo)	double, twice	diplo/blast/ic	pertaining to two germ/embryonic cells
dia-	through, between, part	dia/dermal	cutting through the skin
dis- (ti, to)	separation, away from	dis/infect	to separate or free from infection
dors- (i, o)	to the back, back	dors/al	pertaining to the back
duoden- (o)	duodenum	duoden/ectomy	surgical removal of all or part of the duodenum
dys-	difficult, painful, bad	dys/uria	difficult or painful urination
E			
e- (c)	without	e/dentu/lous	condition of being without teeth
ec- (ti, to)	outside, external	ecto/genous	capable of developing away from the host
-ectasis	expansion, dilation, stretching	bronchi/ectasis	dilation or expansion of air tubes in lungs

(continues)

TABLE 6-1 Word Parts *(continued)*

Word Part	Meaning	Medical Term	Meaning
-ectomy	surgical removal of	hyster/ectomy	surgical removal of the uterus
electr- (o)	electrical	electro/cardio/gram	recording of electrical activity in the heart
-emesis	vomit	hemat/emesis	vomiting blood
-emia	blood	glyc/emia	sugar in the blood
encephal- (o)	brain	encephal/itis	inflammation of the brain
endo-	within, innermost	endo/crine	secrete within
enter- (i, o)	intestine	enter/itis	inflammation of the intestine
epi-	upon, over, upper	epi/gastric	above the stomach
erythro-	red	erythro/cyte	red (blood) cell
-esis	condition of	par/esis	condition of paralysis
-esthesia	sensation, perception, feel	an/esthesia	without feeling
eu-	well, easy, normal	eu/pnea	normal respiration or breathing
ex- (o)	outside of, beyond	exo/path/ic	disease that originates outside the body
F			
faci-	face	facio/plegia	paralysis of the face
-fascia (l)	fibrous band	myo/fascial	muscle fiber
fibr- (a, i, o)	fiber, connective tissue	fibr/oma	tumor of fibrous tissue
fore-	in front of	fore/arm	the front part of the arm
-form	having the form of, shape	uni/form	one shape or form
-fuge	driving away, expelling	centri/fuge	driving away from the center
G			
galacto-	milk, galactose (milk sugar)	galact/orrhea	flow of milk
gast- (i, ro)	stomach	gastr/itis	inflammation of the stomach
-genesis	development, production, creation	fibro/genesis	the development of fibrous tissue
-genetic, -genic	origin, producing, causing	cyto/genic	origin of cells
genito-	organs of reproduction	genito/urinary	organs of reproductive and urinary systems
-genous	kind, type	exo/genous	outside kind or type
geront- (o)	old age, elderly	geront/ology	study of the elderly
gingiv-	gums, gingiva	gingiv/itis	inflammation of the gums
gloss- (o)	tongue	glosso/graph	instrument for recording movements of the tongue
glue- (o)	sweetness, sugar, glucose	gluco/lipid	sugar fat
gly- (c, co)	sugar	glyc/emia	sugar in the blood
-gram	tracing, picture, record	electro/cardio/gram	tracing of the electrical activity in the heart
-graph	diagram, instrument for recording	electro/cardio/graph	instrument for recording electrical activity in the heart
gyn- (ec, o)	woman, female	gynec/ology	the study of women
H			
hem- (a, ato, o)	blood	hemat/ology	study of the blood
hemi-	half	hemi/plegia	paralysis on half of the body
hepat- (o)	liver	hepat/itis	inflammation of the liver
herni-	rupture	hernio/plasty	surgical repair of a rupture
hetero-	other, unlike, different	hetero/genous	different kind or type
hidr-(o)	sweat or sweat gland	hidr/osis	production and excretion of sweat
hist- (o)	tissue	hist/ologist	person who studies tissue
hom- (eo, o)	same, like	homeo/stasis	maintaining a constant level
hydro-	water	hydro/therapy	water treatment
hyper-	excessive, high, over, increased, more than normal	hyper/tension	high blood pressure

(continues)

TABLE 6-1 Word Parts *(continued)*

Word Part	Meaning	Medical Term	Meaning
hypno-	sleep	hypno/sis	process of sleep
hypo-	decreased, deficient, low, under, less than normal	hypo/tension	low blood pressure
hyster- (o)	uterus	hyster/ectomy	surgical removal of the uterus
I			
-ia, -iasis	condition of, abnormal/pathological state	pneumon/ia	abnormal condition of the lung
-ic, -ac	pertaining to	thorac/ic	pertaining to the chest
idio-	peculiar to an individual, self-originating	idio/pathic	disease arising by itself or from an unknown cause
ile- (o, um)	ileum	ileo/stomy	creating an artificial opening into the ileum
infra-	beneath, below	infra/sonic	sound waves below the frequency of the human ear
inter-	between, among	inter/costal	between the ribs
intra-	within, into, inside	intra/ven/ous	into a vein
-ism	condition, theory, state of being	albin/ism	condition of being white
iso-	equal, alike, same	iso/chromatic	constant or same color
-itis	inflammation, inflammation of	pharyng/itis	inflammation of the throat
K			
kary-(o)	nucleus	karyo/lysis	dissolving the cell nucleus
kerat- (o)	cornea of eye	kerato/meter	instrument to measure the curvature of the cornea
-kinesis, -kinetic	motion	dys/kinetic	difficult movement
L			
labi- (a, o)	lip	labio/lingual	pertaining to the lips and tongue
lacrima-	tears	lacrima/tion	secretion of tears
lact- (o)	milk	lacto/genesis	production of milk
lapar- (o)	abdomen, abdominal wall	lapar/otomy	cutting into the abdomen
laryng- (o)	larynx (voice box)	laryng/itis	inflammation of the voice box
latero- (al)	side	ambi/lateral	both sides
-lepsy	seizure, convulsion	narco/lepsy	sleep seizure
leuco, leuko-	white	leuko/cyte	white (blood) cell
lingu- (a, o)	tongue	lingu/al	pertaining to the tongue
lip- (o)	fat, lipids	lipo/cyte	fat cell
lith- (o)	stone, calculus	litho/tripsy	crushing a stone
-logy	study of, science of	bio/logy	study or science of life
lymph- (o)	lymph tissue	lymph/oma	tumor of lymph tissue
-lys (is, o)	destruction, dissolving of	thrombo/lysis	destruction or dissolving of clots
M			
macro-	large	macro/cyte	large cell
mal-	bad, abnormal, disordered, poor	mal/nutrition	poor nutrition
malac- (ia)	softening of a tissue	malac/ia	tissue softening
mamm- (o)	breast, mammary glands	mammo/gram	radiographic (X-ray) image of the breast
-mania	insanity, mental disorder	pyro/mania	individual with the insane desire to start fires
mast- (o)	breast	masto/pathy	disorder of the breast
med- (i, io)	middle, midline	medio/carpal	in the middle of or between the two rows of carpals (wrist bones)
-megaly, mega-	large, enlarged	cardio/megaly	enlarged heart
melan- (o)	black or dark	melan/oma	black or dark cancer
mening- (o)	membranes covering the brain and spinal cord	mening/itis	inflammation of the membranes of the brain and spinal cord

(continues)

TABLE 6-1 Word Parts *(continued)*

Word Part	Meaning	Medical Term	Meaning
meno-	monthly, menstruation	meno/rrhea	monthly flow or discharge
mes- (o)	middle, midline	meso/cephal/ic	condition of having a head of medium proportions
-meter	measuring instrument, measure	urino/meter	instrument to measure (specific gravity of) urine
-metry	measurement	audio/metry	measurement of hearing acuity
micro-	small	micro/scope	instrument to examine small things
mono-	one, single	mono/cyte	single cell
-mortem	death	post/mortem	after death
muc- (o, us)	mucus, secretion of mucous membrane	muco/static	stopping the secretion of mucus
multi-	many, much, a large amount	multi/para	woman who has borne more than one child
my- (o)	muscle	my/algia	muscle pain
myc- (o)	fungus	myco/cide	substance that kills fungus
myel- (o)	bone marrow, spinal cord	myelo/blast	bone marrow cell
myring- (o)	eardrum, tympanic membrane	myring/otomy	cutting into the eardrum
N			
narc- (o)	sleep, numb, stupor	narco/lepsy	sleep seizure
nas- (o)	nose	nas/al	pertaining to the nose
-natal	birth	pre/natal	before birth
necr- (o)	death	necr/osis	condition or process of death
neo-	new	neo/natal	newborn (infant)
neph- (r, ro)	kidney	nephro/lith	kidney stone
neur- (o)	nerve, nervous system	neur/algia	nerve pain
noct- (i)	night, at night	noct/uria	urination at night
non-	no, none	non/toxic	not poison
O			
ocul- (o)	eye	oculo/graph	machine to measure eye (movement)
odont- (o)	tooth	odont/algia	pain in a tooth, toothache
olig- (o)	few, less than normal, small	olig/uria	less than normal (amounts of) urine
-ologist	person who does/studies	radi/ologist	person who studies radiographs
-ology	study of, science of	hemat/ology	study of blood
-oma	tumor, a swelling	carcin/oma	cancerous tumor
onco- (i)	mass, bulk, tumor	oncol/ogist	physician who studies cancer
oophor- (o)	ovary, female egg cell	oophor/ectomy	surgical removal of the ovaries
ophthalm- (o)	eye	ophthalmo/scope	instrument for examining the eye
-opia	vision	dipl/opia	double vision
-opsy	to view	aut/opsy	view internal organs of a dead person
opt- (ic)	vision, eye	optic/al	pertaining to the eye
or- (o)	mouth	or/al	pertaining to the mouth
orch- (ido)	testicle, testes	orch/itis	inflammation of a testis
-orrhea	flow, discharge	rhin/orrhea	flow or discharge from the nose
orth- (o)	normal, straight	ortho/dontics	branch of dentistry involved with aligning or straightening the teeth
ost- (e, eo)	bone	osteo/genesis	formation of bone
-oscopy	diagnostic examination	colon/oscopy	diagnostic examination of the colon or large intestine
-osis	condition, state, process	necr/osis	condition or process of death
ot- (o)	ear	oto/scope	instrument for examining the ear
-otic	pertaining to a condition	leuko/cyt/otic	condition of white blood cells

(continues)

TABLE 6-1 Word Parts *(continued)*

Word Part	Meaning	Medical Term	Meaning
-otomy	cutting into	crani/otomy	cutting into the skull
-ous	full of, containing, pertaining to, condition	ven/ous	pertaining to a vein
ovi-, ovario-	egg, female sex gland, ovary	ovari/ectomy	surgical removal of an ovary
P			
pan-	all, complete, entire	pan/arter/itis	inflammation of all layers of an artery
pancreat- (o)	pancreas	pancreat/itis	inflammation of the pancreas
para-	near, beside, beyond, abnormal, lower half of the body	para/plegia	paralysis of the lower half of the body
paresis	paralysis	hemi/paresis	paralysis on one side of the body
-partum	birth, labor	post/partum	after birth
path- (ia, o, y)	disease, abnormal condition	path/ology	study of disease
ped- (ia)	child	pedia/tric	pertaining to children
-penia	lack of, abnormal reduction in number, deficiency	erythro/cyto/penia	deficiency of red blood cells
pent- (a)	five	penta/dactyl	having five digits (fingers or toes)
-pepsia, -pepsis	digestion	dys/pepsia	difficult digestion (indigestion)
per-	through, by, excessive	per/axillary	through the axilla or armpit
peri-	around	peri/cardi/al	pertaining to area around the heart
-pexy	fixation	gastro/pexy	surgical operation in which the stomach is sutured or fixed to the abdominal wall
phag- (o)	eat, ingest	phago/cyt/osis	process of cells ingesting and destroying microorganisms
-phage, -phagia	to eat, consuming, swallow	dys/phagia	difficult or painful swallowing
pharyng- (o)	pharynx, throat	pharyng/itis	inflammation of the throat or pharynx
-phas, -phasia	speech	a/phasia	without speech
-philia, -philic	affinity for, attracted to	necro/philia	attracted to or unusual interest in death
phleb- (o)	vein	phleb/otomy	cutting into a vein
-phobia	fear	hydro/phobia	fear of water
phon- (o)	sound, voice	phon/asthenia	weakness or hoarseness of the voice
-phylaxis	protection, prevention	pro/phylaxis	for prevention
-plasty	surgical correction or repair	chondro/plasty	surgical repair of cartilage
-plegia	paralysis	hemi/plegia	paralysis of half of the body
pleuro-	side, rib	pleur/itis	inflammation of the pleural membranes lining the side of the thorax
-pnea	breathing	a/pnea	without breathing
pneum- (o, on)	lung, pertaining to the lungs, air	pneumon/ectomy	surgical removal of a lung (or part of a lung)
pod- (e, o)	foot	pod/algia	foot pain
-poiesis	forming, producing, to make	hemo-poiesis	the formation of blood cells
poly-	many, much	poly/uria	much urine (more than normal amounts)
post-	after, behind	post/operative	after an operation
pre-	before, in front of	pre/operative	before an operation
pro-	in front of, forward	pro/cephalic	in front of the head
proct- (o)	rectum, rectal, anus	procto/scope	instrument for examining the rectum
prostat- (o)	prostate gland	Prostat/ectomy	surgical removal of the prostate gland
pseudo-	false	pseudo/appendic/ itis	false inflammation of the appendix
psych- (i, o)	pertaining to the mind	psych/ology	study of the mind
-ptosis	drooping down, sagging, downward displacement	viscero/ptosis	drooping down or displacement of internal organs

(continues)

TABLE 6-1 Word Parts *(continued)*

Word Part	Meaning	Medical Term	Meaning
pulmon- (o)	lung	pulmon/ologist	person who studies the lungs
py- (o)	pus	pyo/genic	producing pus
pyel- (o)	renal pelvis of kidney	pyelo/lith/otomy	surgical incision of the renal pelvis to remove a stone
pyr- (o)	heat, fever	pyro/genic	produced by a fever
Q			
quad- (ra, ri)	four	quadra/plegia	paralysis of four extremities (arms and legs)
R			
radi- (o)	radiographs (X-rays), radiation	radi/ologist	person who studies radiographs
rect- (o)	rectum	recto/cele	rupture of the rectum
ren- (o)	kidney	ren/al	pertaining to the kidney
retro-	backward, in back, behind	retro/lingual	occurring behind or near the base of the tongue
rhin- (o)	nose, pertaining to the nose	rhino/plasty	surgical correction of the nose
-rrhagia	sudden or excessive flow	rhino/rrhagia	sudden flow from the nose (nosebleed)
-rrhaphy	suture of, sewing up of a gap or defect	angio/rrhaphy	sewing (suturing) a gap or defect in a vessel
-rrhea	flow, discharge	meno/rrhea	monthly flow or discharge
-rrhexis	rupture of, bursting	hystero/rrhexis	rupture of the uterus
S			
salping- (i, o)	tube, fallopian tube	salping/ectomy	surgical removal of a fallopian tube
sanguin- (o)	blood	sanguino/purulant	containing blood and pus
sarc- (o)	malignant (cancer) connective tissue	sarc/oma	cancerous tumor of connective tissue
-sarcoma	tumor, cancer	adeno/sarcoma	cancerous tumor of a gland
scler- (o)	hardening	sclero/derma	thickening or hardening of the skin
-sclerosis	dryness or hardness	arterio/sclerosis	hardness of an artery
-scope	examining instrument	oto/scope	instrument for examining the ear
-scopy	observation	procto/scopy	examination of the rectum
-sect	cut	bi/sect	to cut into two parts
semi-	half, part	semi/cartilagin/ous	partly of cartilage
sep- (ti, tic)	poison, rot, infection	septic/emia	blood infection
sinistr- (o)	left	sinistr/ocular	left eye
soma- (t, to)	body	somato/genic	originating in the body
son- (o)	sound	sono/gram	an image produced by sound waves
-spasm	involuntary contraction	myo/spasm	contraction of muscle
sperm- (ato)	spermatozoa, male germ (sex) cell	spermat/uria	discharge of sperm in the urine
splen- (o)	spleen	spleno/megaly	abnormal enlargement of the spleen
-stasis	stoppage, maintaining a constant level	homeo/stasis	maintaining the same constant level
steno-	contracted, narrow	steno/sis	condition of narrowing
stern- (o)	sternum, breast bone	sterno/cost/al	pertaining to the ribs and breastbone (sternum)
stoma- (t)	mouth	stomat/ology	scientific study of the mouth and its disorders
-stomy	artificial opening	colo/stomy	creating an opening into the colon or large intestines
sub-	less, under, below	sub/lingual	under the tongue
sup- (er, ra)	above, upon, over, higher in position	supra/thorac/ic	pertaining to the area in the upper part of the chest
sym-, syn-	joined, fused, together	syn/dactyl	two or more digits (fingers or toes) joined together
T			
tach- (o, y)	rapid, fast	tachy/cardia	fast or rapid heart
ten- (do, don, o)	tendon	tendon/itis	inflammation of a tendon
tetra-	four	tetra/paresis	weakness or paralysis of all four limbs

(continues)

TABLE 6-1 Word Parts *(continued)*

Word Part	Meaning	Medical Term	Meaning
-therapy	treatment	chemo/therapy	treatment with drugs or chemicals
therm- (o, y)	heat	therm/algesia	sensitive to heat
thorac- (o)	thorax, chest	thorac/otomy	cutting into the chest
thromb- (o)	clot, thrombus	thrombo/lysis	dissolving or destruction of clots
thym- (o)	thymus gland	thym/oma	tumor of the thymus gland
thyr- (o, oid)	thyroid gland	thyroid/ologist	individual who studies the thyroid gland
-tome	instrument that cuts	myo/tome	instrument for cutting muscle
-tox (ic)	poison	cyto/toxic	cell poison
trach- (e, i, o)	trachea, windpipe	trache/otomy	cutting into the trachea or windpipe
trans-	across, over, beyond	trans/neural	across a nerve
tri-	three	tri/angle	three angles
trich- (o)	hair	tricho/myo/sis	fungus disease of the hair
-trips (y)	crushing by rubbing or grinding	litho/tripsy	crushing of stone
-trophy	nutrition, growth, development	a/trophy	without nutrition (wasting away)
tympan- (o)	eardrum, tympanic membrane	tympan/itis	inflammation of the eardrum (tympanic membrane)
U			
ultra-	beyond, excess	ultra/sonic	beyond sound waves
uni-	one	uni/ocular	one eye
ur- (in, o)	urine, urinary tract	urino/meter	instrument to measure (specific gravity) urine
ureter- (o)	ureter (tube from kidney to bladder)	uretero/cele	dilation of the ureter into the bladder
urethr- (o)	urethra (tube from bladder to urinary meatus)	urethro/scope	instrument to view the urethra
-uria	urine	hemat/uria	blood in urine
uter- (o)	uterus, womb	utero/vaginal	pertaining to the uterus and vagina
V			
vas- (o)	vessel, duct	vaso/neur/otic	pertaining to blood vessels and nerves
vascul- (o)	blood vessel	vascul-itis	inflammation of a blood vessel
ven- (a)	vein	ven/ous	pertaining to vein
ventro-	to the front, abdomen	ventr/al	pertaining to the front
vertebr- (o)	spine, vertebrae	vertebr/al	pertaining to the spine or vertebrae
vesic- (o)	urinary bladder	vesico/urethral	connecting the urinary bladder and urethra
viscer- (o)	internal organs	viscero/ptosis	drooping or displacement of internal organs
vit- (a)	necessary for life	vit/al	important to life
X			
xanth- (o)	yellow	xantho/derma	yellowish discoloration of the skin
xeno-	strange, abnormal, foreign	xeno/genetic	derived or originating from a foreign species
xer- (o)	dry	xero/derma	dry skin
Z			
zoo-	animal	zo/ology	study of animals
zymo-	enzymes	zymo/gram	picture or tracing of enzymes

check**point**

1. Replace the words in italics with the correct medical term.

Sally has a *fast heart rate* and *fast respiration rate,* and her skin is *blue*. Her lungs are clear, but she is complaining of cranial pain. She feels like she is going to vomit from the pain. Sally is

1 day *after* a *surgical fixation of her nose*. Her doctor recommends *slow breathing* and aspirin.

PRACTICE: Go to the workbook and complete the assignment and evaluation sheets for 6:1, Interpreting Word Parts.

6:2 USING MEDICAL ABBREVIATIONS

Abbreviations are shortened forms of words, usually just letters. Common examples are AM, which means morning, and PM, which means afternoon or evening.

Abbreviations are used in all health care careers. Sometimes they are used by themselves. At other times, several abbreviations are combined to give orders or directions. Consider the following examples:

BR c BRP, FFl qh, VS qid

NPO 8 pm, To Lab for CBC, BUN, and FBS

These examples are short forms for giving directions. The first example is interpreted as follows: bedrest with bathroom privileges, force fluids every hour, vital signs four times a day. The second example is interpreted as follows: nothing by mouth after eight o'clock in the evening, to the laboratory for a complete blood count, blood urea nitrogen, and fasting blood sugar. As these examples illustrate, it is much easier to write using abbreviations than it is to write the corresponding detailed messages.

Table 6-2 contains some of the most commonly used abbreviations. Look at the sample prescription form shown in **Figure 6–3**. Use the table to determine what the prescription says. Different abbreviations may be used in different facilities and in different parts of the country. It is the responsibility of health care providers to learn the meanings of the abbreviations used in the agencies where they are employed.

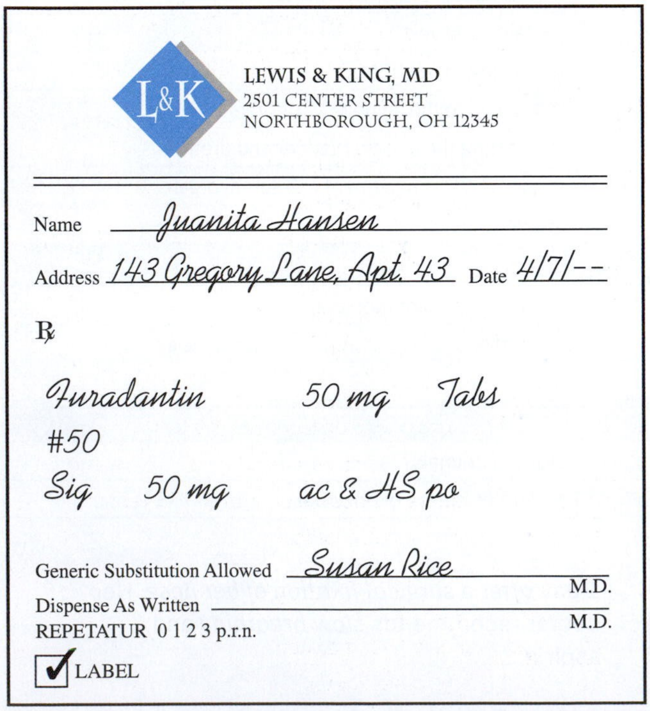

Some agencies are prohibiting the use of specific abbreviations or symbols because they are prone to causing errors. The Joint Commission has adopted an official *Do Not Use* list containing abbreviations and symbols that cause problems. Some common examples include:

- **IU**: abbreviation for international unit; can be mistaken for IV (intravenous) or the number 10; write out "international unit"

- **U or u**: abbreviation for unit; can be mistaken for o (zero), the number 4, or cc; write out "unit"

- **qd, qod,**: abbreviations for every day and every other day, respectively; can be interchanged if written poorly; for example, an every other day order could be done every day; write out "daily" or "every other day"

- **Lack of leading zero (.5 mg)**: decimal point is missed and 10 times the dose is given (5 mg instead of .5 mg); write "0.5 mg" or "0.X mg"

- **Trailing zero (2.0 mg)**: decimal point is missed and 10 times the dose is given (20 milligrams instead of 2 milligrams); write "2 mg" or "X mg"

- **MS**: can mean morphine sulfate or magnesium sulfate; write "morphine sulfate" or "magnesium sulfate"

- **Apothecary unit symbols such as ʒ or ℥**: symbols for dram and ounce; easily mistaken for each other; write "dram" or "ounce" or use metric units

NOTE: *In Table 6-2 these abbreviations and symbols are included because they are still used in some health facilities, especially in computerized electronic records. Because the letters are not written on the records, the chance of error decreases. It is still safer to spell out the words to avoid medical errors. On the lists that follow, an asterisk (*) has been placed in front of the abbreviation or symbol to alert the user that it is on the Do Not Use list.*

Health care team members must use only the abbreviations or symbols approved by the facility in which they are employed. In addition, extreme care must be used while writing abbreviations and symbols so they are legible and readily understood. It is also important to note that texting abbreviations are not allowed on legal documents in a health care facility. For example, b4 is not acceptable for "before" and UR is not acceptable for "you are."

NOTE: *There is a growing trend toward eliminating periods from most abbreviations. Although the table does not show periods, you may work in an agency that chooses to use them. When in doubt, follow the policy of your agency.*

LEWIS & KING, MD
2501 CENTER STREET
NORTHBOROUGH, OH 12345

Name _Juanita Hansen_

Address _143 Gregory Lane, Apt. 43_ Date _4/7/--_

℞

Furadantin   50 mg   Tabs

#50

Sig   50 mg   ac & HS po

Generic Substitution Allowed _Susan Rice_   M.D.

Dispense As Written _____ M.D.

REPETATUR 0 1 2 3 p.r.n.

☑ LABEL

FIGURE 6–3 Can you use the list of abbreviations to interpret the prescription?

TABLE 6-2 Abbreviations

A

@	at
ā	before
A&D	admission and discharge
A&P	anterior and posterior, anatomy and physiology
āā	of each
Ab	abortion
abd	abdomen, abdominal
ABG	arterial blood gas
ABX	antibiotics
ac	before meals
ACLS	advanced cardiac life support
ACTH	adrenocorticotropic hormone
AD	right ear
ADH	antidiuretic hormone
ADHD	attention deficit hyperactivity disorder
ad lib	as desired
ADL	activities of daily living
adm	admission
AED	automated external defibrillation
AHA	American Hospital Association
AIDS	acquired immune deficiency syndrome
AL	assisted living
am, AM	morning, before noon
AMA	American Medical Association, against medical advice
amal	amalgam
amb	ambulate, walk
amt	amount
ANA	American Nurses' Association
ANP	advanced nurse practitioner
ANS	autonomic nervous system
ant	anterior
AP	apical pulse
approx	approximately
aq, aqua	aqueous (water base)
ARC	AIDS-related complex
ARF	acute renal failure
AROM	active range of motion
ART	accredited records technician
AS	left ear
as tol	as tolerated
ASA	aspirin (acetylsalicylic acid)
ASAP	as soon as possible
ASCVD	arteriosclerotic cardiovascular disease
ASHD	arteriosclerotic heart disease
AU	both ears
AV	arteriovenous, atrioventricular
Ax	axilla, axillary, armpit

B

bac	bacteriology
B&B	bowel and bladder training
BBB	bundle branch block
BBS	bilateral breath sounds
BE	barium enema
bid	twice a day
bil	bilateral
Bl	blood
Bl Wk	blood work
BM	bowel movement, bone marrow
BMI	body mass index
BMR	basal metabolic rate
BP	blood pressure
BPH	benign prostatic hypertrophy
BR	bed rest
BRP	bathroom privileges
BS	blood sugar
BSA	body surface area
BSC, bsc	bedside commode
BSE	breast self-examination
BUN	blood urea nitrogen
Bx, bx	biopsy

C

°C	degrees Celsius (Centigrade)
c̄, W/	with
Ca	calcium
CA	cancer
CABG	coronary artery bypass graft
CAD	coronary artery disease
cal	calorie
Cap	capsule
CAT	computerized axial tomography
Cath	catheter, catheterize
CBC	complete blood count
CBET	certified biomedical equipment technician
CBR	complete bed rest
cc	cubic centimeter
CC	chief complaint
CCU	coronary care unit, critical care unit
CDA	certified dental assistant
CDC	Centers for Disease Control and Prevention
CEO	chief executive officer
CEU	continuing education unit
CF	cystic fibrosis
CHD	coronary heart disease
CHF	congestive heart failure
CHO	carbohydrate
chol	cholesterol

(continues)

TABLE 6-2 Abbreviations *(continued)*

CICU	cardiac/coronary intensive care unit
ck	check
Cl	chloride or chlorine
cl liq	clear liquids
cm	centimeter
CMA	certified medical assistant
CMP	comprehensive metabolic panel
CNP	certified nurse practitioner
CNS	central nervous system
co, c/o	complains of
CO	carbon monoxide, coronary occlusion
CO_2	carbon dioxide
Comp	complete, compound
cont	continued
COPD	chronic obstructive pulmonary disease
COTA	certified occupational therapy assistant
CP	cerebral palsy
CPAP	continuous (constant) positive airway pressure
CPK	creatine phosphokinase (cardiac enzyme)
CPR	cardiopulmonary resuscitation
CPT	current procedure terminology
CRTT	certified respiratory therapy technician
CS	central supply or service
C&S	culture and sensitivity
CSF	cerebrospinal fluid
CSR	central supply room
CST	certified surgical technologist
CT	computerized tomography
CVA	cerebral vascular accident (stroke)
CVD	cardiovascular disease
Cx	cervix, complication, complaint
CXR	chest X-ray or radiograph
D	
d	day
D&C	dilatation and curettage
DA	dental assistant
DAT	diet as tolerated
DC	Doctor of Chiropractic
D/C, dc, disc	discontinue, discharge
DDS	Doctor of Dental Surgery
DEA	Drug Enforcement Agency
del	delivery
Dept	department
DH	dental hygienist
DHHS	Department of Health and Human Services
Diff	differential white blood cell count
dil	dilute, dissolve
DM	diabetes mellitus

DMD	Doctor of Dental Medicine
DMS	diagnostic medical sonography
DNA	deoxyribonucleic acid
DNR	do not resuscitate
DO	Doctor of Osteopathic Medicine
DOA	dead on arrival
DOB	date of birth
DOD	date of death
DON	director of nursing
DPM	Doctor of Podiatric Medicine
DPT	diphtheria, pertussis, tetanus
Dr	doctor
dr	dram, drainage
DRG	diagnostic related group
drg, drsg, dsg	dressing
D/S	dextrose in saline
DSD	dry sterile dressing
DTs	delirium tremors
DVM	Doctor of Veterinary Medicine
DVT	deep vein thrombosis
DW	distilled water
D/W	dextrose in water
Dx, dx	diagnosis
E	
EBL	estimated blood loss
ECG, EKG	electrocardiogram
ED	emergency department
EEG	electroencephalogram
EENT	ear, eye, nose, throat
EHR	electronic health record
elix	elixir
EMG	electromyogram
EMR	electronic medical record
EMS	emergency medical services
EMT	emergency medical technician
ENT	ear, nose, throat
EPA	Environmental Protection Agency
ER	emergency room
ESR	erythrocyte sedimentation rate
et, etiol	etiology (cause of disease)
ETT	endotracheal tube
Ex, exam	examination
Exc	excision
Exp	exploratory, expiration
ext	extract, extraction, external
F	
°F	degrees Fahrenheit
FAS	fetal alcohol syndrome
FBS	fasting blood sugar

(continues)

TABLE 6-2 Abbreviations *(continued)*

FBW	fasting blood work
FDA	Food and Drug Administration
Fe	iron
FF, FFl	force fluids
FH	family history
FHR	fetal heart rate
Fl. fl	fluid
FSH	follicle-stimulating hormone
ft	foot
FUO	fever of unknown origin
Fx, Fr	fracture
G	
GA	gastric analysis, general anesthesia
gal	gallon
GB	gallbladder
Gc	gonococcus, gonorrhea
GERD	gastroesophageal reflux disease
GH	growth hormone
GI	gastrointestinal
Gm, g	gram
GP	general practitioner
gr	grain
gtt, gtts	drop, drops
GTT	glucose tolerance test
GU	genitourinary
Gyn	gynecology
H	
H	hydrogen
H&H	hemoglobin and hematocrit
HA	headache, hearing aid
HAI	health care associated infections
H_2O	water
H_2O_2	hydrogen peroxide
HBP	high blood pressure
HBV	hepatitis B virus
HCG	human chorionic gonadotrophin hormone
HCl	hydrochloric acid
hct	hematocrit
HCV	hepatitis C virus
HDL	high-density lipoproteins (healthy type of cholesterol)
Hg	mercury
Hgb, Hb	hemoglobin
HHA	home health assistant/aide
HIE	health information exchange
HIPAA	Health Insurance Portability and Accountability Act
HIV	human immunodeficiency virus (AIDS virus)
HMO	health maintenance organization
HOB	head of bed

HOH	hard of hearing
H&P	history and physical
Hr, hr, H, h	hour, hours
HRT	hormone replacement therapy
HS	hour of sleep (bedtime)
Ht	height
Hx, hx	history
Hyst	hysterectomy
I	
I&D	incision and drainage
I&O	intake and output
ICCU	intensive coronary care unit
ICD	international classification of diseases
ICU	intensive care unit
ID	intradermal, infectious disease
IDDM	insulin-dependent diabetes mellitus
IM	intramuscular
imp	impression
in	inch
inf	infusion, inferior, infection
ing	inguinal
inj	injection
int	internal, interior
IPPB	intermittent positive pressure breathing
irr, irrig	irrigation
Isol, isol	isolation
IT	inhalation therapy
IUD	intrauterine device
IV	intravenous
IVP	intravenous pyelogram
J	
jt	joint
K	
K	potassium
KCl	potassium chloride
Kg, kg	kilogram
KUB	kidney, ureter, bladder X-ray
KVO	keep vein open
L	
L	liter (1,000 milliliters or mL); lumbar
(L), lt, lft	left
L&D	labor and delivery
Lab	laboratory
Lap	laparotomy
lat	lateral
lb	pound
LDH	lactate dehydrogenase (cardiac enzyme)
LDL	low-density lipoprotein (unhealthy type of cholesterol)
lg	large

(continues)

TABLE 6-2 Abbreviations *(continued)*

liq	liquid
LLQ	left lower quadrant
LMP	last menstrual period
LOC	level of consciousness
LP	lumbar puncture
LPN	licensed practical nurse
LS	lumbar sacral
LTAC	long-term assisted care
LTC	long-term care
LUQ	left upper quadrant
LVN	licensed vocational nurse
M	
m	minim
MA	medical assistant
Mat	maternity
mcg	microgram
MD	Medical Doctor, muscular dystrophy, myocardial disease
Med	medical, medicine
mEq	milliequivalent
mg	milligram
Mg	magnesium
MI	myocardial infarction (heart attack)
MICU	medical intensive care unit
min	minute
mL	milliliter
MLT	medical laboratory technician
mm	millimeter
MN	midnight
mod	moderate
MOM	milk of magnesia
MRI	magnetic resonance imaging
MRSA	methicillin-resistant *Staphylococcus aureus*
MS	multiple sclerosis, mitral stenosis, muscular-skeletal
MT	medical technologist
MVA, MVC	motor vehicle accident or collision
N	
N	nitrogen
N/A	not applicable
Na	sodium
NA	nurse aide/assistant
NaCl	sodium chloride (salt)
NB	newborn
N/C	no complaints
neg	negative, none
Neur	neurology
NG, ng, N/G	nasogastric tube
NICU	neurological intensive care unit, neonatal intensive care unit

NIDDM	non-insulin-dependent diabetes mellitus
NIH	National Institutes of Health
NKA	no known allergies
NKDA	no known drug allergies
NO	nursing office
noc, noct	at night, night
NP	nurse practitioner
NPO	nothing by mouth
N/S, NS	normal saline, neurosurgery
NSAIDs	nonsteroidal anti-inflammatory drugs
N/V, N&V	nausea and vomiting
NVD	nausea, vomiting, diarrhea
NVS	neurological vital signs
O	
O_2	oxygen
O&P	ova and parasites
Ob, Obs	obstetrics
OBRA	Omnibus Budget Reconciliation Act
od	overdose
OD	right eye, occular dextra, Doctor of Optometry
oint	ointment
OOB	out of bed
OP	outpatient
OPD, OPC	outpatient department or clinic
opp	opposite
OR	operating room
Ord	orderly
Orth	orthopedics
os	mouth
OS	left eye, occular sinistra
OSHA	Occupational Safety and Health Administration
OT	occupational therapy/therapist
OTC	over the counter
OU	both eyes
OV	office visit
oz	ounce
P	
p̄	after
P	pulse, phosphorus
PA	physician's assistant
PAC	premature atrial contraction
PACU	post anesthesia care unit
PAP	Papanicolaou test (smear)
para	number of pregnancies
Path	pathology
Pb	lead
PBI	protein-bound iodine
pc	after meals
PCA	patient-controlled analgesia

(continues)

TABLE 6-2 Abbreviations *(continued)*

PCC	poison control center
PCP	patient care plan
PCT	patient/personal care technician
PDR	*Physicians' Desk Reference*
PE	physical examination, pulmonary edema, pulmonary embolism
Peds	pediatrics
per	by, through
PET	positron emission tomography
pH	measure of acidity/alkalinity
Pharm	pharmacy
PI	present illness
PID	pelvic inflammatory disease
PKU	phenylketonuria
PM, pm	after noon
PMC	postmortem (afterdeath) care
PMS	premenstrual syndrome
PNS	peripheral nervous system
po	by mouth
PO	phone order
post	posterior, after
post-op	after an operation
PP	postpartum (after delivery)
PPE	personal protective equipment
PPO	preferred provider organization
pre-op	before an operation
prep	prepare
prn	whenever necessary, as needed
PROM	passive range of motion
Psy	psychology, psychiatry
pt	patient, pint (500 mL or cc)
Pt	prothrombin time
PT	physical therapy/therapist
PTT	partial thromboplastin time
PVC	premature ventricular contraction
PVD	peripheral vascular disease
Px	prognosis, physical examination
Q	
q, q̄	every
*qd	every day
qh	every hour
q2h	every 2 hours
q3h	every 3 hours
q4h	every 4 hours
qhs	every night at bedtime
*qid	four times a day
qns	quantity not sufficient
*qod	every other day
qol	quality of life

qs	quantity sufficient
qt	quart
R	
R	respiration, rectal
®, Rt	right
Ra	radium
RBC	red blood cell
RDA	recommended daily allowance
REM	rapid eye movement
RHD	rheumatic heart disease
RICE	rest, ice, compression, and elevation
RLQ	right lower quadrant
RN	registered nurse
RNA	ribonucleic acid
R/O	rule out
RO	reality orientation
ROM	range of motion
RR	recovery room, respiratory rate
RRT	registered respiratory therapist, registered radiologic technologist
RT	respiratory therapy/therapist
RUQ	right upper quadrant
Rx	prescription, take, treatment
S	
s	sacral
s̄, w/o	without
SA	sinoatrial
sc, SC	subcutaneous
SCD	sequential compression device
SGOT, SGPT	transaminase test
SICU	surgical intensive care unit
SIDS	sudden infant death syndrome
Sig	give the following directions
sm	small
SNF	skilled nursing facility
SOB	short of breath
sol	solution
spec	specimen
SpGr, spgr	specific gravity
SPN	student practical nurse
S̄S̄	one-half
S/S, S&S	signs and symptoms
SSE	soap solution enema
staph	staphylococcus infection
stat	immediately, at once
STH	somatotropic hormone
STI	sexually transmitted infection
strep	streptococcus infection

(continues)

TABLE 6-2 Abbreviations *(continued)*

supp	suppository		Vol	volume
Surg	surgery, surgical		vp	venipuncture, venous pressure
susp	suspension		VS	vital signs (TPR & BP)
Sx	symptom, sign		VT	ventricular tachycardia
syp	syrup		**W**	
T			WBC	white blood cell
T&A	tonsillectomy and adenoidectomy		w/c	wheelchair
T, Temp	temperature		WHO	World Health Organization
tab	tablet		WNL	within normal limits
TB	tuberculosis		w/o, wo	without
tbsp	tablespoon		W/P	whirlpool
TCDB	turn, cough, deep breathe		wt	weight
TF	tube feeding		**X**	
TH	thyroid hormone		x	times (2x means do 2 times)
TIA	transient ischemic attack		x-match	cross-match
tid	three times a day		XR	X-ray
TKR	total knee replacement		**Y**	
TLC	tender loving care		y/o, yo	years old
TO	telephone order		YOB	year of birth
tol	tolerated		yr	year
TPN	total parenteral nutrition		YTD	year to date
TPR	temperature, pulse, respiration		**Z**	
tr, tinct	tincture		Zn	zinc
TSH	thyroid-stimulating hormone		**Miscellaneous Symbols**	
tsp	teaspoon		>	greater than
TUR	transurethral resection		<	less than
TWE	tap water enema		↑	higher, elevate, or up
tx	traction, treatment, transplant		↓	lower or down
U			#	pound or number foot or minute
UA, U/A	urinalysis		"	inch or second
Ur, ur	urine		°	degree
URI	upper respiratory infection		♀ or F	female
UTI	urinary tract infection		♂ or M	male
UV	ultraviolet		| or / or T	one
V			|| or // or It	two
Vag	vaginal		V	five
VD	venereal disease		X	ten
VDM	Veterinarian Degree of Medicine		L	fifty
VDRL	serology test for syphilis, Venereal Disease Research Laboratory		C	one hundred
VF	ventricular fibrillation		D	five hundred
VO	verbal order		M	one thousand

Learn the abbreviations in the following way:

- Use a set of index cards to make a set of flashcards of the abbreviations found on the abbreviation list. Print one abbreviation in big letters on each card. Put the abbreviation on the front of the card and the meaning on the back of the card.

- Use the flashcards to study the abbreviations. A realistic goal is to learn all abbreviations for one letter per week. For example, learn all of the *A*s the first week, all of the *B*s the second week, all of the *C*s the third week, and so on until all are learned.

- Follow your instructor's guidelines for tests on the abbreviations. Many instructors give weekly tests. The tests may be cumulative. They may cover the letter of the week plus any letters learned in previous weeks.

Opioids are substances that work in the nervous system of the body or in specific receptors in the brain to reduce the intensity of pain. In the late 1990s, pharmaceutical companies reassured the medical community that patients would not become addicted to opioid pain relievers and health care providers began to prescribe them at greater rates. Increased prescribing of opioid medications led to widespread misuse of both prescription and nonprescription opioids.

In 2017, HHS declared a public health emergency. Roughly 21 to 29 percent of patients prescribed opioids for chronic pain misuse them. Between 8 and 12 percent develop an opioid use disorder. Overdose deaths involving opioids,—including prescription opioids, heroin, and synthetic opioids (like fentanyl)—have increased almost six times since 1999. The crisis has left few untouched, with an average of 115 Americans dying every day from an opioid overdose. Many families are impacted by opioid use disorder, including pregnant women, resulting in rising numbers of infants being born with neonatal abstinence syndrome (NAS) and increased rates of maternal mortality. Children are experiencing trauma as a result of a parent or other family member's substance use disorder (SUD).

According to the American Academy of Pediatrics (AAP) in 2020, the combined members of the American Academy of Family Physicians, American Academy of Pediatrics, American College of Obstetricians and Gynecologists, American College of Physicians, American Osteopathic Association, and American Psychiatric Association joined in urging the country policymakers to address the opioid crisis based on these comprehensive ideas:

1. Align and improve financing incentives to ensure access to evidence-based opioid use disorder treatment. Research shows that medication and therapy together may be more effective than either treatment method alone. Medicare has no SUD treatment benefit. Growing research points to the benefits of keeping families together during treatment for a parent's SUD.

2. Reduce the administrative burden associated with providing patients with effective treatment. Streamline and standardize forms.

3. Incentivize more providers to treat SUD. A critical part of controlling the opioid crisis relates to ensuring an adequate supply of providers. This should include loan forgiveness for substance use and mental health service providers in underserved areas.

4. Advance research to support prevention and treatment of substance use disorders.

5. Address the maternal–child health impact of the opioid crisis. Overdose and suicide directly linked to the rise in the opioid crisis are now the leading cause of maternal mortality in a growing number of states. The rise in untreated opioid use disorder has also led to a troubling increase in newborns experiencing NAS. NAS is a treatable medical condition associated with drug withdrawal in newborns exposed chronically to opioids or other drugs in utero. Greater than one-third of the more than 270,000 children who entered foster care in FY 2016 did so at least in part because of parental substance use.

6. Reduce the stigma related to substance use disorders. Stigma should be addressed with a national prevention strategy, including a public awareness campaign to educate the public and health care providers about addiction as a chronic brain disease that can be effectively treated with evidence-based interventions. Experience with HIV, hepatitis, and other epidemics has demonstrated the capacity of the federal government, if leveraged properly, to raise public awareness.

In 2020, COVID-19 shattered the economy, and joblessness drove some people to addiction. One study found that every percentage point increase in a county's unemployment rate drove up the opioid death rate by 3.6%. To prevent an even more catastrophic rise in addiction and death due to high unemployment rates, the nation needs to rework the recovery networks. The recovery community has been quick to find ways to cope. Narcotics Anonymous and other groups have switched to online and video meetings. Counselors are seeing patients via telemedicine.

checkpoint

Interpret the paragraph below.
1. pt is admitted to a hospital with a dx of pancreatitis, dysphagia, and gastralgia. Sx include NVD and a severe HA. The Dr orders an abd MRI, CBC, NPO except for cl liq, VS q2h, and CBR.

Interpret all these medical abbreviations and terms to determine the patient's condition and plan of treatment.

PRACTICE: Go to the workbook and complete the assignment and evaluation sheets for 6:2, Using Medical Abbreviations.

CHAPTER 6 SUMMARY

- Medical terminology and abbreviations are used in all health care occupations and facilities.

- Medical terminology consists of the use of prefixes, suffixes, and word roots to create words.

- Eponyms—or terms named after people, places, or things—are also used in medical terminology.

- Medical abbreviations are shortened forms of words, usually just letters, that are used to give orders or directions.

REVIEW QUESTIONS

1. True or False
   a. A suffix is added to the beginning of a word root.
   b. "Hyper-" is an example of a prefix.
   c. You need to add the combining vowel when adding a prefix.
   d. You always use a combining vowel when combining two word roots.
   e. A combining form is used when the suffix begins with a consonant.

2. Combine these word parts to form the correct medical term:

   ophthalm/o + -pathy _____

   aden/o + -ectomy _____

   ot/o + -plasty _____

   neur/o + -tripsy _____

   neur/o -ectomy _____

   cardi/o + -ac _____

   gastr/o + enter/o + itis _____

   chir/o + -spasm _____

   hypo- + glyc/o + -emia _____

3. Choose five (5) word roots related to a part of the body. Add different prefixes and/or suffixes to the word root to create at least three (3) different terms for each body part. For example: *cystitis*, *cystoscopy*, and *cystocele.*

4. Identify the individuals or places for whom the following medical terms were named:
   a. Graves' disease
   b. Salk vaccine
   c. Achilles tendon

5. Determine the meaning of the abbreviations *bid*, *tid*, and *qid*. Find prefixes that define the first letters (b, t, and q) of the three abbreviations. Why are these three abbreviations easier to remember when you study them together? Determining associations similar to these will make it easier to learn medical abbreviations.

6. List 20 abbreviations for diagnostic tests, such as blood work or radiology studies.

7. Match each definition with the correct word part.
   a. abnormal hardening
   b. surgical incision
   c. bad, difficult, painful
   d. inflammation

   -itis   __-sclerosis

   -otomy   -algia

   __dys-____   -ostomy

8. Search publisher websites and online sources for medical terminology books and videos. Look for apps available for mobile devices. List two (2) books or videos and two (2) apps. Evaluate different methods of learning medical terminology as presented in these sources.

CRITICAL THINKING

1. Create a story integrating 20 of the medical terms from the week.

2. Using the Kahoot app, construct a game that will help you and your classmates recall the week's medical terms and abbreviations.

3. Research the position of medical scribe. Compose a paper; the first paragraph should be a brief job description. Then write an essay answering the question, "Why is knowledge of medical terminology and abbreviations essential information for a successful medical scribe to possess?" Conclude by naming five (5) different medical fields in which medical terminology skills would also be invaluable.

4. With a partner, interpret and transcribe the meaning for the medical words and conditions in the following case study. Utilize online resources to supplement terms from this book. Create an explanation that would communicate this medical information to the patient and caregivers who may not have an understanding of medical terms; utilize online video and image sources to help illustrate these medical conditions and treatments.

Ms. Mendoza is a 66-year-old obese female with five children. Her Hx is CHF, cardiomyopathy with cardialgia, hypertension, IDDM. She presented to the ER c/o chest pain, dyspnea, bilateral lower extremity edema, BP of 160/98 and was admitted to the hospital. Dr. Benson orders for Ms. Mendoza are 1200cal ADA low Na diet, accu checks ac and hs, activity BRP, AP q4h, monitor VS q2h for 8 h and then q4h, weigh now and in 12 hours.

ACTIVITIES

1. Write the week's medical terms on the board. Divide the class into two teams. The first person on each team gets a flyswatter and stands on a mark on the floor. The scorekeeper reads out a definition, and the two team members hit the corresponding medical term with the flyswatter. The team that gets there first gets a point, and the flyswatter is handed to the next team member.

2. Put medical terms on an inflatable beachball. Have the class form a circle. Toss the ball to each other. The "catcher" must define the term that is closest to their right thumb.

3. In pairs, have a race to see which team can translate the following medical notes first:

Jareed McNeil is a 10 yo African American male and presents to the clinic c/o emesis x 2 days. The RN takes the pt's VS and finds him to be febrile, tachycardic, and hypotensive. Upon taking Mr. McNeil's Hx, the RN finds that he is 6 days post-op tonsillectomy and adenoidectomy. The clinic's pt care tech puts a call in to the otolayngologist. A stat CBC and CMP are ordered and obtained while waiting for the Dr. to arrive. Based on the Hx, Px, S&S, and test results, the Dr. determines the pt has a post-op infection c̄ dehydration. The pt is to be admitted to the hospital for IV fluids and ABX. Jareed McNeil's prognosis is "good."

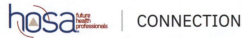 | CONNECTION

Competitive Event: Medical Terminology

Event Summary: Medical Terminology provides members with the opportunity to gain knowledge and skills regarding prefixes, suffixes, roots and anatomy, physiology, pathophysiology and occupations related to the health field. This competitive event consists of a written test and aims to inspire members to learn about terms common to health professions and health specialties.

Details on this competitive event may be found at www.hosa.org/guidelines

ANATOMY AND PHYSIOLOGY

Science

Case Study Investigation

Shanice is a 56-year-old woman who owns a successful bakery that is known for its delicious and beautiful cupcakes. She goes to the doctor because she is concerned about her frequent trips to the bathroom. Shanice states that she is working longer hours because the bakery is so busy, and she has noticed the increased urgency to urinate over the past year. In addition, Shanice drinks a lot more water during the day because she is extremely thirsty. Her physical exam is unremarkable except for a Body Mass Index (BMI) of 30. The score of 30 registers as obese. Tests were ordered which were within normal limits (WNL) except for what is identified in the following chart.

TEST	MARIE'S RESULT/VALUE	NORMAL VALUE
Random blood glucose	205 mg/dl	<140mg/dl
Fasting blood glucose	127 mg/dl	<100mg/dl
Hemoglobin A1c	7%	<5.7%

Shanice is prescribed a hypoglycemic medication, metformin. At the end of this chapter, you will be asked what Shanice's diagnosis is and what clues in this case lead you to this conclusion.

LEARNING OBJECTIVES

After completing this chapter, you should be able to:

- Apply the appropriate terminology to major organs and systems of the human body.
- Identify the major functions of each body system.
- Compare interrelationships of body systems.
- Describe basic diseases affecting each of the body systems.
- Define, pronounce, and spell all key terms.

KEY TERMS

anatomy

cell

cell membrane

centrosome *(sen'-troh-sohm)*

chromatin *(crow'-ma-tin)*

congenital

connective tissue

cytoplasm *(sy'-toe-plaz-um)*

degenerative

dehydration

diagnosis

edema *(eh-dee'-mah)*

endoplasmic reticulum *(en'-doeplaz-mik re-tik'-you-lum)*

epithelial tissue *(ep'-eh-thiel"-e-al tish'-u)*

etiology

genes

genome

Golgi apparatus *(gawl'-jee ap-a-rat'-us)*

homeostasis

infectious

inherited

lysosomes *(ly'-sah-soms)*

meiosis *(my-o'-sis)*

mitochondria *(my-toe-con'-dree-ah)*

mitosis *(my-toe'-sis)*

muscle tissue

nerve tissue

nucleolus *(new"-klee-oh'-lus)*

nucleus

organ

organelles

pathophysiology

physiology *(fizz-ee-all'-oh-gee)*

pinocytic vesicles

prognosis

protoplasm *(pro'-toe-plaz-um)*

stem cells

system

tissue

vacuoles

7:1 BASIC STRUCTURE OF THE HUMAN BODY

OBJECTIVES

After completing this section, you should be able to:

- Identify the six levels of body organization.
- Label a diagram of the main parts of a cell.
- Describe the basic function of the main parts of a cell.
- Compare the four main types of tissue by describing the basic function of each type.
- Explain the relationships among cells, tissues, organs, and systems.
- Define, pronounce, and spell all key terms.

INTRODUCTION

The human body is often described as an efficient, organized machine. When this machine does not function correctly, disease occurs. Before understanding the disease processes, however, the health care worker must first understand the normal functioning of the body. A basic understanding of anatomy and physiology is therefore necessary. **Anatomy** is the study of the form and structure of an organism. **Physiology** is the study of the processes of living organisms, or why and how they work. **Pathophysiology** is the study of how disease occurs and the responses of living organisms to disease processes.

Some different types of diseases include:

- **Congenital**: acquired during development of the infant in the uterus and existing at or dating from birth; examples include club foot, cleft lip and/or palate, fetal alcohol syndrome, and spina bifida
- **Inherited**: transmitted from parents to child genetically; examples include color blindness, hemophilia, cystic fibrosis, and Down syndrome
- **Infectious**: caused by a pathogenic (germ-producing) organism such as a bacteria or virus; examples include the common cold, hepatitis, and sexually transmitted infections
- **Degenerative**: caused by a deterioration of the function or structure of body tissues and organs either by normal body aging or lifestyle choices such as diet and exercise; examples include arteriosclerotic heart disease (ASHD), chronic obstructive pulmonary disease (COPD), and osteoarthritis

Other terms associated with disease include diagnosis, etiology, and prognosis. A **diagnosis** is identifying the disease or stating what it is. **Etiology** refers to the cause of the disease. At times, the etiology is known, such as influenza being caused by a virus. For some diseases, the cause is unknown, or *idiopathic*. When a disease is caused by a prescribed treatment the etiology is *iatrogenic*. Examples include anemia caused by chemotherapy or low potassium levels caused by diuretic medication. **Prognosis** refers to a prediction of the probable course and/or the expected outcome of the disease.

BODY ORGANIZATION

There are six levels of structures that make up body organization. They are chemical, cellular, tissue, organ, organ system, and, finally, the organism level.

Chemical Level

The chemical level consists of the simplest building blocks that make life possible—atoms. *Atoms* are the smallest unit of pure elements like hydrogen, oxygen, carbon, nitrogen, and calcium. Two or more atoms combine to form *molecules* like water, sugars, and protein. These molecules are found in all living things. Molecules are the chemical building blocks of all body structures. They combine to form organelles that form the functional units of life—cells. Molecules can also combine to form *compounds* via a chemical reaction. This reaction is called metabolism. All compounds are either

---

Related Health Careers

Note: A basic knowledge of human anatomy and physiology is essential for almost every health care provider. However, some health careers are related to specific body systems. As each body system is discussed, examples of related health careers are listed. The following health career categories require knowledge of the structure and function of the entire human body and will not be listed in specific body system units.

- Athletic trainer
- Emergency medical careers
- Medical laboratory careers
- Medical assistant
- Medical illustrator
- Nursing careers
- Pharmacy careers
- Physician
- Physician assistant
- Surgical technologist

Specific careers for cells and components of body tissues include:

- Biochemist
- Biologist
- Cytologist
- Forensic scientist
- Genetic engineer

organic (usually carbon and hydrogen) or inorganic (lipids, proteins, carbohydrates). Some compounds dissociate in water and become charged particles or *electrolytes*. For example, a salt solution contains two electrolytes, sodium, and chlorine. Hydrogen ion concentration within the body is called *pH*. pH is basic, acidic, or neutral. Keeping this chemical level in balance is an import part of **homeostasis**, which is a constant state of natural balance within the body.

Cellular Level

The basic substance of all life is **protoplasm**. This material makes up all living things. Although protoplasm is composed of ordinary elements such as carbon, oxygen, hydrogen, sulfur, nitrogen, and phosphorus, scientists are unable to combine such elements to create that characteristic called *life*.

Protoplasm forms the basic unit of structure and function in all living things: the **cell**. Cells are microscopic structures that carry on all the functions of life. They take in food and oxygen; produce heat and energy; move and adapt to their environment; eliminate wastes; perform special functions; and reproduce to create new, identical cells. The human body contains trillions of cells. These cells vary in shape and size, and they perform many different functions.

Most cells have the following basic parts (**Figure 7–1**):

- **Cell membrane**: the outer protective covering of the cell. It is also called the *plasma membrane*. It is semipermeable; that is, it allows certain substances to enter and leave the cell while preventing the passage of other substances. Three main transport mechanisms that allow this transfer of substances to help maintain homeostasis in the body include diffusion, osmosis, and filtration. *Diffusion* is a process

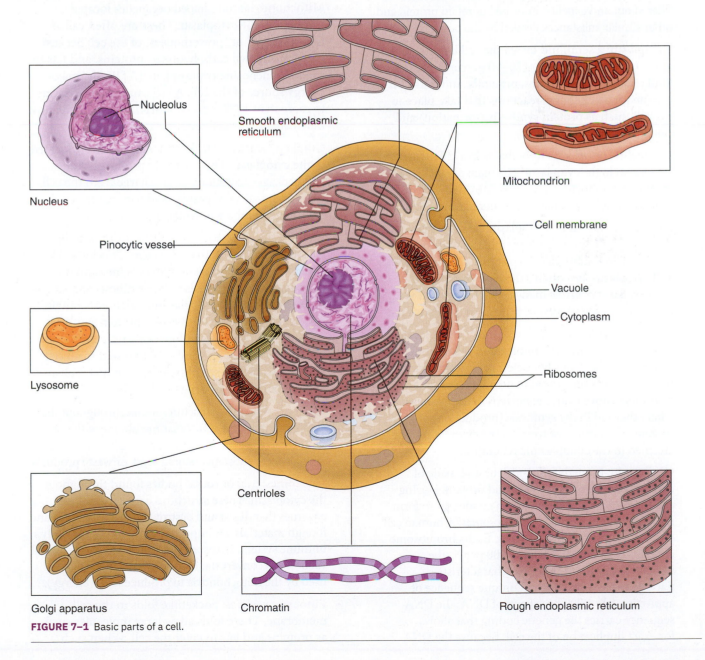

- Nucleolus
- Smooth endoplasmic reticulum
- Mitochondrion
- Nucleus
- Pinocytic vessel
- Cell membrane
- Vacuole
- Cytoplasm
- Lysosome
- Ribosomes
- Golgi apparatus
- Centrioles
- Chromatin
- Rough endoplasmic reticulum

FIGURE 7–1 Basic parts of a cell.

by which molecules of gas, liquids, and solids can pass through a membrane to equalize the concentration of the molecules on both sides of the membrane. Most molecules move from an area of greater concentration to an area of lower concentration. For example, diffusion allows oxygen in the blood to pass into the fluid around a cell and then into the cell itself, where it can be used for cell processes. *Osmosis* is the transfer of water or any solvent through the membrane from an area of higher concentration to an area of lower concentration to equalize the pressure on both sides of the membrane. An example is water entering a cell to neutralize the salt and mineral content that could cause cell damage. *Filtration* is the movement of water and solutes through a membrane as a result of mechanical force such as blood pressure or gravity. The type of membrane determines which molecules will be filtered. For example, the kidneys allow waste materials to be filtered out and expelled in urine but retain protein and other similar substances needed by the body.

- **Cytoplasm**: a semifluid inside the cell but outside the nucleus. It contains water (70–90 percent), proteins, lipids (fats), carbohydrates, minerals, and salts. It is the site for all chemical reactions that take place in the cell, such as protein synthesis (formation) and cellular respiration.

- **Organelles**: or cell structures that help a cell to function, are located in the cytoplasm. The main organelles are the nucleus, mitochondria, ribosomes, lysosomes, centrioles, Golgi apparatus, and endoplasmic reticulum.

- **Nucleus**: a mass in the cytoplasm. It is separated from the cytoplasm by a nuclear membrane that contains pores to allow substances to pass between the nucleus and cytoplasm. It is often called the "brain" of the cell because it controls many cell activities and is important in the process of mitosis or cell division.

- **Nucleolus**: one or more small, round bodies located inside the nucleus, and important in cell reproduction. Ribosomes, made of ribonucleic acid (RNA) and protein, are manufactured in the nucleolus. The ribosomes move from the nucleus to the cytoplasm, where they aid in the synthesis (production) of protein. They can exist freely in the cytoplasm or be attached to the endoplasmic reticulum.

- **Chromatin**: located in the nucleus and made of deoxyribonucleic acid (DNA) and protein. During cell reproduction, the chromatin condenses to form rod-like structures called *chromosomes*. A human cell has 46 chromosomes or 23 pairs. Each chromosome contains between 30,000 to 45,000 **genes**, the structures that carry inherited characteristics. Each gene has a specific and unique sequence of approximately 1,000 base pairs of DNA; the DNA sequence carries the genetic coding that allows for exact duplication of the cell. Because the DNA

sequence on genes is unique for each individual, it is sometimes used as an identification tool similar to fingerprints, but much more exact. A **genome** is the total mass of genetic instruction humans inherit from their parents. It consists of strings of DNA nucleotides. Human beings have about three billion nucleotides in their genome. The order of the nucleotides on the DNA sequences provides instructions for the body to build all of its parts, everything from permanent structures such as teeth and brain cells to short-lived substances such as blood and hormones.

- **Centrosome**: located in the cytoplasm and near the nucleus. It contains two centrioles. During mitosis, or cell division, the centrioles separate. Thin cytoplasmic spindle fibers form between the centrioles and attach to the chromosomes. This creates an even division of the chromosomes in the two new cells.

- **Mitochondria**: rod-shaped organelles located throughout the cytoplasm. These are often called the "furnaces" or "powerhouses" of the cell because they break down carbohydrates, proteins, and fats to produce adenosine triphosphate (ATP), the major energy source of the cell. A cell can contain just one to more than 1,000 mitochondria, depending on how much energy the cell requires.

- **Golgi apparatus**: a stack of membrane layers located in the cytoplasm. This structure produces, stores, and packages secretions for discharge from the cell. Cells of the salivary, gastric, and pancreatic glands have large numbers of Golgi apparatus.

- **Endoplasmic reticulum**: a fine network of tubular structures located in the cytoplasm. This network allows for the transport of materials into and out of the nucleus, and also aids in the synthesis and storage of proteins. Rough endoplasmic reticulum contains *ribosomes*, which are the sites for protein synthesis (production). Smooth endoplasmic reticulum does not contain ribosomes and is not present in all cells. It assists with cholesterol synthesis, fat metabolism, and detoxification of drugs.

- **Vacuoles**: pouchlike structures found throughout the cytoplasm that have a vacuolar membrane with the same structure as the cell membrane. They are filled with a watery substance, stored food, or waste products.

- **Lysosomes**: oval or round bodies found throughout the cytoplasm. These structures contain digestive enzymes that digest and destroy old cells, bacteria, and foreign materials, an important function of the body's immune system. Lysosomes also fuse with stored food vacuoles to convert the food to a form that can be used by the mitochondria to produce ATP (energy).

- **Pinocytic vesicles**: pocketlike folds in the cell membrane. These folds allow large molecules such as proteins and fats to enter the cell. When such molecules are inside the cell, the folds close to form vacuoles or bubbles in the cytoplasm. When the cell needs energy, the vesicles fuse with lysosomes to allow the proteins and fats to be digested and used by the mitochondria to produce ATP (energy).

CELL REPRODUCTION Most cells reproduce by dividing into two identical cells. This process is called **mitosis**, a form of asexual reproduction (**Figure 7–2**). Skin cells, blood-forming cells, and intestinal tract cells reproduce continuously. Muscle cells only reproduce

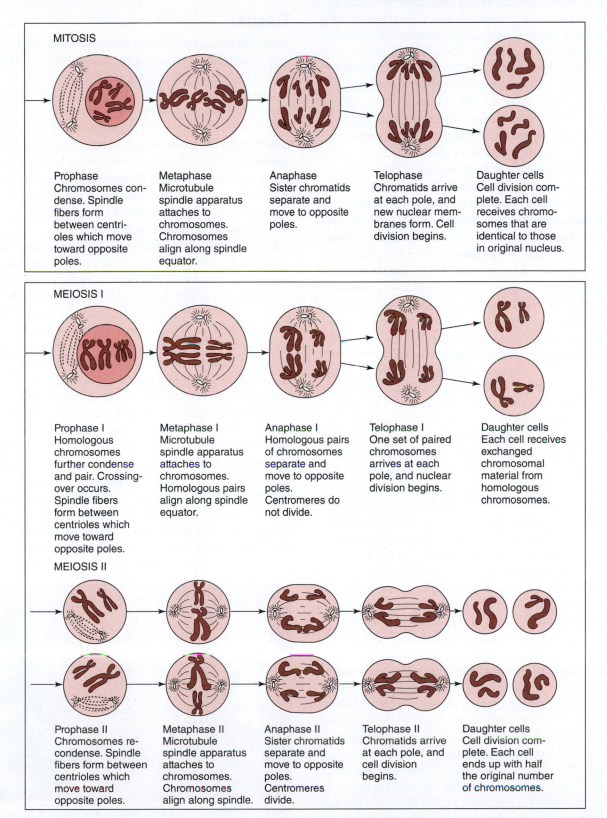

MITOSIS

Prophase
Chromosomes condense. Spindle fibers form between centrioles which move toward opposite poles.

Metaphase
Microtubule spindle apparatus attaches to chromosomes. Chromosomes align along spindle equator.

Anaphase
Sister chromatids separate and move to opposite poles.

Telophase
Chromatids arrive at each pole, and new nuclear membranes form. Cell division begins.

Daughter cells
Cell division complete. Each cell receives chromosomes that are identical to those in original nucleus.

MEIOSIS I

Prophase I
Homologous chromosomes further condense and pair. Crossing-over occurs. Spindle fibers form between centrioles which move toward opposite poles.

Metaphase I
Microtubule spindle apparatus attaches to chromosomes. Homologous pairs align along spindle equator.

Anaphase I
Homologous pairs of chromosomes separate and move to opposite poles. Centromeres do not divide.

Telophase I
One set of paired chromosomes arrives at each pole, and nuclear division begins.

Daughter cells
Each cell receives exchanged chromosomal material from homologous chromosomes.

MEIOSIS II

Prophase II
Chromosomes recondense. Spindle fibers form between centrioles which move toward opposite poles.

Metaphase II
Microtubule spindle apparatus attaches to chromosomes. Chromosomes align along spindle.

Anaphase II
Sister chromatids separate and move to opposite poles. Centromeres divide.

Telophase II
Chromatids arrive at each pole, and cell division begins.

Daughter cells
Cell division complete. Each cell ends up with half the original number of chromosomes.

FIGURE 7–2 Mitosis is a form of asexual reproduction where a cell divides into two identical cells. Meiosis is a process used by sex cells (gametes) to produce four new cells.

every few years, but muscle tissue can be enlarged with exercise. Some specialized cells, such as nerve cells in the brain and spinal cord, do not reproduce after birth. If these cells are damaged or destroyed, others are not formed to replace them.

Prior to mitosis, the chromatin material in the nucleus condenses to form chromosomes, and an exact duplicate of each chromosome is made. Each chromosome then consists of two identical strands, called *chromatids*, joined together by a structure called a *centromere*. When mitosis begins, the two centrioles in the centrosome move to opposite ends of the cell. A spindle of threadlike fibers trails from the centrioles. The nuclear membrane disappears, and the pairs of duplicated chromosomes attach to the spindles at the center of the cell. The chromatids then split from their duplicated halves and move to opposite ends of the cell. Each end now has 46 chromosomes, or 23 pairs. The cytoplasm divides, and a new cell membrane forms to create two new identical cells.

Sex cells (gametes) divide by a process known as **meiosis** (refer to Figure 7–2). This process uses two separate cell divisions to produce four new cells. When female cells (ova) or male cells (spermatozoa or sperm) divide by meiosis, the number of chromosomes is reduced to 23, or one-half the number found in cells created by mitosis. When an ovum and sperm join to create a new life, the zygote, or new cell, has 46 chromosomes: 23 from the ovum and 23 from the sperm. Thus, the zygote has 46 chromosomes, or 23 pairs, the normal number for all body cells except the sex cells.

Immediately after the ovum and sperm join to form a zygote, the zygote begins a period of rapid mitotic division. Within 4–5 days, the zygote is a hollow ball-like mass of cells called a *blastocyst*. Within this blastocyst are embryonic **stem cells**. These stem cells have the ability to transform themselves into any of the body's specialized cells and perform many different functions. A controversial area of research is now concentrated on these stem cells. Scientists are attempting to determine whether stem cells can be transplanted into the body and used to cure diseases such as diabetes mellitus, Parkinson's, heart disease, osteoporosis, arthritis, and spinal cord injuries. The hope is that the stem cells can be programmed to produce new specialized cells that can replace a body's damaged cells and cure a disease. The controversy arises from the fact that a 4–5-day-old embryo, capable of creating a new life, is used to obtain the cells. Right-to-life advocates are strongly opposed to stem cell research if the cells are obtained from embryos. Another source of stem cells is the blood in the discarded umbilical cord and placenta of a newborn. Currently, parents have the option of preserving this blood for its stem cells. The blood is collected and frozen in liquid nitrogen. If the child later develops a disease for which a stem cell transplant can provide a cure, the cells can be harvested from the blood and used for the transplant. The cost of this procedure limits its use, however. Stem cells also exist in adult tissues, such as bone marrow and the liver. Adult stem cells, however, do not have the ability to evolve into every kind of cell; these stem cells evolve into more cells of their own kind. This controversy will continue as scientists expand stem cell research.

Tissue

Although most cells contain the same basic parts, cells vary greatly in shape, size, and special function. When cells of the same type join together for a common purpose, they form a **tissue**. Tissues are 60–99 percent water with various dissolved substances. This water is slightly salty in nature and is called *tissue fluid*. If there is an insufficient amount (not enough tissue fluid), a condition called **dehydration** occurs. When there is an excess amount (too much tissue fluid), a condition called **edema**, or swelling of the tissues, occurs (**Figure 7–3**).

There are four main groups of tissues: epithelial, connective, nerve, and muscle (**Figure 7–4**).

Epithelial tissue covers the surface of the body and is the main tissue in the skin. It forms the lining of the intestinal, respiratory, circulatory, and urinary tracts, as well as that of other body cavities. Epithelial tissue also forms the body glands, where it specializes to produce specific secretions for the body, such as mucus and digestive juices.

Connective tissue is the supporting fabric of organs and other body parts. There are two main classes of connective tissue: soft and hard. One type of soft connective tissue is *adipose*, or fatty, tissue, which stores fat as a food reserve or source of energy, insulates the body, fills the area between tissue fibers, and acts as padding. A second type of soft connective tissue is *fibrous connective tissue*, such as ligaments and tendons, which help hold body structures together. Hard connective tissue includes cartilage and bone. Cartilage is a tough, elastic material that is found between the bones of the spine and at the end of long bones. It acts as a shock absorber and allows for flexibility. It is also found in the nose, ears, and

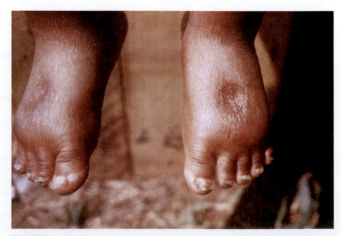

FIGURE 7–3 Edema is an excess amount of tissue fluid that causes swelling of the tissues. CDC/Dr. Lyle Conrad.

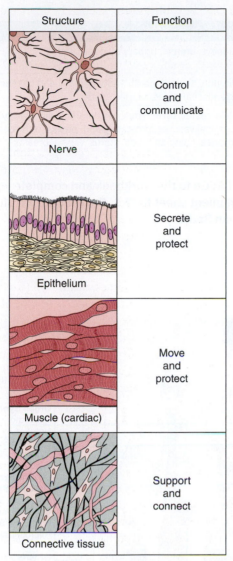

Structure	Function
Nerve	Control and communicate
Epithelium	Secrete and protect
Muscle (cardiac)	Move and protect
Connective tissue	Support and connect

FIGURE 7–4 Four main groups of tissues and their functions.

larynx, or "voice box," to provide form or shaping. Bone is similar to cartilage but has calcium salts, nerves, and blood vessels; it is frequently called *osseous tissue*. Bone helps form the rigid structure of the human body. Blood and lymph are classified as liquid connective tissue, or *vascular tissue*. Blood carries nutrients and oxygen to the body cells and carries metabolic waste away from cells. Lymph transports tissue fluid, proteins, fats, and other materials from the tissues to the circulatory system.

Nerve tissue is made up of special cells called *neurons*. It controls and coordinates body activities by transmitting messages throughout the body. The nerves, brain, and spinal cord are composed of nerve tissue.

Muscle tissue produces power and movement by contraction of muscle fibers. There are three main kinds of muscle tissue: skeletal, cardiac, and visceral (smooth). Skeletal muscle attaches to the bones and provides for movement of the body. Cardiac muscle causes the heart to beat. Visceral muscle is present in the walls of the respiratory, digestive, urinary tract, and blood vessels.

Organs

Two or more tissues joined together to perform a specific function are called an **organ**. Examples of organs include the heart, stomach, and lungs.

Systems

Organs and other body parts joined together to perform a particular function are called a **system**. The basic systems (discussed in more detail in succeeding sections) are the integumentary, skeletal, muscular, circulatory, lymphatic, nervous, respiratory, digestive, urinary (or excretory), endocrine, and reproductive systems. Their functions and main organs are shown in **Table 7–1**.

TABLE 7–1 Systems of the Body

System	Functions	Major Organs/Structures
Integumentary	Protects body from injury, infection, and dehydration; helps regulate body temperature; eliminates some wastes; produces vitamin D	Skin, sweat and oil glands, nails, and hair
Skeletal	Creates framework of body, protects internal organs, produces blood cells, acts as levers for muscles	Bones and cartilage
Muscular	Produces movement, protects internal organs, produces body heat, maintains posture	Skeletal, smooth, and cardiac muscles
Nervous	Coordinates and controls body activities	Nerves, brain, spinal cord
Special Senses	Allow body to react to environment by providing sight, hearing, taste, smell, and balance	Eye, ear, tongue, nose, general sense receptors
Circulatory	Carries oxygen and nutrients to body cells, carries waste products away from cells, helps produce cells to fight infection	Heart, blood vessels, blood, spleen
Lymphatic	Carries some tissue fluid and wastes to blood, assists with fighting infection and body immunity	Lymph nodes, lymph vessels, spleen, tonsils, and thymus gland
Respiratory	Breathes in oxygen and eliminates carbon dioxide	Nose, pharynx, larynx, trachea, bronchi, lungs
Digestive	Digests food physically and chemically, transports food, absorbs nutrients, eliminates waste	Mouth, salivary glands, pharynx, esophagus, stomach, intestine, liver, gallbladder, pancreas

(continues)

TABLE 7-1 Systems of the Body (continued)

System	Functions	Major Organs/Structures
Urinary	Filters blood to maintain fluid and electrolyte balance in the body, produces and eliminates urine	Kidneys, ureters, urinary bladder, urethra
Endocrine	Produces and secretes hormones to regulate body processes	Pituitary, thyroid, parathyroid, adrenal, and thymus glands; pancreas, ovaries, testes
Reproductive	Provides for reproduction	Male: testes, epididymis, vas deferens, ejaculatory duct, seminal vesicles, prostate gland, penis, urethra; female: ovaries, fallopian tubes, uterus, vagina, breasts

Human Organism

In summary, atoms and molecules form cells, cells combine to form tissues, tissues combine to form organs, and organs and other body parts combine to form systems. These systems working together help create the miracle called the human body (**Figure 7–5**).

checkpoint

1. Briefly list and describe the six (6) levels of body structure.

2. Define homeostasis.

3. Define anatomy, physiology, and pathophysiology.

PRACTICE: Go to the workbook and complete the assignment sheet for 7:1, Basic Structure of the Human Body.

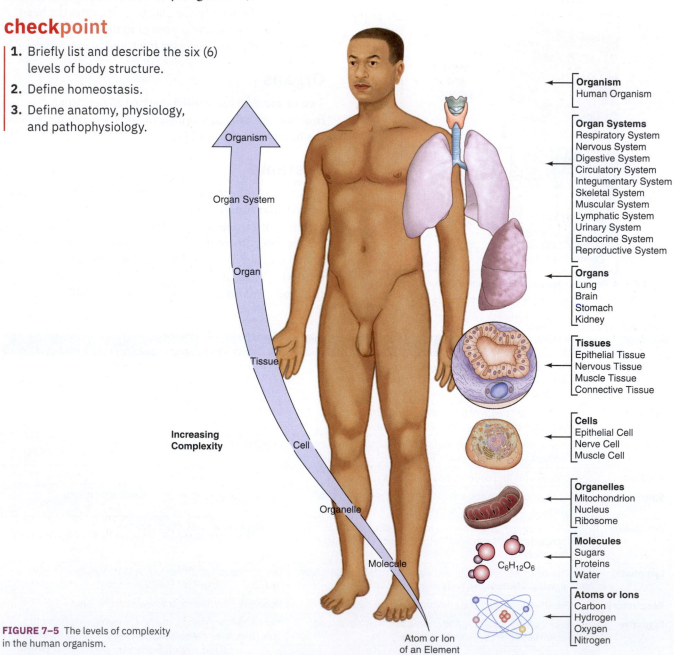

FIGURE 7–5 The levels of complexity in the human organism.

Organism
Organ System
Organ
Tissue
Increasing Complexity
Cell
Organelle
Molecule
Atom or Ion of an Element

Organism
Human Organism

Organ Systems
Respiratory System
Nervous System
Digestive System
Circulatory System
Integumentary System
Skeletal System
Muscular System
Lymphatic System
Urinary System
Endocrine System
Reproductive System

Organs
Lung
Brain
Stomach
Kidney

Tissues
Epithelial Tissue
Nervous Tissue
Muscle Tissue
Connective Tissue

Cells
Epithelial Cell
Nerve Cell
Muscle Cell

Organelles
Mitochondrion
Nucleus
Ribosome

Molecules
Sugars
Proteins
Water
$C_6H_{12}O_6$

Atoms or Ions
Carbon
Hydrogen
Oxygen
Nitrogen

7:2 BODY PLANES, DIRECTIONS, AND CAVITIES

OBJECTIVES

After completing this section, you should be able to:

- Label the names of the planes and the directional terms related to these planes on a diagram of the three planes of the body.

- Label a diagram of the main body cavities.
- Identify the main organs located in each body cavity.
- Locate the nine abdominal regions.
- Define, pronounce, and spell all key terms.

KEY TERMS

abdominal cavity
abdominal regions
anterior
bilateral
body cavities
body planes
buccal cavity
caudal *(kaw'-doll)*
cranial *(kray'-nee-al)*
cranial cavity
deep
distal

dorsal
dorsal cavity
frontal (coronal) plane
inferior
lateral *(lat'-eh-ral)*
medial *(me'-dee-al)*
midsagittal (median) plane *(mid-saj'-ih-tahl)*
nasal cavity
orbital cavity
pelvic cavity
posterior

proximal *(prox'-ih-mahl)*
sagittal plane
spinal cavity
superficial
superior
thoracic cavity *(tho-rass'-ik)*
transverse plane
unilateral
ventral
ventral cavities

Because terms such as *south* and *east* would be difficult to apply to the human body, other directional terms have been developed. These terms are used to describe the relationship of one part of the body to another part. The terms are used when the body is in anatomic position. This means the body is facing forward, standing erect, and holding the arms at the sides with the palms of the hands facing forward.

BODY PLANES

Body planes are imaginary lines drawn through the body at various parts to separate the body into sections. After the body is divided into these body planes, the terms **bilateral** and **unilateral** are used to refer to which sides of the body are affected by certain pathologic conditions. Bilateral conditions affect both sides of the body and unilateral conditions only affect one side. Directional terms are created by these planes. The three main body planes are the transverse, midsagittal, and frontal (**Figure 7–6**).

The **transverse plane** is a horizontal plane that divides the body into a top half and a bottom half. Body parts above other parts are termed **superior**, and body parts

below other parts are termed **inferior**. For instance, the knee is superior to the ankle but inferior to the hip. Two other directional terms related to this plane include **cranial**, which means body parts located near the head, and **caudal**, which means body parts located near the sacral region of the spinal column (also known as the "tail").

The **sagittal plane** divides the body into left and right sections. If a sagittal plane runs down the midline of the body and divides the body into equal halves, it is called a **midsagittal** or **median plane**. Body parts close to the midline, or plane, are called **medial**, and body parts away from the midline are called **lateral**.

The **frontal** or **coronal plane** divides the body into a front section and a back section. Body parts in front of the plane, or on the front of the body, are called **ventral** or **anterior**. Body parts on the back of the body are called **dorsal** or **posterior**.

Proximal and **distal** are terms used to describe the location of the extremities (arms and legs) in relation to the main trunk of the body, generally called the *point of reference*. Body parts close to the point of reference are called *proximal*, and body parts distant from the point of reference are called *distal*. For example, in describing

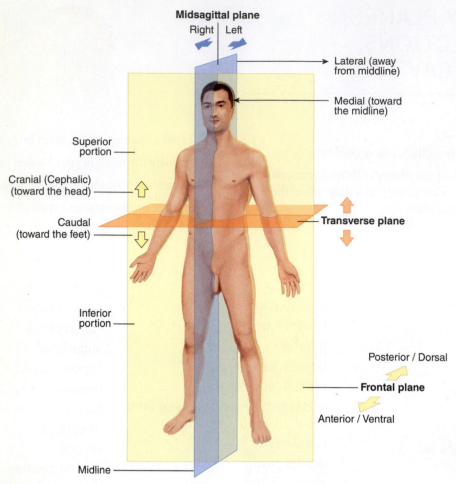

Midsagittal plane
Right | Left

Lateral (away from middline)

Medial (toward the midline)

Superior portion

Cranial (Cephalic) (toward the head)

Caudal (toward the feet)

Transverse plane

Inferior portion

Posterior / Dorsal

Frontal plane

Anterior / Ventral

Midline

FIGURE 7–6 Body planes and directional terms.

the relationship of the wrist and elbow to the shoulder (or point of reference), the wrist is distal and the elbow is proximal to the shoulder.

Terms that relate to structures within the body are **superficial** or *external* to indicate the structures are located near the body surface and **deep** or *internal* to indicate the structures are located away from the body surface.

BODY CAVITIES

Body cavities are spaces within the body that contain vital organs. There are two main body cavities: the dorsal, or posterior, cavity and the ventral, or anterior, cavity (**Figure 7–7**).

The **dorsal cavity** is one long, continuous cavity located on the back of the body. It is divided into two sections: the **cranial cavity**, which contains the brain, and the **spinal cavity**, which contains the spinal cord.

The **ventral cavities** are larger than the dorsal cavities. The ventral cavity is separated into two distinct cavities by the dome-shaped muscle called the *diaphragm*, which is important for respiration (breathing). The **thoracic cavity** is located in the chest and contains the esophagus, trachea, bronchi, lungs, heart, and large blood vessels. The

abdominal cavity, or abdominopelvic cavity, is divided into an upper part and a lower part. The upper **abdominal cavity** contains the stomach, small intestine, most of the large intestine, appendix, liver, gallbladder, pancreas, and spleen. The lower abdominal cavity, or **pelvic cavity**, contains the urinary bladder, the reproductive organs, and the last part of the large intestine. The kidneys and adrenal glands are technically located outside the abdominal cavity because they are behind the peritoneal membrane (peritoneum) that lines the abdominal cavity. This area is called the *retroperitoneal space*.

Three small cavities are the **orbital cavity** for the eyes, the **nasal cavity** for the nose structures, and the **buccal cavity**, or mouth, for the teeth and tongue.

ABDOMINAL REGIONS

The abdominal cavity is so large that it is divided into regions or sections. One method of division is into quadrants, or four sections. As shown in **Figure 7–8**, this results in a right upper quadrant (RUQ), left upper quadrant (LUQ), right lower quadrant (RLQ), and left lower quadrant (LLQ). A more precise method of division is into nine **abdominal regions** (**Figure 7–9**).

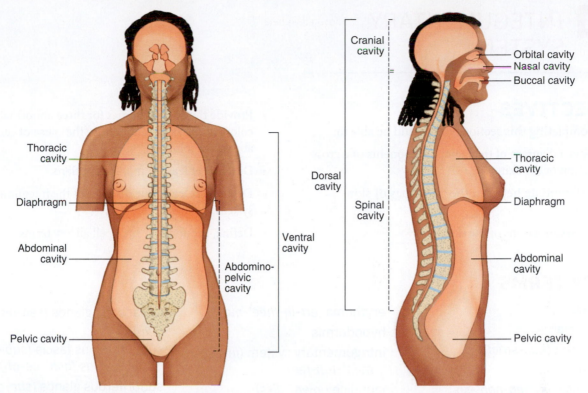

FIGURE 7–7 Body cavities.

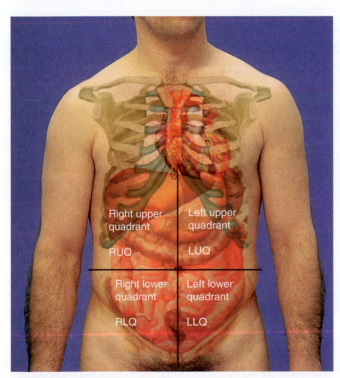

FIGURE 7–8 Abdominal quadrants.

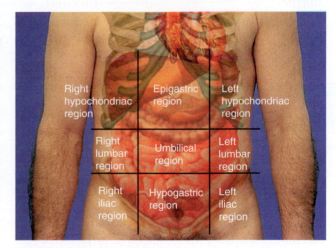

FIGURE 7–9 Nine abdominal regions.

The terms relating to body planes, directions, and cavities are used frequently in the study of human anatomy.

checkpoint

1. Using a balloon to simulate an abdomen, draw and label the nine body regions.
2. Explain why body directions are useful in the study of anatomy.

PRACTICE: Go to the workbook and complete the assignment sheet for 7:2, Body Planes, Directions, and Cavities.

The center regions are the epigastric (above the stomach), umbilical (near the umbilicus or belly button), and hypogastric, or pelvic (below the stomach). On either side of the center the regions are the hypochondriac (below the ribs), lumbar (near the large bones of the spinal cord), and iliac, or inguinal (near the groin).

OBJECTIVES

After completing this section, you should be able to:

- Label a diagram of the major components of a cross section of the skin.

- Differentiate between the two types of skin glands.

- List six functions of the skin.

- Provide the correct names for three abnormal colors of the skin and identify the cause of each abnormal color.

- Describe at least four skin eruptions.

- Describe at least four diseases of the integumentary system.

- Define, pronounce, and spell all key terms.

■ KEY TERMS

albino
alopecia
constrict *(kun-strict')*
crusts
cyanosis *(sy"-eh-noh'-sis)*
cyst
dermis
dilate *(die'-late)*
epidermis *(eh-pih-der'-mis)*

erythema *(err-ih-thee'-ma)*
hypodermis
integumentary system *(in-teg-u-men'-tah-ree)*
jaundice *(jawn'-diss)*
macules *(mack'-youlz)*
melanin
papules *(pap'-Cyoulz)*
pustules *(pus'-tyoulz)*

sebaceous glands *(seh-bay'-shus)*
subcutaneous fascia *(sub-q-tay'-nee-us fash'-ee-ah)*
sudoriferous glands *(sue-de-rif'-eh-rus)*
ulcer
vesicles *(ves'-i-kulz)*
wheals

Related Health Careers

- Allergist
- Dermatologist
- Forensic scientist
- Plastic surgeon

The **integumentary system**, or skin, on an average adult covers more than 3,000 square inches of surface area and accounts for about 15 percent of total body weight.

Three main layers of tissue make up the skin (**Figure 7–10**):

- **Epidermis:** the outermost layer of skin. This layer is actually made of five smaller layers but no blood vessels or nerve cells. Two main layers are the *stratum corneum*, the outermost layer, and the *stratum germinativum*, the innermost layer. The cells of the stratum corneum are constantly shed and replaced by new cells from the stratum germinativum.

- **Dermis**: also called *corium*, or "true skin." This layer has a framework of elastic connective tissue and contains blood vessels, lymph vessels, nerves, involuntary muscle, sweat and oil glands, and hair follicles. The top of the dermis is covered with papillae, which fit into ridges on the stratum

germinativum of the epidermis. These ridges form lines, or striations, on the skin. Because the pattern of ridges is unique to each individual, fingerprints and footprints are often used as methods of identification.

- **Subcutaneous fascia** or **hypodermis**: the innermost layer. It is made of elastic and fibrous connective tissue and adipose (fatty) tissue and connects the skin to underlying muscles.

The integumentary system has two main types of glands: sudoriferous and sebaceous. The **sudoriferous glands** (sweat glands) are coiled tubes that extend through the dermis and open on the surface of the skin at pores. The sweat, or perspiration, eliminated by these glands contains water, salts, and some body wastes. Even though sweat contains body wastes, it is basically odorless. However, when the sweat interacts with bacteria on the skin, body odor occurs. The process of perspiration removes excess water from the body and cools the body as the sweat evaporates into the air. The **sebaceous glands** are oil glands that usually open onto hair follicles. They produce sebum, an oil that keeps the skin and hair from becoming dry and brittle. Because sebum is slightly acidic, it acts as an antibacterial and antifungal secretion to help prevent infections. When an oil gland becomes plugged, the accumulation of dirt and oil results in a blackhead or pimple.

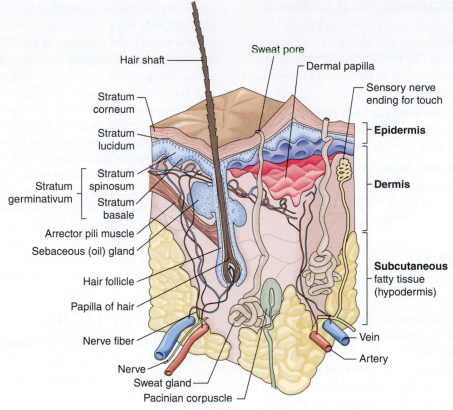

Hair shaft

Sweat pore

Dermal papilla

Sensory nerve ending for touch

Stratum corneum

Epidermis

Stratum lucidum

Stratum germinativum

Stratum spinosum

Stratum basale

Dermis

Arrector pili muscle

Sebaceous (oil) gland

Hair follicle

Subcutaneous fatty tissue (hypodermis)

Papilla of hair

Nerve fiber

Vein

Artery

Nerve

Sweat gland

Pacinian corpuscle

FIGURE 7–10 Cross section of skin.

Two other parts of the integumentary system are the hair and nails. Each hair consists of a root (which grows in a hollow tube called a *follicle*) and a hair shaft. Hair helps protect the body and covers all body surfaces except for the palms of the hands and the soles of the foot. Due to genetics, male (and some female) individuals may experience **alopecia** or baldness, a loss of hair on the scalp. Nails protect the fingers and toes from injury. They are made of dead, keratinized epidermal epithelial cells packed closely together to form a thick, dense surface. They are formed in the nail bed. If lost, nails will regrow if the nail bed is not damaged.

FUNCTIONS

The integumentary system performs the following important functions:

- **Protection**: It serves as a barrier to the sun's ultraviolet rays and the invasion of pathogens, or germs. It also holds moisture in and prevents deeper tissues from drying out.

- **Sensory perception**: The nerves in the skin help the body respond to pain, pressure, temperature (heat and cold), and touch sensations (**Figure 7–11**).

- **Body temperature regulation**: The blood vessels in the skin help the body retain or lose heat. When the blood vessels **dilate** (get larger), excess heat from the blood can escape through the skin. When the blood vessels **constrict** (get smaller), the heat is retained in

the body. The sudoriferous glands also help cool the body through evaporation of perspiration.

- **Storage**: The skin has tissues for temporary storage of fat, glucose (sugar), water, vitamins, and salts. Adipose (fatty) tissue in the subcutaneous fascia is a source of energy.

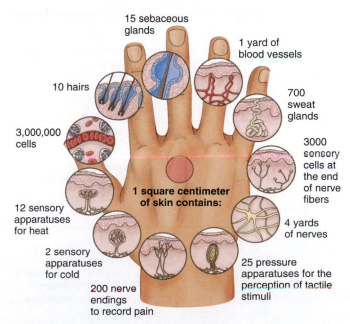

15 sebaceous glands

1 yard of blood vessels

10 hairs

700 sweat glands

3,000,000 cells

1 square centimeter of skin contains:

3000 sensory cells at the end of nerve fibers

12 sensory apparatuses for heat

4 yards of nerves

2 sensory apparatuses for cold

25 pressure apparatuses for the perception of tactile stimuli

200 nerve endings to record pain

FIGURE 7–11 The nerves in the skin allow the body to respond to many different sensations.

- **Absorption**: Certain substances can be absorbed through the skin, such as medications for motion sickness or heart disease and nicotine patches to help stop smoking. The medications are placed on sticky patches and applied to the skin. This is called a *transdermal medication*.

- **Excretion**: The skin helps the body eliminate salt, a minute amount of waste, and excess water and heat through perspiration.

- **Production**: The skin helps in the production of vitamin D by using ultraviolet rays from the sun to form an initial molecule of vitamin D that matures in the liver.

PIGMENTATION

Basic skin color is inherited and is determined by pigments in the epidermis of the skin. A brownish black pigment, **melanin**, is produced in the epidermis by specialized cells called *melanocytes*. Even though everyone has the same number of melanocytes, genes present in each racial group determine the amount of melanin produced. Melanin can lead to a black, brown, or yellow skin tint, depending on the amount of melanin present and racial origin. Ultraviolet light activates the melanocytes to produce more melanin to protect and to tan the skin. Small concentrated areas of melanin pigment form freckles. Carotene, a yellowish red pigment, also helps determine skin color. A person with an absence of color pigments is an **albino**. An albino's skin has a pinkish tint and the hair is pale yellow or white. The person's eyes also lack pigment and are red and very sensitive to light.

Abnormal colors of the skin can indicate disease. **Erythema** is a reddish color of the skin that can be caused by either burns or a congestion of blood in the vessels. **Jaundice**, a yellow discoloration of the skin, can indicate bile in the blood as a result of liver or gallbladder disease. Jaundice also occurs in conjunction with certain diseases that involve the destruction of red blood cells. **Cyanosis** is a bluish discoloration of the skin caused by insufficient oxygen. It can be associated with heart, lung, and circulatory diseases or disorders. Chronic poisoning may cause a gray or brown skin discoloration.

SKIN ERUPTIONS

Skin eruptions can also indicate disease (**Figure 7–12**). The most common eruptions include:

- **Macules**: (macular rash) flat spots on the skin, such as freckles

- **Papules**: (papular rash) firm, raised areas such as pimples and the eruptions seen in some stages of chickenpox and syphilis

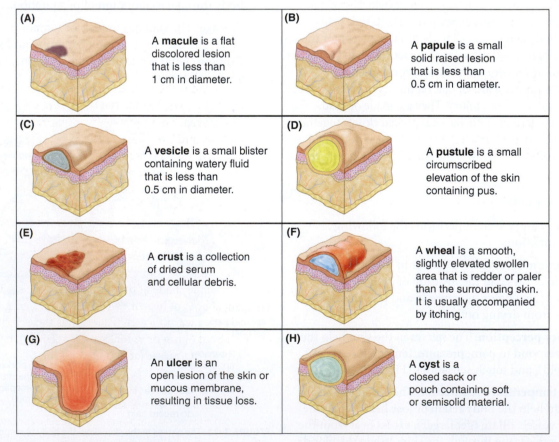

(A) A **macule** is a flat discolored lesion that is less than 1 cm in diameter.

(B) A **papule** is a small solid raised lesion that is less than 0.5 cm in diameter.

(C) A **vesicle** is a small blister containing watery fluid that is less than 0.5 cm in diameter.

(D) A **pustule** is a small circumscribed elevation of the skin containing pus.

(E) A **crust** is a collection of dried serum and cellular debris.

(F) A **wheal** is a smooth, slightly elevated swollen area that is redder or paler than the surrounding skin. It is usually accompanied by itching.

(G) An **ulcer** is an open lesion of the skin or mucous membrane, resulting in tissue loss.

(H) A **cyst** is a closed sack or pouch containing soft or semisolid material.

FIGURE 7–12 Skin eruptions can indicate disease.

- **Vesicles**: blisters, or fluid-filled sacs, such as those seen in chickenpox

- **Pustules**: pus-filled sacs such as those seen in acne, or pimples

- **Crusts**: areas of dried pus and blood, commonly called *scabs*

- **Wheals**: itchy, elevated areas with an irregular shape; hives and insect bites are examples

- **Ulcer**: a deep loss of skin surface that may extend into the dermis; may cause periodic bleeding and the formation of scars

- **Cyst**: a closed sac with a distinct membrane that develops abnormally in a body structure; usually filled with a semisolid material

DISEASES AND ABNORMAL CONDITIONS

Acne Vulgaris

Acne vulgaris is an inflammation of the sebaceous glands. Although the cause is unknown, acne usually occurs at adolescence. Hormonal changes and increased secretion of sebum are probably underlying causes. Symptoms include papules, pustules, and blackheads. These occur when the hair follicles become blocked with dirt, cosmetics, excess oil, and/or bacteria. Treatment methods include frequent, thorough skin washing; avoidance of creams and heavy makeup; topical antimicrobials; oral or topical antibiotics and/or retinoids (vitamin A); and chemical peels. Dermatologists also use light therapy or laser therapy to kill bacteria and decrease the amount of acne.

Athlete's Foot

Athlete's foot is a contagious fungal infection that usually affects the feet. The skin itches, blisters, and cracks into open sores. Treatment involves topical and/or oral antifungal medications and keeping the area clean and dry.

Skin Cancer

Cancer of the skin is the most common type of cancer. There are three main types of skin cancer: basal cell carcinoma, squamous cell carcinoma, and melanoma. *Basal cell carcinoma* is cancer of the basal cells in the epidermis of the skin. It grows slowly and does not usually spread (**Figure 7–13**). The lesions can be pink to yellow-white. They are usually smooth with a depressed center and an elevated, irregular-shaped border.

Squamous cell carcinoma affects the thin cells of the epithelium but can spread quickly to other areas of the body. The lesions start as small, firm, red, flat sores that later scale and crust (**Figure 7–14**). Sores that do not heal are frequently squamous cell carcinomas.

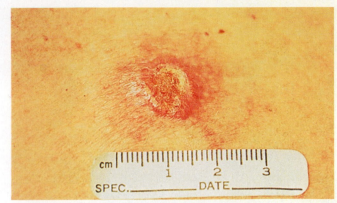

FIGURE 7–13 Basal cell carcinomas usually grow more slowly. Courtesy of Robert A. Silverman, M.D., Clinical Associate Professor, Department of Pediatrics, Georgetown University.

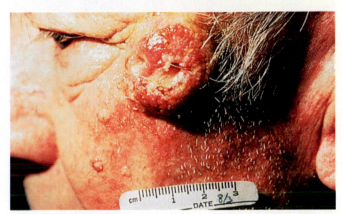

FIGURE 7–14 Squamous cell carcinomas resemble sores that scale and crust. Courtesy of Robert A. Silverman, M.D., Clinical Associate Professor, Department of Pediatrics, Georgetown University.

Melanoma develops in the melanocytes of the epidermis and is the most dangerous type of skin cancer (**Figure 7–15**). The lesions can be brown, black, pink, or multicolored. They are usually flat or raised slightly, asymmetric, and irregular or notched on the edges.

An *ABCDE* method for detecting skin cancer can make it easier to recognize the warning signs of melanoma. The letters and signs include: *A is for Asymmetry:* Most melanomas are asymmetrical. If one draws a line through the middle of the lesion, the two halves are unequal. *B is for Border:* Melanoma borders tend to have ragged edges, while common moles tend to have smoother borders. *C is for Color:* Multiple colors are a warning sign. Moles are usually a single shade of brown; a melanoma may have different shades of brown, tan or black. *D is for Diameter or Dark:* It's a warning sign if a lesion is the size of a pencil eraser (about 6 mm or ¼ inch in diameter or larger). It is also important to look for any lesion, no matter what size, that is darker than others. *E is for Evolving:* Any change in size, shape, color or elevation of a spot on the skin or any new symptom in the area, such as bleeding or itching, may be a warning sign. It is important to see a dermatologist if any of these warning signs are present because skin cancers detected early can usually be cured.

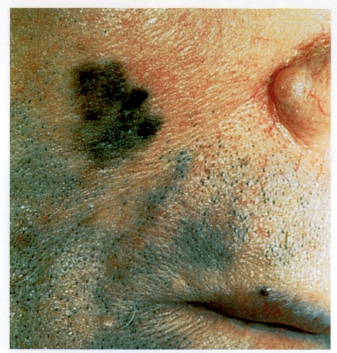

FIGURE 7–15 Melanoma is the most dangerous form of skin cancer.
Courtesy of Robert A. Silverman, M.D., Clinical Associate Professor, Department of Pediatrics, Georgetown University.

Exposure to the sun, prolonged use of tanning beds, irritating chemicals, or radiation are the usual causes of skin cancer. Treatment begins with removal of the lesion. Cryotherapy, or freezing the lesion with liquid nitrogen, is one option. Laser therapy can vaporize growths, but deeper lesions require surgical excision. Removal of the lesion is followed by radiation and/or chemotherapy depending on the degree of metastasis (spreading).

Dermatitis

Dermatitis, an inflammation of the skin, can be caused by any substance that irritates the skin. It is frequently an allergic reaction to detergents, cosmetics, pollen, or certain foods. One example of contact dermatitis is the irritation caused by contact with poison ivy, poison sumac, or poison oak (**Figure 7–16**). Symptoms include dry skin, erythema, itching, edema, maculopapular rashes, and scaling. Treatment is directed at eliminating the cause, especially in the case of allergens. Anti-inflammatory ointments, antihistamines, and/or steroids are also used in treatment.

Eczema

Eczema is a noncontagious, inflammatory dermatitis caused by an allergen or irritant. Diet, cosmetics, soaps, medications, and emotional stress can all cause eczema. Symptoms include dryness, erythema, edema, itching, vesicles that crust or ooze, and scaling. Treatment involves removing the irritant and applying corticosteroids to reduce the inflammatory response. Thick creams with low water content may also be applied to keep the area moist.

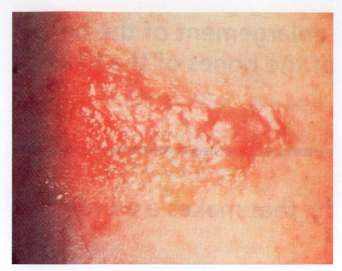

FIGURE 7–16 A contact dermatitis caused by contact with poison oak.
Courtesy of Timothy Berger, M.D., Clinical Professor, Department of Dermatology, University of California, San Francisco.

Impetigo

Impetigo is a highly contagious skin infection usually caused by streptococci or staphylococci organisms (**Figure 7–17**). It mainly affects infants and children. Symptoms include red lesions on the face, especially around the nose and mouth, or on other body surfaces. The lesions rupture and ooze forming a yellowish brown crust. Lesions should be washed with soap and water and kept dry. Antibiotics, both topical and oral, are also used in treatment.

Psoriasis

Psoriasis is a chronic, noncontagious skin disease with periods of exacerbations (symptoms present) and remission (symptoms decrease or disappear). The cause is unknown, but there may be a hereditary link. Stress, cold weather, pregnancy, heavy alcohol consumption,

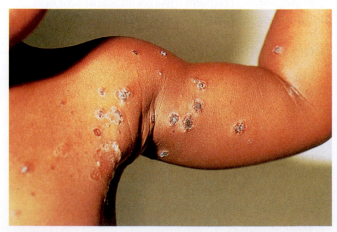

FIGURE 7–17 Impetigo is a highly contagious skin infection usually caused by streptococci or staphylococci organisms. Courtesy of Robert A. Silverman, M.D., Clinical Associate Professor, Department of Pediatrics, Georgetown University.

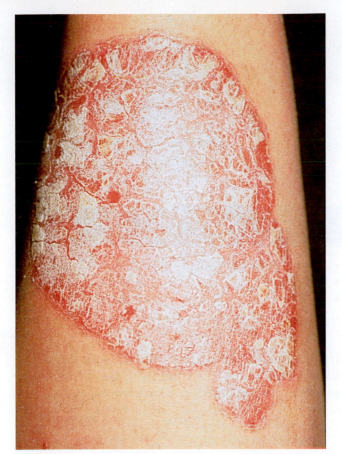

FIGURE 7–18 Psoriasis is characterized by white or silver scales. Courtesy of Robert A. Silverman, M.D., Clinical Associate Professor, Department of Pediatrics, Georgetown University.

or cortisone ointments, topical vitamin D analogs, and phototherapy using natural or artificial UV light to improve symptoms.

Ringworm

Ringworm (tineas) is a highly contagious fungal infection of the skin or scalp. The characteristic symptom is the formation of a flat or raised circular area with a healthy-looking inner area surrounded by an itchy, scaly, or crusty outer ring. Antifungal medications, both oral and topical, are used in treatment.

Verrucae and Warts

Verrucae and warts are caused by the human papilloma virus (HPV). Several different forms exist based on their location: genital, plantar, and palmar. A rough, hard, elevated, rounded surface forms on the skin. Some warts disappear spontaneously, but others must be removed with cryotherapy using liquid nitrogen to freeze the wart, acid (often used in conjunction with duct tape), chemicals, laser therapy, or shave excision (removal with a blade).

checkpoint

1. List the six (6) functions of the integumentary system.
2. If a patient exhibits a warning sign on their *ABCDE* skin screening, what deadly type of skin cancer would the doctor suspect and to what medical specialist would they refer them to?

PRACTICE: Go to the workbook and complete the assignment sheet for 7:3, Integumentary System.

and endocrine changes tend to cause an exacerbation of the disease. Symptoms include thick, red areas covered with white or silver scales (**Figure 7–18**). Although there is no cure, treatment methods include coal/tar

7:4 SKELETAL SYSTEM

OBJECTIVES

After completing this section, you should be able to:

- List five functions of bones.
- Label the parts of a bone on a diagram of a long bone.
- Name the two divisions of the skeletal system and the main groups of bones in each division.
- Identify the main bones of the skeleton.
- Compare the three classifications of joints by describing the type of motion allowed by each.
- Give one example of each joint classification.
- Describe at least four diseases of the skeletal system.
- Define, pronounce, and spell all key terms.

■ KEY TERMS

appendicular skeleton *(ap-pen-dick'-u-lar)*
axial skeleton
carpals
clavicles *(klav'-ih-kulz)*

cranium
diaphysis *(dy-af'-eh-sis)*
endosteum *(en-dos'-tee-um)*
epiphysis *(ih-pif'-eh-sis)*
femur *(fee'-mur)*

fibula *(fib'-you-la)*
fontanels
foramina *(for-ahm'-e-nah)*
humerus *(hue'-mer-us)*
joints

ligaments
medullary canal *(med'-hue-lair-ee)*
metacarpals *(met-ah-car'-pulz)*
metatarsals *(met-ah-tar'-sulz)*
os coxae *(ahs cock'-see)*
patella *(pa-tell'-ah)*
periosteum *(per-ee-os'-tee-um)*

phalanges *(fa-lan'-jeez)*
radius
red marrow
ribs
scapulas
sinuses *(sigh'-nuss-ez)*
skeletal system

sternum
sutures
tarsals
tibia
ulna
vertebrae *(vur'-teh-bray)*
yellow marrow

Related Health Careers

- Athletic trainer
- Chiropractor
- Orthopedist

- Orthoptist
- Osteopathic physician
- Physiatrist

- Physical therapist
- Podiatrist
- Prosthetist

- Radiologic technologist
- Sports medicine physician

The **skeletal system** is made of organs called *bones.* An adult human has 206 bones. These bones work as a system to perform the following functions:

- **Framework**: Bones form a framework to support the body's muscles, fat, and skin.

- **Protection**: Bones surround vital organs to protect them (for example, the skull, which surrounds the brain, and the ribs, which protect the heart and lungs).

- **Levers**: Muscles attach to bones to help provide movement.

- **Production of blood cells**: Bones help produce red and white blood cells and platelets, a process called *hemopoiesis* or *hematopoiesis.*

- **Storage**: Bones store most of the calcium supply of the body in addition to phosphorus and fats.

Bones vary in shape and size depending on their locations within the body. Bones of the extremities (arms and legs) are called *long bones.* The basic parts of these bones are shown in **Figure 7–19**. The long shaft is called the **diaphysis**, and the two extremities, or ends, are each called an **epiphysis**. The **medullary canal** is a cavity in the diaphysis. It is filled with **yellow marrow**, which is mainly a storage area for fat cells. **Yellow marrow** also contains cells that form leukocytes, or white blood cells. The **endosteum** is a membrane that lines the medullary canal and keeps the yellow marrow intact. It also produces some bone growth. **Red marrow** is found in certain bones, such as the vertebrae, ribs, sternum, and cranium, and in the proximal ends of the humerus and femur. Red bone marrow is where a process known as hematopoiesis takes place. *Hematopoiesis* is the way all blood cells are formed, develop, and mature into their final adult

types. A hematopoietic stem cell is a cell isolated from the bone marrow that can renew itself, can differentiate to a variety of specialized cells, can move out of the

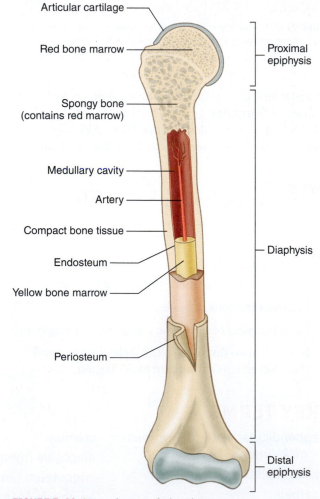

Articular cartilage

Red bone marrow

Spongy bone (contains red marrow)

Medullary cavity

Artery

Compact bone tissue

Endosteum

Yellow bone marrow

Periosteum

Proximal epiphysis

Diaphysis

Distal epiphysis

FIGURE 7–19 Anatomic parts of a long bone.

bone marrow into circulating blood, and can undergo programmed cell death. Red marrow produces red blood cells (erythrocytes), platelets (thrombocytes), and some white blood cells (leukocytes). Because bone marrow is important in the manufacture of blood cells and is involved with the body's immune response, the red marrow is used to diagnose blood diseases and is sometimes transplanted in people with defective immune systems. The outside of bone is covered with a tough membrane, called the **periosteum**, which contains blood vessels, lymph vessels, and *osteoblasts*, special cells that form new bone tissue. The periosteum is necessary for bone growth, repair, and nutrition. A thin layer of articular cartilage covers the epiphysis and acts as a shock absorber when two bones meet to form a joint.

The skeletal system is divided into two sections: the axial skeleton and the appendicular skeleton. The **axial skeleton** forms the main trunk of the body and is composed of the skull, spinal column, ribs, and breastbone. The **appendicular skeleton** forms the extremities and is composed of the shoulder girdle, arm bones, pelvic girdle, and leg bones.

The skull is composed of the cranial and facial bones (**Figure 7–20**). The **cranium** is the spherical structure that surrounds and protects the brain. It is made of eight bones: one frontal, two parietal, two temporal, one occipital, one ethmoid, and one sphenoid. At birth, the cranium is not solid bone. Spaces called **fontanels**, or "soft spots," allow for the enlargement of the skull as brain growth occurs. The fontanels are made of membrane and cartilage, and turn into solid bone by approximately 18 months of age. There are 14 facial bones: 1 mandible (lower jaw), 2 maxilla

(upper jaw), 2 zygomatic (cheek), 2 lacrimal (inner aspect of eyes), 5 nasal, and 2 palatine (hard palate or roof of the mouth). **Sutures** are areas where the cranial bones have joined together. **Sinuses** are air spaces in the bones of the skull that act as resonating chambers for the voice. They are lined with mucous membranes. **Foramina** are openings in bones that allow nerves and blood vessels to enter or leave the bone.

The spinal column is composed of 26 bones called **vertebrae** (**Figure 7–21**). These bones protect the spinal cord and provide support for the head and trunk. They include 7 cervical (neck), 12 thoracic (chest), 5 lumbar (waist), 1 sacrum (back of pelvic girdle), and 1 coccyx (tailbone). Pads of cartilage tissue, called *intervertebral disks*, separate the vertebrae. The disks act as shock absorbers and permit bending and twisting movements of the vertebral column.

There are 12 pairs of **ribs**. They attach to the thoracic vertebrae on the dorsal surface of the body. The first seven pairs are called *true ribs* because they attach directly to the sternum, or breastbone, on the front of the body. The next five pairs are called *false ribs*. The first three pairs of false ribs attach to the cartilage of the rib above. The last two pairs of false ribs are called *floating ribs* because they have no attachment on the front of the body.

The **sternum**, or breastbone, is the last bone of the axial skeleton. It consists of three parts: the manubrium (upper region), the gladiolus (body), and the xiphoid process (a small piece of cartilage at the bottom). The two collarbones, or clavicles, are attached to the manubrium by ligaments. The ribs are attached to the sternum with costal cartilages to form a "cage" that protects the heart and lungs.

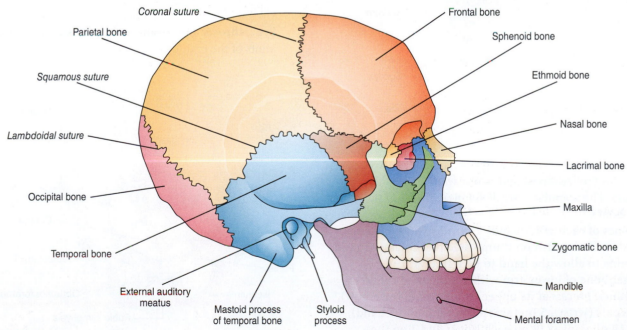

FIGURE 7–20 Bones of the skull.

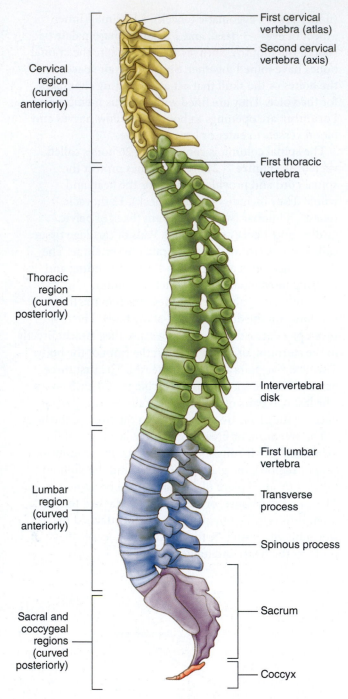

First cervical
vertebra (atlas)

Second cervical
vertebra (axis)

Cervical
region
(curved
anteriorly)

First thoracic
vertebra

Thoracic
region
(curved
posteriorly)

Intervertebral
disk

First lumbar
vertebra

Transverse
process

Lumbar
region
(curved
anteriorly)

Spinous process

Sacral and
coccygeal
regions
(curved
posteriorly)

Sacrum

Coccyx

FIGURE 7–21 Lateral view of the vertebral, or spinal, column.

The pelvic girdle is made of two **os coxae** (coxal, or hip, bones), which join with the sacrum on the dorsal part of the body (**Figure 7–22**). On the ventral part of the body, the os coxae join together at a joint called the *symphysis pubis*. Each os coxae is made of three fused sections: the ilium, the ischium, and the pubis. The pelvic girdle contains two recessed areas, or sockets. These sockets, called *acetabula*, provide for the attachment of the smooth rounded head of the femur (upper leg bone). An opening between the ischium and pubis, called the *obturator foramen*, allows for the passage of nerves and blood vessels to and from the legs.

Each leg consists of 1 **femur** (thigh), 1 **patella** (kneecap), 1 **tibia** (the larger weight-bearing bone of the lower leg commonly called the *shin bone*), 1 **fibula** (the slender smaller bone of the lower leg that attaches to the proximal end of the tibia), 7 **tarsals** (ankle), 5 **metatarsals** (instep of foot), and 14 phalanges (2 on the great toe and 3 on each of the other 4 toes). The heel is formed by the large tarsal bone called the *calcaneous*. The bones of the skeleton are shown in **Figure 7–23**.

Joints

Joints are areas where two or more bones join together. Connective tissue bands, called **ligaments**, help hold long bones together at joints. There are three main types of joints:

- **Diarthrosis** or **synovial**: freely movable; examples include the ball-and-socket joints of the shoulder and hip, or the hinge joints of the elbow and knee

- **Amphiarthrosis**: slightly movable; examples include the attachment of the ribs to the thoracic vertebrae and the symphysis pubis, or joint between the two pelvic bones

- **Synarthrosis**: immovable; examples are the suture joints of the cranium

The shoulder, or pectoral, girdle is made of two **clavicles** (collarbones) and two **scapulas** (shoulder bones). The scapulas provide for attachment of the upper arm bones.

Bones of each arm include 1 **humerus** (upper arm), 1 **radius** (lower arm on thumb side that rotates around the ulna to allow the hand to turn freely), 1 **ulna** (larger bone of lower arm with a projection called the *olecranon process* at its upper end, forming the elbow), 8 **carpals** (wrist), 5 **metacarpals** (palm of the hand), and 14 **phalanges** (3 on each finger and 2 on the thumb).

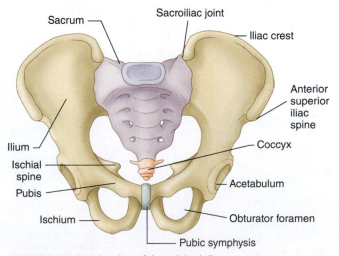

Sacrum

Sacroiliac joint

Iliac crest

Anterior
superior
iliac
spine

Ilium

Ischial
spine

Pubis

Coccyx

Acetabulum

Ischium

Obturator foramen

Pubic symphysis

FIGURE 7–22 Anterior view of the pelvic girdle.

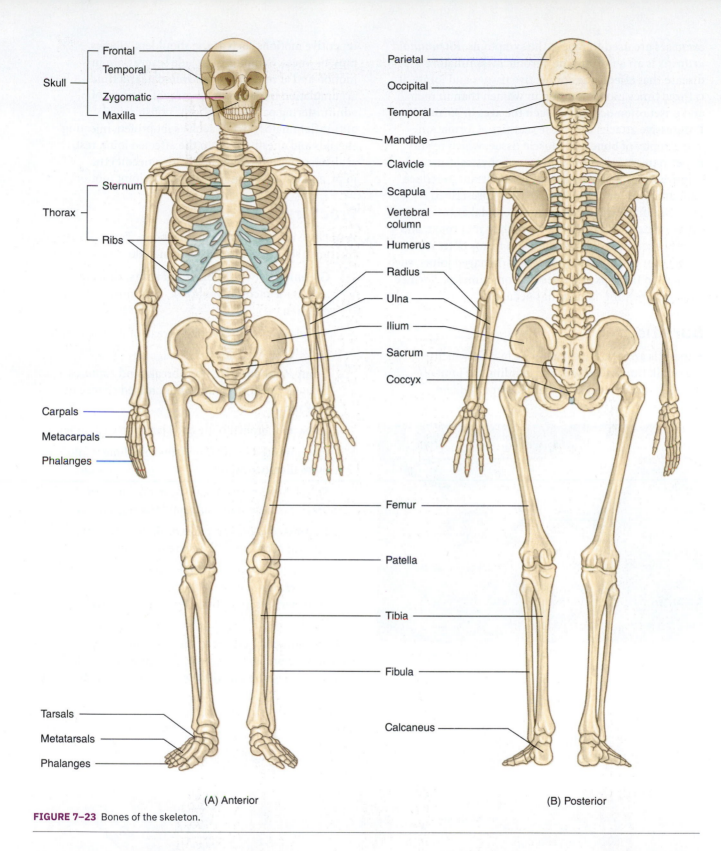

Skull
— Frontal
— Temporal
— Zygomatic
— Maxilla

Parietal
Occipital
Temporal
Mandible
Clavicle
Scapula
Vertebral column

Thorax
— Sternum
— Ribs

Humerus
Radius
Ulna
Ilium
Sacrum
Coccyx

Carpals
Metacarpals
Phalanges

Femur

Patella

Tibia

Fibula

Calcaneus

Tarsals
Metatarsals
Phalanges

(A) Anterior

(B) Posterior

FIGURE 7–23 Bones of the skeleton.

DISEASES AND ABNORMAL CONDITIONS

Arthritis

Arthritis is actually a group of diseases involving inflammation of the joints. The two main types are osteoarthritis and rheumatoid arthritis. *Osteoarthritis,* the most common form, is a chronic disease that usually occurs as a result of aging. It frequently affects the hips, knees, and thumb joints. Symptoms include joint pain, stiffness, aching, and limited range of motion. Although there is no cure, rest, applications of heat and cold, aspirin and anti-inflammatory medications, injection of steroids into the joints, weight control, and special exercises are used to relieve the symptoms. *Rheumatoid arthritis* is an autoimmune chronic inflammatory disease that affects the connective tissues and joints. It is three times more common in women than in men, and onset often occurs between the ages of 35 and 45. Progressive attacks can cause scar tissue formation and atrophy of bone and muscle tissue, which result in permanent deformity and loss of physical function (**Figure 7–24**). Early treatment is important to reduce pain and limit damage to joints. Rest, prescribed exercise, analgesics for pain, nonsteroidal anti-inflammatory drugs (NSAIDs) such as ibuprofen, and careful use of steroids are the main forms of treatment. Surgery, or arthroplasty, to replace damaged joints, such as those in the hips and knees, is sometimes performed when severe joint damage has occurred.

Bursitis

Bursitis is an inflammation of the bursae, which are small, fluid-filled sacs surrounding the joints. It frequently affects joints that perform frequent

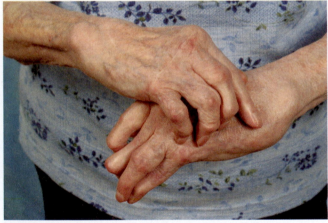

FIGURE 7–24 Rheumatoid arthritis can cause permanent deformity and immobility. ©iStock.com/Stan Rohrer

repetitive motions such as the shoulders, elbows, hips, or knees. Symptoms include severe pain in motion and at rest, limited movement, and fluid accumulation in the joint. Treatment consists of administering pain medications, nonsteroidal anti-inflammatory drugs such as ibuprofen, injecting steroids and anesthetics into the affected joint, rest, aspirating (withdrawing fluid with a needle) the joint, and physical therapy to preserve joint motion.

Fractures

A fracture is a crack or break in a bone. Types of fractures, shown in **Figure 7–25**, include:

- **Greenstick**: bone is bent and splits, causing a crack or incomplete break; common in children

- **Simple** or **closed**: complete break of the bone with no damage to the skin

- **Compound** or **open**: bone breaks and ruptures through the skin; creates an increased chance of infection

- **Impacted**: broken bone ends jam into each other

- **Comminuted**: bone fragments or splinters into more than two pieces

- **Spiral**: bone twists, resulting in one or more breaks; common in skiing and skating accidents

- **Depressed**: a broken piece of skull bone moves inward; common with severe head injuries

- **Colles**: breaking and dislocation of the distal radius that causes a characteristic bulge at the wrist; caused by falling on an outstretched hand

Before a fracture can heal, the bone must be put back into its proper alignment. This process is called *reduction*. *Closed reduction* involves positioning the bone

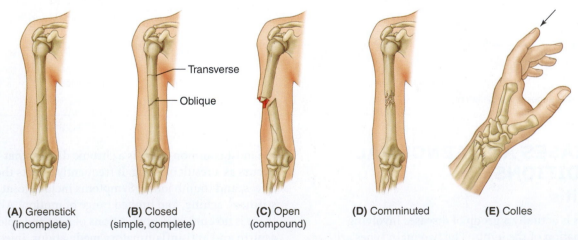

(A) Greenstick (incomplete) **(B) Closed** (simple, complete) **(C) Open** (compound) **(D) Comminuted** **(E) Colles**

Transverse

Oblique

FIGURE 7–25 Types of fractures.

in correct alignment, usually with traction, and applying a cast or splint to maintain the position until the fracture heals. *Open reduction* involves surgical repair of the bone. In some cases, special pins, plates, or other devices are surgically implanted to maintain correct position of the bone.

Dislocation

A dislocation is when a bone is forcibly displaced from a joint. It frequently occurs in shoulders, fingers, knees, and hips. After the dislocation is reduced (the bone is replaced in the joint), the dislocation is immobilized with a splint, a cast, or traction.

Sprain

A sprain occurs when a twisting action tears the ligaments at a joint. The wrists and ankles are common sites for sprains. Symptoms include pain, swelling, discoloration, and limited movement. Treatment methods include rest, elevation, immobilization with an elastic bandage or splint, and/or cold applications.

Osteomyelitis

Osteomyelitis is a bone inflammation usually caused by a pathogenic organism. The infectious organisms cause the formation of an abscess within the bone and an accumulation of pus in the medullary canal. The infection in the bone can impede blood circulation, causing bone death. Symptoms include pain at the site, swelling, chills, and fever. Aggressive antibiotic treatment is required, usually in intravenous (IV) form. Screws, plates, or other "hardware" may be surgically implanted to support damaged bone. If a large part of the bone dies, or the infection is not controlled, amputation may be necessary.

Osteoporosis

Osteoporosis, or increased porosity, is a metabolic disorder caused by a hormone deficiency (especially estrogen in women), prolonged lack of calcium in the diet, and a sedentary lifestyle. The loss of calcium and phosphate from the bones causes the bones to lose density and become porous, brittle, and prone to fracture. Fractures often occur in the weight-bearing bones such as the back or hip. Symptoms include loss of height over time and a stooped posture. Bone density tests lead to early detection and preventative treatment for osteoporosis. Treatment methods include increased intake of calcium and vitamin D, bisphosphonates that act like estrogen to inhibit bone breakdown, medications such as Fosamax and Citracel to increase bone mass, physical therapy to build bone strength and improve posture, and/or estrogen replacement.

Ruptured Disk

A ruptured disk, also called a *herniated* or *slipped disk*, occurs when an intervertebral disk (pad of cartilage separating the vertebrae) ruptures or protrudes out of place and causes pressure on the spinal nerve (**Figure 7–26**). The most common site is at the lumbarsacral area, but a ruptured disk can occur anywhere on the spinal column. Symptoms include severe pain, muscle spasm, impaired movement, numbness, and/or tingling. Pain, anti-inflammatory, and muscle relaxant medications may be used as initial forms of treatment. Other treatments include rest, traction, physical therapy, massage therapy, chiropractic treatment, and/or heat or cold applications. A *laminectomy*, surgical removal of the protruding disk, may be necessary in a small number of severe cases that do not respond to conservative treatment. If pain persists, a spinal fusion may be performed to insert a screw/rod assembly into the spine to permanently immobilize the affected vertebrae.

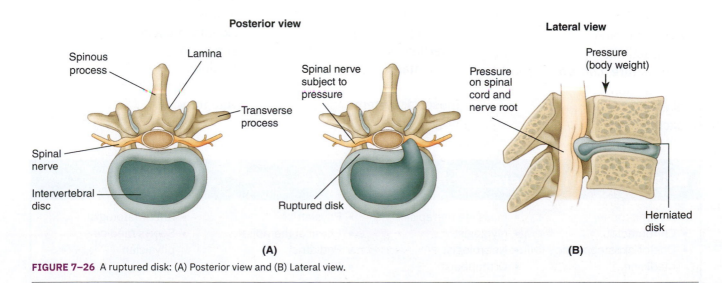

FIGURE 7–26 A ruptured disk: (A) Posterior view and (B) Lateral view.

Spinal Curvatures

Abnormal curvatures of the spinal column include kyphosis, scoliosis, and lordosis (**Figure 7–27**). *Kyphosis*, or "hunchback," is a rounded bowing of the back at the thoracic area. *Scoliosis* is a side-to-side, or lateral, curvature of the spine. *Lordosis*, or "swayback," is an abnormal inward curvature of the lumbar region. Poor posture, congenital (at birth) defects, structural defects of the vertebrae, malnutrition, and degeneration of the vertebrae can all be causes of these defects. Therapeutic exercises, firm mattresses, and/or braces are the main forms of treatment. Severe deformities may require surgical repair.

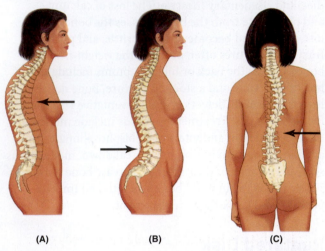

FIGURE 7–27 Abnormal curvatures of the spinal column: (A) Kyphosis, (B) Lordosis, and (C) Scoliosis.

(A)   (B)   (C)

checkpoint

1. Define arthritis and differentiate between the two types. Explain the impact this condition has on lifestyle choices.

2. With a partner, discuss the possible reason(s) why a person may develop each of the spinal curvature conditions.

PRACTICE: Go to the workbook and complete the assignment sheet for 7:4, Skeletal System.

7:5 MUSCULAR SYSTEM

OBJECTIVES

After completing this section, you should be able to:

- Compare the three main kinds of muscle by describing the action of each.

- Differentiate between voluntary muscle and involuntary muscle.

- List at least three functions of muscles.

- Describe the two main ways muscles attach to bones.

- Demonstrate the five major movements performed by muscles.

- Describe at least three diseases of the muscular system.

- Define, pronounce, and spell all key terms.

■ KEY TERMS

abduction *(ab-duck'-shun)*
adduction *(ad-duck'-shun)*
cardiac muscle
circumduction
contractibility
contracture *(con-track'-shur)*
dorsiflexion
elasticity
excitability

extensibility
extension
fascia *(fash'-ee"-ah)*
flexion *(flek'-shun)*
insertion
involuntary
muscle tone
muscular system
origin

plantar flexion
pronation
rotation
skeletal muscle
supination
tendons
visceral (smooth) muscle
voluntary

Related Health Careers

- Athletic trainer
- Chiropractor
- Doctor of osteopathic medicine

- Massage therapist
- Myologist
- Neurologist
- Orthopedist

- Physiatrist
- Physical therapist
- Podiatrist
- Prosthetist

- Rheumatologist
- Sports medicine physician

More than 600 muscles make up the system known as the **muscular system**. Muscles are bundles of muscle fibers held together by connective tissue. All muscles have certain properties or characteristics:

- **Excitability**: irritability, the ability to respond to a stimulus such as a nerve impulse

- **Contractibility**: muscle fibers that are stimulated by nerves contract, or become short and thick, which causes movement

- **Extensibility**: the ability to be stretched

- **Elasticity**: allows the muscle to return to its original shape after it has contracted or stretched

There are three main kinds of muscle: cardiac, visceral, and skeletal (**Figure 7–28**). **Cardiac muscle** forms the walls of the heart and contracts to circulate blood. The microscopic fibers of cardiac muscle are short and branching with indistinct striations and a centrally located nucleus. **Visceral muscle**, also called smooth muscle, is found in the internal organs of the body, such as those of the digestive and respiratory systems, and the blood vessels and eyes. Visceral muscle contracts to cause movement in these organs. The slow, steady contractions allow food to be moved through the digestive system. This muscle action also allows organs to expand as they fill and to shrink when they empty to prevent "flabbiness" in hollow organs. Smooth muscle

fibers are unstriated and don't have the light and dark bands when viewed under a microscope. Cardiac muscle and visceral muscle are **involuntary**, meaning they function without conscious thought or control. **Skeletal muscle** is attached to bones and causes body movement. Microscopically skeletal muscle fibers look striped with alternating light and dark striations. Skeletal muscle is **voluntary** because a person has control over its action. Skeletal muscles perform four important functions:

- Attach to bones to provide voluntary movement.

- Produce heat and energy for the body: Muscles help our bodies keep in a homeostatic temperature range by using energy from *adenosine triphosphate (ATP)*, a compound found in the muscle cell. When a muscle is stimulated, the ATP is released and heat and energy is produced. *Thermogenesis* is the process of producing heat.

- Help maintain posture by holding the body erect.

- Protect internal organs: Muscles in the torso protect internal organs at the front, sides, and back of the body by providing a protective outer covering and by reducing friction and absorbing shock. Smooth muscle also controls the volume of hollow body organs like the stomach.

Skeletal muscles attach to bones in different ways. Some attach by **tendons**, which are strong, tough, fibrous

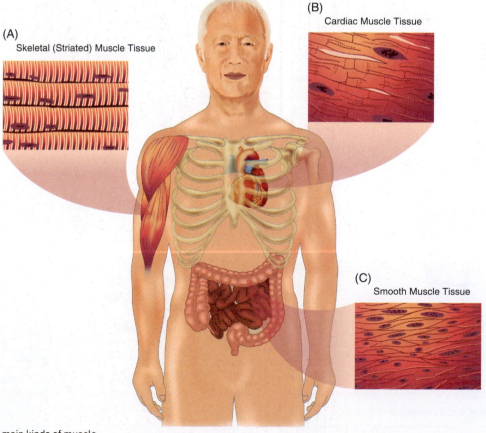

(A) Skeletal (Striated) Muscle Tissue

(B) Cardiac Muscle Tissue

(C) Smooth Muscle Tissue

FIGURE 7–28 Three main kinds of muscle.

connective-tissue cords. An example is the gastrocnemius muscle on the calf of the leg, which attaches to the heelbone by the Achilles tendon. Other muscles attach by **fascia**, a tough, sheetlike membrane that covers and protects the tissue. Examples include the deep muscles of the trunk and back, which are surrounded by the lumbodorsal fascia. When a muscle attaches to a bone, the end that does not move is called the **origin**. The end that moves when the muscle contracts is called the **insertion**. For example, the origin of the shoulder muscle, called the *deltoid*, is by the clavicle and scapula. Its insertion is on the humerus. When the deltoid contracts, the area by the scapula remains stationary, but the area by the humerus moves and abducts the arm away from the body.

A variety of different actions or movements performed by muscles are shown in **Figure 7–29** and are described as follows:

- **Adduction**: moving a body part toward the midline
- **Abduction**: moving a body part away from the midline
- **Flexion**: decreasing the angle between two bones, or bending a body part
- **Extension**: increasing the angle between two bones, or straightening a body part
- **Rotation**: turning a body part around its own axis; for example, turning the head from side to side

- **Circumduction**: moving in a circle at a joint, or moving one end of a body part in a circle while the other end remains stationary, such as swinging an arm in a circle
- **Pronation**: turning a body part downward
- **Supination**: turning a body part upward
- **Dorsiflexion**: bending backward or bending the foot toward the knee
- **Plantar flexion**: bending forward or bending the foot away from the knee

The major superficial muscles of the body are shown in **Figure 7–30**; the locations and actions of the major muscles are noted in **Table 7–2**.

Muscles are partially contracted at all times, even when not in use. This state of partial contraction is called **muscle tone** and is sometimes described as a state of readiness to act. Loss of muscle tone can occur in severe illness such as paralysis. When muscles are not used for a long period, they can *atrophy* (shrink in size and lose strength). Lack of use can also result in a **contracture**, a severe tightening of a flexor muscle resulting in bending of a joint. Foot drop is a common contracture, but the fingers, wrists, knees, and other joints can also be affected.

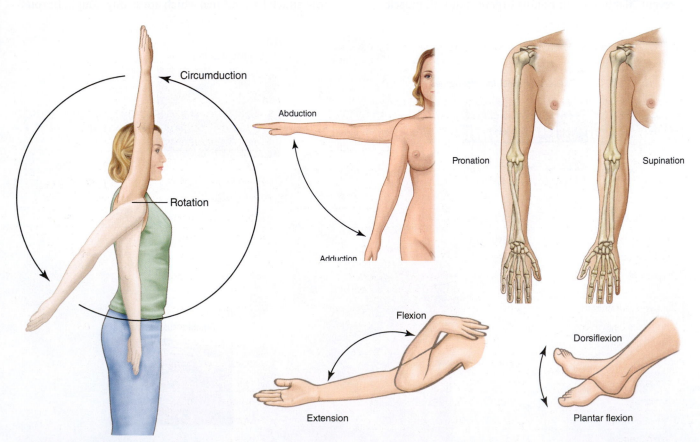

FIGURE 7–29 Types of muscle movement.

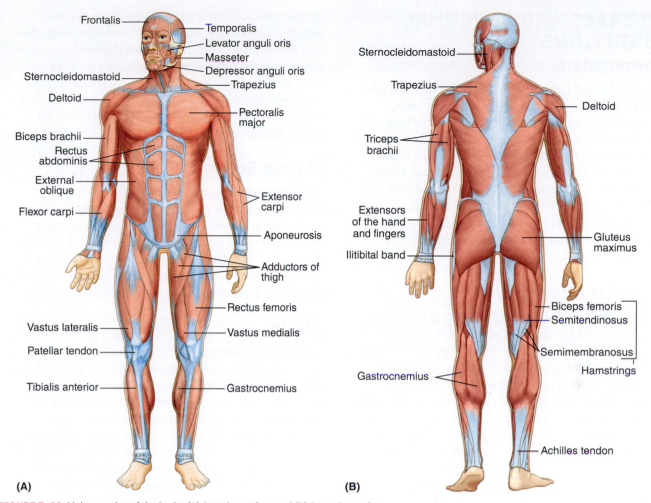

FIGURE 7–30 Main muscles of the body: (A) Anterior surface and (B) Posterior surface.

TABLE 7–2 Locations and Functions of Major Muscles of the Body

Muscle	Location	Function
Sternocleidomastoid	Side of neck	Turns and flexes head
Trapezius	Upper back and neck	Extends head, moves shoulder
Deltoid	Shoulder	Abducts arm, injection site
Biceps brachii	Upper arm	Flexes lower arm and supinates hand
Triceps brachii	Upper arm	Extends and adducts lower arm
Pectoralis major	Upper chest	Adducts and flexes upper arm
Intercostals	Between ribs	Moves ribs for breathing
Diaphragm	Just below the lungs and heart and separates thoracic cavity from abdominal cavity	Contracts as you breathe in and out to help control breathing
Rectus abdominis	Ribs to pubis (pelvis)	Compresses abdomen and flexes vertebral column
Latissimus dorsi	Spine around to chest	Extends and adducts upper arm
Gluteus maximus	Buttocks	Extends and rotates thigh, injection site
Sartorius	Front of thigh	Abducts thigh, flexes leg
Quadriceps femoris	Front of thigh	Extends leg, injection site
Hamstrings	Group of muscles at back of thigh	Flex knee, extend hip
Tibialis anterior	Front of lower leg	Flexes and inverts foot
Gastrocnemius	Back of lower leg	Flexes and supinates sole of the foot

DISEASES AND ABNORMAL CONDITIONS

Fibromyalgia

Fibromyalgia is chronic, widespread musculoskeletal pain. Other symptoms include muscle stiffness, numbness or tingling in the arms or legs, fatigue, sleep disturbances, memory and mood issues, headaches, and depression. The cause is unknown, but stress, weather, and poor physical fitness affect the condition. Treatment is directed toward pain relief and includes physical therapy, massage, exercise, and stress reduction. Pain medications, antidepressants, and muscle relaxers may also be prescribed.

Muscular Dystrophy

Muscular dystrophy is actually a group of inherited diseases that lead to chronic, progressive muscle atrophy. Muscular dystrophy usually appears in early childhood; most types result in total disability and early death. The most common type is Duchenne muscular dystrophy, which is caused by a genetic defect and affects more boys than girls. At birth, the infant is healthy. As muscle cells die, the child loses the ability to move. The onset usually occurs between 2 and 3 years of age. By age 9 to 12, the child is confined to a wheelchair. Eventually, the muscle weakness affects the heart and diaphragm, resulting in respiratory and/or cardiac failure that causes death. The life expectancy is usually from the late 20s to early 30s. Although there is no cure, physical therapy is used to reduce deformities of the joints and spine to maintain mobility as long as possible. Steroids may be given to increase muscle strength and function and to improve lung function. Current research in gene therapy is aimed at reducing the progression of the disease.

Myasthenia Gravis

Myasthenia gravis is a chronic condition where nerve impulses are not properly transmitted to the muscles. This leads to progressive muscular weakness and paralysis. If the condition affects the respiratory muscles, it can be fatal. Although the cause is unknown, myasthenia gravis is thought to be an autoimmune disease, with antibodies attacking the body's own tissues. It can affect any of the muscles that are under voluntary control, but some seem to be affected more than others. The first sign of the disease in many is eye weakness, causing ptosis or drooping of the eyelids (one or both) and/or double vision. Other frequent symptoms include altered speech (soft or nasal sounding) and difficulty chewing or swallowing. There is no cure. Treatments include cholinesterase inhibitors to increase communication between nerves and muscles, corticosteroids to limit antibody production, and immunosuppressants. Plasmapheresis, a treatment similar to hemodialysis, can be done to filter antibodies from the blood. In a small number of people, there is a tumor on the thymus gland that is affecting their immune system. Surgery can be performed to remove the tumor.

Muscle Spasms

Muscle spasms, or cramps, are sudden, painful, involuntary muscle contractions. They usually occur in the legs or feet and may result from overexertion, dehydration, low electrolyte levels, or poor circulation. Prevention includes good hydration and stretching to warm up before physical activity. Gentle pressure and stretching of the muscle are used to relieve the spasm.

Strain

A strain is an overstretching of or an injury to a muscle and/or tendon. Frequent sites include the back, arms, and legs. Prolonged or sudden muscle exertion is usually the cause. Symptoms include myalgia (muscle pain), swelling, and limited movement. Treatment methods include rest, muscle relaxants or pain medications, nonsteroidal anti-inflammatory drugs (NSAIDs) such as ibuprofen, elevating the extremity, using a compression wrap on the site, and alternating hot and cold applications.

Tendonitis

Tendonitis is an inflammation of a tendon, which is a cord that attaches bone to muscle. This condition is usually caused by a constant repetition of a particular movement over a period of time or a sudden injury to a tendon. It frequently affects the shoulder, elbow, knee, or Achilles tendon on the back of the foot, but tendonitis can occur anywhere in the body. Signs and symptoms include pain at site of injury that becomes more severe with movement, a sensation of grating or cracking of the tendon as it moves, swelling, signs of inflammation such as red and hot skin, and reduced function. Treatment is rest of the affected part, cold applications, and NSAIDs (nonsteroidal anti-inflammatory drugs) for pain. Severe injuries may require corticosteroid and pain injections and physical therapy to improve movement.

checkpoint

1. Distinguish three (3) types of muscle tissue.
2. What are two (2) ways muscles attach to bones?

PRACTICE: Go to the workbook and complete the assignment sheet for 7:5, Muscular System.

7:6 NERVOUS SYSTEM

OBJECTIVES

After completing this section, you should be able to:

- Identify the four main parts of a neuron.
- Name the two main divisions of the nervous system.
- Describe the function of each of the five main parts of the brain.
- Explain three functions of the spinal cord.
- Name the three meninges.
- Describe the circulation and function of cerebrospinal fluid.
- Contrast the actions of the sympathetic and parasympathetic nervous systems.
- Describe at least five diseases of the nervous system.
- Define, pronounce, and spell all key terms.

■ KEY TERMS

autonomic nervous system
brain
central nervous system (CNS)
cerebellum (seh"-reh-bell'-um)
cerebrospinal fluid (seh-ree"-broh-spy'-nal fluid)
cerebrum (seh-ree'-brum)
diencephalon
hypothalamus

medulla oblongata (meh-due'-laob-lawn-got'-ah)
meninges (singular: meninx) (meh-nin'-jeez)
midbrain
nerves
nervous system
neuron (nur'-on)
parasympathetic (par"-ah-sim"-pah-thet'-ik)

peripheral nervous system (PNS) (peh-rif'-eh-ral)
pons (ponz)
somatic nervous system
spinal cord
sympathetic
thalamus
ventricles

Related Health Careers

- Acupressurist
- Acupuncturist
- Anesthesiologist
- Chiropractor
- Diagnostic imager
- Doctor of osteopathic medicine
- Electroencephalographic technologist
- Electroneurodiagnostic technologist
- Mental health technician
- Neurologist
- Neurosurgeon
- Nurse anesthetist
- Physical therapist
- Polysomnographic technologist
- Psychiatrist
- Psychologist

The **nervous system** is a complex, highly organized system that coordinates all the activities of the body. This system enables the body to respond and adapt to changes that occur both inside and outside the body.

The basic structural unit of the nervous system is the **neuron**, or nerve cell (**Figure 7–31**). It consists of a cell body containing a nucleus; nerve fibers, called *dendrites* (which carry impulses toward the cell body); and a single nerve fiber, called an *axon* (which carries impulses away from the cell body). Many axons have a lipid (fat) covering called a *myelin sheath*, which increases the rate of impulse transmission and insulates and maintains the axon. The axon of one neuron lies close to the dendrites of many other neurons. The spaces between them are known as *synapses*. Impulses coming from one axon "jump" the synapse to get to

the dendrite of another neuron, which will carry the impulse in the right direction. Special chemicals, called *neurotransmitters*, located at the end of each axon, allow the nerve impulses to pass from one neuron to another. In this way, impulses can follow many different routes.

Nerves are a combination of many nerve fibers located outside the brain and spinal cord. *Afferent*, or sensory, nerves carry messages from all parts of the body to the brain and spinal cord. *Efferent*, or motor, nerves carry messages from the brain and spinal cord to the muscles and glands. These sensory nerves detect stimuli like temperature, pressure, smell, and light and send that information to the spinal cord/brain for interpretation. The brain interprets this information and then immediately directs the correct response. For instance, if you touch a hot stove, sensory nerves immediately

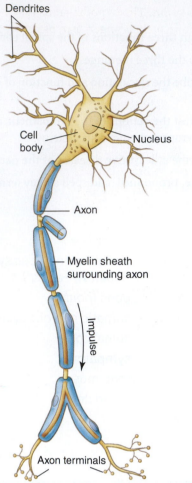

FIGURE 7–31 A neuron, the basic structural unit of the nervous system.

alert the brain. The brain interprets the message and sends an impulse to motor nerves telling muscles to move your hand off of the hot stove. That is how quickly and smoothly the coordination of the nervous system functions. There are also some *associative*, or *internuncial* nerves, that carry both sensory and motor messages.

There are two main divisions to the nervous system: the central nervous system and the peripheral nervous system (**Figure 7–32**). The **central nervous system (CNS)** consists of the brain and spinal cord. The **peripheral nervous system (PNS)** consists of the nerves and has two divisions: the somatic nervous system and the autonomic nervous system. The **somatic nervous system** carries messages between the CNS and the body. The **autonomic nervous system** contains the sympathetic and parasympathetic nervous systems, which work together to control involuntary body functions.

CENTRAL NERVOUS SYSTEM

The **brain** is a mass of nerve tissue well protected by membranes and the cranium, or skull (**Figure 7–33**). Each section or lobe of the brain has different functions (**Figure 7–34**). The main sections include:

- **Cerebrum**: the largest and highest section of the brain. The outer part is arranged in folds, called *convolutions*, and separated into lobes. The lobes include the frontal, parietal, temporal,

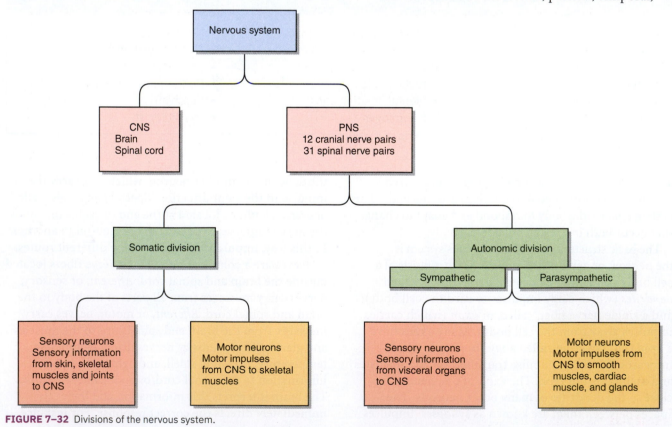

FIGURE 7–32 Divisions of the nervous system.

and occipital, named from the skull bones that surround them (**Figure 7–34**). The cerebrum is responsible for reasoning, thought, memory, judgment, speech, sensation, sight, smell, hearing, and voluntary body movement.

- **Cerebellum**: the section below the back of the cerebrum. It is responsible for muscle coordination, balance, posture, and muscle tone.

- **Diencephalon**: the section located between the cerebrum and midbrain. It contains two structures: the thalamus and hypothalamus. The **thalamus** acts as a relay center and directs sensory impulses to the cerebrum. It also allows conscious recognition of pain and temperature. The **hypothalamus** regulates and controls the autonomic nervous system, temperature, appetite, water balance, sleep, and blood vessel constriction

and dilation. The hypothalamus is also involved in emotions such as anger, fear, pleasure, pain, and affection.

- **Midbrain**: the section located below the cerebrum at the top of the brainstem. It is responsible for conducting impulses between brain parts and for certain eye and auditory reflexes.

- **Pons**: the section located below the midbrain and in the brainstem. It is responsible for conducting messages to other parts of the brain; for certain reflex actions including chewing, tasting, and saliva production; and for assisting with respiration.

- **Medulla oblongata**: the lowest part of the brainstem. It connects with the spinal cord and is responsible for regulating heartbeat, respiration, swallowing, coughing, and blood pressure.

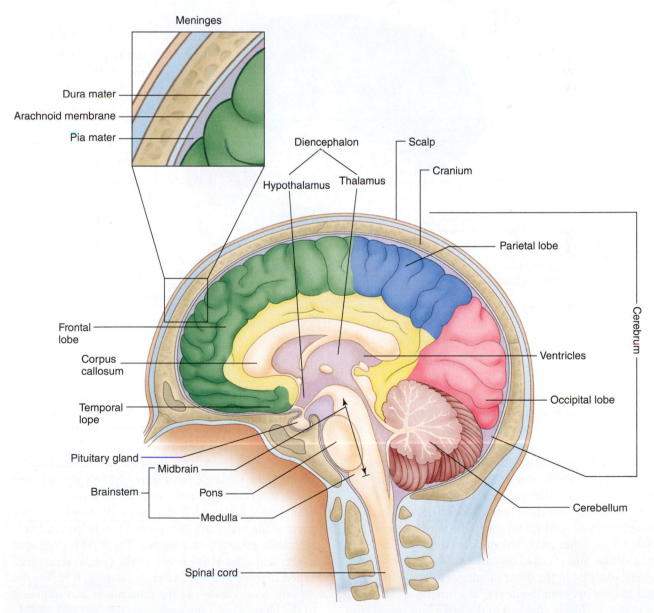

FIGURE 7–33 The brain and spinal cord.

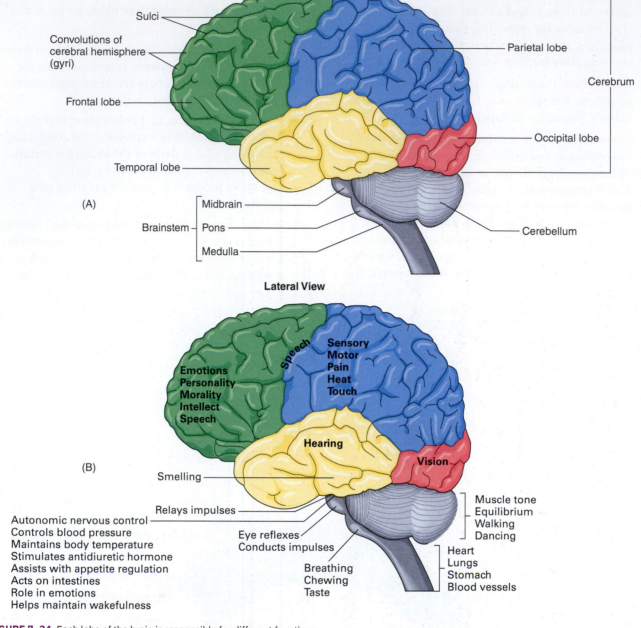

Lateral View

(A)

Sulci
Convolutions of cerebral hemisphere (gyri)
Frontal lobe
Temporal lobe
Midbrain
Brainstem — Pons
Medulla
Parietal lobe
Cerebrum
Occipital lobe
Cerebellum

(B)

Emotions
Personality
Morality
Intellect
Speech

Speech

Sensory
Motor
Pain
Heat
Touch

Hearing

Vision

Smelling
Relays impulses
Autonomic nervous control
Controls blood pressure
Maintains body temperature
Stimulates antidiuretic hormone
Assists with appetite regulation
Acts on intestines
Role in emotions
Helps maintain wakefulness

Eye reflexes
Conducts impulses

Breathing
Chewing
Taste

Muscle tone
Equilibrium
Walking
Dancing

Heart
Lungs
Stomach
Blood vessels

FIGURE 7–34 Each lobe of the brain is responsible for different functions.

The **spinal cord** continues down from the medulla oblongata and ends at the first or second lumbar vertebrae. It is surrounded and protected by the vertebrae. The spinal cord is responsible for many reflex actions and for carrying sensory (afferent) messages up to the brain and motor (efferent) messages from the brain to the nerves that go to the muscles and glands.

The **meninges** are three membranes that cover and protect the brain and spinal cord. The *dura mater* is the thick, tough, outer layer. The middle layer is delicate and weblike, and is called the *arachnoid membrane*. It is loosely attached to the other meninges to allow space for fluid to flow between the layers. The innermost layer, the *pia mater*, is closely attached to the brain and spinal cord, and contains blood vessels that nourish the nerve tissue.

The brain has four **ventricles**, hollow spaces that connect with each other and with the space under the arachnoid membrane (the subarachnoid space). The ventricles are filled with a clear, colorless fluid called **cerebrospinal fluid**. This fluid circulates continually between the ventricles and through the subarachnoid space. It serves as a shock absorber to protect the brain and spinal cord. It also carries nutrients to some parts of the brain and spinal cord and helps remove metabolic products and wastes. The fluid is produced in the ventricles of the brain by the special structures called *choroid plexuses*. After circulating, it is absorbed into the blood vessels of the dura mater and returned to the bloodstream through special structures called *arachnoid villi*.

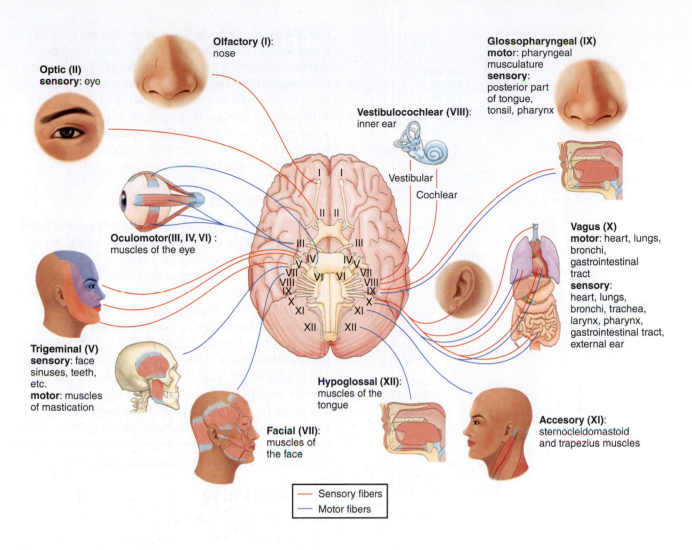

Optic (II)
sensory: eye

Olfactory (I):
nose

Vestibulocochlear (VIII):
inner ear

Vestibular

Cochlear

Glossopharyngeal (IX)
motor: pharyngeal
musculature
sensory:
posterior part
of tongue,
tonsil, pharynx

Oculomotor(III, IV, VI) :
muscles of the eye

Vagus (X)
motor: heart, lungs,
bronchi,
gastrointestinal
tract
sensory:
heart, lungs,
bronchi, trachea,
larynx, pharynx,
gastrointestinal tract,
external ear

Trigeminal (V)
sensory: face
sinuses, teeth,
etc.
motor: muscles
of mastication

Hypoglossal (XII):
muscles of the
tongue

Facial (VII):
muscles of
the face

Accesory (XI):
sternocleidomastoid
and trapezius muscles

I I

II II

III III

V IV   IV V

VII VII

VI VI

VIII VIII

IX IX

X X

XI XI

XII XII

— Sensory fibers
— Motor fibers

FIGURE 7–35 The cranial nerves.

PERIPHERAL NERVOUS SYSTEM

The peripheral nervous system consists of the somatic and the autonomic nervous systems.

Somatic Nervous System

The somatic nervous system consists of 12 pairs of cranial nerves and their branches, and 31 pairs of spinal nerves and their branches. Some of the cranial nerves are responsible for special senses such as sight, hearing, taste, and smell (**Figure 7–35**). Others receive general sensations such as touch, pressure, pain, and temperature, and send out impulses for involuntary and voluntary muscle control. The spinal nerves carry messages to and from the spinal cord and are mixed nerves, both sensory (afferent) and motor (efferent). There are 8 cervical, 12 thoracic, 5 lumbar, 5 sacral, and 1 pair of coccygeal spinal nerves (**Figure 7–36**). Each nerve goes directly to a particular part of the body or networks with other spinal nerves to form a plexus that supplies sensation to a larger segment of the body.

Autonomic Nervous System

The autonomic nervous system is an important part of the peripheral nervous system. It helps maintain a balance in the involuntary functions of the body and allows the body to react in times of emergency. There are two divisions to the autonomic nervous system: the **sympathetic** and **parasympathetic** nervous systems. These two systems usually work together to maintain a balanced state, or *homeostasis*, in the body and to control involuntary body functions at proper rates. In times of emergency, the sympathetic nervous system prepares the body to act by increasing heart rate, respiration, and blood pressure, and by slowing activity in the digestive tract. This is known as the *fight or flight response*. After the emergency, the parasympathetic nervous system counteracts the actions of the sympathetic system by slowing heart rate, decreasing respiration, lowering blood pressure, and increasing activity in the digestive tract.

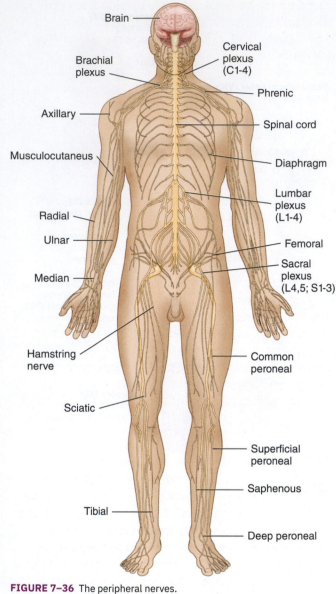

FIGURE 7–36 The peripheral nerves.

Labels on figure:
Brain
Brachial plexus
Cervical plexus (C1-4)
Axillary
Phrenic
Musculocutaneus
Spinal cord
Radial
Diaphragm
Ulnar
Lumbar plexus (L1-4)
Median
Femoral
Sacral plexus (L4,5; S1-3)
Hamstring nerve
Common peroneal
Sciatic
Superficial peroneal
Saphenous
Tibial
Deep peroneal

DISEASES AND ABNORMAL CONDITIONS

Amyotrophic Lateral Sclerosis

Amyotrophic lateral sclerosis (ALS), also known as Lou Gehrig's disease, is a chronic, degenerative neuromuscular disease. The cause is unknown, but genetic or viral-immune factors are suspected. Nerve cells in the CNS that control voluntary movement degenerate, resulting in a weakening and atrophy (wasting away) of the muscles they control. Initial symptoms include muscle weakness, abnormal reflexes, tripping and falling, impaired hand and arm movement, and difficulty in speaking or swallowing. As the disease progresses, more muscles are affected, resulting in total body paralysis. In the later stages, the patient loses all ability to communicate, breathe, eat, and move. Mental acuity is unaffected, so an active mind is trapped inside a paralyzed body. There is no cure for ALS, but drugs such as Riluzole may slow the progress of the disease. Supportive care that includes physical therapy, occupational therapy, and speech therapy is used to relieve symptoms and improve quality of life. ALS life expectancy is 2 to 5 years from time of diagnosis, but some patients with slower rates of progression have survived 10–20 years after the diagnosis of the disease. Only 5 percent live longer than 20 years.

Carpal Tunnel Syndrome

Carpal tunnel syndrome is a progressively painful hand and arm condition that occurs when the medial nerve and tendons that pass through a canal or "tunnel" on their way from the forearm to the hands and fingers are pinched. Repetitive movement of the wrist causes swelling around this tunnel, which puts pressure on the nerves and tendons. Symptoms include pain, muscle weakness in the hand, and impaired movement. A classic symptom is pain, numbness, and tingling in the thumb, ring finger, and middle finger. Initially, carpal tunnel is treated with activity modification, anti-inflammatory medications, analgesics for pain, steroid injections, and splinting to immobilize the joint. Severe cases that do not respond to this treatment may require surgery to enlarge the "tunnel" and relieve the pressure on the nerves and tendons.

Cerebral Palsy

Cerebral palsy is a nonprogressive, noncontagious disturbance in voluntary muscle action and is caused by brain damage. Lack of oxygen to the brain, birth injuries, prenatal rubella (German measles), and infections can all cause cerebral palsy. Of the three forms—spastic, athetoid, and atactic—spastic is the most common. Symptoms include exaggerated reflexes, tense muscles, contracture development, seizures, speech impairment, spasms, tremors, and, in some cases, mental retardation. Although there is no cure, physical, occupational, and speech therapy are important aspects of treatment. Muscle relaxants, anticonvulsive drugs, casts, braces, and/or orthopedic surgery (for severe contractures) are also used. In addition, botulinum toxin (Botox) can be injected directly into affected muscles to decrease spasticity.

Cerebrovascular Accident or Stroke

A cerebrovascular accident (CVA), also called a *stroke*, *brain attack*, or *apoplexy*, occurs when the blood flow to the brain is impaired, resulting in a lack of oxygen and a destruction of brain tissue. There are two main types of stroke: hemorrhagic and ischemic. A *hemorrhagic* stroke occurs when a blood vessel in the brain bursts or bleeds, decreasing blood flow to the brain. This can be the result of hypertension, an aneurysm, anticoagulant use, or trauma. An *ischemic* stroke occurs when a blockage causes a lack of blood flow to the brain. This can be the result of atherosclerosis or a thrombus (blood clot). Factors that increase the risk for a CVA include smoking, a high-fat diet, obesity, hypertension, and a sedentary lifestyle. Symptoms vary depending on the area and amount of brain tissue damaged. Some common symptoms of an acute CVA include loss of consciousness, weakness or paralysis on one side of the body (hemiplegia), dizziness, dysphagia (difficult swallowing), visual disturbances, mental confusion, aphasia (speech and language impairment), and incontinence. A *transient ischemic attack (TIA)*, also known as a ministroke, is caused by the same things as a CVA and has the same symptoms, but the symptoms only last for a few minutes and they do not cause permanent damage. TIAs are often a warning sign of an impending CVA. Prompt diagnosis and treatment of the cause of the TIA is important.

When a CVA occurs, immediate care during the first 3 hours can help prevent brain damage. Computerized tomography (CT) scans (noninvasive computerized X-rays that show cross-sectional views of body tissue) are used to determine the cause of the CVA. If the cause is an ischemic stroke, thrombolytics or "clot busting" drugs such as TPA (tissue plasminogen activator) can be given to dissolve a clot and restore blood flow. If atherosclerosis is the cause, angioplasty of the cerebral arteries may be performed. If the cause is found to be from a hemorrhage, thrombolytic therapy is not an option. In this case, treatment will depend on the cause of the bleed (hypertension, use of anticoagulants, trauma, etc.). In some cases, surgery can be done to stop the bleeding. Neuroprotective agents, or drugs that help prevent injury to neurons, are also used initially to prevent permanent brain damage. Additional treatment depends on symptoms and is directed toward helping the person recover from or adapt to the symptoms that are present. Physical, occupational, and speech therapy are the main forms of treatment.

Concussion

A concussion is a traumatic brain injury that affects brain function. They are usually caused by a blow to the head or a fall. This injury causes the brain to slide back and forth forcefully against the skull. Sometimes violent shaking of the head, especially with young children, can also lead to a concussion. Concussions can be common if you play a contact sport such as football or soccer. As they become more aware of these injuries, sports organizations are taking steps to prevent concussions. Athletes with a suspected concussion should not return to play until they have been medically evaluated. Some concussions cause a loss of consciousness, but most do not. Typical symptoms include headache or a feeling of pressure in the head, confusion, dizziness, ringing in the ears, fatigue, loss of balance, nausea and vomiting, blurred vision, sensitivity to noise or light, and appearing dazed. In most cases, treatment is avoiding any activities that make the symptoms worse, acetaminophen for headache, and rest to allow the brain to recover. Monitoring for bleeding in the brain and making sure brain damage has not occurred is necessary. Repeated concussions can lead to permanent brain damage that affects speech, learning, and body movements, but most people usually recover fully after a concussion.

Encephalitis

Encephalitis is an inflammation of the brain and is caused by a virus, bacterium, chemical agent, or as a complication of measles, chicken pox, or mumps. The virus is frequently contracted from a mosquito bite because mosquitoes can carry the encephalitis virus. Symptoms vary but usually present as flu-like and then escalate, depending on severity of infection. They may include fever, extreme weakness or lethargy, visual disturbances, headaches, vomiting, stiff neck and back, dis-orientation, seizures, coma, and, rarely, death. Treatment methods are supportive and include antiviral drugs, anti-inflammatory drugs, maintenance of fluid and electrolyte balance, antiseizure medication, and monitoring and support of respiratory and kidney function.

Epilepsy

Epilepsy, or seizure syndrome, is a brain disorder associated with abnormal surges in electrical impulses in the neurons of the brain. Although causes can include genetics, brain injury, birth trauma, tumors, toxins such as lead or carbon monoxide, and infections, many cases of epilepsy are idiopathic (spontaneous, or primary). Absence, or petit mal, seizures are milder and are characterized by a loss of consciousness lasting several seconds. They are common in children and frequently disappear by late adolescence. Generalized tonic-clonic, or grand mal, are the most severe seizures. They are characterized by a loss of consciousness lasting several minutes; convulsions accompanied by violent shaking and thrashing movements; hypersalivation, causing foaming at the mouth; and loss of body functions. Some individuals experience an *aura*, such as a particular smell, ringing in the ears, visual disturbances, or tingling in the fingers and/or toes just before a seizure occurs. Anticonvulsant drugs are effective in controlling epilepsy in most people. In conjunction with or in place of medications, a diet high in fat and low in carbohydrates (ketogenic), or vagus nerve stimulation (VNS) may be helpful in controlling seizures. Laser thermal ablation, a minimally invasive procedure, uses a small laser-tipped tube that is inserted into the area of the brain causing the seizure to destroy the tissue. In special cases, brain surgery can be performed to remove the area of the brain causing the seizures.

Hydrocephalus

Hydrocephalus, also known as "water on the brain," is an excessive accumulation of cerebrospinal fluid (CSF) in the ventricles and, in some cases, the subarachnoid space of the brain. It is usually caused by a congenital (at birth) defect, infection, or tumor that obstructs the flow of cerebrospinal fluid out of the brain. Symptoms include an abnormally enlarged head, prominent forehead, bulging eyes, irritability, distended scalp veins, and when pressure prevents proper development of the brain, retardation. If left untreated, it can be fatal. The condition can be treated by the surgical implantation of a shunt (tube) between the ventricles and the veins, heart, or abdominal peritoneal cavity to provide for drainage of the excess fluid. A ventriculostomy can also be performed to create a hole in the bottom of the ventricle to allow CSF to drain toward the base of the brain to be reabsorbed.

Meningitis

Meningitis is an inflammation of the meninges of the brain and/or spinal cord and is caused by a bacterium, virus, fungus, or toxin such as lead or arsenic. Early signs can easily be mistaken as the flu. Symptoms include high fever, headaches, back and neck pain and stiffness, nausea and vomiting, delirium, convulsions, and, if untreated, coma and death. Treatment methods include antibiotics (for bacterial meningitis), antipyretics (for fever), anticonvulsants, and/or medications for pain and cerebral edema. Some forms of bacterial meningitis are preventable with vaccinations.

Multiple Sclerosis

Multiple sclerosis (MS) is a chronic, progressive, disabling condition resulting from a degeneration of the myelin sheath in the CNS. It usually occurs between the ages of 20 and 40 (**Figure 7–37**). The cause is unknown but genetics or an autoimmune disorder in which the body attacks its own tissue (in this case, the myelin sheath) are suspected. The disease progresses at different rates and has periods of remission. Early symptoms include visual disturbances such as diplopia (double vision), weakness, fatigue, poor coordination, and tingling and numbness. As the disease progresses, tremors, muscle spasticity, paralysis, speech impairment, emotional swings, and incontinence occur. There is no cure. Beta interferon medications are being used to slow the rate at which MS progresses. Treatment methods such as physical therapy, muscle relaxants, steroids, and psychological counseling are used to maintain functional ability as long as possible.

Neuralgia

Neuralgia is nerve pain that is experienced without stimulation of the nerve receptor. The pain is caused by nerve damage and is often very difficult to diagnose.

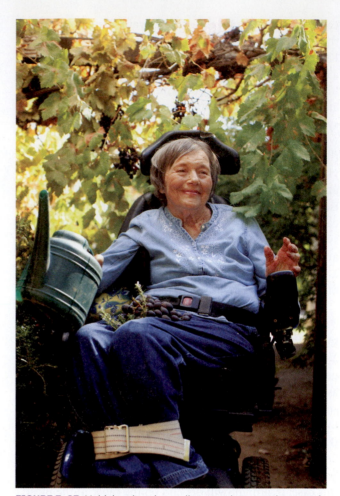

FIGURE 7–37 Multiple sclerosis usually occurs between the ages of 20 and 40. Courtesy, National Multiple Sclerosis Society

It is a form of chronic pain affecting more women than men, and it does not respond well to traditional pain medication. The pain can be so severe that the person is unable to sleep or eat. Antidepressant medications, antiepileptic medication, acupuncture, vitamin or nutritional therapy, hot and cold compresses, and electrical nerve stimulation may also relieve the pain. Studies have shown that the use of medical marijuana (cannabis) may reduce neuropathic pain.

Paralysis

Paralysis is the loss of voluntary muscle movement and coordination in some part of the body. It usually results from a brain or spinal cord injury that destroys neurons and results in a loss of function and sensation below the level of injury. *Hemiplegia* is paralysis on one side of the body and is caused by a tumor, injury, or CVA. *Paraplegia* is paralysis in the lower extremities or lower part of the body and is caused by a spinal cord injury. *Quadriplegia* is paralysis of the arms, legs, and body below the spinal cord injury. Currently, no cure exists, although much research is being directed toward repairing spinal cord damage, including nerve reconstruction. Treatment methods are supportive and include physical and occupational therapy.

Parkinson's Disease

Parkinson's disease is a chronic, progressive condition involving degeneration of brain cells, usually in persons over 50 years of age. Symptoms include tremors, stiffness, muscular rigidity, a forward-leaning position, a shuffling gait, difficulty in stopping while walking, loss of facial expression, drooling, mood swings and frequent depression, and behavioral changes. Although no cure exists, drugs such as levodopa, dopamine agonists, and MAO-B inhibitors are used to relieve the symptoms. Deep brain stimulation (DBS) therapy uses an implantable device that has been proven to reduce some of the symptoms of Parkinson's. In some cases, surgery can be performed to selectively destroy a small area of the brain and control involuntary movements. Physical therapy is also used to limit muscular rigidity.

Shingles

Shingles, or herpes zoster, is an acute inflammation of nerve cells and is caused by the herpes virus, which also causes chicken pox. A person who has shingles can pass the virus to those who have not had chicken pox. This occurs through direct contact with open sores. However, the infected person will develop chicken pox, not shingles. Shingles characteristically occurs in the thoracic area on one side of the body and follows the path of the affected nerves but it can appear anywhere on the body (**Figure 7–38**). Fluid-filled vesicles appear on the skin, accompanied by severe pain, redness, itching, fever, and abnormal skin sensations. In 2006, a Zostavax vaccine to prevent shingles was approved by the FDA. However, it was only 50–70 percent effective. In 2017, a new Shringrix vaccine was approved by the FDA and made available to adults older than the age of 50. The Shringrix vaccine is given in two doses over a 3-month period and has shown 90 percent effectiveness at preventing shingles. Antiviral medications should be started promptly with the first sign of the rash to decrease the severity and duration of the symptoms. Treatment is directed toward relieving pain and itching until the inflammation subsides, usually in 2–6 weeks.

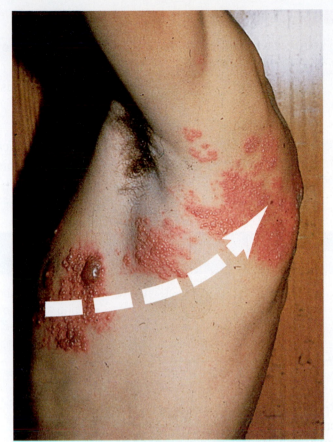

FIGURE 7–38 The vesicles of shingles follow the path of the affected nerves. Courtesy of Robert A. Silverman, M.D., Clinical Associate Professor, Department of Pediatrics, Georgetown University.

checkpoint

1. Distinguish the four (4) main parts of a neuron. What makes a neuron afferent or efferent?

2. Explain the relationship between chicken pox and shingles.

3. List the five (5) parts of the brain and describe their function.

PRACTICE: Go to the workbook and complete the assignment sheet for 7:6, Nervous System.

7:7 SPECIAL SENSES

OBJECTIVES

After completing this section, you should be able to:

- Identify five special senses.
- Label the major parts on a diagram of the eye.
- Trace the pathway of light rays as they pass through the eye.
- Label the major parts on a diagram of the ear.
- Trace the pathway of sound waves as they pass through the ear.
- Explain how the ear helps maintain balance and equilibrium.
- State the locations of the four main taste receptors.
- List at least four general senses located throughout the body.
- Describe at least six diseases of the eye and ear.
- Define, pronounce, and spell all key terms.

aqueous humor *(a'-kwee"-us hue-more)*

auditory canal

auricle *(or'-eh-kul")*

choroid coat *(koh'-royd)*

cochlea *(co'-klee-ah)*

conjunctiva *(kon-junk"-tye'-vah)*

cornea

eustachian tube *(you-stay'-she-en)*

iris

lacrimal glands *(lack'-rih"-mal)*

lens

organ of Corti

ossicles *(os'-ick-uls)*

pinna *(pin'-nah)*

pupil

refracts

retina *(ret'-in-ah)*

sclera *(sklee'-rah)*

semicircular canals

tympanic membrane *(tim-pan'-ik)*

vestibule *(ves'-tih-bewl)*

vitreous humor *(vit'-ree-us hue'-more)*

Related Health Careers

- Allergist
- Audiologist
- Eye, ear, nose, and throat specialist
- Ophthalmic assistant
- Ophthalmic laboratory technician
- Ophthalmic medical technologist
- Ophthalmic technician
- Ophthalmologist
- Optician
- Optometrist
- Otolaryngologist
- Otologist

Special senses allow the human body to react to the environment by providing for sight, hearing, taste, smell, and balance maintenance. There are five types of sensory receptors, each with their area of specialty. *Chemoreceptors* are sensitive to chemical changes; *mechanoreceptors* react to physical interaction like pressure, touch, and itching; *photoreceptors* are sensitive to light changes; *thermoreceptors* respond to temperature fluctuation; and *nociceptors* detect pain. Sensing this information and responding appropriately is possible because the body has structures that receive these sensations, nerves that carry sensory messages to the brain, and a brain that interprets and responds to sensory messages.

THE EYE

The eye is the organ that controls the special sense of sight. It receives light rays and transmits impulses from the rays to the optic nerve, which carries the impulses to the brain, where they are interpreted as vision, or sight.

The eye (**Figure 7–39A**) is well protected. It is partially enclosed in a bony socket of the skull. Eyelids and eyelashes help keep out dirt and pathogens. **Lacrimal glands** in the eye produce tears, which constantly moisten and cleanse the eye. The tears flow across the eye and drain through the nasolacrimal duct into the nasal cavity. A mucous membrane, called the **conjunctiva**, lines the eyelids and covers the front of the eye to provide additional protection and lubrication.

There are three main layers to the eye (**Figure 7–39B**). The outermost layer is the tough connective tissue called the **sclera**. It is frequently referred to as the "white" of the eye. The sclera maintains the shape of the eye. Extrinsic muscles, responsible for moving the eye within the socket, are attached to the outside of the sclera. The **cornea** is a circular, transparent part of the front of the sclera. It allows light rays to enter the eye. The middle layer of the eye, the **choroid coat**, is interlaced with many blood vessels that nourish the eyes. The innermost layer of the eye is the **retina**. It is made of many layers of nerve cells, which transmit the light impulses to the optic nerve. Two of these photoreceptor nerve cells are *cones* and *rods*. Cones are sensitive to color and are used mainly for vision when it is light. Most of the cones are located in a depression located on the back surface of the retina called the *fovea centralis*; this is the area of sharpest vision. Rods are used for vision when it is dark or dim.

The **iris** is the colored portion of the eye. It is located behind the cornea on the front of the choroid coat. The opening in the center of the iris is called the **pupil**. The iris contains two muscles, which control the size of the pupil and regulate the amount of light entering the eye.

Other special structures are also located in the eye. The **lens** is a circular structure located behind the pupil and suspended in position by ligaments. It **refracts** (bends) light rays so the rays focus on the retina. The **aqueous humor** is a clear, watery fluid that fills the space between the cornea and iris. It helps maintain the forward curvature of the eyeball and refracts light rays. The **vitreous humor** is the jellylike substance that fills the area behind the lens. It helps maintain the shape of the eyeball and also refracts light rays. A series of muscles located in the eye provide for eye movement.

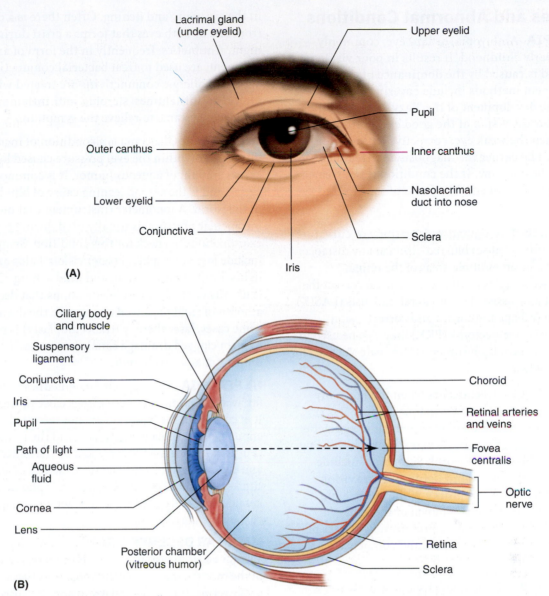

FIGURE 7–39 (A) External view of the eye. (B) Structures of the eye.

When light rays enter the eye, they pass through a series of parts that refract the rays so that the rays focus on the retina. These parts are the cornea, the aqueous humor, the pupil, the lens, and the vitreous humor. In the retina, the light rays (image) are picked up by the rods and cones, changed into nerve impulses, and transmitted by the optic nerve to the occipital lobe of the cerebrum, where sight is interpreted. If the rays are not refracted correctly by the various parts, vision can be distorted or blurred (**Figure 7–40**).

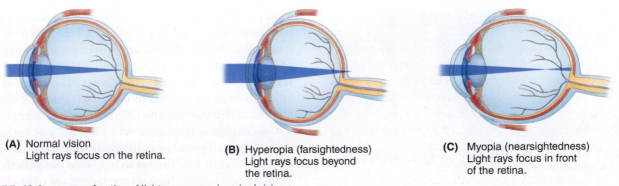

(A) Normal vision
Light rays focus on the retina.

(B) Hyperopia (farsightedness)
Light rays focus beyond the retina.

(C) Myopia (nearsightedness)
Light rays focus in front of the retina.

FIGURE 7–40 Improper refraction of light rays causes impaired vision.

Diseases and Abnormal Conditions

AMBLYOPIA Amblyopia, or lazy eye, commonly occurs in early childhood. It results in poor vision in one eye and is caused by the dominance of the other eye. Treatment methods include covering the good eye to stimulate development of the "lazy" eye, atropine drops to blur the vision of the good eye, exercises to strengthen the weak eye, corrective lenses, and/or surgery. The earlier the diagnosis and treatment, the better the outcome. If the condition is not treated before 8 to 9 years of age, blindness of the affected eye may occur.

ASTIGMATISM Astigmatism is warping or curvature of the cornea that causes blurred vision at any distance. Light rays focus on multiple areas of the retina. Corrective lenses (glasses or contact lenses) correct the condition. Laser-assisted in situ keratomileusis (LASIK) surgery can reshape the cornea and correct vision. Photorefractive keratectomy (PRK) may also be used to reshape the cornea. Both surgeries eliminate the need for glasses or contacts.

CATARACT A cataract occurs when the normally clear lens becomes cloudy or opaque (**Figure 7–41**). This occurs gradually, usually as a result of aging, but may be the result of trauma. Cataracts are the leading cause of blindness in the world. Symptoms include blurred vision, halos around lights, gradual vision loss, and in later stages, a milky-white pupil. Sight is restored by the surgical removal of the lens. An implanted intraocular lens or prescription glasses or contact lenses correct the vision and compensate for the removed lens.

CONJUNCTIVITIS Conjunctivitis, or pink eye, is a highly contagious inflammation of the conjunctiva and is usually caused by a bacterium, virus, or allergen. Symptoms include redness, a gritty sensation

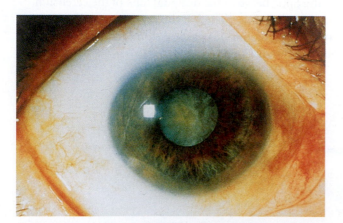

FIGURE 7–41 A cataract occurs when the lens of the eye becomes cloudy or opaque. Courtesy of National Eye Institute, NEI

in the eye, pain, and itching. Often there is a discharge from one or both eyes that forms a crust during the night. Antibiotics, frequently in the form of an eye ointment, are used to treat bacterial conjunctivitis. Viral and allergic conjunctivitis are treated with topical antihistamines, steroids, anti-inflammatories, and decongestants to relieve the symptoms.

GLAUCOMA Glaucoma is a condition of increased intraocular (within the eye) pressure caused by an excess amount of aqueous humor. It is common after age 40 and is the second leading cause of blindness in the world. A tonometer (instrument that measures intraocular pressure) is usually used during regular eye examinations to check for this condition. Symptoms include loss of peripheral (side) vision, halos around lights, limited night vision, and mild aching. Glaucoma is usually controlled with medications that decrease the amount of fluid produced or improve the drainage. In some cases, laser therapy (trabeculoplasty) is performed to open clogged drainage canals and increase the outflow of aqueous humor.

HYPEROPIA Hyperopia is farsightedness. Objects far away are seen clearly but things close up are blurry. It occurs when the light rays are not refracted sharply enough and the image focuses behind the retina (**Figure 7–40**). Vision is corrected by the use of glasses and contact lenses (convex lenses). Laser-assisted in situ keratomileusis (LASIK) surgery or photorefractive keratectomy (PRK) can be performed to reshape the cornea and correct vision.

MACULAR DEGENERATION Macular degeneration, a major cause of vision loss and blindness, is a disease of the macula, the central and most sensitive section of the retina. It is an age-related disorder caused by damage to the blood vessels that nourish the retina. The most common type is *dry macular degeneration* that occurs as fatty deposits decrease the blood supply to the retina, resulting in a gradual thinning of the retina. It progresses slowly and results in blurred, distorted vision with an absence of central vision. Peripheral (side) vision is usually not affected. No cure currently exists, but optical aids such as special lighting or magnifiers may improve vision slightly. A daily intake of high-dose vitamins C and E, beta-carotene, zinc, and copper have been shown to slow progression. Potential new treatments include antioxidant eye drops, implantation of purified human neural stem cells, and fetal cell transplantation. *Wet macular degeneration* is caused by an abnormal growth of blood vessels that leak blood and fluids that damage the retina. Laser treatment (photocoagulation) coagulates or seals the leaking blood vessels and can preserve sight. Medications are also injected directly into the eye to help stop the growth of new blood vessels. New research directed toward creation of an artificial retina or bionic eye may allow individuals with this disease to regain the ability to see light and large objects in the future.

MYOPIA Myopia is nearsightedness. Sight is clear up close, but objects far away are blurry. It occurs when the light rays are refracted too sharply and the image focuses in front of the retina (**Figure 7–40**). Vision is corrected by the use of glasses and contact lenses (concave lenses). Laser-assisted in situ keratomileusis (LASIK) surgery or photorefractive keratectomy (PRK) can be performed to reshape the cornea and correct vision.

PRESBYOPIA Presbyopia is farsightedness caused by a loss of lens elasticity. Light rays focus behind the retina. It results from the normal aging process and usually occurs in the early to mid-40s. It is treated by the use of corrective lenses or "reading" glasses. Laser-assisted in situ keratomileusis (LASIK) surgery or photorefractive keratectomy (PRK) may be performed to correct vision in some cases. A lens implant may be required in other cases.

STRABISMUS Strabismus is a disorder in which the eyes do not move or focus together (**Figure 7–42**). The eyes may move inward (cross-eyed) or outward, or up or down. It is caused by muscle weakness in one or both eyes. Treatment methods include visual training exercises, covering the good eye, corrective lenses, and/or surgery on the muscles that move the eye. Botulinum toxin (Botox) can be injected into the stronger muscle causing temporary paralysis and improving cosmetic appearances. It must be repeated every 3 to 4 months.

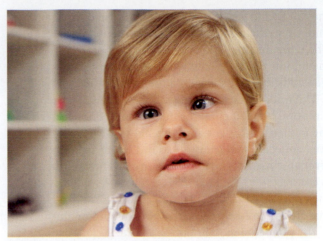

FIGURE 7–42 Strabismus is a disorder in which the eyes do not move or focus together. ©iStock.com/Tea Potocnik

THE EAR

The ear is the organ that controls the special senses of hearing and balance. It transmits impulses from sound waves to the auditory (vestibulocochlear) nerve, which carries the impulses to the brain for interpretation as hearing. The ear is divided into three main sections: the outer ear, the middle ear, and the inner ear (**Figure 7–43**).

The outer ear contains the visible part of the ear, called the **pinna**, or **auricle**. The pinna is elastic cartilage covered by skin. It leads to a canal, or tube, called the *external auditory meatus*, or **auditory canal**. Special glands in this canal produce *cerumen*, a wax that protects

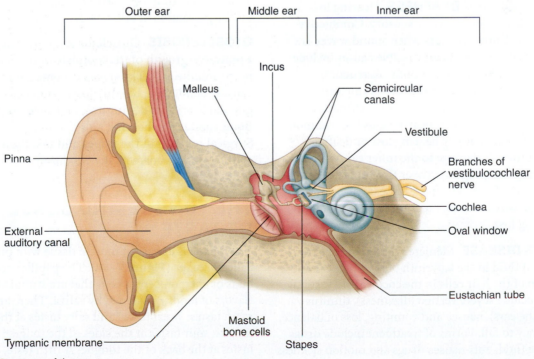

FIGURE 7–43 Structures of the ear.

the ear. Sound waves travel through the auditory canal until they reach the eardrum, or **tympanic membrane**. The tympanic membrane separates the outer ear from the middle ear. It vibrates when sound waves hit it and transmits the sound waves to the middle ear.

The middle ear is a small space, or cavity, in the temporal bone. It contains three small bones (**ossicles**): the malleus, the incus, and the stapes. The bones are connected and transmit sound waves from the tympanic membrane to the inner ear. The middle ear is connected to the pharynx, or throat, by a tube called the **eustachian tube**. This tube allows air to enter the middle ear and helps equalize air pressure on both sides of the tympanic membrane.

The inner ear is the most complex portion of the ear. It is separated from the middle ear by a membrane called the *oval window*. The first section is the **vestibule**, which acts as the entrance to the two other parts of the inner ear. The **cochlea**, shaped like a snail's shell, contains delicate, hairlike mechanoreceptor cells, which compose the **organ of Corti**, a receptor of sound waves. The organ of Corti transmits the impulses from sound waves to the auditory nerve. This nerve carries the impulses to the temporal lobe of the cerebrum, where they are interpreted as hearing. **Semicircular canals** are also located in the inner ear. These canals contain a liquid and delicate, hairlike cells that bend when the liquid moves with head and body movements. Impulses sent from the semicircular canals to the cerebellum of the brain help to maintain our sense of balance and equilibrium.

Diseases and Abnormal Conditions

HEARING LOSS AND DEAFNESS Hearing loss is classified as either conductive or sensory. Conductive hearing loss or deafness occurs when sound waves are not conducted to the inner ear. Possible causes include a wax (cerumen) plug, a foreign body obstruction, otosclerosis, an infection, or a ruptured tympanic membrane. Treatment is directed toward eliminating the cause. Surgery and the use of hearing aids are common forms of treatment. Sensory hearing loss or deafness occurs when there is damage to the inner ear or auditory nerve. Hearing loss progresses over time and can result in permanent deafness. This type of hearing loss usually cannot be corrected, but cochlear implants can improve severe hearing loss.

MÉNIÈRE'S DISEASE Ménière's disease results from a collection of fluid in the labyrinth of the inner ear and a degeneration of the hair cells in the cochlea and vestibule. Symptoms include severe vertigo (dizziness), tinnitus (ringing in the ears), nausea and vomiting, loss of balance, and a tendency to fall. Forms of treatment include drugs to reduce the fluid, anti-nausea drugs and motion sickness medications, draining the fluid, and antihistamines. A diet low in sodium and caffeine and avoidance of alcohol

and nicotine can reduce the symptoms. In severe chronic cases, surgery to destroy the cochlea may be performed; however, this causes permanent deafness.

OTITIS EXTERNA Otitis externa is an inflammation of the external auditory canal. It is caused by a pathogenic organism such as a bacterium or virus. Swimmer's ear is one form. It is caused by swimming in contaminated water. Inserting bobby pins, fingernails, or cotton swabs into the ear or wearing hearing aids or headphones for long periods of time can also cause this condition. Treatment methods include antibiotics; anti-inflammatory drugs; antiseptic ear drops; warm, moist compresses; and/or pain medications.

OTITIS MEDIA Otitis media is an inflammation or infection of the middle ear that is caused by a bacterium or virus. It frequently follows a sore throat because organisms from the throat can enter the middle ear through the eustachian tube. Infants and young children are very susceptible to otitis media because the eustachian tube is angled differently than in adults. Secretions from the nose and throat accumulate in the middle ear, resulting in an inflammatory response that causes the eustachian tube to swell shut. Symptoms include severe pain, fever, vertigo (dizziness), nausea and vomiting, and fluid buildup in the middle ear. A wait-and-see approach is recommended for the first 48 to 72 hours of symptoms because many infections are viral and clear on their own. Treatment usually consists of administering antibiotics and pain medications. At times, a *myringotomy* (incision of the tympanic membrane) is performed, and tubes are inserted to relieve pressure and allow fluid to drain. A pneumococcal conjugate vaccine for the prevention of otitis media is available.

OTOSCLEROSIS Otosclerosis, an inherited disease, is a bony overgrowth of the footplate of the stapes (a bone in the middle ear). The stapes becomes immobile, causing conductive hearing loss. Symptoms include gradual hearing loss, tinnitus, and at times, vertigo. Bone-conduction hearing aids can improve hearing. Surgical removal of the stapes and insertion of an artificial stapes corrects the condition.

THE TONGUE AND SENSE OF TASTE

The tongue is a mass of muscle tissue with projections called *papillae* (**Figure 7–44**). The papillae contain taste buds or chemoreceptor cells that are stimulated by the flavors of foods moistened by saliva. There are four main tastes: sweet tastes and salty tastes at the tip of the tongue; sour tastes at the sides of the tongue; and bitter tastes at the back of the tongue. A fifth taste, *umami*, detects meaty or savory sensations. Taste is influenced by the sense of smell.

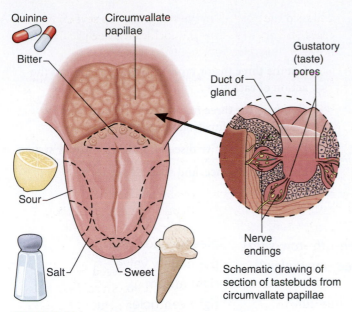

FIGURE 7–44 Locations of taste buds.

THE NOSE AND SENSE OF SMELL

The nose is the organ of smell (**Figure 7–45**). The sense of smell is made possible by olfactory chemoreceptor cells, which are located in the upper part of the nasal cavity. Impulses from these receptors are carried to the brain by the olfactory nerve. The human nose can detect more than 6,000 different smells. The sense of smell is more sensitive than taste, but is closely related to the sense of taste. This is clearly illustrated by the fact that food does not taste as good when you have a head cold and your sense of smell is impaired.

THE SKIN AND GENERAL SENSES

General sense receptors for pressure, heat, cold, touch, and pain are located throughout the body in the skin and connective tissue. Each receptor perceives only one type of sense. For example, the skin contains special thermoreceptors for heat and cold. Mechanoreceptors sense pressure and touch while nociceptors react to pain. Messages from these receptors allow the human body to respond to its environment and help it react to conditions that can cause injury.

checkpoint

1. Describe the four (4) main tastes. Draw a diagram of the tongue with each area of taste labeled.

2. List four (4) general sense receptors that are located throughout the body.

PRACTICE: Go to the workbook and complete the assignment sheet for 7:7, Special Senses.

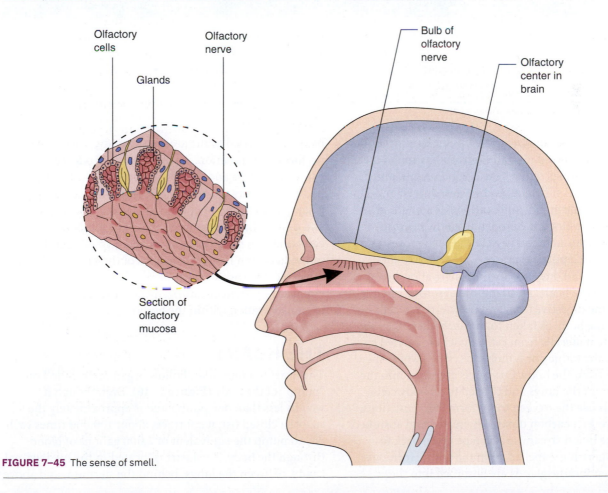

FIGURE 7–45 The sense of smell.

7:8 CIRCULATORY SYSTEM

OBJECTIVES

After completing this section, you should be able to:

- Label the layers, chambers, valves, and major blood vessels on a diagram of the heart.
- Differentiate between systole and diastole by explaining what happens in the heart during each phase.
- List the three major types of blood vessels and the action of each type.
- Compare the three main types of blood cells by describing the function of each.
- Describe at least five diseases of the circulatory system.
- Define, pronounce, and spell all key terms.

KEY TERMS

aortic valve (ay-or'-tick)
arrhythmias
arteries
blood
capillaries (cap'-ih-lair-eez)
circulatory system
diastole (dy-az'-tah-lee")
endocardium (en-doe-car'-dee-um)

erythrocytes (eh-rith'-row-sitez)
hemoglobin (hee'-mow-glow"-bin)
left atrium (ay'-tree-um)
left ventricle (ven' tri"-kul)
leukocytes (lew'-coh-sitez")
mitral valve (my'-tral)
myocardium
pericardium

plasma (plaz'-ma)
pulmonary valve
right atrium
right ventricle
septum
systole (sis"-tah-lee")
thrombocytes (throm'-bow-sitez)
tricuspid valve
veins

Related Health Careers

- Cardiac surgeon
- Cardiologist
- Cardiovascular technologist
- Echocardiographer
- Electrocardiographic technician
- Hematologist
- Internist
- Medical laboratory technologist/technician
- Perfusionist
- Phlebotomist
- Radiology technologist
- Thoracic surgeon

The **circulatory system**, also known as the cardiovascular system, is often referred to as the "transportation" system of the body. It consists of the heart, blood vessels, and blood. It transports nutrients and wastes, oxygen and carbon dioxide, hormones, and antibodies contained in the blood. The blood is pumped from the heart to the aorta and arterial blood vessels and then moves into capillaries. Capillaries are also connected to the venous system, and one-way venous valves allow blood flow return to the heart. Nutrients are absorbed into the blood from the digestive tract and transferred to cells throughout the body or taken to the liver where they are stored. Waste materials from cell activity are carried by the blood to the kidney or lymphatic system, where they are expelled from the body. Oxygen is absorbed into the blood stream in the lungs and carried to all body cells. As body cells use the oxygen to perform their functions, the waste product carbon dioxide is created and absorbed back into the blood stream so it can be taken back to the lungs, where it is expelled from the body. Hormones secreted by endocrine glands are absorbed into the

blood and carried to the area of the body, where they perform their function. Antibodies are produced by white blood cells and the lymphatic system when the body encounters a foreign molecule such as a pathogen. They are circulated by the blood, so they can encounter and destroy the foreign molecules. The antibodies can remain in the blood stream and help protect the individual from further invasions of the same foreign molecule. By working with these other body systems, the circulatory system becomes an extremely efficient system of transportation within the body.

THE HEART

The heart is a muscular, hollow organ often called the "pump" of the body (**Figure 7–46**). Even though it weighs less than one pound and is approximately the size of a closed fist, it contracts about 100,000 times each day to pump the equivalent of 2,000 gallons of blood through the body. The heart is located in the mediastinal cavity, between the lungs, behind the sternum, and above

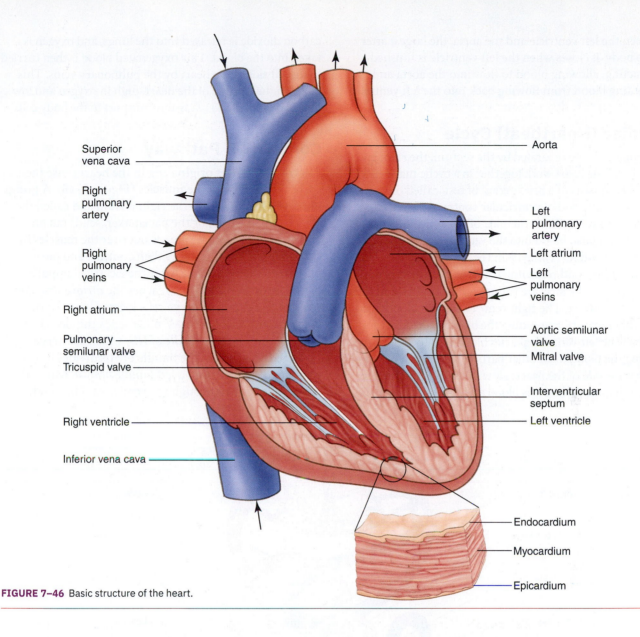

Superior vena cava

Right pulmonary artery

Right pulmonary veins

Right atrium

Pulmonary semilunar valve

Tricuspid valve

Right ventricle

Inferior vena cava

Aorta

Left pulmonary artery

Left atrium

Left pulmonary veins

Aortic semilunar valve

Mitral valve

Interventricular septum

Left ventricle

Endocardium

Myocardium

Epicardium

FIGURE 7–46 Basic structure of the heart.

the diaphragm. Three layers of tissue form the heart. The **endocardium** is a smooth layer of cells that lines the inside of the heart and is continuous with the inside of blood vessels. It allows for the smooth flow of blood. The thickest layer is the **myocardium**, the muscular middle layer. The **pericardium** is a double-layered membrane, or sac, that covers the outside of the heart. A lubricating fluid, pericardial fluid, fills the space between the two layers to prevent friction and damage to the membranes as the heart beats or contracts.

The **septum** is a muscular wall that separates the heart into a right side and a left side. It prevents blood from moving between the right and left sides of the heart. The upper part of the septum is called the *interatrial septum*, and the lower part is called the *interventricular septum*.

The heart is divided into four parts, or chambers. The two upper chambers are called *atria*, and the two lower chambers are called *ventricles*. The **right atrium** receives blood as it returns from the body cells. The **right ventricle** receives blood from the right atrium and pumps

the blood into the pulmonary artery, which carries the blood to the lungs for oxygen. The **left atrium** receives oxygenated blood from the lungs. The **left ventricle** receives blood from the left atrium and pumps the blood into the aorta for transport to the body cells.

One-way valves in the chambers of the heart keep the blood flowing in the right direction. The **tricuspid** valve is located between the right atrium and the right ventricle. It closes when the right ventricle contracts, allowing blood to flow to the lungs and preventing blood from flowing back into the right atrium. The **pulmonary valve** is located between the right ventricle and the pulmonary artery, a blood vessel that carries blood to the lungs. It closes when the right ventricle has finished contracting, preventing blood from flowing back into the right ventricle. The **mitral valve** is located between the left atrium and left ventricle. It closes when the left ventricle is contracting, allowing blood to flow into the aorta (for transport to the body) and preventing blood from flowing back into the left atrium. The **aortic valve** is located between the left ventricle and the aorta, the largest artery in the body. It closes when the left ventricle is finished contracting, allowing blood to flow into the aorta and preventing blood from flowing back into the left ventricle.

Cardiac (Heartbeat) Cycle

Although they are separated by the septum, the right and left sides of the heart work together in a cyclic manner. The cycle consists of a brief period of rest, called **diastole**, followed by a period of ventricular contraction, called **systole** (**Figure 7–47**). At the start of the cycle, the atria contract and push blood into the ventricles. The atria then relax, and blood returning from the body enters the right atrium, while blood returning from the lungs enters the left atrium. As the atria are filling, systole begins, and the ventricles contract. The right ventricle pushes blood into the pulmonary artery, sending the blood to the lungs for oxygen. The left ventricle pushes blood into the aorta, sending the blood to all other parts of the body. The blood in the right side of the heart is low in oxygen and high in carbon dioxide. When this blood arrives in the lungs, the

carbon dioxide is released into the lungs, and oxygen is taken into the blood. This oxygenated blood is then carried to the left side of the heart by the pulmonary veins. This blood in the left side of the heart, high in oxygen and low in carbon dioxide, is ready for transport to the body cells.

Conductive Pathway

Electrical impulses originating in the heart cause the cyclic contraction of the muscles (**Figure 7–48**). A group of nerve cells located in the right atrium and called the *sinoatrial (SA) node*, or the pacemaker, sends out an electrical impulse that spreads out over the muscles in the atria. The atrial muscles then contract and push blood into the ventricles. After the electrical impulse passes through the atria, it reaches the *atrioventricular (AV) node*, a group of nerve cells located between the atria and ventricles. The AV node sends the electrical impulse through the *bundle of His*, which are nerve fibers in the septum. The bundle of His divides into a *right bundle branch* and a *left bundle branch*, which carry the impulse down through the ventricles. The bundle

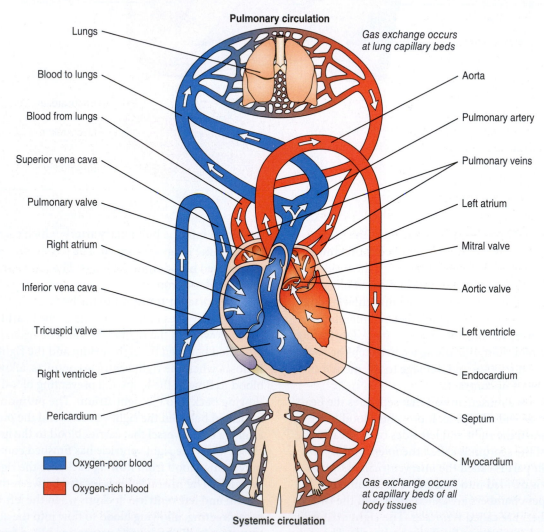

FIGURE 7–47 The pattern of circulation in the cardiovascular system.

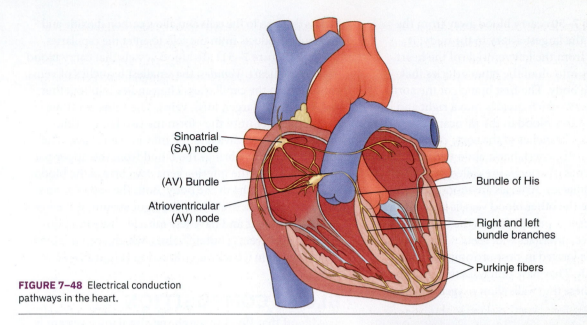

Sinoatrial (SA) node

(AV) Bundle

Atrioventricular (AV) node

Bundle of His

Right and left bundle branches

Purkinje fibers

FIGURE 7–48 Electrical conduction pathways in the heart.

branches further subdivide into the *Purkinje fibers*, a network of nerve fibers throughout the ventricles. In this way, the electrical impulse reaches all the muscle tissue in the ventricles, and the ventricles contract. This electrical conduction pattern occurs approximately every 0.8 seconds. The movement of the electrical impulse can be recorded on an electrocardiogram (ECG) and used to detect abnormal activity or disease.

If something interferes with the normal electrical conduction pattern of the heart, arrhythmias occur. **Arrhythmias** are abnormal heart rhythms and can be mild to life threatening. For example, an early contraction of the atria, or premature atrial contraction (PAC), can occur in anyone and usually goes unnoticed. Ventricular fibrillation, in which the ventricles contract at random without coordination, decreases or eliminates blood output and causes death if not treated. Cardiac monitors and electrocardiograms are used to diagnose arrhythmias. Treatment depends on the type and severity of the arrhythmia. Life-threatening fibrillations are treated with a *defibrillator*, a device that shocks the heart with an electrical current to stop the uncoordinated contraction and allow the SA node to regain control.

At times, it is necessary to use external or internal artificial pacemakers to regulate the heart's rhythm, (**Figure 7–49**). The *pacemaker* is a small, battery-powered device with electrodes. The electrodes are threaded through a vein and positioned in the right atrium and in the apex of the right ventricle. The pacemaker monitors the heart's activity and delivers an electrical impulse through the electrodes to stimulate contraction. Fixed pacemakers deliver electrical impulses at a predetermined rate. Demand pacemakers, the most common type, deliver electrical impulses only when the heart's own conduction system is not responding correctly. For patients that have experienced life-threatening fibrillations, an automatic implantable cardioverter-defibrillator (AICD) is recommended to prevent cardiac

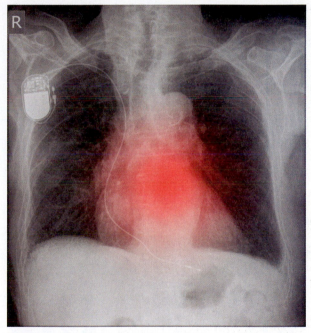

FIGURE 7–49 Artificial pacemakers can help regulate the heart's rhythm. © skyhawk/Shutterstock.com

arrest. The AICD has three elements: pacing/sensing electrodes, defibrillation electrodes, and a pulse generator. Like the pacemaker, it is implanted in the chest wall. When the AICD senses a life-threatening rhythm, it delivers an electrical shock to the heart (defibrillates it) in an attempt to get it to beat normally again.

BLOOD VESSELS

When the blood leaves the heart, it is carried throughout the body in blood vessels. The heart and blood vessels form a closed system for the flow of blood. There are three main types of blood vessels: arteries, capillaries, and veins.

Arteries (**Figure 7–50**) carry blood away from the heart. The aorta is the largest artery in the body; it receives the blood from the left ventricle of the heart. The aorta branches into all of the other arteries that supply blood to the body. The first branch of the aorta is the coronary artery, which divides into a right and left coronary artery to carry blood to the myocardium of the heart. Additional branches of the aorta carry blood to the head, neck, arms, chest, back, abdomen, and legs. The smallest branches of arteries are called *arterioles*. They join with capillaries. Arteries are more muscular and elastic than are the other blood vessels because they receive the blood as it is pumped from the heart.

Capillaries connect arterioles with *venules*, the smallest veins. Capillaries are located in close proximity to almost every cell in the body. They have thin walls that contain only one layer of cells. These thin walls allow oxygen and nutrients to pass through to the cells and allow carbon dioxide and metabolic products from the cells to enter the capillaries.

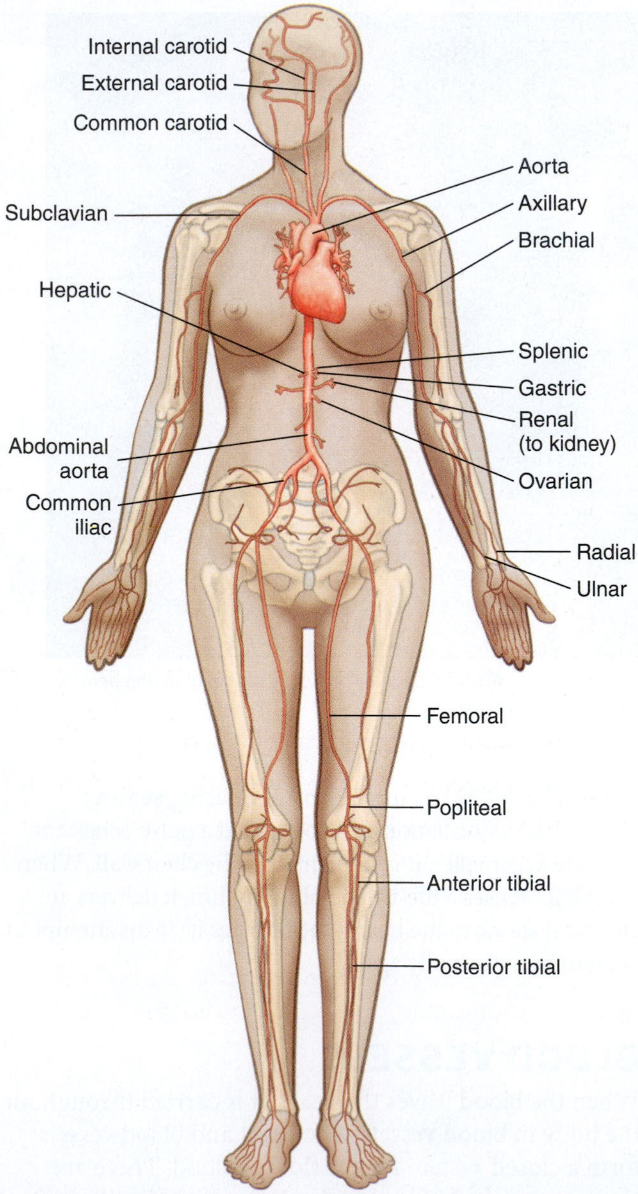

Veins (**Figure 7–51**) are blood vessels that carry blood back to the heart. *Venules*, the smallest branches of veins, connect with the capillaries. The venules join together and, becoming larger, form veins. The veins continue to join together until they form the two largest veins: the superior vena cava and the inferior vena cava. The superior vena cava brings the blood from the upper part of the body, and the inferior vena cava brings the blood from the lower part of the body. Both the superior and inferior vena cava drain into the right atrium of the heart. Veins are thinner and have less muscle tissue than do arteries. Most veins contain valves, which keep the blood from flowing in a backward direction (**Figure 7–52**).

BLOOD COMPOSITION

The **blood** that flows through the circulatory system is often called a *tissue* because it contains many kinds of cells. There are approximately four to six quarts of blood in the average adult. This blood circulates continuously throughout the body. It transports oxygen from the lungs to the body cells, carbon dioxide from the body cells to the lungs, nutrients from the digestive tract to the body cells, metabolic and waste products from the body cells to the organs of excretion, heat produced by various body parts, and hormones produced by endocrine glands to the body organs.

Plasma

Blood is made of the fluid called *plasma* and formed or solid elements called *blood cells* (**Figure 7–53**). **Plasma** is approximately 90 percent water, with many dissolved, or suspended, substances. Among these substances are blood proteins such as fibrinogen and prothrombin (both necessary for clotting); nutrients such as vitamins, carbohydrates, and proteins; mineral salts or electrolytes such as potassium, calcium, and sodium; gases such as carbon dioxide and oxygen; metabolic and waste products; hormones; and enzymes.

Blood Cells

There are three main kinds of blood cells: erythrocytes, leukocytes, and thrombocytes.

The **erythrocytes**, or red blood cells, are produced in the red bone marrow at a rate of about one million per minute. They live approximately 120 days before being broken down by the liver and spleen. There are 4.5 to 6.0 million erythrocytes per cubic millimeter (approximately one drop) of blood, or approximately 25 trillion in the body. The mature form circulating in the blood lacks a nucleus and is shaped like a disk with a thinner central area. The erythrocytes contain **hemoglobin**, a complex protein composed of the protein molecule called *globin* and the iron compound called *heme*. Hemoglobin carries both oxygen and carbon

FIGURE 7–50 Major arteries of the body.

Internal carotid
External carotid
Common carotid
Subclavian
Hepatic
Abdominal aorta
Common iliac

Aorta
Axillary
Brachial
Splenic
Gastric
Renal (to kidney)
Ovarian
Radial
Ulnar
Femoral
Popliteal
Anterior tibial
Posterior tibial

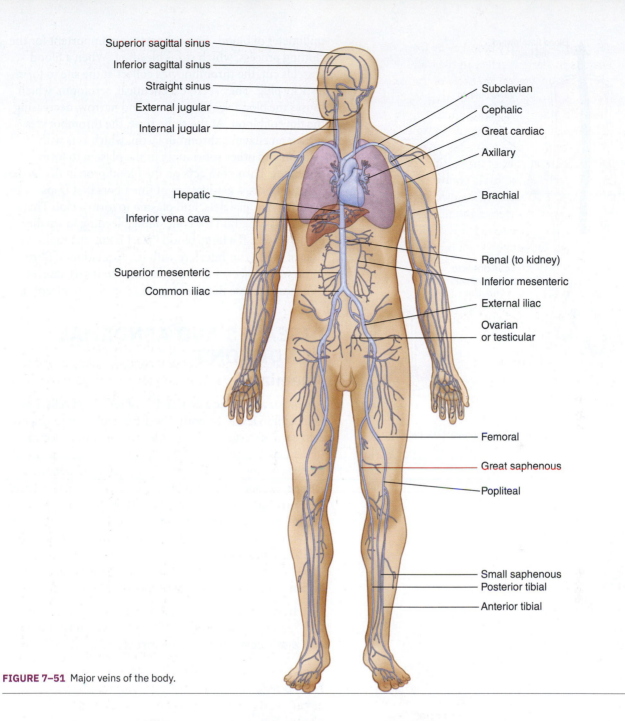

FIGURE 7–51 Major veins of the body.

Superior sagittal sinus
Inferior sagittal sinus
Straight sinus
External jugular
Internal jugular
Hepatic
Inferior vena cava
Superior mesenteric
Common iliac

Subclavian
Cephalic
Great cardiac
Axillary
Brachial
Renal (to kidney)
Inferior mesenteric
External iliac
Ovarian or testicular
Femoral
Great saphenous
Popliteal
Small saphenous
Posterior tibial
Anterior tibial

dioxide. When carrying oxygen, hemoglobin gives blood its characteristic red color. When blood contains a lot of oxygen, it is bright red; when blood contains less oxygen and more carbon dioxide, it is a much darker red with a bluish cast.

Leukocytes, or white blood cells, are not as numerous as are erythrocytes. They are formed in the bone marrow and lymph tissue and usually live about 3–9 days. A normal count is 4,500–11,000 leukocytes per cubic millimeter of blood. Leukocytes can pass through capillary walls and enter body tissue. Their main function is to fight infection. Some do this by engulfing, ingesting, and destroying pathogens, or germs, by a process called *phagocytosis*. The five types of leukocytes and their functions include:

- **Neutrophils**: phagocytize bacteria by secreting an enzyme called lysozyme

- **Eosinophils**: remove toxins and defend the body from allergic reactions by producing antihistamines

- **Basophils**: participate in the body's inflammatory response; produce histamine, a vasodilator, and heparin, an anticoagulant

- **Monocytes**: phagocytize bacteria and foreign materials

- **Lymphocytes**: provide immunity for the body by developing antibodies; protect against the formation of cancer cells

Thrombocytes, also called *platelets*, are usually described as fragments or pieces of cells because they lack nuclei and vary in shape and size. They are formed in the bone marrow and live for about 5–9 days. A normal thrombocyte count is 150,000–400,000 per cubic

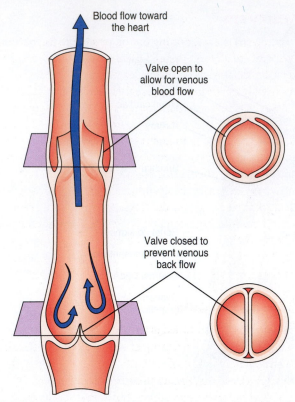

Blood flow toward the heart

Valve open to allow for venous blood flow

Valve closed to prevent venous back flow

FIGURE 7–52 Most veins contain valves to prevent the backflow of blood.

millimeter of blood. Thrombocytes are important for the clotting process, which stops bleeding. When a blood vessel is cut, the thrombocytes collect at the site to form a sticky plug. They secrete a chemical, serotonin, which causes the blood vessel to spasm and narrow, decreasing the flow of blood. At the same time, the thrombocytes release an enzyme, thromboplastin, which acts with calcium and other substances in the plasma to form thrombin. Thrombin acts on the blood protein fibrinogen to form fibrin, a gel-like net of fine fibers that traps erythrocytes, platelets, and plasma to form a clot. This is an effective method for controlling bleeding in smaller blood vessels. If a large blood vessel is cut, the rapid flow of blood can interfere with the formation of fibrin. In these instances, a doctor may have to insert sutures (stitches) to close the opening and control the bleeding.

DISEASES AND ABNORMAL CONDITIONS

Anemia

Anemia is an inadequate number of red blood cells, low hemoglobin levels, or both. The hemoglobin in red blood cells carries oxygen to the tissues and organs. A decrease in hemoglobin or red blood cells can cause *hypoxia*, a lack of oxygen supply. Symptoms include pallor (paleness), fatigue, dyspnea (difficult breathing), and rapid heart rate. Hemorrhage can cause rapid blood loss, resulting in acute blood-loss anemia. Blood transfusions are used to correct this form of anemia. If a blood transfusion is not possible due to medical or religious reasons, hyperbaric oxygen therapy can improve oxygen delivery to the tissues and organs. Some other common types of anemia include:

- **Iron deficiency anemia**: results when there is an inadequate amount of iron to form hemoglobin in erythrocytes. Iron supplements and increased iron

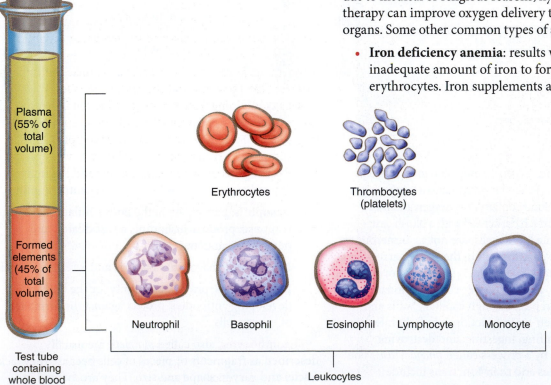

Plasma (55% of total volume)

Formed elements (45% of total volume)

Erythrocytes

Thrombocytes (platelets)

Neutrophil   Basophil   Eosinophil   Lymphocyte   Monocyte

Test tube containing whole blood

Leukocytes

FIGURE 7–53 The major components of blood.

intake in the diet from green leafy vegetables and other foods can correct this condition.

- **Aplastic anemia**: results from injury to or destruction of the bone marrow, leading to poor or no formation of red blood cells. Common causes include chemotherapy, radiation, toxic chemicals, and viruses. Treatment includes eliminating the cause, blood transfusions, and in severe cases, a bone marrow transplant. Unless the damage can be reversed, it is frequently fatal.

- **Pernicious anemia**: results in the formation of erythrocytes that are abnormally large in size but inadequate in number. The cause is a lack of intrinsic factor (a substance normally present in the stomach), which results in inadequate absorption of vitamin B_{12}. Vitamin B_{12} and folic acid are required for the development of mature erythrocytes. Administering vitamin B_{12} injections can control and correct this condition.

- **Sickle cell anemia**: a chronic, inherited anemia. It results in the production of abnormal, crescent-shaped erythrocytes that carry less oxygen, break easily, and block blood vessels (**Figure 7–54**). Sickle cell anemia occurs almost exclusively among African Americans. Treatment methods include transfusions of packed cells and supportive therapy during crisis. Research directed toward bone marrow transplants, stem cell transplants from placental blood, and gene cell therapy may offer a cure for sickle cell anemia in the near future. Genetic counseling can lead to prevention of the disease if carriers make informed decisions not to have children.

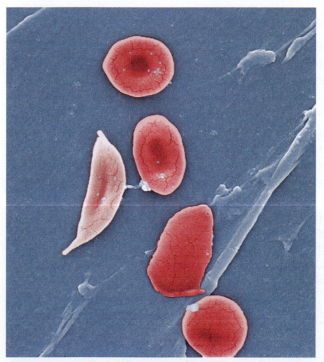

FIGURE 7–54 Sickle cell anemia is characterized by abnormal, crescent-shaped erythrocytes. CDC/Sickle Cell Foundation of Georgia: Jackie George, Beverly Sinclair

Aneurysm

An aneurysm is a ballooning out of, or saclike formation on, the wall of a blood vessel. Disease, high blood pressure, congenital defects, and injuries leading to weakened arterial wall structure can cause this defect. Although some aneurysms cause pain and pressure, others generate no symptoms. Common sites are the cerebral, aortal, and abdominal arteries. If an aneurysm ruptures, hemorrhage, which can cause death, occurs. Since the risks of surgical repair of smaller aneurysms are similar to the risk of rupture, a watchful waiting approach, with control of blood pressure, is often used. If the aneurysm continues to grow or becomes symptomatic, surgery can be performed to remove the damaged area of blood vessel and replace it with a bypass graft or another blood vessel. In some cases, a less invasive endovascular technique can be done.

Arteriosclerosis

Arteriosclerosis, also called arteriosclerotic vascular disease (ASVD), is a hardening or thickening of the arterial walls, resulting in a loss of elasticity and contractility. It commonly occurs as a result of aging. Arteriosclerosis causes high blood pressure, or hypertension, and can lead to an aneurysm or cerebral hemorrhage. The main focus of treatment is lowering blood pressure through the use of diet, medications, or both.

Atherosclerosis

Atherosclerosis occurs when fatty plaques (frequently cholesterol) are deposited on the walls of the arteries. This narrows the arterial opening, which reduces or eliminates blood flow. Lack of blood flow to the heart, brain, or extremities can cause a heart attack, stroke, or gangrene. If plaques break loose, they can circulate through the bloodstream as *emboli*. A low-cholesterol diet, medications to lower blood pressure and cholesterol blood levels (statins), abstaining from smoking, reduction of stress, and exercise are used to prevent atherosclerosis. Angioplasty (**Figure 7–55**) may be used to remove or compress the deposits, or to insert a stent to allow blood flow. Bypass surgery is used when the arteries are completely blocked.

Congestive Heart Failure

Congestive heart failure (CHF) is a condition that occurs when the heart muscles do not beat adequately to supply the blood needs of the body. It may involve either the right side or the left side of the heart. Risk factors include high blood pressure, high cholesterol, obesity, and diabetes. Symptoms include edema (swelling); dyspnea; pallor or cyanosis; distention of the neck veins; a weak, rapid pulse; and a cough accompanied by pink, frothy sputum. Cardiotonic drugs (to slow and strengthen the heartbeat), diuretics (to remove retained body fluids), elastic support hose, oxygen therapy, weight loss, exercise, and/or a low-sodium diet are used as treatment methods.

(A) Conventional balloon angioplasty

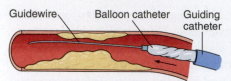

Guidewire   Balloon catheter   Guiding catheter

1. In conventional balloon angioplasty, a guiding catheter is positioned in the opening of the coronary artery. The physician then pushes a thin, flexible guidewire down the vessel and through the narrowing. The balloon catheter is then advanced over this guidewire.

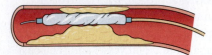

2. The balloon catheter is positioned next to the atherosclerotic plaque.

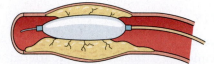

3. The balloon is inflated stretching and cracking the plaque.

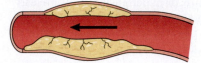

4. When the balloon is withdrawn, blood flow is re-established through the widened vessel.

(B) Coronary atherectomy

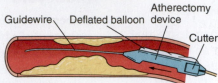

Guidewire   Deflated balloon   Atherectomy device   Cutter

1. In coronary atherectomy procedures, a special cutting device with a deflated balloon on one side and an opening on the other is pushed over a wire down the coronary artery.

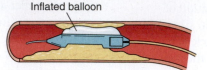

Inflated balloon

2. When the device is within a coronary artery narrowing, the balloon is inflated, so that part of the atherosclerotic plaque is "squeezed" into the opening of the device.

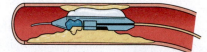

3. When the physician starts rotating the cutting blade, pieces of plaque are shaved off into the device.

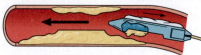

4. The catheter is withdrawn, leaving a larger opening for blood flow.

(C) Coronary stent

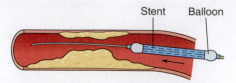

Stent   Balloon

1. To place a coronary stent within a vessel narrowing, physicians use a special catheter with a deflated balloon and the stent at the tip.

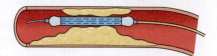

2. The catheter is positioned so that the stent is within the narrowed region of the coronary artery.

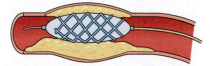

3. The balloon is then inflated, causing the stent to expand and stretch the coronary artery.

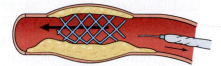

4. The balloon catheter is then withdrawn, leaving the stent behind to keep the vessel open.

FIGURE 7–55 Ways to open clogged arteries: (A) Balloon angioplasty, (B) Coronary atherectomy, and (C) Coronary stent.

Embolus

An embolus is a foreign substance circulating in the bloodstream. It can be air, a blood clot, bacterial clumps, a fat globule, or other similar substances. When an embolus enters an artery or capillary too small for passage, blockage of the blood vessel occurs.

Hemophilia

Hemophilia is an inherited disease that occurs almost exclusively in male individuals but can be carried by female individuals. Most cases are diagnosed by the age of 2, often during circumcision. Because of the lack of a plasma protein required for the clotting process, the blood is unable to clot. A minor cut can lead to prolonged bleeding, and a minor bump can cause internal bleeding. It is a lifelong disease with no cure. Regular infusions of the deficient clotting factor can help control the bleeding. Desmopressin can be given to increase protein clotting factors, and antifibrinolytic therapy may enhance clot stability.

Hypertension

Hypertension is high blood pressure. A systolic pressure above 130 and a diastolic pressure above 80 millimeters of mercury (mmHg) is usually regarded as hypertension stage 1 and a systolic pressure above 140 and a diastolic pressure above 90 mmHg is hypertension stage 2. Risk factors that increase the incidence of hypertension include family history, race (higher in African Americans), obesity, stress, smoking, aging (higher in postmenopausal women), and a diet high in saturated fat. Although there is no cure, hypertension can usually be controlled with antihypertensive drugs, diuretics (to remove retained body fluids), limited stress, avoidance of tobacco, and/or a low-sodium or low-fat diet. If hypertension is not treated, it can cause heart attack, stroke, heart failure, kidney failure, intracerebral hemorrhage, or an aneurysm.

Leukemia

Leukemia is a cancer of the bone marrow or lymph tissue. It results in a high number of immature or abnormal white blood cells that do not function properly to fight infection. There are different types of leukemia, some acute and some chronic. Some types are more common in children and others are more prevalent in adults. Symptoms include fever, frequent infections, pallor, swelling of lymphoid tissues, persistent fatigue, anemia, bleeding gums, excessive bruising, and joint pain. Treatment methods vary with the type of leukemia but can include chemotherapy, radiation, and/or stem cell or bone marrow transplants.

Myocardial Infarction

A myocardial infarction, or heart attack, occurs when a blockage in the coronary arteries cuts off the supply of blood to the heart. The lack of blood flow can cause ischemia, tissue injury, or infarct (tissue death). *Acute coronary syndrome (ACS)* is a term used to identify patients who are suspected of having myocardial ischemia (reduced blood flow to the heart). With myocardial infarction, death can occur immediately. Symptoms vary greatly, especially among men and women, but may include severe crushing pain (angina pectoris) that radiates to the arm, neck, and jaw; pressure in the chest; perspiration and cold, clammy skin; a sense of doom; dyspnea; and a change in blood pressure. If the heart stops, cardiopulmonary resuscitation should be started immediately. Immediate treatment with a thrombolytic or "clot-busting" drug such as streptokinase or tissue plasminogen activator (TPA) may open the blood vessel and restore blood flow to the heart. However, the clot-busting drug must be used within the first several hours, and its use is prohibited if bleeding is present. Additional treatment methods include oxygen therapy, pain medications (morphine), vasodilators (nitroglycerin), beta-blocker drugs (to decrease heart rate and strengthen the heart), anticoagulants (aspirin to prevent additional clots), control of arrhythmias (abnormal heart rhythms), and bed rest. Coronary angioplasty and stenting may be required to open the blocked artery, or coronary artery bypass grafting may be done to bypass the blocked artery. Long-term care includes control of blood pressure, a diet low in cholesterol and saturated fat, avoidance of tobacco and stress, regular exercise, and weight control.

Phlebitis

Phlebitis is an inflammation of a vein, frequently in the leg. If a thrombus, or clot, forms in a vein near the surface of the skin, the condition is termed *thrombophlebitis*. If a thrombus forms in a vein deep within a muscle, it is called a *deep vein thrombosis (DVT)*. These blood clots are often a result of prolonged sitting or immobility. Symptoms include pain, edema, redness, and discoloration at the site. With thrombophlebitis, complications are rare. A DVT poses the risk of a pulmonary embolism, heart attack, or stroke if the clot becomes dislodged and travels to the lungs, coronary artery, or brain. Treatment methods include anticoagulants; clot dissolving drugs; pain medication; elevation of the affected area; antiembolism or support hose; and, if necessary, surgery to remove the clot or bypass the vein. A filter can be inserted into the vena cava to prevent clots from traveling through the body.

Varicose Veins

Varicose veins are gnarled, dilated veins that have lost elasticity and cause stasis, or decreased blood flow. They frequently occur in the legs and result from pregnancy, prolonged sitting or standing, obesity, and hereditary factors. Treatment methods include exercise, antiembolism or support hose, and avoidance of prolonged sitting or standing and tight-fitting or restrictive clothing. Sclerotherapy involves injecting solution into the veins to make them scar and close. Endovenous laser treatment/ablation (ELA) closes off the affected veins. In severe cases, surgery can be performed to remove the vein (vein stripping).

checkpoint

1. List three (3) types of blood cells and describe how they function.

PRACTICE: Go to the workbook and complete the assignment sheet for 7:8, Circulatory System.

7:9 **LYMPHATIC SYSTEM AND IMMUNITY**

OBJECTIVES

After completing this section, you should be able to:

- Explain the function of lymphatic vessels.
- List at least two functions of lymph nodes.
- Identify the two lymphatic ducts and the areas of the body that each drains.
- List at least three functions of the spleen.
- Describe the function of the thymus.
- Define immunity and differentiate between active and passive immunity.
- Describe at least three diseases of the lymphatic system.
- Define, pronounce, and spell all key terms.

cisterna chyli (*sis-tern'-uh-kye'-lee*)
immunity
lacteals
lymph (*limf'*)

lymph nodes
lymphatic capillaries (*lim-fat'-ik*)
lymphatic system
lymphatic vessels
right lymphatic duct

spleen
thoracic duct (*tho-rass'-ik*)
thymus
tonsils

Related Health Careers

- Immunologist
- Internist

- Lymphedema therapist
- Massage therapist

- Oncologist

The **lymphatic system** consists of lymph, lymph vessels, lymph nodes, and lymphatic tissue. This system works in conjunction with the circulatory system to remove wastes and excess fluids from the tissues (**Figure 7–56**). The lymphatic system impacts our **immunity** or ability to resist an infection. It transports, filters, and removes pathogenic or disease-producing microoganisms and produces antibodies and lymphocytes to fight infection. The lymphatic system also works in conjunction with white blood cells to fight infection and provide immunity to disease.

Lymph is a thin, watery fluid composed of *intercellular*, or *interstitial*, fluid, which forms when plasma diffuses into tissue spaces. It is composed of water, digested nutrients, salts, hormones, oxygen, carbon dioxide, lymphocytes, and metabolic wastes such as urea. When this fluid enters the lymphatic system, it is known as lymph.

Lymphatic vessels are located throughout the body in almost all of the tissues that have blood vessels (**Figure 7–57**). Small, open-ended lymph vessels act like drainpipes and are called **lymphatic capillaries**. The lymphatic capillaries pick up lymph at tissues throughout the body. The capillaries then join together to form larger lymphatic vessels, which pass through the lymph nodes. Contractions of skeletal muscles against the lymph vessels cause the lymph to flow through the vessels. Lymphatic vessels also have valves that keep the lymph flowing in only one direction. In the area of the small intestine, specialized lymphatic capillaries, called **lacteals**, pick up digested fats or lipids. When lymph

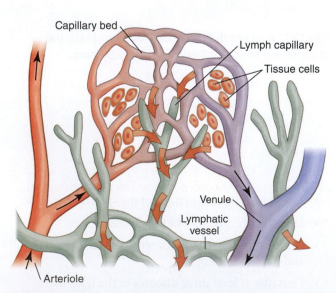

FIGURE 7–56 The lymphatic system works with the circulatory system to remove metabolic waste and excess fluid from the tissues.

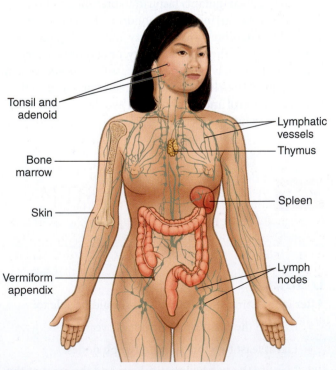

FIGURE 7–57 Main components of the lymphatic system.

is mixed with the lipids it is called *chyle*. The lacteals transport the chyle to the bloodstream through the thoracic duct.

Lymph nodes, popularly called "glands," are located all over the body, usually in groups or clusters. They are small, round, or oval masses ranging in size from that of a pinhead to that of an almond. Lymph vessels bring lymph to the nodes. The nodes filter the lymph and remove impurities such as carbon, cancer cells, pathogens (disease-producing organisms), and dead blood cells. In addition, the lymphatic tissue in the nodes produces lymphocytes (a type of leukocyte, or white blood cell) and antibodies (substances used to combat infection). The purified lymph, with lymphocytes and antibodies added, leaves the lymph node by a single lymphatic vessel.

As lymphatic vessels leave the lymph nodes, they continue to join together to form larger lymph vessels. Eventually, these vessels drain into one of two lymphatic ducts: the right lymphatic duct or the thoracic duct. The **right lymphatic duct** is the short tube that receives all of the purified lymph from the right side of the head and neck, the right chest, and the right arm. It empties into the right subclavian vein, returning the purified lymph to the blood. The **thoracic duct**, a much larger tube, drains the lymph from the rest of the body. It empties into the left subclavian vein. At the start of the thoracic duct, an enlarged pouchlike structure called the **cisterna chyli** serves as a storage area for purified lymph before this lymph returns to the bloodstream. The cisterna chyli also receives chyle from the intestinal lacteals.

In addition to being found in the lymph nodes, lymphatic tissue is located throughout the body. The tonsils, spleen, and thymus are examples of lymphatic tissue.

The **tonsils** are masses of lymphatic tissue that filter interstitial fluid. There are three pairs of tonsils:

- **Palatine tonsils:** located on each side of the soft palate
- **Pharyngeal tonsils:** (also called *adenoids*) located in the nasopharynx (the upper part of the throat)
- **Lingual tonsils:** located on the back of the tongue

The **spleen** is an organ located beneath the left side of the diaphragm and in back of the upper part of the stomach. It produces leukocytes and antibodies, destroys old erythrocytes (red blood cells), stores erythrocytes to release into the bloodstream if excessive bleeding occurs, destroys thrombocytes (platelets), and filters metabolites and wastes from body tissues.

The **thymus** is a mass of lymph tissue located in the center of the upper chest. It atrophies (wastes away) after puberty and is replaced by fat and connective tissue. During early life, it produces antibodies and manufactures lymphocytes to fight infection. Its function is taken over by the lymph nodes.

Immunity

Immunity to a disease is achieved through the presence of antibodies to that disease in a person's system. Antibodies are proteins produced by the body to destroy pathogens. Antibodies are disease specific.

There are two types of immunity:

- **Active immunity** is protection from a specific disease by exposure to the infection—either by contacting the actual disease or by obtaining a vaccine. Both result in the body building up antibodies against disease agents. Vaccines use very small amounts of antigens to build immune system resistance. Vaccine schedules are set by the government and are important to adhere to for public health.
- **Passive immunity** is from actually being given antibodies. This can happen via mother to newborn baby or administration of antibody-containing blood products like immune globulin.

DISEASES AND ABNORMAL CONDITIONS
Adenitis

Adenitis is an inflammation or infection of the lymph nodes. It occurs when large quantities of harmful substances, such as pathogens or cancer cells, enter the lymph nodes and infect the tissue. When the lymph nodes swell, it is termed *lymphadenopathy*. Symptoms include fever and swollen, painful nodes. If the infection is not treated, an abscess may form in the node. Usually treatment methods are antibiotics and warm, moist compresses. If an abscess forms, it is sometimes necessary to incise and drain the node.

Acquired Immune Deficiency Syndrome

Acquired immune deficiency syndrome (AIDS) is caused by a virus called the *human immunodeficiency virus (HIV)*. This virus attacks the body's immune system, rendering the immune system unable to fight off certain infections and diseases, and eventually causing death. The virus is spread through sexual secretions, blood, and body fluids and from an infected mother to her infant during pregnancy or childbirth.

The HIV virus does not live long outside the body and is not transmitted by casual, nonsexual contact. Individuals infected with HIV can remain free of any symptoms for years after infection. During this asymptomatic period, infected individuals can transmit the virus to any other individual with whom they exchange sexual secretions, blood, or blood products. After this initial asymptomatic period, many individuals develop early symptomatic HIV infection, called Class B (formally known as AIDS-related complex or ARC). Symptoms include a positive blood test for antibodies to the HIV virus, lack of infection resistance, appetite loss, weight loss, recurrent fever, night sweats, skin rashes, diarrhea, fatigue, and swollen lymph nodes. When the HIV virus causes a critical low level (less than 200 cells per cubic millimeter of blood) of special leukocytes (white blood cells) called CD4 or T cells, and/or opportunistic diseases appear, AIDS is diagnosed. Three of the most common opportunistic diseases include the rare type of pneumonia called *Pneumocystis jiroveci*, a yeast infection called *Candidiasis*, and the slow-growing cancer called *Kaposi's sarcoma*.

Currently, there is no cure for AIDS, although much research is being directed toward developing a vaccine to prevent and drugs to cure AIDS. Treatment with highly active antiretroviral therapy (HAART), a combination of several drugs called a drug cocktail, is used to slow progression of the disease. Although several experimental drugs are currently being tested, many patients cannot tolerate the side effects and bone marrow toxicity of these drugs. Prevention is the best method in dealing with AIDS. Standard precautions should be followed while handling blood, body secretions, and sexual secretions. High-risk sexual activities, such as having multiple partners, should be avoided. A condom and an effective spermicide should be used to form a protective barrier during intercourse. The use of drugs and sharing of intravenous (IV) needles should be avoided. Females infected with HIV should avoid pregnancy.

Hodgkin's Lymphoma

Hodgkin's lymphoma is a chronic, malignant disease of the lymph nodes. It is the most common form of lymphoma (tumor of lymph tissue). Symptoms include painless swelling of the lymph nodes, fever, night sweats, weight loss, fatigue, and pruritus (itching). Treatment is based on the clinical stage. The majority of cases can be cured. Chemotherapy and radiation are usually effective forms of treatment. The use of stem cell transplantation has also shown positive results.

Lupus

Lupus is a chronic systemic autoimmune disease that occurs when the body's immune system attacks its own healthy tissues, causing chronic inflammation and damage. This can include any organ or system but typically it includes the kidneys, joints, skin, brain, heart, and lungs. There are several different types of lupus, but the most common type is systemic lupus erythematosus (SLE). The etiology is unknown but hormonal, genetic, and environmental factors can have an effect. It is more common in African American, Hispanic, Asian, and Native American women and occurs most frequently between the ages of 15 and 40. It can be difficult to diagnose, but the most distinctive sign of lupus is a "butterfly rash"—a red facial rash that is across the nose and both cheeks. Other symptoms can include severe fatigue; fever with no known cause; joint pain, stiffness, and swelling; muscle pain; photosensitivity (sun sensitivity) that causes lesions on the skin; chest pain; dyspnea (difficult breathing); cold sensitivity that causes poor circulation to the fingers and toes; hair loss; swollen lymph nodes; depression with feelings of anxiety; and headaches, confusion, and memory loss. There is no cure for lupus. Treatment is directed toward the symptoms the individual develops and include corticosteroids to decrease inflammation; NSAIDs for pain, swelling, and fever; immunosuppressants or drugs to suppress the action of the immune system for severe occurrences of inflammation; antimalarial drugs such as Plaquenil to provide long-term control of the progression of the disease; and other medications to treat specific conditions such as heart and kidney medications if these organs have been damaged. With careful treatment directed toward preventing organ damage, most individuals with lupus can live a normal life span.

Lymphangitis

Lymphangitis is an inflammation of lymphatic vessels, usually resulting from a pathogenic organism entering a lymphatic vessel through a skin wound, or a complication from an infection elsewhere. The infection spreads through the lymph channels causing the characteristic red streaks up an arm or leg. Other symptoms include fever, chills, and tenderness or pain. Treatment methods include antibiotics; anti-inflammatory medications; rest; elevation of the affected part; and/or warm, moist compresses. Severe cases may require surgical debridement.

Mononucleosis

Infectious mononucleosis is caused by a virus, most frequently the Epstein-Barr virus. It is commonly called the "kissing disease" because it spreads through saliva. This virus has an incubation period of four to six weeks. The signs and symptoms are fever, sore throat, fatigue, and enlarged lymph nodes and spleen. Treatment is rest and fluids, but if symptoms persist longer than two weeks, a physician should be consulted.

Splenomegaly

Splenomegaly is an enlargement of the spleen. It can be caused by a viral, bacterial, or parasitic infection. Common diseases that can cause the enlargement include infectious mononucleosis, cirrhosis, lymphoma, AIDS, and splenic vein thrombosis. The main symptoms are swelling and abdominal and back pain. A palpable left upper abdominal mass may be present. An increased destruction of blood cells can lead to anemia (low red blood cell count), leukopenia (low white blood cell count), and thrombocytopenia (low thrombocyte count). If the spleen ruptures, intraperitoneal hemorrhage and shock can lead to death. In severe cases, where the underlying cause cannot be treated, a splenectomy (surgical removal of the spleen) is performed.

Tonsillitis

Tonsillitis is an inflammation or infection of the tonsils. Most cases are viral; only a small number are caused by bacteria. It usually involves the pharyngeal (adenoid) and palatine tonsils. Symptoms include throat pain, dysphagia (difficulty swallowing), fever, white or yellow spots of exudate on the tonsils, and swollen lymph nodes near the mandible. Antibiotics are used for bacterial infections. If the infection is viral, symptom relief is the treatment, which includes warm throat irrigations, rest, and analgesics for pain. Chronic, frequent infections; hypertrophy (enlargement) that causes obstruction; and suspicion of neoplasm are indications for a tonsillectomy, or surgical removal of the tonsils.

checkpoint

1. Describe the function of the thymus.
2. Identify two (2) lymphatic ducts and the area of the body that it drains.

PRACTICE: Go to the workbook and complete the assignment sheet for 7:9, Lymphatic System.

7:10 RESPIRATORY SYSTEM

OBJECTIVES

After completing this section, you should be able to:

- Label a diagram of the major parts of the respiratory system.
- List five functions of the nasal cavity.
- Identify the three sections of the pharynx.
- Explain how the larynx helps create sound and speech.
- Describe the function of the epiglottis.
- Compare the processes of inspiration and expiration, including the muscle action that occurs during each process.
- Differentiate between external and internal respiration.
- Describe at least five diseases of the respiratory system.
- Define, pronounce, and spell all key terms.

■ KEY TERMS

alveoli *(ahl-vee'-oh"-lie)*
bronchi *(bron'-kie)*
bronchioles *(bron'-key"-ohlz)*
cellular respiration
cilia *(sil'-lee-ah)*
epiglottis *(ep-ih-glot'-tiss)*
expiration
external respiration

inspiration
internal respiration
larynx *(lar'-inks)*
lungs
nasal cavities
nasal septum
nose
pharynx *(far'-inks)*

pleura
respiration
respiratory system *(res'-peh-reh-tor'-ee)*
sinuses
trachea *(tray'-key"-ah)*
ventilation

Related Health Careers

- Internist
- Otolaryngologist
- Perfusionist
- Pulmonologist
- Respiratory therapist
- Respiratory therapy technician
- Thoracic surgeon

The **respiratory system** consists of the lungs and air passages. This system is responsible for taking in oxygen, a gas needed by all body cells, and removing carbon dioxide, a gas that is a metabolic waste product produced by the cells when the cells convert food into energy. Because the body has only a 4–6-minute supply of oxygen, the respiratory system must work continuously to prevent death.

The parts of the respiratory system are the nose, pharynx, larynx, trachea, bronchi, alveoli, and lungs (**Figure 7–58**).

RESPIRATORY ORGANS AND STRUCTURES

The **nose** consists of a bony framework and cartilage with skin covering this framework. It has two openings, called *nostrils* or *nares*, through which air enters. A wall of cartilage, called the **nasal septum**, divides the nose into two hollow spaces, called **nasal cavities**. The nasal cavities are lined with a mucous

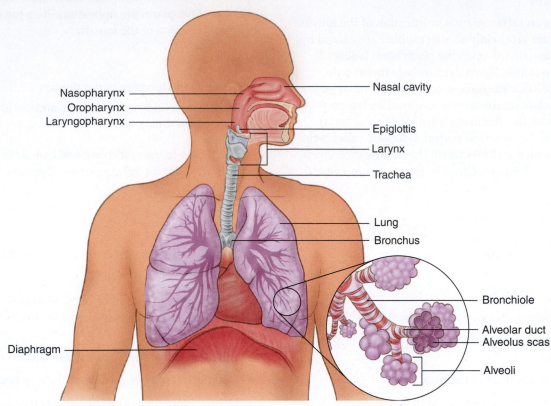

Nasopharynx
Oropharynx
Laryngopharynx
Nasal cavity
Epiglottis
Larynx
Trachea
Lung
Bronchus
Diaphragm
Bronchiole
Alveolar duct
Alveolus scas
Alveoli

FIGURE 7–58 The respiratory system.

membrane and have a rich blood supply. As air enters the cavities, it is warmed, filtered, and moistened. Mucus, produced by the mucous membranes, moistens the air and helps trap pathogens and dirt. Tiny, hairlike structures, called **cilia**, filter inhaled air to trap dust and other particles. The cilia then help move the mucous layer that lines the airways to push trapped particles toward the esophagus, where they can be swallowed. The *olfactory receptors* for the sense of smell are also located in the nose. The *nasolacrimal ducts* drain tears from the eye into the nose to provide additional moisture for the air.

Sinuses are cavities in the skull that surround the nasal area (**Figure 7–59**). They are connected to the nasal cavity by short ducts. The sinuses are lined with a mucous membrane that warms and moistens air. The sinuses also provide resonance for the voice.

The **pharynx**, or throat, lies directly behind the nasal cavities (refer to **Figure 7–59**). As air leaves the nose, it enters the pharynx. The pharynx is divided into three sections. The *nasopharynx* is the upper portion, located behind the nasal cavities. The pharyngeal tonsils, or adenoids (lymphatic tissue), and the eustachian tube (tube to middle ear) openings are located in this section. The *oropharynx* is the middle section, located behind the oral cavity (mouth). This section receives both air from the nasopharynx and food and air from the mouth. The *laryngopharynx* is the bottom section of the pharynx. The

esophagus, which carries food to the stomach, and the trachea, which carries air to and from the lungs, branch off the laryngopharynx.

The **larynx**, or voice box, lies between the pharynx and trachea. It has nine layers of cartilage. The largest, the thyroid cartilage, is commonly called the *Adam's apple*. The larynx contains two folds, called *vocal cords*. The opening between the vocal cords is called the *glottis*. As air leaves the lungs, the vocal cords vibrate and produce sound. The tongue and lips act on the sound to produce speech. The **epiglottis**, a special leaflike piece of cartilage, closes the opening into the larynx during swallowing. This prevents food and liquids from entering the respiratory tract.

The **trachea** (windpipe) is a tube extending from the larynx to the center of the chest. It carries air between the pharynx and the bronchi. A series of C-shaped cartilages (which are open on the dorsal, or back, surfaces) help keep the trachea open.

The trachea divides into two **bronchi** near the center of the chest, a right bronchus and a left bronchus. The right bronchus is shorter, wider, and extends more vertically than the left bronchus. Each bronchus enters a lung and carries air from the trachea to the lung. In the lungs, the bronchi continue to divide into smaller and smaller bronchi until, finally, they divide into the smallest branches, called **bronchioles**. The smallest bronchioles, called *terminal bronchioles*, end in air sacs, called *alveoli*.

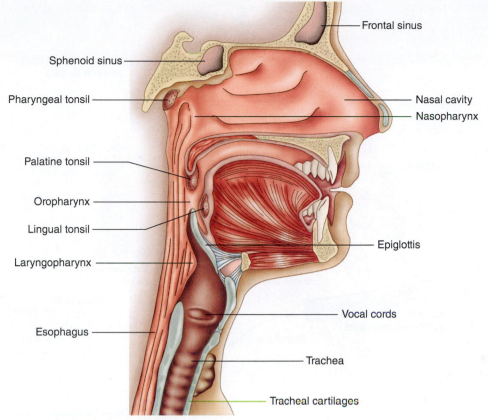

FIGURE 7–59 Respiratory structures in the head and throat.

The **alveoli** resemble a bunch of grapes. An adult lung contains approximately 500 million alveoli. They are made of one layer of squamous epithelial tissue and contain a rich network of blood capillaries. The capillaries allow oxygen and carbon dioxide to be exchanged between the blood and the lungs. The inner surfaces of the alveoli are covered with a lipid (fatty) substance, called *surfactant*, to help prevent them from collapsing.

The divisions of the bronchi and the alveoli are found in organs called **lungs**. The right lung has three sections, or lobes: the superior, the middle, and the inferior. The left lung has only two lobes: the superior and the inferior. The left lung is smaller because the heart is located toward the left side of the chest. Each lung is enclosed in a membrane, or sac, called the **pleura**. The pleura consists of two layers of serous membrane: a *visceral pleura* attached to the surface of the lung, and a *parietal pleura* attached to the chest wall. A pleural space, located between the two layers, is filled with a thin layer of pleural fluid that lubricates the membranes and prevents friction as the lungs expand during breathing. Both of the lungs, along with the heart and major blood vessels, are located in the thoracic cavity.

PROCESS OF BREATHING

Ventilation is the process of breathing. It involves two phases: inspiration and expiration. **Inspiration** (inhalation) is the process of breathing in air. The diaphragm (dome-shaped muscle between the thoracic and abdominal cavities) and the intercostal muscles (between the ribs) contract and enlarge the thoracic cavity to create a vacuum. Air rushes in through the airways to the alveoli, where the exchange of gases takes place. When the diaphragm and intercostal muscles relax, the process of **expiration** (exhalation) occurs. Air is forced out of the lungs and air passages. This process of inspiration and expiration is known as **respiration**. The process of respiration is controlled by the respiratory center in the medulla oblongata of the brain. An increased amount of carbon dioxide in the blood, or a decreased amount of oxygen as seen in certain diseases (asthma, congestive heart failure, or emphysema), causes the respiratory center to increase the rate of respiration. Although this process is usually involuntary, a person can control the rate of breathing by breathing faster or slower.

STAGES OF RESPIRATION

There are two main stages of respiration: external respiration and internal respiration (**Figure 7–60**). **External respiration** is the exchange of oxygen and carbon dioxide between the lungs and bloodstream. Oxygen, breathed in through the respiratory system, enters the alveoli. Because the

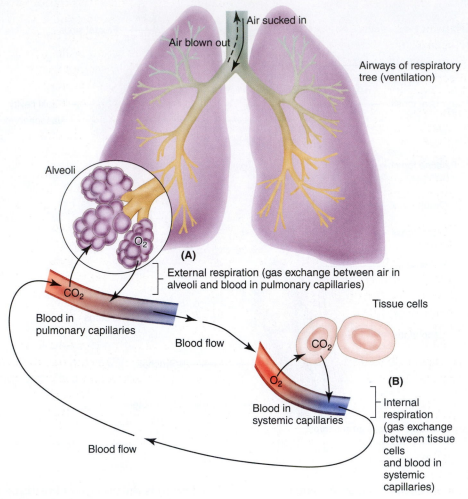

Air sucked in

Air blown out

Airways of respiratory
tree (ventilation)

Alveoli

O_2

(A)

External respiration (gas exchange between air in
alveoli and blood in pulmonary capillaries)

CO_2

Blood in
pulmonary capillaries

Blood flow

Tissue cells

CO_2

O_2

Blood in
systemic capillaries

(B)

Internal
respiration
(gas exchange
between tissue
cells
and blood in
systemic
capillaries)

Blood flow

FIGURE 7–60 External and internal respiration.

oxygen concentration in the alveoli is higher than
the oxygen concentration in the blood capillaries,
oxygen leaves the alveoli and enters the capillaries
and the bloodstream. Carbon dioxide, a metabolic
waste product, is carried in the bloodstream. Because
the carbon dioxide concentration in the capillaries
is higher than the carbon dioxide concentration
in the alveoli, carbon dioxide leaves the capillaries
and enters the alveoli, where it is expelled from the
body during exhalation. **Internal respiration** is the
exchange of carbon dioxide and oxygen between the
tissue cells and the bloodstream. Oxygen is carried
to the tissue cells by the blood. Because the oxygen
concentration is higher in the blood than in the
tissue cells, oxygen leaves the blood capillaries and
enters the tissue cells. The cells then use the oxygen
and nutrients to produce energy, water, and carbon
dioxide. This process is called **cellular respiration**.
Because the carbon dioxide concentration is higher
in tissue cells than in the bloodstream, carbon
dioxide leaves the cells and enters the bloodstream
to be transported back to the lungs, where external
respiration takes place.

DISEASES AND ABNORMAL CONDITIONS
Asthma

Asthma is a chronic inflammatory disorder of the
airways, usually caused by a sensitivity to an allergen
such as dust, pollen, an animal, medications, or a food.
Stress, overexertion, and infection can also cause an
asthma attack, during which bronchospasms narrow
the openings of the bronchioles, mucus production
increases, and edema develops in the mucosal lining.
Symptoms of an asthma attack include dyspnea (difficult
breathing), wheezing, coughing accompanied by
expectoration of sputum, and tightness in the chest.
Treatment methods include bronchodilators (to enlarge
the bronchioles), anti-inflammatory medications, allergy
shots and medications, epinephrine, and oxygen therapy.
In severe cases, bronchial thermoplasty may be helpful.
An electrode is used to heat the inside of the airways
to reduce smooth muscle and lessen the ability of the
airway to tighten. Identification and elimination of or
desensitization to allergens are important in preventing
asthma attacks.

Bronchitis

Bronchitis is an inflammation of the bronchi and bronchial tubes. *Acute bronchitis* is very common and frequently develops from a cold or the flu. It is usually caused by a viral infection. It is caused by bacteria in only about 10 percent of the cases. It is characterized by a productive cough, dyspnea, rales (bubbly or noisy breath sounds), chest pain, and fever. If it is bacterial, it is treated with antibiotics. Other treatments include expectorants (to remove excessive mucus), nonsteroidal anti-inflammatory drugs (for fever and sore throat), decongestants, cough suppressants, rest, and drinking large amounts of water. *Chronic bronchitis* results from frequent attacks of acute bronchitis and long-term exposure to pollutants or smoking. It is characterized by chronic inflammation, damaged cilia, and enlarged mucous glands. Symptoms include excessive mucus resulting in a productive cough, wheezing, dyspnea, chest pain, and prolonged air expiration. Although there is no cure, antibiotics (for bacterial infections), bronchodilators, and/or respiratory therapy (including breathing exercises) are used in treatment.

Chronic Obstructive Pulmonary Disease

Chronic obstructive pulmonary disease (COPD) is a term used to describe any chronic lung disease that results in obstruction of the airways and limitation of airflow. Disorders such as chronic asthma, chronic bronchitis, emphysema, and tuberculosis lead to COPD. Smoking is the primary cause, but allergies and chronic respiratory infections are also factors. Symptoms include shortness of breath, wheezing, chest tightness, chronic cough, and physical impairment. Treatment methods include bronchodilators, mucolytics (to loosen mucus secretions), cough medications, supplemental oxygen, and pulmonary rehabilitation to optimize respiratory function. The flu and pneumonia vaccines should always be given to prevent infections and exacerbation of COPD. The prognosis is poor because damage to the lungs causes a deterioration of pulmonary function, leading to respiratory failure and death.

Emphysema

Emphysema is a noninfectious, chronic respiratory condition that occurs when the walls of the alveoli deteriorate and lose their elasticity, resulting in an abnormal and permanent enlargement of the airspaces. Carbon dioxide remains trapped in the alveoli, and there is poor exchange of gases. The most common causes are heavy smoking and prolonged exposure to air pollutants. Symptoms include dyspnea, a feeling of suffocation, pain, barrel chest, chronic cough, cyanosis, rapid respirations accompanied by prolonged expirations, and eventual respiratory failure and death. Although there is no cure, treatment methods include bronchodilators, inhaled steroids, breathing exercises, prompt treatment of respiratory infections, oxygen therapy, respiratory therapy, and avoidance of smoking. In advanced cases, lung volume reduction surgery (LVRS) can be done to remove areas of diseased lung. In severe cases, a lung transplant may be an option.

Epistaxis

Epistaxis, or a nosebleed, occurs when capillaries in the nose become congested and bleed. It can be caused by an injury or blow to the nose, hypertension, chronic infection, anticoagulant drugs, nose-picking, dry or cold air, and blood diseases such as hemophilia and leukemia. Compressing the nostrils toward the septum; elevating the head and tilting it slightly forward; and applying cold compresses will usually control epistaxis. A local vasoconstrictive agent can be used to reduce bleeding time. Sometimes it is necessary to insert nasal packs or cauterize (burn and destroy) the bleeding vessels. Treatment of any underlying cause, such as hypertension, is important in preventing epistaxis.

Influenza

Influenza, or flu, is a highly contagious viral infection of the upper respiratory system. Onset is sudden, and symptoms include chills, fever, a cough, sore throat, runny nose, muscle pain, and fatigue. Treatment methods include bed rest, fluids, analgesics (for pain), and antipyretics (for fever). Antiviral medications (Tamiflu), should be started with the onset of symptoms. These drugs can injure the virus and fight the infection, shortening the duration and severity of the illness. Antibiotics are not effective against the viruses that cause influenza, but they are sometimes given to prevent secondary infections such as pneumonia. The CDC recommends that everyone 6 months and older receive an annual flu vaccine. Because many different viruses cause influenza, vaccines are developed each year to immunize against the most common viruses identified.

Laryngitis

Laryngitis is an inflammation of the larynx and vocal cords. It can be caused by a viral infection, vocal cord strain (screaming), or irritation. It frequently occurs in conjunction with other respiratory infections. Symptoms include hoarseness or loss of voice, sore throat, and dysphagia (difficult swallowing). Treatment methods include rest, limited voice use, fluids, corticosteroids (to decrease vocal cord swelling), and salt water gargles. Almost all cases are viral and will not be cured with antibiotics.

Lung Cancer

Lung cancer is the leading cause of cancer death in both men and women, and is the most common type of cancer worldwide (**Figure 7–61**). It is a preventable disease because the main cause is exposure to carcinogens in tobacco, either through smoking or through exposure to "secondhand" smoke. Other causes include environmental toxins (asbestos) and radiation from treatment of another cancer. Three common types of lung cancer include small cell, squamous cell, and adenocarcinoma. In the early stages, there are no symptoms. In later stages, symptoms include a chronic cough, hemoptysis (coughing up blood-tinged sputum), dyspnea, fatigue, weight loss, and chest pain. The prognosis (outcome) for lung cancer patients is poor because the disease is usually advanced before it is diagnosed. Treatment includes surgical removal of the cancerous sections of the lung, radiation, and/or chemotherapy.

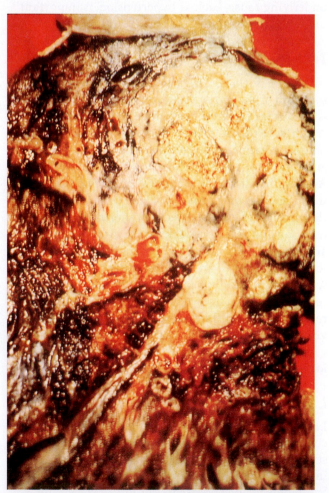

FIGURE 7–61 Lung cancer is the most common type of cancer worldwide, and it is a preventable disease. Courtesy of the National Cancer Institute

Pleurisy

Pleurisy is an inflammation of the pleura, or membranes, of the lungs. The double-membrane pleura layers rub when inflamed, causing a sharp, stabbing pain while breathing. It usually occurs in conjunction with pneumonia or other lung infections and is usually viral. Other symptoms include crepitation (grating sounds in the lungs), dyspnea, and fever. Treatment methods include rest and medications to relieve pain and inflammation. If fluid collects in the pleural space, a *thoracentesis* (withdrawal of fluid through a needle) is performed to remove the fluid and prevent compression of the lungs.

Pneumonia

Pneumonia is an inflammation or infection of the lungs characterized by exudate (a buildup of fluid) in the alveoli. It is usually caused by bacteria, viruses, protozoa, or chemicals. It often mimics the flu with symptoms being chills, fever, chest pain, productive cough, dyspnea, muscle pain, and fatigue. Treatment methods include bed rest, oxygen therapy, fluids, antibiotics (if indicated), respiratory therapy, and/or pain medication. The flu and pneumonia vaccines are both helpful in preventing pneumonia.

Rhinitis

Rhinitis is an inflammation of the nasal mucous membrane, resulting in a runny nose, watery eyes, sneezing, soreness, and congestion. Common causes are viral respiratory infections and allergens. Treatment consists of administering fluids and medications to relieve congestion and inflammation. Rhinitis is usually self-limiting.

Sinusitis

Sinusitis is an inflammation of the mucous membrane lining the sinuses. One or more sinuses may be affected. Sinusitis is usually caused by a virus, and less often by a bacteria. Symptoms include headache, facial or teeth pain and pressure, dizziness, thick nasal discharge, congestion, and loss of voice resonance. Treatment methods include analgesics (for pain), antibiotics (if indicated), decongestants (medications to loosen secretions), and moist inhalations. In more serious cases, balloon sinuplasty can be performed to expand the opening of the sinuses and improve drainage. Functional endoscopic sinus surgery (FESS) can be done to remove obstructions and allow for normal sinus drainage.

Sleep Apnea

Sleep apnea is a condition in which an individual stops breathing while asleep, causing a measurable decrease in blood oxygen levels. There are two main kinds of sleep apnea: obstructive and central. *Obstructive sleep apnea* is caused by a blockage in the air passage that occurs when the muscles that keep the airway open relax and allow the tongue and palate to block the airway. *Central sleep apnea* is caused by a disorder in the respiratory control center of the brain. The condition is more common in men. Factors such as obesity, hypertension, smoking, alcohol ingestion, and/or the use of sedatives may increase the severity. Sleep apnea is diagnosed when more than five periods of apnea lasting at least 10 seconds each occur during 1 hour of sleep. The periods of apnea reduce the blood oxygen level. This causes the brain to awaken the individual, who then gasps for air and snores loudly. This interruption of the sleep cycle leads to excessive tiredness and drowsiness during the day. Treatment involves losing weight, abstaining from smoking and the use of alcohol or sedatives, and sleeping on the side or stomach. An oral appliance or mouth piece designed to maintain airway patency may be helpful if worn while sleeping. In more severe cases of obstructive sleep apnea, a continuous positive airway pressure, or CPAP (pronounced see-pap), is used to deliver pressure to the airway to keep the airway open while the individual sleeps (**Figure 7–62**). The CPAP consists of a mask that is fit securely against the face. Tubing connects the mask with a blower device that can be adjusted to deliver air at different levels of pressure. If other treatments are ineffective, a maxillomandibular advancement surgery (MMA) may be performed to move the jaw forward. The obstructing tissue may be surgically removed by uvulopalatopharyngoplasty (UPPP). In severe life-threatening cases, a tracheostomy (surgical opening in the neck) must be performed. Treatment of central sleep apnea usually involves the use of medications to stimulate breathing.

Tuberculosis

Tuberculosis (TB) is an infectious lung disease caused by the bacterium *Mycobacterium tuberculosis*. At times, white blood cells surround the invading TB organisms and wall them off, creating nodules, called *tubercles*, in the lungs. The TB organisms remain dormant in the tubercles but can cause an active case of TB later, if body resistance is lowered (as with HIV or cancer). Symptoms of an active case of TB include fatigue, fever, night sweats, weight loss, hemoptysis (coughing up blood-tinged sputum), and chest pain. Treatment includes administering drugs for one or more years to destroy the bacteria. In cases where there is massive hemoptysis, bronchial artery embolization may be required. Good nutrition and rest are also important. In recent years, a new strain of the TB bacteria resistant to drug therapy has created concern that TB will become a widespread infectious disease again.

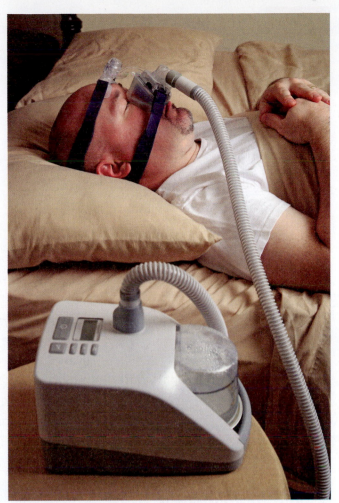

FIGURE 7–62 The continuous positive airway pressure (CPAP) mask attaches to a blower device that uses air pressure to keep the airway open and prevent sleep apnea. © iStockphoto/Amy Walters

Upper Respiratory Infection

An upper respiratory infection (URI), or common cold, is an inflammation of the mucous membrane lining the upper respiratory tract. Caused by viruses, URIs are highly contagious. Symptoms include fever, runny nose, watery eyes, congestion, sore throat, and hacking cough. There is no cure, and symptoms usually last approximately one week. Analgesics (for pain), antipyretics (for fever), rest, vitamin C, increased fluid intake, and antihistamines (to relieve congestion) are used to treat the symptoms.

checkpoint

1. What are five (5) functions of the nasal cavity?
2. Describe three (3) sections of the pharynx.
3. Describe the function of the epiglottis.

PRACTICE: Go to the workbook and complete the assignment sheet for 7:10, Respiratory System.

OBJECTIVES

After completing this section, you should be able to:

- Label the major organs on a diagram of the digestive system.
- Identify at least three organs that are located in the mouth and aid in the initial breakdown of food.
- Cite two functions of the salivary glands.
- Describe how the gastric juices act on food in the stomach.
- Explain how food is absorbed into the body by the villi in the small intestine.
- List at least three functions of the large intestine.
- List at least four functions of the liver.
- Explain how the pancreas helps digest foods.
- Describe at least five diseases of the digestive system.
- Define, pronounce, and spell all key terms.

■ KEY TERMS

alimentary canal (ahl-ih-men'-tar"-ee)
anus
colon (coh'-lun)
digestive system
duodenum (dew-oh-deh'-num)
esophagus (ee"-sof'-eh-gus)
gallbladder
hard palate

ileum (ill'-ee"-um)
impaction
jejunum (jeh-jew'-num)
large intestine
liver
mouth
pancreas (pan'-cree"-as)
peristalsis (pair"-ih-stall"-sis)
pharynx (far'-inks)

rectum
salivary glands
small intestine
soft palate
stomach
teeth
tongue
vermiform appendix
villi (vil'-lie)

Related Health Careers

- Dental assistant
- Dental hygienist
- Dentist
- Dietetic assistant
- Dietitian
- Enterostomal RN, technician, or therapist
- Gastroenterologist
- Hepatologist
- Internist
- Proctologist

The **digestive system**, also known as the *gastrointestinal system*, is responsible for the breakdown of food so that it can be taken into the bloodstream and used by body cells and tissues. There are two major ways food is broken down—physical and chemical. *Physical* breakdown occurs when mechanical forces such as chewing and muscle action break the food into smaller components. *Chemical* breakdown occurs when the digestive enzymes break food down into simpler nutrients that can be used by the cells.

The system consists of the alimentary canal and accessory organs (**Figure 7–63**). The **alimentary canal** is a long, muscular tube that begins at the mouth and includes the mouth (oral cavity), pharynx, esophagus, stomach, small intestine, large intestine, and anus. The accessory organs are the salivary glands, tongue, teeth, liver, gallbladder, and pancreas. Along the alimentary canal, the four basic processes of *ingestion* (eating and drinking), *digestion* (breaking down food into nutrients),

absorption (blood or lymph capillaries picking up the digested nutrients), and *excretion* (eliminating waste from the body) are carried out.

PARTS OF THE ALIMENTARY CANAL

The **mouth**, also called the *buccal cavity* (**Figure 7–64**), receives food as it enters the body. While food is in the mouth, it is tasted, broken down physically by the teeth, lubricated and partially digested by saliva, and swallowed. The **teeth** are special structures in the mouth that physically break down food by chewing and grinding. This process is called *mastication*. The **tongue** is a muscular organ that contains special receptors called *taste buds*. The taste buds allow a person to taste sweet, salty, sour, and bitter sensations, in addition to a fifth taste, *umami*, that detects meaty or savory sensations.

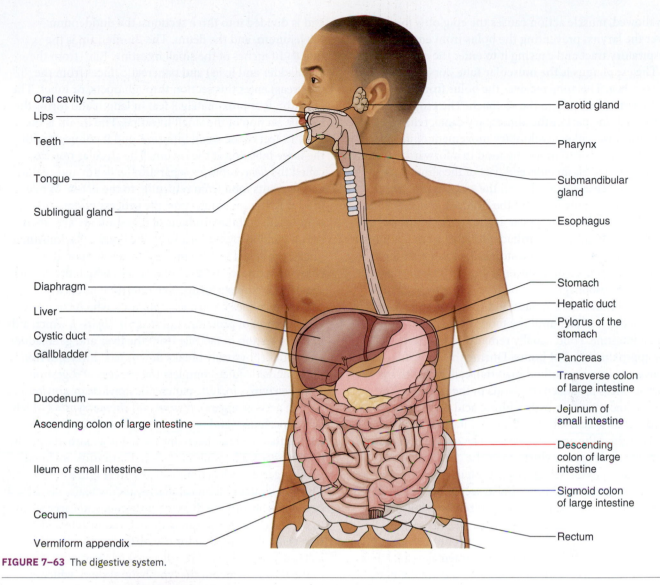

Oral cavity
Lips
Teeth
Tongue
Sublingual gland

Parotid gland
Pharynx
Submandibular gland
Esophagus

Diaphragm
Liver
Cystic duct
Gallbladder
Duodenum
Ascending colon of large intestine
Ileum of small intestine
Cecum
Vermiform appendix

Stomach
Hepatic duct
Pylorus of the stomach
Pancreas
Transverse colon of large intestine
Jejunum of small intestine
Descending colon of large intestine
Sigmoid colon of large intestine
Rectum

FIGURE 7–63 The digestive system.

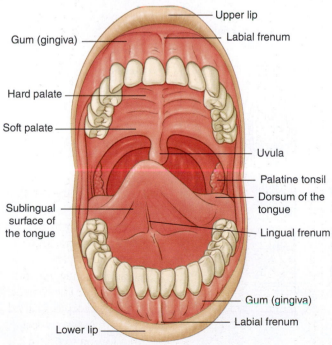

Gum (gingiva)

Hard palate

Soft palate

Sublingual surface of the tongue

Upper lip
Labial frenum

Uvula
Palatine tonsil
Dorsum of the tongue
Lingual frenum

Gum (gingiva)
Labial frenum

Lower lip

FIGURE 7–64 Parts of the oral cavity, or mouth.

The tongue also aids in chewing and swallowing food. The **hard palate** is the bony structure that forms the roof of the mouth and separates the mouth from the nasal cavities. Behind the hard palate is the **soft palate**, which separates the mouth from the nasopharynx. The *uvula*, a cone-shaped muscular structure, hangs from the middle of the soft palate. It prevents food from entering the nasopharynx during swallowing. Three pairs of **salivary glands**—the parotid, sublingual, and submandibular—produce a liquid called *saliva*. Saliva lubricates the mouth during speech and chewing and moistens food so that it can be swallowed easily. Saliva also contains an enzyme (a substance that speeds up a chemical reaction) called *salivary amylase*, formerly known as *ptyalin*. Salivary amylase begins the chemical breakdown of carbohydrates, or starches, into sugars that can be taken into the body.

After the food is chewed and mixed with saliva, it is called a *bolus*. When the bolus is swallowed, it enters the **pharynx** (throat). The pharynx is a tube that carries both air and food. It carries the air to the trachea, or windpipe, and food to the esophagus. When a bolus is being swallowed, muscle action causes the epiglottis to close over the larynx, preventing the bolus from entering the respiratory tract and causing it to enter the esophagus.

The **esophagus** is the muscular tube dorsal to (behind) the trachea. This tube receives the bolus from the pharynx and carries the bolus to the stomach. The esophagus, like the remaining part of the alimentary canal, relies on a rhythmic, wavelike, involuntary movement of its muscles called **peristalsis** to move the food in a forward direction.

The **stomach** is an enlarged part of the alimentary canal. It receives the food from the esophagus. The mucous membrane lining of the stomach contains folds, called *rugae*. These disappear as the stomach fills with food and expands. The cardiac sphincter, a circular muscle between the esophagus and stomach, closes after food enters the stomach and prevents food from going back up into the esophagus. The pyloric sphincter, a circular muscle between the stomach and small intestine, keeps food in the stomach until the food is ready to enter the small intestine. Food usually remains in the stomach for approximately 2–4 hours. During this time, food is converted into a semifluid material, called *chyme*, by gastric juices produced by glands in the stomach. The gastric juices contain hydrochloric acid and enzymes. Hydrochloric acid kills bacteria, facilitates iron absorption, and activates the enzyme pepsin. The enzymes in gastric juices include lipase, which starts the chemical breakdown of fats, and pepsin, which starts protein digestion. In infants, the enzyme rennin is also secreted to aid in the digestion of milk. Rennin is not present in adults.

When the food, in the form of chyme, leaves the stomach, it enters the small intestine. The **small intestine** is a coiled section of the alimentary canal. It is approximately 20 feet in length and 1 inch in diameter,

and is divided into three sections: the duodenum, the jejunum, and the ileum. The **duodenum** is the first 9–10 inches of the small intestine. Bile (from the gallbladder and liver) and pancreatic juice (from the pancreas) enter this section through ducts, or tubes. The **jejunum** is approximately 8 feet in length and forms the middle section of the small intestine. The **ileum** is the final 12 feet of the small intestine, and it connects with the large intestine at the cecum. The circular muscle called the *ileocecal valve* separates the ileum and cecum and prevents food from returning to the ileum. While food is in the small intestine, the process of digestion is completed, and the products of digestion are absorbed into the bloodstream for use by the body cells. Intestinal juices, produced by the small intestine, contain the enzymes maltase, sucrase, and lactase, which break down sugars into simpler forms. The intestinal juices also contain enzymes known as *peptidases*, which complete the digestion of proteins, and *steapsin (lipase)*, which aids in the digestion of fat. Bile from the liver and gallbladder emulsifies (physically breaks down) fats. Enzymes from the pancreatic juice complete the process of digestion. These enzymes include pancreatic *amylase* or *amylopsin* (which acts on sugars), *trypsin* and *chymotrypsin* (which act on proteins), and *lipase* or *steapsin* (which acts on fats). After food has been digested, it is absorbed into the bloodstream. The walls of the small intestine are lined with fingerlike projections called **villi** (**Figure 7–65**). The villi contain blood capillaries and lacteals. The blood capillaries absorb the digested nutrients and carry them to the liver, where they are either stored or released into general circulation for use by the body cells. The lacteals absorb most of the digested fats and carry them to the thoracic duct in the lymphatic system, which

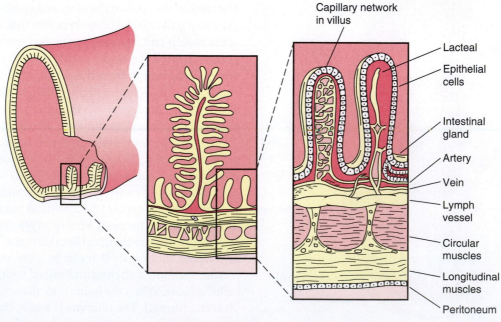

FIGURE 7–65 Lymphatic and blood capillaries in the villi of the small intestine provide for the absorption of the products of digestion.

releases them into the circulatory system. When food has completed its passage through the small intestine, only wastes, indigestible materials, and excess water remain.

The **large intestine** is the final section of the alimentary canal. It is approximately 5 feet in length and 2 inches in diameter. Functions include absorption of water and any remaining nutrients; storage of indigestible materials before they are eliminated from the body; synthesis (formation) and absorption of some B-complex vitamins and vitamin K by bacteria present in the intestine; and transportation of waste products out of the alimentary canal. The large intestine is divided into a series of connected sections. The *cecum* is the first section and is connected to the ileum of the small intestine. It contains a small projection, called the **vermiform appendix**. The next section, the **colon**, has several divisions. The *ascending colon* continues up on the right side of the body from the cecum to the lower part of the liver. The *transverse colon* extends across the abdomen, below the liver and stomach and above the small intestine. The *descending colon* extends down the left side of the body. It connects with the *sigmoid colon*, an S-shaped section that joins with the rectum. The **rectum** is the final 6–8 inches of the large intestine and is a storage area for indigestibles and wastes. It has a narrow canal, called the *anal canal*, which opens at a hole, called the **anus**. Fecal material, or stool, the final waste product of the digestive process, is expelled through this opening.

ACCESSORY ORGANS

The **liver** (**Figure 7–66**) is the largest gland in the body and is an accessory organ to the digestive system. It is located under the diaphragm and in the upper right quadrant of the abdomen. The liver secretes bile, which is used to emulsify fats in the digestive tract. Bile also makes fats water soluble, which is necessary for absorption. The liver stores sugar in the form of glycogen. The glycogen is converted to glucose and released into the bloodstream when additional blood sugar is needed. The liver also stores iron and certain vitamins. It produces heparin, which prevents clotting of the blood; blood proteins such as fibrinogen and prothrombin, which aid in clotting of the blood; and cholesterol. Finally, the liver detoxifies (renders less harmful) substances such as alcohol and pesticides and destroys bacteria that have been taken into the blood from the intestine.

The **gallbladder** is a small, muscular sac located under the liver and attached to it by connective tissue. It stores and concentrates bile, which it receives from the liver. When the bile is needed to emulsify fats in the digestive tract, the gallbladder contracts and pushes the bile through the cystic duct into the common bile duct, which drains into the duodenum.

The **pancreas** is a glandular organ located behind the stomach. It produces pancreatic juices, which contain enzymes to digest food. These juices enter the duodenum

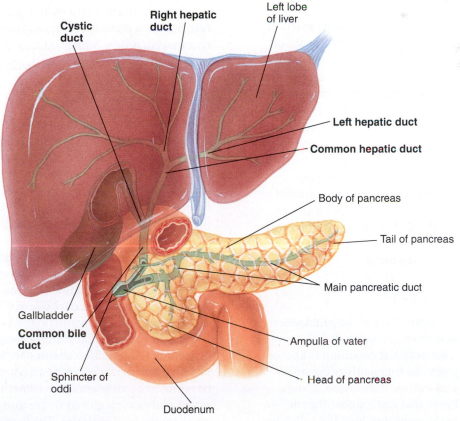

FIGURE 7–66 The liver, gallbladder, and pancreas.

through the pancreatic duct. The enzymes in the juices include pancreatic amylase or amylopsin (to break down sugars), trypsin and chymotrypsin (to break down proteins), and lipase or steapsin (to act on fats). The pancreas also produces insulin, which is secreted into the bloodstream. Insulin regulates the metabolism, or burning, of carbohydrates to convert glucose (blood sugar) to energy.

DISEASES AND ABNORMAL CONDITIONS

Appendicitis

Appendicitis is an acute inflammation of the appendix, usually resulting from an obstruction and infection. Symptoms include generalized abdominal pain that later localizes at the lower right quadrant, nausea and vomiting, mild fever, and elevated white blood cell count. If the appendix ruptures, the infectious material will spill into the peritoneal cavity and cause peritonitis, a serious condition. Appendicitis is treated by an appendectomy (surgical removal of the appendix). Since the appendix has no known essential purpose, postoperative prognosis is good. The appendix can be removed with an open surgery (in cases where there was a rupture) or, in less complicated cases, it can removed with minimally invasive laparoscopic surgery.

Celiac Disease

Celiac disease is a chronic genetic immune reaction to eating gluten, which is a group of proteins found in wheat, barley, and rye. Over time, this chronic inflammation damages the villi in the small intestine and results in the inability to absorb nutrients. The symptoms are diarrhea with pale, foul-smelling stools, excessive flatulence (gas), bloating, abdominal swelling or pain, fatigue, and weight loss. If the condition is not treated, it can cause anemia, osteoporosis, dermatitis, failure to thrive in children, and other diseases associated with malnutrition. The main treatment is a lifelong gluten-free diet. Vitamin and mineral supplements may be added to the diet if needed. After several months on the diet, the villi will begin to heal, and nutrient absorption can occur.

Cholecystitis

Cholecystitis is an inflammation of the gallbladder. When gallstones form from crystallized cholesterol, bile salts, and bile pigments, the condition is known as *cholelithiasis*. Symptoms frequently occur after eating fatty foods and include indigestion, nausea and vomiting, and pain that starts under the rib cage and radiates to the right shoulder. If a gallstone blocks the bile ducts, the gallbladder can rupture and cause peritonitis. Gallbladder rupture is rare but life threatening. Treatment methods include a low-fat diet, pain medications, lithotripsy (shock waves that are used to shatter the gallstones), and/or a cholecystectomy (surgical removal of the gallbladder). In less serious cases, a minimally invasive laparoscopic surgery can be performed.

Cirrhosis

Cirrhosis is a chronic destruction of liver cells accompanied by the formation of fibrous connective and scar tissue. When the liver is injured, it attempts to repair itself which creates scar tissue. If the damage is mild, the liver can continue to function effectively. With advanced cirrhosis, the scar tissue can prevent proper functioning of the liver. Causes include hepatitis, bile duct disease, nonalcoholic fatty liver (associated with obesity and diabetes), chemical toxins, and malnutrition associated with alcoholism. The liver is a vital organ with many functions. Symptoms of liver failure vary and become more severe as the disease progresses. Some common symptoms are liver enlargement, anemia, indigestion, nausea, edema in the legs and feet, hematemesis (vomiting blood), nosebleeds, jaundice (yellow discoloration), and ascites (an accumulation of fluid in the abdominal peritoneal cavity). When the liver fails, disorientation, hallucinations, hepatic coma, and death occur. Treatment is directed toward preventing further damage to the liver. Alcohol avoidance, proper nutrition, vitamin supplements, diuretics (to reduce ascites and edema), rest, infection prevention, and appropriate exercise are encouraged. A liver transplant may be performed if too much of the liver is destroyed.

Constipation

Constipation is when fecal material remains in the colon too long, causing excessive reabsorption of water. The feces or stool becomes hard, dry, and difficult to eliminate. Causes include poor bowel habits, chronic laxative use leading to a "lazy" bowel, a diet low in fiber, use of opioids (pain killers), diuretics, and certain digestive diseases. The condition is usually corrected by a high-fiber diet, adequate fluids, and exercise. Probiotics (beneficial bacteria) can improve gastric motility, and lubricants and stool softeners make stool easier to pass. Although laxatives are sometimes used to stimulate defecation, frequent laxative use may be habit forming and lead to chronic constipation. An **impaction** is a large, hard mass of fecal material lodged in the intestine or rectum. Oil-retention enemas are frequently ordered to soften the impaction so it can be expelled. If it cannot be removed by an enema, it is sometimes necessary to insert a lubricated, gloved finger into the rectum to break up the fecal material. The licensed supervisor or advanced care provider usually performs this procedure.

Crohn's Disease

Crohn's disease is a chronic inflammatory autoimmune disease of the digestive track that leads to destruction of healthy tissue in any area of the alimentary canal. Etiology is unknown, but genetics may be a factor. Symptoms include diarrhea that may be watery or bloody, a sudden and frequent need to defecate even when the bowel is empty, fever, fatigue, anorexia (loss of appetite), weight loss, abdominal cramping and pain, blood in the stool or rectal bleeding, and mouth ulcers. This inflammation can affect deep bowel areas and be very painful. Crohn's disease is characterized by periods of exacerbation when symptoms are present and periods of remission when symptoms disappear. Treatment includes NSAIDs (nonsteroidal anti-inflammatory drugs) for pain, a low-residue diet to decrease diarrhea, antibiotics for abscesses or infection, corticosteroids to decrease inflammation, and immunosuppressants or drugs to suppress the action of the immune system for severe inflammation. Dietary restrictions, exercise, and controlling stress is part of treatment as well. In extreme cases with repeated infections, surgery may be indicated to remove the damaged section of the digestive tract.

Diarrhea

Diarrhea is a condition characterized by frequent watery stools. Causes include infection (viral, bacterial, or parasitic), stress, diet, an irritated colon, and toxic substances. Diarrhea can be extremely dangerous in infants and small children because of the excessive fluid loss. Treatment is directed toward eliminating the cause, providing adequate fluid intake, and modifying the diet. Anti-motility agents can be used to slow down the movement of stool, and probiotics help the intestine recolonize with nonpathogenic flora. An aggressive type of diarrhea is caused by the bacterium *Clostridium difficile* (*C. diff*). Use of high-dose or multiple antibiotics is usually the cause of *C. diff* infections. Hospitalization and severe illness are also risk factors for contracting *C. diff*. Symptoms include frequent watery diarrhea, abdominal cramping, dehydration, weight loss, and, in severe cases, organ failure and death. Treatment usually consists of discontinuing the current antibiotics and starting another one, probiotics, and hydration. Recent research has found that fecal microbiota transplantation (FMT) is more effective and less costly than antibiotics for the treatment of *C. diff*. Fecal transplants are done by taking stool from a healthy donor and placing it in the colon of patients with *C. diff* via a colonoscopy or enema. More recently, an oral pill has been developed. The healthy bacteria (microbiota—formerly called gut flora) in the donor stool helps restore the normal flora in the colon of the *C. diff* patient.

Diverticulitis

Diverticulitis is an inflammation of the diverticula, pouches (or sacs) that form in the intestine as the mucosal lining pushes through the surrounding muscle. When fecal material and bacteria become trapped in the diverticula, inflammation occurs. This can result in an abscess or rupture, leading to peritonitis. Symptoms vary depending on the amount of inflammation but may include abdominal pain, irregular bowel movements, flatus (gas), constipation or diarrhea, abdominal distention (swelling), low-grade fever, and nausea and vomiting. Treatment methods include antibiotics, stool-softening medications, pain medications, probiotics (beneficial bacteria), high-fiber diet, and in severe cases, surgery to remove the affected section of the colon.

Gastroenteritis

Gastroenteritis, commonly called the stomach flu, is an inflammation of the mucous membrane that lines the stomach and intestinal tract. Causes include food poisoning, infection, and toxins. Symptoms include abdominal cramping, nausea, vomiting, fever, and diarrhea. Usual treatment methods are rest and increased fluid intake. In severe cases, antibiotics, intravenous fluids, antiemetics (for vomiting), and medications to slow peristalsis may be used. Probiotics may be helpful for prevention.

Gastroesophageal Reflux Disease (GERD)

Gastroesophageal reflux disease, or GERD, is a chronic disease of the digestive tract. It occurs when acid from the stomach flows back up into the esophagus through the lower esophageal sphincter. This occurs when the sphincter becomes weak and opens spontaneously or does not close properly. This reflux of acid into the esophagus causes irritation, inflammation, and damage to the lining of the esophagus. Symptoms include chest burning or pain (heartburn), a sour taste in the mouth, and dysphagia (difficulty swallowing). GERD is diagnosed if these symptoms are experienced at least twice a week. Risk factors include obesity, pregnancy, hiatal hernia, and smoking. Chronic inflammation of the lining can cause scar tissue to form, creating esophageal strictures. These strictures narrow the esophagus, making it difficult for food to pass through. The chronic inflammation can also cause esophageal ulcers (open sores) that may bleed. In addition, tissue changes from the chronic inflammation can lead to Barrett's esophagus, a precancerous condition. Lifestyle changes including losing weight, wearing loose-fitting clothes, eating smaller meals, and staying upright after eating can reduce symptoms. Medications are used to neutralize stomach acid and reduce or block stomach acid production to prevent further damage. Prokinetics are used to strengthen the sphincter and speed gastric emptying. If other treatments are not effective, Nissen fundoplication surgery can be performed to tighten the sphincter by wrapping the upper stomach around it. In many cases, this can be done with a minimally invasive laparoscopic procedure.

Hemorrhoids

Hemorrhoids are painful dilated or varicose veins of the rectum and/or anus. They may be caused by straining to defecate, constipation, pressure during pregnancy, insufficient fluid intake, laxative abuse, and prolonged sitting or standing. Symptoms include pain, itching, and bleeding. Treatment methods include a high-fiber diet; increased fluid intake; stool softeners; sitz baths or warm, moist compresses; and creams or medicated pads containing witch hazel or hydrocortisone. Rubber band ligation using tiny rubber bands that are placed around the hemorrhoid cuts off the blood supply, thus killing the tissue. Sclerotherapy is done by injecting the hemorrhoid with a solution that shrinks it. The use of infrared or laser treatment causes the hemorrhoid to harden and shrivel. In some cases, a hemorrhoidectomy (surgical removal of the hemorrhoid) is necessary.

Hepatitis

Hepatitis is a viral inflammation of the liver. *Type A*, *HAV* or infectious hepatitis, is highly contagious and is transmitted in food or water contaminated by the feces of an infected person. It is the most benign form of hepatitis and is usually self-limiting. A vaccine is available to prevent hepatitis A. *Type B*, *HBV* or serum hepatitis, is transmitted by body fluids including blood, serum, saliva, urine, semen, vaginal secretions, and breast milk. It is more serious than type A and can lead to chronic hepatitis or to cirrhosis of the liver. A vaccine developed to prevent hepatitis B is recommended for all health care providers. *Type C*, or *HCV*, is also spread through contact with blood or body fluids. The main methods of transmission include sharing needles while injecting drugs, getting stuck with a contaminated needle or sharps while on the job, or passing the virus from an infected mother to the infant during birth. Hepatitis C is much more likely to progress to chronic hepatitis, cirrhosis, or both. There is no vaccine for type C. Antiviral medications such as interferons and ribavirin have been the main forms of treatment. However, directly acting antiviral agents (DAAs), like teleprevir and boceprevir, have been found to be more effective in treating hepatitis C. In October 2014, the FDA approved Harvoni, a combination pill that does not require interferon or ribavirin to be administered with it. It has had a great success rate. Other strains of the hepatitis virus that have been identified include types D and E. Symptoms include fever, anorexia (lack of appetite), nausea, vomiting, fatigue, dark-colored urine, clay-colored stool, myalgia (muscle pain), enlarged liver, and jaundice. Treatment methods include rest and a diet high in protein and calories and low in fat. A liver transplant may be necessary if the liver is severely damaged.

Hernia

A hernia, or rupture, occurs when an internal organ pushes through a weakened area or natural opening in a body wall. A hiatal hernia is when the stomach protrudes through the diaphragm and into the chest cavity through the opening for the esophagus (**Figure 7–67**). Symptoms include heartburn, stomach distention, chest pain, and dysphagia (difficult swallowing). Treatment methods include a bland diet; small, frequent meals; staying upright after eating; and surgical repair. An inguinal hernia is when a section of the small intestine protrudes through the inguinal rings of the lower abdominal wall. If the hernia cannot be reduced (pushed back in place), a herniorrhaphy (surgical repair) is performed. In uncomplicated cases, a minimally invasive laparoscopic surgery can be performed.

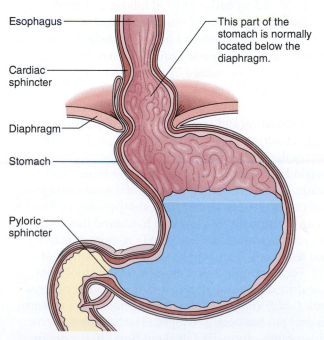

Esophagus

Cardiac sphincter

Diaphragm

Stomach

Pyloric sphincter

This part of the stomach is normally located below the diaphragm.

FIGURE 7–67 A hiatal hernia occurs when the stomach protrudes through the diaphragm.

Pancreatitis

Pancreatitis is an inflammation of the pancreas. The pancreatic enzymes begin to digest the pancreas itself, and the pancreas becomes necrotic, inflamed, and edematous. If the damage extends to blood vessels in the pancreas, hemorrhage and shock occur. The most common cause of pancreatitis is gallstones blocking the pancreatic ducts. It may also be a result of trauma or excessive alcohol consumption. Some cases are *idiopathic*, or of unknown cause. Symptoms include severe abdominal pain that radiates to the back, nausea, vomiting, diaphoresis (excessive perspiration), and jaundice if swelling blocks the common bile duct. Treatment depends on the cause. A cholecystectomy, removal of the gall bladder, is performed if gallstones are the cause. Analgesics for pain, nutritional support, and treatment for alcohol dependence are used if the cause of pancreatitis is alcoholism or idiopathic. This type of pancreatitis has a poor prognosis and often results in death.

Peritonitis

Peritonitis, an inflammation of the abdominal peritoneal cavity, usually occurs when a rupture in the intestine allows the intestine contents to enter the peritoneal cavity. Any rupture in the abdominal cavity (appendix, gallbladder, or stomach) can cause peritonitis, and it can be life threatening if the infection spreads to the blood and throughout the body. Symptoms include abdominal pain and distention, fever, nausea, and vomiting. Treatment methods include antibiotics and, if necessary, surgery for exploration and repair of the cause.

Ulcer

An ulcer is an open sore on the lining of the digestive tract. Peptic ulcers include gastric (stomach) ulcers and duodenal ulcers. The major cause is a bacterium, *Helicobacter pylori* (*H. pylori*), that burrows into the stomach membranes, allowing stomach acids and digestive juices to create an ulcer. In addition, regular use of some medications can irritate the lining of the stomach or intestine and cause an ulcer. Symptoms include burning pain, indigestion, hematemesis (bloody vomitus), and melena (dark, tarry stool). Usual treatment methods are antacids, a bland diet, decreased stress, and avoidance of irritants such as alcohol, fried foods, tobacco, and caffeine. If the *H. pylori* bacteria are present, treatment with antibiotics and a bismuth preparation, such as Pepto-Bismol, usually cures the condition. In addition, a proton pump inhibitor (such as Prilosec) is often prescribed. In severe cases, surgery is performed to remove the affected area.

Ulcerative Colitis

Ulcerative colitis is a severe inflammation of the colon accompanied by the formation of ulcers and abscesses (**Figure 7–68**). The exact cause is unknown. An autoimmune reaction is a possible cause. Stress, genetics, and food allergies or intolerances may aggravate the condition. The main symptom is diarrhea containing blood, pus, and mucus. Other symptoms include weight loss, weakness, abdominal pain, anemia, and anorexia. Periods of remission and exacerbation are common. Treatment is directed toward controlling inflammation (corticosteroids), immune system suppressors, reducing stress with mild sedation, pain relief, maintaining proper nutrition, and avoiding foods or substances that aggravate the condition. In some cases, surgical removal of the affected colon and creation of a colostomy (an artificial opening in the colon that allows fecal material to be excreted through the abdominal wall) is necessary. Another surgical procedure, ileoanal anastomosis, eliminates the need for the abdominal wall bag and allows for waste to be expelled more normally.

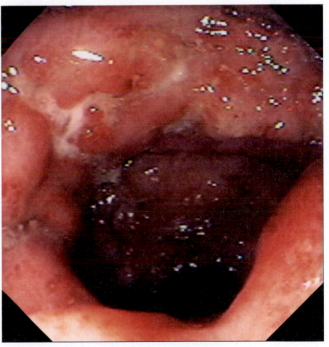

FIGURE 7–68 A colon with ulcerative colitis has a red, inflamed surface with ulcerations. Courtesy of Dr. David M. Martin/Science Photo Library

checkpoint

1. List two (2) functions of the salivary glands.
2. List three (3) functions of the liver.
3. Describe how food is absorbed into the body by the villi in the small intestine.

PRACTICE: Go to the workbook and complete the assignment sheet for 7:11, Digestive System.

OBJECTIVES

After completing this section, you should be able to:

- Label a diagram of the major parts of the urinary system.

- Explain the action of the following parts of a nephron: glomerulus, Bowman's capsule, convoluted tubule, and collecting tubule.

- State the functions of the ureter, bladder, and urethra.

- Explain why the urethra is different in male and female individuals.

- Interpret at least five terms used to describe conditions that affect urination.

- Describe at least three diseases of the urinary system.

- Define, pronounce, and spell all key terms.

■ KEY TERMS

bladder

Bowman's capsule

cortex *(core'-tex)*

excretory system *(ex'-kreh-tor"-ee)*

glomerulus *(glow"-mare'-you-luss)*

hilum

homeostasis

kidneys

medulla *(meh-due'-la)*

nephrons *(nef'-ronz)*

renal pelvis

ureters *(you'-reh"-turz)*

urethra *(you"-wreath'-rah)*

urinary meatus *(you'-rih-nah-ree" me-ate'-as)*

urinary system

urine

void

Related Health Careers

- Dialysis technician
- Medical laboratory technologist/technician
- Nephrologist
- Urologist

The **urinary system**, also known as the **excretory system**, is responsible for removing certain wastes and excess water from the body and for maintaining the body's acid–base or pH balance. It is one of the major body systems that maintains **homeostasis**, a state of equilibrium or constant state of natural balance in the internal environment of the body. The urinary system influences homeostasis by regulating volume and composition of blood. It filters out blood waste products but reabsorbs components such as glucose, proteins, vitamins, and electrolytes like sodium needed by the body. It keeps the pH of the blood and urine correct. Blood volume is also affected by the hormonal regulation of urine. These hormones respond to the amount of water and substances in the blood stream to determine what should be retained and what should be expelled in the urine. For example, if the glucose level is high in the blood, glucose is expelled in the urine. If the glucose level is low, glucose is reabsorbed and retained in the blood stream. The delicate balance of hormone levels, pH, and fluid volume is how

the urinary system functions to maintain correct blood volume levels and keep the body in a normal homeostatic range. The parts of the urinary system are two kidneys, two ureters, one bladder, and one urethra (**Figure 7–69**).

The **kidneys** (**Figure 7–70**) are two bean-shaped organs located on either side of the vertebral column, behind the upper part of the abdominal cavity, and separated from this cavity by the peritoneum. Their location is often described as retroperitoneal. The kidneys are protected by the ribs and a heavy cushion of fat. Connective tissue helps hold the kidneys in position. Each kidney is enclosed in a mass of fatty tissue, called an *adipose capsule*, and covered externally by a tough, fibrous tissue, called the *renal fascia*, or *fibrous capsule*.

Each kidney is divided into two main sections: the cortex and the medulla. The **cortex** is the outer section of the kidney. It contains most of the nephrons, which aid in the production of urine. The **medulla** is the inner section of the kidney. It contains most of the collecting tubules, which carry the urine from the nephrons through the kidney. Each kidney has a **hilum**, a notched or indented area through which the ureter, nerves, blood vessels, and lymph vessels enter and leave the kidney.

Nephrons (**Figure 7–71**) are microscopic filtering units located in the kidneys. There are more than one million nephrons per kidney. Each nephron consists of a glomerulus, a Bowman's capsule, a proximal convoluted tubule, a distal convoluted tubule, and a

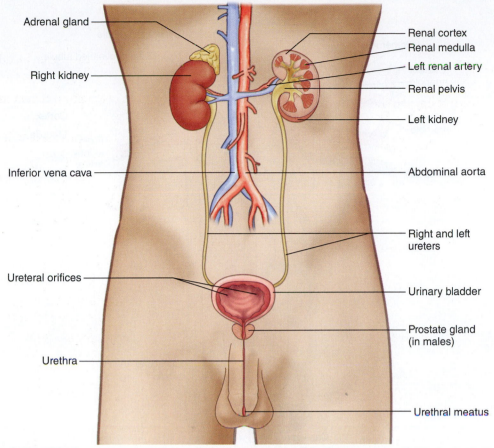

Adrenal gland

Right kidney

Inferior vena cava

Ureteral orifices

Urethra

Renal cortex
Renal medulla
Left renal artery
Renal pelvis

Left kidney

Abdominal aorta

Right and left
ureters

Urinary bladder

Prostate gland
(in males)

Urethral meatus

FIGURE 7–69 The urinary system.

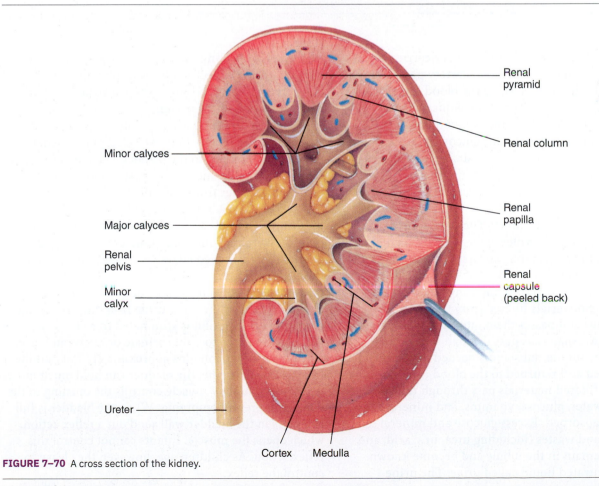

Minor calyces

Major calyces

Renal
pelvis

Minor
calyx

Ureter

Cortex   Medulla

Renal
pyramid

Renal column

Renal
papilla

Renal
capsule
(peeled back)

FIGURE 7–70 A cross section of the kidney.

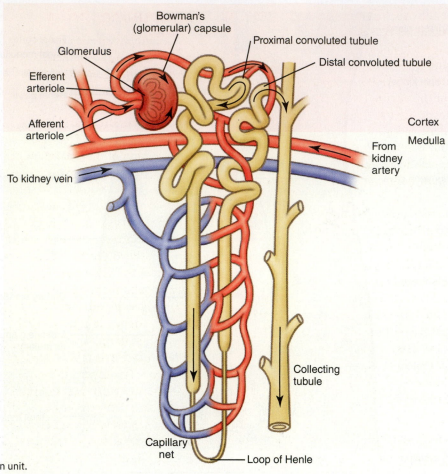

FIGURE 7–71 A nephron unit.

collecting duct (tubule). The renal artery carries blood to the kidney. Branches of the renal artery pass through the medulla to the cortex, where the blood enters the first part of the nephron, the **glomerulus**, which is a cluster of capillaries. As blood passes through the glomerulus, water, mineral salts, glucose (sugar), metabolic products, and other substances are filtered out of the blood. Red blood cells and proteins are not filtered out. The filtered blood leaves the glomerulus and eventually makes its way to the renal vein, which carries it away from the kidney. The substances filtered out in the glomerulus enter the next section of the nephron, the **Bowman's capsule**. The Bowman's capsule is a C-shaped structure that surrounds the glomerulus and is the start of the convoluted tubule. It picks up the materials filtered from the blood in the glomerulus and passes them into the convoluted tubule. As these materials pass through the various sections of the tubule, substances needed by the body are reabsorbed and returned to the blood capillaries. By the time the filtered materials pass through the tubule, most of the water, glucose, vitamins, and mineral salts have been reabsorbed. Excess glucose and mineral salts, some water, and wastes (including urea, uric acid, and creatinine) remain in the tubule and become known as the concentrated liquid called *urine*. The urine

then enters collecting ducts, or tubules, located in the medulla. These collecting ducts empty into the **renal pelvis** (renal basin), a funnel-shaped structure that is the first section of the ureter.

The **ureters** are two muscular tubes approximately 10–12 inches in length. One extends from the renal pelvis of each kidney to the bladder. Peristalsis (a rhythmic, wavelike motion of muscle) moves the urine through the ureter from the kidney to the bladder.

The **bladder** is a hollow, muscular sac that lies behind the symphysis pubis and at the midline of the pelvic cavity. It has a mucous membrane lining arranged in a series of folds, called *rugae*. The rugae disappear as the bladder expands to fill with urine. Three layers of visceral (smooth) muscle form the walls of the bladder, which receives the urine from the ureters and stores the urine until it is eliminated from the body. Although the urge to **void** (urinate or micturate) occurs when the bladder contains approximately 250 milliliters (mL) (1 cup) of urine, the bladder can hold much more. A circular sphincter muscle controls the opening to the bladder to prevent emptying. When the bladder is full, receptors in the bladder wall send out a reflex action, which opens the muscle. Infants cannot control this reflex action. As children age, however, they learn to control the reflex.

The **urethra** is the tube that carries the urine from the bladder to the outside. The external opening is called the **urinary meatus**. The urethra is different in female individuals and male individuals. In females, it is a tube approximately 3.75 cm (1.5 inches) in length that opens in front of the vagina and carries only urine to the outside. In males, the urethra is approximately 20 cm (8 inches) in length and passes through the prostate gland and out through the penis. It carries both urine (from the urinary system) and semen (from the reproductive system), although not at the same time.

Urine is the liquid waste product produced by the urinary system. It is approximately 95 percent water. Waste products dissolved in this liquid are urea, uric acid, creatinine, mineral salts, and various pigments. **Table 20-1** may be referenced for a complete list of the components of urine. Excess useful products, such as sugar, can also be found in the urine, but their presence usually indicates disease. Approximately 1,500–2,000 milliliters (mL) (1.5–2 quarts) of urine are produced daily from the approximately 150 quarts of liquid that is filtered through the kidneys.

Terms used to describe conditions that affect urination include:

- **Polyuria**: excessive urination
- **Oliguria**: below normal amounts of urination
- **Anuria**: absence of urination
- **Hematuria**: blood in the urine
- **Pyuria**: pus in the urine
- **Nocturia**: urination at night
- **Dysuria**: painful urination
- **Retention**: inability to empty the bladder
- **Incontinence**: involuntary urination
- **Proteinuria**: protein in the urine
- **Albuminuria**: albumin (a blood protein) in the urine

DISEASES AND ABNORMAL CONDITIONS

Cystitis

Cystitis is an inflammation of the bladder, usually caused by pathogens (most commonly *Escherichia coli* or *E. coli*) entering the urinary meatus. When it is caused by a bacterial infection, it is called a urinary tract infection (UTI). It is more common in female individuals because of the shortness of the urethra. Symptoms include frequent urination, dysuria, a burning sensation during urination, hematuria, lower back pain, bladder spasm, and fever. Treatment methods are antibiotics and increased fluid intake.

Glomerulonephritis

Glomerulonephritis, or nephritis, is an inflammation of the glomerulus of the kidney. *Acute glomerulonephritis* usually follows a streptococcal infection such as strep throat, scarlet fever, or rheumatic fever. Symptoms include chills, fever, fatigue, edema, oliguria, hematuria, and albuminuria (protein in the urine). Treatment methods include rest, restriction of salt, maintenance of fluid and electrolyte balance, antipyretics (for fever), diuretics (for edema), and antibiotics for bacterial infections. With treatment, kidney function is usually restored, and the prognosis is good. Repeated attacks can cause a chronic condition. *Chronic glomerulonephritis* is a progressive disease that causes scarring and sclerosing of the glomeruli. Early symptoms include hematuria, albuminuria, and hypertension. As the disease progresses and additional glomeruli are destroyed, edema, fatigue, anemia, hypertension, anorexia (loss of appetite), weight loss, congestive heart failure, pyuria, and, finally, renal failure and death occur. Treatment is directed at treating the symptoms, and treatment methods include a low-sodium diet, antihypertensive drugs, maintenance of fluids and electrolytes, and hemodialysis (removal of the waste products from the blood by a hemodialysis machine) (**Figure 7–72**). When both kidneys are severely damaged, a kidney transplant can be performed.

Pyelonephritis

Pyelonephritis, a type of UTI, is an inflammation of the kidney tissue and renal pelvis (upper end of the ureter), usually caused by pyogenic (pus-forming) bacteria. The infection usually starts in the urethra or bladder and travels to the kidneys, but can also be caused by an infection somewhere else in the body that travels in the bloodstream to the kidneys. It can cause permanent damage to the kidneys or spread to the bloodstream, creating a life-threatening condition. Symptoms include chills, fever, abdominal pain that radiates to the back, fatigue, a frequent strong persistent urge to void, hematuria, and pyuria (pus in the urine). Treatment methods are antibiotics targeted at the specific invading organism and increased fluid intake. In severe cases that do not respond to antibiotics, a nephrectomy (removal of the kidney) may be necessary.

Renal Calculus

A renal calculus, renal lithiasis, or urinary calculus is a kidney stone. A calculus is formed when minerals and salts in the urine precipitate (settle out of solution). Some small calculi may be eliminated in the urine, but

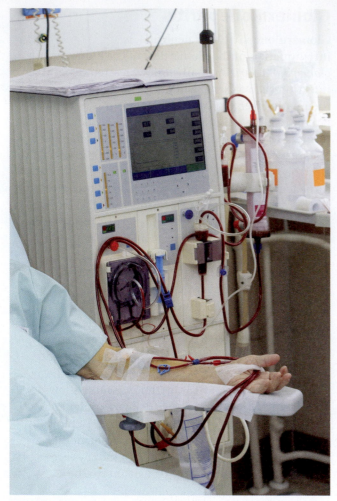

FIGURE 7–72 A hemodialysis machine helps remove waste products from the blood when the kidneys are not functioning correctly.
© Picsfive/www.Shutterstock.com

larger stones often become lodged in the renal pelvis or ureter. Symptoms include sudden, intense pain (renal colic); hematuria; nausea and vomiting; a frequent urge to void; and, in some cases, urinary retention. Initial treatment consists of increasing fluids, providing pain medication, antispasmodic agents, and straining all urine through gauze or filter paper to determine whether stones are being eliminated. Extracorporeal shock-wave lithotripsy is a procedure where high-energy pressure waves are used to crush the stones so that they can be eliminated through the urine. An ureteroscopic lithotripsy with laser probes can be done to break up the stones. In some cases, stones can be removed surgically using a minimally invasive laparoscopic procedure. Open surgical stone removal is rarely needed.

Renal Failure

Renal failure is when the kidneys stop functioning. *Acute renal failure (ARF)* can be caused by hemorrhage, shock, hypotension, injury, poisoning, nephritis, a surgical procedure during which the kidneys were deprived of blood flow for long periods (cardiac bypass), or dehydration. Symptoms include oliguria or anuria, headache, an ammonia odor to the breath, edema, cardiac arrhythmia, and uremia. Prompt treatment involving dialysis, restricted fluid intake, strict blood pressure control, and correction of the condition causing renal failure results in a good prognosis. *Chronic renal failure (CRF)* results from the progressive loss of kidney function. It can be caused by chronic glomerulonephritis, hypertension, toxins, and endocrine disease such as diabetes mellitus. Long-term substance abuse and alcoholism can also lead to renal failure. Waste products accumulate in the blood and affect many body systems. Symptoms include nausea, vomiting, diarrhea, weight loss, decreased mental ability, convulsions, muscle irritability, an ammonia odor to the breath, uremic frost (deposits of white crystals on the skin), and, in later stages, coma, prior to death. Treatment methods are dialysis, diet modifications and restrictions, strict blood pressure control, careful skin and mouth care, and control of fluid intake. A kidney transplant is the only cure.

Uremia

Uremia, also called *azotemia*, is a toxic condition that occurs when the kidneys fail and urinary waste products are present in the bloodstream. It can result from any condition that affects the proper functioning of the kidneys, such as renal failure, chronic glomerulonephritis, and hypotension. If treated quickly, permanent damage can be prevented. Untreated or poorly managed uremia can result in irreversible damage. Symptoms include headache, dizziness, nausea, vomiting, an ammonia odor to the breath, oliguria or anuria, mental confusion, convulsions, coma, and, eventually, death. Treatment consists of a restricted diet, cardiac medications to increase blood pressure and cardiac output, and dialysis. A kidney transplant could be required.

Urethritis

Urethritis is an inflammation of the urethra, usually caused by bacteria (such as gonococcus), viruses, or chemicals (such as bubble bath solutions). It is more common in male than female individuals. Symptoms include frequent and painful urination, redness and itching at the urinary meatus, and a purulent (pus) discharge. Treatment methods include sitz baths or warm, moist compresses; antibiotics; and/or increased fluid intake.

Urinary Tract Infection (UTI)

A urinary tract infection (UTI) is an infection in any part of the urinary system—ureters, kidneys, urethra, or bladder. It typically is caused from bacteria entering the urinary tract through the urethra and multiplying in the bladder. Sometimes cystitis or urethritis lead to a UTI. Symptoms may include a burning sensation when urinating; passing small amount of urine frequently; strong smelling urine, urine that is a red, pink, or dark color; pelvic pain; and fever. Treatment is antibiotics and pain medication. Drinking plenty of fluids helps to flush any bacteria from the urinary tract and may help to prevent UTIs.

checkpoint

1. Explain to a partner why a urethra is different in male and female individuals.

2. Distinguish the functions of the ureter, bladder, and urethra.

PRACTICE: Go to the workbook and complete the assignment sheet for 7:12, Urinary System.

7:13 ENDOCRINE SYSTEM

OBJECTIVES

After completing this section, you should be able to:

- Differentiate between exocrine and endocrine glands.

- Label a diagram of the main endocrine glands.

- Describe how hormones influence various body functions.

- Describe at least five diseases of the endocrine glands.

- Define, pronounce, and spell all key terms.

■ KEY TERMS

adrenal glands (ah "-dree'-nal)
endocrine glands
endocrine system (en'-doh"-krin)
exocrine glands
hormones

ovaries
pancreas (pan'-kree"-as)
parathyroid glands
pineal body (pin'-knee"-ahl)
pituitary gland (pih"-too'-ih-tar-ee)

placenta
testes (tess'-tees)
thymus
thyroid gland

Related Health Careers

- Dietitian
- Endocrinologist
- Nuclear medicine technologist

There are two types of glands: exocrine and endocrine. **Exocrine glands** secrete substances into ducts that lead to targeted tissues and include glands such as sudoriferous glands that excrete sweat directly onto the skin or salivary glands that excrete saliva into the mouth to aid in the digestion of food. **Endocrine glands** secrete substances directly into the bloodstream. The **endocrine system** consists of a group of these ductless (without tubes) endocrine glands that secrete substances directly into the bloodstream. These substances are called *hormones*. The endocrine system consists of the pituitary gland, thyroid gland, parathyroid gland, adrenal glands, pancreas, ovaries, testes, thymus, pineal body, and placenta (**Figure 7–73**).

Hormones, chemical substances produced and secreted by the endocrine glands, are frequently called "chemical messengers." They are transported throughout the body by the bloodstream and perform many functions, including:

- Stimulate exocrine glands (glands with ducts, or tubes) to produce secretions
- Stimulate other endocrine glands
- Regulate growth and development
- Regulate metabolism
- Maintain fluid and chemical balance
- Control various sex processes

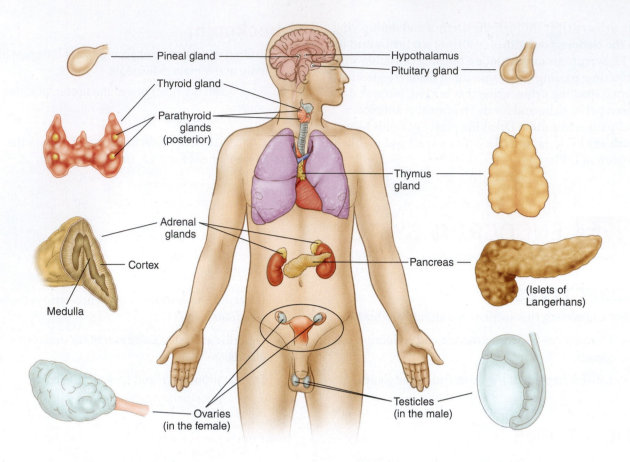

FIGURE 7–73 The endocrine system.

Table 7–3 lists the main hormones produced by each endocrine gland and the actions they perform.

PITUITARY GLAND

The **pituitary gland** is often called the "master gland" of the body because it produces many hormones that affect other glands. It is located at the base of the brain in the sella turcica, a small, bony depression of the sphenoid bone. It is divided into two sections, or lobes: the anterior lobe and the posterior lobe. Each lobe secretes certain hormones, as shown in **Table 7–3**.

Diseases and Abnormal Conditions

ACROMEGALY Acromegaly results from an oversecretion of somatotropin (growth hormone) in an adult (after normal bone growth has stopped) and is usually caused by a benign (noncancerous) tumor of the pituitary called an *adenoma*. There is a slow progression of signs over many years. Bones of the hands, feet, and face enlarge and create a grotesque appearance. The skin and tongue thicken, and slurred speech develops. Treatment includes medications that decrease growth hormone secretion or inhibit its action. Surgical removal and/or radiation of the

tumor is the treatment of choice, but the tumor frequently recurs. Acromegaly eventually causes cardiovascular and respiratory diseases that shorten life expectancy.

GIGANTISM Gigantism is a rare disorder resulting from an oversecretion of somatotropin before puberty, when the bones are still growing (**Figure 7–74**). The most common cause is a benign tumor of the pituitary gland, an adenoma. It causes excessive growth of long bones, extreme tallness, decreased sexual development, and, at times, retarded mental development. If a tumor of the pituitary is the cause, surgical removal or radiation is the treatment. Medications that reduce growth hormone release and hormone levels are also used.

DIABETES INSIPIDUS Diabetes insipidus is caused by decreased secretion of vasopressin, or antidiuretic hormone (ADH). Risk factors include pituitary surgery, trauma, encephalopathy, or an autoimmune disorder. A low level of ADH prevents water from being reabsorbed in the kidneys. Symptoms include polyuria (excessive urination), polydipsia (excessive thirst), dehydration, weakness, constipation, and dry skin. The condition is corrected by administering ADH.

TABLE 7–3 Hormones Produced by the Endocrine Glands and Their Actions

Gland	Hormone	Action
Pituitary		
Anterior lobe	ACTH—adrenocorticotropic	Stimulates growth and secretion of the cortex of the adrenal gland
	TSH—thyrotropin	Stimulates growth and secretion of the thyroid gland
	GH—somatotropin	Growth hormone, stimulates normal body growth
	FSH—follicle stimulating	Stimulates growth and hormone production in the ovarian follicles of female individuals, production of sperm in male individuals;
	LH—luteinizing (female) *or* ICSH—interstitial cell stimulating (male)	Causes ovulation and secretion of progesterone in female individuals Stimulates testes to secrete testosterone
	LTH—lactogenic or prolactin	Stimulates secretion of milk from mammary glands after delivery of an infant
	MSH—melanocyte stimulating	Stimulates production and dispersion of melanin pigment in the skin
Posterior lobe	ADH—vasopressin	Antidiuretic hormone, promotes reabsorption of water in kidneys, constricts blood vessels
	Oxytocin (pitocin)	Causes contraction of uterus during childbirth, stimulates milk flow from the breasts
Thyroid		
	Thyroxine and triiodothyronine	Increase metabolic rate; stimulate physical and mental growth; regulate metabolism of carbohydrates, fats, and proteins
	Thyrocalcitonin (calcitonin)	Accelerates absorption of calcium by the bones and lowers blood calcium level
Parathyroid		
	Parathormone (PTH)	Regulates amount of calcium and phosphate in the blood, increases reabsorption of calcium and phosphates from bones, stimulates kidneys to conserve blood calcium, stimulates absorption of calcium in the intestine
Adrenal		
Cortex	Mineralocorticoids Aldosterone	Regulate the reabsorption of sodium in the kidney and the elimination of potassium, increase the reabsorption of water by the kidneys
	Glucocorticoids Cortisol-hydrocortisone Cortisone	Aid in metabolism of proteins, fats, and carbohydrates; increase amount of glucose in blood; provide resistance to stress; and depress immune responses (anti-inflammatory)
	Gonadocorticoids	Act as sex hormones
	Estrogens	Stimulate female sexual characteristics
	Androgens	Stimulate male sexual characteristics
Medulla	Epinephrine (adrenaline)	Activates sympathetic nervous system, acts in times of stress to increase cardiac output and increase blood pressure
	Norepinephrine	Activates body in stress situations
Pancreas		
	Insulin	Used in metabolism of glucose (sugar) by promoting entry of glucose into cells to decrease blood glucose levels, promotes transport of fatty acids and amino acids (proteins) into the cells
	Glucagon	Maintains blood level of glucose by stimulating the liver to release stored glycogen in the form of glucose
Ovaries		
	Estrogen	Promotes growth and development of sex organs in female individuals
	Progesterone	Maintains lining of uterus
Testes		
	Testosterone	Stimulates growth and development of sex organs in male individuals, stimulates maturation of sperm
Thymus		
	Thymosin (thymopoietin)	Stimulates production of lymphocytes and antibodies in early life

(continues)

Gland	Hormone	Action
Pineal		
	Melatonin	May delay puberty by inhibiting gonadotropic (sex) hormones, may regulate sleep/wake cycles
	Adrenoglomerulotropin	May stimulate adrenal cortex to secrete aldosterone
	Serotonin	May prevent vasoconstriction of blood vessels in the brain, inhibits gastric secretions
Placenta		
	Estrogen	Stimulates growth of reproductive organs
	Chorionic gonadotropin	Causes corpus luteum of ovary to continue secretions
	Progesterone	Maintains lining of uterus to provide fetal nutrition

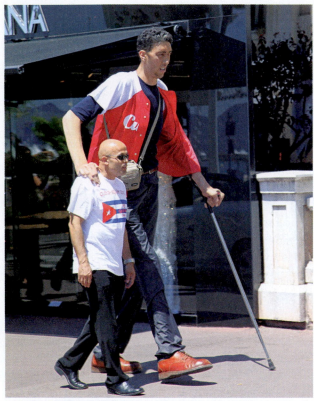

FIGURE 7-74 Gigantism results when the pituitary gland secretes excessive amounts of somatotropin (growth hormone) before puberty. Courtesy of UPI/David Silpa/Newscom

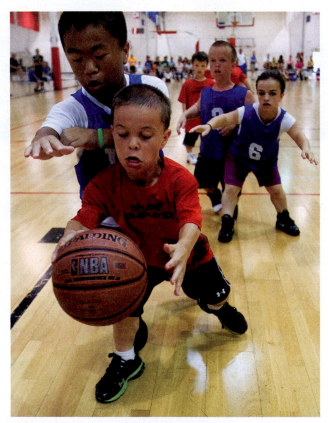

FIGURE 7-75 Dwarfism results from an undersecretion of somatotropin (growth hormone). Courtesy of Zuma Press/Newscom

DWARFISM Dwarfism results from an undersecretion of somatotropin (**Figure 7-75**). A random genetic mutation is the cause of most dwarfism. It can also be caused by a tumor, infection, or injury. It is characterized by an adult height less than 4 feet 10 inches, small body size, short extremities, and lack of sexual development. Mental development is usually normal. If the condition is diagnosed early, it can be treated with injections of somatotropic hormone for 5 or more years until long bone growth is complete.

THYROID GLAND

The **thyroid gland** synthesizes hormones that regulate the body's metabolism and control the level of calcium in the blood. It is located in front of the upper part of the trachea (windpipe) in the neck. It has two lobes, one on either side of the larynx (voice box), connected by the isthmus, a small piece of tissue. To produce its hormones, the thyroid gland requires iodine, which is obtained from certain foods and iodized salt. The hormones secreted by the thyroid gland are shown in Table 7-3.

Diseases and Abnormal Conditions

GOITER A goiter is an enlargement of the thyroid gland. Causes can include a hyperactive thyroid, an iodine deficiency, an oversecretion of thyroid-stimulating hormone on the part of the pituitary gland, or a tumor. Symptoms include thyroid enlargement, dysphagia (difficult swallowing), dyspnea (difficult breathing), a cough, and a choking sensation. Treatment is directed toward eliminating the cause. For example, iodine is given if a deficiency exists. Surgery may be performed to remove very large goiters. Radioiodine therapy for goiter volume reduction can be used if surgery is not an option.

HYPERTHYROIDISM Hyperthyroidism is an overactivity of the thyroid gland, which causes increased production of thyroid hormones and increased basal metabolic rate (BMR). Symptoms include extreme nervousness, tremors, irritability, rapid pulse, diarrhea, diaphoresis (excessive perspiration), heat intolerance, polydipsia (excessive thirst), goiter formation, and hypertension. An excessive appetite with extreme weight loss is a classic symptom. Treatment consists of antithyroid medications to decrease the amount of hormone produced, beta-blockers to decrease symptoms, radioactive iodine to destroy much of the thyroid gland, or a thyroidectomy (surgical removal of the thyroid). If the thyroid is removed, or destroyed, thyroid hormones are given for the lifetime of the individual.

GRAVES' DISEASE Graves' disease is a severe form of hyperthyroidism more common in women than men. Symptoms include a strained and tense facial expression, exophthalmia (protruding eyeballs), goiter, nervous irritability, emotional instability, tachycardia, a tremendous appetite accompanied by weight loss, and diarrhea. Treatment methods include medication to inhibit the synthesis of thyroxine, beta-blockers to decrease symptoms, radioactive iodine to destroy thyroid tissue, and/or a thyroidectomy.

HYPOTHYROIDISM Hypothyroidism is an underactivity of the thyroid gland and a deficiency of thyroid hormones. Two main forms exist: *cretinism* and *myxedema*. Cretinism develops in infancy or early childhood and results in a lack of mental and physical growth, leading to mental retardation and an abnormal, dwarfed stature. If diagnosed early, oral thyroid hormone can be given to minimize mental and physical damage. Myxedema occurs in later childhood or adulthood. Symptoms include coarse, dry skin; slow mental function; fatigue; weakness; intolerance of cold; weight gain; edema; puffy eyes; and a slow pulse. Treatment consists of administering oral thyroid hormone to restore normal metabolism. In some countries where iodized salt is not available, myxedema may be caused by an iodine deficiency. Adding iodine to the diet corrects this type of myxedema.

PARATHYROID GLANDS

The **parathyroid glands** are four small glands located behind and attached to the thyroid gland. Their hormone, parathormone, regulates the amount of calcium in the blood (see Table 7–3). It stimulates bone cells to break down bone tissue and release calcium and phosphates into the blood, causes the kidneys to conserve and reabsorb calcium, and activates intestinal cells to absorb calcium from digested foods. Although most of the body's calcium is in the bones, the calcium circulating in the blood is important for blood clotting, the tone of heart muscle, and muscle contraction. Because there is a constant exchange of calcium and phosphate between the bones and blood, the parathyroid hormone plays an important function in maintaining the proper level of circulating calcium.

Diseases and Abnormal Conditions

HYPERPARATHYROIDISM Hyperparathyroidism is an overactivity of the parathyroid gland resulting in an overproduction of parathormone. This results in hypercalcemia (increased calcium in the blood), which leads to renal calculi (kidney stones) formation, lethargy, gastrointestinal disturbances, and calcium deposits on the walls of blood vessels and organs. Because the calcium is drawn from the bones, they become weak, deformed, and likely to fracture.

This condition is often caused by an adenoma (glandular tumor), and removal of the tumor usually results in normal parathyroid function. Surgery is the treatment of choice, with a 90 percent cure rate. Other treatments include surgical removal of the parathyroids followed by administration of parathormone. A minimally invasive parathyroidectomy (MIP) is the procedure of choice. Diuretics to increase the excretion of water and calcium, and a low-calcium diet can be used as an adjunct therapy.

HYPOPARATHYROIDISM Hypoparathyroidism is an underactivity of the parathyroid gland, which causes a low level of calcium and a high level of phosphorous in the blood. Causes include the surgical removal of or injury to the parathyroid and/or thyroid glands. Symptoms include tetany (a sustained muscular contraction), hyperirritability of the nervous system, convulsive twitching, and patchy hair loss. Death can occur if the larynx and respiratory muscles are involved. The condition is easily treated with calcium, vitamin D (which increases the absorption of calcium and increases elimination of phosphorous), and parathormone.

ADRENAL GLANDS

The **adrenal glands** are frequently called the *suprarenal* glands because one is located above each kidney. Each gland has two parts: the outer portion, or cortex, and the inner portion, or medulla. The adrenal cortex secretes many steroid hormones, which are classified into three groups: mineralocorticoids, glucocorticoids, and gonadocorticoids. The groups and the main hormones in each group are listed in Table 7–3. The adrenal medulla secretes two main hormones: epinephrine and norepinephrine. These hormones are sympathomimetic; that is, they mimic the sympathetic nervous system and cause the fight or flight response.

Diseases and Abnormal Conditions

ADDISON'S DISEASE Addison's disease is caused by decreased secretion of aldosterone on the part of the adrenal cortex. This interferes with the reabsorption of sodium and water and causes an increased level of potassium in the blood. Symptoms include dehydration, diarrhea, fatigue, hypotension (low blood pressure), anorexia (lack of appetite), weight loss, muscle weakness, edema, excessive pigmentation leading to a "bronzing" (yellow-brown color) of the skin, hypoglycemia (low blood sugar), mental lethargy, and, in severe cases, coma and death. Treatment methods include administering corticosteroid hormones, controlled intake of sodium, and fluid regulation to combat dehydration.

CUSHING'S SYNDROME Cushing's syndrome results from an oversecretion of glucocorticoids on the part of the adrenal cortex. It can be caused by a tumor of the adrenal cortex, excess production of ACTH on the part of the pituitary gland, or overuse of injectable corticosteroids (for joint or back pain). Symptoms include hyperglycemia (high blood sugar), hypertension, muscle weakness, fatigue, hirsutism (excessive growth and/or an abnormal distribution of hair), poor wound healing, a tendency to bruise easily, a "moon" face, a fatty hump between the shoulders, and obesity (**Figure 7–76**). If a tumor is causing the disease, treatment is removal of the tumor. Radiation can also be used to stop the growth of abnormal cells. If the glands are removed, hormonal therapy is required to replace the missing hormones. If the disease is caused by long-term steroid use, these patients must be monitored closely, and steroid therapy must be reduced gradually.

PANCREAS

The **pancreas** is a fish-shaped organ located behind the stomach. It is both an exocrine gland and an endocrine gland. As an exocrine gland, it secretes pancreatic juices, which are carried to the small intestine by the pancreatic duct to aid in the digestion of food. Special B, or beta, cells located throughout the pancreas in patches of tissue

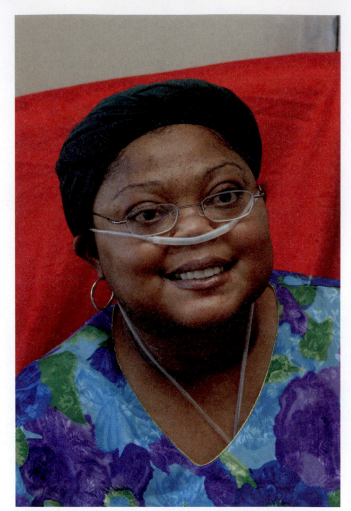

FIGURE 7–76 Symptoms of Cushing's Syndrome include hypertension, muscle weakness, fatigue, poor wound healing, a "moon" face, and obesity.

called *islets of Langerhans* produce the hormone insulin, which is needed for the cells to absorb sugar from the blood. Insulin also promotes the transport of fatty acids and amino acids (proteins) into the cells. Alpha, or A, cells produce the hormone glucagon, which increases the glucose level in blood (refer to Table 7–3).

Disease

DIABETES MELLITUS Diabetes mellitus is a chronic disease caused by decreased secretion of insulin or by body cells resistant to the effect of insulin. The metabolism of carbohydrates, proteins, and fats is affected. There are two main types of diabetes mellitus, named according to the need for insulin. *Insulin-dependent diabetes mellitus* (IDDM), or *Type 1*, usually occurs early in life, is more severe, and requires insulin. *Noninsulin-dependent diabetes mellitus* (NIDDM), or *Type 2* is the form of diabetes mellitus that may be treated with oral hypoglycemic (lower-blood-sugar) medication or insulin. It frequently occurs in obese adults and is sometimes controlled with diet and exercise. Another type of diabetes is *gestational diabetes* that occurs during pregnancy and disappears after the birth of the child. The main symptoms of diabetes include hyperglycemia (high blood sugar), polyuria (excessive urination), polydipsia (excessive thirst), polyphagia (excessive hunger), glycosuria (sugar in the urine), weight loss, fatigue, slow healing of skin infections, and vision changes. If the condition is not treated, diabetic coma and death may occur. Treatment methods are a carefully regulated diet to control the blood sugar level, regulated exercise, and oral hypoglycemic drugs or insulin injections. Newer medications that increase insulin production, increase the sensitivity to insulin, or slow the absorption of glucose into cells are also available. External and implantable insulin pumps that monitor blood glucose levels and deliver the required amount of insulin can be used to replace insulin injections (**Figure 7–77**). New research is being done with stem cells.

Estimates by the World Health Organization (WHO) indicate that 422 million people worldwide have diabetes. Researchers have proved that weight control (avoiding obesity) and moderate exercise can reduce the risk for development of diabetes by as much as 55–70 percent. Preventing diabetes is important because diabetes can cause atherosclerosis; myocardial infarctions (heart attacks); cerebrovascular accidents (strokes); peripheral vascular disease leading to poor wound healing and gangrene in the legs and feet, with possible amputations; diabetic retinopathy causing blindness; and kidney disease or failure.

OTHER ENDOCRINE GLANDS

The **ovaries** are the gonads, or sex glands, of the female. They are located in the pelvic cavity, one on each side of the uterus. They secrete hormones that regulate menstruation and secondary sexual characteristics (see Table 7–3).

The **testes** are the gonads of the male. They are located in the scrotal sac and are suspended outside the body. They produce hormones that regulate sexual characteristics of the male (see Table 7–3).

The **thymus** is a mass of tissue located in the upper part of the chest and under the sternum. It contains lymphoid tissue. The thymus is active in early life, activating cells in the immune system, but atrophies (wastes away) during puberty, when it becomes a small mass of connective tissue and fat. It produces one hormone, thymosin (see Table 7–3).

The **pineal body** is a small structure attached to the roof of the third ventricle in the brain. Knowledge regarding the physiology of this gland is limited. The three main hormones secreted by this gland are listed in Table 7–3.

The **placenta** is a temporary endocrine gland produced during pregnancy. It acts as a link between the mother and infant, provides nutrition for the developing infant, and promotes lactation (the production of milk in the breasts). It is expelled after the birth of the child (when it is called *afterbirth*). The three hormones secreted by this gland are listed in Table 7–3.

checkpoint

| **1.** Distinguish between endocrine and exocrine glands.

PRACTICE: Go to the workbook and complete the assignment sheet for 7:13, Endocrine System.

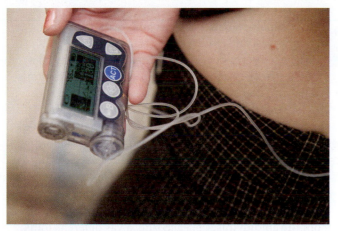

FIGURE 7–77 Insulin pumps that monitor blood glucose levels and deliver the required amount of insulin can be used to replace insulin injections. © iStockphoto/Mark Hatfield

7:14 REPRODUCTIVE SYSTEM

OBJECTIVES

After completing this section, you should be able to:

- Label a diagram of the male reproductive system.
- Trace the pathway of sperm from where they are produced to where they are expelled from the body.
- Identify at least three organs of the male reproductive system that secrete fluids added to semen.
- Label a diagram of the female reproductive system.
- Describe how an ovum is released from an ovary.
- Explain the action of the endometrium.
- Describe at least six diseases of the reproductive systems.
- Define, pronounce, and spell all key terms.

KEY TERMS

Bartholin's glands *(Bar'-tha-lens)*

breasts

Cowper's (bulbourethral) glands *(Cow'-purrs)*

ejaculatory ducts *(ee-jack'-you-lah-tore"-ee)*

endometrium *(en"-doe-me'-tree-um)*

epididymis *(eh"-pih-did'-ih-muss)*

fallopian tubes *(fah-low'-pea"-an)*

fertilization *(fur"-til-ih-zay'-shun)*

labia majora *(lay'-bee"-ah mah"-jore'-ah)*

labia minora *(lay'-bee"-ah ma-nore'-ah)*

ovaries

penis

perineum *(pear"-ih-knee'-um)*

prostate gland

reproductive system

scrotum *(skrow'-tum)*

seminal vesicles *(sem'-ih-null ves'-ik-ullz)*

testes *(tes'-tees)*

urethra

uterus

vagina *(vah-jie'-nah)*

vas (ductus) deferens *(vass deaf'-eh-rens)*

vestibule

vulva *(vull'-vah)*

Related Health Careers

- Embryologist
- Genetic counselor
- Geneticist
- Gynecologist
- Midwife
- Obstetrician
- Ultrasound technologist (sonographer)

The function of the **reproductive system** is to produce new life. Although the anatomic parts differ in male and female individuals, the reproductive systems of both have the same types of organs: gonads (sex glands), ducts (tubes) to carry the sex cells and secretions, and accessory organs.

MALE REPRODUCTIVE SYSTEM

The male reproductive system consists of the testes, epididymis, vas deferens, seminal vesicles, ejaculatory ducts, urethra, prostate gland, Cowper's glands, and penis (**Figure 7–78**).

The male gonads are the **testes**. The two testes are located in the **scrotum**, a sac suspended between the thighs. The testes are where *spermatogenesis* or production of the male *gamete* (sex cell), called *sperm* or *spermatozoa*, happens. The germ cell undergoes a two-part cell division called meiosis. Meiosis produces sperm with one-half the number of chromosomes as a parent cell (detailed information on the process of meiosis can be found in Section 7:1 and Figure 7-2). Testes produce the sperm in seminiferous tubules located within each testis. Because the scrotum is located outside the body, the temperature in the scrotum is lower than that inside the body. This lower temperature is essential for the production of sperm. The testes also produce male hormones. The main hormone is testosterone, which aids in the maturation of the sperm and also is responsible for the secondary

male sex characteristics such as body hair, facial hair, large muscles, and a deep voice.

After the sperm develop in the seminiferous tubules in the testes, they enter the **epididymis**. The epididymis is a tightly coiled tube approximately 20 feet in length and located in the scrotum and above the testes. It stores the sperm while they mature and become motile (able to move by themselves). It also produces a fluid that becomes part of the semen (fluid released during ejaculation). The epididymis connects with the next tube, the vas deferens.

The **vas (ductus) deferens** receives the sperm and fluid from the epididymis. On each side, a vas deferens joins with the epididymis and extends up into the abdominal cavity, where it curves behind the urinary bladder and joins with a seminal vesicle. Each vas deferens acts as both a passageway and a temporary storage area for sperm. The vas deferens are also the tubes that are cut during a *vasectomy* (procedure to produce sterility in the male).

The **seminal vesicles** are two small, pouchlike tubes located behind the bladder and near the junction of the vas deferens and the ejaculatory ducts. They contain a glandular lining. This lining produces a thick, yellow fluid that is rich in sugar and other substances and provides nourishment for the sperm. This fluid composes a large part of the semen.

The **ejaculatory ducts** are two short tubes formed by the union of the vas deferens and the seminal vesicles. They carry the sperm and fluids known collectively as *semen* through the prostate gland and into the urethra.

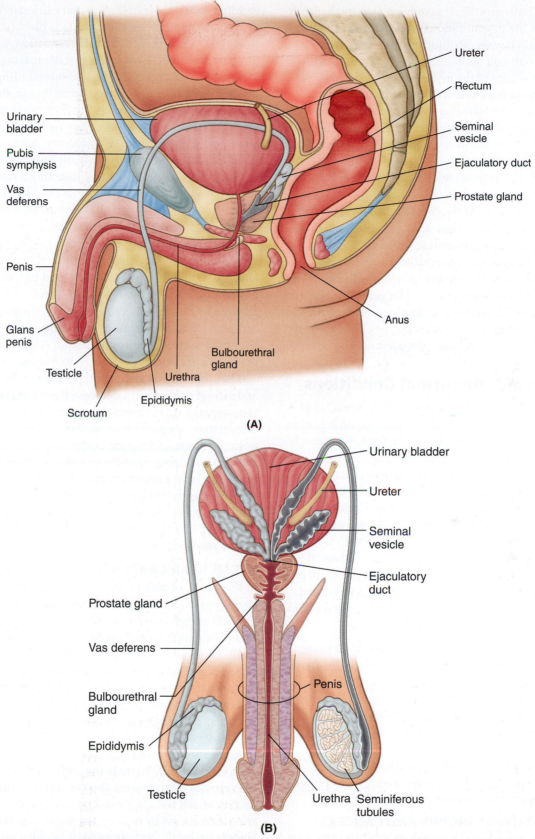

Urinary
bladder

Pubis
symphysis

Vas
deferens

Penis

Glans
penis

Testicle

Scrotum

Urethra

Epididymis

Bulbourethral
gland

Ureter

Rectum

Seminal
vesicle

Ejaculatory duct

Prostate gland

Anus

(A)

Urinary bladder

Ureter

Seminal
vesicle

Ejaculatory
duct

Prostate gland

Vas deferens

Bulbourethral
gland

Epididymis

Testicle

Penis

Urethra Seminiferous
tubules

(B)

FIGURE 7–78 The male reproductive system. (A) Lateral view. (B) Anterior view.

The **prostate gland** is a doughnut-shaped gland located below the urinary bladder and on either side of the urethra. It produces an alkaline secretion that both increases sperm motility and neutralizes the acidity in the vagina, providing a more favorable environment for the sperm. The muscular tissue in the prostate contracts during ejaculation (expulsion of the semen from the body) to aid in the expulsion of the semen into the urethra. When the prostate contracts, it also closes off the urethra, preventing urine passage through the urethra.

Cowper's (bulbourethral) glands are two small glands located below the prostate and connected by small tubes to the urethra. They secrete mucus, which serves as a lubricant for intercourse, and an alkaline fluid, which decreases the acidity of the urine residue in the urethra, providing a more favorable environment for the sperm.

The **urethra** is the tube that extends from the urinary bladder, through the penis, and to the outside of the body. It carries urine from the urinary bladder and semen from the reproductive tubes.

The **penis** is the external male reproductive organ and is located in front of the scrotum. At the distal end is an enlarged structure, called the *glans penis*. The glans penis is covered with a prepuce (foreskin), which is sometimes removed surgically in a procedure called *circumcision*. The penis is made of spongy, erectile tissue. During sexual arousal, the spaces in this tissue fill with blood, causing the penis to become erect. The penis functions as the male organ of copulation, or intercourse; deposits the semen in the vagina; and provides for the elimination of urine from the bladder through the urethra.

Diseases and Abnormal Conditions

EPIDIDYMITIS Epididymitis is an inflammation of the epididymis, usually caused by a pathogenic organism such as gonococcus, streptococcus, or staphylococcus. It frequently occurs with a urinary tract or prostate infection, mumps, or sexually transmitted infections (most commonly, chlamydia). If epididymitis is not treated promptly, it can cause scarring and sterility. Symptoms include intense pain in the testes, swelling, and fever. Treatment methods include antibiotics, cold applications, scrotal support, and pain medication. If an abscess is present, a procedure to drain the pocket of pus may be performed. In severe cases that do not respond to other treatments, an epididymectomy (removal of the epididymis) may be necessary.

ORCHITIS Orchitis is an inflammation of the testes, usually caused by the virus that causes mumps, bacterial infections from sexually transmitted infections, or injury. It can lead to atrophy of the testes and cause sterility. Symptoms include swelling of the scrotum, pain, and fever. Treatment methods include antibiotics (if indicated), antipyretics (for fever), scrotal support, and pain medication. Prevention methods include mumps vaccinations and observing measures to prevent sexually transmitted infections (STIs).

PROSTATIC HYPERTROPHY AND CANCER
Prostatic hypertrophy, or hyperplasia, is an enlargement of the prostate gland. Common in men over age 50, prostatic hypertrophy can be a benign condition—caused by inflammation, a tumor, or a change in hormonal activity—or a malignant (cancerous) condition. Symptoms of prostatic hypertrophy include difficulty in starting to urinate, frequent urination, nocturia

(voiding at night), dribbling, urinary infections, and urinary retention when the urethra is blocked. Initial treatment methods include fluid restriction, antibiotics (for bacterial infections), and prostatic massage. Medications that relax the muscle surrounding the urethra, keep the prostate from growing, or shrink the prostate make voiding easier. When hypertrophy causes urinary retention, a prostatectomy (surgical removal of all or part of the prostate) is necessary. A transurethral resection of the prostate (TURP), or removal of part of the prostate, is performed by inserting a scope into the urethra and resecting, or removing, the enlarged area. A prostatectomy can also be done by a perineal, or suprapubic (above the pubis bone), incision.

Prostatic carcinoma (cancer) can have the same symptoms as prostatic hypertrophy or it may not have any symptoms. A screening blood test, called a *prostatic-specific antigen (PSA) test*, can detect a substance released by cancer cells and aid in an early diagnosis. A digital rectal examination (DRE) may show a hard, abnormal mass in the prostate gland. A tissue biopsy of the prostate is usually performed to diagnose cancer.

If the condition is malignant, prostatectomy, radiation, and estrogen therapy (to decrease the effects of testosterone) are the main treatments. In some cases, an orchiectomy, surgical removal of the testes, is performed to stop the production of testosterone. Radioactive seeds can also be implanted in the prostate to destroy the cancerous cells without affecting the organs and tissue surrounding the prostate. If prostate cancer is detected early, the prognosis (expected outcome) is good. All men older than 50 years (earlier for high-risk patients) are encouraged to have annual prostate examinations.

TESTICULAR CANCER Testicular cancer, or cancer of the testes, occurs most frequently in men from ages 15 to 35. It is a highly malignant form of cancer and can metastasize, or spread, rapidly. Symptoms include a painless swelling of the testes, a heavy feeling, and an accumulation of fluid. Treatment includes an *orchiectomy*, or surgical removal of the testis, chemotherapy, and/or radiation. With proper treatment, it is one of the most curable cancers, with a 95 percent 5-year survival rate. It has been recommended that male individuals begin monthly testicular self-examinations at the age of 15. To perform the examination, the male individuals should examine the testicles after a warm shower when scrotal skin is relaxed. Each testicle should be examined separately with both hands by placing the index and middle fingers under the testicle and the thumbs on top. The testicle should be rolled gently between the fingers to feel for lumps, nodules, or extreme tenderness. In addition, the male should examine the testes for any signs of swelling or changes in appearance. If any abnormalities are noted, the male should be examined by a physician as soon as possible.

FEMALE REPRODUCTIVE SYSTEM

The female reproductive system consists of the ovaries, fallopian tubes, uterus, vagina, Bartholin's glands, vulva, and breasts (**Figure 7–79**).

The **ovaries** are the female gonads (**Figure 7–80**). They are small, almond-shaped glands located in the pelvic cavity and attached to the uterus by ligaments. The ovaries are where *oogenesis* or production and maturation of the female *gamete* called an *ovum* happens. After Meiosis I (cell division, discussed in detail in Section 7:1 and Figure 7-2), it will not continue to develop unless the egg cell or ovum is fertilized by a sperm. The ovaries contain thousands of small sacs called *follicles*. Each follicle contains an

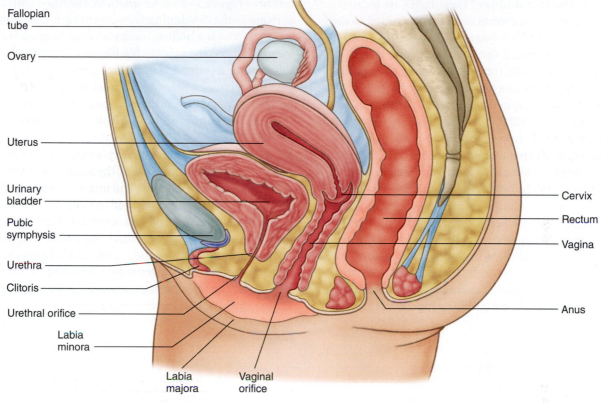

Fallopian tube
Ovary
Uterus
Urinary bladder
Pubic symphysis
Urethra
Clitoris
Urethral orifice
Labia minora
Labia majora
Vaginal orifice
Cervix
Rectum
Vagina
Anus

FIGURE 7–79 The female reproductive system.

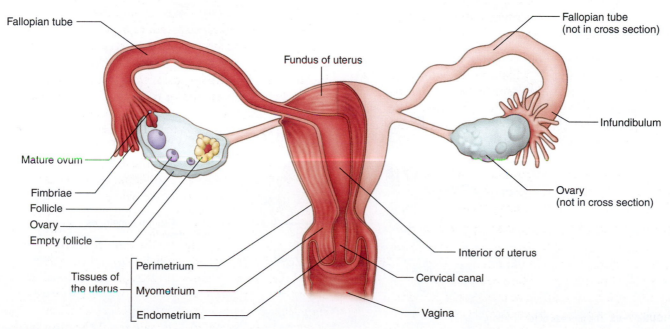

Fallopian tube
Fundus of uterus
Fallopian tube (not in cross section)
Infundibulum
Mature ovum
Fimbriae
Follicle
Ovary
Empty follicle
Ovary (not in cross section)
Interior of uterus
Tissues of the uterus
Perimetrium
Myometrium
Endometrium
Cervical canal
Vagina

FIGURE 7–80 Anterior view of the female reproductive system.

immature ovum, or female sex cell. When an ovum matures, the follicle enlarges and then ruptures to release the mature ovum. This process, called *ovulation*, usually occurs once every 28 days. The ovaries also produce hormones like estrogen and progesterone that aid in the development of the reproductive organs and produce secondary sexual characteristics as the female matures.

The **fallopian tubes** are two tubes, each approximately 5 inches in length and attached to the upper part of the uterus. The lateral ends of these tubes are located above the ovaries but are not directly connected to the ovaries. These ends have fingerlike projections, called *fimbriae*. The fimbriae help move the ovum, which is released by the ovary, into the fallopian tube. Each fallopian tube serves as a passageway for the ovum as the ovum moves from the ovary to the uterus. The muscle layers of the tube move the ovum by peristalsis. *Cilia*, hairlike structures on the lining of the tubes, also keep the ovum moving toward the uterus. **Fertilization**, the union of the ovum and a sperm to create a new life, takes place in the fallopian tubes. During sexual intercourse, or *coitus*, millions of sperm are deposited in the female vagina, where they travel through the uterus to the fallopian tubes. If an ovum is present in the fallopian tubes, the sperm surround the ovum and try to penetrate the outer wall (**Figure 7–81**). When a sperm enters the ovum, the sperm nucleus combines with the ovum nucleus to form a *zygote* or fertilized egg

cell. The zygote has received 23 chromosomes from each of the gametes and now has 23 pairs of chromosomes containing the deoxyribonucleic acid (DNA) that carries the genetic code from each parent. The zygote now travels to the uterus where it is implanted in the endometrial lining of the uterus and develops rapidly into an *embryo* and then a *fetus* (**Figure 7–82**). As the development occurs, a placenta forms, which provides the embryo and fetus with nourishment from the mother (**Figure 7–83**). An *amniotic sac* filled with fluid surrounds the developing fetus to cushion and protect it.

The **uterus** is a hollow, muscular, pear-shaped organ located behind the urinary bladder and in front of the rectum. It is divided into three parts: the *fundus* (the top section, where the fallopian tubes attach); the body, or *corpus* (the middle section); and the *cervix* (the narrow, bottom section, which attaches to the vagina). The uterus is the organ of menstruation, allows for the development and growth of the fetus, and contracts to aid in expulsion of the fetus during birth. The uterus has three layers. The inner layer is called the **endometrium**. This layer of specialized epithelium provides for implantation of a fertilized ovum and aids in the development of the fetus. If fertilization does not occur, the endometrium deteriorates and causes the bleeding known as *menstruation*. The middle layer of the uterus, the *myometrium*, is a muscle layer. It allows for the expansion of the uterus during pregnancy and

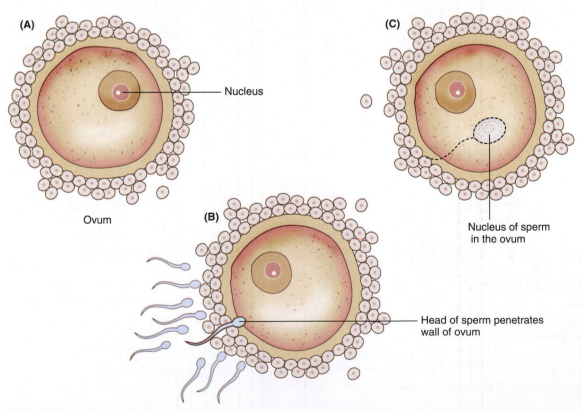

FIGURE 7–81 The process of fertilization.

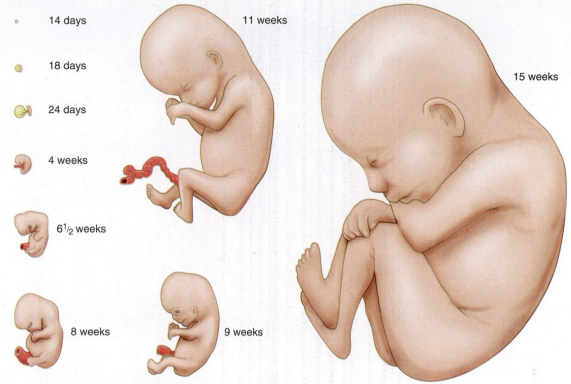

FIGURE 7–82 Growth of an embryo into a fetus once fertilization has occurred.

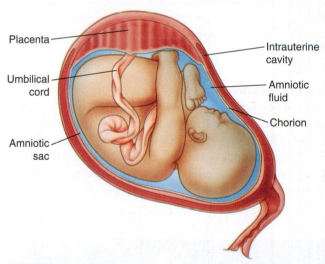

FIGURE 7–83 A normal pregnant uterus with a view of the fetus.

contracts to expel the fetus during birth. The outer layer, the *perimetrium*, is a serous membrane.

The **vagina** is a muscular tube that connects the cervix of the uterus to the outside of the body. It serves as a passageway for the menstrual flow, receives the sperm and semen from the male, is the female organ of copulation, and acts as the birth canal during delivery of the infant. The vagina is lined with a mucous membrane arranged in folds called *rugae*. The rugae allow the vagina to enlarge during childbirth and intercourse.

Bartholin's glands, also called *vestibular glands*, are two small glands located one on each side of the vaginal opening. They secrete mucus for lubrication during intercourse.

The **vulva** is the collective name for the structures that form the external female genital area (**Figure 7–84**). The *mons veneris*, or mons pubis, is the triangular pad of fat that is covered with hair and lies over the pubic area. The **labia majora** are the two large folds of fatty tissue that are covered with hair on their outer surfaces; they enclose and protect the vagina. The **labia minora** are the two smaller hairless folds of tissue that are located within the labia majora. The area of the vulva located inside the labia minora is called the **vestibule**. It contains the openings to the urethra and the vagina. An area of erectile tissue, called the *clitoris*, is located at the junction of the labia minora. It produces sexual arousal when stimulated directly or indirectly during intercourse. The **perineum** is defined as the area between the vagina and anus in the female body, although it can be used to describe the entire pelvic floor in both the male and female individual.

The **breasts**, or mammary glands, contain lobes separated into sections by connective and fatty tissue. Milk ducts located in the tissue exit on the surface at the nipples. The main function of the glands is to secrete milk (lactate) after childbirth.

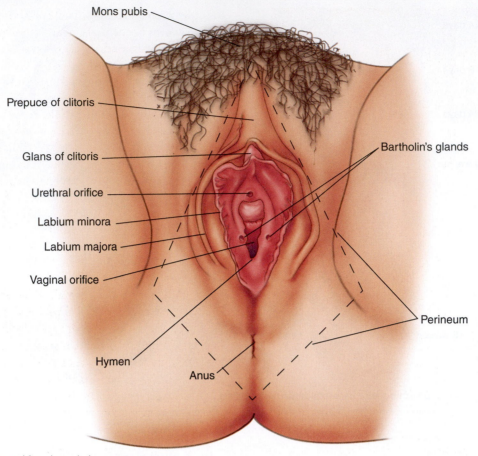

FIGURE 7–84 The external female genital area.

Mons pubis

Prepuce of clitoris

Glans of clitoris

Urethral orifice

Labium minora

Labium majora

Vaginal orifice

Hymen

Anus

Bartholin's glands

Perineum

Diseases and Abnormal Conditions

BREAST TUMORS Breast tumors can be benign or malignant. Symptoms include a lump or mass in the breast tissue, a change in breast size or shape (flattening or bulging of tissue), and a discharge from the nipple. Breast self-examination (BSE) can often detect tumors early (**Figure 7–85**). The American Cancer Society recommends that an adult woman should do a BSE every month at the end of menstruation, or on a scheduled day of the month after menopause. The breasts should be examined in front of a mirror to observe for changes in appearance, in a warm shower after soaping the breasts, and while lying flat in a supine position. A physician should be contacted immediately if any abnormalities are found. A clinical breast exam (CBE) is recommended every 3 years for women in their 20s and 30s and every year for women 40 and older. In addition, the American Cancer Society recommends that women have a yearly mammogram starting at age 40. Mammograms and ultrasonography can often detect tumors or masses up to 2 years before the tumor or mass could be felt. Treatment methods for breast tumors include a lumpectomy (removal of the tumor), a simple mastectomy (surgical removal of the breast), or a radical mastectomy (surgical removal of the breast tissue, underlying muscles, and axillary lymph nodes). Some women are candidates for breast-conserving therapy (BCT), in which the tumor is removed and the cosmetic appearance of the breast is spared. If the tumor is malignant, chemotherapy and/or radiation are usually used in addition to surgery.

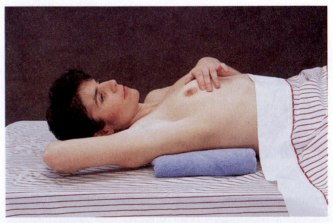

FIGURE 7–85A For a breast self-examination (BSE), a woman should lie down and use the tips of the fingers to press the breast tissue against the chest wall to feel for thickening or lumps.

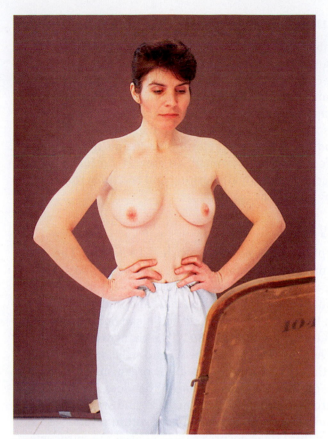

FIGURE 7-85B The woman should also stand in front of a mirror to check the breasts for symmetry (same form or shape) and to observe any change in appearance.

CERVICAL OR UTERINE CANCER Cancer of the cervix and/or uterus is common in women. Cervical cancer can be detected early by a Pap smear. The most common cause of uterine cancer is the human papillomavirus (HPV). Symptoms of cervical cancer include abnormal vaginal discharge and bleeding. Symptoms of uterine cancer include an enlarged uterus, a watery discharge, and abnormal bleeding. If cervical cancer is in the early stages, some fertility-sparing treatments may be an option. In these cases, just a portion of the cervix is removed. Other treatment methods include a hysterectomy (surgical removal of the uterus and cervix) or panhysterectomy (surgical removal of the uterus, ovaries, and fallopian tubes); chemotherapy; and/or radiation. A vaccine is available to prevent infection by the human papillomavirus (HPV). The Centers for Disease Control and Prevention (CDC) recommends that all children ages 11 and 12 should receive the three dose series of HPV vaccine. If children do not receive the vaccine at this age, young women can be vaccinated through age 26 and young men can be vaccinated through age 21.

ENDOMETRIOSIS Endometriosis is the abnormal growth of endometrial tissue outside the uterus. The tissue can be transferred from the uterus by the fallopian tubes, blood, or lymph, or during surgery. It usually becomes embedded in a structure in the pelvic area, such as the ovaries or the peritoneal tissues, and constantly grows and sheds. Endometriosis can cause sterility if the fallopian tubes become blocked with scar tissue. Symptoms include pelvic pain, abnormal bleeding, and dysmenorrhea (painful menstruation). Treatment methods vary with the age of the patient and the degree of abnormal growth but can include hormonal therapy, pain medications, and/or surgery. Conservative therapy can be done to remove just the endometrial growths and scar tissue. In severe cases, a hysterectomy (surgical removal of the uterus) may be necessary.

OVARIAN CANCER Ovarian cancer is one of the most common causes of cancer deaths in women due to its difficult diagnosis. It frequently occurs between ages 40 and 65. Risk factors include family history, race (more common in white females), never being pregnant, and early onset of menstrual periods. Initial symptoms are vague and include abdominal discomfort and mild gastrointestinal disturbances such as constipation and/or diarrhea. As the disease progresses, pain, abdominal distention, nausea, anorexia, and urinary frequency occur. Due to vague symptoms and difficult diagnoses, the majority of women are not diagnosed until they have advanced disease. Treatment includes surgical removal of all of the reproductive organs and affected lymph nodes, chemotherapy, and radiation in some cases.

PELVIC INFLAMMATORY DISEASE Pelvic inflammatory disease (PID) is an inflammation of the cervix (cervicitis), the endometrium of the uterus (endometritis), fallopian tubes (salpingitis), and at times, the ovaries (oophoritis). It is usually caused by pathogenic organisms such as bacteria (commonly from a sexually transmitted infection), viruses, and fungi. Symptoms include pain in the lower abdomen, fever, chills, and a purulent (pus) vaginal discharge. Treatment methods include antibiotics (for bacterial infections), increased fluid intake, rest, and/or pain medication.

PREMENSTRUAL SYNDROME Premenstrual syndrome (PMS) is actually a group of symptoms that appear 3–14 days before menstruation. A large percentage of women experience some degree of PMS. Symptoms usually peak in the late 20s and early 30s. The cause is unknown but may be related to a hormonal or biochemical imbalance, poor nutrition, or stress. Symptoms vary and may include nervousness, irritability, depression, headache, edema, backache, constipation, abdominal bloating, food cravings, temporary weight gain, and breast tenderness and enlargement. Treatment is geared mainly toward relieving symptoms, and methods include diet modification, exercise, massage, light therapy, stress reduction, diuretics to remove excess fluids, analgesics for pain, and/or medications to relieve the emotional symptoms.

SEXUALLY TRANSMITTED INFECTIONS

Sexually transmitted infections (STIs) affect both men and women. The incidence of these infections has increased greatly in recent years. If not treated, STIs can cause serious chronic conditions and, in some cases, sterility or death. In addition to the following STIs, AIDS is considered an STI and is discussed in detail in Section 7:9.

Chlamydia

Chlamydia (klah,-mid-e-ah) is one of the most frequently occurring STIs and is caused by several strains of the chlamydia organism, a specialized bacterium that lives as an intracellular parasite. Chlamydia can also be spread from mother to baby during childbirth and can cause serious eye infections or pneumonia. Symptoms are similar to those of gonorrhea. Male individuals experience burning when urinating and a mucoid discharge. Female individuals are frequently asymptomatic, although some may have a vaginal discharge. The infection frequently causes pelvic inflammatory disease and sterility in women, if not treated. Chlamydia can be treated with tetracycline or erythromycin antibiotics.

Gonorrhea

Gonorrhea (gon-oh,-re-ah), frequently called "the clap," is caused by the gonococcus bacterium *neisseria gonorrhoeae*. Symptoms in male individuals include a greenish yellow discharge, burning when urinating, sore throat, and swollen glands. Female individuals are frequently asymptomatic but may experience dysuria, pain in the lower abdomen, and greenish-yellow vaginal discharge. An infected woman can transmit the gonococcus organism to her infant's eyes during childbirth, causing blindness. To prevent this, a drop of silver nitrate or antibiotic is routinely placed in the eyes of newborn babies. Gonorrhea is treated with large doses of antibiotics, either by mouth or injection.

Herpes

Herpes is a viral infection caused by the herpes simplex virus type II. Symptoms include a burning sensation, fluid-filled vesicles (blister-like sores) that rupture and form painful ulcers, and painful urination. After the sores heal, the virus becomes dormant. Many people have repeated attacks, but the attacks are milder. There is no cure; the virus remains in the body for life. Treatment is directed toward promoting healing and easing discomfort. Chronic suppressive therapy with antiviral medications are used to decrease the number and severity of recurrences.

Pubic Lice

Pubic lice ("crabs") are parasites that are usually transmitted sexually, although they can be spread by contact with clothing, bed linen, or other items containing the lice. Symptoms include an intense itching and redness of the perineal area. Pubic lice can also spread to other areas with hair, such as armpits and eyelashes. Topical lotions or creams that kill the lice are used as treatment. To prevent a recurrence, it is essential to wash all clothing and bed linen to destroy any lice or nits (eggs).

Syphilis

Syphilis is caused by a spirochete bacterium. The symptoms occur in stages. During the primary stage, a painless chancre (shang,-ker), or sore, appears, usually on the penis of the male and in the vulva or on the cervix of the female, but it can occur anywhere on the body (**Figure 7–86**). This chancre heals within several weeks. During the second stage, which occurs if the chancre is not treated, the organism enters the bloodstream and causes a rash that does not itch, a sore throat, a fever, headache, malaise, and swollen glands. These symptoms also disappear within several weeks. The third stage occurs years later after the spirochete has damaged vital organs. Damage to the heart and blood vessels causes cardiovascular disease; damage to the spinal cord causes a characteristic gait and paralysis; and brain damage causes mental disorders, deafness, and blindness. At this stage, damage is irreversible, and death occurs. Early diagnosis and treatment with antibiotics can cure syphilis during the first two stages.

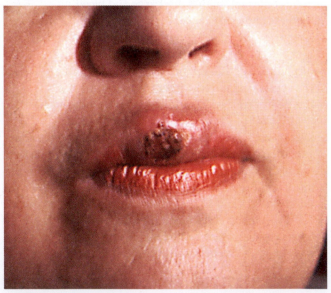

FIGURE 7–86 A painless chancre, or sore, can appear anywhere on the body during the primary stage of syphilis. CDC

Trichomoniasis

Trichomoniasis is caused by a parasitic protozoan, *Trichomonas vaginalis*. The main symptom is a large amount of a frothy, yellow-green, foul-smelling discharge. Men may experience urethral itching, but are frequently asymptomatic, and in some cases may expel the parasite without treatment. The antiparasitic oral medications Flagyl or Tinidazole (which may be better tolerated) are used to treat this infection. Both sexual partners must be treated to prevent reinfection.

checkpoint

1. Identify three (3) organs that secrete fluids added to semen.
2. Describe the pathway of sperm from where they are produced to where they are expelled from the body.
3. Describe how an ovum is released from an ovary.

PRACTICE: Go to the workbook and complete the assignment sheet for 7:14, Reproductive System.

Today's Research   Tomorrow's Health Care

Body Organs That Are Grown in the Laboratory?

Organ transplants have become a common type of surgery. Hearts, lungs, livers, kidneys, and many other organs are transplanted daily to save lives. The big problem is the major shortage of organs to transplant. Today, almost 114,000 Americans are on the national waiting list for an organ. Statistics show that every day 20 people will die before they can receive an organ.

Researchers are trying to grow human organs by using a patient's own cells. Initially, researchers in Boston created a urinary bladder that functioned in dogs. They molded a biodegradable material (substance that will dissolve inside the body) in the shape of a bladder. They then coated the outside of the structure with layers of muscle cells and the inside with layers of urothelial cells obtained from a dog's bladder. After the cells grew and multiplied, the dog's own bladder was removed, and the new artificial organ was transplanted. Within a month, the organ performed like a normal urinary bladder, storing urine until it was expelled to the outside. The chance of the dog rejecting the new organ was also slim because the cells that produced it were the dog's own cells.

Using this technology, researchers led by Dr. Atala at Wake Forest University in North Carolina replaced the bladders of many patients. They later created new urethras (tube that transports urine out of the body from the bladder) and transplanted them into patients. The bladders and urethras function well. Dr. Atala's team is now working to grow 20 different tissues and organs in the laboratory including bone, cartilage, and muscle tissue. Recently, doctors in Sweden replaced the cancerous trachea (windpipe) of a Maryland man with a new trachea grown in the lab with stem cells from the man's bone marrow. Another group of doctors in Spain created a trachea by using a trachea obtained from a man who died. They removed the donor's cells from the trachea with antibiotics and enzymes. They then seeded the outside and inside of the donor trachea with stem cells taken from the bone marrow of a woman whose own trachea was severely damaged by tuberculosis. The new trachea was implanted in the woman, who recovered quickly from the surgery and has shown no signs of rejecting the trachea. Many similar tracheal implants using the patient's own stem cells have been performed successfully since this first transplant. Bioprinting research is being conducted at the University of Missouri. A team of researchers led by Dr. Forgacs is using a 3-D printer to create blood vessels that branch the way real veins and arteries do. The team hopes to make replacement blood vessels that can be used in surgery in addition to creating other tissues and eventually more complex organs.

Even though tissue engineering is still in its infancy, the National Science Foundation estimates that it has attracted more than $3.5 billion in investments for research. It will take many more years before complex organs such as the heart and kidney can be created in a laboratory. However, the future for individuals needing transplants will be much better when scientists can "grow" the organs the individuals need.

Did you decide on a diagnosis for Shanice? Why does she have to urinate so frequently? Why is she so thirsty? How does the hypoglycemic medication impact her condition? Remember that hypotheses are tentative and testable statements that you can support with observable evidence. Support your opinion/hypothesis of Shanice's diagnosis with evidence.

CHAPTER 7 SUMMARY

- A health care provider must understand normal functioning of the human body (anatomy and physiology) to understand disease processes (pathophysiology).

- There are six structural levels that comprise the human body. Chemical, cellular, tissue, organs organ systems, and organism.

- Chemical building blocks construct cells, cells join together to form tissues. Tissues form organs, and organs work together to form body systems.

- Systems work together to provide for proper functioning of the human body. They work as a unit to maintain a constant balance (homeostasis) within the human body. When disease occurs, this homeostatic state is disturbed.

REVIEW QUESTIONS

1. Differentiate between congenital, inherited, infectious, and degenerative diseases. Give four (4) examples of each type of disease.

2. Draw a sketch of the body with all body cavities identified. List the organs in each body cavity on the side. Use a smaller piece of paper to overlay the abdomen and label the quadrants. What organs are in each quadrant?

3. Describe at least five (5) skin eruptions.

4. Identify the main bones or groups of bones in both the axial and the appendicular skeleton.

5. Differentiate between voluntary muscle and involuntary muscle. Give an example of each.

6. Contrast the actions of the sympathetic and parasympathetic nervous systems. Why do we need both systems?

7. Describe a cerebrovascular accident; etiology, signs and symptoms, and treatment.

8. Trace the path of light rays as they pass through the eye.

9. What is tinnitus and what condition can cause it?

10. Describe these circulatory system diseases:
    a. Anemia (all four listed in the book)
    b. Congestive heart failure
    c. Aneurysm
    d. Atherosclerosis
    e. Myocardial infarction

11. Explain the function of lymph vessels.

12. Describe chronic pulmonary obstructive disease (COPD).

13. Explain how the pancreas helps digest food.

14. Define these terms that describe conditions that affect urination:
    a. Oliguria
    b. Polyuria
    c. Nocturia
    d. Incontinence
    e. Pyuria
    f. Albuminuria

15. What is the "master gland," and why is it considered to be a master gland?

16. Evaluate three sexually transmitted infections (STIs), and describe how symptoms are the same or different in male versus female individuals.

■ CRITICAL THINKING

1. Body systems are interrelated and work together to perform specific functions. For example, the circulatory and respiratory systems perform a joint function of obtaining oxygen for the body and eliminating carbon dioxide. Describe five (5) other examples of interrelationships between body systems.

2. Create a patient information brochure. Choose one disease. State the definition, etiology, how it is diagnosed, prognosis, and treatment. Include two pictures and one Internet link connecting the patient to a support group or blog.

3. In a small group, create a song or jingle to name all the parts of the alimentary canal in order. Begin in the mouth.

■ ACTIVITIES

1. With a partner, use your cell phone or iPad to record a short video describing and demonstrating examples of ten (10) actions or movements of muscles.

2. Each student creates a Play-Doh heart. Each heart must include each chamber, valves, aorta, ascending and descending vena cava, pulmonary arteries, and veins. Each student then demonstrates with a piece of yarn or butcher string the pathway of a drop of blood through the heart; starting from the right atrium.

3. Create a mobile: Each small group gets a coat hanger. At the top is the organism body. Students will create an image of each body system (10) with the systems' function and organs written on the other side. They then will hang each image from the coat hanger with an "end piece" of the word homeostasis at the bottom. This depiction of the human body should all balance just like the miracle of our body!

4. In a small group, pick a spot on the sidewalk and outline a teammate's body, and then list as many body directions, planes, and cavities as you can. A large piece of butcher paper can be used instead.

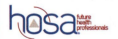 | CONNECTION

Competitive Event: Pathophysiology

Event Summary: Pathophysiology provides members with the opportunity to gain knowledge and skills regarding pathophysiology concepts. This competitive event consists of a written test with a tie-breaker essay question. This event aims to inspire members to learn about the anatomy and physiology of human diseases impacting the health community.

Details on this competitive event may be found at www.hosa.org/guidelines

Case Study Investigation

You are the nurse practitioner at the pediatric office where Jennifer and Charlie Schmidt take their beautiful baby boy Collin. As the months go by, Collin achieves all of the major milestones for his age. When he is 2, Collin stops talking, starts flapping his hands and will not look at Jennifer when she calls his name. He starts crying inconsolably when he is in the car and complains that the sun is burning his eyes. At the end of the chapter you will be asked to identify what diagnosis these signs and symptoms might indicate for Collin. What should Charlie and Jennifer do for their son? What are some treatments?

■ LEARNING OBJECTIVES

After completing this chapter, you should be able to:

- Identify at least two physical, mental, emotional, and social developments that occur during each of the seven main life stages.

- Explain the causes and treatments for chemical abuse.

- Identify methods used to prevent suicide and list common warning signs.

- Recognize ways that life stages affect an individual's needs.

- Describe the five stages of grieving that occur in the dying patient and the role of the health care provider during each stage.

- List two purposes of hospice care and provide justifications for the "right to die."

- Create examples for each of Maslow's Hierarchy of Needs.

- Name the two main methods people use to meet or satisfy needs.

- Create a situation that shows the use of each of the following defense mechanisms: rationalization, projection, displacement, compensation, daydreaming, repression, suppression, denial, and withdrawal.

- Define, pronounce, and spell all key terms.

■ KEY TERMS

acceptance

adolescence

affection

Alzheimer's disease *(Altz″ -high-merz)*

anger

arteriosclerosis *(ar-tear″ -ee-oh-skleh-row′ -sis)*

bargaining

chemical abuse

cognitive

compensation *(cahm″ -pen-say′ -shun)*

daydreaming

defense mechanisms

denial

depression

development

displacement

early adulthood

early childhood

emotional

esteem

growth

hospice *(hoss′ -pis)*

infancy

late adulthood

late childhood

life stages

mental

middle adulthood

motivated

needs

physical

physiological needs *(fizz″ -ee-oh-lodg′ -ih-kal)*

projection

puberty *(pew″ -burr′ -tee)*

rationalization *(rash″ -en-nal-ih-zay′ -shun)*

regression

repression

right to die

safety

satisfaction

self-actualization

sexuality

social

suicide

suppression

tension

terminal illness

withdrawal

INTRODUCTION

Human growth and development is a process that begins at birth and does not end until death. **Growth** refers to the measurable physical changes that occur throughout a person's life. Examples include height, weight, body shape, head circumference, physical characteristics, development of sexual organs, and dentition (dental structure). **Development** refers to the changes in intellectual, mental, emotional, social, and functional skills that occur over time. Development is more difficult to measure but usually proceeds from simple to complex tasks as maturation, or the process of becoming fully grown and developed, occurs. During all stages of growth and development, individuals have certain tasks that must be accomplished and needs that must be met. A health care provider must be aware of the various life stages and of individual needs to provide quality health care. (**Figure 8–1**).

8:1 LIFE STAGES

Even though individuals differ greatly, each person passes through certain stages of growth and development from birth to death. These stages are frequently called **life stages**. A common method of classifying life stages is as follows:

- **Infancy**: birth to 1 year
- **Early childhood**: 1–6 years
- **Late childhood**: 6–12 years
- **Adolescence**: 12–18 years
- **Early adulthood**: 19–40 years
- **Middle adulthood**: 40–65 years
- **Late adulthood**: 65 years and older

As individuals pass through these life stages, four main types of growth and development occur: physical, mental or cognitive, emotional, and social. **Physical** refers to body growth and includes height and weight changes, muscle and nerve development, and changes in body organs. **Mental** or **cognitive** refers to intellectual development and includes learning how to solve problems, make judgments, and deal with situations. **Emotional** refers to feelings and includes dealing with love, hate, joy, fear, excitement, and other similar feelings. **Social** refers to interactions and relationships with other people. Relationships with family, friends, and peers affect our emotional and physical health.

Each stage of growth and development has its own characteristics and has specific developmental tasks that an individual must master. These tasks progress from the simple to the more complex. For example, an individual first learns to sit, then crawl, then stand, then walk, and then, finally, run. Each stage establishes the foundation for the next stage. In this way, growth and development proceeds in an orderly pattern. It is important to remember, however, that the rate of progress varies among individuals. Some children master speech early; others master it later. Similarly, an individual may experience a sudden growth spurt and then maintain the same height for a period of time.

Erik Erikson, a psychoanalyst, has identified eight stages of psychosocial development. His eight stages of development, the basic conflict or need that must be resolved at each stage, and ways to resolve the conflict are shown in **Table 8–1**. Erikson believes that if an individual is not able to resolve a conflict at the appropriate stage, the individual will struggle with the same conflict later in life. For example, if a toddler is not allowed to learn to develop autonomy and become independent by mastering

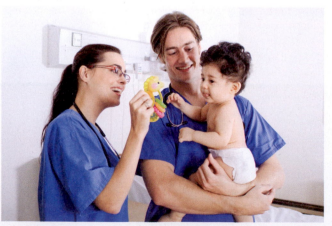 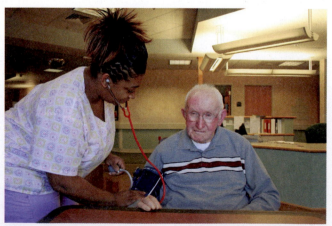

FIGURE 8–1 An understanding of life stages is important for the health care provider, who may provide care to individuals of all ages, from the very young (left) to the elderly (right). © Andrew Gentry/Shutterstock.com; © michaeljung/Shutterstock.com

basic tasks, the toddler may develop a sense of doubt in his or her abilities. Giving a toddler some simple limited choices, such as choosing between two shirts, allows the toddler to practice autonomous decision making. If these preparation sessions are not available to the child, a sense of doubt will interfere with later attempts at mastering independence and a sense of self-governance.

Jean Piaget, a developmental biologist, identified cognitive stages of development based on how an organism adapts to its environment. His basic concept is that infants are born with reflexes that the infant uses to adapt to the environment. Through *assimilation*, a process by which a person's mind takes in information from the environment, and *accommodation*, the process of changing cognitive ideas based on the new information, the person learns to maintain *equilibrium*, or a balance with the environment. Piaget's four stages of cognitive development are shown in **Table 8–2**. During each level, Piaget believes new abilities are learned that prepare the individual for the next level.

Health care providers must understand that each life stage creates certain needs in individuals. Likewise, other factors can affect life stages and needs. An individual's race, heredity (factors inherited from parents, such as hair color and body structure), gender identity and sexual orientation; culture, life experiences, and health status can influence needs. Injury or illness usually has a negative effect and can change needs or impair development.

INFANCY
Physical Development

The most dramatic and rapid changes in growth and development occur during the first year of life. A newborn baby usually weighs approximately 6–8 pounds (2.7–3.6 kg) and measures 18–22 inches (46–55 cm) (**Figure 8–2**). By the end of the first year of life, weight has usually tripled, to 21–24 pounds (9.5–11 kg), and height has increased to approximately 29–30 inches (74–76 cm).

Muscular system and nervous system developments are also dramatic. The muscular and nervous systems are very immature at birth. Certain reflex actions present

TABLE 8–1 Erikson's Eight Stages of Psychosocial Development

Stage of Development	Basic Conflict	Major Life Event	Ways to Resolve Conflict
Infancy Birth to 1 year Oral–Sensory	Trust versus mistrust	Feeding	Infant develops trust in self, others, and the environment when caregiver is responsive to basic needs and provides comfort; if needs are not met, infant becomes uncooperative and aggressive and shows a decreased interest in the environment
Toddler 1–3 Years Muscular–anal	Autonomy versus shame/ doubt	Toilet training	Toddler learns control while mastering skills such as feeding, toileting, and dressing when caregivers provide reassurance but avoid overprotection; if needs are not met, toddler feels ashamed and doubts own abilities, which leads to lack of self-confidence in later stages
Preschool 3–6 years Locomotor	Initiative versus guilt	Independence	Child begins to initiate activities in place of just imitating activities; uses imagination to play; learns what is allowed and what is not allowed while beginning to develop a conscience; caregivers must allow child to be responsible and develop autonomy while providing reassurance; if needs are not met, child feels guilty and thinks everything he or she does is wrong, which leads to a hesitancy to try new tasks in later stages
School-Age 6–12 years Latency	Industry versus inferiority	School	Child becomes productive by mastering learning and obtaining success; child learns to deal with academics, group activities, and friends when others show acceptance of actions and praise success; if needs are not met, child develops a sense of inferiority and incompetence, which hinders future relationships and the ability to deal with life events
Adolescence 12–18 years	Identity versus role confusion	Peer	Adolescent searches for self-identity by making choices about occupation, sexual orientation, lifestyle, and adult role; relies on peer group for support and reassurance to create a self-image separate from parents; if needs are not met, adolescent experiences role confusion and loss of self-belief
Young Adulthood 19–40 years	Intimacy versus isolation	Love relationships	Young adult learns to make a personal commitment to others and share life events with others; if self-identity is lacking, adult may fear relationships and isolate self from others
Middle Adulthood 40–65 years	Generativity versus stagnation	Parenting	Adult seeks satisfaction and obtains success in life by using career, family, and civic interests to provide for others and the next generation; if adult does not deal with life issues, feels lack of purpose to life and sense of failure
Older Adulthood 65 years to death	Ego integrity versus despair	Reflection on and acceptance of life	Adult reflects on life in a positive manner, feels fulfillment with his or her own life and accomplishments, deals with losses, and prepares for death; if fulfillment is not felt, adult feels despair about life and fear of death

at birth allow the infant to respond to the environment. These include the Moro, or startle, reflex to a loud noise or sudden movement; the rooting reflex, in which a slight touch on the cheek causes the mouth to open and

TABLE 8–2 Piaget's Four Stages of Cognitive Development

Stage	Characteristic Behavior
Sensorimotor Birth–2 years	Initially uses simple reflexes such as sucking and grasping
	Recognizes self as causing an action and repeats action intentionally
	Begins to understand that objects are permanent even when they can't be seen
	Explores new possibilities and discovers ways to get different results
	Begins to recognize cause-and-effect relationships
Preoperational 2–7 years	Begins to use words and images to represent objects
	Tends to be egocentric (self-centered)
	Classifies objects in simple ways, such as shape, color, or important features
	Reacts to all similar objects as though they are identical
	By age 4, begins to understand concepts but has limited logic
	By age 6 to 7, understands the difference between reality and fantasy
Concrete Operational 7–11 years	Egocentrism decreases and speech becomes more socialized
	Thinks logically about events, objects, and the environment
	Still experiences difficulty with abstract or hypothetical concepts
	Understands reversibility, or an ability to retrace mental steps to solve problems
	Classifies objects and can position them in a series based on specific features
Formal Operational Older than 11 years	Thinks logically about abstract propositions and hypotheses to solve problems
	Becomes less dependent on concrete reality and is able to reason contrary to facts
	Develops ability to become concerned with ideological problems and the future

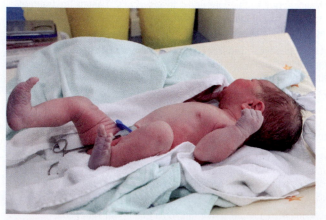

FIGURE 8–2 A newborn baby usually weighs approximately 6-8 pounds and measures 18-22 inches in length. © Philip Lange/Shutterstock.com

the head to turn; the sucking reflex, caused by a slight touch on the lips; and the grasp reflex, in which infants can grasp an object placed in the hand (**Figure 8–3**). Muscle coordination develops in stages. At first, infants are able to lift the head slightly. By 2–4 months, they can usually roll from side to back, support themselves on their forearms when prone, and grasp or try to reach objects. By 4–6 months, they can turn the body completely around, accept objects handed to them, grasp stationary objects such as a bottle, and with support, hold the head up while sitting. By 6–8 months, infants can sit unsupported, grasp moving objects, transfer objects from one hand to the other, and crawl on the stomach. By 8–10 months, they can crawl using their knees and hands, pull themselves to a sitting or standing position, and use good hand–mouth coordination to put things in their mouths. By 12 months, infants frequently can walk without assistance, grasp objects with the thumb and fingers, and throw small objects.

Other physical developments are also dramatic. Most infants are born without teeth but usually have 10–12 teeth by the end of the first year of life. At birth, vision is poor and may be limited to black and white, and eye movements are not coordinated. By 1 year of age, however, close vision is good, in color, and can readily focus on small objects. Sensory abilities such as those of smell, taste, sensitivity to hot and cold, and hearing, while good at birth, become more refined and exact. Positive interaction with family and caregivers and the stimulation they provide promote accomplishing these physical milestones.

Mental Development

Mental development is also rapid during the first year. Newborns respond to discomforts such as pain, cold, or hunger by crying. As their needs are met, they gradually become more aware of their surroundings and begin to recognize individuals associated with their care. As infants respond to stimuli in the environment, learning activities grow. At birth, they are unable to speak. By 2–4 months, they coo or babble when spoken to, laugh out loud, and squeal with pleasure. By 6 months of age, infants understand some words and can make basic sounds, such as "mama" and "dada." By 12 months, infants understand many words and use single words in their vocabularies.

Emotional Development

Emotional development is observed early in life. Newborns show excitement. By 4–6 months of age, distress, delight, anger, disgust, and fear can often be seen. By 12 months of age, elation and affection for family and caregivers is evident. Events and relationships that occur in the first year of life when these emotions are first exhibited can have a strong influence on an individual's emotional behavior during adulthood.

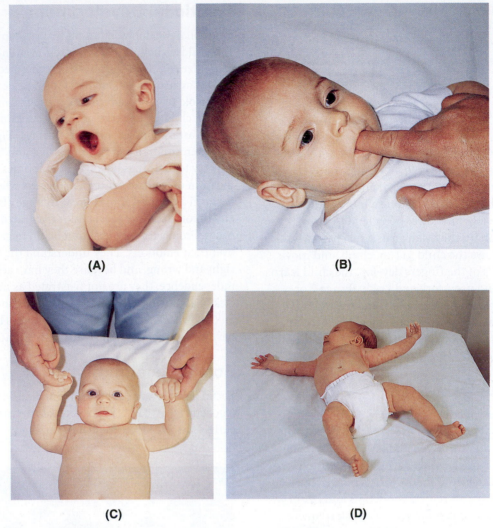

(A) (B)

(C) (D)

FIGURE 8–3 Some reflex actions an infant has at birth include (A) rooting, (B) sucking, (C) grasp, and (D) Moro.

Social Development

Social development progresses gradually from the self-centeredness concept of the newborn to the recognition of others in the environment. By 4 months of age, infants recognize their caregivers, smile readily, and stare intently at others (**Figure 8–4**). By 6 months of age, infants watch the activities of others, show signs of possessiveness, and may become shy or withdraw when in the presence of strangers. By 12 months of age, infants may still be shy with strangers, but they socialize freely with familiar people, and mimic and imitate gestures, facial expressions, and vocal sounds.

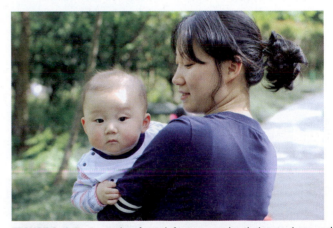

FIGURE 8–4 By 4 months of age, infants recognize their caregivers and stare intently at others. © Bendao/Shutterstock.com

Needs and Care

Infants are dependent on others for all needs. Food, cleanliness, and rest are essential for physical growth. Love and security are essential for emotional and social growth. Stimulation is essential for mental growth.

While caring for infants, a health care provider should give the parents or guardians support and reassurance and involve them in the infant's care. Promoting these positive relationships will ensure the appropriate amount of stimulation for infant development in physical and emotional ways. Providing information on nutrition, growth, development, sleep patterns, meeting needs, and creating a healthy environment will promote wellness in the infant. Care must be taken at all times to ensure the infant's safety. Preventing the transmission of infection by washing hands thoroughly and observing standard precautions is also essential during care.

EARLY CHILDHOOD
Physical Development

During early childhood, from 1–6 years of age, physical growth is slower than during infancy. By age 6, the average weight is 45 pounds (20.4 kg), and the average height is 46 inches (116 cm). Skeletal and muscle development helps the child assume a more adult appearance. The legs and lower body tend to grow more rapidly than do the head, arms, and chest. Muscle coordination allows the child to run, climb, and move freely. As muscles of the fingers develop, the child learns to write, draw, and use a fork and knife. By age 2 or 3, most primary teeth have erupted, and the digestive system is mature enough to handle most adult foods. Between 2 and 4 years of age, most children learn bladder and bowel control.

Mental Development

Mental development advances rapidly during early childhood. Verbal growth progresses from the use of several words at age 1 to a vocabulary of 1,500–2,500 words at age 6. Two-year-olds have short attention spans but are interested in many different activities (**Figure 8–5**). They can remember details and begin to understand concepts. Four-year-olds ask frequent questions and usually recognize letters and some words. They begin to make decisions based on logic rather than on trial and error. By age 6, children are very verbal and want to learn how to read and write. Memory has developed to the point where the child can make decisions based on both past and present experiences.

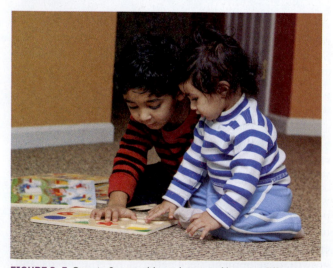

FIGURE 8–5 One- to 2-year-olds are interested in many different activities, but they have short attention spans. © Ami Parikh/Shutterstock.com

Emotional Development

Emotional development also advances rapidly. At ages 1–2, children begin to develop self-awareness and to recognize the effect they have on other people and things. Limits are usually established for safety, leading the 1- or 2-year-old to either accept or defy such limits. By age 2, most children begin to gain self-confidence and are enthusiastic about learning new things (**Figure 8–6**). However, children can feel impatient and frustrated as they try to do things beyond their abilities. Anger, often in the form of "temper tantrums," occurs when they cannot perform as desired. Children at this age also like routine and become stubborn, angry, or frustrated when changes occur. From ages 4–6, children begin to gain more control over their emotions. They understand the concept of right and wrong, and because they have achieved more independence, they are not frustrated as much by their lack of ability. By age 6, most children also show less anxiety when faced with new experiences because they have learned they can deal with new situations.

Social Development

Social development expands from a self-centered (egocentric) 1-year-old to a sociable 6-year-old. In the early years, children are usually strongly attached to

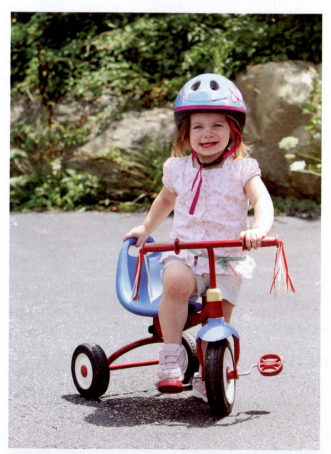

FIGURE 8–6 By age 2, most children begin to gain some self-confidence and are enthusiastic about learning new things. © Stuart Monk/Shutterstock.com

their parents (or to the individuals who provide their care), and they fear any separation. They begin to enjoy the company of others, but are still very possessive. Playing alongside other children is more common than playing with other children (**Figure 8–7**). Gradually, children learn to put "self" aside and begin to take more of an interest in others. They learn to trust other people and make more of an effort to please others by becoming more agreeable and social. Friends of their own age are usually important to 6-year-olds.

Autism

Autism, or autism spectrum disorder, is a broad range of conditions that impairs the ability to communicate and interact. It is characterized by challenges with social skills, repetitive behaviors, speech, and nonverbal communication. According to the Centers for Disease Control, autism affects an estimated 1 in 54 children in the United States today and affects boys four times more than girls. Factors pointing to autism usually appear by ages 2 or 3. Some development delays can appear even earlier, and it can sometimes be diagnosed as early as 18 months.

Signs and symptoms of autism include:

- Avoiding eye contact
- Difficulty understanding other people's feelings
- Delayed language development
- Persistent repetition of words or phrases; repetitive behaviors (flapping, rocking)
- Resistance to changes in routine
- Intense reactions to sounds, smells, tastes, textures, light, colors

Research shows that early intervention leads to positive outcomes later in life for people with autism. Many children affected also benefit from other interventions such as speech and occupational therapy. Applied behavior analysis is the most researched and commonly used behavioral intervention for autism.

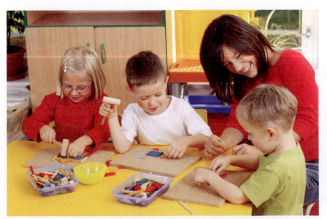

FIGURE 8–7 Playing alongside and with other children allows preschoolers to learn how to interact with others. © matka_Wariatka/Shutterstock.com

Needs and Care

The needs of early childhood still include food, rest, shelter, protection, love, and security. In addition, children need routine, order, and consistency in their daily lives. They must be taught to be responsible and must learn how to conform to rules. This can be accomplished by making reasonable demands based on the child's ability to comply.

While caring for toddlers, a health care provider must be sensitive to the child's fears and anxiety when dealing with strangers. Enlisting the help of parents or guardians, using a calm but firm approach, establishing rapport with the child, using play to alleviate fear, providing simple explanations to gain cooperation, allowing the child to participate in care by providing one or two choices, and reassuring the child are all ways to make care easier. Building these positive family relationships allows the child to develop self-control and participate fully in the larger community. After a painful procedure, it is essential to comfort the child. At all times, it is important to maintain a safe environment and prevent the transmission of infection.

While caring for preschoolers, many of the same techniques can be used. Because the child is older, encouraging verbalization of fears, answering questions, allowing the child to make choices such as what color cast to use to splint a fractured bone, praising the child for cooperating, making health education fun, and listening to the child's requests and trying to fulfill them are additional techniques that can be used.

LATE CHILDHOOD
Physical Development

The late childhood life stage, which covers ages 6–12, is also called *preadolescence*. Physical development is slow but steady. Weight gain averages 4–7 pounds (2.3–3.2 kg) per year, and height usually increases approximately 2–3 inches (5–7.5 cm) per year. Muscle coordination is well developed, and children can engage in physical activities that require complex motor-sensory coordination. During this age, most of the primary teeth are lost, and permanent teeth erupt. The eyes are well developed, and visual acuity is at its best. During ages 10–12, secondary sexual characteristics begin to develop in some children.

Mental Development

Mental development increases rapidly because much of the child's life centers around school. Speech skills develop more completely, and reading and writing skills are learned. Children learn to use information to solve problems, and the memory becomes more complex. They begin to understand more abstract concepts such as loyalty, honesty, values, and morals. Children use more active thinking and become more adept at making judgments.

Emotional Development

Emotional development continues to help the child achieve a greater independence and a more distinct personality. At age 6, children are often frightened and uncertain as they begin school. Reassuring parents and success in school help children gain self-confidence. Role-playing also allows a child to control fears and gain self-confidence (**Figure 8–8**). Gradually, fears are replaced by the ability to cope. Emotions are slowly brought under control and dealt with in a more effective manner. By ages 10–12, sexual maturation and changes in body functions can lead to periods of depression followed by periods of joy. These emotional changes can cause children to be restless, anxious, and difficult to understand.

Social Development

Social changes are evident during these years. Seven-year-olds tend to like activities they can do by themselves and do not usually like group activities. However, they want the approval of others, especially their parents and friends. Children from ages 8 to 10 tend to be more group oriented, and they typically form groups with members of their own sex. They are more ready to accept the opinions of others and learn to conform to rules and standards of behavior followed by the group. Toward the end of this period, children tend to make friends more easily, and they begin to develop relationships with others of both sexes. As children spend more time with others their own age, their dependency on their parent(s) lessens, as does the time they spend with their parents. During this time, constructive peer relationships start to become important. As these relationships develop, a sense of being part of a wider community develops.

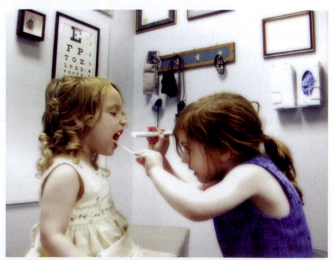

FIGURE 8–8 Role-playing allows a child to control fears and gain self-confidence. © Lisa Eastman/Shutterstock.com

Needs and Care

Needs of children in this age group include the same basic needs of infancy and early childhood, together with the need for reassurance, parental approval, and peer acceptance. Hopefully family relationships have been built to support the child.

Because this age group is prone to accidents and minor infections, health care providers must stress safety and healthy living principles. Information should be provided about nutrition, personal hygiene, sleep patterns, exercise, dental hygiene, preventing infection, and puberty. It is also important to encourage independence and to allow the child to make his or her own decisions whenever possible. Health care providers and caregivers must be sensitive to the child's need for privacy but should make every effort to encourage the child to discuss his or her concerns by using a nonjudgmental approach.

ADOLESCENCE
Physical Development

Adolescence, ages 12 to 18, is often a traumatic life stage. Physical changes occur most dramatically in the early period. A sudden "growth spurt" can cause rapid increases in weight and height. A weight gain of up to 25 pounds (11 kg) and a height increase of several inches can occur in a period of months. Muscle coordination does not advance as quickly. This can lead to awkwardness or clumsiness in motor coordination. This growth spurt usually occurs anywhere from ages 11 to 13 in girls and ages 13 to 15 in boys.

The most obvious physical changes in adolescents relate to the development of the sexual organs and secondary sexual characteristics, frequently called **puberty**. Secretion of sex hormones leads to the onset of menstruation in girls and the production of sperm and semen in boys. Secondary sexual characteristics in females include growth of pubic hair, development of breasts and wider hips, and distribution of body fat leading to the female shape. The male develops a deeper voice; attains more muscle mass and broader shoulders; and grows pubic, facial, and body hair.

Mental Development

Since most of the foundations have already been established, mental development primarily involves an increase in knowledge and a sharpening of skills. Adolescents learn to make decisions and to accept responsibility for their actions. At times, this causes conflict because they are treated as both children and adults, or are told to "grow up" while being reminded that they are "still children."

Emotional Development

Emotional development is often stormy and conflicted. As adolescents try to establish their identities and independence, they are often uncertain and feel inadequate and insecure. They worry about their appearance, their abilities, and their relationships with others. They frequently respond more and more to peer group influences. At times, this leads to changes in attitude and behavior and conflict with values previously established via family relationships. Toward the end of adolescence, self-identity has been established. At this point, teenagers feel more comfortable with who they are and turn attention toward what they may become. They gain more control of their feelings and become more mature emotionally.

Social Development

Social development usually involves spending less time with family and more time with peer groups. As adolescents attempt to develop self-identity and independence, they seek security in groups of people their own age who have similar problems and conflicts (**Figure 8–9**). If these peer relationships help develop self-confidence through the approval of others, adolescents become more secure and satisfied. Peer relationships that are considerate and supportive allow the adolescent to have more confidence in their choices. Toward the end of this life stage, adolescents develop a more mature attitude and begin to develop patterns of behavior that they associate with adult behavior or status.

Needs and Care

In addition to basic needs, adolescents need reassurance, support, and understanding. Many problems that develop during this life stage can be traced to the conflict and feelings of inadequacy and insecurity that adolescents experience. Examples include eating disorders, drug and alcohol abuse, and suicide. Even

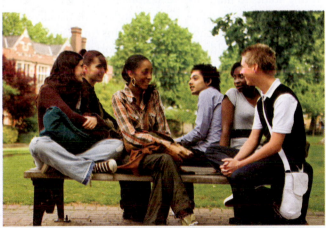

FIGURE 8–9 Adolescents use the peer group as a safety net as they try to establish their identities and independence. ©iStock.com/Chris Schmidt

though these types of problems also occur in earlier and later life stages, they are frequently associated with adolescence.

Eating disorders often develop from an excessive concern with appearance. Three common eating disorders are *anorexia nervosa*, *bulimia*, and *bulimarexia*. These disorders are discussed in detail in Section 11:5, Weight Management. All three conditions are more common in female than male individuals. Psychological or psychiatric help is usually needed to treat these conditions.

Chemical abuse is the use of substances such as alcohol or drugs and the development of a physical and/or mental dependence on these chemicals. Chemical abuse can occur in any life stage, but it frequently begins in adolescence. Reasons for using chemicals include anxiety or stress relief, peer pressure, escape from emotional or psychological problems, experimentation with feelings the chemicals produce, desire for "instant gratification," hereditary traits, and cultural influences. Chemical abuse can lead to physical and mental disorders and disease. Treatment is directed toward total rehabilitation that allows the chemical abuser to return to a productive and meaningful life.

Suicide, found in many life stages, is one of the leading causes of death in adolescents. Suicide is always a permanent solution to a temporary problem. Reasons for suicide include depression, grief over a loss or love affair, failure in school, inability to meet expectations, influence of suicidal friends, or lack of self-esteem. The risk for suicide increases with a family history of suicide; a major loss or disappointment; previous suicide attempts; and/or the recent suicide of friends, family, or role models (heroes or idols). The impulsive nature of adolescents also increases the possibility of suicide. Most individuals who are thinking of suicide give warning signs such as verbal statements like "I'd rather be dead" or "You'd be better off without me." Other warning signs include:

- Sudden changes in appetite and sleep habits
- Withdrawal, depression, and moodiness
- Excessive fatigue or agitation
- Neglect of personal hygiene
- Alcohol or drug abuse
- Losing interest in hobbies and other aspects of life
- Preoccupation with death
- Injuring one's body
- Giving away possessions
- Social withdrawal from family and friends

These individuals are calling out for attention and help and usually respond to efforts of assistance. Their direct and indirect pleas should never be ignored. Support, understanding, and psychological or psychiatric counseling are used to prevent suicide.

Because of the many conflicts adolescents experience, health care providers must be nonjudgmental to establish rapport while providing care. It is essential to listen to the adolescent's concerns, be sensitive to their nonverbal behavior, involve them in decision making, and answer questions as honestly and completely as possible. It is also important to provide education about hygiene, nutrition, developmental changes, sexually transmitted diseases, and substance abuse. Encouraging and upbeat relationships between peers, family, and friends not only impacts the individuals' physical and emotional health but promotes healthy relationships with the entire community as the adolescent moves into adulthood.

EARLY ADULTHOOD
Physical Development

Early adulthood, ages 19–40, is frequently the most productive life stage. Physical development is basically complete, muscles are developed and strong, and motor coordination is at its peak. This is also the prime child-bearing time and usually produces the healthiest babies (**Figure 8–10**). Both male and female sexual development is at its peak.

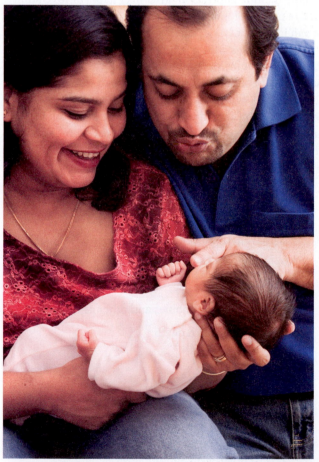

FIGURE 8–10 Early adulthood is the prime childbearing time and usually produces the healthiest babies. © Rohit Seth/Shutterstock.com

Mental Development

Mental development usually continues throughout this stage. Many young adults pursue additional education to establish and progress in their chosen careers. Frequently, formal education continues for many years. The young adult often also deals with independence, makes career choices, establishes a lifestyle, selects a marital partner, starts a family, and establishes values, all of which involve making many decisions and forming many judgments.

Emotional Development

Emotional development usually involves preserving the stability established during previous stages. Young adults are subjected to many emotional stresses related to career, marriage, family, and other similar situations. If emotional structure is strong, most young adults can cope with these worries. They find satisfaction in their achievements, take responsibility for their actions, and learn to accept criticism and to profit from mistakes.

Social Development

Social development frequently involves moving away from the peer group. Instead, young adults tend to associate with others who have similar ambitions and interests, regardless of age. The young adult often becomes involved with a mate and forms a family. Young adults do not necessarily accept traditional sex roles and frequently adopt nontraditional roles. For example, male individuals fill positions as nurses and secretaries, and female individuals enter administrative or construction positions. Such choices have caused and will continue to cause changes in the traditional patterns of society.

Needs and Care

Needs of early adulthood include the same basic needs as other age groups. In addition, young adults need independence, social acceptance, self-confidence, and reassurance.

During care, information must be provided to allow young adults to make wise decisions regarding their health status and wellness goals. Even though this is usually the healthiest life stage, choices made at this time can affect both middle and old age. It is also important to listen to what the person is saying and to observe nonverbal behavior. Individuals in this age group frequently experience stress due to their responsibilities. Positive relationships continue to be essential because sensitive supportive care is necessary during periods of stress.

MIDDLE ADULTHOOD
Physical Development

Middle adulthood, ages 40–65, is frequently called *middle age*. Physical changes begin to occur during these years. The hair tends to gray and thin, the skin begins to wrinkle, muscle tone tends to decrease, hearing loss starts, visual acuity declines, and weight gain occurs. Women experience *menopause*, or the end of menstruation, along with decreased hormone production that causes physical and emotional changes. Men also experience a slowing of hormone production. This can lead to physical and psychological changes, a period frequently referred to as the *male climacteric*. However, except in cases of injury, disease, or surgery, men never lose the ability to produce sperm or to reproduce.

Mental Development

Mental ability can continue to increase during middle age, a fact that has been proved by the many individuals in this life stage who seek formal education. Middle adulthood is a period when individuals have acquired an understanding of life and have learned to cope with many different stresses. This allows them to be more confident in making decisions and to excel at analyzing situations.

Emotional Development

Emotionally, middle age can be a period of contentment and satisfaction, or it can be a time of crisis. The emotional foundation of previous life stages and the situations that occur during middle age determine emotional status during this period. Job stability, financial success, the end of child rearing, and good health can all contribute to emotional satisfaction (**Figure 8–11**). Stress—created by loss of job, fear of aging, loss of youth and vitality, illness, marital problems, problems with children, or aging parents—can contribute to emotional feelings of depression, insecurity, anxiety, and even anger. Therefore, emotional status varies in this age group and is largely determined by events that occur during this period.

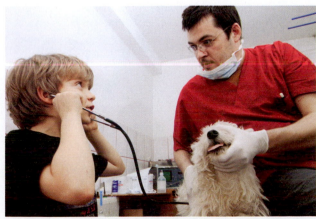

FIGURE 8–11 Job stability and enjoyment during middle adulthood contribute to emotional satisfaction. © Nagy Melinda/Shutterstock.com

Social Development

Social relationships also depend on many factors. Family relationships often see a decline as children begin lives of their own and parents die. Work relationships frequently replace family. Relationships between husband and wife can become stronger as they have more time together and opportunities to enjoy success. However, divorce rates are also high in this age group, as couples who have remained together "for the children's sake" now separate. Friendships are usually with people who have the same interests and lifestyles.

Needs and Care

Needs of middle adulthood include the same basic needs as other age groups. In addition, these individuals need self-satisfaction, a sense of accomplishment, autonomy, and supportive social relationships. Peer and friend relationships continue to be important as these adults establish a healthy role in their community.

Health care providers must encourage middle-aged adults to identify risk factors to their health status and to make changes to promote wellness. Increasing exercise, improving nutrition, avoiding obesity, quitting smoking, eliminating or decreasing alcohol intake, and other similar actions can improve health status and increase longevity. At this life stage, individuals begin to see the physical signs of aging. With proper guidance, they can learn how to practice better health principles that will help establish a pattern for later years of life. Nonjudgmental supportive care is important while helping individuals to establish and meet health goals.

LATE ADULTHOOD
Physical Development

Late adulthood, age 65 and older, has many different terms associated with it. These include "elderly," "senior citizen," "golden ager," and "retired citizen." Much attention has been directed toward this life stage in recent years because people are living longer, and the number of people in this age group is increasing daily.

Physical development is on the decline. All body systems are usually affected. The skin becomes dry, wrinkled, and thinner. Brown or yellow spots (frequently called "age spots") appear. The hair becomes thin and frequently loses its luster or shine. Bones become brittle and porous and are more likely to fracture or break. Cartilage between the vertebrae thins and can lead to a stooping posture. Muscles lose tone and strength, which can lead to fatigue and poor coordination. A decline in the function of the nervous system leads to hearing loss, decreased visual acuity, and decreased tolerance for temperatures that are too hot or too cold. Memory loss can occur, and reasoning ability can diminish. The heart is less efficient, and circulation decreases. The kidney and bladder are less efficient. Breathing capacity decreases and causes shortness of breath. However, it is important to note that these changes usually occur slowly over a long period. Many individuals, because of better health and living conditions, do not show physical changes of aging until their 70s and even 80s.

Mental Development

Mental abilities vary among individuals. Elderly people who remain mentally active and are willing to learn new things tend to show fewer signs of decreased mental ability (**Figure 8–12**). Although some 90-year-olds remain alert and well oriented, other elderly individuals show decreased mental capacities at much earlier ages. Short-term memory is usually first to decline. Many elderly individuals can clearly remember events that occurred 20 years ago but do not remember yesterday's events. Diseases such as **Alzheimer's disease** can lead to irreversible loss of memory, deterioration of intellectual functions, speech and gait disturbances, and disorientation. **Arteriosclerosis**, a thickening and hardening of the walls of the arteries, can also decrease the blood supply to the brain and cause a decrease in mental abilities. These diseases are discussed in greater detail in Section 9:4.

Emotional Development

Emotional stability also varies among individuals in this age group. Some elderly people cope well with the stresses presented by aging and remain happy and able to enjoy life. Others become lonely, frustrated, withdrawn, and depressed. Emotional adjustment is necessary throughout this cycle. Retirement, death of a spouse and friends, physical disabilities, financial problems, loss of independence, and knowledge that life must end all can cause emotional distress. The adjustments that the individual makes during this life stage are similar to those made throughout life.

Social Development

Social adjustment also occurs during late adulthood. Retirement can lead to a loss of self-esteem, especially if work is strongly associated with self-identity: "I am a teacher," instead of "I am Sandra Jones." Less contact with team members and a more limited circle of friends usually occur. Many elderly adults engage in other activities and continue to make new social contacts (**Figure 8–13**). Others limit their social relationships. Death of a spouse and friends and moving to a new environment can also cause changes in social relationships. Development of new social contacts is important at this time. Senior centers, golden age groups, churches, and many other organizations help provide the elderly with the opportunity to find new social roles.

Needs and Care

Needs of this life stage are the same as those of all other life stages. In addition to basic needs, the elderly need a sense of belonging, self-esteem, financial security, social acceptance, and love.

While caring for older adults, health care providers must use a nonjudgmental, supportive approach. Encourage them to talk; allow them as much independence as possible; recognize achievements they have accomplished; provide required health care information as illnesses occur; help them adjust and adapt to physical and mental changes; allow them to express fears and regrets, but remind them of positive accomplishments; and help them find support systems and social networks. The family and friends in their

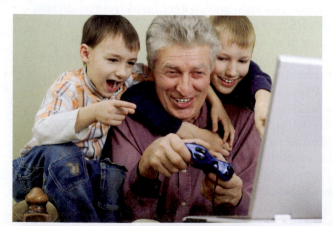

FIGURE 8–12 Elderly individuals who are willing to learn new things show fewer signs of decreased mental ability. © privilege/Shutterstock.com

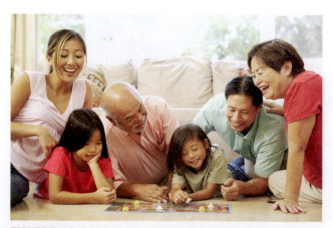

FIGURE 8–13 Social contacts and activities are important during late adulthood. © Monkey Business Images/Shutterstock.com

community they have established throughout their lifetime will continue to bring comfort and support to them. Providing a safe environment and preventing infection are also essential.

checkpoint

1. What are the seven (7) main life stages?
2. Identify two (2) physical, mental, emotional, and social developments that occur during each of the life stages.

PRACTICE: Go to the workbook and complete the assignment sheet for 8:1, Life Stages.

8:2 DEATH AND DYING

Death is often referred to as "the final stage of growth." It is experienced by everyone and cannot be avoided. In our society, the young tend to ignore its existence. It is usually the elderly, having lost spouses and/or friends, who begin to think of their own deaths.

When a patient is told that he or she has a **terminal illness**, a disease that cannot be cured and will result in death, the patient may react in different ways. Some patients react with fear and anxiety. They fear pain, abandonment, and loneliness. They fear the unknown. They become anxious about their loved ones and about unfinished work or dreams. Anxiety diminishes in patients who feel they have had full lives and who have strong religious beliefs regarding life after death. Some patients view death as a final peace. They know it will bring an end to loneliness, pain, and suffering.

STAGES OF DYING AND DEATH

Dr. Elisabeth Kübler-Ross has done extensive research on the process of death and dying, and is known as a leading expert on this topic. Because of her research, most medical personnel now believe patients should be told of their approaching deaths. However, patients should be left with "some hope" and the knowledge that they will "not be left alone." It is important that all staff members who provide care to the dying patient know both the extent of information given to the patient and how the patient reacted.

Dr. Kübler-Ross has identified five stages of grieving that dying patients and their families/friends may experience in preparation for death. The stages may not occur in order, and they may overlap or be repeated several times. Some patients may not progress through all of the stages before death occurs. Other patients may be in several stages at the same time. The five stages are denial, anger, bargaining, depression, and acceptance.

Denial is the "No, not me!" stage, which usually occurs when a person is first told of a terminal illness. It occurs when the person cannot accept the reality of death or when the person feels loved ones cannot accept the truth. The person may make statements such as "The doctor does not know what he is talking about" or "The tests have to be wrong." Some patients seek second medical opinions or request additional tests. Others refuse to discuss their situations and avoid any references to their illnesses. It is important for patients to discuss these feelings. The health care provider should listen to a patient and try to provide support without confirming or denying. Statements such as "It must be hard for you" or "You feel additional tests will help?" will allow the patient to express feelings and move on to the next stage.

Anger occurs when the patient is no longer able to deny death. Statements such as "Why me?" or "It's your fault" are common. Patients may strike out at anyone who comes in contact with them and become hostile and bitter. They may blame themselves, their loved ones, or health care personnel for their illnesses. It is important for the health care provider to understand that this anger is not a personal attack; the anger is caused by the situation the patient is experiencing. Providing understanding and support, listening, and making every attempt to respond to the patient's demands quickly and with kindness is essential during this stage. This stage continues until the anger is exhausted or the patient must attend to other concerns.

Bargaining occurs when patients accept death but want more time to live. Frequently, this is a period when patients turn to religion and spiritual beliefs. At this point, the will to live is strong, and patients fight hard to achieve goals set. They want to see their children graduate or get married, they want time to arrange care for their families, they want to hold new grandchildren, or other similar desires. Patients make promises to God in order to obtain more time. Health care providers must again be supportive and be good listeners. Whenever possible, they should help patients meet their goals.

Depression occurs when patients realize that death will come soon and they will no longer be with their families or be able to complete their goals. They may express these regrets, or they may withdraw and become quiet (**Figure 8–14**). They experience great sadness and, at times, overwhelming despair. It is important for health care providers to let patients know that it is "OK" to be depressed. Providing quiet understanding, support, and/or a simple touch, and allowing patients to cry or express grief are important during this stage.

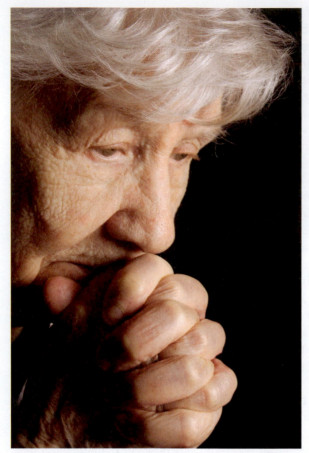

FIGURE 8–14 Depression can be a normal stage of grieving in a dying patient. © Voronin76/Shutterstock.com

Acceptance is the final stage. Patients understand and accept the fact that they are going to die. Patients may complete unfinished business and try to help those around them deal with the oncoming death. Gradually, patients separate themselves from the world and other people. At the end, they are at peace and can die with dignity. During this final stage, patients still need emotional support and the presence of others, even if it is just the touch of a hand (**Figure 8–15**).

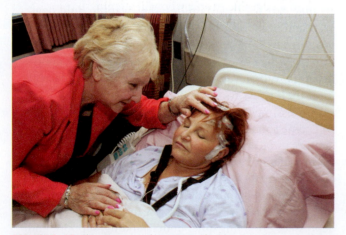

FIGURE 8–15 The support and presence of others is important to the dying person. ©iStock.com/Jodi Jacobson

HOSPICE CARE

Providing care to dying patients can be very difficult but very rewarding. Providing supportive care when families and patients require it most can be one of the greatest satisfactions a health care provider can experience. To be able to provide this care, however, health care providers must first understand their own personal feelings about death and come to terms with these feelings. Feelings of fear, frustration, and uncertainty about death can cause providers to avoid dying patients or provide superficial, mechanical care. With experience, health care providers can find ways to deal with their feelings and learn to provide the supportive care needed by the dying.

Hospice care can play an important role in meeting the needs of the dying patient. Hospice care offers *palliative care*, or care that provides support and comfort. It can be offered in hospitals, medical centers, and special facilities, but most frequently, it is offered in the patient's home. Hospice care is not limited to a specific time period in a patient's life. Usually it is not started until a physician declares that the patient has 6 months or less to live, but it can be started sooner. Most often patients and their families are reluctant to begin hospice care because they feel that this action recognizes the end of life. They seem to feel that if they do not use hospice care until later, death will not be as near as it actually is.

The philosophy behind hospice care is to allow the patient to die with dignity and comfort. Using palliative measures of care and the philosophy of death with dignity provides patients and families with many comforts and provides an opportunity to find closure. Some of the comforts provided by hospice may include providing hospital equipment such as beds, wheelchairs, and bedside commodes; offering psychological, spiritual, social, and financial counseling; and providing free or less expensive pain medication. Pain is controlled so that the patient can remain active as long as possible. In medical facilities, personal care of the patient is provided by the staff; in the home situation, this care is provided by home health aides and other health care professionals. Specially trained volunteers are an important part of many hospice programs. They make regular visits to the patient and family, stay with the patient while the family leaves the home for brief periods of time, and help provide the support and understanding that the patient and family need. When the time for death arrives, the patient is allowed to die with dignity and in peace. After the death of the patient, hospice personnel often maintain contact with the family during the initial period of mourning.

RIGHT TO DIE

Legal

The **right to die** is another issue that health care providers must understand. Because health care providers are ethically concerned with promoting life, allowing patients to die can cause conflict. However, a large number of surveys have shown that most people feel that an individual who has a terminal illness with no hope of being cured or is suffering from unrelenting pain that limits their quality of life should be allowed to refuse measures that would prolong life. A federal law called the *Patient Self-Determination Act* mandates that every individual has the right to make decisions regarding medical care, including the right to refuse treatment and the right to die. Adults who have terminal illnesses or have a low quality of life may instruct their doctors, in writing, to withhold treatments that might prolong life. The law involves the use of advance directives, discussed in Section 5:4. Under this law, specific actions to end life cannot be taken. However, the use of respirators, pacemakers, and other medical devices can be withheld, and the person can be allowed to die with dignity.

Death with Dignity laws have been passed by District of Columbia (DC) and eight states: California, Colorado, Hawaii, Maine, New Jersey, Oregon, Washington, and Vermont. Other states such as Nevada and New Mexico have approved laws through legal court decisions. These laws allow for *assisted suicide*, where a physician or other authorized individual provides medications the patient can use to end his/her own life. The laws do not allow *euthanasia*, where a physician or other individual administers the lethal medication. To qualify for assisted suicide, a person must be a resident of the state, mentally competent, and have a terminal illness. Most of the laws require the consent of two doctors who have examined the patient, a written request by the individual for the lethal medication, and a waiting period before the medication is dispensed. The patient can then decide whether or not to take the medication when he/she is ready to die. Many other states are considering *Death with Dignity* acts to allow individuals to have assistance with their right to die.

Caring Connections, a program of the National Hospice and Palliative Care Organization (NHPCO), created a national LIVE campaign to encourage individuals to make decisions about end-of-life care and services through the LIVE promise. This promise encourages individuals to:

- Learn about end-of-life services and care
- Implement plans or advance directives to ensure wishes are honored
- Voice decisions
- Engage others in conversations about end-of-life care options

Health care providers must be aware that a dying person has rights that must be honored. A Dying Person's Bill of Rights was created at a workshop sponsored by the Southwestern Michigan Inservice Education Council. This bill of rights states:

- I have the right to be treated as a living human being until I die.
- I have the right to maintain a sense of hopefulness, however changing its focus may be.
- I have the right to be cared for by those who can maintain a sense of hopefulness, however challenging this might be.
- I have the right to express my feelings and emotions about my approaching death in my own way.
- I have the right to participate in decisions concerning my care.
- I have the right to expect continuing medical and nursing attention even though "cure" goals must be changed to "comfort" goals.
- I have the right not to die alone.
- I have the right to be free from pain.
- I have the right to have my questions answered honestly.
- I have the right not to be deceived.
- I have the right to have help from and for my family in accepting my death.
- I have the right to die in peace and with dignity.
- I have the right to retain my individuality and not be judged for my decisions, which may be contrary to the beliefs of others.
- I have the right to discuss and enlarge my religious and/or spiritual experiences, whatever these may mean to others.
- I have the right to expect that the sanctity of the human body will be respected after death.
- I have the right to be cared for by caring, sensitive, knowledgeable people who will attempt to understand my needs and will be able to gain some satisfaction in helping me face my death.

Health care providers deal with death and with dying patients because death is a part of life. By understanding the process of death and by thinking about the needs of dying patients, the health care provider will be able to provide the special care needed by these individuals.

checkpoint

1. What are the five (5) stages of grieving, and who first described them?

PRACTICE: Go to the workbook and complete the assignment sheet for 8:2, Death and Dying.

8:3 HUMAN NEEDS

Needs are frequently defined as "a lack of something that is required or desired." From the moment of birth to the moment of death, every human being has needs. Needs motivate the individual to behave or act so that these needs will be met, if at all possible.

Certain needs have priority over other needs. For example, at times a need for food may take priority over a need for social approval, or the approval of others. If individuals have been without food for a period of time, they will direct most of their actions toward obtaining food. Even though they want social approval and the respect of others, they may steal for food, knowing that stealing may cause a loss of social approval or respect.

MASLOW'S HIERARCHY OF NEEDS

Abraham Maslow, a noted psychologist, developed a hierarchy of needs (**Figure 8–16**). According to Maslow, the lower needs should be met before an individual can strive to meet higher needs. Only when satisfaction has been obtained at one level is an individual motivated toward meeting needs at a higher level. The levels of needs include physiological needs, safety, affection, esteem, and self-actualization.

Physiological Needs

Physiological needs are often called "physical," "biological," or "basic" needs. These needs are required by every human being to sustain life. They include food, water, oxygen, elimination of waste materials, sleep, and protection from extreme temperatures. These needs must be met for life to continue. If any of these needs goes unmet, death will occur. Even among these needs, a priority exists. For example, because lack of oxygen will cause death in a matter of minutes, the need for oxygen has priority over the need for food. A patient with severe lung disease who is gasping for every breath will not be concerned with food intake. This individual's main concern will be to obtain enough oxygen to live through the next minute.

Other physiological needs include sensory and motor needs. If these needs are not met, individuals may not die, but their body functions will be affected. Sensory needs include hearing, seeing, feeling, smelling, tasting, and mental stimulation. When these needs are met, they allow the individual to respond to the environment. If these needs are not met, the person may lose contact with the environment or with reality. An example is motor needs, which include the ability to move and respond to the individual's environment. If muscles are not stimulated, they will atrophy (waste away), and function will be lost.

Many of the physiological needs are automatically controlled by the body. The process of breathing is usually not part of the conscious thought process of

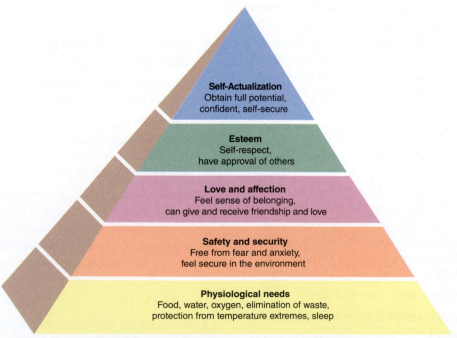

FIGURE 8–16 Maslow's Hierarchy of Needs: The lower needs should be met before the individual can try to meet higher needs. Adaptation based on Maslow's Hierarchy of Needs

the individual until something occurs to interfere with breathing. Another example is the functioning of the urinary bladder. The bladder fills automatically, and the individual only becomes aware of the bladder when it is full. If the individual does not respond and go to the restroom to empty the bladder, eventually control will be lost and the bladder will empty itself.

Health care providers must be aware of how an illness interferes with meeting physiological needs. A patient scheduled for surgery or laboratory tests may not be allowed to eat or drink before the procedure. Anxiety about an illness may interfere with a patient's sleep or elimination patterns. Medications may affect a patient's appetite. Elderly individuals are even more likely to have difficulty meeting physiological needs. A loss of vision or hearing due to aging may make it difficult for an elderly person to communicate with others. A decreased sense of smell and taste can affect appetite. Deterioration of muscles and joints can lead to poor coordination and difficulty in walking. Any of these factors can cause a change in a person's behavior. If health care providers are aware that physiological needs are not being met, they can provide understanding and support to the patient and make every effort to help the patient satisfy the needs.

Safety

Safety becomes important when physiological needs have been met. **Safety** needs include the need to be free from anxiety and fear, and the need to feel secure in the environment. The need for order and routine is another example of an individual's effort to remain safe and secure. Individuals often prefer the familiar over the unknown. New environments, a change in routine, marital problems, job loss, injury, disease, and other similar events can threaten an individual's safety.

Illness is a major threat to an individual's security and well-being. Health care providers are familiar with laboratory tests, surgeries, medications, and therapeutic treatments. Patients are usually frightened when they are exposed to them and their sense of security is threatened. If health care providers explain the reason for the tests or treatments and the expected outcomes to the patient, this can frequently alleviate the patient's anxieties. Patients admitted to a health care facility or long-term care facility must adapt to a strange and new environment. They frequently experience anxiety or depression. Patients may also experience depression over the loss of health or loss of a body function. Health care providers must be aware of the threats to safety and security that patients are experiencing and must make every effort to explain procedures, provide support and understanding, and help patients adapt to the situation.

Love and Affection

The need for love and **affection**, a warm and tender feeling for another person, occupies the third level of Maslow's Hierarchy of Needs. When an individual feels safe and secure, and after all physiological needs have been met, the individual next strives for social acceptance, friendship, and to be loved. The need to belong, to relate to others, and to win approval of others motivates an individual's actions at this point. The individual may now attend a social function that was avoided when safety was more of a priority. Individuals who feel safe and secure are more willing to accept and adapt to change and are more willing to face unknown situations. The need for love and affection is satisfied when friends are made, social contacts are established, acceptance by others is received, and the individual is able to both give and receive affection and love (**Figure 8–17**).

Maslow states that sexuality is both a part of the need for love and affection, as well as a physiological need. **Sexuality** in this context is defined by people's feelings concerning their masculine/feminine natures, their abilities to give and receive love and affection, and finally, their roles in reproduction of the species. It is important to note that in all three of these areas, sexuality involves a person's feelings and attitudes, not just the person's sexual relationships.

It is equally important to note that a person's sexuality extends throughout the life cycle. At conception, a person's sexual organs are determined. Following birth, a person is given a name, at least generally associated with the person's gender. Studies have shown that children receive treatment according to gender from

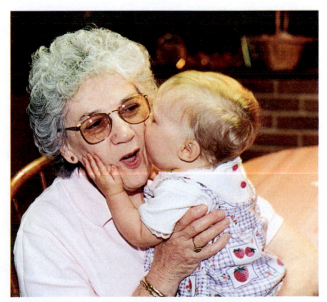

FIGURE 8–17 Individuals of all ages need love and affection.
Courtesy of Sandy Clark

early childhood and frequently are rewarded for behavior that is deemed "gender appropriate." With the onset of puberty, adolescents become more aware of their emerging sexuality and of the standards that society places on them. During both childhood and adolescence, much of what is learned about sexuality comes from observing adult role models. As the adolescent grows into young adulthood, society encourages a reexamination of sexuality and the role it plays in helping to fulfill the need for love and affection. In adulthood, sexuality develops new meanings according to the roles that the adult takes on. Sexuality needs do not cease in late adulthood. Long-term care facilities are recognizing this fact by allowing married couples to share a room. Even after the death of a spouse, an individual may develop new relationships. Determining what role sexuality will play in a person's life is a dynamic process that allows people to meet their need for love and affection throughout their life.

Sexuality, in addition to being related to the satisfaction of needs, is also directly related to an individual's moral values. Issues such as the appropriateness of sex before marriage, the use of birth control, how to deal with pregnancy, and how to deal with sexually transmitted diseases all require individuals to evaluate their moral beliefs. These beliefs then serve as guidelines to help people reach decisions on their behaviors.

Some individuals use sexual relationships as substitutes for love and affection. Individuals who seek to meet their needs only in this fashion cannot successfully complete Maslow's third level.

Esteem

Maslow's fourth level includes the need for esteem. **Esteem** includes feeling important and worthwhile. When others show respect, approval, and appreciation, an individual begins to feel esteem and gains self-respect. The self-concept—or beliefs, values, and feelings people have about themselves—becomes positive. Individuals will engage in activities that bring achievement, success, and recognition in an effort to maintain their need for esteem. Failure in an activity can cause a loss of confidence and lack of esteem. When esteem needs are met, individuals gain confidence in themselves and begin to direct their actions toward becoming what they want to be.

Illness can have a major effect on esteem. When self-reliant individuals, competent at making decisions, find themselves in a health care facility and dependent on others for basic care such as bathing, eating, and elimination, they can experience a severe loss of esteem. They may also worry about a lack of income, possible job loss, the well-being of their family, and/or the possibility of permanent disability or death. Patients may become angry and frustrated or quiet and withdrawn. Health care providers must recognize this loss of esteem and make

every attempt to listen to the patient, encourage as much independence as possible, provide supportive care, and allow the person to express anger or fear.

Self-Actualization

Self-actualization, frequently called *self-realization*, is the final need in Maslow's hierarchy. All other needs must be met, at least in part, before self-actualization can occur. **Self-actualization** means that people have obtained their full potentials, or that they are what they want to be. People at this level are autonomous, confident, and willing to express their beliefs and stick to them. They feel so strongly about themselves that they are willing to reach out to others to provide assistance and support.

MEETING NEEDS

When needs are felt, individuals are **motivated** (stimulated) to act. If the action is successful and the need is met, **satisfaction**, or a feeling of pleasure or fulfillment, occurs. If the need is not met, **tension**, or frustration, an uncomfortable inner sensation or feeling, occurs. Several needs can be felt at the same time, so individuals must decide which needs are stronger. For example, if individuals need both food and sleep, they must decide which need is most important, because an individual cannot eat and sleep at the same time.

Individuals feel needs at different levels of intensity. The more intense a need, the greater the desire to meet or reduce the need. Also, when an individual first experiences a need, the individual may deal with it by trying different actions in a trial-and-error manner, a type of behavior frequently seen in very young children. As they grow older, children learn more effective means of meeting the need and are able to satisfy the need easily.

METHODS OF SATISFYING HUMAN NEEDS

Needs can be satisfied by direct or indirect methods. Direct methods work at meeting the need and obtaining satisfaction. Indirect methods work at reducing the need or relieving the tension and frustration created by the unmet need.

Direct Methods

Direct methods include:

- Hard work
- Realistic goals
- Situation evaluation
- Cooperation with others

All these methods are directed toward meeting the need. Students who constantly fail tests but who want to pass a course have a need for success. They can work harder by listening more in class, asking questions on points they do not understand, and studying longer for the tests. They can set realistic goals that will allow them to find success. By working on one aspect of the course at a time, by concentrating on new material for the next test, by planning to study a little each night rather than studying only the night before a test, and by working on other things that will enable them to pass, they can establish goals they can achieve. They can evaluate the situation to determine why they are failing and to try to find other ways to pass the course. They may determine that they are always tired in class and that by getting more sleep, they will be able to learn the material. They can cooperate with others. By asking the teacher to provide extra assistance, by having parents or friends question them on the material, by asking a counselor to help them learn better study habits, or by having a tutor provide extra help, they may learn the material, pass the tests, and achieve satisfaction by meeting their need.

Indirect Methods

Indirect methods of dealing with needs usually reduce the need and help relieve the tension created by the unmet need. The need is still present, but its intensity decreases. **Defense mechanisms**, unconscious acts that help a person deal with an unpleasant situation or socially unacceptable behavior, are the main indirect methods used. Everyone uses defense mechanisms to some degree. Defense mechanisms provide methods for maintaining self-esteem and relieving discomfort. Some use of defense mechanisms is helpful because it allows individuals to cope with certain situations. However, defense mechanisms can be unhealthy if they are used all the time and individuals substitute them for more effective ways of dealing with situations. Being aware of the use of defense mechanisms and the reason for using them is a healthy use. This allows the individual to relieve tension while modifying habits, learning to accept reality, and striving to find more efficient ways to meet needs.

Examples of defense mechanisms include:

- **Rationalization**: This involves using a reasonable excuse or acceptable explanation for behavior to avoid the real reason or true motivation. For example, a patient who fears having laboratory tests performed may tell the health provider, "I can't take time off from my job," rather than admit fear.

- **Projection**: This involves placing the blame for one's own actions or inadequacies on someone else or on circumstances rather than accepting responsibility for the actions. Examples include, "The teacher failed me because she doesn't like me," rather than "I failed because I didn't do the work"; and "I'm late because the alarm clock didn't go off," rather than "I forgot to set the alarm clock, and I overslept." When people use projection to blame others, they avoid having to admit that they have made mistakes.

- **Displacement**: This involves transferring feelings about one person to someone else. Displacement usually occurs because individuals cannot direct the feelings toward the person who is responsible. Many people fear directing hostile or negative feelings toward their bosses or supervisors because they fear job loss. They then direct this anger toward team members and/or family members. The classic example is the man who is mad at his boss. When the man gets home, he yells at his wife or children. In such a case, a constructive talk with the boss may solve the problem. If not, or if this is not possible, physical activity can help work off hostile or negative feelings.

- **Compensation**: This involves the substitution of one goal for another goal to achieve success. If a substitute goal meets needs, this can be a healthy defense mechanism. For example, Joan wanted to be a doctor, but she did not have enough money for a medical education. So she changed her educational plans and became a physician's assistant. Compensation was an efficient defense mechanism because she enjoyed her work and found satisfaction.

- **Daydreaming**: This is a dreamlike thought process that occurs when a person is awake. Daydreaming provides a means of escape when a person is not satisfied with reality. If it allows a person to establish goals for the future and leads to a course of action to accomplish those goals, it is a good defense mechanism. However, if daydreaming is a substitute for reality, and the dreams become more satisfying than actual life experiences, it can contribute to a poor adjustment to life. For example, if a person dreams about becoming a dental hygienist and takes courses and works toward this goal, daydreaming is effective. If the person dreams about the goal but is satisfied by the thoughts and takes no action, the person will not achieve the goal and is simply escaping from reality.

- **Repression**: This involves the transfer of unacceptable or painful ideas, feelings, and thoughts into the unconscious mind. An individual is not aware that this is occurring. When feelings or emotions become too painful or frightening for the mind to deal with, repression allows the individual to continue functioning and to "forget" the fear or feeling. Repressed feelings do not vanish, however. They can resurface in dreams or affect behavior. For example, a person is terrified of heights but does not know why. It is possible that a frightening experience regarding heights happened in early childhood and that the experience was repressed.

- **Suppression**: This is similar to repression, but the individual is aware of the unacceptable feelings or thoughts and refuses to deal with them. The individual may substitute work, a hobby, or a project to avoid the situation. For example, a woman ignores a lump in her breast and refuses to go to a doctor. She avoids thinking about the lump by working overtime and joining a health club to exercise during her spare time. This type of behavior creates excessive stress, and eventually the individual will be forced to deal with the situation.

- **Regression**: This involves retreating to a previous developmental level that provided more safety and security than the current level an individual is experiencing. For example, an 8-year-old child might scream at being separated from parents or start sucking his or her thumb as a result of a hospitalization or serious illness. The child is regressing to the comfort of parents or thumb sucking to avoid the conflicts and stress of the illness or hospitalization.

- **Denial**: This involves disbelief of an event or idea that is too frightening or shocking for a person to cope with. Often, an individual is not aware that denial is occurring. Denial frequently occurs when a terminal illness is diagnosed. The individual will say that the doctor is wrong and will seek another opinion. When the individual is ready to deal with the event or idea, denial becomes acceptance.

Today's Research   Tomorrow's Health Care

A Microchip to Cure Diabetic Retinopathy?

Diabetes mellitus is a chronic disease caused by a decreased secretion of insulin, a hormone that is needed by body cells to absorb glucose (sugar) from the blood. According to the National Institutes for Health (NIH) approximately 30.3 million or 9.4 percent of the people in the United States have diabetes, 22 million diagnosed and 8.3 million undiagnosed. A common complication of diabetes is diabetic retinopathy, a disorder of the retina, or nerve-sensitive layer of the eye that provides vision. Diabetic retinopathy affects approximately 28 to 30 percent of people with diabetes and is the leading cause of blindness.

Treatment for diabetic retinopathy has its limitations. Laser therapy is used, but it can cause diminished peripheral (side) and night vision and cause laser burns that damage the eyes. A cancer drug, docetaxel, is effective, but the high dosages required to produce the desired effect cause toxic damage to other tissues in the body. Now a team of researchers in Canada has created a microelectromechanical system, commonly called a "MEMS," that can be implanted behind the eyes to release docetaxel on command using an external magnet. The team made the device from a reservoir loaded with docetaxel, sealed in place with an elastic magnetic membrane. By applying a magnetic field, the team was able to trigger the release of a specific amount of docetaxel into the back of the eye, similar to a squirt bottle. The team also found that the MEMS device lasted for more than two months without significant leakage of the medication. Dr. Mu Chiao, the head of research at the University of British Columbia (UBC) MEMS and nanotechnology department, does recognize two problems with current technologies. One problem is that they are either battery operated or too large for use in the eye. The second problem is that they rely on diffusion, which means the drug-release rates cannot be stopped, and, therefore, it is difficult to deliver the dosage the patient requires. Dr. Chiao also admits there are still many challenges that must be overcome before the mechanical device can be designed to treat specific diseases.

Many other researchers are trying to develop MEMS to treat specific diseases. Some researchers are evaluating MEMS that secrete blood-clotting factors for individuals with hemophilia. Others are trying to develop MEMS that will carry dopamine to treat Parkinson's disease. Think of a future in which tiny capsules floating or implanted in the body will cure chronic diseases and allow individuals to live long and healthy lives.

- **Withdrawal**: There are two main ways withdrawal can occur: individuals can either cease to communicate or remove themselves physically from a situation (**Figure 8–18**). Withdrawal is sometimes a satisfactory means of avoiding conflict or an unhappy situation. For example, if you are forced to work with an individual you dislike and who is constantly criticizing your work, you can withdraw by avoiding any and all communication with this individual, quitting your job, or asking for a transfer to another area. At times, however, interpersonal conflict cannot be avoided. In these cases, an open and honest communication with the individual may lead to improved understanding in the relationship.

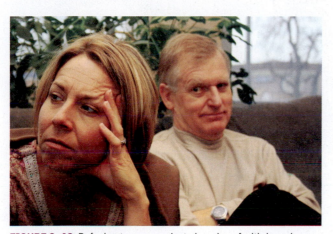

FIGURE 8–18 Refusing to communicate is a sign of withdrawal.
©iStock.com/Brad Killer

It is important for health care providers to be aware of both their own and patients' needs and be able to express them. In order to provide empathetic care, health care team members must recognize needs and understand the actions individuals take to meet needs. Efficient and higher-quality care can be provided when needs are known and communicated. Health care providers will be better able to understand their own behavior and the behavior of others.

checkpoint

1. What are the two (2) main methods people use to meet or satisfy needs?

PRACTICE: Go to the workbook and complete the assignment sheet for 8:3, Human Needs.

Case Study Investigation Conclusion

What can you conclude about the signs and symptoms that Collin is exhibiting? Why did this not manifest earlier? Is early intervention indicated or should you wait for a different life stage? Evaluate Collin's symptoms and formulate your own hypothesis regarding his diagnosis and what you would recommend for his treatment. Support your opinion with evidence from the chapter.

CHAPTER 8 SUMMARY

- Human growth and development is a process that begins at birth and does not end until death.

- Each life stage has its own characteristics and has specific developmental tasks that an individual must master. Each stage also establishes the foundation for the next stage.

- Death is often called "the final stage of growth."

- There are five stages that dying patients may experience before death. These stages are denial, anger, bargaining, depression, and acceptance. The health care provider must be aware of these stages to provide supportive care to the dying patient.

- Abraham Maslow, a noted psychologist, developed a hierarchy of needs used to classify and define the needs experienced by human beings. The needs are classified into five levels: physiological, safety and security, love and affection, esteem, and self-actualization.

- Needs are met or satisfied by direct and indirect methods. Direct methods meet and eliminate a need. Indirect methods, usually the use of defense mechanisms, reduce the need and help relieve the tension created by the unmet need.

REVIEW QUESTIONS

1. Differentiate between growth and development.

2. Describe the five (5) stages of grieving that occur in the dying patient. What role does the health care member have in each of these stages?

3. Differentiate between euthanasia and assisted suicide.

4. What are two (2) purposes of hospice care?

5. What signs might you interpret as a warning of suicide? Based upon this evidence, what methods would you recommend to prevent suicide?

6. As a health care provider, why is it important to understand human needs?

CRITICAL THINKING

1. You are an oncologist practicing at MD Anderson in Houston. You have two patients that have cancer that are no longer responding to anything you can offer them. They are facing death within 4 months. Patient 1 is Danielle, a 15-year-old volleyball player, and patient 2 is Roxanne, a 6-year-old first grader that has just learned to read. How would you explain what is happening to each girl? How would your explanation be adjusted because of each individual's life stage?

2. Justin Ballton is a 22-year-old baseball player that has just signed with the minor league team that feeds the St. Louis Cardinals. He is excited to finish his college ball days and move into the next phase. Justin is doing well as the starting pitcher for his team when he starts noticing his grip has changed and it's starting to affect his pitching accuracy. He goes to the doctor and is diagnosed with ALS or Lou Gehrig's Disease.

   Research this disease and review the "right to die." Do you think that Justin might eventually come to consider this option? State your case and provide justification for the "right to die" option for Justin.

3. Reflect on how you obtain the things you need. What are two (2) methods you use to meet or satisfy your needs?

4. Using an unlined sheet of paper, create a symbolic representation for Maslow's Hierarchy, such as a building, pile of books, or anything else to make the analogy. Based upon your idea, label each level, and list a health care-based example of each level of needs.

ACTIVITIES

1. The teacher will form seven groups. With your group, create a brochure for patient education for families in your clinic where you are a physician's assistant. These brochures will include your evaluation of the factors that impact growth and development in the physical, mental, emotional, and social areas for the stage of life your teacher assigns to your group. The brochure must also contain an illustration or summary paragraph analyzing how each of these factors contributes to the health and wellness of individuals in this stage of life.

2. Lisa Tran is a 16-year-old junior in high school that has severe asthma. She has been hospitalized an average of six times a year, for a week at a time, throughout her life. She is an average student, has low physical endurance, and is not part of any groups or organizations at school or in the community. She has three friends, and they are all freshmen that live on her street. Lisa is in a meeting with her counselor, Ms. Coronado, complaining that she does not feel a part of her high school or community and needs help to understand her options.

   In a small group, create a dialogue between Lisa and Ms. Coronado that would illustrate her use of each defense mechanism: rationalization, projection, displacement, compensation, daydreaming, repression, suppression, denial, and withdrawal as Lisa reacts to Ms. Coronado's suggestions.

3. With a partner, create a flow chart explaining the causes and treatment for chemical abuse. Include healthy choices instead of turning to chemical abuse.

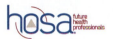 | CONNECTION

Competitive Event: Human Growth and Development

Event Summary: Human Growth & Development provides members with the opportunity to gain knowledge and skills regarding biophysical, mental/cognitive, social, and emotional development in the human life span. This competitive event consists of a written test with a tie-breaker essay question.

This event aims to inspire members to learn more about growth and development as a whole across the life span.

Details on this competitive event may be found at www.hosa.org/guidelines

Case Study Investigation

Peyton is living with and taking care of her 87-year-old grandmother, Jessica, while she is in nursing school. Her grandmother has lost her hearing; her eyesight is dimming; and she is losing weight, strength, and endurance. She loves to be with people, but her husband and many of her friends have passed away. She has become forgetful and no longer drives; she misses going out to eat with her church friends. At the end of the chapter, you will be asked to list the ways that Jessica is experiencing the physical and emotional changes associated with aging.

◼ LEARNING OBJECTIVES

After completing this chapter, you should be able to:

- Differentiate between the myths and facts of six aspects of aging.
- Identify at least two physical changes of aging in each body system.
- Demonstrate methods of providing care to the elderly individual who is experiencing physical changes of aging.
- List five factors that cause psychosocial changes of aging.
- Describe at least six methods to assist an elderly individual in adjusting to psychosocial changes.
- Recognize the causes and effects of confusion and disorientation in the elderly.
- Create a reality orientation program.
- Justify the importance of respecting cultural and spiritual differences.
- Explain the role of an ombudsman.
- Define, pronounce, and spell all key terms.

■ KEY TERMS

Alzheimer's disease (AD) *(Altz'-high-merz)*

arteriosclerosis *(ar-tear-ee-o-skleh-row'-sis)*

arthritis

atherosclerosis *(ath-eh-row"-skleh-row'-sis)*

autonomy

bronchitis

cataracts

cerebrovascular accident

culture

delirium

dementia *(d-men'-she-a)*

disability

disease

dysphagia *(dis-fay'-gee-ah)*

emphysema

geriatric care

gerontology *(jer-un-tahl'-oh-gee)*

glaucoma *(glaw-ko'-mah)*

incontinence

myths

nocturia *(nok-tur'-ee-ah)*

ombudsman

osteoporosis *(os-tee'-oh-pour-oh'-sis)*

reality orientation (RO)

senile lentigines *(seen'-ile len-ti'-jeans)*

spiritual

thrombus

transient ischemic attacks (TIAs) *(tran'-z-ent is-ke'mik)*

INTRODUCTION

Just as they experienced the "baby boom," the United States and most other countries are now experiencing an "aging boom." In 1900, most individuals died before age 60, and there were only 3.1 million people older than 65 in the United States. In 2010, according to statistics from the U.S. Census Bureau, 38.6 million Americans were older than 65 and 5.8 million were older than 85. This means that the over-65 age group represented approximately 13 percent of the population in the United States, a figure that is projected to increase to 21 percent by 2050. This is supported by statistics from 2018 that showed 52 million Americans were older than 65, which was approximately 16 percent of the population. Projections on aging by the U.S. Administration on Aging are shown in **Figure 9–1**. These statistics truly indicate an "aging boom."

Today, most individuals can expect to live into their 70s, and many individuals enjoy healthy and happy lives as 80- and 90-year-olds. This age group uses health care services frequently, so it is essential for a health care provider to understand the special needs of the elderly population.

9:1 MYTHS ON AGING

Aging is a process that begins at birth and ends at death. It is a normal process and leads to normal changes in body structure and function. Even though few people want to grow old, it is a natural event in everyone's life. **Gerontology** is the scientific study of aging and the problems of the old. **Geriatric care** is care provided to older individuals. Through the study of the aging process and the elderly, many facts on aging have been established. However, many **myths**, or false beliefs, still exist regarding aging and elderly individuals. It is essential for the health care provider to be able to distinguish fact from myth when providing geriatric care.

- **Myth**: Anyone over a certain set age, such as 65, is "old."

- **Fact**: Old is determined less by the number of years lived and more by how an individual thinks, feels, and behaves. For example, to a 10-year-old, a 35-year-old is old. It is important to remember that many individuals are active, productive, and self-sufficient into their 80s and even 90s. Too often, the term *old* becomes synonymous with *worthless* or *worn-out*. Better terms would be *experienced* or *mature*.

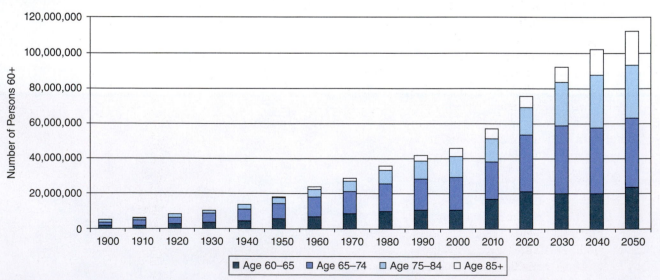

FIGURE 9–1 The "aging boom" is evident from the U.S. Administration on Aging projections through 2050. Courtesy U.S. Bureau of the Census

- **Myth**: Elderly people are incompetent and incapable of making decisions or handling their own affairs.

- **Fact**: Even though some experience confusion and disorientation, the majority of elderly individuals remain mentally competent until they die. In fact, older individuals may make better decisions and judgments because they frequently base their decisions on many years of experience and knowledge. In addition, studies have proved that older people are able to concentrate, learn new skills, and evaluate new information. Colleges and adult education programs recognize this fact and often provide tuition-free access that allows elderly individuals to participate in a wide variety of educational programs.

- **Myth**: All elderly people live in poverty.

- **Fact**: Recent statistics provided by the U.S. government show that less than 12 percent of adults older than 65 live at the poverty level. Even though many older individuals have limited incomes, most also have comparatively low expenses. Many own their own homes, and their children are raised and out on their own. With social security, savings, retirement pensions, and other sources of income, some elderly individuals are financially secure and enjoy comfortable lifestyles. Although it is true that some elderly individuals live in poverty, this is true of some individuals in all age groups. The financial status of the elderly varies just as the financial status of young or middle-aged people varies.

- **Myth**: Most elderly individuals are cared for in institutions or long-term care facilities (more detailed information on facilities can be found in Section 2:1 of this text).

- **Fact**: Only approximately 5 percent of the elderly population lives in long-term care facilities. Most elderly individuals live in their own homes or apartments, or with other family members (**Figure 9–2**). Others may choose to live in retirement communities or in independent-living or assisted-living facilities. These facilities provide assistance with meals, transportation, housekeeping, social activities, and medical care. By purchasing or renting a home or apartment in one of these facilities, the individual can obtain the degree of assistance needed while still living independently.

- **Myth**: Older people are unhappy and lonely.

- **Fact**: Studies have shown that most elderly individuals live with someone and/or associate frequently with friends or family members. Many elderly individuals are active in civic groups, charities, social activities, and volunteer programs. Others provide care for grandchildren and remain active as heads of extended families (**Figure 9–3**).

Although it is true that some elderly individuals are lonely and unhappy, the percentage is small, and many social agencies exist to assist these individuals.

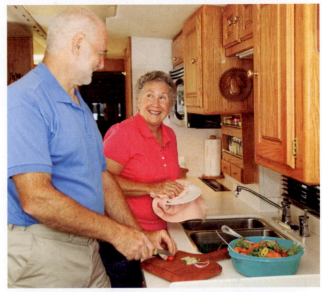

FIGURE 9–2 Most elderly individuals live in their own homes or apartments. © iStock.com/Lisa F. Young

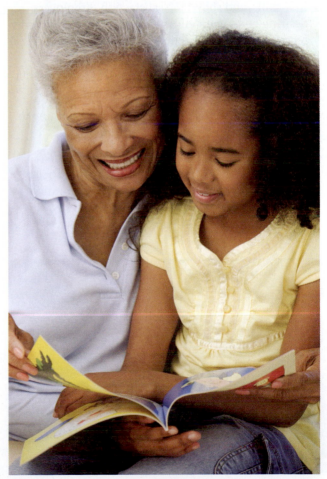

FIGURE 9–3 Caring for grandchildren is a very satisfying social relationship for many elderly individuals. © Monkey Business Images/Shutterstock.com

- **Myth**: Being old means being sick or disabled.

- **Fact**: Because of healthier lifestyles, better nutrition, regular exercise, preventive health care, new medications, and technological advances, most elderly individuals are in general good health. Medicare provides for health insurance and assists with the cost of medications (Medicare is discussed in greater detail in Section 2:5 of this text). Having good access to health care, stress reduction, maintaining a proper body weight, and avoiding or limiting alcohol and smoking are additional factors that can help slow the aging process. Advancements in diagnosing and treating heart disease, hypertension, diabetes, and similar chronic conditions have also improved the general health of the elderly. Today, many individuals in their 80s and 90s have no major disabilities or illnesses.

- **Myth**: Elderly individuals do not want to work—that is, the goal of the elderly is to retire and, prior to retirement, they lose interest in work.

- **Fact**: Many individuals remain employed and productive into their 70s and even 80s (**Figure 9–4**). Studies have shown that the older employee has good attendance, performs efficiently, readily learns new skills, and shows job satisfaction. Employers, desiring good work ethics and experience, frequently recruit and hire older employees. Many retired individuals do not want a full-time job, but they return to part-time positions or serve as consultants or volunteers.

- **Myth**: Retired people are bored and have nothing to do with their lives.

- **Fact**: Many retired people enjoy full and active lives. They engage in travel, hobbies, sports, social activities, family events, and church or community activities. In fact, many retired individuals say, "I don't know how I found time to work."

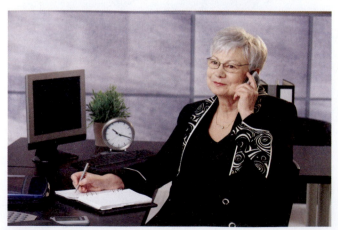

FIGURE 9–4 Many individuals remain employed and productive into their 70s and even 80s. © StockLite/Shutterstock.com

Many other myths also exist. It is important for the health care provider both to recognize problems that do exist for the elderly and to understand that the needs of the elderly vary according to many circumstances. Even the fact that only 5 percent of the elderly are in long-term care facilities means that more than 3.5 million people will be in these facilities by the year 2030. Many health care team members at all levels will provide needed services for these individuals. Geriatric care is and will continue to be a major aspect of health care.

checkpoint

1. Is the number of people 65 years and older in the United States predicted to increase or decrease through the year 2050?
2. Define gerontology.

PRACTICE: Go to the workbook and complete the assignment sheet for 9:1, Myths on Aging.

9:2 PHYSICAL CHANGES OF AGING

As aging occurs, certain physical changes also occur in all individuals (**Figure 9–5**). These changes are a normal part of the aging process. It is important to note that most of the changes are gradual and take place over a long period. In addition, the rate and degree of change varies among individuals. Physical structures and functions are affected by disease and can increase the speed and degree of the changes. Lifestyle, nutrition, economic status, social environment, and limited access to medical care can also have effects.

Most physical changes of aging involve a decrease in the function of body systems. Body processes slow down. There is a corresponding decrease in energy level. If an individual can recognize these changes as a normal part of aging, the individual can usually learn to adapt to and cope with the changes.

INTEGUMENTARY SYSTEM

Some of the most obvious effects of aging are seen in the integumentary system (**Figure 9–6**). Production of new skin cells decreases with age. The sebaceous (oil) and sudoriferous (sweat) glands become less active. Circulation to the skin decreases and causes coldness, dryness, and poor healing of injured tissue. The hair loses color, and hair loss occurs.

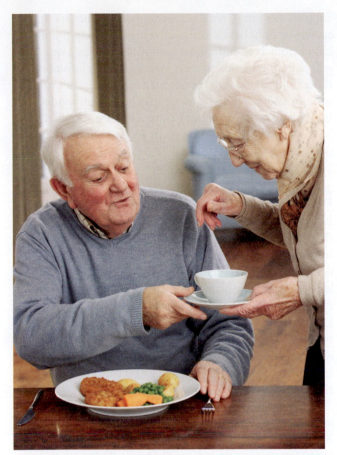

FIGURE 9–5 Note the physical signs of aging. © iStock.com/Catherine Yeulet

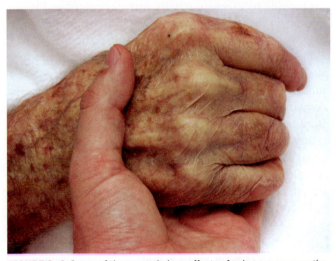

FIGURE 9–6 Some of the most obvious effects of aging are seen on the skin. © Marcin Moryc/Shutterstock.com

The decreases in body function lead to the physical or structural changes. The skin becomes dry, less elastic, and fragile, making it prone to skin tears and injury. Itching is common. Dark yellow or brown colored spots, called **senile lentigines**, appear. Although these are frequently called "liver spots," they are not related to the liver. When the structure of the fatty tissue layer of the skin diminishes, lines and wrinkles develop. The nails become

thick, tough, and brittle. A decrease in fatty tissue and poor circulation causes the older adult to frequently feel cold. Hypothermia, a below-normal body temperature, can be a serious problem for the elderly.

Good skin, nail, and hair care are essential. Mild soaps should be used because many soaps cause dryness. Frequently, bath oils or moisturizing lotions are recommended to combat dryness and itching. Daily baths can also contribute to dry, itchy skin; baths or showers two or three times a week with partial baths on other days are recommended. Brushing of the hair helps stimulate circulation and production of oil. Shampooing is usually done less frequently, but should be done as often as needed for cleanliness and comfort. Any sores or injuries to the skin should be cared for immediately. It is important to keep injured areas clean and free from infection. When elderly people notice sores or injuries that do not heal, they should get medical help. Frequently, the elderly person requires a room temperature that is higher than normal and free from drafts. Socks, sweaters, lap blankets, and layers of clothing can all help alleviate the feeling of coldness. The use of hot water bottles or heating pads is not recommended because the decreased sensitivity to temperature can result in burns.

Proper diet, exercise, good hygiene, decreased sun exposure, use of sunscreen while outdoors, and careful skin care can help slow and even decrease the normal physical changes in the integumentary system.

MUSCULOSKELETAL SYSTEM

As aging occurs, muscle structures lose tone, volume, and strength. **Osteoporosis**, a condition in which calcium and other minerals are lost from the bones, causes the bones to become brittle and more likely to fracture or break. **Arthritis**, an inflammation of the joints, causes the joints to become stiff, less flexible, and painful. The rib cage becomes more rigid, and the bones in the vertebral column press closer together (compress).

These physical and structural changes cause the elderly individual to experience a gradual loss in height, decreased muscular function and mobility, and weakness. Movement is slower, and the sense of balance is less sure. Falls occur easily and often result in fractures of the hips, arms, and/or legs. Fine finger movements, such as those required when buttoning clothes or tying shoes, are often difficult for the elderly individual.

Elderly individuals should be encouraged to exercise as much as their physical conditions permit (**Figure 9–7**). This helps keep muscles active and joints as flexible as possible. Even slow, daily walks help maintain muscle tone. Range-of-motion exercises can also maintain muscle strength. A diet rich in protein, calcium, and vitamins can slow the loss of minerals from the bones and maintain muscle structure. Medications such as Fosamax and Evista along with a daily intake of calcium

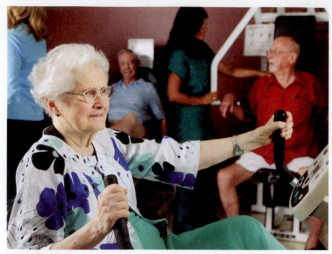

FIGURE 9–7 Elderly individuals should be encouraged to exercise as much as their physical condition permits. © iStock.com/Rich Legg

and vitamin D can slow the progress of osteoporosis. Extra attention must be paid to the environment so it is safer for the elderly person. Grab bars in the bathroom, hand rails in halls and on stairs, and other similar devices aid in ambulation. When the sense of balance is poor, an elderly person may need assistance and support during ambulation. The use of walkers and quad canes is frequently recommended. In addition, well-fitting shoes with nonslip soles and flat heels can help prevent falls. Self-stick strips and bands can replace buttons and shoestrings to make dressing easier. A consultation with a physician, physical therapist, and/or occupational therapist can provide an elderly individual with information on the latest and most effective adaptive devices to maintain independence.

CIRCULATORY SYSTEM

In the circulatory system, the heart muscle becomes less efficient at pushing blood into the arteries, and cardiac output decreases with aging. Structurally, the blood vessels narrow and become less elastic. Blood flow to the brain and other vital organs may decrease. Blood pressure may increase or decrease.

Many elderly individuals do not notice any changes while at rest. They are more aware of functional changes when exercise, stress, excitement, illness, and other similar events call for increases in the body's need for oxygen and nutrients. During these periods, they experience weakness, dizziness, numbness in the hands and/or feet, and a rapid heart rate.

Elderly individuals who experience circulatory structural and functional changes should avoid strenuous exercise or overexertion. They need periods of rest during the day. Moderate exercise, according to the individual's ability to tolerate it, does stimulate circulation and help prevent the formation of a **thrombus**, or blood clot.

Support stockings, antiembolism hose, and not using garters or tight bands around the legs also help prevent blood clots. If an individual is confined to a bed or wheelchair, range-of-motion exercises help circulation. If high blood pressure is present, a diet low in salt or sodium and, in some cases, fat may be recommended. Individuals with circulatory system disease should follow the diet and exercise plans recommended by their doctors.

RESPIRATORY SYSTEM

Respiratory muscles become weaker with age. The rib cage becomes more rigid. The alveoli, or air sacs in the lungs, become thinner and less elastic, which decreases the exchange of gases between the lungs and bloodstream. The bronchioles, or air tubes in the lungs, also lose elasticity. Structural changes in the larynx lead to a higher-pitched and weaker voice. Chronic conditions such as **emphysema**, in which the alveoli lose their elasticity, or **bronchitis**, in which the bronchioles become inflamed, decrease the efficiency and function of the respiratory system even more severely.

These structural changes frequently cause the elderly individual to experience *dyspnea*, or difficult breathing. Breathing becomes more rapid, and they have difficulty coughing up secretions from the lungs. This makes them more susceptible to respiratory infections such as colds and pneumonia.

Learning to alternate activity with periods of rest is important to avoid dyspnea. Proper body alignment and positioning can also ease breathing difficulties. The elderly individual with respiratory problems frequently sleeps in a semi-Fowler's position with two or three pillows elevating the upper body to make breathing easier. Avoiding polluted air, such as that in smoke-filled rooms, is essential. Breathing deeply and coughing at frequent intervals helps clear the lung passages and increase lung capacity. Elderly individuals with chronic respiratory functional issues often use oxygen on a continuous basis. Portable oxygen units allow many individuals to continue to lead active lives.

NERVOUS SYSTEM

Physical changes to the structures in the nervous system affect many body functions. Blood flow to the brain decreases, and there is a progressive loss of brain cells. This loss of structural functioning interferes with thinking, reacting, interpreting, and remembering. The senses of taste, smell, vision, and hearing diminish. Nerve endings are less sensitive, and there is a decreased ability to respond to pain and other stimuli.

As these structural and functional changes occur, the elderly individual may experience memory loss. Short-term memory is usually affected. For example, an individual may not remember what he or she ate for breakfast, but does remember the entire menu from his or her retirement party. Long-term memory and intelligence do not always decrease. It may take elderly individuals longer to react, but given enough time, they can think and react appropriately. Individuals who remain mentally active and involved in current events usually show fewer mental changes (**Figure 9–8**). Studies have shown that most elderly adults remain mentally competent throughout their life-spans.

Changes in vision cause problems in reading small print or seeing objects at a distance. There is a decrease in peripheral (side) vision and night vision. The eyes take longer to adjust from light to dark, and there is an increased sensitivity to glare. Elderly individuals are also more prone to the development of **cataracts**, where the normally transparent lens of the eye becomes cloudy or opaque. **Glaucoma**, a condition in which the intraocular pressure of the eye increases and interferes with vision, is also more common in the elderly. Proper eye care, prescription glasses/lenses, medical treatment of cataract or glaucoma, and proper lighting can all improve vision (**Figure 9–9**).

Hearing loss usually occurs gradually in the elderly. The individual may speak more loudly than usual, ask for words to be repeated, and not hear high-frequency sounds such as the ringing of a telephone. Problems may be more apparent when there is a lot of background noise. For example, an elderly person may not hear well in a crowded restaurant where music is playing and many other people are talking. A hearing aid can help resolve some hearing problems. However, in cases of severe structural nerve damage, a hearing aid will not eliminate the problem. In addition, many individuals resist using hearing aids. If a person wears a hearing aid, it is important to keep the aid in good working condition by changing batteries, keeping the aid clean, and checking to make sure the individual is wearing it correctly. When a person has a hearing impairment, it is important to talk slowly and clearly.

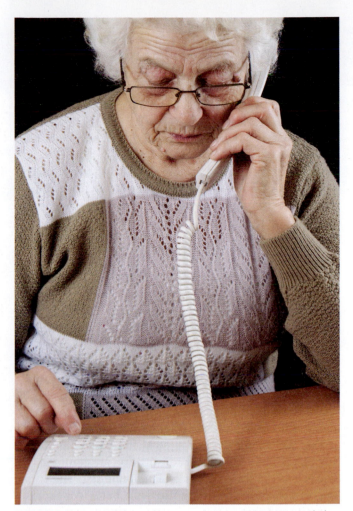

FIGURE 9–9 Good lighting and large numbers on a telephone can help improve vision. © Hunor83/Shutterstock.com

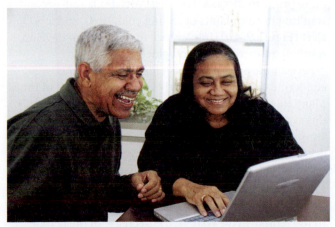

FIGURE 9–8 Individuals who remain mentally active usually show fewer mental changes. © Rob Marmion/Shutterstock.com

Avoid yelling or speaking excessively loud. Facing individuals while talking to them also helps in many situations. Eliminating background noise, such as that produced by a radio or television, also increases the ability to hear.

The decrease in the sense of taste and smell frequently affects the appetite. Elderly individuals often complain that food is tasteless and add sugar, salt, or pepper. Attractive foods with a variety of textures and tastes may help stimulate the appetite. The decrease in the sense of smell may also make the elderly individual less sensitive to the smell of gas, chemicals, smoke, and other dangerous odors. A smoke detector, chemical detectors, and careful monitoring of the environment can help eliminate this danger.

Decreased sensation of pain and other stimuli can lead to injuries. The elderly are more susceptible to burns, frostbite, cuts, fractures, muscle strain, and many other injuries. At times, elderly people are not even aware of injury or disease because they do not sense pain. It is important for elderly individuals to handle hot or cold items with extreme care, and to be aware of dangers in the environment.

Changes in the structure and function of the nervous system usually occur gradually over a long period of time. This allows an individual time to adapt to the changes and learn to accommodate them. However, it is sometimes necessary for someone else to assist when the changes become severe. For example, many elderly individuals continue to drive cars. Because of slower reaction times, however, these individuals may be more prone to having automobile accidents. When an elderly person shows impaired driving ability, it often becomes necessary for a family member or the law to prevent the individual from driving.

DIGESTIVE SYSTEM

Physical changes in the digestive system occur when fewer digestive juices and enzymes are produced, the function of muscle action becomes slower and peristalsis decreases, teeth are lost, and liver function decreases.

Dysphagia, or difficult swallowing, is a frequent complaint of the elderly. Less saliva and a slower gag reflex contribute to this problem. In addition, the structural loss of teeth or use of poor-fitting dentures makes it more difficult to chew food properly. Another common complaint is indigestion, which results from slower digestion of foods caused by decreased digestive juices. Flatulence (gas) and constipation are common because of decreased peristalsis and poor diet. The decreased sensation of taste also contributes to a poor appetite and diet.

Good oral hygiene, repair or replacement of damaged teeth, and a relaxed eating atmosphere can contribute to better chewing and digestion of food. Most elderly people find it is best to avoid dry, fried, and/or fatty foods because such foods are difficult to chew and digest. High-fiber and high-protein foods with different tastes and textures are recommended. Careful use of seasonings and herbs to improve taste also increases appetite. It is important to avoid excessive seasonings because they can cause indigestion. Because metabolism slows, fewer calories are needed to maintain body weight. Careful monitoring of weight is important to prevent obesity. Increasing fluid intake makes swallowing easier, helps prevent constipation, and aids kidney function.

URINARY SYSTEM

With aging, the kidneys structure decreases in size and become less efficient at producing urine. Poor circulation to the kidneys and a decrease in the number of nephrons result in a functional loss of ability to concentrate the urine, which causes a loss of electrolytes and fluids. The ability of the bladder to hold urine decreases. Sometimes the bladder does not empty completely and urine is retained in the bladder, a major cause of bladder infections.

The elderly person may find it necessary to urinate more frequently. Nocturia, or urination at night, is common and disrupts the sleep pattern. Retention of urine in the bladder causes bladder infections. Men frequently experience enlargement of the prostate gland, which makes urination difficult and causes urinary retention. Loss of muscle tone results in incontinence, or the inability to control urination. Incontinence may also result from treatment for prostatic hypertrophy (enlargement of the prostate gland) or for prostate cancer.

Many elderly individuals decrease fluid intake to cut down on the frequent need to urinate. This can cause dehydration, constipation, kidney disease, and infection. Elderly individuals should be encouraged to increase fluid intake to improve kidney function. To decrease incidents of nocturia, most fluids should be taken before evening. Regular trips to the bathroom, wearing easy-to-remove clothing, and using absorbent pads as needed can help the individual who has mild incontinence. Bladder training programs can also help increase bladder capacity and lead to more control over urination in incontinent persons. An indwelling catheter may be needed if all urinary control is lost.

When structural changes in the urinary system cause poor functioning of the kidneys, waste substances can build up in the bloodstream and cause serious illness. Therefore, it is important to keep the kidneys functioning as efficiently as possible.

ENDOCRINE SYSTEM

Changes in the endocrine system result in increased production of some hormones, such as parathormone and thyroid-stimulating hormone, and decreased production of other hormones, such as thyroxin, estrogen, progesterone, and insulin. The actions of these hormones are listed in **Table 7–3** of Section 7:13 of this text.

Because hormones affect many body functions, several physical changes may occur. The immune system of the body functions less effectively, and elderly individuals are more prone to disease. The basal metabolic rate decreases, resulting in complaints of feeling cold, tired, and less alert (**Figure 9–10**). Intolerance to glucose can develop, resulting in increased blood glucose levels.

As with the other body systems, changes in the endocrine system occur slowly over a long period of time. Many elderly individuals are not as aware of changes in this system. Proper exercise, adequate rest, medical care for illness, a balanced diet, and a healthy lifestyle all help decrease the effects caused by changes in hormone activity.

REPRODUCTIVE SYSTEM

In the reproductive system, the decrease of the female hormones, estrogen and progesterone causes a thinning of the vaginal walls and a decrease in vaginal secretions.

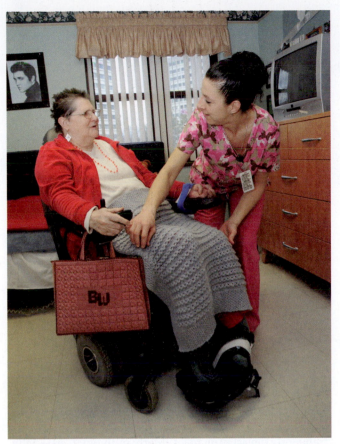

FIGURE 9–10 A lap blanket can help when an elderly person complains of feeling cold.

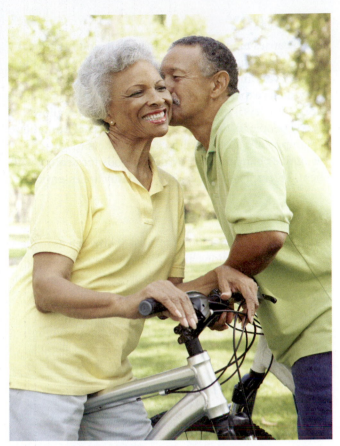

FIGURE 9–11 Elderly individuals still experience a need for companionship and sexuality. © Monkey Business Images/Shutterstock.com

Vaginal infections or inflammations become more common. In some cases, a weakness in its supporting tissues causes the uterus to sag downward, a condition known as *prolapsed uterus*. The breasts sag when fat is redistributed.

Slowly decreasing levels of the male hormone testosterone slow the production of sperm. Response to sexual stimulation of the penis is slower, and ejaculation may take longer. The testes become smaller and less firm. The seminal fluid becomes thinner, and smaller amounts are produced.

Sexual desire and need do not necessarily diminish with age (**Figure 9–11**). Many elderly individuals are sexually active. Studies have shown that sex improves muscle tone and circulation. Even pain from arthritis seems to decrease after sexual activity, probably because of increased hormone levels. When elderly individuals are in long-term care facilities, it is important for the health care provider to understand both the physical and psychological sexual needs of the resident. Long-term care facilities now allow married couples to live together in the same room. The health care provider must respect the privacy of these residents and allow them to meet their sexual needs (**Figure 9–12**).

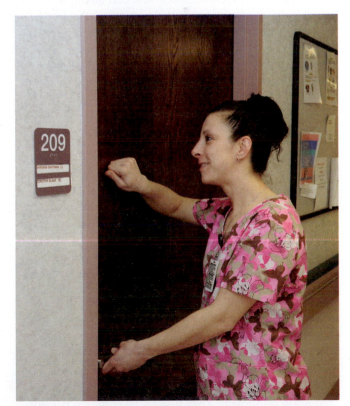

FIGURE 9–12 To respect the right to privacy, always knock before entering a resident's room.

SUMMARY

Aging causes many physical, structural, and functional changes in all body systems. The rate and degree of the changes vary in different individuals, but all elderly individuals experience some degree of change. Providing means of adapting to and coping with changes allows elderly people to enjoy life even with physical limitations. It is important for all health care providers to learn to recognize changes and provide methods for dealing with them. Tolerance, patience, and empathy are essential.

checkpoint

1. Give two (2) specific examples of how the nervous system's functions are affected because of structural changes affecting blood flow to the brain.

PRACTICE: Go to the workbook and complete the assignment sheet for 9:2, Physical Changes of Aging.

9:3 PSYCHOSOCIAL CHANGES OF AGING

In addition to physical changes, elderly individuals also experience psychological and social changes. Some individuals cope with these changes effectively, but others experience extreme frustration and mental distress. It is important for the health care provider to be aware of the psychosocial changes and stresses experienced by the elderly.

WORK AND RETIREMENT

Most adults spend a large portion of their days working. Many associate their feelings of self-worth with the jobs they perform. They are proud to state that they are nurses, electricians, teachers, lawyers, or administrative assistants. In addition, social contact while working is a major form of interaction with others.

Retirement is often viewed as an end to the working years. Many individuals are able to enjoy retirement and find other activities to replace job roles. Some individuals find part-time or consultant-type jobs after retirement from their primary jobs. Other individuals become active in volunteer work or take part in community or club activities. These individuals find satisfactory replacements for the feelings of self-worth once provided by their jobs.

However, some elderly individuals feel a major sense of loss upon retirement. They lose social contacts, develop feelings of uselessness, and, in some cases, experience financial difficulties. This causes them to experience stress, and they frequently become depressed. Until other sources of restoring the individual's sense of self-worth are found, these elderly individuals can have difficulty coping with life.

SOCIAL RELATIONSHIPS

Social relationships change throughout life. Among the elderly, these changes may occur more frequently. Often, children marry and move away. This brings about a loss of contact with the family. If a spouse dies, the "couple" image is replaced by one of "widow" or "widower." As a person ages, more friends and relatives die, and social contacts decrease.

Some elderly individuals are able to adjust to these changes by making new friends and establishing new social contacts (**Figure 9–13**). Church and community groups provide many social activities for the elderly. By taking part in these activities, individuals who made friends readily throughout their lives can continue to do so as they grow older.

Some elderly individuals cannot cope with the continuous loss of friends and relatives. They become withdrawn and depressed. They avoid social events and isolate themselves from others. The death of a spouse is frequently devastating to an elderly individual, especially when a couple has had a close relationship for many years. A surviving spouse may even attempt suicide. Psychological help is essential in these cases.

LIVING ENVIRONMENTS

Changes in living environments create psychosocial changes. Most elderly individuals prefer to remain in their own homes. They feel secure surrounded by familiar environments. Many elderly individuals express fear at the thought of losing their homes.

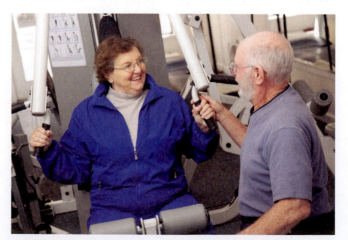

FIGURE 9–13 After the death of a spouse, the elderly individual sometimes may adjust by making new social contacts. © Andy Dean Photography/Shutterstock.com

Some elderly people leave their homes by personal choice. They find the burden of maintaining their homes too great and move to apartments or retirement communities. The elderly individual may even move to another state with a better climate. These individuals often cope well with the change in living environment and feel the change is beneficial.

Financial problems or physical disabilities may force some people to move from their homes, sometimes to retirement communities or apartments. If they can maintain their independence, coping is usually good. In other cases, an elderly individual may be forced to move in with a son or daughter. This move creates a change in roles, in which the dependent becomes the caretaker and vice versa. This can be a very difficult adjustment, and it affects everyone in the household. It can put a strain on marriages and other relationships. The help and support of others in the family (both in the household and those living elsewhere) can make the transition easier. If the elderly person feels welcome and secure in this situation, coping occurs much easier. However, if the elderly person feels unwanted or useless, conflicts and tension may develop.

Moving to a long-term care facility often creates stress in elderly individuals. They feel a loss of independence and become frightened by their lack of control over their environment. The loss of **autonomy**, self-governance or the ability to decide for oneself by making choices and pursuing a course of action, can be frustrating and upsetting. Many elderly individuals view long-term care facilities as "places to die," even when they may require the use of the facility for only a short period. For this reason, it is important to allow individuals to create their own "home" environments in the facility (**Figure 9–14**). Most long-term care facilities refer to the individuals as "residents." They allow the residents to bring favorite pieces of furniture, pictures, televisions, radios, and personal items. By being allowed choices in the arrangement of their items, residents are able to create comfortable, homelike environments. Factors such

as these allow the elderly individual to adjust to the new environment and to cope with the changes it brings.

INDEPENDENCE

Most individuals want to be independent and self-sufficient. Even 2-year-olds begin to learn autonomy as they assert their right to choose and strive to be independent. Just as children learn that there are limits to independence, the elderly learn that independence can be threatened with age. Physical disability, illness, decreased mental ability, and other factors can all lead to a loss of independence in the elderly.

Individuals who once were autonomous and took care of themselves find it necessary to ask others for assistance. After driving for a lifetime, elderly individuals might find that they can no longer drive safely. They may have stopped driving or no longer have personal transportation. They have to depend on others to take them where they need to go. The restrictions of public transportation may be unfamiliar and feel limiting. In addition, physical limitations prevent them from mowing lawns, cooking meals, washing, cleaning, and, in some cases, even taking care of themselves. Frustration, anger, and depression can develop.

Any care provided to elderly individuals should allow as much independence and autonomy as possible. Assistance should be provided as needed for the individual's safety, but the individual should be encouraged to do as much as possible. For example, a health care team member should encourage elderly persons to choose their clothing and dress themselves, even if this takes longer. Self-stick strips can replace buttons to make the task of dressing easier and to provide more independence. This helps the elderly individual retain a feeling of autonomy, adapt to the situation, and maintain a sense of self-worth. At all times, elderly individuals should be allowed as much choice as possible to help them maintain their individuality (**Figure 9–15**).

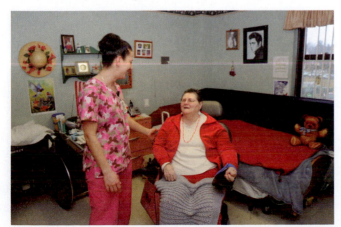

FIGURE 9–14 It is important to allow residents to create their own "home" environments in the long-term care facility.

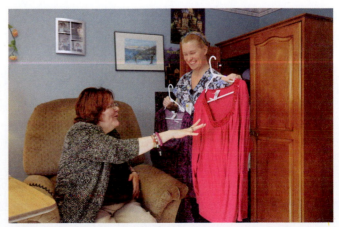

FIGURE 9–15 To promote independence, encourage elderly individuals to make as many decisions as possible.

DISEASE AND DISABILITY

Elderly people are more prone to disease and disability. **Disease** is usually defined as any condition that interferes with the normal function of the body. Common examples in the elderly include diabetes, heart disease, chronic obstructive pulmonary disease (COPD), arthritis, and osteoporosis. A **disability** is defined as a physical or mental defect or handicap that interferes with normal functions. Hearing impairments, visual defects, or the inability to walk caused by a fractured hip are examples. Diseases sometimes cause permanent disabilities. For example, a cerebrovascular accident, or stroke, can result in permanent paralysis of one side of the body, or *hemiplegia*.

When disease or disability affects the functioning of the body, an individual may experience psychological problems. When this occurs in an elderly individual already stressed by other changes or circumstances, it can be traumatic. A fractured hip can cause an elderly individual who had been living independently in his or her own home to be admitted to a long-term care facility. Disease or disability frequently occurs suddenly and does not allow for gradual adjustment, causing coping to be much more difficult.

Sick people often have fears of death, chronic illness, loss of function, and pain. These are normal fears, and these individuals need time to adjust to their situations. Listen to them as they express these fears, and be patient and understanding. If they cannot discuss their feelings, accept this and provide supportive care (**Figure 9–16**).

SUMMARY

Psychosocial changes can be major sources of stress in the elderly. As changes occur, the individual must learn to accommodate the changes and function in new situations. It is important to remember that older adults have survived many crises in their lives and have learned many different coping methods. These individuals must be encouraged to use their existing strengths and coping skills. With support, understanding, and patience, the health care provider can assist elderly individuals as they learn to adapt.

checkpoint

1. What are three (3) ways elderly people can retain their autonomy?

PRACTICE: Go to the workbook and complete the assignment sheet for 9:3, Psychosocial Changes of Aging.

9:4 CONFUSION AND DISORIENTATION IN THE ELDERLY

Although most elderly individuals remain mentally alert until death, some experience periods of confusion and disorientation. Signs of confusion or disorientation include talking incoherently, not knowing their own names, not recognizing others, wandering aimlessly, lacking awareness of time or place, displaying hostile and combative behavior (**Figure 9–17**), hallucinating, regressing in behavior, paying less attention to personal hygiene, and being unable to respond to simple commands or follow instructions.

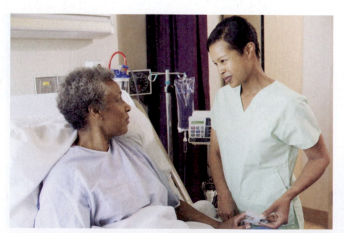

FIGURE 9–16 Provide supportive care and listen to sick individuals as they express their fears. © Monkey Business Images/Shutterstock.com

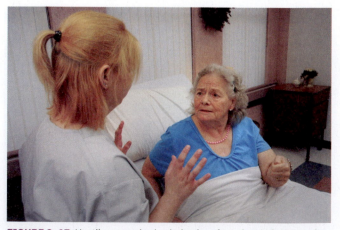

FIGURE 9–17 Hostile or combative behavior often signals feelings of frustration or confusion.

CAUSES OF CONFUSION AND DISORIENTATION

Delirium is the term used when confusion or disorientation is a temporary condition caused by a treatable condition. Stress and/or depression caused by physical or psychosocial changes is one possible cause. Use of alcohol or chemicals is another. Kidney disease, which interferes with electrolyte balance; respiratory disease, which decreases oxygen; and liver disease, which interferes with metabolism, are other causes. Elderly individuals are also more sensitive to medications, and drugs can sometimes accumulate in the body and cause confusion and disorientation. Even poor nutrition or lack of fluid intake can interfere with mental ability. Frequently, identification and treatment of any of these conditions decreases and even eliminates the confusion and disorientation. For example, changing a medication or giving it in smaller doses may restore normal function.

Disease and/or damage to the brain can sometimes result in chronic confusion or disorientation. A **cerebrovascular accident**, or stroke, which damages brain cells, is one possible cause. A blood clot can obstruct blood flow to the brain, or a vessel can rupture and cause hemorrhaging in the brain. **Arteriosclerosis**, a condition in which the walls of blood vessels become thick and lose their elasticity, is common in elderly individuals. If the vessels become narrow because of deposits of fat and minerals, such as calcium, the condition is called **atherosclerosis.** These conditions can cause **transient ischemic attacks (TIAs)**, or ministrokes, which result in temporary periods of diminished blood flow to the brain. Each time an attack occurs, more damage to brain cells results.

Dementia, also called *brain syndrome*, is a loss of mental ability characterized by a decrease in intellectual ability, loss of memory, impaired judgment, personality change, and disorientation. When the symptoms are caused by high fever, kidney infection, dehydration, hypoxia (lack of oxygen), drug toxicity, or other treatable conditions, the condition is called *delirium* or, in some cases, *acute dementia*. When the symptoms are caused by permanent irreversible damage to brain cells, the condition is called *chronic dementia*. Cerebrovascular accidents, arteriosclerosis, and TIAs can be contributing causes to chronic dementia. One modern theory suggests that chronic dementia is caused by either a complete lack or an inadequate amount of an enzyme. Whatever the cause, chronic dementia is usually regarded as a progressive, irreversible disease.

Alzheimer's disease (AD) is a form of dementia that causes progressive changes in brain cells. Individuals with AD lack a neurotransmitter, or chemical, that allows messages to pass between nerve cells in the brain. This results in the death of neurons and the development of amyloid plaques (deposits of protein) and neurofibrillary tangles. Alzheimer's disease can occur in individuals as young as 40 years of age but frequently occurs in those in their 60s and 70s. The cause is unknown, but there are many theories currently being researched. A genetic defect, a missing enzyme, toxic effects of aluminum, a virus, and the faulty metabolism of glucose have all been implicated as possible causes. Whatever the cause, AD is viewed as a terminal, incurable brain disease usually lasting from 3 to 10 years.

In the early stages, the individual exhibits self-centeredness, a decreased interest in social activities, memory loss, mood and personality changes, anxiety, agitation, depression, poor judgment, confusion regarding time and place, and an inability to plan and follow through with many activities of daily living (**Figure 9–18**). As the disease progresses, nighttime restlessness and wandering occur, mood swings become frequent, personal hygiene is ignored, confusion and forgetfulness become severe, perseveration or repetitious behavior occurs, the ability to understand others and/or speak coherently decreases, weight fluctuates, paranoia and hallucinations increase, and full-time supervision becomes necessary. In the terminal stages, the individual experiences total disorientation regarding person, time, and place; becomes incoherent and is unable to communicate with words; loses control of bladder and bowel functions; develops seizures; loses weight despite eating a balanced diet; becomes totally dependent; and finally, lapses into a coma and dies. Death is frequently caused by pneumonia, infections, complications from falls, and kidney failure. Progress through the various stages of this disease varies among individuals.

Diagnosing AD is difficult and can only be confirmed when amyloid plaques are found during an autopsy after death. Testing for AD is based on individual situations. Usually, a brain scan (CT scan or MRI) is done to rule out other conditions that may mimic the symptoms—such

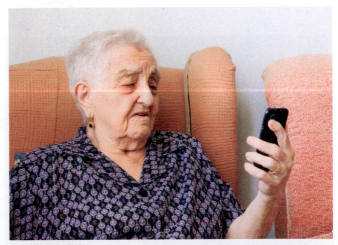

FIGURE 9–18 A patient with Alzheimer's disease may forget how common objects are used and have problems with normal activities of daily living. © Ramon Espelt Photography/Shutterstock.com

as a neoplasm, hematoma, or cerebrovascular disease. Blood tests may also be done to determine if a chemical or hormonal imbalance or vitamin deficiency is causing the behavior. Clinical assessment using diagnostic mental testing that evaluates how questions are answered and tasks are performed provides diagnostic accuracy in many cases. The Montreal Cognitive Assessment (MoCA) is a sensitive and brief tool used to diagnose AD. The Mini-Mental State Exam (MMSE) documents the presence and progression of the disease. Although there is no cure for AD, several different medications have shown promise in improving memory and thinking skills in the earlier stages of the disease. Other drugs that act to increase blood flow to the brain and clear away the amyloid plaques are currently being tested. In addition, medications that treat common symptoms of AD, such as depression or anxiety, may be prescribed. Early diagnosis and intervention is essential.

CARING FOR CONFUSED OR DISORIENTED INDIVIDUALS

⚠️ Safety

Whatever the cause of confusion or disorientation, certain courses of care should be followed. A primary concern is to provide a safe and secure environment. Dangerous objects such as drugs, poisons, scissors, knives, razors, guns, power tools, cleaning solutions, and matches and lighters should be kept out of reach and in a locked area. If the individual tends to wander, doors and windows should be secure. In severe cases, special sensors may be attached to the leg or wrist of the disoriented individual (**Figure 9–19**). The sensors alert others if the individual starts to leave a specific area. Many of the sensors also have GPS tracking abilities.

Following the same routine is also important. Meals, baths, dressing, walks, and bedtime should each occur at approximately the same time each day. Any change in routine can cause stress and confusion. Even though the individual should be encouraged to be as active as possible, activities should be kept simple and last for short periods of time (**Figure 9–20**). A calm, quiet environment is also important. Loud noises, crowded rooms, and excessive commotion can cause the individual to become agitated and even more disoriented.

Reality orientation (RO) consists of activities that help promote awareness of person, time, and place. The activities can be followed by anyone caring for the confused individual, whether the care is in the home or in a long-term care facility. Some aspects of reality orientation are the following:

- Be calm and gentle when approaching the individual.
- Address the person by the name they prefer, for example, "Mr. Smith" or "Mike."
- Avoid terms such as "sweetie," "baby," and "honey."
- State your name and correct the person if they call you a wrong name. For example, if a patient thinks you are their daughter, say, "I am not your daughter Lisa. I am Mrs. Simmers, your nurse for today."
- Make constant references to day, time, and place. "It is 8:00 Tuesday morning and time for breakfast."
- Use clocks, calendars, and information boards to point out time, day, and activities (**Figure 9–21**).
- Maintain a constant, limited routine.
- Keep the individual oriented to day-night cycles. During the day, encourage the person to wear regular clothes. Also, open the curtains and point out the sunshine. At night, close the curtains, use night lights if necessary, and promote quiet and rest.
- Speak slowly and clearly, and ask clear and simple questions.
- Never rush or hurry the individual.
- Repeat instructions patiently. Allow time for the individual to respond.

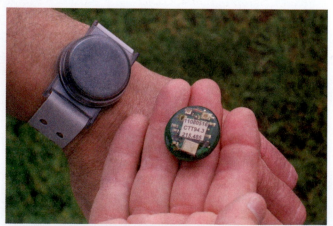

FIGURE 9–19 Special sensors may be attached to the leg or wrist of a wandering or disoriented individual. Courtesy Care Trak International, Inc.

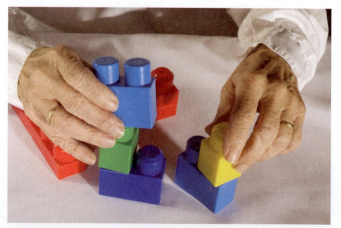

FIGURE 9–20 Activities for an individual who is confused or disoriented should be kept simple and last for short periods of time. © Ivonne Wierink/Shutterstock.com

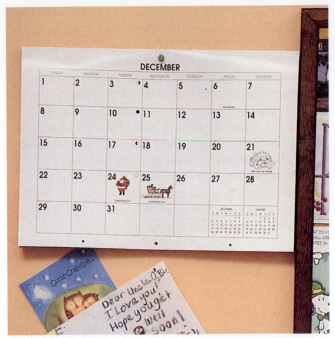

FIGURE 9–21 A large calendar may help orient a person to days and special events.

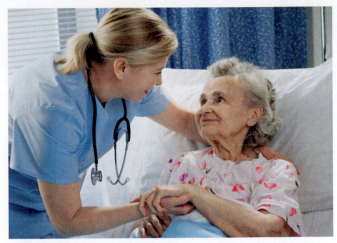

FIGURE 9–22 Do not hesitate to use touch, if culturally appropriate, to communicate with an individual who is disoriented. © Alexander Raths/Shutterstock.com

- Encourage conversations about familiar things.
- Allow the person to reminisce or remember past experiences.
- Encourage the use of a television or radio, but avoid overstimulating the individual.
- Make sure the individual uses sensory aids such as glasses and hearing aids (if needed), and that the devices are in good working order.
- Keep familiar objects and pictures within view. Avoid moving the person's furniture or belongings.
- Do not argue with incorrect statements. Gently provide correct information if the person is able to accept the information without agitation. For example, when a person states it is time to dress for work, say, "You don't have to go to work today. You retired seven years ago."
- Do not hesitate to use appropriate touch to communicate with the person, unless this causes agitation (**Figure 9–22**).
- Avoid arguments or recriminations. When you find an elderly resident in the wrong area, do not say, "You know you are not supposed to be here." Instead, say, "Let me show you how to get to your room."
- Encourage independence and self-help whenever possible.
- Always treat the person with respect and dignity.

Reality orientation is usually effective during the early stages of confusion or disorientation. In later stages, when the individual is not able to respond, it can cause

increased anxiety and agitation. When patient assessment shows that this is occurring, avoid confronting the patient with reality. For example, do not tell a patient who wants to see her husband that her husband died 10 years ago. Instead, ask her to tell you about her husband and allow her to reminisce. Provide supportive care to allow the patient to maintain dignity and express feelings.

Caring for a confused or disoriented individual can be frustrating and even frightening at times. Continual assessment of the individual's abilities and problems is needed to design a health care program that will allow the individual to function within the level of their ability. Patience, consistency, and sincere caring are essential on the part of the health care provider.

check**point**

1. List five (5) methods of reality orientation used when caring for confused patients.

PRACTICE: Go to the workbook and complete the assignment sheet for 9:4, Confusion and Disorientation in the Elderly.

9:5 MEETING THE NEEDS OF THE ELDERLY

Providing care to the elderly can be a challenging but rewarding experience. It is important to remember that the needs of the elderly do not differ greatly from the needs of any other individual. They have the same physical and psychological needs as any person at any age. However, these needs are sometimes intensified by physical or psychosocial changes that disrupt the normal life pattern. When this occurs, the elderly individual needs understanding, acceptance, and the knowledge that someone cares.

A few other factors must be considered when caring for elderly individuals. One is the importance of meeting cultural needs. **Culture** can be defined as the values, beliefs, ideas, customs, and characteristics that are passed from one generation to the next. An individual's culture can affect language, food habits, dress, work, leisure activities, and health care. Culture creates differences in individuals. For example, a person may speak a different language or have specific likes or dislikes about food or dress. It is important for the health care provider to learn about a person's culture and about the person's likes, dislikes, and beliefs. This allows the health care provider to administer care that shows a respect and acceptance of the cultural differences. (Cultural diversity is discussed in greater detail in Chapter 10 of this text.)

Spiritual needs are another important aspect of care. This can be defined as the beliefs and practices of an individual. Like culture, spiritual beliefs can affect the lifestyle of an individual. Diet, days of worship, practices relating to birth and death, and even acceptance of medical care can be affected. It is important to accept an individual's beliefs without bias. It is equally important that health care team members do not force their own spiritual beliefs on the individuals for whom they provide care. For example, if a patient asks, "Do you believe in life after death?" a health care team member may respond by saying, "How do you feel?" or "You have been thinking about the meaning of life." This allows patients to express their own feelings and thoughts. Other ways the health care team member can show respect and consideration for a person's spiritual beliefs include respectful treatment of spiritual articles, such as a Bible or Koran; enabling a person to observe religious holidays or participate in spiritual services; honoring a patient's requests for special foods; and providing privacy during clergy visits (**Figure 9–23**).

 Freedom from abuse is another important aspect of care. Abuse of the elderly can be physical, verbal, psychological, or sexual. Handling the individual roughly; denying food, water, or medication; yelling or screaming at the person; or causing fear are all forms of abuse. Abuse is sometimes difficult to prove. Frequently, the abuser is a family member or caretaker. Elderly individuals may want to protect the abuser or may even feel that they deserve the abuse. All state governments have enacted laws impacting the health care industry by requiring the reporting of any suspected abuse. It is important for any health care team member who sees or suspects abuse of the elderly to report it to the proper agency.

 A final aspect of meeting the needs of the elderly is to respect and follow the patient's rights. Patients' rights are discussed in Section 5:3 in this text. These rights assure the elderly individual of "kind and considerate care" and provide for meeting individual needs. One program the federal government developed that impacts the health care industry is the Ombudsman Program. It exists to ensure the rights of the elderly. (**Figure 9–24**). It was

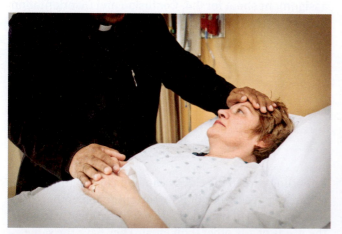

FIGURE 9–23 Respect religious needs and provide privacy while a resident is visiting with a member of the clergy. © iStock.com/nano

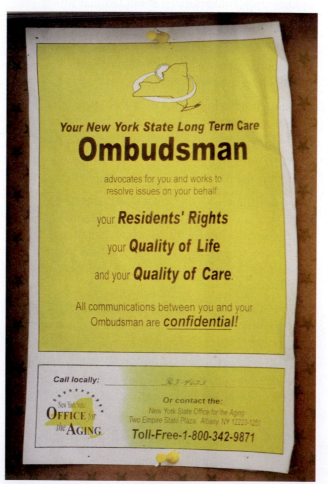

FIGURE 9–24 The Ombudsman Program, established by the federal government in the Older Americans Act, ensures the rights of elderly individuals.

People Living to 200 Years of Age?

Aging has always been considered a normal deterioration of the human body. This concept changed when Cynthia Kenyon, a geneticist at the University of California, discovered a set of genes in worms that seemed to regulate aging. By suppressing the action of one of the genes, Kenyon was able to increase a worm's life-span by six times and keep it young.

Research started with a mutant tiny nematode worm, about 1 millimeter long, that appeared to live about 50 percent longer than other nematode worms. By looking for mutant genes, Kenyon discovered the *daf-2* gene, a gene that controls the aging process. Further research showed that the *daf-2* gene is a protein that allows body tissues to respond to hormones. The mutant *daf-2* gene reduced this activity, making the tissue less responsive to hormones and allowing it to delay the aging process. A second gene, the *daf-16* gene, was identified as the "fountain of youth" gene because it promotes youthfulness. These genes allowed the mutant worms not only to delay the aging process but also to remain youthful, similar to a 95-year-old functioning like a 45-year-old. The research showed that aging is regulated by genetics. Kenyon and other researchers are now working with roundworms, organisms as small as commas that get old and wrinkled in only 10 days and rarely live longer than 2 weeks. By altering the worm's DNA *daf-2* gene, the researchers were able to increase the roundworm's life-span to as much as 10 to 12 weeks. Additional studies throughout the world have shown that people living more than 100 years were more likely to have this same genetic mutation. If additional research can lead to an application of these factors in humans, aging can be postponed, and age-related diseases can be prevented. This is because age is the largest risk factor for many diseases. An individual is much more likely to experience development of a cancerous tumor at age 70 than at age 30.

Other researchers using this information are extending the life-span of mice by more than 30 percent and are continuing to experiment with other mammals that have genes similar to those of humans. Their goal is to develop drugs that mimic the effects of the genes in the long-lived animals. If they succeed, many of the age-related diseases may be preventable, and individuals may remain youthful and productive throughout their life-spans.

---

developed by the federal government in its Older Americans Act. Each state government has its own program designed to meet federal standards. Basically, an **ombudsman** is a specially trained individual who works with the elderly and their families, health care providers, and other concerned individuals to improve quality of care and quality of life. The ombudsman may investigate and try to resolve complaints, suggest improvements for health care, monitor and enforce state and/or federal regulations, report problems to the correct agency, and provide education for individuals involved in the care of the elderly. Although the role of the ombudsman may vary from state to state, it is important for the health care team member to cooperate and work effectively with the ombudsman government program to ensure that the needs of the elderly are met and therefore positively impact the health care industry.

check**point**

1. Name one government law that impacts the health science industry.

PRACTICE: Go to the workbook and complete the assignment sheet for 9:5, Meeting the Needs of the Elderly.

Case Study Investigation Conclusion

Were you able to name several physical and emotional changes that Jessica is experiencing as a part of aging? What are some ways Peyton can help support Jessica's efforts to remain autonomous and involved?

CHAPTER 9 SUMMARY

- Geriatric care is care provided to elderly individuals.
- This age group is increasing in numbers and uses health care services frequently.
- Many myths, or false beliefs, exist regarding elderly individuals.
- Physical changes occur in all individuals as a normal part of the aging process.
- The health care provider should be aware of these changes and provide individuals with ways to remain as autonomous as possible.

- Psychosocial changes also create special needs in the elderly. Retirement, death of a spouse, new living environments, and disease and disability can cause stress.
- Although most elderly individuals remain mentally alert until death, some have periods of confusion and disorientation. Providing a safe and secure environment is of paramount importance.
- It is important for health care providers to respect and follow the "rights" of elderly individuals and to protect the elderly from abuse.

REVIEW QUESTIONS

1. What measures can be taken to help an individual adapt to or cope with the impaired functioning because of these physical/structural changes of aging?
   a. Dry, itching skin
   b. Decreased muscle tone
   c. Hearing loss and the inability to hear high-frequency sounds
   d. Difficulty in chewing and a decreased sense of taste
   e. Indigestion, flatulence, and constipation
   f. Weakness, dizziness, and dyspnea while exercising

2. Differentiate between disease and disability.

3. List four (4) factors that cause psychosocial changes in aging. For each factor, provide at least two (2) examples of ways an individual can be helped to adapt or cope with the change.

4. Differentiate between acute dementia (delirium) and chronic dementia. Identify four (4) causes for each type of dementia.

5. Identify factors that can decrease the speed and degree of physical changes of aging. Identify factors that can cause an increase.

6. Why is it important to respect an individual's cultural and spiritual beliefs?

7. What is an ombudsman? Why is their role important to elderly people?

8. Why is it important for a health care provider to differentiate between myths and facts of aging?

CRITICAL THINKING

1. Mrs. Lopez is an 83-year-old mother of eight and grandmother of 21. Her family is very close and loves to visit at her house every Sunday. They have a meal and talk and play games. Mrs. Lopez fell and fractured her hip. She had surgery and is now in a rehabilitation unit at Serene Meadows, the local long-term care facility. She has started to lose weight because she doesn't like the food at Serene Meadows. Maddie is her PT and has studied geriatric care. What changes can Maddie make for her rehab routine and what might she suggest to the dietary department and other staff to promote Mrs. Lopez's healing?

2. When a loved one becomes confused and disoriented, it impacts everyday life for both the individual and the individual's family. The financial, mental, and emotional burden can be heavy. Analyze this influence and create three (3) ways families can cope in a positive way with this new reality.

■ ACTIVITIES

1. With a partner, create a display that differentiates between six myths and facts of aging. Use three (3) pictures or graphs to further demonstrate these aging facts.

2. In groups of four, do the following:

   A. Don a pair of vision-altering glasses, put one cotton ball in each ear, use a tie to bind one arm to chest to simulate mobility impairment, and put on thick leather work gloves.

   At your table, complete the following tasks:
   a. Text your friend.
   b. Read a newspaper article,
   c. Shuffle and play cards with your group mates.
   d. Take two yellow candies (to simulate medicine pills) from a childproof container.
   e. Play Bingo with your instructor calling numbers.

   B. After these activities are completed, write a one-page essay answering the following questions: What are the top three (3) things that made accomplishing the everyday tasks the most aggravating? What interventions could your health care provider implement to address these concerns while supporting your autonomy?

   C. In your group, consider this question: "If I was an assisted living facility administrator, what would be the top five (5) methods of providing care for the residents that I would insist my staff implement?" Be ready to present to class.

3. With a small group, use a shoebox to create the perfect memory care facility. Incorporate at least three (3) reality orientation considerations to the physical building. Write a short essay explaining details of your reality orientation program and how this building supports those goals.

4. Bernice Jones is an 86-year-old woman that has lived in Cedar Park Home for the last 12 years. She is hard of hearing and wears glasses. She is very lonesome. She never married and has no children. Her sisters and brothers have all passed away, and her extended family has moved out of state. Many of her friends are no longer able to come and visit her with the regularity they once did. Her clergy comes every week, and for the last two visits, has found Bernice very much changed, Instead of being up, dressed and ready for the day, she has been in dirty clothes and appeared to be extra hungry for the afternoon snack they usually shared. How might Maria Ortiz, a 32-year-old ombudsman, help Bernice? Create a role play for the interaction that may take place between Bernice and Maria taking into consideration their differences in age and background.

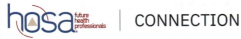 | CONNECTION

Competitive Event: Home Health Aide

Event Summary: Home Health Aide provides members with the opportunity to gain knowledge and skills required for supporting patients in their homes. This competitive event consists of 2 rounds. Round one is a written, multiple choice test and the top scoring competitors will advance to Round Two for the skills assessment. This event aims to inspire members to be proactive future health professionals and be equipped to serve patients in a home health setting.

Details on this competitive event may be found at

www.hosa.org/guidelines

Case Study Investigation

Leticia and Rosa met in nursing school and became good friends. After graduating from a small nursing school in central Texas and becoming RNs, they decided to move to New York City and work in a big hospital. They both found jobs on the medical floor of the largest hospital in the city. Leticia and Rosa were anxious to provide the best care they could to an unfamiliar, diverse patient population. Leticia and Rosa did some research in order to better understand the cultural and ethnic diversity they encountered. At the end of this chapter, you will be asked how Leticia and Rosa's research impacted the nursing care they delivered.

■ LEARNING OBJECTIVES

After completing this chapter, you should be able to:

- List the four basic characteristics of culture.
- Differentiate between culture, ethnicity, and race.
- Identify some of the major ethnic groups in the United States.
- Provide an example of acculturation in the United States.
- Create an example of how a bias, prejudice, or stereotype can cause a barrier to effective relationships with others.
- Describe at least five ways to avoid bias, prejudice, and stereotyping.
- Differentiate between a nuclear family and an extended family.
- Identify ways in which language, personal space, touching, eye contact, and gestures are affected by cultural diversity.
- Compare and contrast the diverse health beliefs of different ethnic/cultural groups.
- List five ways health care providers can show respect for an individual's religious beliefs.
- Identify methods that can be used to show respect for cultural diversity.
- Define, pronounce, and spell all key terms.

KEY TERMS

acculturation

agnostic

atheist

bias

cultural assimilation

cultural diversity

culture

ethnicity

ethnocentric

extended family

holistic care

matriarchal *(may'-tree-ar"-kel)*

monotheist

nuclear family

patriarchal *(pay'-tree-ar"-kel)*

personal space

polytheist

prejudice

race

religion

sensitivity

spirituality

stereotyping

transcultural health care

10:1 CULTURE, ETHNICITY, AND RACE

Health care providers must work with and provide care to many different people. At the same time, they must respect the individuality of each person. Therefore, every health care provider must be aware of the factors that cause each individual to be unique. Uniqueness is influenced by many things including physical characteristics (gender, body size, and hair, eye, and skin color), family life, socioeconomic status, religious beliefs, geographical location, education, occupation, and life experiences. A major influence on any individual's uniqueness is the person's cultural/ethnic heritage.

Culture is defined as the values, beliefs, attitudes, languages, symbols, rituals, behaviors, and customs unique to a particular group of people and passed from one generation to the next. It is often defined as a set of rules because culture provides an individual with a blueprint or general design for living. Family relations, child rearing, education, occupational choice, social interactions, spirituality, religious beliefs, food preferences, health beliefs, and health care are all influenced by culture. Culture is not uniform among all members within a cultural group, but it does provide a foundation for behavior. Even though differences exist between cultural groups and in individuals within a cultural group, all cultures have four basic characteristics:

- **Culture is learned**: Culture does not just happen. It is taught to others. For example, children learn patterns of behavior by imitating adults and developing attitudes accepted by others.
- **Culture is shared**: Common practices and beliefs are shared with others in a cultural group.
- **Culture is social in nature**: Individuals in the cultural group understand appropriate behavior based on traditions that have been passed from generation to generation.
- **Culture is dynamic and constantly changing**: New ideas may generate different standards for behavior. This allows a cultural group to meet the needs of the group by adapting to environmental changes.

Ethnicity is a classification of people based on national origin and/or culture. Members of an ethnic group may share a common heritage, geographic location, social customs, language, and beliefs. Even though every individual in an ethnic group may not practice all of the beliefs of the group, the individual is still influenced by other members of the group. There are many different ethnic groups in the United States (**Figure 10–1**). Examples of some of the common ethnic groups and their possible countries of origin include:

- **African American**: Central and South African countries, Dominican Republic, Haiti, and Jamaica
- **Asian/Pacific American**: Australia, Cambodia, China, Guam, Hawaii, India, Indonesia and Pacific

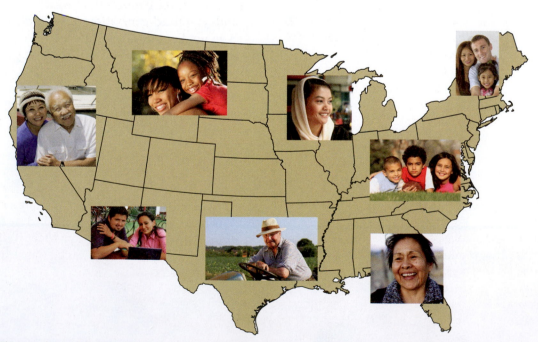

FIGURE 10–1 The many faces of the United States. Clockwise from left, © bikeriderlondon/www.Shutterstock.com, © Jenkedco/www.Shutterstock.com, © Peter Nadolski/www.Shutterstock.com, © iStockphoto/James Pauls, © Studio 1One/www.Shutterstock.com, © William Casey/www.Shutterstock.com, © erwinova/www.Shutterstock.com, © Studio 1One/www.Shutterstock.com

Island countries, Japan, Korea, Laos, Malaysia, New Zealand, Pakistan, Philippines, Samoa, Taiwan, Thailand, and Vietnam

- **European American**: Austria, Czech Republic, Denmark, England, France, Germany, Greece, Hungary, Ireland, Italy, the Netherlands, Norway, Poland, Portugal, Russia, Scotland, Sweden, and Switzerland
- **Hispanic American**: Cuba, Mexico, Puerto Rico, Spain, and Spanish-speaking countries in Central and South America
- **Middle Eastern/Arabic American**: Egypt, Iran, Iraq, Israel, Jordan, Kuwait, Lebanon, Palestine, Saudi Arabia, Syria, Turkey, Yemen, and other North African and Middle Eastern countries
- **Native American**: more than 500 tribes of American Indians and Eskimos such as Apache, Choctaw, Cherokee, Chippewa, Navajo, Seminole, and Sioux

It is important to recognize that within each of the ethnic groups, there are numerous subgroups, each with its own lifestyle and beliefs. For example, the European American group includes Italians and Germans, two groups with different languages and lifestyles.

Race is a classification of people based on physical or biological characteristics such as the color of skin, hair, and eyes; facial features, blood type, and bone structure. People may share many of the same physical characteristics, but they can have different cultural beliefs and values. In addition, there are different races present in most ethnic groups.

Culture and ethnicity can influence an individual's behavior, self-perception, judgment of others, and interpersonal relationships. These differences based on cultural and ethnic factors are called **cultural diversity**. It is important to remember that differences exist within ethnic/cultural groups and in individuals within a group. In previous times, the United States has often been called a "melting pot" to represent the absorption of many cultures into the dominant culture through a process called **cultural assimilation**. Cultural assimilation requires that the newly arrived cultural group alter unique beliefs and behaviors and adopt the ways of the dominant culture. In reality, the United States is striving to be more like a "salad bowl" where cultural differences are appreciated and respected. The simultaneous existence of various ethnic/cultural groups gives rise to a "multicultural" society that must recognize and respect many different beliefs.

Acculturation, or the process of learning the beliefs and behaviors of a dominant culture and assuming some of the characteristics, does occur. However, acculturation occurs slowly over a long period, usually many years. Recent immigrants to the United States are more likely to use the language and follow the patterns

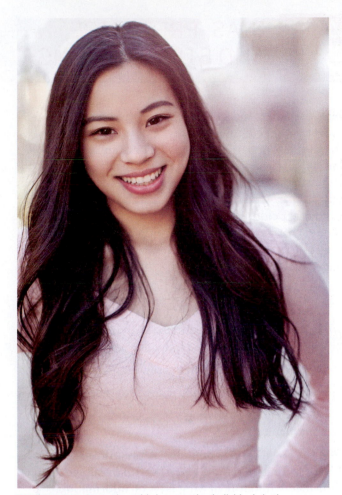

FIGURE 10–2 Second- or third-generation individuals in the same ethnic/cultural group may adopt many patterns of behavior dominant in the United States. © arek_malang/www.Shutterstock.com

of behavior of the country from which they emigrated. Second- and third-generation Americans are more likely to use English as their main language and follow the patterns of behavior prevalent in the United States (**Figure 10–2**).

Because they provide care to culturally diverse patients in a variety of settings, health care providers must be aware of these factors and remember that *no* individual is 100 percent anything! Every individual has and will continue to create new and changing blends of values and beliefs. **Sensitivity**, the ability to recognize and appreciate the personal characteristics of others, is essential in health care. For example, in some cultures, calling an adult by a first name is not acceptable except for close friends or relatives. Sensitive health care providers will address patients by their last names unless they are asked to use a patient's first name.

checkpoint

1. Define culture.
2. Define ethnicity.

10:2 BIAS, PREJUDICE, AND STEREOTYPING

Bias, prejudice, and stereotyping can interfere with acceptance of cultural diversity. A **bias** is a preference that inhibits impartial judgment. For example, individuals who believe that their cultural values are better than the cultural values of others are called **ethnocentric**. They may antagonize and alienate people from other cultures because they think other cultures should change to be like theirs. Individuals may also be biased with regard to other factors. Examples of common biases include:

- **Age**: Young people are physically and mentally superior to older people.
- **Education**: College-educated individuals are superior to uneducated individuals.
- **Economic**: Rich people are superior to poor people.
- **Physical size**: Obese and short people are inferior.
- **Occupation**: A physician is superior to an auto mechanic.

Prejudice means to prejudge. A prejudice is a strong feeling or belief about a person or subject that is formed without reviewing facts or information. Prejudiced individuals regard their ideas or behavior as right and other ideas or behavior as wrong. They are frequently afraid of things that are different. Prejudice causes fear and distrust and interferes with interpersonal relationships. Every individual is prejudiced to some degree. We all want to feel that our beliefs are correct. In health care, however, it is important to be aware of our prejudices and to make every effort to obtain as much information about a situation as possible. This allows us to learn about other individuals, understand their beliefs, and communicate successfully with them.

Stereotyping occurs when an assumption is made that everyone in a particular group is the same. A stereotype ignores individual characteristics and "labels" an individual. A classic example is "All blondes are dumb." This stereotype has been perpetuated by "blonde jokes" that are detrimental to individuals who have light-colored hair. Similar stereotypes exist with regard to race, sex, body size (thin, obese, short, or tall), occupation, and ethnic/cultural group. It is essential to remember that each person is a unique individual. Each person will have different life experiences and exposure to other cultures and ideas. This allows a person to develop a unique personality and lifestyle.

Bias, prejudice, and stereotyping are barriers to effective relationships with others. Health care providers must be alert to these barriers and make every effort to avoid them. Some ways to avoid bias, prejudice, and stereotyping include:

- Know and be consciously aware of your own personal and professional values and beliefs.
- Obtain as much information as possible about different ethnic/cultural groups.
- Be sensitive to behaviors and practices different from your own.
- Remember that you are not being pressured to adopt other beliefs but that you must respect them.
- Develop friendships with a wide variety of people from different ethnic/cultural groups.
- Ask questions and encourage questions from others to share ideas and beliefs.
- Evaluate all information before you form an opinion.
- Be open to differences.
- Avoid jokes that may offend.
- Remember that mistakes happen. Apologize if you hurt another person, and forgive if another person hurts you.

checkpoint

1. List two (2) ways to avoid bias, prejudice, and stereotyping.

10:3 UNDERSTANDING CULTURAL DIVERSITY

The cultural and ethnic beliefs of an individual can affect the behavior of the individual. Health care providers must be aware of these beliefs in order to provide **holistic care**, that is, care that provides for the well-being of the whole person and meets not only physical needs, but also social, emotional, and mental needs. Some areas of cultural diversity include family organization, language, personal space, touching, eye contact, gestures, health care beliefs, spirituality, and religion.

FAMILY ORGANIZATION

Family organization refers to the structure of a family and the dominant or decision-making person in a family. Families vary in their composition and in the roles assumed by family members. A **nuclear family** usually consists of one or two parents and a child or children (**Figure 10–3**). An **extended family** includes the nuclear family plus grandparents, aunts, uncles, and cousins

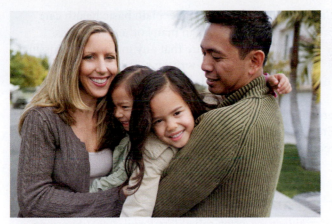

FIGURE 10–3 A nuclear family usually consists of a mother, father, and children. © StockLite/www.Shutterstock.com

(Figure 10–4). In some extended families, several different generations may live in the same household. Family structure is important in many aspects. One aspect is its effect on the care of children, the sick, and the elderly. In extended family cultures, families usually take care of their children and sick or elderly relatives in their home. They have great respect for their elders and consider it a privilege to care for them. In other family cultures, because of jobs and other obligations the parents have, people outside the family may care for children and sick or elderly relatives. Health care providers should never assume anything about a family's organization. It is important to ask questions and observe the family.

Some families are **patriarchal** and the father or oldest male is the authority figure. In a **matriarchal** family, the mother or oldest female is the authority figure. This also affects health care. In a patriarchal family, the dominant male will make most health care decisions for all family members. In these families, men have the power and authority and women are expected to

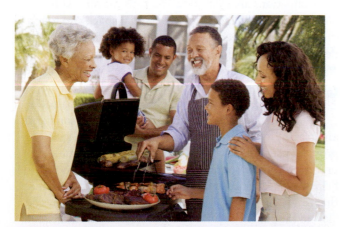

FIGURE 10–4 An extended family includes grandparents, aunts, uncles, and cousins in addition to the nuclear family. © Monkey Business Images/www.Shutterstock.com

be obedient. Husbands frequently accompany their wives to medical appointments and expect to make all the medical care decisions. In a matriarchal family, the dominant female may assume this responsibility. For example, if the mother or other female is the dominant figure in a family, they will make the health care decisions for all members of the family. In many families, both the mother and father share the decisions. Regardless of who the decision maker is, respect for the individual and the family must be the primary concern for the health care team members. Health care providers must respect patients who state, "I have to check with my husband (wife) before I decide if I should have the surgery."

Recognition and acceptance of family organization is essential for health care providers. Patients who have extended families as basic units may have many visitors in a hospital or long-term care center. Everyone will be concerned with the care provided, and all family members may help make decisions regarding care. At times, family members may even insist on providing basic personal care for the patient, such as bathing or hair care. Health care providers must adapt to these situations and allow the family to assist as much as possible.

Comm

To determine a patient's family structure and learn about a patient's preferences, the health care provider should talk with the patient or ask questions. Examples of questions that can be asked include:

- Who are the members of your family?
- Do you have any children? Who will care for them while you are sick?
- Do you have extended family? For example, aunts, uncles, cousins, nephews, nieces?
- Who will be caring for you while you are sick?
- What do you and your family do together for recreation?
- Do you have family members who will be visiting you? (If patient is admitted to a health care facility)

LANGUAGE

Comm

In the United States, the dominant language is English, but many other languages are also spoken. Statistics from the U.S. Census Bureau verified that more than 22 percent of the population younger than age 65 speaks a language other than English at home. There are even variations within a language caused by different dialects. For example, the German taught in school may differ from the language spoken by Germans from different areas of Germany. Health care providers frequently encounter patients who do not use English as a dominant language. The health care provider must determine the patient's ability to communicate by talking with the patient or a relative and asking questions such as:

- Do you speak English as your primary language?
- What language is spoken at home?
- Do you read English? Do you read another language?
- Do you have a family member or friend who can help us communicate?

Whenever possible, try to find an interpreter who speaks the language of the patient (**Figure 10–5**). Frequently, another health care provider, a consultant, or a family member may be able to assist in the communication process. Most health care facilities have a roster of employees who speak other languages.

 When providing care to people who have limited English-speaking abilities, speak slowly, use simple words, use gestures or pictures to clarify
Comm the meaning of words, and use nonverbal communication in the form of a smile or gentle touch if it is culturally appropriate. Avoid the tendency to speak louder because this does not improve comprehension. Whenever possible, try to obtain feedback from the patient to determine whether the patient understands the information that has been provided.

Most patients appreciate it when a health care provider can speak even a few words in the patient's language. Make every attempt to try to learn some words or phrases in the patient's language. Even a few words allow you to show the patient that you are trying to communicate. If you work with many patients who speak a common language, such as Spanish, try to master the basics of that language by taking an introductory course, using resources on the Internet, or learning words of the language through an app.

Other resources are also available to help a health care provider meet the needs of a non-English-speaking patient. Many health care facilities have health care information or questions printed in several languages.

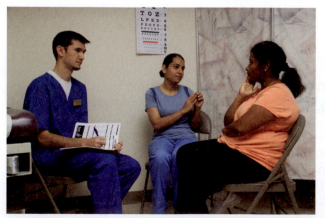

FIGURE 10–5 Whenever possible, try to find an interpreter to assist in communicating with a non-English-speaking patient.

Cards can be purchased that explain basic health care procedures or treatments in many other languages.

 Most states require that any medical permission form requiring a written signature be printed in
Legal the patient's language to ensure that the patient understands what they are signing. Health care providers must be aware of legal requirements for non-English-speaking patients and make sure that these requirements are met.

PERSONAL SPACE AND TOUCH

Personal space, often called *territorial space*, describes the distance people require to feel comfortable while interacting with others. This varies greatly among different ethnic/cultural groups. Some cultures are called "close contact" and others are called "distant contact." Individuals from close-contact cultures are comfortable standing very close to and even touching the person with whom they are interacting. They may use hugs, handshakes, and even kisses to greet others. Individuals from distant-contact cultures are more comfortable with space between them and the person with whom they are interacting and they may avoid touching others. In some cultures, kissing or hugging is reserved for intimate relationships and never done in public. Other cultures may believe that members of the opposite sex should never touch each other in public, not even brothers and sisters. In some cases, males are prohibited from touching females who are not family members, and females in these cultures may refuse personal health care from a male health care provider. Some believe the head of a child is sacred and should only be touched by a parent or an elderly relative.

Even within different cultural groups, there are variations. For example, women tend to stand closer together than men do, and children stand closer together than adults do. The type of relationship also has an effect. For example, friends usually have closer contact than strangers or coworkers. It is important to understand that these situations are examples. You must never assume anything about an individual's personal space and touch preferences. You need to question the individual to determine their preferences.

 Health care providers have to use touch and invade personal space to give many types of care. For
Comm example, taking blood pressure involves palpation of arteries, wrapping a cuff around a person's arm, and placing a stethoscope on the skin. If a health care provider uses a slow, relaxed approach, explains the procedure, and encourages the patient to relax, this may help alleviate fear and eliminate the discomfort and panic that can occur when personal space is invaded. Always be alert to the patient's verbal and nonverbal communication, as well as inconsistencies between them. For example, a patient may give verbal permission for a procedure, but may seem anxious when personal space is invaded and

demonstrate nonverbal behavior such as tensing muscles, turning or pulling away, or shaking when touched. An alert health care provider can try to move away from the patient periodically to give the patient "breathing room" and encourage the patient to relax.

Comm
When personal care must be administered to a patient, the health care provider should determine the patient's preferences by talking with the patient or asking questions. Examples of questions that may be asked include:

- Do you prefer to do as much of your own personal care as possible, or would you like assistance?
- Would you like a family member to assist with your personal care?
- Are there any special routines you would like followed while receiving personal care?
- Do you prefer to bathe in the morning or evening?
- Is there anything I can do to make you more comfortable?

TIME ORIENTATION

Time orientation refers to the manner in which an individual responds to the past, present, or future passage of time. Some cultural groups seem to be *past-oriented* because they value tradition and tend to do things the way they have always been done. These individuals may be hesitant to try new procedures and may prefer to treat medical conditions the way they have always been treated.

Other cultural groups may be *present-oriented* and concentrate on what is happening now. These individuals are more prone to seek instant gratification and not worry about how current behaviors will affect them later. They are often unconcerned about the future and may neglect preventive health care measures. If they are ill, they will seek treatment, but may ignore a follow-up visit if they recover. In many cases, they also ignore the past and feel that it has no implication in their lives.

Cultural groups who are *future-oriented* set long-term goals, try to anticipate measures that can be followed to prevent future problems, and tend to be willing to take risks to achieve their goals. They are more likely to take preventive health care measures to ensure better health as they age.

In most cases, health care systems function on a present-oriented time structure with scheduled appointments, routines that must be observed, prescribed treatments at specific times, and organized care. Health care providers must be aware of conflicting time orientations that can cause problems with the delivery of health care. Even though no individuals or cultures will be exclusively past, present, or future-oriented, their general time-orientation will affect their behavior. For example, if a patient tends to always be late or miss appointments, a health care provider may have to schedule this patient at the end of the day to allow minimal disruption to the appointment schedule. In addition, sending frequent reminders about the importance of the appointment to the patient may motivate the patient to keep the appointment. Health care providers must make every effort to recognize time orientation problems and find ways to motivate patients.

EYE CONTACT

Eye contact is also affected by different cultural beliefs. Many people regard eye contact during a conversation as indicative of interest and trustworthiness. They feel that individuals who look away are either not trustworthy or not paying attention. Other people consider direct eye contact to be rude. They may use peripheral (side) vision or look down to avoid direct eye contact. They may regard direct stares as hostile and threatening. Some people may use brief eye contact, but then look away to indicate respect and attentiveness. In a few cultures, women may avoid eye contact as a sign of modesty. In other cultures, people of different socioeconomic classes may avoid eye contact with each other. The many different beliefs regarding eye contact can lead to misunderstandings when people of different cultures interact.

Health care providers must be alert to the comfort levels of patients while using direct eye contact and must recognize the cultural diversity that exists. Lack of eye contact is often interpreted as "not listening," when in reality, it can indicate respect.

GESTURES

Gestures are used to communicate many things. A common gesture is nodding the head up and down for "yes," and side to side for "no," but in some countries the head motions for "yes" and "no" are the exact opposite. Pointing at someone may be used to stress a specific idea but this can represent a strong threat to some people. Even the hand gesture for "OK" can be found insulting to some individuals.

Again, health care providers must be aware of how patients respond to hand gestures. If a patient seems uncomfortable with hand gestures, they should be avoided.

HEALTH CARE BELIEFS

Career
The most common health care system in the United States is the biomedical health care system or the "Western" system. This system of health care bases the cause of disease on such things as microorganisms, diseased cells, and the process of aging. When the cause of disease is determined, health care is directed toward eliminating the microorganisms, conquering the disease process, and/or preventing the effects of aging. Some beliefs of this system of care include encouraging patients to learn as much as possible

about their illnesses, informing patients about terminal diseases, teaching self-care, using medications and technology to cure or decrease the effects of a disease or illness, and teaching preventive care.

It is important to note that health care beliefs vary greatly. These beliefs can affect an individual's response to health care. Most cultures have common traditional conceptions regarding the cause of illness, ways to maintain health, the appropriate response to pain, and effective methods of treatment. Some of the possible beliefs for a few different cultures are shown in **Table 10–1** as examples. *It is essential to remember that not all individuals in a specific ethnic/cultural group will believe and follow all of the customs.* The customs, however, might still influence an individual's response to a different type of care.

Health care providers must understand that every culture has a system for health care based on values and beliefs that have existed for generations. Individuals may use herbal remedies, religious rites, and other forms of ethnic/cultural health care even while receiving biomedical health care. A major change in the practice of health care in the United States is the increase in the use of alternative health care methods. Many individuals are using alternative health care in addition to, or as a replacement for, biomedical care. Some types of treatments discussed in more detail in Table 1–8 of Section 1:2 include:

- **Nutritional methods**: organic foods, herbs, vitamins, and antioxidants
- **Mind and body control methods**: relaxation, meditation, biofeedback, hypnotherapy, and imagery

- **Energetic touch therapy**: massage, acupuncture, acupressure, and therapeutic touch
- **Body-movement methods**: chiropractic, yoga, and tai chi
- **Spiritual methods**: faith healing, prayer, and spiritual counseling

Legal

Comm

It is important to remember that every individual has the right to choose the type of health care system and method of treatment they feel is best. Health care providers must respect this right. To determine a patient's health care preferences, the health care provider should talk with the patient and ask questions. Examples of questions that may be asked include:

- What do you do to stay healthy?
- Except for this current illness, do you feel that you are reasonably healthy?
- What do you feel is a healthy diet? Do you try to follow this diet?
- What do you do for exercise?
- Is there anything else that you do to stay healthy?
- Why do you think people become ill?
- What health care treatment method do you use when you are ill?
- Why do you think you have become ill?

When health care providers become aware of how cultural preferences influence behavior, they will make more of an effort to provide care that is

TABLE 10–1 Possible Traditional Health Care Beliefs

NOTE: These are examples of a few different cultures. It is essential to remember that not all individuals in a specific cultural group will believe and follow all of the customs.

Culture	Health Concepts	Cause of Illness	Traditional Healers	Methods of Treatment
South African	Maintain harmony of body, mind, and spirit Harmony with nature Illness can be prevented by diet, rest, and cleanliness	Supernatural cause Spirits and demons Punishment from God Conflict or disharmony in life	Root doctor Folk practitioners (community "mother" healer, spiritualist) Sangoma Voodoo healer	Restore harmony Prayer or meditation Herbs, roots, poultices, and oils Religious rituals Charms, talismans, and amulets Healthy diet and cleanliness
Asian	Health is a state of physical and spiritual harmony with nature Balance of two energy forces: yin (cold) and yang (hot)	Imbalance between yin and yang Supernatural forces such as God, evil spirits, or ancestral spirits Unhealthy environment	Herbalist Physician Shaman healer (physician–priest)	Cold remedies if yang is overpowering and hot remedies if yin is overpowering Herbal remedies Acupuncture and acupressure Energy to restore balance between yin and yang Tai chi Meditation
European	Health can be maintained by diet, rest, and exercise Immunizations and preventive practices help maintain health Good health is a personal responsibility	Outside sources such as germs, pollutants, or contaminants Punishment for sins Lack of cleanliness Self-abuse (drugs, alcohol, tobacco)	Physician Nurse Alternative health care practitioners	Medications and surgery Diet and exercise Home remedies and self-care for minor illnesses Prayer and religious rituals Alternative treatments

(continues)

TABLE 10–1 Possible Traditional Health Care Beliefs (continued)

Culture	Health Concepts	Cause of Illness	Traditional Healers	Methods of Treatment
Hispanic	Health is a reward from God Health is good luck Balance between "hot" and "cold" forces	Punishment from God for sins Susto (fright), mal ojo (evil eye), or envidia (envy) Imbalance between hot and cold	Native healers (Curandero, Espiritualista, Yerbero or herbalist, Brujo or witchcraft) Shaman (physician–priest) Partera (midwife)	Hot and cold remedies to restore balance Prayers, medals, candles, and religious rituals Herbal remedies, especially teas Massage Anointing with oil Wearing an Azabache (black stone) to ward off the evil eye Amulets
Middle Eastern	Health is caused by spiritual forces Good health is a great blessing Cleanliness essential for health Usually male individuals make the decisions on health care	Spiritual forces Punishment for sins Evil spirits or evil "eye"	Traditional healers Physicians Faith healers Alternative health care practitioners	Meditation and prayers Charms and amulets with verses of the Koran Medications and surgery Cupping and cautery Herbal remedies Prefer that male health professionals be prohibited from touching or examining female patients
Native American	Health is harmony between man and nature Balance among body, mind, and spirit Spiritual powers control body's harmony	Supernatural forces and evil spirits Violation of a taboo Imbalance between man and nature	Shaman Medicine man	Rituals, charms, and masks Prayer and meditation to restore harmony with nature Plants and herbs Medicine bag or bundle filled with herbs and blessed by medicine man Burning sacred herbs such as sage or sweetgrass Sweat lodges or total immersion in water to purify body and regain harmony

directed to meeting the needs of the patient. The term **transcultural health care**, or care based on the cultural beliefs, emotional needs, spiritual feelings, and physical needs of a person, can be used to describe this method of holistic care. In addition to providing the biomedical aspects of care, it recognizes the use of alternative methods of care, the healing ability of the mind, the effect of spirituality, and how emotional responses will influence care.

SPIRITUALITY AND RELIGION

Spirituality and religion may be an inherent part of every ethnic or cultural group. **Spirituality** is defined as the beliefs individuals have about themselves, their connections with others, and their relationship with a higher power. It is also described as an individual's need to find meaning and purpose in life (**Figure 10–6**). When a person's spiritual beliefs are firmly established, the individual has a basis for understanding life, finding sources of support when they are needed, and drawing on inner and/or external resources and strength to deal with situations that arise. Spirituality is often expressed through religious practices, but spirituality and religion are different. Spirituality is an individualized and

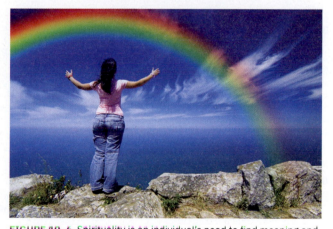

FIGURE 10–6 Spirituality is an individual's need to find meaning and purpose in life. © Mario Lopes/www.Shutterstock.com

personal set of beliefs and practices that evolves and changes throughout an individual's life.

Religion is an organized system of belief in a higher power. Religious beliefs and practices are usually associated with a particular form or place of worship. Beliefs about birth, life, illness, and death may have a religious origin. Some of the more common traditional religious beliefs are shown in **Table 10–2**.

TABLE 10–2 Traditional Religious Beliefs

NOTE: It is essential to remember that not all individuals will believe and follow all of the customs of their religion.

Religion	Beliefs About Birth	Beliefs About Death	Health Care Beliefs	Special Symbols, Books, and Religious Practices
Amish (Subgroup of Mennonites)	No infant baptism Baptism usually between ages of 16 and 25 when a person makes a commitment to church Many give birth at home with husband or other Amish woman assisting, but will use birthing centers and hospitals Birth control not forbidden but most do not use because of belief that large families are a gift from God Prohibits abortion but some groups will allow only to save the life of the mother	No last rites. Body may be embalmed, but it is buried in plain coffin in grave dug by hand by other members of Amish church No eulogy or flowers at funeral Life support is a personal decision but many refuse it Organ donation allowed if it is for the health and welfare of the recipient Autopsy only when required by law Cremation not used	Believe in living a simple life in harmony with nature Use hard work to please God Important to keep body pure and spotless Avoid contaminating influence of worldly aspects of life and remain clustered with members of their church and relatives Do not buy health insurance; church establishes a mutual aid fund to assist any member with health care expenses Accept standard treatments such as blood transfusions, surgery, and chemotherapy but will also use a variety of alternative treatments Immunizations and preventive practices not prohibited, but very few use them Many refuse prescription medicines and rely on herbal remedies	Believe in God the Father, Jesus Christ as the son of God, and the Holy Spirit Churches are small groups of Amish in a particular locale Bible is the authoritative word of God Church services are held every other Sunday in the home of one of the members Services are led by a bishop, deacons, and several ministers who are all members of the group Ordnung, or the rules of the church, must be observed by every member and vary between different groups of Amish The Ordnung cover all aspects of day-to-day living, including the type of clothing to be worn, and prohibits the use of modern technology such as electricity, cars, telephones, and computers Reject Hochmut (pride and arrogance) and place high value on Demut (humility) and Gelassenheit (calmness and composure) Ausbund is the hymnal used but it contains only words, no musical notes Faith prohibits the swearing of oaths in courts; they make affirmations of truth instead
Baptist	No infant baptism Baptism after person reaches age of understanding Abortion usually not allowed Birth control is an individual's decision	Clergy provides prayer and counseling to patient and family Autopsy, organ donation, and cremation are an individual's choice Removal of life support allowed No last rites	Some believe in the healing power of "laying on of hands" May respond passively to medical treatment, believing that illness is "God's will" Physician is instrument for God's intervention	Believe in God the Father, Jesus Christ as the son of God, and Holy Spirit Bible is holy book Rite of Communion important Baptism by full immersion in water after a person reaches an age of understanding and accepts Jesus Christ Some use cross as symbol
Buddhism	No infant baptism but have infant presentation to dedicate child to Buddha Oppose abortion unless it is to save mother's life Birth control is an individual's decision	Believe in reincarnation Desire calm environment and limited touching during the process of death Desire that body not be touched or handled immediately after death so life force can leave peacefully Buddhist priest must be present at death whenever possible Last rites chanted at bedside immediately after death Autopsy and organ donation are controversial but usually regarded as an individual's choice Removal of life support is allowed in specific conditions Cremation is common	Suffering is an inevitable part of life Illness is the result of negative Karma (a person's acts and their ethical consequences) Cleanliness is important to maintain health May refuse medications that affect mental alertness because a mindful awareness of all of life's experiences is essential	Belief in Buddha, the "enlightened one" Tripitaka, three collections of writings, are Buddhist canon Nirvana, the state of greater inner freedom, is the goal of existence Emphasize practice and personal enlightenment rather than doctrine or study of scripture May use pictures or statues of Buddha as religious symbols Some wear mala beads around the left wrist that may be removed only if absolutely necessary

TABLE 10–2 Traditional Religious Beliefs *(continued)*

Religion	Beliefs About Birth	Beliefs About Death	Health Care Beliefs	Special Symbols, Books, and Religious Practices
Christian Scientist	No infant baptism Believe baptism is an individual spiritual experience with no rites or ceremony Abortion discouraged as being incompatible with faith Birth control is an individual's decision	No last rites Autopsy only when required by law Organ donation discouraged but can be an individual's decision Removal of life support is an individual's decision Cremation acceptable	Illness can be eliminated through prayer and spiritual understanding May not use medicine or surgical procedures May refuse blood transfusions Most will accept legally mandated immunizations	Believe in God the Father, Jesus Christ as the son of God, and Holy Spirit Bible is holy book Rite of Communion important *Science and Health* by Mary Baker Eddy is basic textbook of Christian Science Prayer and faith will maintain health and prevent disease
Episcopal	Infant baptism (may be performed by anyone in an emergency) Abortion opposed Birth control is an individual's decision	Some observe prayer ritual at time of death Autopsy and organ donation encouraged but can be an individual's decision Removal of life support is allowed in specific conditions Cremation is an individual's choice	May use Holy Unction or anointing of the sick with oil or laying on of hands as a healing sacrament	Believe in God the Father, Jesus Christ as the son of God, and Holy Spirit Bible is holy book Rite of Communion important Book of Common Prayer Use cross as symbol May use prayer beads
Hinduism	No ritual at birth Naming ceremony is performed 10–11 days after birth to obtain blessings from gods and goddesses Abortion allowed only to save the life of the mother Birth control allowed but the duty of having a family is stressed	Believe in reincarnation as humans, animals, or even plants Ultimate goal is freedom from the cycle of rebirth and death Priest ties thread around the neck or wrist of the deceased and may pour holy water in the mouth Only family and friends may touch and wash the body Autopsy and organ donation discouraged because it disfigures the body Removal of life support allowed if life no longer meaningful Embalming forbidden Cremation preferred	Some believe illness is punishment for sins Some believe in faith healing Will accept most medical interventions	Vedas (four books) are the sacred scripture Brahma is principal source of universe and center of all things All forms of nature and life are sacred Person's Karma is determined by accumulated merits and demerits that result from all the actions the soul has committed in its past life or lives Cows are sacred and feeding a cow is an act of worship May use symbols such as statues of various gods, flat stones, incense, or sandalwood
Islam (Muslim)	Believe that first words an infant should hear at birth are "There is no God but Allah, and Mohammed is His prophet." Circumcision performed routinely at or near birth, but before 7 days old Birth control generally permitted Abortion prohibited except to save life of mother and forbidden after 120 days, when fetus is ensouled; father must give permission	Family must be with dying person Dying person must confess sins and ask forgiveness Only family touches or washes body after death Body is turned toward Mecca after death Autopsy only when required by law Organ donation is controversial but permitted if it helps recipient and will not harm donor Removal of life support allowed in specific conditions Cremation not permitted	Illness is an atonement for sins May face city of Mecca (southeast direction if in the United States) five times a day to pray to Allah Ritual washing before and after prayer May take medications with right hand since left hand considered dirty Use Halal diet with no pork, shellfish, or alcohol	Allah is supreme deity Mohammed, founder of Islam, is chief prophet Holy Day of Worship is sunset Thursday to sunset Friday Koran is holy book of Islam (do not touch or place anything on top) Prayer rug is sacred Fast during daylight hours in month of Ramadan and during other religious holidays May wear item with words from Koran on arm, neck, or waist; do not remove or allow item to get wet An Imam is a Muslim preacher and teacher

(continues)

TABLE 10–2 Traditional Religious Beliefs *(continued)*

Religion	Beliefs About Birth	Beliefs About Death	Health Care Beliefs	Special Symbols, Books, and Religious Practices
Jehovah's Witness	No infant baptism Baptism by immersion done when child or adult accepts beliefs Birth control is a personal decision Abortion allowed only to save the life of the mother	No last rites Autopsy only when required by law and body parts may not be removed Organ donation discouraged due to transmission of blood, but decision is an individual's choice All organs and tissues must be drained of blood before transplantation Removal of life support allowed but is an individual's decision Cremation permitted	Prohibited from receiving blood or blood products Elders of church will pray and read scriptures to promote healing Medications accepted if not derived from blood products	Name for God is Jehovah Jesus Christ died to redeem mankind Bible is holy book: New World Bible Rite of Communion important Church elders provide guidance Each witness is a minister who must spread the group's teachings Acknowledge allegiance only to kingdom of Jesus Christ and refuse allegiance to any government
Judaism (Orthodox)	No infant baptism Male circumcision performed on 8th day after birth by Mohel (circumcisor), child's father, or Jewish physician Birth control allowed Abortion permitted only in specific circumstances	Person should never die alone Body is ritually cleaned after death May bury dead before sundown on day of death and usually within 24 hours Autopsy only when required by law and all body parts must be buried together Organ donation permitted only after consultation with rabbi Removal of life support allowed in specific conditions Cremation forbidden	May refuse surgical procedure or diagnostic tests on Sabbath or holy days Family may want surgically removed body parts for burial Ritual handwashing upon awakening and prior to eating May ask for kosher food with no pork or shellfish	Lord God Jehovah is the one Lord Sabbath is sunset Friday to sunset Saturday Sabbath is devoted to prayer, study, and rest Torah is basis of religion (five books of Moses) Rabbi is spiritual leader Cantor often leads prayer services, performs marriages, and conducts funerals Star of David is symbol of Judaism Fast (no food or drink) during some holy days Men may wear kippah or yarmulke (small cap) and a tallith (prayer shawl)
Lutheran	Infant baptism by sprinkling (may be performed by any baptized Christian in an emergency) Birth control allowed Abortion discouraged but allowed in specific conditions	No last rites Autopsy and organ donation allowed Removal of life support allowed Cremation permitted	Communion often administered by clergy to sick or prior to surgery	Believe in God the Father, Jesus Christ as the son of God, and Holy Spirit Bible is holy book Rite of Communion important Use cross as symbol
Methodist (United)	Infant baptism Birth control allowed Abortion discouraged but allowed in specific conditions	No last rites Organ donations encouraged Removal of life support allowed Cremation permitted	May request communion before surgery or while ill	Believe in God the Father, Jesus Christ as the son of God, and Holy Spirit Bible is holy book Rite of Communion important Religion is a matter of personal belief and provides a guide for living Use cross as symbol
Mormon (Latter Day Saints)	Infant blessed by clergy in church as soon as possible after birth Baptism at 8 years of age Abortion prohibited Birth control is discouraged but is an individual's decision	May want church elders present at death No last rites or rituals Autopsy and organ donation is individual's decision Removal of life support is individual's or family's decision Cremation discouraged	May believe in divine healing with "laying on of hands" or blessing by church elders Anointing with oil can promote healing	Mormon refers to the four holy books: The Bible, *The Book of Mormon*, *The Doctrine and Covenants*, and *Pearl of Great Price* Jesus Christ is the redeemer and savior of the world Special undergarment may be worn to symbolize dedication to God and should not be removed unless necessary Fast on first Sunday of each month Avoid medications containing alcohol or caffeine

TABLE 10–2 Traditional Religious Beliefs *(continued)*

Religion	Beliefs About Birth	Beliefs About Death	Health Care Beliefs	Special Symbols, Books, and Religious Practices
Presbyterian	Infant baptism Birth control allowed Abortion discouraged but allowed in specific conditions	No last rites Autopsy and organ donation permitted Removal of life support allowed Cremation permitted	Prayer and counseling are an important part of healing May request communion while ill or before surgery	Believe in God the Father, Jesus Christ as the son of God, and Holy Spirit Bible is holy book Rite of Communion important Salvation is a gift from God Use cross as symbol
Roman Catholic	Infant baptism mandatory Baptism necessary for salvation (any baptized Christian may perform an emergency baptism) Birth control prohibited except for natural methods Abortion prohibited	Sacrament of the Sick may be performed by priest Autopsy and organ donation permitted Removal of life support allowed if condition is hopeless Cremation permitted	Sacrament of the Sick and anointing with oil Life is sacred: abortion and contraceptive use prohibited Believe embryos are human beings and should not be destroyed or used for research	Believe in God the Father, Jesus Christ as the son of God, and Holy Spirit Bible is holy book Rite of Holy Eucharist (Communion) important May use prayer books, crucifix, rosary beads, religious medals, pictures, and statues of saints Confession used as a rite for forgiveness of sins Use cross as symbol
Russian Orthodox	Infant baptism by priest Birth control prohibited Abortion prohibited	Last rites by ordained priest mandatory Arms of deceased are crossed Autopsy only if required by law Organ donations not encouraged Removal of life support allowed Cremation prohibited	Holy Unction and anointing body with oil used for healing Will accept most medical treatments but believe in divine healing	Believe in God the Father, Jesus Christ as the son of God, and Holy Spirit Bible is holy book Rite of Communion important May wear a cross necklace that should not be removed unless absolutely necessary Use cross as symbol
Seventh Day Adventist	No infant baptism (baptize individuals when they reach the age of accountability) Birth control is an individual's decision Therapeutic abortions permitted as an individual's decision	No last rites Autopsy only when required by law Organ donation is an individual's decision Removal of life support is a personal decision Cremation permitted	May avoid over-the-counter medications and caffeine May anoint body with oil Use prayer for healing Some believe only in divine healing Will accept required immunizations	Believe in God the Father, Jesus Christ as the son of God, and Holy Spirit Literal acceptance of Holy Bible Rite of Communion important Sabbath worship is sunset on Friday to sunset on Saturday

Even though a religion may establish certain beliefs and rituals, it is important to remember that *not* everyone follows all of the beliefs or rituals of their own religion. Some individuals are **monotheists** and believe in the existence of one God, a characteristic of Judaism, Christianity, and the Islamic religion. Other individuals are **polytheists** and worship and believe in many gods, a characteristic of Hinduism and some believers of Buddhism. In addition, some individuals are nonbelievers. For example, an **atheist** is a person who does not believe in any deity. An **agnostic** is an individual who believes that the existence of God cannot be proved or disproved. Health care providers must determine what an individual personally believes to be important and respect that individual's beliefs.

Comm

To determine an individual's spiritual and religious needs, the health care provider should talk with the patient and ask questions. Examples of questions that may be asked include:

- Do you have a religious affiliation?
- Are there any spiritual practices that help you feel better (prayer, meditation, reading scriptures)?
- Do you normally pray at certain times of the day?
- Would you like a visit from a representative of your religion?
- Do you observe any special religious days?
- Do you wear clothing or jewelry with a religious significance?
- Do you have any religious objects that require special care?
- Do your beliefs restrict any specific food or drink?
- Do you fast or abstain from eating certain foods?
- Should food be prepared in a certain way?
- Do you prefer certain types of foods (vegetarian diet, diet free from pork)?

As long as it will not cause harm, every effort must be made to allow an individual to express their beliefs, practice any rituals, and/or follow a special diet.

To show respect for an individual's beliefs and practices, the health care provider should:

- Be a willing listener.
- Provide support for spiritual and religious practices.
- Respect religious symbols and books (**Figure 10–7**).
- Allow privacy for the patient during clergy visits or while the patient is observing religious customs such as communion, prayer, and meditation.
- Refrain from imposing their own beliefs on the patient.

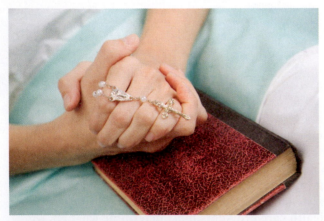

FIGURE 10–7 Always respect the patient's religious symbols and books. © iStockphoto/Rafal Ulicki

checkpoint

1. List five (5) ways to be respectful of a patient's religious beliefs and practices.

10:4 RESPECTING CULTURAL DIVERSITY

The key to respecting cultural diversity is to regard each person as a unique individual. Every individual adopts beliefs and forms a pattern of behavior based on culture, ethnicity, life experiences, spirituality, and religion. Even though this pattern of behavior and beliefs may change based on new exposures and experiences, they are still an inherent part of the individual.

Health care team members must be aware of the needs of each individual in order to provide total care. They must learn to appreciate and respect the personal characteristics of others. Some ways to achieve this goal include:

- Listen to patients as they express their beliefs.
- Appreciate differences in people.
- Learn more about the cultural and ethnic groups that you see frequently.
- Recognize and avoid bias, prejudice, and stereotyping.
- Ask questions to determine a person's beliefs.
- Evaluate all information before forming an opinion.
- Allow patients to practice and express their beliefs as much as possible.
- Remember that you are not expected to adopt another's beliefs, just accept and respect them.
- Recognize and promote the patient's positive interactions with family.
- Be sensitive to how patients respond to eye contact, touch, and invasion of personal space.
- Respect spirituality, religious beliefs, symbols, and rituals.

checkpoint

1. List three (3) ways to respect cultural diversity and the unique personal characteristics of others.

PRACTICE: Go to the workbook and complete the assignment sheet for Chapter 10, Cultural Diversity.

A Computer Microchip That Uses an Individual's Cultural and Genetic Factors to Determine What Medication the Person Needs?

Every individual has a unique genetic makeup based on both cultural and inherited factors. Because of this, individuals react to medications in different ways. Some individuals need large amounts of pain medication but others need smaller quantities. A blood pressure medication works well for one individual but is not effective for another patient. An antibiotic cures an infection in one person but causes an allergic reaction that kills another person. This causes a major problem in determining what drug and what dosage should be used for a patient. *Pharmacogenetics*, or prescribing medicine based on a person's unique genetic makeup, is the start of a revolution in personalizing treatment for a particular individual.

Researchers are using genetic information about individuals to try to determine their reactions to different medications. Currently, researchers are working to catalog as many genetic variations as possible. These variations, or SNPs (pronounced "snips"), can be used to predict a person's response to a drug. The SNPs control how a drug is absorbed, used, and eliminated. By examining a person's DNA, doctors can determine the presence of specific SNPs. Until recently, testing the DNA of an individual was slow and expensive. Now DNA microarrays, or DNA chips, are being developed that will allow doctors to examine a patient's DNA quickly and economically. At present, the ones that have been developed allow for clinical diagnostic tests for some diseases. Additional research is directed at developing more generalized DNA chips for a variety of tests. When this technology has been perfected and approved, SNP screening in a doctor's office will become a common practice prior to prescribing any medication. Because of this technology, a physician will be able to prescribe the exact medication and dosage that would be most beneficial to a patient.

Imagine a future where people will have a computer chip that contains all of their genetic information. Before any medication is given to a patient, the genetic information will be scanned to make sure it is compatible with the chemical properties of the medication. A computer will analyze the information and determine the exact dosage needed by the patient. Even though this process raises concerns about patient confidentiality, privacy, and legal regulations, it has the potential to save lives. If a medicine given to a patient is based on that person's specific needs, diseases will be cured because they will be treated correctly.

Case Study Investigation Conclusion

What different cultures and ethnicities might Leticia and Rosa have researched? How might each culture respond differently to the health care system? What interpersonal interactions could the women identify as possibly being affected by culture? How would this research and sensitivity on the part of Leticia and Rosa make their patients more comfortable?

CHAPTER 10 SUMMARY

- Health care providers work with and care for many different people and they must be aware of the factors that cause each individual to be unique. These factors include culture and ethnicity. The differences among people resulting from cultural and ethnic factors are called *cultural diversity*. Health care providers must show sensitivity, or recognize and appreciate the personal characteristics of others.

- Bias, prejudice, and stereotyping can interfere with acceptance of cultural diversity. Bias, prejudice, and stereotyping are barriers to effective relationships with others. Health care providers must be alert to these barriers and make every effort to avoid them. An understanding of cultural diversity allows health care providers to give holistic or transcultural care; that is, care that provides for the well-being of the whole person and meets not only physical, but also social, emotional, and mental needs.

- The key to respecting cultural diversity is to regard each person as a unique individual. Health care providers must learn to appreciate and respect the personal characteristics of others.

REVIEW QUESTIONS

1. List the four (4) basic characteristics of culture.

2. Identify four (4) common ethnic groups in the United States.

3. What is an example of acculturation in the United States?

4. Differentiate between a nuclear and an extended family.

5. Differentiate between culture, ethnicity, and race.

6. Why is it important for a health care provider to have an awareness of a patient's religious beliefs while caring for them?

7. You are preparing a patient for a surgical procedure and know that all jewelry must be removed. The patient is wearing a bracelet and states she is not allowed to remove it. What do you do?

8. List six (6) specific ways to respect cultural diversity.

   NOTE: The cultural assessment questions presented in this unit were adapted from Joan Luckmann's *Transcultural Communication in Health Care* (2000), which adapted them from Fong's CONFHER model and Rosenbaum.

CRITICAL THINKING

1. Do you feel acculturation occurs in the United States? Why or why not?

2. Describe and draw a sketch of your family structure. Is it a nuclear or an extended family or neither? Is it patriarchal or matriarchal or neither? Why?

3. Identify five (5) methods that can be used to show respect for cultural diversity. Give an example in a health care setting of how these methods impact:
   a. Patient satisfaction
   b. Customer service
   c. Civility in general

4. With a partner, develop a public service announcement for your school, a poster for the hallway, or a brochure to inform students about an alternative medicine like acupuncture and herbal treatments. It must include general information, purported benefits, use in the United States, side effects or risks, relevant research, cost, and links to more information. Cite evidence from print and digital resources such as research journals, the National Institute of Health, the Mayo Clinic, and Medline Plus. (You may use Table 1–8 in Section 1:2 for other reference sources.)

ACTIVITIES

1. Create a flow chart defining and showing the differentiation between culture, ethnicity, and race.

2. In a small group, create a role-play script to model examples of how a bias, prejudice, and stereotype may interfere with providing quality health care. Describe five (5) ways to avoid bias, prejudice, and stereotyping in the health care setting. Include how interaction between generations may impact communication.

3. Set up a "Cultural Awareness Day" at your school. To prepare, work with a partner to research and differentiate between five (5) ethnic/cultural groups' health care beliefs. Create a poster, trifold, or visual aid to illustrate these differences. Set up a table to display the class projects.

4. As a class, identify the ethical issues and some of their health care implications related to these topics: euthanasia, in vitro fertilization, organ donation, defining scope of practice, and how ethics committees impact health care law. Debate Day: Pick a side for each of these topics and with your team research supporting data for your opinion of each topic. Prepare for a debate with an opposing view team.

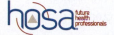 | CONNECTION

Competitive Event: Cultural Diversity and Disparities in Healthcare

Event Summary: Cultural Diversity & Disparities in Healthcare provides members with the opportunity to gain knowledge and skills regarding cultural competence in the promotion of better health. This competitive event consists of a written test with a tie-breaker essay question. This event aims to inspire members to learn about cultural diversity, identify disparities in healthcare, and understand cultural differences.

Details on this competitive event may be found at www.hosa.org/guidelines.

CHAPTER 11 NUTRITION AND DIETS

Case Study Investigation

Denise loves her new job as Lakeside Assisted Living dietician. She enjoys getting to know the residents and learning about their dietary likes and dislikes in order to design a meal plan for them. She must keep in mind disease process, cognition, and physical limitations as well. Mrs. Washington has been living at Lakeside Assisted Living for three years. She has a BMI of 34, a history of stroke, hypertension, diabetes mellitus, and has recently broken her lower denture. At the end of this chapter you will be asked what considerations Denise needs to keep in mind as she creates a meal plan for Mrs. Washington.

LEARNING OBJECTIVES

After completing this chapter, you should be able to:

- Define the term *nutrition* and list the effects of good and bad nutrition.
- Name the six groups of essential nutrients and their functions and sources.
- Differentiate between the processes of digestion, absorption, and metabolism.
- Create a sample daily menu using the five major food groups and recommendations on *MyPlate.*
- Use the body mass index (BMI) graph or calculator to determine an individual's BMI.
- Calculate an individual's daily required caloric intake to maintain current weight.
- Name, describe, and explain the purposes of at least eight therapeutic diets.
- Define, pronounce, and spell all key terms.

KEY TERMS

absorption

anorexia nervosa *(an-oh-rex'-see"-ah ner-voh'-sah)*

antioxidants

atherosclerosis *(ath-eh-row"-skleh-row'-sis)*

basal metabolic rate (BMR) *(base'-al met"-ah-ball'-ik)*

bland diet

body mass index (BMI)

bulimarexia *(byou-lee"-mah'-rex'-ee-ah)*

bulimia *(byou-lee'-me-ah)*

calorie

calorie-controlled diets

carbohydrates

cellulose

cholesterol *(co'-less'-ter-all)*

diabetes mellitus

diabetic diet

digestion

essential nutrients

fat-restricted diets

fats

fiber diets

hypertension *(high"-purr-ten'-shun)*

lipids

liquid diets

low-cholesterol diet

malnutrition

metabolism *(meh-tab'-oh-liz"-em)*

minerals

nutrition

nutritional status

obesity

osteoporosis *(os-tee'-oh-pour"-oh'-sis)*

overweight

peristalsis *(per-eh-stall'-sis)*

protein diets

proteins

regular diet

sodium-restricted diets

soft diet

therapeutic diets *(ther"-ah-pew'-tick)*

underweight

vitamins

wellness

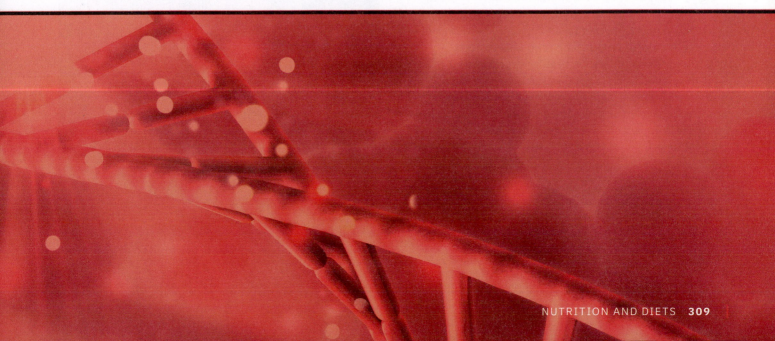

Related Health Careers

- Athletic trainer
- Behavioral disorder counselor
- Dietetic assistant
- Dietetic technician
- Dietitian
- Gastroenterologist
- Health educator
- Naturopathic physician
- Personal trainer
- Wellness coach

11:1 FUNDAMENTALS OF NUTRITION

People enjoy food and like to discuss it. Most people know that there is an important relationship between food and good health. However, many people do not know which nutrients are needed or why they are necessary. They are not able to select proper foods in their daily diets in order to promote optimum health. Therefore, it is important for every health care provider to have a solid understanding of basic nutrition. With this understanding, the health care provider can both practice and promote good nutrition.

Nutrition includes all body processes relating to food. These include digestion, absorption, metabolism, circulation, and elimination. These processes allow the body to use food for energy, maintenance of health, and growth. **Nutritional status** refers to the state or condition of one's nutrition. The goal is, of course, to be in a state of good nutrition and to maintain **wellness**, a state of good health with optimal body function. To do this, one must choose foods that are needed by the body, not just foods that taste good.

Nutrition plays a large role in determining height, weight, strength, skeletal and muscular development, physical agility, resistance to disease, appetite, posture, complexion, mental ability, and emotional and psychological health. The immediate effects of good nutrition include a healthy appearance, a well-developed body, a good attitude, proper sleep and bowel habits, a high energy level, enthusiasm, and freedom from anxiety. In addition, the effects of good nutrition accumulate throughout life and may prevent or delay diseases or conditions such as the following:

- **Hypertension**: high blood pressure; may be caused by an excess amount of fat or salt in the diet; can lead to diseases of the heart, blood vessels, and kidneys

- **Atherosclerosis**: condition in which arteries are narrowed by the accumulation of fatty substances on their inner surfaces; thought to be caused by a diet high in saturated fats and cholesterol; can lead to heart attack or stroke

- **Osteoporosis**: condition in which bones become porous (full of tiny openings) and break easily; one cause is long-term deficiencies of calcium, magnesium, and vitamin D

- **Diabetes mellitus**: metabolic disease caused by an insufficient secretion or use of insulin leading to an increased level of glucose (sugar) in the blood; heredity, obesity, lack of exercise, and diets high in carbohydrates and sugars contribute to individuals developing this disease

- **Malnutrition**: the state of poor nutrition; may be caused by poor diet or illness. Symptoms include fatigue, depression, poor posture, being overweight or under-weight, poor complexion, lifeless hair, and irritability (**Figure 11–1**); It can cause deficiency diseases, poor muscular and skeletal development, reduced mental abilities, and even death. Malnutrition is most likely to affect individuals living in extreme poverty, patients undergoing drug therapy, such as treatments for cancer, infants, young children, adolescents, and the elderly. Obesity is a form of malnutrition caused by excess food consumption.

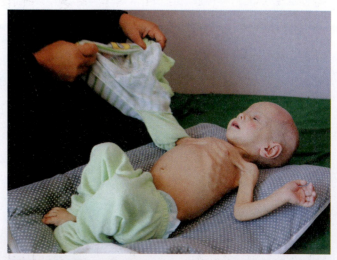

FIGURE 11–1 This child shows many of the signs of severe malnutrition.
Courtesy of the Centers for Disease Control Public Health Image Library

checkpoint

1. Define *nutrition*.
2. List four (4) diseases that may be avoided by good nutrition.

11:2 ESSENTIAL NUTRIENTS

Essential nutrients are composed of chemical elements found in food. They are used by the body to perform many different body functions. As the body uses these elements, they are replaced by elements in the food one eats. The essential nutrients are divided into six groups. The six groups and the specific functions of each group are shown in **Table 11–1**.

CARBOHYDRATES

Carbohydrates are the major source of readily usable human energy. They are commonly called *starches* or *sugars*. Carbohydrates are a cheaper source of energy than proteins and fats because they are mainly produced by plants. They are easily digested, grow well in most climates, and keep well without refrigeration. They are made of carbon, hydrogen, and oxygen.

The main sources of carbohydrates are breads, cereals, noodles or pastas, crackers, potatoes, corn, peas, beans, grains, fruits, sugar, and syrups.

TABLE 11–1 The Six Essential Nutrient Groups

Nutrient Group	Functions
Carbohydrates	Provide heat and energy Supply fiber for good digestion and elimination
Lipids (Fats)	Provide fatty acids needed for growth and development Provide heat and energy Carry fat-soluble vitamins (A, D, E, and K) to body cells
Proteins	Build and repair body tissue Provide heat and energy Help produce antibodies
Vitamins	Regulate body functions Build and repair body tissue
Minerals	Regulate body functions Build and repair body tissue
Water	Carries nutrients and wastes to and from body cells Regulates body functions

Cellulose is the fibrous, indigestible form of plant carbohydrate. It is important because it provides bulk in the digestive tract and causes regular bowel movements. The best sources of cellulose are bran, whole-grain cereals, and fibrous fruits and vegetables.

LIPIDS (FATS)

Lipids, commonly called **fats** and oils, are organic compounds. Three of the most common lipids found in both food and the human body are *triglycerides* (fats and fatty acids), *phospholipids* (lecithin), and *sterols* (cholesterol). Lipids also are made of carbon, hydrogen, and oxygen, but they contain more oxygen than carbohydrates do. Fats provide the most concentrated form of energy but are a higher calorie option source of energy than carbohydrates. Fats also maintain body temperature by providing insulation, cushion organs and bones, aid in the absorption of fat-soluble vitamins, and provide flavor to meals. The main sources of fats include butter, margarine, oils, cream, fatty meats, cheeses, and egg yolks.

Fats are also classified as saturated or polyunsaturated. *Saturated fats* are usually solid at room temperature and are found in animal-based foods. Examples include the fats in meats, eggs, whole milk, cream, butter, and cheeses. *Polyunsaturated fats* are usually soft or oily at room temperature and are found in plant-based foods. Examples include vegetable oils, margarines and other products made from vegetable oils, fish, and peanuts. One type of polyunsaturated fat that seems to decrease the risk of coronary artery disease is *omega-3 fatty acid*. It is found in fatty fish such as salmon, tuna, trout, mackerel, sardines, and herring.

Cholesterol is a sterol lipid found in body cells and animal products. It is used in the production of steroid hormones, vitamin D, and bile acids. Cholesterol is also a component of cell membranes. Common sources are egg yolks, fatty meats, shellfish, butter, cream, cheeses, whole milk, and organ meats (liver, kidney, and brains). In addition, cholesterol is synthesized (manufactured) by the liver. Cholesterol is transported in the bloodstream mainly by two carrier molecules called *lipoproteins*. They are known as HDL and LDL, or high-density and low-density lipoprotein. HDL, commonly called "good" cholesterol, tends to transport cholesterol back to the liver and prevents plaque from accumulating on the walls of arteries. LDL, commonly called "bad" cholesterol, tends to contribute to plaque buildup, and an excess amount leads to atherosclerosis. Consequently, it is advisable to limit the intake of foods that contain fats from animal sources.

PROTEINS

Proteins are the basic components of all body cells. They are essential for building and repairing tissue, regulating body functions, producing antibodies that help prevent infection and disease, and providing energy and heat. They are made of carbon, hydrogen, oxygen, and nitrogen, and some also contain sulfur, phosphorus, iron, and iodine.

Proteins are made up of 22 "building blocks" called *amino acids*. Nine of these amino acids are essential to life. The proteins that contain all nine essential amino acids are called *complete proteins*. The best sources of complete proteins are animal foods such as meats, fish, poultry, milk, cheeses, and eggs. Proteins that contain any of the remaining 13 amino acids and some of the nine essential amino acids are called *incomplete proteins*. Sources of incomplete proteins are usually plant foods such as cereals, soybeans, dry beans, peas, corn, and nuts. Choosing plant foods carefully can provide a mixture of amino acids from incomplete proteins that contain all the essential amino acids. It is important for a vegetarian to select foods that meet these dietary needs.

VITAMINS

Vitamins are organic compounds that are essential to life. They are important for metabolism, tissue building, and regulation of body processes. They allow the body to use the energy provided by carbohydrates, fats, and proteins. Only small amounts of vitamins are required, and a well-balanced diet usually provides the required vitamins. An excess amount of vitamins or a deficiency of vitamins can cause poor health.

Some vitamins are **antioxidants**, organic molecules that help protect the body from harmful chemicals called *free radicals*. In the body, oxygen used during metabolism causes free radicals to form. Free radicals can damage tissues, cells, and even genes in the same way that oxygen causes metals to rust or apples to become brown. Research indicates that free radicals can lead to the development of chronic diseases such as cancer, heart disease, and arthritis. Antioxidants, found mainly in fruits and vegetables, deactivate the free radicals and prevent them from damaging body cells. The main antioxidant vitamins are vitamins A, C, and E.

Vitamins are usually classified as water soluble or fat soluble. *Water-soluble* vitamins dissolve in water; are not normally stored in the body; and are easily destroyed by cooking, air, and light. *Fat-soluble* vitamins dissolve in fat; can be stored in the body; and are not easily destroyed by cooking, air, and light. Some of the vitamins along with their sources and functions are listed in **Table 11–2**.

MINERALS

Minerals are inorganic (nonliving) elements found in all body tissues. They regulate body fluids, assist in various body functions, contribute to growth, and aid in building tissues. Some minerals—such as selenium, zinc, copper, and manganese—are antioxidants. **Table 11–3** lists some of the minerals essential to life, their sources, and their main functions.

WATER

Water is found in all body tissues. It is essential for the digestion (breakdown) of food, makes up most of the blood plasma and cytoplasm of cells, helps body tissues absorb nutrients, and helps move waste material through the body. Total daily intake of water includes water that is found in all foods and beverages. Dietary guidelines state that thirst should be the main indicator of how much water an individual drinks. High external temperatures and a great amount of exercise or physical activity also increase the need for water. A general guideline is that the average person should drink six to eight glasses of water each day to provide the body with the water it needs.

checkpoint

1. List the six (6) groups of essential nutrients.
2. According to general guidelines, how much water should the average person drink a day?

11:3 UTILIZATION OF NUTRIENTS

Before the body is able to use nutrients, it must break down the foods that are eaten to obtain the nutrients and then absorb them into the circulatory system. These processes are called *digestion* and *absorption* (**Figure 11–2**). The actual use of the nutrients by the body is called *metabolism*. These processes are discussed in greater detail in Section 7:11 of this textbook.

DIGESTION

Digestion is the process by which the body breaks down food into smaller parts, changes the food chemically, and moves the food through the digestive system.

TABLE 11–2 Vitamins

Vitamins	Best Sources	Functions
Fat-Soluble Vitamins		
Vitamin A (Retinol)	Liver, fatty fish Butter, margarine Whole milk, cream, cheese Egg yolks Leafy green and yellow vegetables	Growth and development Health of eyes Structure and function of the cells of the skin and mucous membranes Antioxidant to protect cells from free radicals
Vitamin D (Calciferol)	Sunshine (stimulates production in skin) Fatty fish, liver Egg yolks Butter, cream, fortified milk	Growth Regulates calcium and phosphorous absorption and metabolism Builds and maintains bones and teeth
Vitamin E (Tocopherol)	Vegetable oils, butter, margarine Peanuts Egg yolks Dark green leafy vegetables Soybeans and wheat germ	Necessary for protection of cell structure, especially red blood cells and epithelial cells Antioxidant to inhibit breakdown of vitamin A and some unsaturated fatty acids
Vitamin K	Spinach, kale, cabbage, broccoli Liver Soybean oil Cereals	Normal clotting of blood Formation of prothrombin
Water-Soluble Vitamins		
Thiamine (B$_1$)	Enriched breads and cereals Liver, heart, kidney, lean pork Potatoes, legumes	Carbohydrate metabolism Promotes normal appetite and digestion Normal function of nervous system
Riboflavin (B$_2$)	Milk, cheese, yogurt, eggs Enriched breads and cereals Dark green leafy vegetables Liver, kidney, heart, fish	Carbohydrate, fat, and protein metabolism Health of mouth tissue Healthy eyes
Niacin (Nicotinic Acid, B$_3$)	Meats (especially organ meats) Poultry and fish Enriched breads and cereals Peanuts and legumes	Carbohydrate, fat, and protein metabolism Healthy skin, nerves, and digestive tract
Pantothenic Acid (B$_5$)	Organ meats and poultry Broccoli and kale Avocados Whole grain cereals	Metabolism of energy Production of hormones and cholesterol
Pyridoxine (B$_6$)	Liver, kidney, pork Poultry and fish Enriched breads and cereals	Protein synthesis and metabolism Production of antibodies
Biotin (B$_7$)	Liver and organ meats Egg yolks Milk Whole grain cereals	Healthy bones and hair Metabolism of energy Synthesis of niacin
Vitamin B$_{12}$ (Cobalamin)	Liver, kidney, muscle meats, seafood Milk, cheese Eggs	Metabolism of proteins Production of healthy red blood cells Maintains nerve tissue
Vitamin C (Ascorbic Acid)	Citrus fruits, pineapple Melons, berries, tomatoes Cabbage, broccoli, green peppers	Healthy gums Aids in wound healing Aids in absorption of iron Formation of collagen
Folic Acid (Folacin, Folate, B$_9$)	Green leafy vegetables Citrus fruits Organ meats, liver Whole-grain cereals, yeast	Protein metabolism Maturation of red blood cells Formation of hemoglobin Synthesis of DNA Reduces risk for neural tube defect (spina bifida) in fetus—important for pregnant women to consume recommended daily amount

TABLE 11–3 Minerals

Minerals	Best Sources	Functions
Calcium (Ca)	Milk and milk products Cheese Salmon and sardines Some dark green leafy vegetables	Develops/maintains bones and teeth Clotting of the blood Normal heart and muscle action Nerve function
Phosphorus (P)	Milk and cheese Meat, poultry, fish Nuts, legumes Whole-grain cereals	Develops/maintains bones and teeth Maintains blood acid–base balance Metabolism of carbohydrates, fats, and proteins Constituent of body cells
Magnesium (Mg)	Meat, seafood Nuts and legumes Milk and milk products Cereal grains Fresh green vegetables	Constituent of bones, muscles, and red blood cells Healthy muscles and nerves Metabolism of carbohydrates and fats
Sodium (Na)	Salt Meat and fish Poultry and eggs Milk, cheese	Fluid balance, acid–base balance Regulates muscles and nerves Glucose (sugar) absorption
Potassium (K)	Meat Milk and milk products Vegetables Oranges, bananas, prunes, raisins Cereals	Fluid balance Regular heart rhythm Cell metabolism Proper nerve function Regulates contraction of muscles
Chlorine (Cl) (Chloride)	Salt Meat, fish, poultry Milk, eggs	Fluid balance Acid–base balance Formation of hydrochloric acid
Sulfur (S)	Meat, poultry, fish Eggs	Healthy skin, hair, and nails Activates energy-producing enzymes
Iron (Fe)	Liver, muscle meats Dried fruits Egg yolks Enriched breads and cereals Dark green leafy vegetables	Formation of hemoglobin in red blood cells Part of cell enzymes Aids in production of energy
Iodine (I)	Saltwater fish Iodized salt	Formation of hormones in thyroid gland Regulates basal metabolic rate
Copper (Cu)	Liver, organ meats, seafood Nuts, legumes Whole-grain cereals	Utilization of iron Component of enzymes Formation of hemoglobin in red blood cells
Fluorine (Fl) (Fluoride)	Fluoridated water Fish, meat, seafood	Healthy teeth and bones
Zinc (Zn)	Seafood, especially oysters Eggs Milk and milk products	Component of enzymes and insulin Essential for growth and wound healing
Selenium (Se)	Organ meats Seafood	Metabolism of fat Acts as an antioxidant

There are two types of digestive action: mechanical and chemical. During *mechanical digestion*, food is broken down by the teeth and moved through the digestive tract by a process called **peristalsis**, a rhythmic, wavelike motion of the muscles. During *chemical digestion*, food is mixed with digestive juices secreted by the mouth, stomach, small intestine, and pancreas. The digestive juices contain enzymes, which break down the food chemically so the nutrients can be absorbed into the blood.

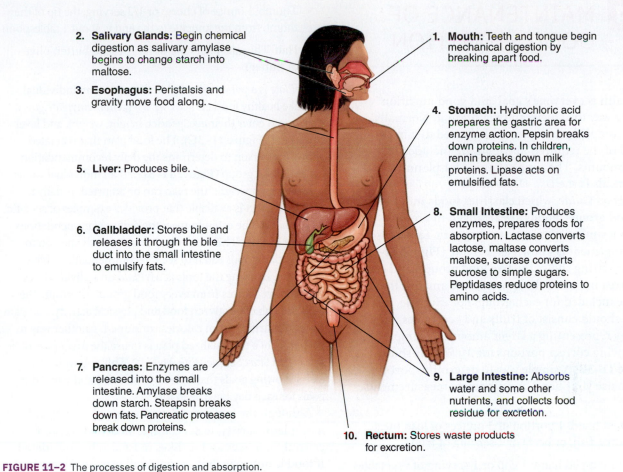

2. Salivary Glands: Begin chemical digestion as salivary amylase begins to change starch into maltose.

3. Esophagus: Peristalsis and gravity move food along.

5. Liver: Produces bile.

6. Gallbladder: Stores bile and releases it through the bile duct into the small intestine to emulsify fats.

7. Pancreas: Enzymes are released into the small intestine. Amylase breaks down starch. Steapsin breaks down fats. Pancreatic proteases break down proteins.

1. Mouth: Teeth and tongue begin mechanical digestion by breaking apart food.

4. Stomach: Hydrochloric acid prepares the gastric area for enzyme action. Pepsin breaks down proteins. In children, rennin breaks down milk proteins. Lipase acts on emulsified fats.

8. Small Intestine: Produces enzymes, prepares foods for absorption. Lactase converts lactose, maltase converts maltose, sucrase converts sucrose to simple sugars. Peptidases reduce proteins to amino acids.

9. Large Intestine: Absorbs water and some other nutrients, and collects food residue for excretion.

10. Rectum: Stores waste products for excretion.

FIGURE 11–2 The processes of digestion and absorption.

ABSORPTION

After the food is digested, absorption occurs. **Absorption** is the process in which blood or lymph capillaries pick up the digested nutrients. The nutrients are then carried by the circulatory system to every cell in the body. Most absorption occurs in the small intestine, but water, salts, and some vitamins are absorbed in the large intestine.

METABOLISM

After nutrients have been absorbed and carried to the body cells, **metabolism** occurs. This is the process in which nutrients are used by the cells for building tissue, providing energy, and regulating various body functions.

During this process, nutrients are combined with oxygen, and energy and heat are released. Energy is required for voluntary work, such as swimming or housecleaning, and for involuntary work, such as breathing and digestion. The rate at which the body uses energy just for maintaining its own tissue, without doing any voluntary work, is called the **basal metabolic rate**, or **BMR**. The body needs energy continuously, so it stores some nutrients for future use. These stored nutrients are used to provide energy when food intake is not adequate for energy needs.

checkpoint

1. Define *peristalsis*.
2. Where in the body does most of the absorption of nutrients occur?

MAINTENANCE OF GOOD NUTRITION

- Thumb: 1 ounce of cheese or 1/2 serving; the tip of the thumb from the knuckle to the end is about 1 tablespoon
- Half-Thumb: 1 serving of fat (peanut butter, olive oil, or butter)

Good health is everyone's goal, and good nutrition is the best way to achieve and maintain it. Normally, this is accomplished by eating a balanced diet in which all of the required nutrients are included in correct amounts. The simplest guide for planning healthy meals is the *U.S. Department of Agriculture (USDA) Food Guide*, which classifies foods into five major food groups. Foods are arranged in groups containing similar nutrients, as shown in **Table 11–4**. This arrangement is known as *MyPlate* (**Figure 11–3A**). The place setting shows the five food groups, and each colored area indicates the approximate amount that should be included for each group. For example, half of the plate should consist of fruits and vegetables, with vegetables representing a larger amount. A sample meal showing correct portions for *MyPlate* is shown in **Figure 11–3B**. A simple way to determine portion sizes is to use your hand. Approximate measurements include:

- Palm of hand: 1 portion or 3 ounces of lean meat (poultry, fish, or beef) or 1 serving of fruit
- Fist or cupped hand: 1 cup or 1 serving of vegetables or starchy carbohydrates (pasta, potatoes, or rice)

MyPlate is a personalized plan that allows an individual to make healthy food choices. At *www.choosemyplate.gov*, a person can enter their age, gender, height, weight, and level of exercise (**Figure 11–3C**). The food plan that is created allows the person to determine the daily recommendation for each food group (**Figure 11–3D**). If an individual wants to lose or gain weight, the plan can be adjusted. A daily food plan worksheet is available that provides examples of specific foods that can be eaten to meet the daily recommendations (**Figure 11–3E**). This worksheet also allows the person to keep track of foods eaten to see if recommendations have been met. By using the tools at *MyPlate*, an individual can make smart choices from every food group, determine the required balance between food and physical activity, and gain optimal nutrition from calories consumed. Another way to keep tract of a personalized plan is to use the *MyPlate* mobile app called *Start Simple With MyPlate*. This app will send alerts showing goals that have been selected and when the goals for each day have been met.

Although the major food groups are a key to healthy meal plans, variety, taste, color, aroma, texture, and general food likes and dislikes must also be considered. If food is not appealing, people will usually not eat it even though it is healthy.

TABLE 11–4 Nutrients in Food

Food Group	Average Recommended Portion Size	Nutrient Content
Grains: Breads, Cereals, Rice, and Pasta	1 slice bread 1/2 bagel or English muffin 1/2 cup cooked cereal 1/2 cup cooked pasta or rice 1 cup dry cereal	Carbohydrates; phosphorus; magnesium; potassium; iron; vitamins B and K and folic acid
Vegetables	1 cup raw leafy vegetables 1/2 cup cooked vegetables 3/4 cup vegetable juice	Carbohydrates; iron; calcium; potassium; magnesium; vitamins A, B, C, E, and K and folic acid
Fruits	1 medium-sized piece of fruit 1/2 cup canned/cooked fruit 1/4 cup dried fruit 1 cup fruit juice 1 cup fresh fruit	Carbohydrates; potassium; vitamin C and folic acid
Dairy: Milk, Milk Products, Yogurt, and Cheese	1 cup milk, yogurt, pudding 1 1/2 ounces cheese 1 cup cottage cheese 1 cup ice cream	Protein; carbohydrate; fat; calcium; potassium; sodium; magnesium; phosphorus; vitamins A, B_{12}, D, biotin, and riboflavin
Protein: Meats, Fish, Poultry, Dry Beans, Eggs, and Nuts	1 ounce meat, fish, or poultry 1/4 cup dry beans 1/2 cup cooked beans 1 egg 1 tablespoon peanut butter 1/2 ounce nuts	Proteins; fats; iron; sulfur; copper; iodine; sodium; magnesium; zinc; potassium; phosphorus; chlorine; fluorine; vitamins A, B, and D

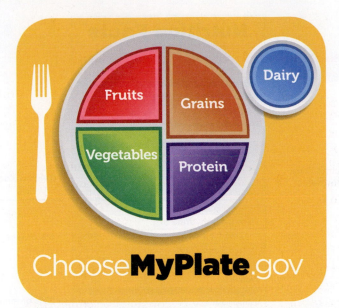

FIGURE 11-3A *MyPlate* provides the guidelines for a healthier you.
Courtesy of the USDA. USDA does not endorse any products, services, or organizations.

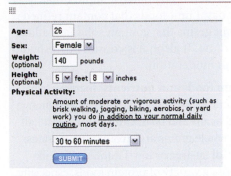

FIGURE 11-3C By using the *Daily Food Plan* on *www.choosemyplate. gov*, an individual can find personal recommendations for recommended daily food intake by entering their height, weight, age, and physical activity level. Courtesy of the USDA. USDA does not endorse any products, services, or organizations.

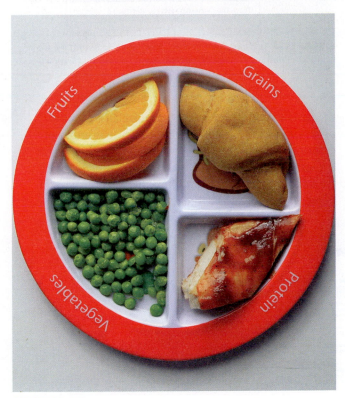

FIGURE 11-3B A sample meal following *MyPlate* guidelines shows the correct portion sizes. Courtesy of Superhealthykids.com

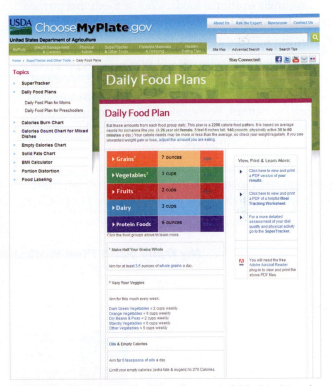

FIGURE 11-3D The *Daily Food Plan* allows an individual to determine daily recommended requirements for a healthy diet. Courtesy of the USDA. USDA does not endorse any products, services, or organizations.

Sound and sensible nutritional principles can be found in the booklet published by the U.S. Department of Agriculture (USDA) entitled *Dietary Guidelines for Americans*, or on the Internet at *www.dietaryguidelines. gov*. Some guidelines discussed in greater detail in the booklet or on the Internet include:

- **Balance calories to manage weight**: Improve eating and physical activity behaviors to reduce obesity.

Control total calorie intake to manage body weight. Increase physical activity. Maintain an appropriate caloric balance during each life stage.

- **Reduce certain foods and food components**: Reduce daily sodium (salt) intake to less than 2,300 milligrams (mg) and to less than 1,500 mg for people who are age 51 and older and for those of any age who have hypertension, diabetes, or chronic kidney disease. Consume less than 10 percent of calories from saturated fats. Keep trans-fatty acid consumption as low as possible. Reduce the calories from solid fats and added sugars. Consume less than 10 percent of calories from added sugars, limiting sugar to about 50 grams or approximately 12 teaspoons per day. Limit foods that contain refined grains, and limit grains that contain solid fats, added sugars, and sodium. If alcohol is consumed, it should be consumed in moderation.

- **Increase certain foods and nutrients**: Increase fruit and vegetable intake, especially dark green and orange vegetables, and beans and peas. Consume at least half of all grains as whole grains and avoid refined grains. Increase intake of fat-free or low-fat milk and milk products. Choose a variety of protein foods, especially seafood, lean meat, poultry, eggs, beans, soy products, and unsalted nuts and seeds. Limit red and processed meats. Eat unsaturated fats found in fish, nuts, and vegetable oils in place of saturated fats that occur naturally in animal foods. Choose foods that provide more potassium, dietary fiber, calcium, and vitamin D.

- **Build healthy eating patterns**: Select an eating pattern that meets nutrient needs and appropriate calorie levels. Account for all foods and beverages consumed and assess how they fit within a healthy eating pattern. Follow all safety recommendations when preparing and eating foods to reduce the risk of foodborne illnesses.

It is also important to read food labels to find the facts you need to know about the foods you eat. Most foods have a Nutrition Facts label (**Figure 11–4**). Check

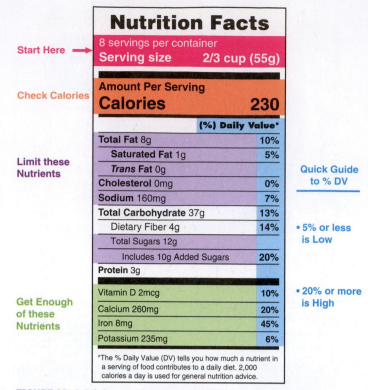

FIGURE 11–4 It is important to check food labels to determine the caloric and nutrient content of the food. Adapted from the US Food and Drug Administration

the label to determine the serving size and number of servings in the container. Evaluate the number of calories per serving to determine whether the food is a low- or high-calorie food. Calculate the amount of fat and try to keep total fat intake between 20 and 35 percent of total caloric intake. Look at the daily value

My Daily Food Plan Worksheet

Check how you did today and set a goal to aim for tomorrow

Write in Your Food Choices for Today	Food Group	Tip	Based on a 2200 Calorie pattern. Your Goals Are:	Match Your Food Choices with Each Food Group	Estimate Your Total
	GRAINS	Make at least half your grains whole grains	**7 ounce equivalents** (1 ounce equivalent is about 1 slice bread; 1 ounce ready-to-eat cereal; or ½ cup cooked rice, pasta, or cereal)		ounce equivalents
	VEGETABLES	Aim for variety every day; pick vegetables from several subgroups: Dark green, red & orange, beans & peas, starchy, and other veggies	**3 cups** (1 cup is 1 cup raw or cooked vegetables, 2 cups leafy salad greens, or 1 cup 100% vegetable juice)		cups
	FRUITS	Select fresh, frozen, canned, and dried fruit more often than juice	**2 cups** (1 cup is 1 cup raw or cooked fruit, ½ cup dried fruit, or 1 cup 100% fruit juice)		cups
	DAIRY	Include fat-free and low-fat dairy foods every day	**3 cups** (1 cup is 1 cup milk, yogurt, or fortified soy beverage; 1½ ounces natural cheese; or 2 ounces processed cheese)		cups
	PROTEIN FOODS	Aim for variety—choose seafood, lean meat & poultry, beans, peas, nuts, and seeds each week	**6 ounce equivalents** (1 ounce equivalent is 1 ounce lean meat, poultry, or seafood; 1 egg; 1 Tbsp peanut butter; ¼ cup cooked beans or peas; or ½ ounce nuts or seeds)		ounce equivalents
	PHYSICAL ACTIVITY	Be active every day. Choose activities that you like and fit into your life.	Be physically active for at least **150 minutes** each week.	Some foods and drinks, such as sodas, cakes, cookies, donuts, ice cream, and candy, are high in fats and sugars. Limit your intake of these.	minutes

How did you do today? ☐ Great ☐ So-So ☐ Not so Great

My food goal for tomorrow is: _____

My activity goal for tomorrow is: _____

FIGURE 11–3E The *Daily Food Plan Worksheet* provides examples of foods that meet the daily recommended requirements and allows an individual to keep a record of foods consumed. Courtesy of the USDA. USDA does not endorse any products, services, or organizations.

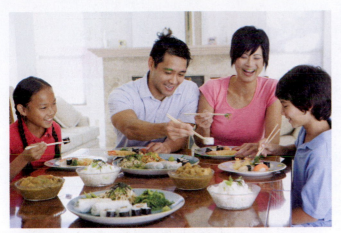

FIGURE 11–5 Cultural or religious beliefs influence food preferences and affect nutrition. © Monkey Business Images/Shutterstock.com

percentage for each nutrient listed to determine whether the food is nutritious and worth eating. Avoid empty calories or high-caloric foods with no vitamins, minerals, carbohydrates, and/or proteins.

Food habits also affect nutrition. Habits are sometimes based on cultural or religious beliefs. Different cultures may have certain food preferences (**Figure 11–5**). Some religions require certain dietary restrictions that must be observed. Of course, not all people follow their religions customs. However, if an individual states that they cannot eat certain foods because of a cultural or religious belief, a health care provider must respect this belief and try to find an appropriate replacement.

Food habits should be evaluated using the five major food groups as a guide. When habits do need to be changed in order to improve nutrition, the person making the suggestions must use tact, patience, and imagination and try to find compromise. Many food habits are formed during youth, and changing them is a difficult and slow process.

checkpoint

1. How many food groups are there? Name them.
2. What body part can you use to help determine portion size?

11:5 WEIGHT MANAGEMENT

Math

Good nutrition and adequate exercise allow an individual to maintain a body weight that is in proportion to body height. Most research has shown that the best indication of an individual's health status is body mass index. **Body mass index (BMI)** is a calculation that measures weight in relation to height

and correlates this with body fat. It is determined by dividing a person's weight in kilograms by height in meters squared. A graphic chart showing BMI ranges is the easiest way to determine BMI (**Figure 11–6**). A calculator to determine BMI is also available at the National Institutes of Health (NIH) Internet site for the National Heart, Lung, and Blood Institute, *www.nhlbi.nih.gov/health/educational/ lose_wt/BMI/bmi-m.htm*. The ideal range is 18.5 to 24.9. A BMI less than 18.5 indicates the individual is underweight. A BMI from 25 to 29.9 indicates the individual is overweight and has increased health risks. A BMI of 30 and above indicates obesity and much higher health risks.

UNDERWEIGHT AND OVERWEIGHT

Weight management is used to achieve and maintain the desired body weight. The major conditions that occur due to poor nutrition and improper exercise are underweight, overweight, and obesity.

Underweight is a body weight that is 10 to 15 percent less than the average recommended weight for a person's height, or a BMI less than 18.5. Underweight individuals are much more likely to have nutritional deficiencies. Causes can include an inadequate supply of or intake of food, excessive exercise, severe infections, and diseases and/or treatments that cause anorexia (lack of appetite) such as chemotherapy for cancer. However, the most common cause is eating disorders, which can lead to severe malnutrition and even death. Individuals who develop eating disorders may start by dieting to lose weight but then become obsessed with controlling the amount of food they consume. A poor self-image, emotional stress, unsatisfactory social relationships, peer pressure, the desire to resemble slim fashion models, obsessive-compulsive personality traits, an extreme drive for perfectionism, and even genetic influences may cause an individual to develop eating disorders. Eating disorders are more common in females and often develop during adolescence or early adulthood. Some of the most common eating disorders include:

- **Anorexia nervosa**: commonly called *anorexia*; a psychological disorder in which a person drastically reduces food intake or refuses to eat at all

- **Bulimia**: a psychological disorder in which a person alternately binges (eats excessively) and then fasts, or refuses to eat at all; in some cases, a person will exercise excessively after binging

- **Bulimarexia**: a psychological disorder in which a person alternately binges and then induces vomiting or uses laxatives to get rid of food that has been eaten

Physical symptoms of eating disorders include excessive weight loss, extreme weakness and fatigue, irregular heart rhythms, low blood pressure, amenorrhea (absence

Body Mass Index Table

Height (inches)	Normal						Overweight					Obese										Extreme Obesity														
BMI	19	20	21	22	23	24	25	26	27	28	29	30	31	32	33	34	35	36	37	38	39	40	41	42	43	44	45	46	47	48	49	50	51	52	53	54
													Body Weight (pounds)																							
58	91	96	100	105	110	115	119	124	129	134	138	143	148	153	158	162	167	172	177	181	186	191	196	201	205	210	215	220	224	229	234	239	244	248	253	258
59	94	99	104	109	114	119	124	128	133	138	143	148	153	158	163	168	173	178	183	188	193	198	203	208	212	217	222	227	232	237	242	247	252	257	262	267
60	97	102	107	112	118	123	128	133	138	143	148	153	158	163	168	174	179	184	189	194	199	204	209	215	220	225	230	235	240	245	250	255	261	266	271	276
61	100	106	111	116	122	127	132	137	143	148	153	158	164	169	174	180	185	190	195	201	206	211	217	222	227	232	238	243	248	254	259	264	269	275	280	285
62	104	109	115	120	126	131	136	142	147	153	158	164	169	175	180	186	191	196	202	207	213	218	224	229	235	240	246	251	256	262	267	273	278	284	289	295
63	107	113	118	124	130	135	141	146	152	158	163	169	175	180	186	191	197	203	208	214	220	225	231	237	242	248	254	259	265	270	278	282	287	293	299	304
64	110	116	122	128	134	140	145	151	157	163	169	174	180	186	192	197	204	209	215	221	227	232	238	244	250	256	262	267	273	279	285	291	296	302	308	314
65	114	120	126	132	138	144	150	156	162	168	174	180	186	192	198	204	210	216	222	228	234	240	246	252	258	264	270	276	282	288	294	300	306	312	318	324
66	118	124	130	136	142	148	155	161	167	173	179	186	192	198	204	210	216	223	229	235	241	247	253	260	266	272	278	284	291	297	303	309	315	322	328	334
67	121	127	134	140	146	153	159	166	172	178	185	191	198	204	211	217	223	230	236	242	249	255	261	268	274	280	287	293	299	306	312	319	325	331	338	344
68	125	131	138	144	151	158	164	171	177	184	190	197	203	210	216	223	230	236	243	249	256	262	269	276	282	289	295	302	308	315	322	328	335	341	348	354
69	128	135	142	149	155	162	169	176	182	189	196	203	209	216	223	230	236	243	250	257	263	270	277	284	291	297	304	311	318	324	331	338	345	351	358	365
70	132	139	146	153	160	167	174	181	188	195	202	209	216	222	229	236	243	250	257	264	271	278	285	292	299	306	313	320	327	334	341	348	355	362	369	376
71	136	143	150	157	165	172	179	186	193	200	208	215	222	229	236	243	250	257	265	272	279	286	293	301	308	315	322	329	338	343	351	358	365	372	379	386
72	140	147	154	162	169	177	184	191	199	206	213	221	228	235	242	250	258	265	272	279	287	294	302	309	316	324	331	338	346	353	361	368	375	383	390	397
73	144	151	159	166	174	182	189	197	204	212	219	227	235	242	250	257	265	272	280	288	295	302	310	318	325	333	340	348	355	363	371	378	386	393	401	408
74	148	155	163	171	179	186	194	202	210	218	225	233	241	249	256	264	272	280	287	295	303	311	319	326	334	342	350	358	365	373	381	389	396	404	412	420
75	152	160	168	176	184	192	200	208	216	224	232	240	248	256	264	272	279	287	295	303	311	319	327	335	343	351	359	367	375	383	391	399	407	415	423	431
76	156	164	172	180	189	197	205	213	221	230	238	246	254	263	271	279	287	295	304	312	320	328	336	344	353	361	369	377	385	394	402	410	418	426	435	443

FIGURE 11–6 Body mass index (BMI) helps individuals determine healthy weight ranges.

of menstruation), thin or brittle hair that falls out, an intolerance to cold, dehydration, constipation, dry skin, metabolic disturbances, and osteoporosis. Individuals with a disorder may refuse to eat or lie about eating habits, monitor weight constantly, exercise excessively, withdraw from social situations, use laxatives or diet aids frequently, and have a distorted body image. Death can occur if the condition is not treated. Treatments for eating disorders include medical intervention for severe physical symptoms such as irregular heart rhythms and metabolic disturbances, and psychotherapy or counseling to allow the individual to develop behavioral patterns that maintain a healthy weight.

Overweight is a body weight that is 10 to 20 percent greater than the average recommended weight for a person's height, or a BMI from 25 to 29.9. **Obesity** is excessive body weight 20 percent or more above the average recommended weight, or a BMI equal to or greater than 30. Obesity has become a major health concern in the United States according to the following statistics provided by the Centers for Disease Control and Prevention (CDC):

- More than four-tenths, or 42.4 percent, of adults are obese. This means that more than 140 million adults in the United States are obese.

- More than 18.5 percent of 13.7 million young people aged 2–19 are obese.

- Health problems associated with overweight and obesity have a significant economic impact on the U.S. health care system, with current estimates of expenses ranging from $176 billion to more than $210 billion per year.

The main causes of obesity are excessive calorie consumption and inadequate physical activity. Genetic, psychological, and biochemical (metabolic) factors can also contribute to this condition. Treatment involves modifying eating habits and increasing physical activity. In more severe cases, medical intervention with medications, counseling, and even surgery may be necessary. If obesity is not controlled, an individual is at high risk for development of hypertension, diabetes mellitus, coronary heart disease, high cholesterol, cerebrovascular accident (stroke), osteoarthritis, gallbladder disease, breathing problems such as sleep apnea, certain types of cancer such as breast and colon cancer, and many other similar conditions. Research has also shown that obesity decreases life span and causes many early deaths.

Following the principles shown on *MyPlate* and in the USDA dietary guidelines is the easiest way to manage weight. Every person should become familiar with these principles and make every attempt to follow them on a daily basis. Even though poor food habits are hard to break, it can be done if an individual is motivated to change their behavior.

MEASURING FOOD ENERGY

Foods vary in the amount of energy they contain. For example, a candy bar provides more energy than an apple does. When the body metabolizes nutrients to produce energy, heat is also released. The amount of heat produced during metabolism is the way the energy content of food is measured. This heat is measured by a unit called a **calorie**. The number of calories in a certain food is known as that food's *caloric value*. Carbohydrates and proteins provide four calories per gram. Fat provides nine calories per gram. Vitamins, minerals, and water do not provide any calories.

An individual's caloric requirement is the number of calories needed by the body during a 24-hour period. Caloric requirements vary from person to person, depending on activity, age, size, sex, physical condition, and climate. The amount of physical activity or exercise is usually the main factor determining caloric requirement because energy used must be replaced. An individual who wants to gain weight can decrease activity and increase caloric intake. An individual who wants to lose weight can increase activity and decrease caloric intake.

MANAGING WEIGHT

Most people know that maintaining desired body weight can lead to a longer and healthier life. For this reason, people try many different types of diets to lose weight and/or remain healthy. Examples of some popular diets are shown in **Table 11–5**. Research has shown that even though these diets might be beneficial or lead to weight loss, they usually do not allow an individual to maintain their weight when the diet is no longer used. Most fad diets require eating specific foods, limiting certain food groups, eating large amounts of one type of food, or using liquid supplements in place of food. When individuals resume their normal eating habits, the weight that was lost is quickly regained.

The best method for weight control is to make desired changes slowly. Research has shown that gradual weight loss with a change in habits is much healthier and more likely to be sustained. For example, a person never exercises but knows that it is important. Initially, the person may walk at a slow pace for 15 minutes every day. Gradually, the time and rate can be increased until the person is walking at a brisk pace for 30 minutes 5 days a week. At the same time that the amount of exercise increases, the number of calories consumed must change.

Before starting any diet or weight management plan, a physician should be consulted. The physician may perform a physical examination, order blood or other laboratory tests to check for diseases that could affect weight, run an electrocardiogram, or order a stress test to determine cardiovascular fitness. The physician can then recommend a nutrition plan and exercise program that is customized to the individual's needs.

TABLE 11–5 Popular Diets

Name of Diet	Basic Principles
Atkins Diet	Based on a very low carbohydrate intake that avoids foods with refined flour or sugar and encourages the use of lean protein and low-starch vegetables; divided into four phases, with each phase becoming less restrictive
DASH Diet (Dietary Approaches to Stop Hypertension)	Focuses on eating low-fat dairy, fruits, vegetables, lean meats, and whole grains while limiting salty foods and processed foods; promoted as a heart-healthy diet to lower hypertension (high blood pressure)
Gluten-free Diet	Used as treatment for individuals with celiac disease or a sensitivity to gluten; others promote it as a diet to improve health, lose weight, and increase energy; eliminates gluten-grains such as wheat, barley, rye, and triticale; allows fruits, vegetables, beans, nuts, eggs, lean meats, fish, poultry, and most low-fat dairy products
Ketogenic Diet	Focuses on eating a high-fat, adequate protein, but very low-carbohydrate diet to lose weight; forces body into ketosis where fats and proteins are burned for energy instead of carbohydrates; encourages avoiding foods such as low-fat dairy, most fruits, grains, pasta, rice, starchy vegetables, beans, and foods high in sugar or sweeteners
Mediterranean Diet	Promoted as a heart-healthy diet that emphasizes vegetables, fruits, whole grains, beans, nuts, fish, and olive oil; encourages moderate consumption of poultry, cheese, and eggs; suggests eating red meats and sweets only on special occasions
Nutrisystem Diet	Commercial diet that allows clients to choose prepared meals from a list; the number and types of meals are selected based on the client's body build and weight loss goal; meals stress healthy carbohydrates and lean proteins; more expensive than other diets
Paleo Diet	Also called the Caveman Diet because it concentrates on basic foods eaten by primitive humans; encourages eating fresh fruits and vegetables, seafood, lean meat, and healthy fats
Probiotic Diet	Encourages foods rich in probiotics or healthy bacteria; main sources are cultured foods such as yogurt and buttermilk, fermented vegetables such as pickled beets and sauerkraut, and microalgae or ocean-based plants such as chlorella and blue-green algae; promoted as a diet that can improve digestion, boost the immune system, and possibly reduce the risk of cancer
SlimFast Diet	Commercial diet that provides shakes and meal bars for two meals and two or three snacks each day; only one additional 500-calorie meal is eaten per day
South Beach Diet	Focuses on replacing bad carbohydrates and fats with good carbohydrates and fats; encourages eating lots of vegetables, fish, eggs, lean meats such as chicken, whole grains, and low-fat dairy products; divided into three phases, with each phase becoming less restrictive
Volumetrics Diet	Based on classifying foods into four density levels that range from low-density foods in level 1 such as fruits, vegetables, and nonfat milk to high-density foods in level 4 such as cookies, butter, and candy; encourages concentrating on foods in the lower density levels
Weight Watchers	Uses a point system to track foods eaten; encourages a balanced diet but stresses fruits, vegetables, lean meat, and low-fat dairy; provides group support to help an individual achieve their weight goal
Zone Diet	Stresses five to six meals with smaller quantities; suggests that each meal contains 40 percent carbohydrates, 30 percent protein, and 30 percent healthy fat

A general guideline for weight loss or gain is that 1 pound of body fat equals approximately 3,500 calories. To lose 1 pound, a decrease of 3,500 calories is required, either by consuming 3,500 fewer calories or by using 3,500 calories through increased exercise. To gain 1 pound, an increase of 3,500 calories is required. A general guideline to maintain weight is that a person consumes 15 calories per pound per day. For example, if a person weighs 120 pounds, maintaining this weight would require a daily intake of 15 × 120, or 1,800, calories daily. By decreasing caloric intake by 500 calories per day, a person would lose 1 pound per week (500 calories per day times 7 days equals 3,500 calories, or 1 pound of fat). By increasing caloric intake by 500 calories per day, a person would gain 1 pound per week. It is important to note that increasing or decreasing exercise along with controlling calorie intake is essential. Also, a slow, steady gain or loss of 1–2 pounds per week is an efficient and safe form of weight control.

The USDA *Dietary Guidelines* recommendations for managing weight include:

- Balance calories from foods and beverages with calories expended

- Prevent gradual weight gain by making small decreases in daily calories and small increases in physical activity

- Engage in at least 30 minutes or more of moderate-intensity physical activity most days of the week with a weekly goal of at least 150 minutes

- Consume less than 10 percent of calories from saturated fatty acids

- Keep daily total fat intake to between 20 and 35 percent of calories consumed

- Select lean, low-fat, or fat-free foods whenever possible

- Eat more fiber-rich fruits, vegetables, and whole grains

- Limit foods high in sugar and salt

Following these recommendations can help an individual obtain and maintain a healthy weight. This will help reduce the risk for heart disease, hypertension, diabetes mellitus, high cholesterol, osteoarthritis, certain cancers, and many other diseases. It will also allow the individual to enjoy a longer and healthier life span.

checkpoint

| **1.** What is the best method for weight control?

11:6 THERAPEUTIC DIETS

Therapeutic diets are modifications of the normal diet and are used to improve specific health conditions. They are normally prescribed by a doctor and planned by a dietitian. These diets may change the nutrients, caloric content, or texture of the normal diet. They may seem strange and even unpleasant to patients. In addition, a patient's appetite may be affected by anorexia (loss of appetite), weakness, illness, loneliness, self-pity, and other factors. Therefore, it is essential that the health care provider use patience and tact to convince the patient to eat the foods on the diet. An understanding of the purposes of the various diets will also help the health care provider give simple explanations to patients.

REGULAR DIET

A **regular diet** is a balanced diet usually used for the patient with no dietary restrictions. At times, it has a slightly reduced calorie content. Foods such as rich desserts, cream sauces, salad dressings, and fried foods may be decreased or omitted.

LIQUID DIETS

Liquid diets include both clear liquids and full liquids. Both are nutritionally inadequate and should be used only for short periods of time. All foods served must be liquid at body temperature. Foods included on the clear-liquid diet are mainly carbohydrates and water, including apple or grape juices, fat-free broths, plain gelatin, fruit ice, ginger ale, and tea or black coffee with sugar. The full-liquid diet includes the liquids allowed on the clear-liquid diet plus strained soups and cereals, fruit and vegetable juices, yogurt, hot cocoa, custard, ice cream, pudding, sherbet, milk, and eggnog. These diets may be used after surgery, for patients with acute infections or digestive problems, to replace fluids lost by vomiting or diarrhea, and before some X-rays of the digestive tract.

SOFT DIET

A **soft diet** is similar to the regular diet, but foods must require little chewing and be easy to digest. Foods to avoid include meat and shellfish with tough connective tissues (most meat is ground), coarse cereals, spicy foods, rich desserts, fried foods, raw fruits and vegetables, nuts, and coconut. This diet may be used following surgery or for patients who have infections, digestive disorders, dysphagia (difficulty in swallowing), or chewing problems. At times, if an individual cannot chew food or has dysphagia, a soft diet is *pureed* to create a thick liquid with more nutrients than a full-liquid diet can provide (**Figure 11–7**).

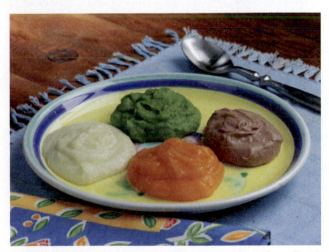

FIGURE 11–7 A pureed diet can provide more nutrients than a liquid diet if a patient cannot chew or has dysphagia. Courtesy of Polara Studios

DIABETIC DIET

A **diabetic diet** is used for patients with diabetes mellitus. In this condition, the body does not produce enough of the hormone insulin to metabolize carbohydrates. Patients frequently take insulin by injection. The diet is called a *carbohydrate-controlled diet* because patients must calculate the amount of carbohydrates in each meal. Usually approximately 40–60 percent of calories are from carbohydrates. In some cases, calorie levels are controlled in addition to the amount of carbohydrates. Sugar-heavy foods such as candy, soft drinks, desserts, cookies, syrup, honey, condensed milk, chewing gum, and jams and jellies are usually avoided.

CALORIE-CONTROLLED DIETS

Calorie-controlled diets include both low-calorie and high-calorie diets. Low-calorie diets are frequently used for patients who are overweight. High-calorie foods are either prohibited or very limited. Examples of such foods are butter, cream, whole milk, cream soups or gravies, sweet soft drinks, alcoholic beverages, salad dressings, fatty meats, candy, and rich desserts. High-calorie diets are used for patients who are underweight or have anorexia nervosa, hyperthyroidism (overactivity of thyroid gland), or cancer. Extra proteins and carbohydrates are included. High-bulk foods such as green salads, watermelon, and fibrous fruits are avoided because they fill up the patient too soon. High-fat foods such as fried foods, rich pastries, and cheesecake are avoided because they digest slowly and spoil the appetite.

LOW-CHOLESTEROL DIET

A **low-cholesterol diet** restricts foods that contain cholesterol and usually limits fats to less than 50 grams (g) daily. It is used for patients who have atherosclerosis and heart disease. Foods high in saturated fat—such as beef, liver, pork, lamb, egg yolks, cream cheese, natural cheeses, shellfish (crab, shrimp, lobster), and whole milk—are limited, as are coconut and palm oil products.

FAT-RESTRICTED DIETS

Fat-restricted diets, also called *low-fat diets*, usually limit fats to less than 50 grams (g) daily. Examples of foods to avoid include cream, whole milk, cheeses, fats, fatty meats, rich desserts, chocolate, nuts, coconut, fried foods, and salad dressings. Fat-restricted diets may be used for obese patients or patients who have gallbladder and liver disease or atherosclerosis.

SODIUM-RESTRICTED DIETS

Sodium-restricted diets are also called *low-sodium* or *low-salt diets*. Frequently, patients use low-sodium-diet lists that provide the amount of sodium present in a specific food. Patients should avoid or limit adding salt to food and avoid smoked meats or fish, processed foods, pickles, olives, sauerkraut, and some processed cheeses. This diet reduces salt intake for patients who have cardiovascular diseases (such as hypertension or congestive heart failure), kidney disease, and edema (retention of fluids).

PROTEIN DIETS

Protein diets include both low-protein and high-protein diets. Protein-rich foods include meats, fish, milk, cheeses, and eggs. These foods would be limited or decreased in low-protein diets and increased in high-protein diets. Low-protein diets are ordered for patients who have certain kidney or renal diseases and certain allergic conditions. High-protein diets may be ordered for children and adolescents, if growth is delayed; for pregnant or lactating (milk-producing) women; before and/or after surgery; and for patients suffering from burns, fevers, or infections.

BLAND DIET

A **bland diet** consists of easily digested foods that do not irritate the digestive tract. Foods to be avoided include coarse foods, fried foods, highly seasoned foods, pastries, candies, raw fruits and vegetables, alcoholic and carbonated beverages, smoked and salted meats or fish, nuts, olives, avocados, coconut, whole-grain breads and cereals, and usually coffee and tea. This diet is used for patients who have gastric (stomach) disorders, colitis, and other diseases of the digestive system.

FIBER DIETS

Fiber diets are usually classified as high fiber or low fiber. A high-fiber diet usually provides at least 30 grams (g) of fiber without seeds or nuts. It is used to stimulate activity in the digestive tract. A *low-fiber or low-residue* diet containing less than 10–15 grams of fiber per day eliminates or limits foods that are high in bulk and fiber. It is used for patients who have digestive and rectal diseases, such as colitis or diarrhea. Examples of high-fiber foods include raw fruits and vegetables, whole-grain breads and cereals, nuts, seeds, beans, peas, coconut, and fried foods.

OTHER DIETS

Other therapeutic diets that restrict or increase certain nutrients may also be ordered. The health care provider should always check the prescribed diet and ask questions if foods seem incorrect. Every effort should be made to include foods the patient likes if they are allowed on a particular diet. If a patient will not eat the foods on a prescribed therapeutic diet, the diet will not contribute to good nutrition.

check**point**

| **1.** What is the difference between a regular diet and a therapeutic diet?

PRACTICE: Go to the workbook and complete the assignment sheet for Chapter 11, Nutrition and Diets.

A Daily Pill That Prevents Cardiovascular Disease and Alzheimer's Disease?

Cardiovascular (heart and blood vessels) disease is the main cause of death in the United States. The American Heart Association estimates that every year in the United States, there are 2 million heart attacks and strokes, and 800,000 people die. The Alzheimer's Association estimates that 5.8 million people of all ages are affected by Alzheimer's disease and that one out of every ten persons aged 65 or older is affected.

Scientists at the University of Chester in the United Kingdom and at Kent State University in Ohio have developed two new vitamin compounds that could reduce the risk of these diseases. Working as an international team, they are evaluating the effectiveness of the vitamins in reducing elevated blood levels of an amino acid, homocysteine. Homocysteine is acquired mainly by eating meat. It increases the risk of cardiovascular disease and Alzheimer's disease

because it produces large amounts of free radicals that interfere with the way body cells use oxygen. Even though vitamin B_{12} and folic acid are somewhat effective in breaking down the homocysteine in the body, researchers have found that the new compounds are four times more effective. Tests were carried out using human vascular cells in a model cell system. Results indicated that the compounds reduced the inflammation caused by the homocysteine in vascular cells. Clinical trials will have to be conducted to determine if there are any adverse effects from the compounds. If the trials are successful, the researchers estimate that in 5–6 years a new vitamin medication could be available.

In addition to cardiovascular disease and Alzheimer's disease, elevated blood levels of homocysteine may be associated with osteoporosis (bones become porous), pregnancy complications, and other inflammatory disorders. If a vitamin compound could reduce the risk of these conditions, thousands of lives could be saved each year.

Case Study Investigation Conclusion

Mrs. Washington has several medical conditions that Denise will have to address when she makes her dietary recommendations. What other physical restrictions should she consider? Should Denise give

Mrs. Washington's food preferences any consideration? What other things do you think will impact Denise's menu plan?

CHAPTER 11 SUMMARY

- An understanding of basic nutrition is essential for health care providers.

- Good nutrition helps maintain wellness, a state of good health with optimal body function.

- There are six groups of essential nutrients: carbohydrates, fats, proteins, vitamins, minerals, and water.

- The simplest guide for planning healthy meals that provide the required essential nutrients is to eat a variety of foods from the five major food groups.

- Weight management is used to achieve and maintain the desired body weight. Good weight management reduces the risks for many diseases and allows an individual to enjoy a longer and healthier life span.

- Therapeutic diets are modifications of the normal diet. They are used to improve specific health conditions.

REVIEW QUESTIONS

1. List the six (6) essential nutrients and the main function of each nutrient.

2. Differentiate between the processes of digestion, absorption, and metabolism.

3. Differentiate between overweight and obesity. List six (6) conditions that can develop as a result of obesity.

4. Calculate the number of calories you require per day to maintain your present weight. How many calories should you ingest per day to gain 1 pound per week? How many calories should you ingest per day to lose 1 pound per week?

5. Identify the type of therapeutic diet that may be ordered for patients with the following conditions:
   a. Gallbladder or liver disease
   b. Diabetes mellitus
   c. Hypertension or heart disease
   d. Gastric disorders, colitis, or diseases of the digestive tract
   e. Pregnant or lactating women
   f. Severe nausea, vomiting, or diarrhea
   g. Kidney disease
   h. Poor dentition

CRITICAL THINKING

1. You are planning your family's meals. It is important that everyone eat a balanced diet and about 1,800 calories a day to maintain a healthy weight. Based on those criteria, create a sample menu for three (3) meals and two (2) snacks. Don't forget to include beverages.

2. You have an 88-year-old male patient who is from Mexico in the hospital recovering from a left hip fracture. It is day 4; he has lost 8 pounds and doesn't like the hospital food. As the hospital's dietician, what are three (3) questions you might ask this patient in order to provide balanced nutrition and the food he will eat?

3. Using the data from **Table 11–1**, list what kind of nutrient group each patient needs to increase based on their medical condition:
   a. A 16-year-old with anorexia
   b. An 8-month-old with dysentery
   c. An underweight 78-year-old with cancer
   d. A 19-year-old burn victim
   e. A 26-year-old with the flu that has been vomiting for 2 days who can't start an IV
   f. A 6-year-old undergoing a fourth major surgery to correct congenital problems

■ ACTIVITIES

1. a. Define *BMI*. Using the BMI graph or calculator, determine your BMI. What does your number indicate?
    b. List everything you ate yesterday. Don't forget to include snacks, coffee, water, candy, and gum. Determine how many servings of each nutrient you consumed. Show this on the *MyPlate* tool. Calculate your calories.
    c. Based upon your BMI, calorie intake, and *MyPlate* food distribution, answer these questions:

    1. Do I need to change my total caloric intake? Raise, lower, or remain the same. If you need to adjust, by how much?

    2. Do I need to change the types of foods I eat? Do I eat fruit? Do I eat enough vegetables for a balance diet?

2. In a small group, create a patient education oral presentation that will include:
    a. A poster, trifold, or commercial promoting healthy eating and nutrition
    b. A brochure on a disease that poor eating habits impact. This brochure must include signs and symptoms of the disease, major associated physical concerns, preventive measures, treatment, and support systems. Include at least three (3) resources. Be ready to present to the class or the public at a health fair.

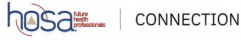 | CONNECTION

Competitive Event: Nutrition

Event Summary: The Nutrition test provides HOSA members with the opportunity to explore and learn about the relationship of nutrition and wellness and to assess knowledge common in this health field. This competitive event consists of a written test with a tie-breaker essay question. This event aims to inspire members to be proactive future health professionals and to apply and analyze information related to nutrition and health.

Details on this event may be found at

www.hosa.org/guidelines

COMPUTERS AND TECHNOLOGY IN HEALTH CARE

Technology

Case Study Investigation

Ricardo Galvez is a team member of technology support at the University Hospital System. Jessica is a nurse in ICU. Jessica has a new patient that has come up from the emergency room. She is having trouble pulling up the patient's ER intake report, radiology and lab results, and the medication and dietary orders. Jessica calls the help desk and Ricardo answers. After giving Jessica some instructions and running a preliminary diagnostic check, Ricardo determines that he will need to come to the ICU to teach Jessica how to access the patient information and to make sure there are no other problems. While he is there, Ricardo will also update the computer and install a shielding security screen. At the end of this chapter, you will be asked about troubleshooting and patient confidentiality as it relates to computer technology.

■ LEARNING OBJECTIVES

After completing this chapter, you should be able to:

- Describe the areas in health care where computer and technology applications are currently being used.
- Describe a situation showing how at least six different health care personnel in a health care facility use computers and technology as information systems.
- Identify at least four diagnostic tools that use computers and technology.
- Describe at least six treatments using computers and technology.
- Discuss how computers and technology are used for health science education and research.
- Illustrate how computers and technology have improved health care communication.
- Determine the validity and reliability of Internet sites while conducting research on a specific topic.
- Identify precautions that must be taken to maintain the confidentiality of patient information.
- Differentiate between antivirus and firewall software, and explain how each helps to provide computer security.
- Define, pronounce, and spell all key terms.

■ KEY TERMS

adenosine stress test

computer literacy *(come-pew'-tur lit'-er-ass-see)*

computer-aided design (CAD)

computer-assisted instruction (CAI)

computerized tomography (CT) *(com-pew'-tur-eyesd toe-mawg'-rah-fee)*

database

dobutamine stress test

echocardiogram

electrocardiogram (ECG)

electronic health record (EHR)

electronic mail

ergonomics

exercise stress test

fields

file

firewalls

health information exchange (HIE)

image-guided surgery (IGS)

Internet

lasers

magnetic resonance imaging (MRI) *(mag-net'-ik rez'-oh-nance im'-adj-ing)*

mainframe computer

microcomputer

networks

nuclear stress test

patient portals

personal computer

positron emission tomography (PET) *(pahs'-ih'-tron ee-miss'-shun toe-mawg'-rah-fee)*

radiation therapy

record

robotic surgery

spreadsheet

telemedicine

telepharmacies

ultrasonography *(ul-trah-sawn-ahg'-rah-fee)*

uninterrupted power supply (UPS)

virtual learning

viruses

Computers and technology have become essential in almost every aspect of health care. They are used in many different areas:

- **Information systems**: managing budgets, equipment inventories, patient information, electronic health records (EHRs), laboratory reports, operating room and personnel scheduling, and general records; two common systems in use are hospital information systems (HIS) and medical information systems (MIS)

- **Diagnostic testing**: analyzing blood, performing medical laboratory analyses, and scanning or viewing body parts by computerized tomography (CT scan), magnetic resonance imaging (MRI), positron emission tomography (PET), and ultrasonography

- **Treatment**: lasers, robotic surgery, image-guided surgery, cancer treatment, dispensing medications, and rehabilitation

- **Patient monitoring**: monitors are used for cardiac, critical care, neurological, neonatal, and surgical patients; also used for premature infants and patients who have dementia or Alzheimer's disease

- **Educational tools**: computer-assisted instruction (CAI) for professional nurses, physicians, and other allied health personnel, virtual learning, patient simulator manikins, and web conferences

- **Research**: statistical analysis of data

- **Communication**: use of a network or the Internet to communicate with other health care personnel in the same agency or other agencies, insurance companies, financial institutions, research networks, and patients; also includes electronic mail, telemedicine, and telepharmacies

No matter what career you choose in health care, a working knowledge of computers and an understanding of technology is essential. This working knowledge is sometimes called computer literacy. **Computer literacy** means a basic understanding of how a computer works and the applications used in your field or profession. Computer literacy also means feeling comfortable using a computer for your job needs. Practice and experience in using a computer are essential in order to develop computer literacy.

Basic troubleshooting is something to become familiar with when computer issues occur. Checking the power connections and restarting the computer is one of the first things to investigate. Sometimes, simply refreshing the browser or double-checking the settings is all it takes to restore the computer. If a particular software program is not functioning correctly, shutting it down and restarting it may correct the problem. At times, the computer may freeze and it will not allow any way to exit a program or restart the computer. Holding down the Ctl + Alt + Delete (control, alternate, and delete) keys at the same time will bring up the task manager and provide a way to exit the program and restart the computer. If the computer is running slowly, it is wise to run a virus scanner to detect any viruses and malware so they can be removed. In addition, deleting programs that are not used may increase the operating speed. If difficulties still occur after running through basic troubleshooting techniques, you will need to implement your facility's procedure for accessing technology help from the IT or information technology department. Each workplace will have a method of contacting this department and placing a work order. Health care providers need to be familiar with this process at their health care facility.

Different types of computers are used in health care, and they vary in size. Computer size can range anywhere from a **microcomputer**, such as a handheld tablet, smartphone, or personal digital assistant (PDA), to a laptop in a compact case (**Figure 12–1**) to a **personal computer**, which can sit on a desktop, to a very large **mainframe computer** that can control the launch of a rocket to outer space.

Using a computer for long periods can cause injuries. **Ergonomics** is an applied science used to promote an

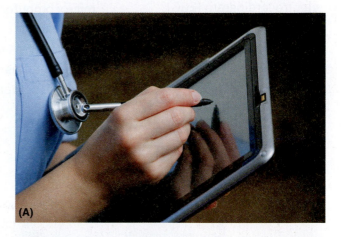

(A)

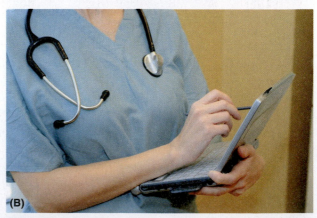

(B)

FIGURE 12–1 Microcomputers include (A) handheld tablets and (B) laptops in compact cases. ©iStock.com/Mutlu Kurtbas ©iStock.com/Sam Sefton

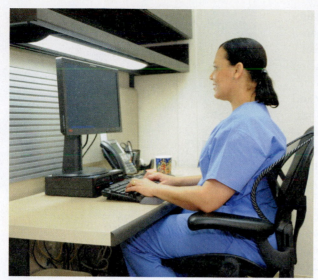

Top of monitor at or just below eye level

Head and neck balanced and in-line with torso

Shoulders relaxed

Elbows close to body and supported

Lower back supported

Wrists and hands in-line with forearms

Adequate room for keyboard and mouse

Feet flat on the floor

FIGURE 12–2 Good ergonomics and proper posture are essential while using a computer.

individual's safety and well-being by adapting to the environment and using techniques to prevent injuries. Ergonomic techniques for computer use include proper lighting, correct positioning of the computer keyboard and monitor, a chair that provides good support, and proper posture (**Figure 12–2**).

checkpoint

1. Name four (4) areas in health care where computers and technology applications are used.
2. Define *computer literacy*.

12:2 INFORMATION SYSTEMS

Today's health care providers use computers and technology to manage information in every health care facility. Computers are used for:

- **Word processing**: This includes writing letters, memos, reports, policies, and procedures, creating patient care plans, and documenting care on a patient's record. Documents created by word processing software can be edited and corrected, stored for future use, and printed or sent by electronic mail or fax.

- **Compiling databases**: This includes creating information records for patients and employees. A **database** is an organized collection of information. Information is entered into areas called **fields**. For example, the database may contain information such as name, address, telephone, e-mail address,

insurance information, social security number, place of employment, and medical history. Each type of information is a field. Within the database, each collection of related information is called a **record**. For example, when all of the fields for a particular patient are combined, the information on the patient is the record. All records can be edited and corrected, stored for future use, and printed or sent by e-mail or fax. When a group of related records is combined, this is called a **file**. For example, all of the patient records in a dental office are a file. A database allows a user to locate records quickly, compile statistics and reports, enter additional information and changes readily, and store information more efficiently than paper files. A primary concern while using databases is security of the information. Most databases that contain patient records are access limited or password protected to maintain patient confidentiality.

- **Creating and transferring electronic health records (EHRs)**: An **electronic health record (EHR)** is a computerized version of a patient's medical information that may include statistical data (name, address, telephone number, insurance information, etc.), diagnoses, medical history, treatments, medications taken, tests performed, and any other information that could be included in a patient's paper record. The U.S. government has provided funding and guidance for creating a national **health information exchange (HIE)** that allows all health care agencies to readily transfer patient electronic health records (EHRs) between agencies in a national network. The Office of the National Coordinator for Health Information Technology (ONC) is establishing policies and standards to ensure that health care personnel can exchange records through a coordinated system. The purpose of the HIE is to improve the speed, quality, and safety of patient care by providing health care personnel with quick access to a patient's medical history. If a person is injured or ill, and unconscious or confused, the health care provider would have immediate access to the person's health history and a record of any diseases or allergies the person has. In addition, the HIE allows patients to have access to their EHRs to monitor their health, identify incorrect information, and share the information with others. To facilitate this access **patient portals** or secure online websites are established by a physician, health care facility, or other health care provider. Patients are given an access code to register for the portal so they can log in anytime to see their personal health information. The portals allow easy communication between the health care provider and patient and can be used to view medical history, treatments, and laboratory test results, request prescription refills, update insurance information, make payments, send messages to the health care provider, view educational material, download and complete forms, schedule appointments, and many other similar tasks. Concerns about the HIE system are the security of the networks used to transfer the records and the compatibility of the software systems used by different health care agencies to interpret the data.

- **Scheduling**: Scheduling is recording appointments for patients and creating work schedules for employees.

- **Maintaining financial records**: This includes processing charges, billing patients, recording payments, completing insurance forms, maintaining accounts, and calculating payrolls for employees.

- **Maintaining inventories and ordering supplies**: Inventory maintenance includes ordering and tracking supplies and equipment, as well as coding supplies with bar codes for billing purposes. For example, a pharmacist might scan a bar code on a medication to maintain an inventory, order the medication from a supply company, or bill a patient's account (**Figure 12–3**). Many scanning systems allow the user to enter the quantity needed for an inventory, order additional supplies, or charge an account by inserting a number on a touch screen. Other scanners connect directly to software on a computer where the inventory, order, or billing charge is compiled.

- **Developing spreadsheets**: A **spreadsheet** uses special software to perform high-speed math calculations. The user enters formulas to tell the computer to perform specific math functions (addition, subtraction, multiplication, division, percentage) with numerical data. This allows the user to process bills, maintain accounts, create budgets, develop statistical reports, analyze finances, tabulate nutritional value of foods, evaluate treatments, and

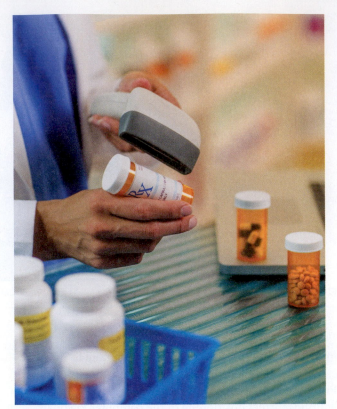

FIGURE 12–3 A pharmacist can scan a bar code on a medication to maintain an inventory, place an order, or bill a patient account.
©iStock.com/stevecoleimages

project future needs. In addition, once a spreadsheet has been created, the numerical data and statistics can be displayed as a graph or chart (**Figure 12–4**).

An example of how information systems operate occurs when a patient is admitted to a hospital. Some of the different health care providers who use computers and technology to record the patient's information include:

- **Health information technician (admitting officer or clerk)**: obtains the patient's name, age, and all other vital information to enter, process, and store in the computer's memory; establishes an electronic database so that the information about the patient can be retrieved whenever it is needed; creates an electronic health record (EHR) for the patient or retrieves the patient's EHR from a health information exchange

- **Physician**: uses word processing or dictation to enter all the findings of the initial admitting physical examination; orders all of the patient's medications from the pharmacy; orders laboratory tests, including blood and urine studies; orders an electrocardiogram or radiographs; specifies dietary restrictions; and identifies specific nursing care

- **Pharmacist**: checks the database regularly for new orders, supplies the nursing departments with ordered medications, warns physicians of drug interactions, and monitors pharmacy inventory

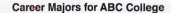

Career Majors for ABC College

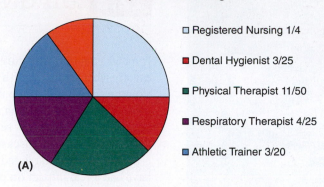

☐ Registered Nursing 1/4

■ Dental Hygienist 3/25

■ Physical Therapist 11/50

■ Respiratory Therapist 4/25

■ Athletic Trainer 3/20

(A)

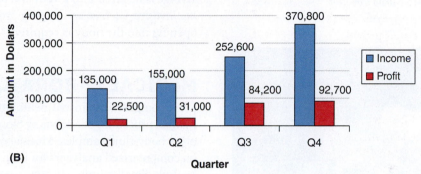

Gental Dentistry Group Income and Profit-Year

(B)

FIGURE 12–4 The numerical data and statistics on a spreadsheet can be displayed as graphs or charts.

- **Dietitian**: checks the dietary restrictions and creates a spreadsheet to show a nutritional analysis of the prescribed diet

- **Laboratory technician**: checks the database for new or revised orders; when any test or procedure is completed, records the results in the patient's electronic health record

- **Environmental service worker (central/sterile supply/service technician)**: maintains an inventory of all supplies in the facility, orders required supplies, and provides information for billing supplies. Many facilities use bar codes on each supply item. When the item is used for a particular patient, the bar code is scanned into the patient's record for automatic billing to the patient.

After each health care provider inputs information into the patient's record, the information is then immediately accessible to the medical, nursing, and allied health teams. These teams no longer have to wait for the results of tests to be printed and hand delivered to the patient care area. Nurses no longer have to manually transcribe physicians' orders or nurses' notes. Because patient care plans are electronic records, they can be easily updated. This use of the computer decreases the time health care providers spend on paperwork and away from patient care.

Many health care facilities are using bar codes on patient identification bands. Small scanners are used to scan the band and verify that a treatment or medication is being given to the correct patient. The bar codes are extremely useful for disoriented or unconscious patients.

Handheld or tablet computers are used in many health care facilities. The terminal device contains a miniature keyboard or touch screen with a wireless link to the nurse's station. With this small terminal, the health care provider is able to record data at a patient's bedside (**Figure 12–5**). Patient information, such as temperature, heart rate, and respirations, is recorded and immediately available to other health care providers.

HIPAA

Eventually, this will lead to a "paperless" patient record, and only an electronic health record (EHR) will be used. All information will be stored in a computer database and sent electronically to insurance companies, pharmacies, and other health care facilities that require the information. Massive filing systems with tons of paper charts will no longer be necessary. Safeguards have to be installed in the computers and networks, however, to meet Health Insurance Portability and Accountability Act (HIPAA) requirements (discussed in Sections 5:1 and 12:10) and to protect the privacy of patient information.

Legal

Confidentiality of patient information must be strictly enforced. This is usually done by means of access codes, special passwords, fingerprints

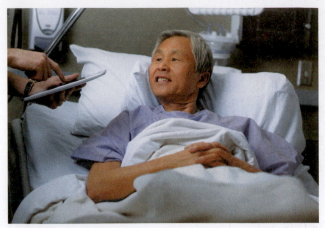

FIGURE 12–5 Handheld or tablet computers with a wireless link can be used to record information at a patient's bedside. ©iStock.com/Nicole Waring

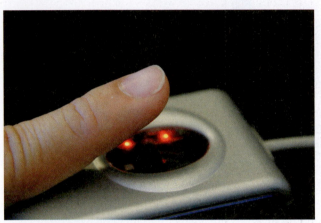

FIGURE 12–6 Fingerprints are often used as an identifying factor for computer access. ©iStock.com/Mike Liu

(**Figure 12–6**), or iris identification (visualization of the eye). Computer users must employ the required access code to enter or retrieve information. Only authorized users are given access to the system. Health care providers must keep their required access code confidential to protect themselves and the patient.

A contingency backup plan is always essential when computers are used. At times, a computer must be shut down for reprogramming or adding additional or new software. At other times, power or computer failure will shut down the computer system. When the computer is not functioning, manual recording of all information is required and an alternative plan must be used to avoid losing essential information. Most facilities make frequent or continuous backups of the data onto external hard drives, disks, flash drives, secure clouds, or off-site servers to prevent a loss of information when computer failure occurs.

checkpoint

| **1.** What is a HIE?

12:3 DIAGNOSTICS

A major goal of health care and medicine is determining exactly what is wrong with the patient, or making a diagnosis. The first step in the process is taking a medical history and doing a physical examination. Based on these findings, several tests may be ordered to diagnose or rule out disease.

Several computer-related technological diagnostic tests have had a real impact on patient care. These diagnostic aids or specialized technological tools are quite varied. They may be *invasive*, such as a blood test where a syringe is inserted into a vein and blood is removed, or *noninvasive*, such as an imaging procedure where no opening into the body is required.

MEDICAL LABORATORY TESTS

Some computerized instruments automate the step-by-step manual procedure of analyzing blood, urine, serum, and other body-fluid samples. Most laboratories rely heavily on computerized analyzers for both blood and urine analysis. Smaller units are now used in many medical offices and other health care facilities. These computerized instruments can analyze a drop of serum, blood, urine, or body fluid placed on a slide or in special tubes at rates of 50 to more than 2,000 specimens per hour. Such systems are also reliable for clinical chemistry evaluations, and many analyzers can perform hundreds of different tests. In larger facilities, laboratories have different analyzers that are interconnected. When one analyzer completes the testing of a specimen, it automatically transfers the specimen to another analyzer so additional tests can be performed. Computers and technology have changed the way medical laboratories function.

CARDIAC TESTS

Computers and technology have also revolutionized cardiac care. Examples include:

- **Electrocardiogram (ECG)**: a computerized interpretation system that produces visual pictures on a computer monitor and a printout of the electrical activity of a patient's heart; gives important information concerning the spread of electrical impulses to the heart chambers and assists in diagnosing heart disease

- **Exercise stress test**: an ECG run while the patient is exercising (**Figure 12–7**); usually involves walking a treadmill or riding an exercise bike until a target heart rate is reached; allows the physician to evaluate the function of the patient's heart during activity

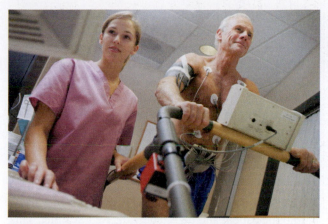

FIGURE 12–7 Computers are used to perform stress tests to evaluate the function of a patient's heart during exercise. ©Monkey Business Images/Shutterstock.com

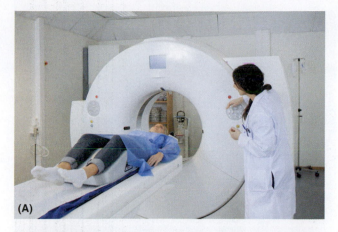

(A)

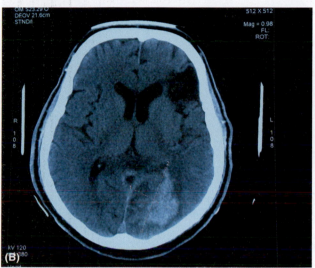

(B)

FIGURE 12–8 (A) A computerized tomography (CT) scanner uses a pencil-thin beam of radiation to create clear, cross-sectional views of both bone and body tissues. (B) This CT scan shows bleeding in the right hemisphere of the brain. Top image, ©iStock.com/Mark Kostich and bottom image, ©iStock.com/atbaei

- **Nuclear stress test**: a small amount of a radioactive substance such as thallium is given intravenously; a special camera is used to identify the rays emitted from the substance while the patient is at rest and then during exercise; allows the physician to evaluate which parts of the heart are healthy and function normally and which parts are not because a less-than-normal amount of the radioactive substance will be seen in areas of the heart with a decreased blood supply

- **Dobutamine** or **adenosine stress test**: used for patients who cannot exercise; a medication that simulates the effect of exercise is given to increase the blood flow and heart rate; physician can determine how heart responds to stress

- **Echocardiogram**: uses technology to direct ultrahigh-frequency sound waves through the chest wall and into the heart; a computer then converts the reflection of the waves into an image of the heart; usually a reading is taken while the patient is at rest and then another reading is taken after exercise when the heart rate rises to a target level; used to evaluate cardiac function, reveal valve irregularities, show defects in the heart walls, and visualize the presence of fluid between the layers of the pericardium (membrane that surrounds the outside of the heart)

IMAGING TECHNOLOGY

Medical imaging using technology and computers has allowed for better diagnosis and treatment. Examples of imaging devices include:

- **Computerized tomography (CT)**: Introduced in 1972, this noninvasive, computerized X-ray (**Figure 12-8A**) permits physicians to see clear, cross-sectional views of both bone and body tissues and to find abnormalities such as tumors or bleeding

(**Figure 12–8B**). The CT scanner shoots a pencil-thin beam of radiation through any part of the body and from many different angles. The computer then creates a cross-sectional image of the body part on a screen. There is a concern about radiation exposure from CT scans, especially in children, so newer, low-dose CT scans are now in use.

- **Magnetic resonance imaging (MRI)**: This computerized, body-scanning method uses nuclear magnetic resonance instead of X-ray radiation. Magnetic resonance imaging alters the magnetic position of hydrogen atoms to produce an image. The patient is placed in a large circular magnet, which uses the magnetic field to measure the activity of hydrogen atoms within the body (**Figure 12–9A**). A computer translates that activity into cross-sectional images of the body (**Figure 12–9B**). For example, a lung tumor can be more easily detected by scanning with MRI than by scanning with

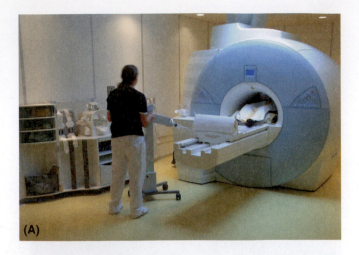

(A)

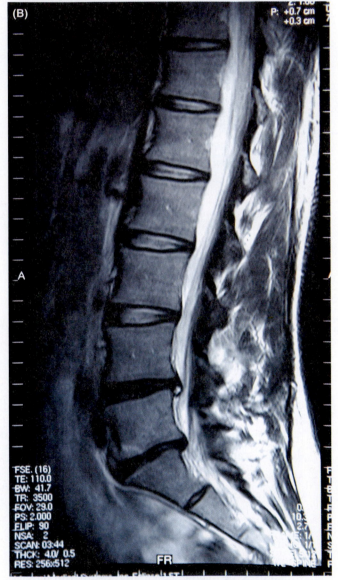

(B)

FIGURE 12–9 (A) For magnetic resonance imaging (MRI), the patient is placed in the center of a large magnet that measures the activity of hydrogen ions inside the body and creates an image of the body. (B) This MRI scan shows a herniated disc between the fifth lumbar and first sacral (L5/S1) vertebrae in the spine. Top image, ©iStock.com/Dr. Heinz Linke and bottom image, ©iStock.com/Lorraine Kourafas

X-rays or CT. Magnetic resonance imaging allows physicians to see blood moving through veins and arteries, to see a swollen joint shrink in response to medication, and to see the reaction of cancerous tumors to treatment. Because of the strong magnetic field in the MRI scanner, patients with pacemakers or metal implants cannot receive an MRI unless the devices are certified as MRI safe. In addition, extreme caution must be taken to make sure that no loose metal objects are in the room.

- **Positron emission tomography (PET):** To perform a PET scan, a slightly radioactive substance is injected into the patient and detected by the PET scanner. This radioactive tracer travels through the body and is picked up by body cells. If there is a poor blood supply, there will be a decreased amount of tracer. This aids in the diagnosis of heart disease or other circulatory problems. In addition, cancer cells have a much higher metabolic rate than normal cells so they will pick up larger amounts of the tracer. This allows the physician to detect cancer, check for metastasis, or see if treatment is working by decreasing the tumor size. The device's computer composes a three-dimensional image from the radiation detected (**Figure 12–10**). The image allows the doctor to see any body part from all sides. In this way, a PET image is similar to a model that can be picked up and examined.

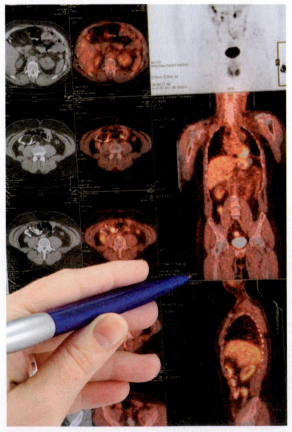

FIGURE 12–10 A PET scan composes a three-dimensional image from the radiation detected. ©iStock.com/Ivan Ivanov

- **Ultrasonography**: This is a noninvasive scanning method that uses high-frequency sound waves that bounce back as an echo when they hit different tissues and organs inside the body (**Figure 12–11A**). A computer then uses the sound wave signals to create a picture of the body part, which can be viewed on a computer screen or processed on a photographic film that resembles a radiograph. Ultrasonography can be used to detect tumors, locate aneurysms and blood vessel abnormalities, and examine the shape and size of internal organs. During pregnancy, when radiation can harm the fetus, ultrasonography is used to detect multiple pregnancies and to determine the size, position, sex, and even abnormalities of the fetus (**Figure 12–11B**). A more recent development in sonography is the three-dimensional (3-D) sonogram. This type of ultrasound uses a specialized machine that allows technicians to store 5 seconds' worth of images in a computer. The technician can then create a 3-D colored picture similar to a portrait of the infant in the uterus. Physicians use the 3-D ultrasound to detect birth defects that are not always visible on a standard sonogram and to determine the severity of a birth defect. The newest ultrasound is a 4-D

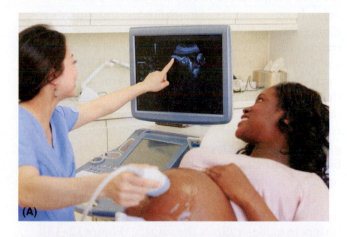

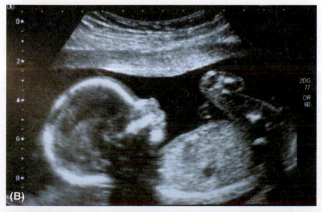

FIGURE 12–11 (A) Ultrasonography is used during pregnancy to determine the size, position, sex, and even abnormalities of the fetus. (B) This ultrasound shows a fetus at 22 weeks. Top image, ©iStock.com/Bojan Fatur and bottom image, ©iStock.com/Isabelle Limbach

ultrasound that actually creates a live video similar to a movie. It allows physicians to study the motion of various moving organs in the body.

- **Dental digital radiography**: This has replaced conventional radiographs or X-rays in dental offices. A small electronic sensor is placed in the patient's mouth. The sensor uses imaging techniques to transfer the image to a computer monitor where it can be seen immediately. It can be saved as an electronic file in the patient's record. Because the patient is exposed to less radiation than a conventional radiograph, it is safer for the patient. Digital imaging is environmentally friendly because it eliminates the need for X-ray film and developing solutions. Storage of the images is easier, and images can be sent electronically to another dentist for a consultation. The digital images can also be enlarged and the contrast can be enhanced (lighter or darker) to visualize dental disease, something that cannot be done with standard dental radiographs. The disadvantage of digital radiography in a dental office is the cost of the system and software.

- **Computer-aided detection (CADe) and computer-aided diagnosis (CADx)**: CADe and CADx are systems that use artificial intelligence to aid in the detection and diagnosis of disease. These technological tools have proven beneficial as basic screening methods, but their reliability for constant accurate diagnoses has not been perfected. For example, CADe or CADx may be used to initially scan mammogram images. The computer can be programmed to identify conspicuous structures such as dense areas in the breast tissue, calcification clusters, or abnormal shading that may indicate tumors. The radiologist is then alerted to examine these areas on the mammogram image carefully. In the same manner, CADe or CADx may be used to initially screen a series of Pap test slides, chest radiographs, or other similar diagnostic tools. These systems do not replace the physician, but they do play a supporting role in identifying potential conditions or diseases that require a more thorough evaluation.

SUMMARY

Computers and technology have made diagnosing diseases easier and more precise. Manual laboratory tests and simple radiographs that were the only methods used to diagnose disease 30 years ago have been replaced by more exacting tests or imaging techniques. As technology improves, new techniques and diagnostic tests will be developed.

checkpoint

1. List five (5) diagnostic tools that use computers and technology.

12:4 TREATMENT

Many different types of treatment use technology and computers. **Lasers**, or light beams that can be focused precisely, are one example. A laser scalpel using a highly focused light beam will cut an incision at the same, constant depth because the light beam gives off the same amount of energy every second. A surgeon using a regular scalpel might cut deeper into some tissues than others. The laser light beam heats the targeted cells until they burst open. At the same time, the heat in the beam cauterizes, or seals off, smaller blood vessels such as those in the skin. This results in less bleeding at the surgical site. Another advantage is that cells in human tissue are poor heat conductors, so tissues close to the laser site are not affected by the beam. This allows surgeons to operate on tiny areas without disturbing the surrounding healthy tissues and organs. One of the most common uses for lasers is reshaping the cornea of the eye to correct vision defects (**Figure 12–12**). Precise measurements programmed into a computer direct the laser beam to shape the cornea so the patient has correct vision. Another common use of lasers is to remove plaque from arteries, a procedure called laser angioplasty. A very small optic fiber with a sensor is inserted into an artery. When the fiber reaches the area of plaque accumulation, the plaque is destroyed by laser pulses and the artery is "unclogged." The patient recovers quickly because the procedure is minimally invasive. Lasers are also used to remove warts, moles, birthmarks, scars, and even tattoos. They can be used by cosmetic surgeons to remove skin wrinkles, hair, dilated blood vessels, and other blemishes. Pediatric surgeons use lasers to perform circumcisions. Dentists use lasers to remove carious lesions (decay) in teeth, because the decayed material is much softer than the enamel of the tooth.

The laser is set at a power that is strong enough to destroy the carious lesion but preserve the healthy tooth tissue. This allows a dentist to avoid the use of a dental handpiece (drill) and provides a less painful procedure for the patient. As new technology occurs, many other uses for lasers will be developed.

Robotic surgery, also called *computer-assisted surgery*, is another major technological advance. A robot is a mechanical device that is computer controlled. Most systems include a camera arm with mechanical arms that attach to surgical instruments. The surgeon is seated at a computer console that provides 3-D magnified images of the surgical site. At times, the maneuvers the robot will perform are preprogrammed into the system, and the surgeon supervises. At other times, the surgeon will operate the robot. There are two main methods for operating the robot: a telemanipulator, a device similar to a joystick that the surgeon uses to perform the movements that the robot carries out, or a computerized control. Both methods allow a surgeon to have more precise control over the surgical instruments and to eliminate human inconsistencies such as hand tremors. The computerized method also allows the surgeon to operate from a distance, from anywhere in the world. Some robots are even programmed to respond to the surgeon's voice. Robotic surgery is more precise, movements are more controlled, tissues and organs experience less trauma, incisions are smaller, bleeding is decreased, and recovery is faster. However, the cost of the robot, instruments, computer, and software is much higher than that of standard operatory equipment. In addition, the surgeon needs advanced training to operate the robot. Robotic surgery is used in many fields, including gynecology (female reproductive), urology (kidney and bladder), cardiac (heart), thoracic (chest and lungs), and oncology (cancer).

Image-guided surgery (IGS) is a surgical procedure in which a surgeon uses preoperative and intraoperative images to guide or direct the surgery (**Figure 12–13**). Before the surgery, CTs or MRIs are taken of the surgical area. Using computerized technology, the images are converted into three-dimensional (3-D) images that show precise details of the organs and tissues. The images allow the surgeon to create a precise plan for the surgery: where to make the incision, how deep the incision should be, critical areas to be avoided, basic required instruments, and, in some cases, determine whether or not the surgery will be beneficial. During the surgery, the 3-D images are synchronized with LED (light emitting diode) cameras that project current images of the surgery. The surgeon can see the path of the instruments, identify the surgical area such as the tumor being removed, avoid critical areas, make minute adjustments to achieve the best results, and prevent damage to healthy tissues and organs. Because

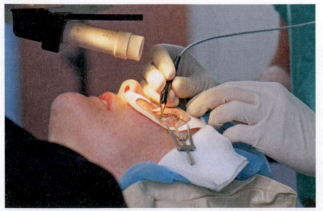

FIGURE 12–12 Lasers are used to reshape the cornea of the eye to correct vision defects. ©iStock.com/David Kevitch

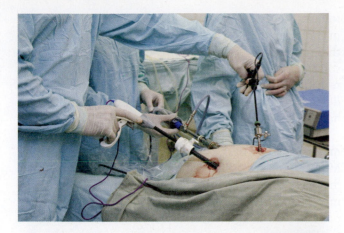

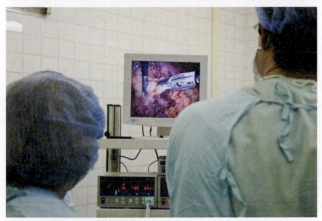

FIGURE 12–13 Image-guided surgery allows the surgeon to see three-dimensional images of the operative site during the procedure. Top image, © Farferros/Shutterstock.com and bottom image, © Farferros/Shutterstock.com

of the high degree of precision that can be obtained with image-guided surgery, there is minimal invasion, incisions are smaller, critical structures are avoided to prevent postoperative impairments, tumors or surgeries once considered "inoperable" now may be an option, and patient recovery is faster. This technology was first developed for brain tumors, but it is now used for sinus surgeries, biopsies or resections of tumors, neurological (nerve) procedures, spinal injury repairs, reconstructive orthopedic (bone) surgery, and many other types of surgeries.

Radiation therapy uses high-energy particles to decrease the size of tumors and treat cancer. There are two major types of this therapy: external-beam and brachytherapy. External-beam radiation usually uses photon beams (either X-rays or gamma rays) to kill cancer cells by destroying their DNA or genetic structures. When the DNA is destroyed, the cancer cells stop reproducing and die. Before radiation treatment, CTs, MRIs, PETs, or even ultrasound scans are taken to produce a detailed image of the patient's tumor and the tissues surrounding it. A radiation oncologist uses sophisticated computers and technology to design an individualized treatment plan that shows the exact area to be treated, the total dose of radiation that will

be used, the safest angle for delivery of the radiation to limit the destruction of healthy tissue, and the number of treatments needed. In many cases, masks or body moldings are custom-made for a patient to ensure that the patient will not move during the treatment and that the radiation is delivered to the exact same spot for each treatment (**Figure 12–14A**). For each radiation treatment, the radiation machine is programmed and positioned at the precise angle required to administer the calculated dose of radiation (**Figure 12–14B**). Brachytherapy uses radioactive isotopes that are sealed inside tiny pellets or "seeds." Using imaging and computerized programs, the exact location for the placement of the pellets is determined. They are then inserted into the patient using needles, catheters, or specialized probes. They can be inserted interstitially (directly into the tumor), intracavity (into a cavity such as the uterus or chest), or systemically (into the blood stream; for example, radioactive iodine to destroy thyroid tissue). Radiation therapy can be given to cure cancer by destroying all the cancer cells or, in cases where this is not possible, as a palliative treatment to improve the quality of a person's life by reducing pain and suffering.

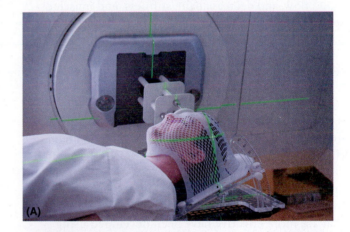

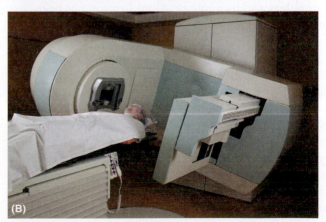

FIGURE 12–14 (A) Special masks may be used to prevent patient movement and ensure that the radiation is delivered to the exact same spot for each treatment. (B) The radiation machine is programmed and positioned at the precise angle required to administer the calculated dose of radiation. Top image, ©iStock.com/Mark Kostich and bottom image, ©iStock.com/Mark Kostich

Computer-aided design (CAD), originally used by engineers and designers, has also found a place in therapeutic treatment. Using three-dimensional imaging models, individuals who make prosthetics, or artificial parts, can custom design individualized prosthetics such as hands, legs, fingers, and other body parts that will precisely match the physical requirements of the individual for whom they are designed. Dentists use CAD to form perfect images of crowns, dental implants, or bridges to replace damaged or destroyed teeth. Plastic surgeons use CAD to show patients how surgery will change their physical appearance. By using CAD, the surgeons can determine tissue that has to be replaced or removed for optimal effect. In the field of biomedicine, CAD is used to create models that can be duplicated as precisely as possible for research or functioning models of body parts.

Ultrasound, the use of high-frequency sound waves, is a therapeutic device in addition to a method of imaging. Ultrasound is used by physical therapists and chiropractors as a form of deep heat therapy. When applied to soft tissues and joints, the sound waves use heat and gentle massage to reduce swelling, increase blood flow, and decrease pain, stiffness, and muscle spasms. High-intensity or high-frequency ultrasound uses focused ultrasound at a high frequency to heat and destroy pathogenic (diseased) tissue by ablation (vaporization or erosion). Ultrasound is also used to enhance the delivery of drugs or medications. It enhances the absorption of drugs through the skin, promotes gene therapy to tissues, directs chemotherapy to tumors, and delivers thrombolytic drugs into blood clots to dissolve or destroy the clots.

Hearing assistive technology has provided many enhancements for individuals who have hearing impairments. Cochlear implants and hearing aids that are more effective have been developed using computers and technology. Amplification has been increased in phones, doorbells, alarms, and many other devices. Infrared systems are used to transmit sounds using infrared light waves. The sounds are transmitted to the patient's receiver, which can be adjusted to a volume that the patient desires. An infrared system can be installed in an individual's home or in meeting areas and theaters. Induction loop systems are used in large meeting rooms, group areas, theaters, and homes. An induction loop wire is permanently installed in the room, usually in the ceiling or on the floor. The wire connects to a microphone that is used by the speaker or to devices such as a television in a home. This creates an electromagnetic field in the room. An individual who has a hearing impairment can adjust their hearing aid to a telecoil or telephone mode that picks up the electromagnetic signal and allows the individual to hear the speaker without hearing other noises in the room. Other large areas have technology that transmits a speaker's words onto a computer screen that can be read by anyone in the room. As technology and computers advance, many other devices will be developed to assist individuals who have hearing impairments.

Computers and technology have provided major advances in the distribution of medications. Medications are used as a treatment for many diseases. An error in the administration of a medication can result in injury and even death to a patient. New drug distribution systems are designed to eliminate as many medication errors as possible. There are many different systems available for use. *Automated drug dispensing systems (ADDS)* may be used in large pharmacies, such as those found in hospitals. These devices use automated storage and dispensing cabinets or carts, commonly called ADCs (**Figure 12–15A**). The carts contain unit doses of medications that are maintained at the proper temperature and lighting conditions. When a medication is ordered for a patient, the pharmacist notes the order. Many facilities use a computerized prescribing program to eliminate errors associated with poor handwriting, incorrect transcription of dosage or name, and other similar problems. The computerized program can also check the patient's record to make sure that the new medication is compatible with other medications, that no allergies are present, and that the dosage and method of administration are correct. The medication is then prepared for the patient and usually put in single-dose packets. In most systems, the patient's individualized bar code is placed on the packet. When a nurse administers the medication, they use a scanner on the bar code on the packet to verify the patient's name and the name and dose of the medication (**Figure 12–15B**). Before administering the medication, the nurse scans the bar code on the patient's identification band to verify that the medication is being given to the correct individual (**Figure 12–15C**). Some systems allow the nurse to use the scanner to verify that the medication has been given. The ADDS then automatically records this information on the patient's record and bills the dose to the patient's account. Security of and limited access to the ADCs is critical. Most facilities use secure passwords, frequently changed codes, or fingerprint or iris identification to limit access to the carts.

These are just a few of the therapies that use technology and computers. However, it is obvious that advances in technology and computers have enhanced the treatment for many diseases and conditions and will continue to do so in the future of health care.

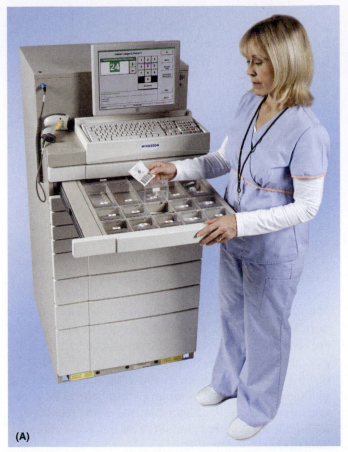

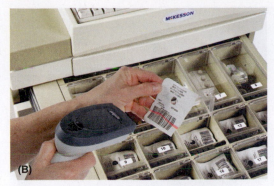

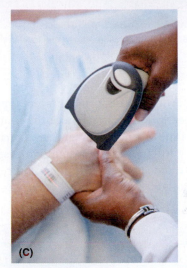

(A) (B) (C)

FIGURE 12–15 (A) Automated dispensing cabinets or carts (ADCs) store unit doses of medications at the correct temperature and lighting conditions. (B) When the unit dose is removed from the ADC, the bar code on the label is scanned to identify the patient and medication. (C) Before administering the medication to a patient, the scanner is used to scan the bar code on the patient's identification band to ascertain that the medication is being given to the correct individual. Courtesy of McKesson Automation Solutions/Courtesy of McKesson Automation Solutions/Courtesy of McKesson Automation Solutions

check**point**

1. List two (2) ways lasers are used in the medical field.

2. How is hearing assisted with technology?

12:5 PATIENT MONITORING

Patient monitoring is another major field that uses computers and technology. Monitors that measure and display vital signs such as pulse, blood pressure, respiratory rate, and heart rhythms are used in critical care units, cardiac care, emergency care, surgery, and many other areas (**Figure 12–16**). The monitors record information from sensors placed on or in the patient's body. Specific information, such as an abnormal heart rhythm, can also be printed for a hard-copy record or transferred to a patient's electronic record. Some monitors also measure pulmonary blood pressure or intracranial pressure (pressure inside the skull against the brain).

Pulse oximeters are used to monitor the oxygen level of the blood. They usually consist of a sensor that is placed on a finger or, in the case of infants, on the heel,

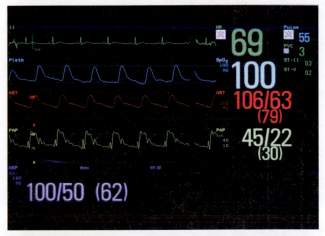

FIGURE 12–16 Monitors are used to measure and display vital signs such as pulse, blood pressure, and heart rhythms. ©iStock.com/aaM Photography, Ltd

and a monitor that displays the reading (**Figure 12–17**). Many of the monitors have alarm systems that are programmed to sound an alert to health care providers when abnormalities occur. A normal range is usually 90 to 100 percent and levels below 90 are considered to be hypoxia, or a deficiency of oxygen reaching the tissues. Low levels can indicate a need for supplemental oxygen.

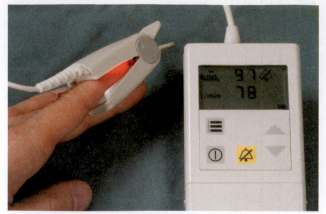

FIGURE 12–17 Pulse oximeters measure the oxygen level in the blood.
©iStock.com/Photomick

Obstetrical departments use many different types of monitors. Fetal heart monitors can check the heart rate of the infant any time during the pregnancy. During labor and delivery, monitors can constantly measure the fetal heart rate and at the same time monitor the strength of the mother's contractions (**Figure 12–18**).

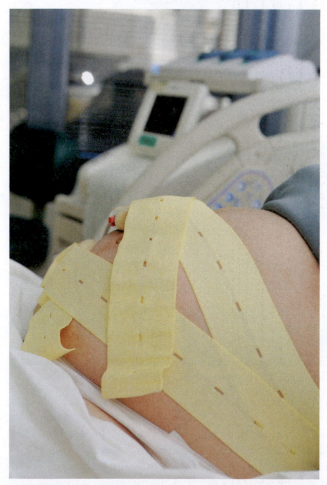

FIGURE 12–18 During labor and delivery, monitors can be used to measure and display the fetal heart rate and the strength of contractions. ©iStock.com/dblight

This allows the obstetrician and staff to determine the progress of labor and approximate the time of birth. Infants born prematurely are placed in incubators that constantly monitor temperature, humidity, oxygen levels, and many other factors to provide the infant with optimal conditions for survival. Some incubators even have computer-controlled photo (light) therapy for infants with jaundice, a yellow discoloration of the skin and eyes (**Figure 12–19**). Jaundice is a common condition in premature infants and usually occurs because the baby's liver is too immature to eliminate bilirubin (a product from the destruction of red blood cells or erythrocytes) from the blood. The condition usually corrects itself as the liver begins to function more efficiently.

A newer method of monitoring is *electrical impedance tomography (EIT)*. EIT is an imaging technique that creates images by measuring the electrical conductivity of body tissues using sensors placed on the skin. It is now being used to monitor the lungs of patients who are on mechanical ventilators for breathing. Ventilators can cause injury to the lungs by uneven distribution of air. The EIT monitor image shows the air volumes in different regions of the lungs. By using the EIT measurements, the ventilator controls can be regulated to provide the required amount of air but avoid injury to lung tissue.

Wearable monitors or sensors are another technology that is advancing quickly. They consist of a device that can be worn on the body, such as a wrist band or strip that adheres to a body part. Other sensors can be implanted in the body and even bioelectric tattoos are being evaluated. These sensors can be used to monitor fitness, blood pressure, heart rhythms, body temperature, blood oxygen saturation, gait and posture, chemical balance, stress, and many other similar physiological activities in the body. Some of the monitors simply alert the wearer to the body's response to exercise, the amount

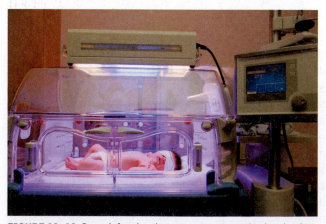

FIGURE 12–19 Some infant incubators use computerized technology to provide photo (light) therapy for infants with jaundice. ©iStock.com/stockstudioX

of exercise obtained, or even an abnormal reading such as a high blood pressure or blood sugar level. Others are used to transmit information obtained to health care providers for interpretation. This usually involves the use of a smartphone to collect the information and transmit it or the use of a cloud-based software system that receives the information through a wireless network. The continuous and remote monitoring can alert health care providers instantly and allow them to respond to emergencies such as a heart attack. However, the use of these monitors and transmission of information must meet all HIPAA requirements for security and confidentiality of patient information and follow ethical guidelines.

GPS (global positioning satellites) technology is being used to monitor patients who have dementia and Alzheimer's disease. A wrist or ankle bracelet is used to track and find these individuals if they wander away. As computerized technological advances occur, many new types of monitors will be used in health care.

checkpoint

1. List three (3) ways technology assists medical providers in monitoring patients.

12:6 EDUCATION

Computers and technology have become commonplace educational tools. Research has shown that computer-based learning decreases time on the task and increases achievement and retention of knowledge. Therefore, it comes as no surprise to find computer-based learning in most schools of medicine, nursing, and allied health.

Computer-assisted instruction (CAI) is educational computer programming designed for individualized use. It is user paced, user friendly, and proceeds in an orderly, organized fashion from topic to topic. It may use video, animated graphics, color, and sound. It may be a drill-and-practice program for learning to calculate medication doses, or it may take the form of a tutorial for learning concepts about the heart. In addition, it can be a simulation that allows the learner to do a clinical procedure, such as taking a patient's blood pressure or drawing blood from a vein (venipuncture), while sitting in front of the computer. Computer programs have even been developed to allow a user to perform a simulated physical examination or operation on a patient.

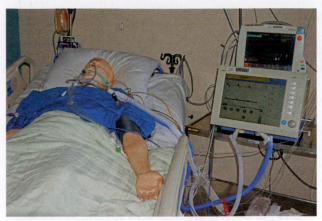

FIGURE 12–20 A simulator manikin can be monitored and programmed to react in a positive or negative manner when treated.

New technology has produced patient simulator manikins that have been programmed to provide lifelike learning experiences for health care providers. Actual emergency situations are created to allow health care providers to learn how to "treat" the patient. Depending on the treatment provided, the manikin is programmed to react in a positive or negative manner (**Figure 12–20**). The simulation programs and manikins have become more specific as technology has improved. We now have infant simulators, pregnant manikins that deliver a baby, surgical manikins that can have surgery and even "die" if the anesthesia is incorrect, and manikins that can be monitored, intubated, and receive CPR. Instructors can change the manikin response based on the actions of the student to provide an even more individualized experience. This provides instant feedback to the learner and prepares the learner to treat patients more effectively. Research has shown that this technology greatly enhances learning and retention.

Patient-education software is available for the patient who has osteoarthritis (inflammation of the joints), obesity (overweight), and many other diseases. Software is even available to teach people how to manage stress.

Technology has even improved the availability and storage of knowledge. Books and entire reference libraries can be downloaded onto wireless devices, decreasing the need for massive libraries holding volumes of books. Internet search engines can identify vast amounts of information about any given topic. Technology and computers have created an information age to make knowledge readily accessible to anyone. Technology has also improved the storage of data. Electronic health records (EHRs) have become a part of every aspect of health care but this creates the problem of securely storing and protecting a large amount of data. Cloud storage has helped solve this problem. Cloud storage consists of a data server that a user connects with through the Internet. The hardware for this data server can be located anywhere and basically it serves as a massive file cabinet for electronic data with unlimited storage space. When data is sent it is duplicated and readily available if computer failure or a natural disaster such as a tornado causes a loss of data. It is essential to use a secure and reliable cloud storage provider to ensure the privacy of the data and to have strict security methods for accessing the cloud storage.

The Internet offers an approach to education called **virtual learning**. Virtual learning is an online teaching and learning environment that uses computers and the Internet to allow teachers to present information and activities and, at times, even engage and interact with students. Students can access a wide variety of courses over the Internet. This allows them to complete the courses in their own homes at times convenient to them. Many health care providers use the Internet to obtain continuing education units (CEUs) or to complete college courses to advance in their professions. Refresher courses to prepare for licensure are also available for many health care careers. In addition, many tests for licensure are now taken on computers. This allows for immediate grading of the licensure examination. Examples include the licensure tests for registered nurses and physicians.

Web conferences are online meetings between two or more people in different locations using an online service, special software, a computer, and Internet. Simple examples are Facebook and Skype. Now online services offer teleconferencing services that allow meetings, presentations, visual and verbal contact with all participants, and even sharing of information on computer screens. After subscribing to a service by paying a monthly fee, a host will contact participants and ask them to download the software for the service. Each participant is given a phone number to call or an identifying code so they can enter the meeting at an established time. This provides security and privacy for the meeting or presentation because access is limited to the invited participants. Web conferencing is an efficient way of hosting meetings and doing presentations when participants live in different parts of the country or even the world. Examples of some of the main online conferencing services are *GoToMeeting, Zoom, Google Meet,* and *Microsoft Meeting Teams.*

The educational opportunities provided by technology will continue to advance and progress as more individuals learn to utilize these services.

checkpoint

1. List two (2) ways education can be improved because of better technology.

12:7 RESEARCH

Today, health care research without the use of computers is almost nonexistent. A major source used to help health care providers analyze statistics and obtain information is the National Library of Medicine (NLM) database, MEDLINE.

The main topics covered by MEDLINE are biomedicine and health, including all areas of life sciences, behavioral sciences, chemical sciences, biophysics, and bioengineering. Free access to the MEDLINE database is available at PubMed (*www.pubmed.gov*). At this site, there are over 30 million citations for biomedical literature with more added on a daily basis. PubMed has easy-to-follow directions to search for topics by subject, author names, title words or phrases, or journal names. An advanced search mode allows the user to specify data fields, such as age groups, gender, or human or animal study. A search can even be directed to find specific information about a disease, such as the etiology (cause), criteria for diagnosis, symptoms, prognosis (expected outcome), or treatment. The database immediately displays references that pertain to the search topic. The search results can be viewed on a monitor or downloaded in different formats.

MedlinePlus (*www.medlineplus.gov.*) is another service offered by the NLM. It provides consumer-oriented health information. It combines information from the NLM, the National Institutes of Health (NIH), other U.S. government agencies, and health-related organizations. MedlinePlus contains health topics, a medical encyclopedia containing information about diseases and wellness issues, a medical dictionary, drug information, herbal and dietary supplement information, health news and press releases, directories of health care providers, videos of surgeries and medical procedures, tutorials that use animation and sound to explain medical conditions and procedures, a service that links patients or providers in electronic health record (EHR) systems to related information in MedlinePlus, and even a mobile site to provide information to mobile Internet users. It is an excellent source of information for research.

Research using computer technology is being conducted for almost every disease, infection, or abnormal health condition that exists. Examples include genetic diseases, heart conditions, diabetes, arthritis, patient management systems, and speech recognition patterns. Information acquired during research is frequently organized into large databases and shared with other researchers throughout the world. This process, known as *bioinformatics*, allows for rapid scientific progress through the sharing of information. In addition, the high speeds and increased capabilities of computers

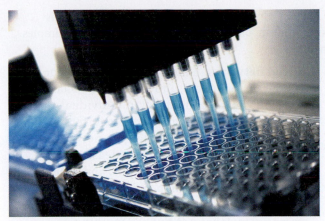

FIGURE 12–21 Robots can be used in research to fill pipettes with the correct amount of solution. ©iStock.com/David Gray

allow scientific researchers to analyze huge amounts of data and run statistical analyses quickly and accurately. They are also able to run simulations and build electronic models to facilitate research.

Technologies such as imaging devices, lasers, and robotics have also enhanced research, especially in bio-technology. For example, robots can be used in laboratory experiments to decrease the need for manual labor (**Figure 12–21**). These technologies are used in gene therapy, creating artificial organs, developing new medications, evaluating cancer cells to find methods that destroy them, and many other similar areas.

In addition, clinical researchers are now using technology to help people who have severe spinal cord injuries. Different systems have been evaluated. Some use electrodes that are placed on the body. A computer-controlled program sends electrical impulses to the electrodes to stimulate movement of the person's muscles. Other systems implant sensors that detect and enhance the person's ability to move. The implanted sensors provide information to the computerized program that stimulates movement. Small computer chips have even been implanted under the skin as a method of directing muscle movement and coordination. Another field of research is directed toward stimulating the spinal cord to generate new cells and repair itself. In time, researchers will find a way to reverse paralysis. Even today, people who are quadriplegics (paralyzed from the neck down) can operate computers by simple movements, voice commands, eye signals such as blinking, or even tongue movements. Brain-interfacing using small implants to detect signals associated with movements is a major area of current research. It will allow the person to just think about a movement and the implanted sensor will interface with the computer or other device and cause the movement to occur. As technology and computers advance, researchers will develop new technologies to assist people who have spinal cord injuries.

checkpoint

1. List two (2) ways research is facilitated because of advances in technology and computer use.

12:8 COMMUNICATION

Computers have enhanced communication for health care providers in multiple ways. Through the use of systems called **networks**, computers can be linked together. A network can consist of three or four computers linked together in a medical office, hundreds of computers linked together in a large health care facility, or the ultimate networked system, the **Internet**, which links millions of computers throughout the world. Networks allow multiple users to share the same data or information at the same time. They also allow rapid communication between individuals. Examples of communication methods that use networks include electronic mail, telemedicine, telepharmacies, and virtual communities.

Electronic mail, or e-mail, is the process of sending messages from one computer to another. It allows health care providers to quickly send messages, memos, announcements, reports, and other data to one or more persons. Files created in word-processing programs, insurance forms completed with insurance software, financial data compiled in spreadsheets, radiographic images, and photographs, can be sent electronically. For example, all claims for Medicare and Medicaid must be submitted electronically. The claim form is usually completed on specialized insurance software and filed electronically as a claim. Electronic messages should follow the same professional standards as for any written document. The message should be clear and concise, correct grammar and spelling must be used, and slang or codes should be avoided. It is also important for all health care personnel to understand that all e-mail messages belong to the employer or owner of the computer. The messages may be stored in backup files, and employers have the legal right to read and monitor any messages. Health care personnel should never send or receive personal e-mail correspondence at their place of employment.

Telemedicine, discussed in detail in Section 1:2, involves the use of video, audio, and computer systems to provide medical or health care services. For example, radiographs or electrocardiograms can be transmitted electronically from one physician to another for consultation. A cardiologist can use specialized software to check the functioning of a patient's pacemaker and the patient's heart rhythm using a patient's telephone line or computer. A surgeon can direct the work of another surgeon, or even a robotic arm, by watching the procedure on video. Telemedicine also allows patients to communicate with physicians or health care specialists at a distance, transmit medical information to a physician, or be monitored by health care professionals. A recent advance in telemedicine is a computerized device that has sensors to remind a patient to take medications at specific times and a touch screen medicine cabinet that recognizes faces and can determine that the patient is taking the correct medication.

Electronic medicine is another growing practice that allows patients to communicate with a physician by e-mail to ask routine medical questions, ask for renewals of prescriptions, obtain the results of laboratory tests, or obtain financial information about their account. In most cases, the physician and patient form a contract to use electronic medicine. In most cases, a *patient portal* or secure online website is used for this transmission of information. Most physicians do not charge for prescription renewals or information about billing or laboratory results. However, physicians may charge for assisting with routine medical problems or evaluating health information sent by patient monitors. The term *Web visit* has been used to describe this interaction between patient and physician. It allows physicians to handle routine medical problems in a quick and efficient manner. If the patient's problems seem more complex, physicians can recommend an office visit.

 Electronic health records (EHRs) and the **health information exchange (HIE)** have also simplified communication between different health care providers. Previously if medical records had to be transferred between physicians or health care agencies, they were faxed, mailed, or manually carried by the patient. Now EHRs containing all of a patient's medical information can be electronically transferred by the HIE to any other health care facility or provider. However, this system does require the software systems in the different health care agencies to be compatible and able to interpret the data. In addition, the networks used to transfer the records must be secure, and every precaution must be taken to ensure the privacy of the information.

Telepharmacies allow for rapid dispensing of medications. Prescriptions are sent electronically to a computerized dispensing unit. The unit prepares and dispenses the ordered prescription, which is then mailed or sent by a carrier service to the patient or health care facility. A telepharmacy can also be used in areas where patients may not have access to a pharmacist. It allows the pharmacist to use telecommunications through a computer or telephone line to counsel patients regarding medications and to monitor drug usage.

Virtual communities are another way individuals communicate on the Internet. Some common examples include:

- **Social networks**: Examples include Facebook, Instagram, Snapchat, and Twitter. A social network usually consists of an individual's profile, including interests, hobbies, family, work, and other similar data. The network allows this individual to share ideas, activities, interests, photographs, and other information with friends and family. While using a social network, it is important for the user to remember not to post anything on the page that could cause embarrassment or show a lack of respect for others. Employers frequently check social networks before hiring an individual, and if the potential employee uses poor judgment in postings, it could cost the individual the job.

- **Professional networks**: These are used by people in professional occupations to maintain contact with other professionals, post a resume, research potential job or career opportunities, and obtain answers to questions from other professionals. Examples include LinkedIn, Meetup, and Xing.

- **Blogs**: Blogs are usually maintained by one or more individuals to provide information about certain topics. Most blogs are interactive and allow others to leave comments. Some blogs contain links to other sites. For example, a neurosurgeon specializing in cancerous tumors of the brain might start a blog with information they have acquired. Other neurosurgeons or health personnel could monitor the blog and add comments or ask questions.

- **Discussion groups**: These sites allow participants to communicate with each other electronically to discuss shared interests. These may consist of chat rooms or even gaming communities. Technology now allows individuals to see and speak with each other online through web conferencing. This is an ideal method for conducting a meeting when participants live in different areas because it eliminates the need for all participants to travel to a meeting site.

- **Automatic mailings**: These are also part of the online communities. An individual can subscribe to newspapers, drug company alerts, medical alerts, sources for continuing education units (CEUs), and many other topics. When information is released, the subscriber receives it immediately. An example is LISTSERV. Health care providers can receive health information through LISTSERV mailing lists. These automated systems send e-mail messages about specific topics, similar to receiving a newsletter or magazine. Some health care LISTSERVs are free, while others charge monthly or annual fees.

🔒 **HIPAA** Even though technology and computers have enhanced the communication options for health care personnel and facilities, it is essential to remember that professional standards must be observed at all times while using these technologies. Safeguards must be used to ensure the privacy of patient information and to meet the requirements of the Health Insurance Portability and Accountability Act (HIPAA).

checkpoint

| **1.** What is a telepharmacy?

12:9 USING THE INTERNET

A network of computer users can be found on the Internet. Many types of services and sources of information are offered. Through the Internet, health care professionals can readily contact others for medical updates, information about new procedures, aid in making diagnoses, and many other kinds of information.

One major use of the Internet in health care relates to organ transplants. When an individual needs a transplant, vital information regarding that individual is recorded on the transplant network. The network monitors all organs as they become available and can immediately notify the online facility when an organ is suitable for a particular patient. This allows the most expedient use of donor organs and ensures that organs are given to the most compatible recipient. It is another example of modern technology providing a service that saves lives.

Because the Internet contains a wealth of information, every health care provider should be familiar with how to use the Internet as a research tool. In order to do this, the health care provider must first become familiar with search engines. A search engine can be defined as a database of Internet files. It usually consists of three parts:

- **Search program**: commonly called a spider, wanderer, crawler, robot, or worm, the search program explores different sites and identifies and reads pages
- **Index**: the search program creates a main database that contains copies of all the information obtained

- **Retrieval program**: a program that searches the database for specific information, lists all sources of the information, and, in most cases, ranks the sources with the most relevant first

There are many different search engines available. Some common examples include Google, Bing, and Yahoo. To find relevant material on the Internet, it is important to develop a strategy to efficiently and effectively locate information about a specific topic. Searching for information about a topic such as "Does smoking or drinking alcohol during pregnancy increase the chance of a premature birth?" can result in hundreds or even thousands of listings. Some of the listings may be relevant; others will not be. Various techniques can be used to limit the search and produce only information that is specific to the topic. Basic steps that should be followed include:

- **Identify key words**: Always try to determine the main words that pertain to the information you desire. In the example above, the key words are *smoking*, *alcohol*, *pregnancy*, and *premature birth*. Other words that are alternative ways of expressing the key words might include *cigarettes*, *premature infants*, and *alcoholism*.

- **Use an advanced search**: Most search engines provide for an advanced search. By putting key words in quotation marks or specifying related fields such as "medical" or "health", results from the search will be more specific and relevant to the topic.

- **Use different search engines**: If one search engine does not locate pertinent information, try different search engines. No search engine has access to all the information on the Internet.

- **Evaluate the source of all information**: The Internet can provide a wealth of information to health care providers, but individuals using it must also evaluate the information. Not all data are accurate or current. It is important to check the source of any information (universities, government agencies, and national organizations are usually reliable sources); the author (the person should have the proper education and credentials); the date of publication, if provided (information should be recent and up-to-date); and references, if they are listed. For example, a search for *diabetes mellitus* will provide many journal articles, newsletters, organizational reports, and similar data. If material is published by an organization such as the American Diabetic Association, the information should be accurate. If material is published by an individual who states he has diabetes but can eat any and all sweets, it would be wise to discount this information.

Health care providers can research many topics on the Internet. They can obtain current health care information; learn about new diagnostic tests; research diseases, medications, therapies, and other health concerns; and communicate with other health care providers. The Internet is an excellent learning tool and another example of how technology has enhanced health care. Some reliable sources for medical information on the Internet include:

- **www.aap.org**: American Academy of Pediatrics
- **www.ada.org**: American Dental Association
- **www.alz.org**: Alzheimer's Association
- **www.ama-assn.org**: American Medical Association
- **www.cancer.gov**: National Cancer Institute
- **www.cdc.gov**: Centers for Disease Control and Prevention
- **www.diabetes.org**: American Diabetes Association
- **www.emedicinehealth.com**: provides health, medical, lifestyle, and wellness information for all age groups
- **www.familydoctor.org**: American Academy of Family Physicians
- **www.fda.gov**: Food and Drug Administration
- **www.healthfinder.gov**: health information from the U.S. Department of Health and Human Services
- **www.healthinaging.org**: American Geriatrics Society's Health in Aging Foundation
- **www.healthypeople.gov**: a health information site provided by the U.S. government
- **www.heart.org**: American Heart Association
- **www.lung.org**: American Lung Association
- **www.mayoclinic.com**: Mayo Clinic site that provides health and medical information; also has "Ask a specialist" feature people can use to obtain specific health information
- **www.medicinenet.com**: medical information site that includes an "ask the experts" feature
- **www.medlineplus.gov**: consumer information from National Library of Medicine (NLM), National Institutes of Health (NIH), other government agencies, and health-related organizations
- **www.medscape.com**: a news service that has full-text medical articles
- **https://www.nccih.nih.gov/**: National Center for Complementary and Alternative Medicine (NCCAM)
- **www.netwellness.org**: consumer health website with excellent search resources
- **www.nih.gov**: National Institutes of Health
- **www.pdrhealth.com**: Physician's Desk Reference; provides information about prescription and nonprescription medications
- **www.pubmed.gov**: National Library of Medicine's database or Medline
- **www.rxlist.com**: information about prescription and nonprescription drugs, herbs, and supplements
- **www.samhsa.gov**: Substance Abuse and Mental Health Services Administration
- **www.stroke.org**: National Stroke Association
- **www.webmd.com**: provides health and medical news supplied by physicians

checkpoint

1. Identify a website you would use to find out more about heart health.

12:10 COMPUTER PROTECTION AND SECURITY

The widespread use of electronic records in health care has created the need to protect and secure the information. Electrical surges, power outages, viruses, and hackers (individuals who use the Internet or networks to obtain unauthorized access to computers) can all result in a loss of information and/or damage to a computer's software and hardware.

To protect a computer from electrical surges and power outages, an **uninterrupted power supply (UPS)** device should be used. The computer is plugged into the UPS, which has a surge protector and a battery backup. If an electrical failure occurs, the computer operates on the battery backup in the UPS. Even when a UPS is used, it is still important to back up data on the computer frequently. A computer crash can cause a loss of all data and programs. Most health care facilities perform frequent backups onto optical disks (DVDs or CDs), flash drives, or external hard drives (**Figure 12–22**). To protect against loss by fire, natural disasters, or theft, the backups should be stored in a safe and secure location outside the health care facility. Most health care facilities contract with computer

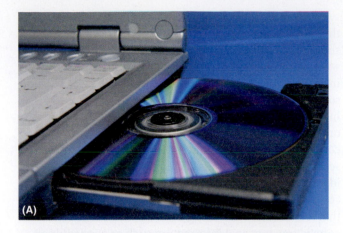

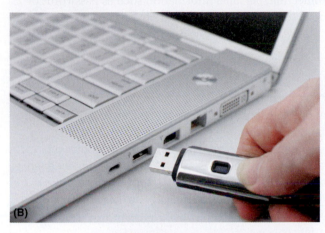

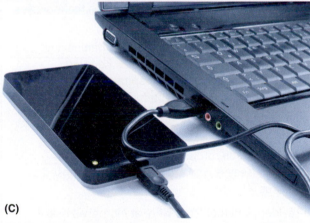

FIGURE 12–22 Data from a computer can be transferred to (A) an optical disk, (B) a flash drive, or (C) an external hard drive. ©iStock.com/Tom Gufler ©iStock.com/Angelo Arcadi ©iStock.com/Inga Nielsen

security companies to have backups performed continuously and stored in an off-site facility or secure cloud.

Viruses are programs that contain instructions to alter the operation of the computer programs, erase or scramble data on the computer, or allow access to information on the computer. Viruses can enter a computer through files downloaded from the Internet, opened e-mails, or the use of disks or flash drives that

contain viruses. Antivirus software must be installed on every computer to protect against these invasive programs. This software should also be updated on a daily basis. When the software issues a virus alert, the computer user should follow the software's recommendations.

Firewalls are protective programs that limit the ability of other computers to access a computer. A firewall alert will usually inform the user that an outside program is trying to access the computer. A strong firewall will prevent some programs and hackers from entering the database, but no firewall is entirely secure. The best way to prevent access to the database is to use only a specific dedicated computer to communicate with an outside network or the Internet and to block access to the Internet on other computers. Computers that contain the databases should be networked only within the health care facility. When information must be transferred to an outside source, the information can be copied, placed on the dedicated computer, and then sent to the correct recipient.

 Security to protect confidential patient information is essential for any health care facility. Most facilities limit access to information by means of access codes, special passwords, fingerprints, or iris identification (visualization of the eye). Computer users must employ the required access code to enter or retrieve information. Only authorized users are given access to the system. Health care providers must keep their required access code confidential to protect themselves and the patient. Guidelines to protect patient privacy have been established by many health care organizations, including the American Medical Association and the American Health Information Management Association. In addition, specific standards have been established through the Privacy Rule of the Health Insurance Portability and Accountability Act (HIPAA). HIPAA is discussed in detail in Section 5:1. The main requirements established by HIPAA to protect the confidentiality of health care information include:

- Develop and implement a security plan to ensure compliance with HIPAA policies and procedures.

- Prepare documents that patients sign to stipulate consent for the use and dissemination of health information.

- Establish a certification process and educational program to ascertain that all employees understand the security plan.

- Require individuals to sign a contract verifying that they will follow the security and privacy regulations.

- Determine the level of security necessary for each job classification.

- Establish access levels that provide authorization to confidential information on a need-to-know basis.

- Create a system that identifies the date, time, and name of the individual who enters information into any database.

- Incorporate periodic password expirations.

- Secure workstations, record storage areas, and computer hardware.

- Use encryption technology when health care information is transmitted electronically.

- Create a system to destroy duplicate or obsolete records (electronic and hard copy).

Wireless technology used to connect with networks or the Internet also creates security risks. A security code should be installed on the network to prevent access to the wireless connection. Encryption programs that secure the information on the database are also available. Encryption software uses *cryptography*, or the converting of data into a code or symbols, to protect digital information on computers and the information that is sent to other computers. This prevents unauthorized people from seeing the data if it is intercepted. In addition, the wireless identifier, usually a number or name for the wireless connection, can be suppressed so others are not aware that it is in use. When using a public wireless or WiFi connection, personal information such as passwords or social security numbers should not be used.

Issues in Health Care

Telemedicine

The World Health Organization (WHO) defines telemedicine as "healing from a distance." Telemedicine gives people the opportunity to get expert medical treatment without going to a clinic. Using telemedicine, people can receive a diagnosis, learn their treatment options, and get a prescription. Health care providers can even monitor readings from medical devices remotely to monitor patients' conditions. There are three common types of telemedicine:

- Interactive medicine: physicians and patients communicate in real-time

- Remote patient monitoring: allows caregivers to monitor patients who use mobile medical equipment to collect data on things like blood pressure, blood sugar levels, and so on

- Store and forward: providers can share a patient's health information with other healthcare professionals or specialists

Telemedicine isn't appropriate for emergency situations like a heart attack or broken bones that require X-rays and casts. Anything that requires immediate, hands-on care should be handled in person. However, telemedicine is very useful for simple issues. For instance, if a patient suspects that a cut may be infected, they can schedule a virtual consultation with a health care provider to discuss their symptoms. If a patient is on vacation and thinks that they are coming down with strep throat, they can communicate with a physician. It is helpful for a variety of other health issues including psychotherapy and dermatology, which offers consultations of moles, rashes, and so on.

In 2020, as the COVID-19 virus started wreaking havoc with the health care system, telemedicine was used to help caregivers respond to the needs of people who had contracted the virus as well as people who needed to touch base with their providers for other health issues. Telemedicine made a very positive contribution to health care during the pandemic and was used in a variety of ways.

There were three main roles for telehealth technologies during the COVID-19 crisis:

- To screen patients remotely rather than having them visit the practice or hospital. Keeping infected individuals out of hospitals and doctors' offices, the health care system could lower the risk of transmission to other patients and health care staff.

- To help provide routine care for patients with chronic diseases who are at high risk if exposed to the virus.

- Providers and their staff were at increased risk for contracting COVID-19 due to their continuous exposure to infected patients. Once tested and confirmed, these providers were quarantined and technologies in place, quarantined providers had the option to continue to see patients.

Telemedicine also can reduce health care costs. It can increase efficiency of care delivery, cut the cost of transporting patients, and can keep patients out of the hospital. In fact, one study showed that telemedicine care had 19 percent savings over inpatient care. It seems that telemedicine is here to stay and grow as a useful health care tool.

Health care providers must make every effort to protect and secure computerized records. Passwords should be kept confidential and never given to any other individual. When a password is keyed into a computer, no other individual should be able to see the keyboard. Other individuals should not be able to read the computer screen when confidential patient information is on the screen. Monitor screens that contain confidential data should be cleared before leaving the work area. E-mails or files from unknown parties must never be opened or downloaded onto the computer. If a virus or firewall alert occurs, instructions provided by the program should be followed. Discarded hard copies or printouts should be shredded. If every team member in a health care facility follows the established security and privacy policy, the confidentiality of patient information will be protected.

checkpoint

1. How should a provider dispose of hard copies of health care documents?
2. How do firewalls keep computer information secure from Internet viruses and hackers?
3. Why is encryption technology used when transmitting information electronically?

PRACTICE: Go to the workbook and complete the assignment sheet for Chapter 12, Computers and Technology in Health Care.

Case Study Investigation Conclusion

What might Ricardo advise Jessica to do before he sends a staff member to her floor? What confidentiality concerns must they be aware of before they access this patient files?

CHAPTER 12 SUMMARY

- The use of computers and technology in health care has become a necessity. All health care providers should have basic computer literacy.

- Computers are used to provide patient information, schedule personnel, manage financial records, and maintain records and inventory.

- Computers are used as diagnostic tools to perform blood tests or view body parts. Technology, such as lasers, robotics, image-guided surgery, radiation therapy, ultrasound, hearing-assistive devices, and medication-dispensing systems, have provided efficient methods of treatment.

- Patient monitoring also uses computerized technology.

- Computers and technology are major educational tools.

- Computers are critical components in health care research.

- The Internet is used by almost every health care team member. It is important to ensure that any information obtained is from reliable sources.

- The widespread use of computers in health care makes it essential to protect and secure the data to maintain patient confidentiality. Uninterrupted power supply devices, antivirus programs, firewalls, encryption, and strict control of access to computers can help protect both the computer and the information it contains.

REVIEW QUESTIONS

1. List six (6) different health care personnel that use computer technology as information systems.

2. Briefly describe the main uses of the following imaging techniques:
   a. computerized tomography (CT)
   b. magnetic resonance imaging (MRI)
   c. positron emission tomography (PET)
   d. ultrasonography

3. As part of a research project, you are conducting an Internet search for information about the following research question: "Does hypertension affect some cultures or age groups more readily than others?"
   a. Identify the key words in the question.
   b. List at least two (2) possible search phrases.
   c. Which search engine will you use? Why?
   d. Using correct formatting, create a paragraph based on the results of your research.

4. When researching the COVID-19 pandemic, list three (3) ways to identify a valid and reliable website.

5. List five (5) ways a health care provider can help meet HIPAA standards for maintaining the confidentiality of patient information while using computer technology.

6. Why is a contingency backup plan essential when computers are used to record information?

CRITICAL THINKING

1. Why are lasers, robotic surgery, and image-guided surgery more efficient than standard types of surgery?

2. How do HIPAA standards impact computer use?

3. Differentiate between an antivirus program and a firewall program. How do they help provide computer security?

■ ACTIVITIES

1. In a small group, create two (2) brochures; each describing a treatment using computers and technology.

2. Using the following scenarios, create a flow chart illustrating how computer technologies have improved communication and therefore improved patient care.

   2a. Tracy Hoang is expecting her first child and has developed high blood pressure. Her doctor has ordered complete bedrest and blood pressure medication, but Tracy needs to be monitored for spikes in blood pressure, premature contractions, and personal stress levels.

   2b. Anthony Johnson is a 58-year-old man that is suffering from kidney failure and is currently on dialysis while awaiting a kidney transplant. He has developed Type 2 diabetes mellitus and is having difficulty stabilizing his diabetes.

 | CONNECTION

Competitive Event: Exploring Medical Innovation

Event Summary: Exploring Medical Innovation provides HOSA members with the opportunity to gain knowledge regarding a medical innovation that impacted the future of health or the delivery of healthcare. This competitive event consists of a display and presentation, and each team consists of 2–4 people. This event aims to inspire members to be proactive future health professionals and understand and research the value of medical innovation.

Details on this competitive event may be found at:

www.hosa.org/guidelines

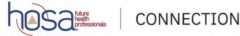 | CONNECTION

Bioengineering

The goal of the Academic Testing Center is to provide as many International Leadership Conference HOSA delegates as space permits with the opportunity to demonstrate their basic knowledge in preparation to become future health professionals.

The series of events in the Academic Testing Center are written tests based on items from the identified text specific to each event. Competitors will recognize, identify, define, interpret, and apply knowledge in a 50-item multiple choice test with a tie-breaker question. The written test will measure knowledge and understanding at the recall, application and analysis levels. Higher-order thinking skills, will be incorporated.

Details on this event may be found at

www.hosa.org/guidelines

Case Study Investigation

Laura is a brand-new Certified Nursing Assistant at Oak Village, a long-term care facility. She is assigned to pick up trays after lunch. She has to record fluid intake and estimate the percentage of food patients consume. Laura had difficulty with percentages in school, but fractions were easy for her to understand. What concepts in math could she use? At the end of the chapter, you will be asked how you would help Laura to calculate this information.

*This chapter has been adapted from Dakota Mitchell and Lee Haroun's textbook entitled *Introduction to Health Care*, 2/E, Cengage Learning, 2007. Our sincere thanks to these authors for allowing the use of their material in this textbook.

LEARNING OBJECTIVES

After completing this chapter, you should be able to:

- Perform basic math calculations on whole numbers, decimals, fractions, percentages, and ratios.
- Convert between the following numerical forms: decimals, fractions, percentages, and ratios.
- Round off numbers correctly.
- Solve mathematical problems with proportions.
- Express numbers using Roman numerals.
- Estimate angles from a reference plane.
- Use household, metric, and apothecary units to express length, volume, and weight.
- Convert between the Fahrenheit and Celsius temperature scales.
- Express time using the 24-hour clock (military time).
- Define, pronounce, and spell all key terms.

KEY TERMS

angles	Fahrenheit	percentages
apothecary system (ah-pa'-the-ker-E)	fractions	proportion
	household system	ratios
Celsius	improper fractions	reciprocal (ree-si'-pre-kal)
centigrade	metric system	reference plane
decimals	military time	Roman numerals
degrees	nomenclature (no'-men-kla-shure)	rounding numbers
estimating		whole numbers

INTRODUCTION

Working in health care requires the use of math skills to measure and perform various types of calculations. There are applications in all types of occupations:

- Calculating medication dosages
- Taking height and weight readings
- Measuring the amount of intake (fluids consumed or infused) and output (fluids expelled, e.g., urine, vomit)
- Billing and bookkeeping tasks
- Performing lab tests
- Mixing cleaning solutions

 Safety Errors in math can have negative effects on patients. For example, administering the wrong dosage of medication is a serious mistake and can harm the patient. Health care providers must strive for 100 percent accuracy. *If there is any doubt, it is essential to ask your supervisor or a qualified team member to double-check calculations.*

13:1 BASIC CALCULATIONS

To work safely in health care, it is essential to be able to add, subtract, multiply, and divide whole numbers, decimals, fractions, and percentages. Health care providers also need to understand equivalents when using decimals, fractions, and percentages (**Figure 13–1**).

Many health care providers use small calculators to assist them with calculations. During your health science studies, some instructors will allow the use of calculators, and others will not. It is always best to know how to do the basic functions by "long hand" (without a calculator). Calculators can quit working at any time during a test or at the workplace. In addition, some professional examinations required for licensure or certification do not allow the use of calculators.

WHOLE NUMBERS

Whole numbers are what we traditionally use to count (1, 2, 3, …). They do not contain fractions or decimals. For example, 30 is a whole number, while 30½ and 30.5 are not. Health care providers must be able to accurately add, subtract, multiply, and divide whole numbers.

Addition of Whole Numbers

Addition is adding two or more numbers together to find the *sum*, or total. A few examples of how addition is used in health care include:

- Counting and totaling supplies for an inventory
- Adding oral (by mouth) intake
- Adding intravenous or IV (into a vein) intake
- Measuring and totaling output from the body such as amounts of urine
- Completing statistical information such as the total number of patients diagnosed with lung cancer or the total number of surgeries performed in a hospital in a 1-year period

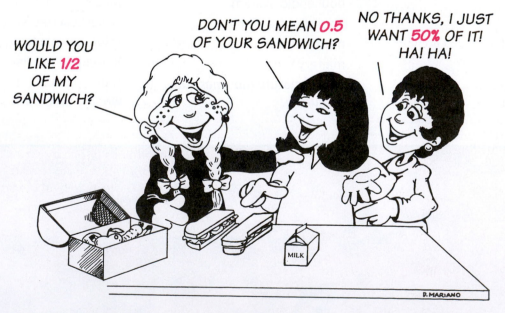

FIGURE 13–1 An easy way to remember how to convert decimals, percentages, and fractions is to think of this humorous cartoon.

To add whole numbers together, the numbers are placed in a column and lined up on the right side of the column. The columns are then added together starting with the column on the right.

Example: A nurse assistant must encourage a patient to drink large amounts of fluid. For lunch, the patient drank 240 milliliters (mL) of milk, 120 mL of coffee, 45 mL of water, and 60 mL of juice. What is the total amount of fluids the patient drank?

$$
\begin{array}{r}
^{+1}2\,4\,0 \\
1\,2\,0 \\
4\,5 \\
+\ \ 6\,0 \\
\hline
4\,6\,5
\end{array}
$$

Answer: The patient drank 465 mL of fluid.

Subtraction of Whole Numbers

Subtraction is the process of taking a number away from another number to find the *difference*, or *remainder*, between the numbers. A few examples of how subtraction is used in health care include:

- Determining weight loss or gain
- Maintaining an inventory of supplies
- Calculating a pulse deficit (difference between the number of times a heart beats and the actual pulse it creates)
- Performing laboratory tests
- Reporting statistical information such as number of deaths from a particular disease

To subtract whole numbers, the number to be subtracted *(subtrahend)* is placed under the number from which it is to be subtracted *(minuend)*. Both numbers must be lined up on the right-hand column. Starting at the right side, the bottom number is subtracted from the top number.

Example: A patient with a heart condition is on a weight-reduction plan. Last month, the patient weighed 214 pounds. This month, the patient weighs 195 pounds. How much weight did the patient lose?

$$
\begin{array}{r}
^{1}2\ ^{0}1\ 4 \\
-1\ 9\ 5 \\
\hline
1\ 9
\end{array}
$$

Answer: The patient lost 19 pounds.

Multiplication of Whole Numbers

Multiplication is actually a simple method of addition. For example, if three *7s* are added together, the answer or sum is *21* (7 + 7 + 7 = 21). If the number *7* is multiplied by *3*,

the answer or product is *21* (7 × 3 = 21). A few examples of how multiplication is used in health care include:

- Maintaining payroll records including hours worked and salary earned
- Performing laboratory tests
- Determining the magnification power of a microscope
- Calculating prescription amounts such as the number of pills a patient should receive for a 30-day supply of medication
- Calculating caloric requirement based on body weight

To multiply whole numbers, write the number to be multiplied *(multiplicand)* first. If possible, use the largest number as the multiplicand. Under the multiplicand, write the number of times it is to be multiplied *(multiplier)*, making sure the numbers are lined up on the right side. Then multiply every number in the multiplicand by every number in the multiplier. After all of the multipliers are used, the products obtained are added together to get the answer.

Example 1: A pharmacy technician is preparing a prescription for a patient. The physician ordered a dosage of 2 tablets after meals and at bedtime every day. How many tablets should the technician dispense for a 30-day supply of the medication?

First, it is necessary to determine how many tablets the patient would require each day. The patient would take 2 tablets of the medication 4 times daily, once after 3 meals and once at bedtime.

$$
\begin{array}{r}
2 \\
\times\ 4 \\
\hline
8
\end{array}
$$

The patient needs 8 tablets a day for 30 days.

$$
\begin{array}{r}
3\,0 \\
\times\ \ 8 \\
\hline
2\,4\,0
\end{array}
$$

Answer: The pharmacy technician would dispense 240 tablets of the medication to the patient.

Example 2: A medical laboratory technician is preparing agar slant tubes. The tubes are used to grow microorganisms so the cause of a disease can be identified. The technician needs a total of 24 tubes. For each tube, 30 milliliters (mL) of broth and 15 mL of agar is needed (**Figure 13–2**). What is the total amount of broth needed and the total amount of agar needed?

$$
\begin{array}{r}
3\,0 \\
\times\ 2\,4 \\
\hline
1\,2\,0 \\
+\ 6\,0 \\
\hline
7\,2\,0
\end{array}
\qquad
\begin{array}{r}
1\,5 \\
\times\ 2\,4 \\
\hline
6\,0 \\
+\ 3\,0 \\
\hline
3\,6\,0
\end{array}
$$

Answer: The laboratory technician needs 720 mL of broth and 360 mL of agar to prepare 24 agar slant tubes.

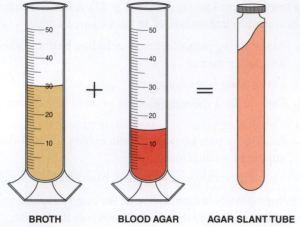

FIGURE 13–2 How much broth and agar is needed to fill 24 agar slant tubes?

BROTH   BLOOD AGAR   AGAR SLANT TUBE

Division of Whole Numbers

Division is a simple method used to determine how many times one number is present in another number. A few examples of how division is used in health care include:

- Calculating diets and amounts of nutrients allowed
- Determining cost per item while ordering bulk supplies or equipment
- Performing laboratory tests
- Compiling statistics on diseases and death rates
- Calculating budgets and salaries

Division involves the use of two numbers: a dividend and a divisor. The number to be divided is the *dividend*. The *divisor* is the number of times the dividend is to be divided. It is important to position these numbers correctly to obtain an answer, or *quotient*.

Example: A student doing research learns that statistics show 569,484 people die of cancer each year. On average, how many people die of cancer each month? (*Hint:* Remember that there are 12 months in a year.)

$$
\begin{array}{r}
47457 \\
12\overline{\smash{)}569484} \\
-\,48 \\
\hline
89 \\
-\,84 \\
\hline
54 \\
-\,48 \\
\hline
68 \\
-\,60 \\
\hline
84 \\
-\,84 \\
\hline
0
\end{array}
$$

Answer: On average, 47,457 people die of cancer each month.

DECIMALS

Decimals are one way of expressing parts of numbers or anything else that has been divided into parts. The parts are expressed in units of 10. That is, decimals represent the number of tenths, hundredths, thousandths, and so on that are available. For example, 0.7 represents 7 of the 10 parts into which something has been divided. When reading decimals verbally, it is necessary to know the place values for the decimals (digits to the right of the decimal point) and that the decimal point is read as "and" (**Figure 13–3**). For example:

- 0.5 is read "five tenths"
- 1.5 is read "one and five tenths"
- 1.50 is read "one and fifty hundredths"
- 1.500 is read "one and five hundred thousandths"
- 1.5000 is read "one and five thousand ten thousandths"

Note that a zero is placed to the left of the decimal point if the number begins to the right of the point. This is necessary to prevent errors from occurring if the decimal point is not seen.

Decimals are added, subtracted, multiplied, and divided in the same way as whole numbers. The most common mistake is incorrect placement of the decimal point (**Table 13–1**).

A few examples of how decimals are used in health care include:

- Determining medication dosages
- Performing laboratory tests
- Calculating dietary requirements or restrictions
- Measuring respiratory function
- Maintaining payroll records
- Billing charges on patient accounts
- Determining exposure to radiation
- Totaling the cost of supplies and equipment orders

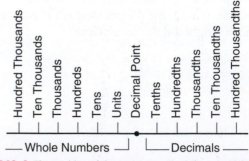

FIGURE 13–3 The position of the number to the left or the right of the decimal point is its place value. The value of each place left of the decimal point is 10 times that of the place to its right. The value of each place right of the decimal point is one-tenth the value of the place to its left.

TABLE 13-1 Working with Decimals

Function	Example	Key Points
Add: (+)	1.5 + 2.25 —— 3.75	1. Line up the decimal points. 2. Add the numbers. 3. Bring the decimal point straight down.
Subtract: (−)	3.75 − 1.25 —— 2.50	1. Line up the decimal points. 2. Subtract the numbers. 3. Bring the decimal point straight down.
Multiply: (×)	2.5 × 2.5 —— 125 + 50 —— 6.25	1. Multiply the numbers. 2. Count the total number of digits to the right of the decimal points in the numbers you are multiplying. In this example, there are two decimal points total, one decimal point in the multiplicand of 2.5 and one decimal point in the multiplier of 2.5. 3. Count the same number of places in your answers. Start to the right of the last digit in your answer and move that number of places to the left. This is where the decimal point is placed. In this example, the decimal point was moved two places to the left.

Divide: (÷)	2.5)‾50.5‾
	
	25.)‾505.0‾
	
	 20.2
	25)‾505.0‾
	 −50
	 ——
	  5
	  −0
	  ——
	  50
	  −50
	  ——
	   0
		1. Move the decimal point to the right in the number you are dividing by (divisor) to make it a whole number. In this example, the decimal point is moved one place to the right to change 2.5 to 25.
		2. Move the decimal point the same number of places to the right in the number being divided (dividend). Add zeros if necessary. In this example, the decimal point in the dividend is moved one place to the right (50.5 to 505.0) because the decimal point was moved one place to the right in the divisor.
		3. Divide the numbers.
		4. Place the decimal point in the answer by moving it straight up from the dividend, or number that was divided.

Example: A dietitian is teaching teenagers about the high levels of fat in fast food. She notes that there are 44.51 grams (g) of fat in a bacon cheeseburger, 18.3 g in a large serving of fries, and 13.83 g in a milkshake. How many grams of fat does this meal contain? (Remember to line up the decimal points to add the numbers together.)

$$
\begin{array}{r}
44.51 \\
18.30 \\
+\,13.83 \\
\hline
76.64
\end{array}
$$

This meal contains 76.64 g of fat. If the recommended daily allowance for fat grams is 60 g in an 1,800-calorie diet, how many extra grams of fat are present in just this one meal? To solve this, subtract the recommended daily allowance from the total number of fat grams in the meal. Add zeros to the right of the decimal point to make it easier to subtract the numbers.

$$
\begin{array}{r}
76.64 \\
-\,60.00 \\
\hline
16.64
\end{array}
$$

Answer: This fast-food meal contains 76.64 g of fat, which is 16.64 g more than is recommended for an entire day of meals.

FRACTIONS

Fractions are another way of expressing numbers that represent parts of a whole. A few examples of how fractions are used in health care include:

- Measuring solutions for laboratory tests
- Calculating height and weight
- Measuring head circumference on an infant
- Mixing solutions such as disinfectants for infection control
- Preparing dental materials and trimming dental models
- Mixing infant formulas or tube feedings
- Calculating dosages for certain medications

A fraction has a *numerator* (top number) and a *denominator* (bottom number). An example of a fraction is $\frac{3}{10}$, where 3 is the numerator and 10 is the denominator.

The 3 tells how many parts are present. The 10 tells how many parts make up the whole (**Figure 13–4**). The fraction $\frac{3}{10}$ has been *reduced* to its lowest terms because no number can be divided evenly into both the numerator and denominator.

Some fractions must be *reduced* to their lowest terms. An example is $\frac{4}{8}$. Both the numerator and denominator can be divided evenly by 4: $4 ÷ 4 = 1$ and $8 ÷ 4 = 2$. As a result, $\frac{4}{8} = \frac{1}{2}$.

TABLE 13–2 Working with Fractions

Function	Example	Key Points
Add: (+)	$\dfrac{1}{5} = \dfrac{6}{30}$ $+\dfrac{1}{6} = \dfrac{5}{30}$ $= \dfrac{11}{30}$	1. If the denominators are not the same, find a number both denominators divide into evenly. 2. Multiply the numerators by the number of times the old denominators divide into the new denominator. 3. Add the numerators. 4. Place the new numerator over the denominator. 5. Reduce the fraction, if necessary.
Subtract: (−)	$\dfrac{1}{5} = \dfrac{6}{30}$ $-\dfrac{1}{6} = \dfrac{5}{30}$ $= \dfrac{1}{30}$	1. If the denominators are not the same, find a number both denominators divide into evenly. 2. Multiply the numerators by the number of times the old denominators divide into the new denominator. 3. Subtract the numerators. 4. Place the new numerator over the denominator. 5. Reduce the fraction, if necessary.
Multiply: (×)	$\dfrac{1}{5} \times \dfrac{1}{6} = \dfrac{1}{30}$	1. Multiply numerators. 2. Multiply denominators. 3. Reduce the fraction, if necessary.
Divide: (÷)	$\dfrac{1}{5} \div \dfrac{1}{6} = \dfrac{1}{5} \times \dfrac{6}{1} = \dfrac{6}{5} = 1\dfrac{1}{5}$	1. Invert the dividing fraction. 2. Multiply numerators. 3. Multiply denominators. 4. Reduce the fraction, if necessary.

Improper fractions have numerators that are larger than the denominators. To reduce these fractions, divide the denominator into the numerator. The result will be a whole number or a mixed number (whole number and a fraction). For example:

- The fraction $^{12}\!/_4$ would be reduced to the whole number 3 ($12 \div 4 = 3$)
- The fraction $^{11}\!/_4$ would be reduced to the mixed number $2\,^3\!/_4$ ($11 \div 4 = 2\,^3\!/_4$)

Performing calculations with fractions is not difficult, but it does require following a series of steps. These are described in **Table 13–2**. When adding and subtracting

fractions, it is necessary to change all the denominators to the same number to perform the calculations. This is known as *converting the fractions*. To do this, find a number that each denominator can divide into evenly. Then, adjust the numerators to maintain an equivalent fraction. For example, to add $\frac{1}{2} + \frac{1}{3}$, convert both fractions to sixths = $\frac{3}{6} + \frac{2}{6} = \frac{5}{6}$. The denominators 2 and 3 both divide into 6 evenly, so 6 is the new denominator. Then multiply the numerator by the number of times the old denominator divides into the new denominator (2 divides into 6 three times, so 1×3 then creates the new fraction of $\frac{3}{6}$; 3 divides into 6 two times, so 1×2 then creates the new fraction of $\frac{2}{6}$).

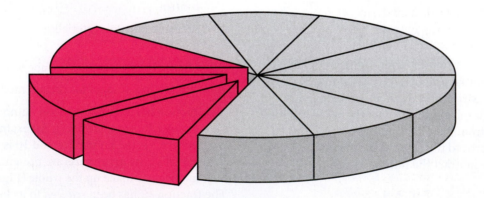

$$\frac{\text{Part or Numerator}}{\text{Whole or Denominator}} = \frac{3}{10}$$

FIGURE 13–4 A fraction is a comparison of parts (numerator) to a whole (denominator).

Multiplying fractions is straightforward. First, multiply the two numerators and then the two denominators. For example, $\frac{2}{3} \times \frac{2}{5}$ is $\frac{4}{15}$ ($2 \times 2 = 4$ and $3 \times 5 = 15$).

Dividing fractions requires the dividing fraction to be *inverted* (turned upside down). The new, upside-down fraction is called the **reciprocal**. The numerators and denominators are then multiplied to get the answer. For example, $\frac{1}{2} \div \frac{2}{3} = \frac{1}{2} \times \frac{3}{2} = \frac{3}{4}$.

Study the examples in Table 13–2 to see how to add, subtract, multiply, and divide fractions. Then review these examples:

Example 1: A dental assistant has $\frac{1}{2}$ ounce of disinfectant solution in one bottle and $\frac{2}{3}$ ounce in a second bottle. Can the two bottles be combined in a $1\frac{1}{2}$-ounce bottle? To solve this, add $\frac{1}{2}$ and $\frac{2}{3}$ together using the following steps:

First think of a number that both *2* and *3* divide into evenly. The answer is 6.

$$6 \div 2 = 3 \qquad 6 \div 3 = 2$$

Then multiply the numerator by the number of times the old denominator goes into 6.

$$1 \times 3 = 3 \quad \frac{1}{2} = \frac{3}{6}$$
$$2 \times 2 = 4 \quad \frac{2}{3} = \frac{4}{6}$$

Now add the two numerators together and place the answer over the common denominator.

$$\frac{3}{6} + \frac{4}{6} = \frac{7}{6}$$

The fraction $\frac{7}{6}$ is an improper fraction because the numerator is larger than the denominator. Divide the denominator into the numerator.

$$7 \div 6 = 1\frac{1}{6} \text{ ounces}$$

Will $1\frac{1}{6}$ ounces fit into a $1\frac{1}{2}$-ounce bottle? Change the $\frac{1}{2}$ to sixths.

$$6 \div 2 = 3 \quad 3 \times 1 = 3 \quad \frac{1}{2} = \frac{3}{6}$$

Answer: The bottle will hold $1\frac{3}{6}$ ounces, so $1\frac{1}{6}$ ounces will fit into the bottle.

Example 2: A pharmacy technician must prepare 24 ounces of a tube feeding for a patient. The mixture is $\frac{1}{3}$ formula and $\frac{2}{3}$ water. How much formula should she use? How much water?

To determine the amount of formula, multiply 24 (write as the fraction $\frac{24}{1}$) by $\frac{1}{3}$:

$$\frac{24}{1} \times \frac{1}{3} = ?$$

Multiply the numerators: $24 \times 1 = 24$.
Multiply the denominators: $1 \times 3 = 3$.
Put the new numerator over the new denominator: $\frac{24}{3}$.
Reduce the improper fraction by dividing the denominator into the numerator: $24 \div 3 = 8$.

Answer: The pharmacy technician will need 8 ounces of formula. To determine the amount of water, multiply 24 by $\frac{2}{3}$:

$$\frac{24}{1} \times \frac{2}{3} = ?$$

Multiply the numerators: $24 \times 2 = 48$.
Multiply the denominators: $3 \times 1 = 3$.
Put the new numerator over the new denominator: $\frac{48}{3}$.
Reduce the improper fraction by dividing the denominator into the numerator: $48 \div 3 = 16$.

Answer: The pharmacy technician will need 16 ounces of water.

To check the answers, add $8 + 16 = 24$. The answers are correct because 24 ounces is the total amount of tube feeding needed.

PERCENTAGES

Percentages are used to express either a whole or part of a whole. The whole is expressed as 100 percent (100%). Refer to **Figure 13–4** and imagine this as a hot apple pie sliced into 10 equal pieces. The 10 slices together equal the whole, or 100%, of the pie. 100 divided by 10 equals 10. Therefore, each slice represents 10% of the pie. If each slice is 10%, then three slices represent 30% of the pie.

A few examples of how percentages are used in health care include:

- Recording statistics such as the percentage of people who die of lung cancer
- Preparing solutions for laboratory tests
- Mixing solutions for infection control such as a 10 percent bleach solution
- Calculating the amount of tax that must be subtracted from a salary check
- Determining dietary requirements or calculating special (therapeutic) diets

When working with percentages, it is easier to convert the percentage to a decimal and then perform the addition, subtraction, multiplication, and division. Converting percentages to decimals is explained in **Table 13–3**.

Look at the pie chart in **Figure 13–5** that shows emergency department admissions for a one-month period. Then use this information to find the answers to the following questions on percentages.

Example 1: What is the total percentage of people admitted due to heart attacks or respiratory problems?

The percentage admitted for heart attacks was 11.8%.

The percentage admitted for respiratory problems was 8.8%.

These two percentages can be added together by lining up the decimal points:

$$\begin{array}{r} 11.8\% \\ + 8.8\% \\ \hline 20.6\% \end{array}$$

TABLE 13–3 Converting Decimals, Fractions, and Percentages

Converting	Example	Key Points
Decimals to fractions	$0.75 = 75/100$ $\dfrac{75}{100} = \dfrac{75}{100} \div \dfrac{25}{25} = \dfrac{3}{4}$	1. Drop the decimal point. 2. Position the number over its placement value (Figure 13–3). 3. If necessary, reduce the fraction.
Decimals to percentages	$5.275 = 5.275 \times 100 = 527.5$ 527.5%	1. Move the decimal point two places to the right because percentages are based on 100. This is the same as multiplying by 100. 2. Add the percentage sign.
Fractions to decimals	$3/5 = 3 \div 5 = 0.6$	1. Divide the numerator by the denominator.
Fractions to percentages	$7/8 = 7 \div 8 = 0.875$ $0.875 \times 100 = 87.5$ 87.5%	1. Divide the numerator by the denominator. 2. Move the decimal point two places to the right because percentages are based on 100. This is the same as multiplying by 100. 3. Add the percentage sign.
Percentages to decimals	$125.5\% = 125.5$ $125.5 \div 100 = 1.255$	1. Remove the percentage sign. 2. Move the decimal point two places to the left because percentages are based on 100. This is the same as dividing by 100.
Percentages to fractions	$5\% = 5$ $\dfrac{5}{100} = \dfrac{5 \div 5}{100 \div 5} = \dfrac{1}{20}$	1. Remove the percentage sign. 2. Place the number over 100. 3. If appropriate, reduce the fraction to its lowest terms.
Percentages to ratios	$75\% = 75$ 75:100	1. Remove the percentage sign. 2. Create a ratio using the former percentage and the number 100. 3. Insert a colon (:) between the numbers.
Ratios to percentages	$1:2 = 1 \div 2 = 0.5$ $0.5 \times 100 = 50$ $50 = 50\%$	1. Divide the number on the left of the colon or ratio sign by the number on the right of the ratio sign. 2. Move the decimal point two places to the right. Add zero(s) if necessary. This is the same as multiplying by 100. 3. Add the percentage sign.

Answer: 20.6 percent of the people were admitted with heart attacks or respiratory problems.

Example 2: If a total of 364 patients were admitted to the emergency department during the one-month period, how many people were admitted because of an auto accident?

Check the pie chart: 26.1 percent of the admissions were for auto accidents.

First convert the 26.1 percent to decimals:

$26.1\% = 26.1$ (Remove percent sign)

$26.1 \div 100 = 0.261$ (Divide by 100 to convert to a decimal)

EMERGENCY DEPARTMENT ADMISSIONS

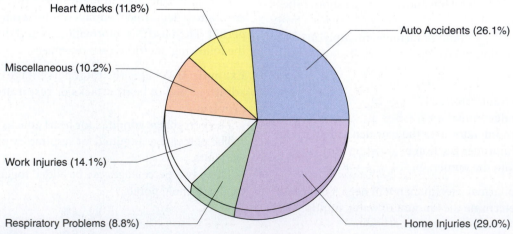

Heart Attacks (11.8%)
Miscellaneous (10.2%)
Work Injuries (14.1%)
Respiratory Problems (8.8%)
Auto Accidents (26.1%)
Home Injuries (29.0%)

FIGURE 13–5 Causes for emergency department admissions in a one-month period.

Now multiply the total number of patients, or 364, by 0.261:

$$
\begin{array}{r}
364 \\
\times\,0.261 \\
\hline
364 \\
2184 \\
728 \\
\hline
95004. = 95.004 = 95
\end{array}
$$

Starting at the right side, move the decimal point the same number of places to the left as it is in the multiplier. Because 0.261 has three decimal places, 95.004 is the correct answer.

Answer: A total of 95 people were admitted to the emergency department because of auto accidents. Note that the 4 at the end of the answer was ignored. When percentages are calculated, answers are often rounded to whole numbers.

RATIOS

Ratios show relationships between numbers or like values: how many of one number or value is present as compared with the other. For example, a bleach and water solution with a 1:2 ratio means that one part of bleach is added for every two parts of water. This relationship applies regardless of the units used:

- 1 cup of bleach and 2 cups of water
- 1 quart of bleach and 2 quarts of water
- ½ cup of bleach and 1 cup of water
- ¼ cup of bleach and ½ cup of water

The use of ratios to express the strength of a solution is commonly seen in health care. Solution strengths are also frequently expressed as percentages. A 50 percent bleach solution is the same as the 1:2 ratio. Conversions between ratios and percentages are explained in the next section.

CONVERTING DECIMALS, FRACTIONS, PERCENTAGES, AND RATIOS

Decimals, fractions, and percentages all express parts of a whole. The cartoon in **Figure 13–1** humorously portrayed how they are related: the fraction ½, the decimal 0.5, and the percentage 50% all represent the same amount of the sandwich. The steps used to convert between these numerical forms are shown in **Table 13–3**.

ROUNDING NUMBERS

Rounding numbers means changing them to the nearest ten, hundred, thousand, and so on. Deciding which to use depends on the size of the original number and the degree of accuracy required. Deciding whether to round up or round down depends on the digits (numbers) located to the right of the value chosen for rounding. The following examples illustrate how these rules are applied:

Example 1: When rounding to the nearest 10: look at the digit to the right of the tens place (the ones place). If the number is 5 or greater, round up. If it is less than 5, round down.

88 rounds up to 90

83 rounds down to 80

Example 2: When rounding to the nearest 100, look at the digit to the right of the hundreds place (the tens place). If the number is 5 or greater, round up. If it is less than 5, round down.

67 rounds up to 100

133 rounds down to 100

668 rounds up to 700

621 rounds down to 600

Example 3: When rounding to the nearest 1,000, look at the digit to the right of the thousands place (the hundreds place). If the number is 5 or greater, round up. If it is less than 5, round down.

7777 rounds up to 8,000

7355 rounds down to 7,000

All numbers can be rounded. Review **Figure 13–3** and study the examples in **Table 13–4**.

SOLVING PROBLEMS WITH PROPORTIONS

A **proportion** is a statement of equality between two ratios. For example, the proportion 2:6 = 3:9 means that 2 is related to 6 in the same way that 3 is related to 9. It is verbalized as "two is to six as three is to nine."

Proportions are used to solve many math problems in health care. Some common examples include:

- Calculating height to feet and inches
- Calculating weight to pounds and ounces
- Determining the proper dosage of a medicine
- Calculating a flow rate for IV (intravenous, or into a vein) solutions
- Determining measurements to mix solutions
- Interpreting laboratory test results

Proportions are useful for determining an amount needed when three of the terms in the proportion are known.

TABLE 13–4 Rounding Numbers

Round the Number 1,234.5678 to the Nearest:	Result	Comments
Whole number	1,234.5678 = 1,235	The digit to the right of the whole number (1,234) is 5, so you round up one number.
Tens	1,234.5678 = 1,230	The digit to the right of the tens place is 4, so you round down.
Hundreds	1,234.5678 = 1,200	The digit to the right of the hundreds place is 3, so you round down.
Thousands	1,234.5678 = 1,000	The digit to the right of the thousands place is 2, so you round down.
Tenths	1,234.5678 = 1,234.6	The digit to the right of the tenths place is 6, so you round up.
Hundredths	1,234.5678 = 1,234.57	The digit to the right of the hundredths place is 7, so you round up.
Thousandths	1,234.5678 = 1,234.568	The digit to the right of the thousandths place is 8, so you round up.
Ten thousandths	1,234.56780 = 1,234.5678	No change.

Example 1: A pharmacy technician has to prepare 500 milliliters (mL) of a 5% boric acid solution. How many grams (g) of boric acid crystals will he use?

First, calculate that a 5% boric acid solution equals 0.05 or 5/100 or 5:100 or 5 g of boric acid in every 100 mL of solution. Three of the terms in the proportion are known:

- 5 g of boric acid crystal
- 100 mL of solution
- 500 mL of solution required

The proportion is set up as follows:

$$\frac{5 \text{ g}}{x \text{ g}} = \frac{100 \text{ mL}}{500 \text{ mL}}$$

Note that the unit measurements on each side of the equation are the same (grams per milliliter).

To solve this problem, follow these steps:
Cross multiply:

$$\frac{5 \text{ g}}{x \text{ g}} = \frac{100 \text{ mL}}{500 \text{ mL}}$$

$$5 \times 500 = 100 \times x \quad 2,500 = 100 \, x$$

Divide each side by the number in front of x:

$$100x \div 100 = x \text{ and } 2,500 \div 100 = 25$$

$$x = 25 \text{ g}$$

The complete proportion is:

$$\frac{5 \text{ g}}{25 \text{ g}} = \frac{100 \text{ mL}}{500 \text{ mL}}$$

Answer: The pharmacy technician must use 25 g of boric acid crystals to prepare 500 mL of a 5% boric acid solution.

Converting units of measurement is another common application of proportions. When a patient's height is measured, the height bar on most medical scales provides the measurement in inches. This must be converted to feet and inches.

Example 2: A medical assistant measures the height of a small child at 36 inches. How many feet are in 36 inches? Three of the terms in the proportion are known:

- 36 inches
- 12 (the number of inches in 1 foot)
- 1 foot

The proportion is set up as follows:

$$\frac{1 \text{ foot}}{x \text{ feet}} = \frac{12 \text{ inches}}{36 \text{ inches}}$$

To solve this problem, follow these steps:
Cross multiply:

$$\frac{1 \text{ foot}}{x \text{ feet}} = \frac{12 \text{ inches}}{36 \text{ inches}}$$

$$12 \times x = 1 \times 36 \quad 12x = 36$$

Divide each side by the number in front of x:

$$12x \div 12 = x \text{ and } 36 \div 12 = 3$$

$$x = 3 \text{ feet}$$

The completed proportion is:

$$\frac{1 \text{ foot}}{3 \text{ feet}} = \frac{12 \text{ inches}}{36 \text{ inches}}$$

Answer: The small child is 3 feet tall.

NOTE: *If a child is 38 inches tall, 12 would divide into 38 three times with a remainder of 2. The child's height would be recorded as 3 feet, 2 inches tall.*

Another common application of proportions in health care is to find the value of an unknown when calculating the dosage of medications.

Example 3: A physician orders a patient to have 50 milligrams (mg) of a medication. When the nurse checks, he notes that the medication is only available in 12.5-mg tablets. How many tablets should he give the patient?

Set up the proportion with the three known facts:

$$\frac{1 \text{ tablet}}{x \text{ tablets}} = \frac{12.5 \text{ mg}}{50 \text{ mg}}$$

Cross multiply:

$$\frac{1 \text{ tablet}}{x \text{ tablets}} = \frac{12.5 \text{ mg}}{50 \text{ mg}}$$

$$12.5 \times x = 1 \times 50 \quad 12.5x = 50$$

Divide each side by the number in front of x:

$$12.5x \div 12.5 = x \text{ and } 50 \div 12.5 = 4$$
$$x = 4 \text{ tablets}$$

The complete proportion is:

$$\frac{1 \text{ tablet}}{4 \text{ tablets}} = \frac{12.5 \text{ mg}}{50 \text{ mg}}$$

Answer: 4 tablets are needed to equal 50 mg.

Example 4: A pharmacy technician reviews a prescription that orders amoxicillin suspension 300 milligrams (mg) by mouth three times a day. The amoxicillin suspension that is available is labeled 400 mg/2 mL. How many mL must be dispensed for a 10-day supply?

First, calculate the amount of amoxicillin that is required for a single dose. Three of the terms in the proportion are known:

- 300 mg of amoxicillin
- 400 mg of amoxicillin
- 2 mL of suspension

The proportion is set up as follows:

$$\frac{400 \text{ mg}}{300 \text{ mg}} = \frac{2 \text{ mL}}{x \text{ mL}}$$

To solve this problem, follow these steps:

Cross multiply:

$$\frac{400 \text{ mg}}{300 \text{ mg}} = \frac{2 \text{ mL}}{x \text{ mL}}$$

$$2 \times 300 = 400 \times x \quad 600 = 400x$$

Divide each side by the number in front of x:

$$400x \div 400 = x \text{ and } 600 \div 400 = 1.5$$
$$x = 1.5 \text{ mL}$$

The completed proportion is:

$$\frac{400 \text{ mg}}{300 \text{ mg}} = \frac{2 \text{ mL}}{1.5 \text{ mL}}$$

Answer: The amount of amoxicillin required for a single dose of 300 mg is 1.5 mL.

Now, calculate the number of mL needed per day. Since the patient is taking the medication 3 times a day, multiply by 3:

$$3 \times 1.5 \text{ mL} = 4.5 \text{ mL}$$

Finally, calculate how many mL will be needed for a 10-day supply. Multiply the 4.5 mL daily dose by 10:

$$10 \times 4.5 \text{ mL} = 45 \text{ mL}$$

Answer: The pharmacy technician must dispense 45 mL of the amoxicillin suspension for a 10-day supply.

checkpoint

| **1.** Define *whole number*.

13:2 ESTIMATING

Health care providers must work carefully and thoughtfully when performing calculations. An important skill to help check work is anticipating the results. This involves **estimating**—calculating the approximate answer—and judging if the calculated results seem reasonable. If calculations are performed without thought and answers simply accepted, errors can go unnoticed. It is easy for mistakes to occur when you're working in a hurry. Numbers can be placed in the wrong order, decimal points misplaced, or operations carried out incorrectly. Knowing when an answer "just doesn't look right" serves as an alert to double-check the results. Working on "automatic pilot" is not acceptable when using math in the workplace.

Learning to estimate and detect incorrect answers takes practice and thought. There are a few guidelines to make estimating useful. First, use rounding to get numbers that are easier to mentally compute.

- For example, when multiplying 47 times 83, round 47 up to 50 and 83 down to 80. Multiplying 50 times 80 is much easier to multiply mentally than the original numbers.

- Second, watch place values carefully. In the 50 times 80 example, if 5 is multiplied times 8, two zeros must be added to the quick result of 40. This means the result must be approximately 4,000, *not* 40 or 400.

- Third, look at the size of the answer. Does it make sense? For example, when multiplying whole numbers, the answer should be larger than either of the numbers in the problem. When dividing numbers, it should be smaller.

- Fourth, be careful about placing decimal points. Remember that everything to the right of the point is a fraction. Even 0.99999 does not equal 1.0.

Estimates can also be useful in planning at health care agencies. For example, an estimate can be made for the approximate number of slides a cytologist (an individual who studies cells on slides) could examine in an 8-hour day. If a cytologist examines 12 slides the first hour,

16 slides the second hour, 11 slides the third hour, and 14 slides the fourth hour, an average number of slides per hour can be calculated. By adding the four numbers together and dividing by 4, an average of 13.25 slides per hour is the result. In an 8-hour period, the cytologist could examine 106 (8 × 13.25) slides. This estimate could be used to plan the daily workload of the cytologist. This does not mean that the cytologist will examine 106 slides in one day. She may examine more or fewer slides. However, the estimate is a good approximation of what could occur and allows the health care agency to determine employees needed and workloads that can be completed.

checkpoint

1. What is estimating?

13:3 ROMAN NUMERALS

The traditional numbering system we use every day is referred to as Arabic numerals (1, 2, 3, …). In health care, it is necessary to know Roman numerals because they are used for some medications, solutions, and ordering systems. You may also see some files or materials organized using Roman numerals. When using **Roman numerals**, remember the following key points:

- All numbers can be expressed by using seven key numerals:

  I = 1

  V = 5

  X = 10

  L = 50

  C = 100

  D = 500

  M = 1000

- If a smaller numeral is placed in front of a larger numeral, the smaller numeral is *subtracted* from the larger numeral. For example:

  IV = 1 is placed before the 5, so it is subtracted (5 − 1 = 4)

- If a smaller numeral is placed after a larger numeral, the smaller numeral is *added* to the larger numeral. For example:

  VI = 1 is placed after the 5, so it is added (5 + 1 = 6)

- When the same numeral is placed next to itself, it is added. For example:

  III = 1 + 1 + 1 = 3

  XX = 10 + 10 = 20

XIX = this has two of the same numerals with a smaller numeral in the middle, but the rules still apply (10 + 10 − 1 = 19 OR 10 + (10 − 1) = 10 + 9 = 19)

- The same numeral is *not* placed next to itself more than three times. For example:

  XXX = 30

  XL = 40 (XXXX is not correct)

  To express 40, subtract 10 from the 50 symbol to get XL

- When Roman numerals are used with medication dosages, the lowercase (i, v, x, l, c, d, m) may be used rather than uppercase (capital letters). For example, ii = 2, iv = 4, xix = 19.

Study **Table 13–5** to practice converting between Arabic and Roman numerals.

TABLE 13–5 Arabic and Roman Numeral Conversion Chart

Arabic	Roman	Arabic	Roman
1	I	23	XXIII
2	II	24	XXIV
3	III	25	XXV
4	IV	26	XXVI
5	V	27	XXVII
6	VI	28	XXVIII
7	VII	29	XXIX
8	VIII	30	XXX
9	IX	40	XL
10	X	50	L
20	XX	100	C
21	XXI	500	D
22	XXII	1000	M

checkpoint

1. A cornerstone on a building is engraved with MCMLXXVI. What year was the building built?

13:4 ANGLES

Angles are used in health care when injecting medications, describing joint movement, and indicating bed positions. **Angles** are always defined by comparison to a **reference plane**, a real or imaginary flat surface from which the angle is measured. The distance between the plane and the line of the angle is measured in units called **degrees**. For example, if a flat stick is placed on a table (the reference plane), the angle is at 0 degrees. If the stick is moved to a straight up position (perpendicular to the table), there is a 90-degree angle to the table. Moving the stick halfway between these two positions creates a 45-degree angle. Rotating the stick all the way around the arc and returning to the reference point creates a complete circle and represents 360 degrees (**Figure 13–6**). The following examples illustrate how angles are used in health care:

Example 1: Angles for injecting needles vary, depending on the type of medication or procedure being performed (**Figure 13–7**). Note that in this case the reference plane is the surface of the skin.

Example 2: When describing the angle of extremities (arms and legs), the body in a full upright position is the reference plane (**Figure 13–8**). Each joint (e.g., elbow,

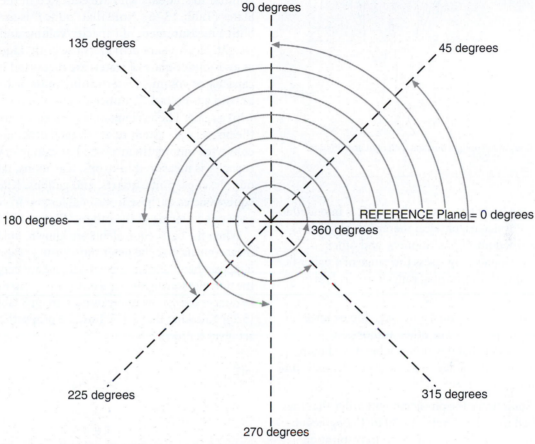

FIGURE 13–6 All angles are expressed in relation to a real or imaginary reference plane.

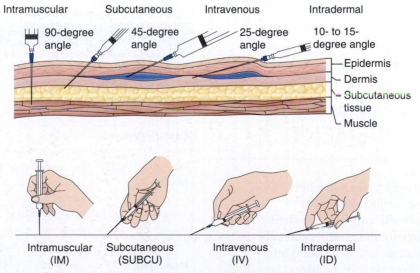

FIGURE 13–7 The correct angle must be used when inserting needles for administration of injections.

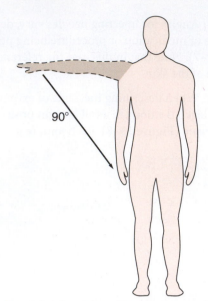

90°

FIGURE 13–8 Body in full upright position with right arm lifted to 90-degree angle.

knee, hip) in the body has a normal range it is intended to move within. Physicians, physical therapists, physician's assistants, certified nurse practitioners, and other qualified professionals may assess the range of a patient's joint compared with this normal range to chart loss of function or progress of recovery.

Example 3: After surgery on a joint (e.g., hip or knee replacement), the physician or other authorized individual will order that the joint not be moved more than a certain number of degrees to prevent the new joint from "popping" out of place.

Example 4: Sometimes the physician will order that the head of the bed must be elevated by 30 to 45 degrees at all times. This is usually ordered to aid in respiration or to prevent aspiration (stomach contents entering the lungs). In this situation, the bed in the flat position is the reference plane.

checkpoint

| **1.** Define *reference plane*.

13:5 SYSTEMS OF MEASUREMENT

Basic skills in calculation are applied when learning and using the various systems of measurement used in health care. Each system has its own terminology for designating distance (length), capacity (volume), and mass (weight). Converting between these systems requires the use of the skills presented in this chapter. The

three systems used in health care are household, metric, and apothecary. Each system has its own **nomenclature** (method of naming).

HOUSEHOLD SYSTEM

The **household system**, or U.S. customary or English system, is probably the method of measurement most familiar to students who are educated in the United States (**Table 13–6**). Note that "ounce" is used as both a measurement of capacity/volume and mass/weight. Health care providers use both. Liquids, such as an 8-ounce glass of water, are measured in terms of capacity or volume. Determining mass or weight, such as with a 6-pound 12-ounce infant, is done by weighing with a scale. The various units of measurements in the household system relate to each other and can be converted among themselves. For example, volume/capacity is measured in drops, teaspoons, tablespoons, ounces, cups, pints, quarts, and gallons. Knowing the equivalencies of these units enables you to calculate each one in terms of the others (**Figure 13–9**).

When the basic equivalents are known, unknown measurements can be determined using proportions. Suppose that 3 tablespoons of a liquid are needed, but the only measuring device available is a cup marked in ounces (oz). How many ounces are in 3 tablespoons (3 T)? Knowing that 2 T = 1 oz, the proportion would be set up as follows:

$$\frac{2\,T}{3\,T} = \frac{1\,oz}{x\,oz}$$

$$2x = 3$$
$$2x \div 2 = 3 \div 2$$
$$x = 1.5\,oz$$

Answer: There are 1.5 ounces in 3 tablespoons.

TABLE 13–6 Household Measurement System

Type of Measurement	Nomenclature	Common Equivalents
Distance/Length	inch (″ or in)	
	foot (′ or ft)	12 in = 1 ft
	yard (yd)	3 ft = 1 yd
	mile (mi)	1,760 yds = 1 mi
Capacity/Volume	drop (gtt)	
	teaspoon (t or tsp)	60 gtts = 1 t
	tablespoon (T or tbsp)	3 t = 1 T
	ounce (oz)	2 T = 1 oz
	cup (C)	8 oz = 1 C
	pint (pt)	2 C = 1 pt
	quart (qt)	2 pt = 1 qt
	gallon (gal)	4 qt = 1 gal
Mass/Weight	ounce (oz)	
	pound (lb)	16 oz = 1 lb

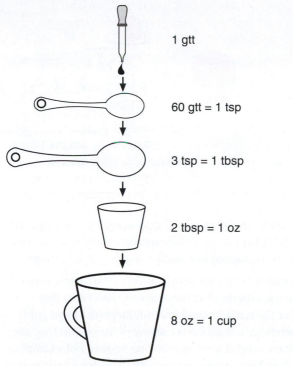

1 gtt

60 gtt = 1 tsp

3 tsp = 1 tbsp

2 tbsp = 1 oz

8 oz = 1 cup

FIGURE 13–9 Common household measurements used in health care.

The next example involves measurement of height. If a patient is 63 inches tall and asks how many feet that is, the calculation would use the following proportion:

$$\frac{12\ \text{inches}}{63\ \text{inches}} = \frac{1\ \text{foot}}{x\ \text{feet}}$$

$$12x = 63$$
$$12x \div 12 = 63 \div 12$$
$$x = 5.25\ \text{feet}$$

Because most people do not say they are 5.25 feet tall, the decimal of 0.25 feet can be converted to inches. The following proportion can be used:

$$\frac{1\ \text{foot}}{0.25\ \text{ft}} = \frac{12\ \text{inches}}{x\ \text{inches}}$$

Cross multiply:

$$1 \times x = 1x \qquad 12 \times 0.25 = 3$$

Divide both by 1 to find the value of x:

$$1x \div 1 = x \qquad 3 \div 1 = 3$$

The value of x is 3 inches. The patient is 5 feet 3 inches tall.

METRIC SYSTEM

The **metric system**, frequently called the International System of Units or simply SI, is more accurate than the household system. Converting between numbers is easier because everything is based on a unit of 10. The nomenclature for the metric units is as follows:

- Distance/length: meter (m)
- Capacity/volume: liter (L)
- Mass/weight: gram (g)

The meter, liter, and gram are modified by adding the appropriate prefix to express larger or smaller units (**Table 13–7**).

Because metric units are based on multiples of 10, conversions within the metric system are calculated by multiplying or dividing by 10, 100, 1,000, and so on:

- 1 *kilo*liter = 1,000 × 1 liter = 1,000 liters
- 1 *hecto*liter = 100 × 1 liter = 100 liters
- 1 *deca*liter = 10 × 1 liter = 10 liters
- 1 *deci*liter = 0.1 × 1 liter = 0.1 liter
- 1 *centi*liter = 0.01 × 1 liter = 0.01 liter
- 1 *milli*liter = 0.001 × 1 liter = 0.001 liter

A shortcut for performing these operations is to move the decimal point the number of places indicated by the prefix. Here are three examples:

Example 1: Multiplying by 10 means moving the decimal point one place to the right. This may require adding one or more zeros. Multiplying 4.2 by 10 = 42. Dividing by 10 means moving the decimal point one place to the left. Dividing 4.2 by 10 = 0.42.

TABLE 13–7 Common Prefixes of the Metric System

Prefix	Meaning	Examples	Meaning of Examples
kilo	1,000 times	kilogram	1,000 grams
		kilometer	1,000 meters
		kiloliter	1,000 liters
hecto	100 times	hectogram	100 grams
deca (also "deka")	10 times	decaliter	10 liters
meter, liter, gram	Whole units of measurement		
deci	1/10	decigram	1/10 of a gram
centi	1/100	centimeter	1/100 of a meter
milli	1/1,000	milliliter	1/1,000 of a liter
micro	1/1,000,000	microgram	1/1,000,000 of a gram

Example 2: Multiplying by 100 means moving the decimal point two places to the right. This may require adding one or more zeros. Multiplying 4.2 by 100 = 420. Dividing by 100 means moving the decimal point two places to the left. Dividing 4.2 by 100 = 0.042.

Example 3: Multiplying by 1,000 means moving the decimal point three places to the right. This may require adding one or more zeros. Multiplying 4.2 by 1,000 = 4,200. Dividing by 1,000 means moving the decimal point three places to the left. Dividing 4.2 by 1,000 = 0.0042.

Converting units within the metric system is accomplished by moving the decimal point. See **Figure 13–10** for a visual representation of decimal placement. Examples of how this is used in health care include:

Example 1: A physician orders 2 grams (g) of a medication. The medication is available in 1,000-milligram (mg) tablets. The 2 g must be changed to milligrams. The conversion is made as follows:

- *Milli* is in the third place to the right of *gram*. Move the decimal point three places to the right toward milligrams: 2 = 2,000
- Change unit name to milligrams: 2,000 milligrams.
- The proper dose would be 2,000 mg, or two 1,000-mg tablets.

Example 2: A physical therapist measures a distance at 1,000 centimeters, but must know the distance in kilometers to check a patient's progress. The conversion is made as follows:

- *Centi* is five decimal places to the right of *kilo*, so move the decimal point five places to the left *toward* kilo. Add zeros as needed: 1,000 = 0.01.
- Change unit name to kilometers: 0.01 kilometer.
- 1,000 centimeters equals 0.01 kilometer.

In addition to moving the decimal point the correct number of places, it is critical that it be moved in the correct direction. This can be confusing. The easiest way is to determine whether the answer should be a larger or smaller number and then just move the decimal point accordingly:

- If converting from a larger to a smaller prefix (e.g., *kilo* to *milli*), the answer will be larger. It takes more smaller units to make up the larger unit.

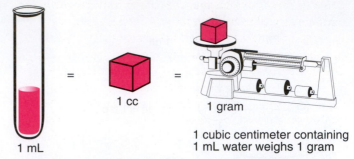

FIGURE 13–11 The metric units that measure weight and volume are related.

- If converting from a smaller to a larger prefix (e.g., *milli* to *kilo*), the answer will be smaller. Many small units can be contained in a smaller number of large units.

A common health care application of the metric system is in the measurement of medications. Two units that represent the same amount are milliliters (mL) and cubic centimeters (cc). Both units measure volume and they are often interchanged when dispensing liquids. For example, 1mL = 1cc, 2 mL = 2cc, and so forth. It is also worth noting that 1 mL or cc has a weight of 1 g (**Figure 13–11**). In most health care careers, milliliters (mL) are the unit of choice.

APOTHECARY SYSTEM

The **apothecary system** is the oldest and least used of the three systems of measurement presented. Even though it is used very infrequently, it is still necessary to be familiar with these units of measurements (**Table 13–8**).

TABLE 13–8 Apothecary Measurement System

Type of Measurement	Nomenclature	Common Equivalents
Distance/Length	N/A	N/A
Capacity/Volume	minim m fluid-dram (fl dr) fluid ounce (fl oz) pint (pt) quart (qt)	1 minim = 1 drop 60 minims = 1 fl dr 8 fl dr = 1fl oz 16 fl oz = 1 pt 2 pt = 1qt
Mass/Weight	grain (gr) dram (dr) ounce (oz)	60 gr = 1dr 480 gr = 1 oz

PREFIX	KILO-	HECTO-	DEKA-	BASE	DECI-	CENTI-	MILLI-	DECIMILLI-	CENTIMILLI-	MICROMILLI-
Common Units	kilogram			gram liter meter		centimeter	milligram milliliter millimeter			microgram
Value to Base	**1,000**	100	10	**1.0**	0.1	**0.01**	**0.001**	0.0001	0.00001	0.000001

FIGURE 13–10 Comparison of common metric units used in health care.

Health care providers must be able to convert within the system as well as to convert to the metric system.

Roman numerals can be used in conjunction with the apothecary system, and may be seen in uppercase or lowercase. If lowercase is used, the Roman numeral for 1 is written with a line and a dot or as $\overline{i}$. The Roman numeral for 2 is written as $\overline{ii}$. A commonly used abbreviation that originated with the apothecary system is $\overline{ss}$, which means "half." For example, 2½ would be written as $\overline{iiss}$.

CONVERTING SYSTEMS OF MEASUREMENT

Health care work sometimes requires that units from one system of measurement are converted to those of another. This requires knowledge of the equivalencies between the units of the systems. There are frequently no exact equivalents, so when converting between systems, the answer is considered to be a close approximation (see **Table 13–9**).

Using the appropriate equivalencies, a proportion is set up to identify and solve for the unknown quantity. The following steps are used for performing conversions:

- Identify an equivalent between the two systems.
- Set up a proportion so unit measurements on each side of the equation are the same.
- Use x for the unknown value being calculated.
- Cross multiply.
- Solve for x.
- Verify that the answer is reasonable.
- If converting from a smaller unit to a larger unit, the answer will be smaller. For example, when converting 10 mL to teaspoons, the result will be smaller than 10 because a milliliter is a smaller unit than a teaspoon. Because there are 5 mL in 1 teaspoon, 10 mL = 2 teaspoons.
- If converting from a larger unit to a smaller unit, the answer will be larger. For example, when converting 2 grains to milligrams, the result will be a larger unit than 2 because a grain is a larger unit than a milligram. Because there are 60 mg in every grain, 2 grains = 120 mg.

The following examples illustrate how to perform conversions:

Example 1: Convert 19 inches to centimeters:

- Identify the equivalency: 1 inch = 2.5 centimeters
- Set up a proportion with the same units on each side of the equation. Use x for the unknown.

$$\frac{1 \text{ in}}{19 \text{ in}} = \frac{2.5 \text{ cm}}{x \text{ cm}}$$

- Cross multiply:

$$1 \times x = 2.5 \times 19 \qquad 1x = 47.5$$

- Solve for x:

$$1x \div 1 = 47.5 \div 1$$
$$x = 47.5 \text{ cm}$$

- Verify that the answer is reasonable: It takes a larger number of centimeters (2½ times) to measure the same distance as 1 inch. Therefore, it makes sense that the answer is larger than 19.

Answer: There are 47.5 centimeters in 19 inches.

Example 2: Convert 1.5 meters to inches:

- Identify the equivalency: 39.4 inches = 1 meter
- Set up a proportion with the same units on each side of the equation. Use x for the unknown.

$$\frac{39.4 \text{ in}}{x \text{ in}} = \frac{1 \text{ m}}{1.5 \text{ m}}$$

- Cross multiply:

$$1 \times x = 1.5 \times 39.4 \qquad 1x = 59.1$$

- Solve for x:

$$1x \div 1 = 59.1 \div 1$$
$$x = 59.1 \text{ inches}$$

- Verify that the answer is reasonable: It takes many inches to measure the distance designated by 1 meter. Therefore, the answer 59.1 makes sense.

Answer: There are 59.1 inches in 1.5 meters.

Example 3: Convert 5 teaspoons to milliliters:

$$\frac{1 \text{ tsp}}{5 \text{ tsp}} = \frac{5 \text{ ml}}{x \text{ ml}}$$
$$1 \times x = 5 \times 5 \quad 1x = 25$$
$$x = 25 \text{ ml}$$

Answer: There are 25 milliliters in 5 teaspoons.

TABLE 13–9 Approximate Equivalents Between Measuring Systems

Distance/Length	Capacity/Volume	Mass/Weight
1 in = 2.5 cm	1 tsp = 5 mL = 5 cc	1 lb = 0.454 kg
39.4 in = 1 m	1 oz = 30 mL = 30 cc	2.2 lb = 1 kg
1.094 yards (yd) = 1 m	1 pt = 500 mL = 500 cc	1 grain = 60 mg
0.621 mile (Mi) = 1 km	1 qt = 1,000 mL = 1000 cc	15 grains = 1 g

Example 4: Convert 75 milliliters to ounces:

$$\frac{1 \text{ oz}}{x \text{ oz}} = \frac{30 \text{ mL}}{75 \text{ mL}}$$

$30x = 75$ (Note that in solving for x, each side is divided by 30.)

$$x = 2.5 \text{ oz}$$

Answer: There are 2.5 ounces in 75 milliliters.

Example 5: Convert 120 pounds to kilograms:

$$\frac{2.2 \text{ lb}}{120 \text{ lb}} = \frac{1 \text{ kg}}{x \text{ kg}}$$

$2.2x = 120$ (Note that in solving for x, each side is divided by 2.2.)

$$x = 54.5 \text{ kg (rounded to nearest tenth)}$$

Answer: There are 54.5 kilograms in 120 pounds.

Example 6: Convert 15 grains to milligrams:

$$\frac{1 \text{ gr}}{15 \text{ gr}} = \frac{60 \text{ mg}}{x \text{ mg}}$$

$$x = 900 \text{ mg}$$

Answer: There are 900 milligrams in 15 grains.

Example 7: Convert 2 grams to grains:

$$\frac{15 \text{ gr}}{x \text{ gr}} = \frac{1 \text{ g}}{2 \text{ g}}$$

$$x = 30 \text{ gr}$$

Answer: There are 30 grains in 2 grams.

Example 8: Convert 60 kilograms to ounces:

$$\frac{2.2 \text{ lb}}{x \text{ oz}} = \frac{1 \text{ kg}}{60 \text{ kg}}$$

This problem cannot be solved using this proportion, because the unit measurements on the left side of the equation are not the same size (pound and ounce). To solve this problem, pounds must first be converted to ounces. Refer back to the household system and **Table 13–6**:

$$\frac{16 \text{ oz}}{x} = \frac{1 \text{ lb}}{2.2 \text{ lb}}$$

$$x = 35.2 \text{ oz}$$

Knowing that 2.2 pounds = 35.2 ounces = 1 kilogram allows the appropriate proportion to be set up:

$$\frac{35.2 \text{ oz}}{x \text{ oz}} = \frac{1 \text{ kg}}{60 \text{ kg}}$$

$$x = 2,2112 \text{ oz}$$

Answer: There are 2,112 ounces in 60 kilograms.

checkpoint

| **1.** What is meant by nomenclature?

13:6 TEMPERATURE CONVERSION

Thermometers using **Fahrenheit (F)** as the measuring unit are more familiar to people living in the United States. The **Celsius (C)** or **centigrade (C)** system of measurement, however, is frequently seen in medical practice and in other countries. One way to start understanding the difference between the two systems is to compare how each one expresses the boiling and freezing points of water:

Boiling points: 212°F = 100° C
Freezing points: 32°F = 0° C

See **Figure 13–12** for a comparison of Fahrenheit (F) and Celsius (C) thermometers and **Table 13–10** for a conversion chart. Health care providers may have to convert between the Fahrenheit and Celsius systems when a conversion chart is not available. **Table 13–11** contains the formulas for conversion. There is a fraction and a decimal approach that give the same results. Deciding which to use depends on whether you have stronger skills working with fractions or decimals. All the formulas include parentheses. These are used to indicate that the enclosed calculation must be performed first. For example, the steps to solve the formula $(°F - 32) \times \frac{5}{9} = °C$ are to first subtract 32 from the value for °F and *then* multiply that value by $\frac{5}{9}$.

TABLE 13–10 Fahrenheit–Celsius Conversion Chart

Fahrenheit	Celsius
32 (freezing point)	0 (freezing point)
95	35
96	35.6
97	36.1
97.4	36.3
98	36.7
98.6	37
99	37.2
99.4	37.4
100	37.8
101	38.3
102	38.9
103	39.4
104	40
212 (boiling point)	100 (boiling point)

checkpoint

| **1.** Name the two (2) systems used to measure temperature.

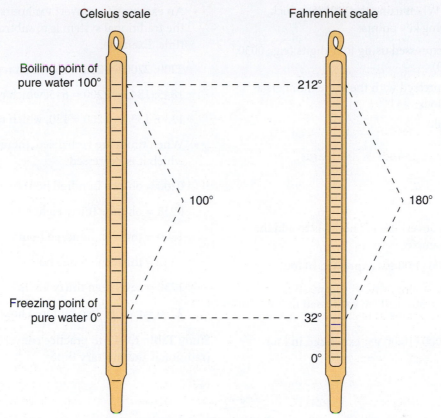

Celsius scale | Fahrenheit scale

Boiling point of pure water 100° — 212°

100° — 180°

Freezing point of pure water 0° — 32°

0°

FIGURE 13–12 Comparison of Fahrenheit and Celsius (Centigrade) temperature scales.

TABLE 13–11 Temperature Scale Conversion Formulas

Convert From	Fraction Formula	Decimal Formula
Celsius to Fahrenheit	(°C × 9/5) + 32 = °F Example: 37°C (37 × 9/5) + 32 = °F 333/5 + 32 = °F 66.6 + 32 = 98.6°F	(°C × 1.8) + 32 = °F Example: 37°C (37 × 1.8) + 32 = °F 66.6 + 32 = 98.6°F
Fahrenheit to Celsius	(°F − 32) × 5/9 = °C Example: 101°F (101 − 32) × 5/9 = °C 69 × 5/9 = °C 345/9 = 38.3°C (rounded to nearest tenth)	(°F − 32) × 0.55565 = °C OR (°F − 32) ÷ 1.8 = °C Example: 101°F (101 − 32) × 0.5556 = °C 69 × 0.5556 = 38.3°C (rounded to nearest tenth) OR (101 − 32) ÷ 1.8 = °C 69 ÷ 1.8 = 38.3°C (rounded to nearest tenth)

13:7 MILITARY TIME

Military time is frequently used in health care to avoid the confusion created by the AM and PM used in the traditional system to designate the correct time. The problem with the traditional system is that if the AM or PM is omitted or misread, an error of 12 hours is made. Errors in recording times are unacceptable in health care. For example, accuracy is critical when entering data on a patient chart, reporting when medications are given, or signing off on physician orders.

When **military time** is the standard used, all time designations are made with the 24-hour clock. The 12th hour is at 12 noon, or 12 PM, and the 24th hour is at 12 midnight, or 12 AM. At 12 midnight, the clock starts again at zero since there are 24 hours in a day.

See **Figure 13–13**. When using the 24-hour clock, remember the following key points:

- Time is always expressed using four digits (e.g., 0030, 0200, 1200, 1700)
- AM hours are expressed with the same numbers as the traditional clock:

  12 Midnight: 0000

  1 AM: 0100

  5:30 AM: 0530

  10 AM: 1000

  12 Noon: 1200

- An easy way to convert the PM hours is to add the time to 1200. Example:

  1 PM: 1200 + 0100 (1:00 PM expressed in four digits) = 1300

  5:30 PM: 1200 + 0530 (5:30 PM expressed in four digits) = 1730

  10 PM: 1200 + 1000 (10:00 PM expressed in four digits) = 2200

- An easy way to convert PM hours in military time to the traditional system is to subtract 1200 from the time. Example:

  2200: 2200 – 1200 = 10, which represents 10 PM

  1845: 1845 – 1200 = 645, which represents 6:45 PM

  1330: 1330 – 1200 = 130, which represents 1:30 PM

- When times are verbalized, there is a specific way in which it is expressed:

  0200 = oh two hundred hours

  0938 = oh nine thirty eight hours

  1300 = thirteen hundred hours

  1301 = thirteen oh one hours

  1730 = seventeen thirty hours

  2200 = twenty-two hundred hours

Study **Table 13–12** to practice converting between traditional and military times.

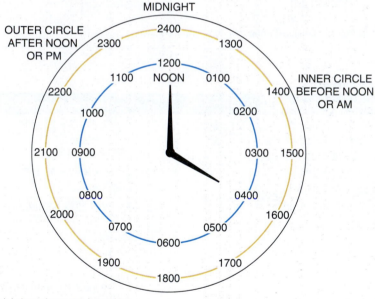

FIGURE 13–13 The military clock is based on a 24-hour day.

TABLE 13–12 Military (24-Hour Clock) and Traditional Time Conversion Chart

Traditional	24-Hour Time	Traditional	24-Hour Time	Traditional	24-Hour Time	Traditional	24-Hour Time
12:01 AM	0001	6:00 AM	0600	12:01 PM	1201	6:00 PM	1800
12:30 AM	0030	7:00 AM	0700	12:30 PM	1230	7:00 PM	1900
1:00 AM	0100	8:00 AM	0800	1:00 PM	1300	8:00 PM	2000
2:00 AM	0200	9:00 AM	0900	2:00 PM	1400	9:00 PM	2100
3:00 AM	0300	10:00 AM	1000	3:00 PM	1500	10:00 PM	2200
4:00 AM	0400	11:00 AM	1100	4:00 PM	1600	11:00 PM	2300
5:00 AM	0500	12:00 noon	1200	5:00 PM	1700	12:00 midnight	2400

Scorpions and Snakes to Cure Cancer?

Eighty percent of cancerous brain tumors are gliomas and they affect more than 26,000 people every year in the United States. Gliomas grow at a rapid rate and can kill a person in a matter of weeks. In most cases, surgical removal of the tumors will destroy too much brain tissue or the tumors grow back quickly if they are surgically removed, so treatment is extremely limited. Few patients live more than 6 to 12 months after the tumor is diagnosed.

Now there is hope for people with gliomas. Dr. Harald Sontheimer, working with a research team at the University of Alabama at Birmingham, initially discovered that a giant Israeli golden scorpion secretes a venom that is safe to humans but paralyzes muscles of a cockroach. The toxic molecules of the venom target a specific protein on the muscles of the cockroach, killing the cockroach. Through research, Sontheimer found that the same protein is present on the cancerous glioma cells. Researchers were then able to develop TM-601, a synthetic version of the venom. In the first clinical trials conducted at Cedars-Sinai Medical Center in California, 18 patients with advanced reoccurring gliomas had the tumors removed. Then a single low dose of radioactive iodine attached to TM-601 was injected into a small tube inserted in the surgical area where the tumor was removed. The TM-601 attached to the glioma cells and the radioactive iodine was able to target the specific cancer cells. Very few side effects were noted. While most patients survived approximately 6 to 10 months, the main result seemed to show the venom stopped the spread of any remaining cancer cells.

Using this initial research, Dr. James Olson for the Fred Hutchinson Cancer Research in Seattle found that the scorpion venom binds to brain tumor cells but not normal cells and actually illuminates the cancer cells. Dr. Olson felt that this "tumor paint" would help a surgeon remove all cancer cells while removing a brain tumor. A major problem was the quick regrowth of the brain tumor if any cancer cells were left behind. Brain surgery was performed on 80 people including 20 children after they were given the tumor paint intravenously. Surgeons found the tumor stays lit for several days and they could readily identify all cancer cells. Additional research has shown that it is also effective for breast, colon, prostate, lung, skin, and other cancers. If this venom allows surgeons to see and remove all cancerous cells, it decreases the chance of reoccurrence and metastasis of the cancer. Clinical trials are currently being established with the FDA. Other medical researchers are evaluating if the scorpion venom is effective for treating neurological conditions such as epilepsy or seizure disorders.

Snake venom is also a major area of research. Some scientists are trying to use snake venom to destroy the blood vessels that supply cancerous tumors with nourishment and fluid. If access to nourishment is restricted, tumors will not be able to grow. A research team at the University of South California is using mice to determine if a protein in copperhead snake venom can inhibit the growth of breast cancer. Initial studies showed a 60 to 70 percent reduction in the growth rate of breast tumors in the mice treated with the protein. However, it will be several years before the venom protein will be available for human tests. Finally, researchers are studying snake venom from the prairie rattler and rear-fanged snakes to determine if it is effective against melanoma (skin), colon, or breast cancer. One of the leading causes of death will be eliminated if research finds that readily available venom from scorpions and snakes can cure a cancerous tumor.

checkpoint

1. Why do we use military time in the health care field?

PRACTICE: Go to the workbook and complete the assignment sheet for Chapter 13, Medical Math.

Case Study Investigation Conclusion

Laura may just need to be reminded of basic math concepts. To get the amount consumed in order to record intake, she would need to convert from ounces to mL.

She may be more comfortable working with fractions than percentages. How can that knowledge impact her estimation of food consumed by her residents?

CHAPTER 13 SUMMARY

- Work in health care requires the use of math skills to measure and perform various types of calculations.

- An important skill to help check work is anticipating the results. Learning to estimate and detect incorrect answers takes practice and thought.

- Roman numerals are used in health care for some medications, solutions, and ordering systems. Angles are used when injecting medications, describing joint movement, and indicating bed positions.

- The three systems of measurement used in health care are household, metric, and apothecary.

- Military time is frequently used in health care to avoid the confusion created by the AM and PM used in the traditional system.

- Health care providers must work carefully and thoughtfully when performing calculations. Errors in math can have serious effects on the patient; therefore, health care providers must strive for 100 percent accuracy.

REVIEW QUESTIONS

1. A patient's oral intake is being measured. For breakfast, he drinks 240 milliliters (mL) of coffee, 120 mL of juice, and 60 mL of water. What is the total fluid intake?

2. A patient is on a diet to lose weight. Last month, she weighed 172 pounds. This month, she weighs 159 pounds. How many pounds did she lose? How many kilograms did she lose?

3. A physical therapist is buying elastic bandages. Each roll costs $3.25. How much would 30 rolls cost?

4. A central supply worker orders 12 new stethoscopes for a total cost of $108.48. How much does each stethoscope cost?

5. A pharmacy technician reviews a prescription for an antibiotic. The patient must take 2½ tablets 3 times a day for 7 days. Using the method of rounding, how many tablets should the technician dispense?

6. A surgical nurse works 1¼ hours in preoperative (before surgery) care, 2½ hours in the operating room, and 3¾ hours in the recovery room. What is the total number of hours worked?

7. An electrocardiograph technician knows that one small block on electrocardiographic paper represents $\frac{1}{25}$ of a second. How many seconds are represented by 150 small blocks?

8. A laboratory technician counts 7,742 leukocytes (white blood cells). If 36% of the leukocytes are lymphocytes, how many lymphocytes are present?

9. A pharmacy technician must prepare 250 mL of a 2.5% dextrose solution. How many grams of dextrose are needed?

10. A doctor orders 500 mg of Sumycin for a patient. Sumycin, an antibiotic, is available in 250-mg capsules. How many capsules should be given to the patient?

11. A cough medicine is ordered for a child. The child must take 1 teaspoon every 4 hours. How many ounces should be dispensed for an 8-day supply of cough medicine?

12. A medical assistant orders MM pairs of gloves. How many gloves were ordered?

13. How many liters are in 2.5 kiloliters?

14. A patient drinks 90 mL of water. How many ounces did the patient drink?

15. A doctor orders a saline irrigation with 2,000 mL. How many quarts of solution must be used?

16. An emergency medical technician must report to work at 1830. What does this mean in traditional time?

17. Convert 70 degrees Fahrenheit to Celsius.

18. Convert 28 degrees Celsius to Fahrenheit.

19. Mr. Washington hurt his right arm and shoulder. The physical therapist would like him to work toward moving his right shoulder at a 90-degree angle from his body. Draw a sketch depicting what achieving that goal would look like.

20. James was walking down the street and a person jumped out of the shadows and stabbed him. The hospital ER doctor said that he would have to stitch his 3-centimeter-long cut. How many inches long was James's wound?

CRITICAL THINKING

Peak Months For Influenza

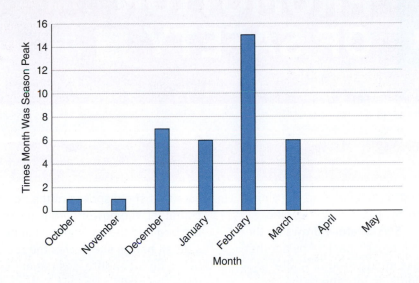

1. What is the subject of the graph?

2. What information is given on the vertical scale?

3. Which month has the most cases of influenza?

4. How many cases are reported for the month of December?

ACTIVITIES

1. In a small group, research a medical topic (i.e. incidents of flu in your county, medication errors in a hospital in your area, the rate of obesity in your community by age) and create a graph, pie chart, or table to illustrate the results of your research.

2. With a partner, focus on one math concept. Develop a plan to teach that concept to the appropriate-level math class. Use a table, chart, or graph to illustrate a medical application of this concept. Formulate five (5) problems for your students to solve.

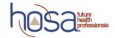 | CONNECTION

Competitive Event: Medical Math

Event Summary: Medical Math provides members with the opportunity to gain knowledge and skills required to identify, solve, and apply mathematical principles. This competitive event consists of a written test with tie-breaker questions. This event aims to inspire members to learn about the integration of mathematics in health care, including temperature, weights, and measures used in the health community.

Details on this competitive event may be found at:

www.hosa.org/guidelines

CHAPTER 14

PROMOTION OF SAFETY

Safety   OBRA

Case Study Investigation

Sylvia is a nurse at Metro Hospital. She is giving an insulin injection to her patient, Andre, who has diabetes mellitus. She carefully draws up the correct dose and has it cross-checked by another nurse. When she walks into the room, Andre asks her if she can help him into the bathroom before she gives him the insulin because he can't maneuver around the power cord for the bed. After she assists him to the bathroom, Sylvia removes her gloves and washes her hands before administering Andre's medication. She makes sure that she disposes of the needle in the sharps container, the power cord is tucked safely under the bed and the call light is clipped to the bed's siderail before she leaves the room. What does Sylvia do that addresses patient safety? How does she make sure that Andre's environment is safe and equipment is correctly maintained? At the end of this chapter, you will be asked about the basic safety techniques Sylvia needs to be aware of in order to keep both herself and her patient safe.

LEARNING OBJECTIVES

After completing this chapter, you should be able to:

- Define body mechanics.
- Use correct body mechanics while performing procedures in the laboratory or clinical area.
- Observe all safety standards established by OSHA, especially the Occupational Exposure to Hazardous Chemicals Standard and the Bloodborne Pathogen Standard.
- Follow safety regulations stated while performing in the laboratory area.
- Observe all regulations for patient safety while performing procedures on a student partner in the laboratory or classroom area, or on a patient in any area.
- List the five main classes of fire extinguishers.
- Relate each class of fire extinguisher to the specific fire(s) for which it is used.
- Simulate the operation of a fire extinguisher by following the directions on the extinguisher and specific measures for observing fire safety.
- Describe the operation of the nearest fire alarm.
- Describe in detail the active shooter plan for your classroom area according to established school policy.
- Define, pronounce, and spell all key terms.

KEY TERMS

base of support
Bloodborne Pathogen Standard
body mechanics
ergonomics
fire extinguishers

Occupational Exposure to
  Hazardous Chemicals
  Standard
Occupational Safety and Health
  Administration (OSHA)

radiation exposure
Safety Data Sheet (SDS)
safety standards

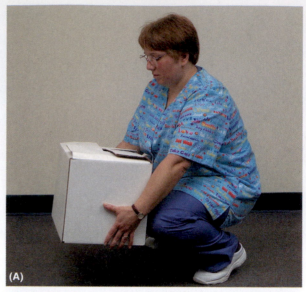

FIGURE 14–1A Bend from the hips and knees to get close to an object.

14:1 USING BODY MECHANICS

To prevent injury to yourself and others while working in the health care field, it is important that you observe good body mechanics and maintain correct posture.

Body mechanics refers to the way in which the body moves and maintains balance while making the most efficient use of all its parts. Basic rules for body mechanics are provided as guidelines to prevent strain and help maintain muscle strength.

There are four main reasons for using good body mechanics:

- Muscles work best when used correctly.
- The correct use of muscles makes lifting, pulling, and pushing easier.
- The correct application of body mechanics prevents unnecessary fatigue and strain and saves energy.
- The correct application of body mechanics prevents injury to self and others.

Eight basic rules of good body mechanics include:

- Maintain a broad **base of support** by keeping the feet 8–10 inches apart, placing one foot slightly forward, balancing weight on both feet, and pointing the toes in the direction of movement.
- Bend from the hips and knees to get close to an object, and keep your back straight (**Figure 14–1A**). Do not bend at the waist.
- Use the strongest muscles to do the job. The larger and stronger muscles are located in the shoulders, upper arms, hips, and thighs. Back muscles are weak.
- Use the weight of your body to help push or pull an object. Whenever possible, push, slide, or pull rather than lift.
- Carry heavy objects close to the body (**Figure 14–1B**). Also, stand close to any object or person being moved.

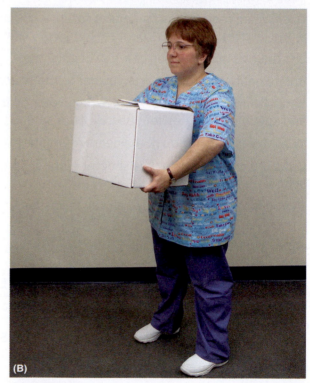

FIGURE 14–1B Maintain a broad base of support while carrying objects close to the body.

- Avoid twisting your body as you work. Turn with your feet and entire body when you change direction of movement.
- Avoid bending for long periods.
- If a patient or object is too heavy for you to lift alone, always get help. Mechanical lifts, transfer (gait) belts, wheelchairs, and other similar types of equipment are also available to help lift and move patients.

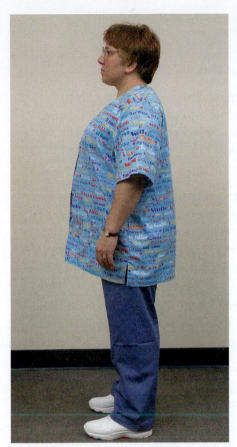

FIGURE 14–2 Correct posture puts less stress on muscles and prevents fatigue.

Good posture is also an essential part of correct body mechanics. Aligning the body correctly puts less stress on muscles and prevents fatigue (**Figure 14–2**). Basic principles include standing straight with stomach muscles pulled in, shoulders relaxed and pulled back, weight balanced equally on each foot and aligned with the shoulders, and chest and chin held up.

Some health care facilities may require health care providers to wear back supports while lifting or moving patients. These supports are supposed to help prevent back injuries, but their use is controversial. Back supports may provide a false sense of security as an individual tries to lift heavier loads. It is important to remember that a back brace does not increase strength. Back supports may also cause sweating, skin irritation, and increased abdominal pressure. They do remind the wearer to use good body mechanics. If a back support is used, it should be the correct size to provide the maximum benefit. When the worker is performing strenuous tasks, the support should fit snugly. At other times, it should be loosened to decrease abdominal pressure.

checkpoint

| **1.** Define body mechanics.

PRACTICE: Go to the workbook and complete the assignment sheet for 14:1, Using Body Mechanics. Then return and continue with the procedure.

Procedure 14:1

Using Body Mechanics

Equipment and Supplies

Heavy book, bedside stand, bed with wheel locks

Procedure

1. Assemble equipment.

2. Practice correct posture. Stand straight with your feet aligned with your shoulders and your weight supported equally on each foot. Pull in your stomach muscles. Relax your shoulders and pull them back. Hold your chin and chest up. Notice how this helps maintain your spine in a straight line while it also balances all parts of your body.

3. Compare using a narrow base of support to using a broad base of support. Stand on your toes, with your feet close together. Next, stand on your toes with your feet farther apart. Then, stand with your feet flat on the floor but close together. Finally, stand with your feet flat on the floor but approximately 8–10 inches apart and with one foot slightly forward. Balance your weight on both

feet. You should feel the best support in the final position because the broad base supports your body weight.

4. Place the book on the floor. Bend from the hips and knees (not the waist) and keep your back straight to pick up the book. Return to the standing position.

5. Place the book between your thumb and fingers, but not touching the palm of your hand, and hold your hand straight out in front of your body. Slowly move your hand toward your body, stopping several times to feel the weight of the book in different positions. Finally, hold the book with your entire hand and bring your hand close to your body. The final position should be the most comfortable.

   NOTE: This illustrates the need to carry heavy objects close to your body and to use the strongest muscles to do the job.

6. Stand at either end of the bed. Release the wheel locks on the bed. Position your feet to provide a broad base of support. Get close to the bed. Use the weight of your body to push the bed forward.

(continues)

7. Place the book on the bed. Pick up the book and place it on the bedside stand. Avoid twisting your body. Turn with your feet to place the book on the stand.

    NOTE: Remember that holding the book close to your body allows you to use the strongest muscles.

8. Practice the rules of body mechanics by setting up situations similar to those listed in the previous steps. Continue until the movements feel natural to you.

9. Replace all equipment used.

PRACTICE: Use the evaluation sheet for 14:1, Using Body Mechanics, to practice this procedure. When you believe you have mastered this skill, sign the sheet and give it to your instructor for further action.

✅ **FINAL EVALUATION:** Using the criteria listed on the evaluation sheet, your instructor will grade your performance.
Check

14:2 PREVENTING ACCIDENTS AND INJURIES

 The **Occupational Safety and Health Administration (OSHA)**, a division of the Department of Labor, establishes and enforces **safety standards** for the workplace. Two main standards affect health care providers:

OBRA

- The Occupational Exposure to Hazardous Chemicals Standard
- The Bloodborne Pathogen Standard

CHEMICAL HAZARDS

The **Occupational Exposure to Hazardous Chemicals Standard** requires that employers inform employees of all chemicals and hazards in the workplace. In addition, all manufacturers must provide **Safety Data Sheets (SDSs)**, formerly known as Material Safety Data Sheets (MSDSs), with any hazardous products they sell (**Figure 14–3**). The SDSs contain 16 standard sections that make it easy to locate and understand information about how to properly and safely handle hazardous chemicals. The SDSs must always be readily accessible and provide the following information:

- Section 1: Identification: identifies the chemical, its recommended uses, and contact information for the supplier
- Section 2: Hazard(s) Identification: identifies the hazards of the chemical and other warning information
- Section 3: Composition/Information on Ingredients: identifies the ingredients of the chemical

- Section 4: First-Aid Measures: describes the initial care required for people exposed to the chemical
- Section 5: Fire-Fighting Measures: identifies the best way to extinguish a fire caused by the chemical
- Section 6: Accidental Release Measures: recommends how to clean up and contain a spill
- Section 7: Handling and Storage: recommends how to safely handle and store the chemical
- Section 8: Exposure Controls/Personal Protection: indicates the maximum exposure limit, engineering controls (ventilation, containment, etc.), and what personal protective equipment is required
- Section 9: Physical and Chemical Properties: identifies physical properties such as look and smell
- Section 10: Stability and Reactivity: describes stability and reactivity hazards of the chemical
- Section 11: Toxicology Information: identifies the health effects of exposure and amount of toxicity
- Section 12: Ecological Information: identifies the environmental impact of an exposure
- Section 13: Disposal Considerations: identifies how to safely dispose of the chemical
- Section 14: Transport Information: provides guidance on how the chemical can be safely transported
- Section 15: Regulatory Information: identifies other safety, health, and environmental regulations for the chemicals that are not indicated elsewhere in SDS
- Section 16: Other Information: states when this SDS was prepared or revised

Chemicals must also be labeled with a hazardous category classification according to the National Fire Protection Association's (NFPA) color code (**Figure 14–4**). This code alerts the user to health, fire, reactivity, or other specific hazards of the chemical.

MERCURY
Safety Data Sheet
according to the federal final rule of hazard communication revised on 2012 (HazCom 2012)

Date of issue: 11/19/2013

SECTION 1: Identification of the substance/mixture and of the company/undertaking

1.1. Product identifier

Trade name	:	MERCURY
CAS No	:	7439-97-6
Other means of identification	:	Colloidal Mercury, Quick Silver, Liquid Silver, NCI-C60399, Hydrargyrum

1.2. Relevant identified uses of the substance or mixture and uses advised against

Use of the substance/mixture   : Variety of industrial, analytical and research applications.

1.3. Details of the supplier of the safety data sheet

ABC Pharmaceuticals

1234 Chemcial Way
Amalgam Center, AL 31313

1.4. Emergency telephone number

Emergency number   : 1-800-555-5656

SECTION 2: Hazards identification

2.1. Classification of the substance or mixture

GHS-US classification

Acute Tox. 1 (Inhalation:dust,mist)	H330
Repr. 1B	H360
STOT RE 1	H372
Aquatic Acute 1	H400
Aquatic Chronic 1	H410

2.2. Label elements

GHS-US labelling

Hazard pictograms (GHS-US)   :

GHS06   GHS08   GHS09

Signal word (GHS-US)	:	Danger
Hazard statements (GHS-US)	:	H330 - Fatal if inhaled
		H360 - May damage fertility or the unborn child
		H372 - Causes damage to organs through prolonged or repeated exposure
		H400 - Very toxic to aquatic life
		H410 - Very toxic to aquatic life with long lasting effects
Precautionary statements (GHS-US)	:	P201 - Obtain special instructions before use
		P202 - Do not handle until all safety precautions have been read and understood
		P260 - Do not breathe vapors, gas
		P264 - Wash skin, hands thoroughly after handling
		P270 - Do not eat, drink or smoke when using this product
		P271 - Use only outdoors or in a well-ventilated area
		P273 - Avoid release to the environment
		P280 - Wear eye protection, protective clothing, protective gloves, Face mask
		P284 - [In case of inadequate ventilation] wear respiratory protection
		P304+P340 - IF INHALED: Remove person to fresh air and keep comfortable for breathing
		P308+P313 - IF exposed or concerned: Get medical advice/attention
		P310 - Immediately call a POISON CENTER/doctor/...
		P314 - Get medical advice and attention if you feel unwell
		P320 - Specific treatment is urgent (see First aid measures on this label)
		P391 - Collect spillage
		P403+P233 - Store in a well-ventilated place. Keep container tightly closed
		P405 - Store locked up
		P501 - Dispose of contents/container to comply with applicable local, national and international regulation.

2.3. Other hazards

other hazards which do not result in classification   : When inhaled, Mercury will be rapidly distributed throughout the body. During this time, Mercury will cross the blood-brain barrier, and become oxidized to the Hg (II) oxidation state. The oxidized species of Mercury cannot cross the blood-brain barrier and thus accumulates in the

FIGURE 14–3 Read the Safety Data Sheet (SDS) before using any chemical product. LabChem

(continues)

MERCURY
Safety Data Sheet
according to the federal final rule of hazard communication revised on 2012 (HazCom 2012)

brain. Mercury in other organs is removed slowly from the body via the kidneys. The average half-time for clearance of Mercury for different parts of the human body is as follows: lung: 1.7 days; head: 21 days; kidney region: 64 days; chest: 43 days; whole body: 58 days. Mercury can be irritating to contaminated skin and eye. Prolonged contact may lead to ulceration of the skin. Allergic reactions (i.e. rashes, welts) may occur in sensitive individuals. Mercury can be irritating to contaminated skin and eyes. Short-term over-exposures to high concentrations of mercury vapors can lead to breathing difficulty, coughing, acute, and potentially fatal lung disorders. Depending on the concentration of inhalation over-exposure, heart problems, damage to the kidney, liver or nerves and effects on the brain may occur.

| 2.4. | Unknown acute toxicity (GHS-US) |

No data available

SECTION 3: Composition/information on ingredients

| 3.1. | Substance |

Not applicable

Full text of H-phrases: see section 16

| 3.2. | Mixture |

Name	Product identifier	%	GHS-US classification
Mercury	(CAS No) 7439-97-6	100	Acute Tox. 2 (Inhalation), H330 Repr. 1B, H360 STOT RE 1, H372 Aquatic Acute 1, H400 Aquatic Chronic 1, H410

SECTION 4: First aid measures

| 4.1. | Description of first aid measures |

First-aid measures general	:	Never give anything by mouth to an unconscious person. If exposed or concerned: Get medical advice/attention.
First-aid measures after inhalation	:	Remove to fresh air and keep at rest in a position comfortable for breathing. Assure fresh air breathing. Allow the victim to rest. Immediately call a POISON CENTER or doctor/physician. In case of irregular breathing or respiratory arrest provide artificial respiration.
First-aid measures after skin contact	:	Wash immediately with lots of water (15 minutes)/shower. Remove affected clothing and wash all exposed skin area with mild soap and water, followed by warm water rinse. Seek immediate medical advice.
First-aid measures after eye contact	:	Rinse immediately and thoroughly, pulling the eyelids well away from the eye (15 minutes minimum). Keep eye wide open while rinsing. Seek medical attention immediately.
First-aid measures after ingestion	:	Immediately call a POISON CENTER or doctor/physician. Rinse mouth. If conscious, give large amounts of water and induce vomiting. Give water or milk if the person is fully conscious. Obtain emergency medical attention.

| 4.2. | Most important symptoms and effects, both acute and delayed |

Symptoms/injuries after inhalation	:	Short-term over-exposures to high concentrations of mercury vapors can lead to breathing difficulty, coughing, acute, chemical pneumonia, and pulmonary edema (a potentially fatal accumulation of fluid in the lungs). Depending on the concentration of over-exposure, cardiac abnormalities, damage to the kidney, liver or nerves and effects on the brain may occur. Long-term inhalation over-exposures can lead to the development of a wide variety of symptoms, including the following: excessive salivation, gingivitis, anorexia, chills, fever, cardiac abnormalities, anemia, digestive problems, abdominal pains, frequent urination, an inability to urinate, diarrhea, peripheral neuropathy (numbness, weakness, or burning sensations in the hands or feet), tremors (especially in the hands, fingers, eyelids, lips, cheeks, tongue, or legs), alteration of tendon reflexes, slurred speech, visual disturbances, and deafness. Allergic reactions (i.e. breathing difficulty) may also occur in sensitive individuals.
Symptoms/injuries after skin contact	:	Symptoms of skin exposure can include redness, dry skin, and pain. Prolonged contact may lead to ulceration of the skin. Allergic reactions (i.e. rashes, welts) may occur in sensitive individuals. Dermatitis (redness and inflammation of the skin) may occur after repeated skin exposures.
Symptoms/injuries after eye contact	:	Symptoms of eye exposure can include redness, pain, and watery eyes. A symptom of Mercury exposure is discoloration of the lens of the eyes.
Symptoms/injuries after ingestion	:	If Mercury is swallowed, symptoms of such over-exposure can include metallic taste in mouth, nausea, vomiting, central nervous system effects, and damage to the kidneys. Metallic mercury is not usually absorbed sufficiently from the gastrointestinal tract to induce an acute, toxic response. Damage to the tissues of the mouth, throat, esophagus, and other tissues of the digestive system may occur. Ingestion may be fatal, due to effects on gastrointestinal system and kidneys.
Chronic symptoms	:	Long-term over-exposure can lead to a wide range of adverse health effects. Anyone using Mercury must pay attention to personality changes, weight loss, skin or gum discolorations, stomach pains, and other signs of Mercury over-exposure. Gradually developing syndromes ("Erethism" and "Acrodynia") are indicative of potentially severe health problems. Mercury can cause the development of allergic reactions (i.e. dermatitis, rashes, breathing difficulty) upon prolonged or repeated exposures. Refer to Section 11 (Toxicology Information) for additional data.

MERCURY

Safety Data Sheet
according to the federal final rule of hazard communication revised on 2012 (HazCom 2012)

4.3.	Indication of any immediate medical attention and special treatment needed

Treatment for Mercury over-exposure must be given. The following treatment protocol for ingestion of Mercury is from Clinical Toxicology of Commercial Products (5th Edition, 1984).

SECTION 5: Firefighting measures

5.1.	Extinguishing media

Suitable extinguishing media	: Foam. Dry powder. Carbon dioxide. Water spray. Sand.
Unsuitable extinguishing media	: Do not use a heavy water stream.

5.2.	Special hazards arising from the substance or mixture

Fire hazard	: Not flammable. Mercury vapors and oxides generated during fires involving this product are toxic.
Reactivity	: Stable. Reacts with (some) metals. Mercury can react with metals to form amalgams.

5.3.	Advice for firefighters

Firefighting instructions	: Use water spray or fog for cooling exposed containers. Exercise caution when fighting any chemical fire. Prevent fire-fighting water from entering environment. Do not allow run-off from fire fighting to enter drains or water courses.
Protective equipment for firefighters	: Do not enter fire area without proper protective equipment, including respiratory protection.
Other information	: Decontaminate all equipment thoroughly after the conclusion of fire-fighting activities.

SECTION 6: Accidental release measures

6.1.	Personal precautions, protective equipment and emergency procedures

General measures	: Uncontrolled release should be responded to by trained personnel using pre-planned procedures. Evacuate area. Evacuate personnel to a safe area.

6.1.1.	For non-emergency personnel

Emergency procedures	: Evacuate unnecessary personnel.

6.1.2.	For emergency responders

Protective equipment	: Equip cleanup crew with proper protection. In the event of a release under 1 pound: the minimum level "C" Personal Protective Equipment is needed. Triple-gloves (rubber gloves and nitril gloves over latex gloves), chemical resistant suit and boots, hard-hat, and Air-Purifying Respirator with Cartridge appropriate for Mercury. In the event of a release over 1 pound or when concentration of oxygen in atmosphere is less than 19.5% or unknown, the level "B" Personal Protective Equipments which includes Self-Contained Breathing Apparatus must be worn.
Emergency procedures	: Ventilate area.

6.2.	Environmental precautions

Prevent entry to sewers and public waters. Notify authorities if liquid enters sewers or public waters. Avoid release to the environment.

6.3.	Methods and material for containment and cleaning up

For containment	: For larger spills, dike area and pump into waste containers. Put into a labelled container and provide safe disposal.
Methods for cleaning up	: There are a variety of methods which can be used to clean-up Mercury spills. Use a commercially available Mercury Spill Kit for small spills. A suction pump with aspirator can also be used during clean-up operations. For larger release, a Mercury vacuum can be used. Calcium polysulfide or excess sulfur can be also used for clean-up. Mercury can migrate into cracks and other difficult-to-clean areas; calcium polysulfide and sulfur can be sprinkled effectively into these areas. Decontaminate the area thoroughly. The area should be inspected visually and with colorimetric tubes for Mercury to ensure all traces have been removed prior to re-occupation by non-emergency personnel. Decontaminate all equipment used in response thoroughly. If such equipments cannot de adequately decontaminated, it must be discarded with other spill residue. Place all spill residues in an appropriate container, seal immediately, and label appropriately. Dispose of in accordance with federal, state, and local hazardous waste disposal requirements. (Refer to Section 13 of this SDS).

6.4.	Reference to other sections

See Heading 8. Exposure controls and personal protection.

SECTION 7: Handling and storage

7.1.	Precautions for safe handling

Additional hazards when processed	: Supervisors and responsible personnel must be aware of personality changes, weight loss, or other sign of Mercury over-exposure in employees using this product; These symptoms can develop gradually and are indicative of potentially severe health effects related to Mercury contamination.

(continues)

MERCURY
Safety Data Sheet
according to the federal final rule of hazard communication revised on 2012 (HazCom 2012)

Precautions for safe handling	: As with all chemicals, avoid getting Mercury ON YOU or IN YOU. Do not handle until all safety precautions have been read and understood. Obtain special instructions before use. Wash hands and other exposed areas with mild soap and water before eating, drinking or smoking and when leaving work. Provide good ventilation in process area to prevent formation of vapor. Report all Mercury releases promptly. Open container slowly on a stable surface. Drums, flasks and bottles of this product must be properly labeled. Empty containers may contain residual amounts of Mercury and should be handled with care.
Hygiene measures	: Do not eat, drink or smoke when using this product. Always wash hands and face immediately after handling this product, and once again before leaving the workplace. Remove contaminated clothing immediately.

7.2.   Conditions for safe storage, including any incompatibilities

Technical measures	: Follow practice indicated in Section 6. Make certain that application equipment is locked and tagged-out safely. Always use this product in areas where adequate ventilation is provided. Decontaminate equipment thoroughly before maintenance begins.
Storage conditions	: Keep container tightly closed. Store drums, flasks and bottles in a cool, dry location, away from direct sunlight, source of intense heat, or where freezing is possible. Store away from incompatible materials. Material should be stored in secondary container or in a diked area, as appropriate.
Incompatible materials	: Acetylene and acetylene derivatives, amines, ammonia, 3-bromopropyne, boron diiodophosphide, methyl azide, sodium carbide, heated sulfuric acid, methylsilane/oxygen mixtures, nitric acid/alcohol mixtures, tetracarbonylnickel/oxygen mixtures, alkyne/silver perchlorate mixtures, halogens and strong oxidizers. Mercury can attack copper alloys. Mercury can react with many metals (i.e. calcium, lithium, potassium, sodium, rubidium, aluminum) to form amalgams.
Prohibitions on mixed storage	: Mercury can attack copper alloys. Mercury can react with many metals (i.e. calcium, lithium, potassium, sodium, rubidium, aluminum) to form amalgams.
Storage area	: Storage area should be made of fire-resistant materials.
Special rules on packaging	: Inspect all incoming containers before storage to ensure containers are properly labeled and not damaged.

7.3.   Specific end use(s)

No additional information available

SECTION 8: Exposure controls/personal protection

8.1.   Control parameters

Mercury (7439-97-6)

USA ACGIH	ACGIH TWA (mg/m³)	0,025 mg/m³
USA OSHA	OSHA PEL (Ceiling) (mg/m³)	0,1 mg/m³

8.2.   Exposure controls

Appropriate engineering controls	: Ensure adequate ventilation. Ensure exposure is below occupational exposure limits (where available). Emergency eye wash fountains and safety showers should be available in the immediate vicinity of any potential exposure.
Personal protective equipment	: Avoid all unnecessary exposure. Gloves. Protective clothing. Safety glasses. Mist formation: aerosol mask.

Hand protection	: Wear neoprene gloves for routine industrial use. Use triple gloves for spill response, as stated in Section 6 of this SDS.
Eye protection	: Splash goggles or safety glasses. For operation involving the use of more than 1 pound of Mercury, or if the operation may generate a spray of Mercury, the use of a faceshield is recommended.
Skin and body protection	: Wear suitable protective clothing.
Respiratory protection	: Maintain airborne contaminants concentration below provided exposure limits. If respiratory protection is needed, use only protection authorized in 29 CFR 1910.134 or applicable state regulations. Use supplied air respiration protection if oxygen levels are below 19.5% or are unknown.
Other information	: Do not eat, drink or smoke during use.

SECTION 9: Physical and chemical properties

9.1.   Information on basic physical and chemical properties

Physical state	: Liquid
Colour	: Silver white.

MERCURY
Safety Data Sheet
according to the federal final rule of hazard communication revised on 2012 (HazCom 2012)

Odor	:	Odorless.
Odor threshold	:	Not applicable
pH	:	Not applicable
Relative evaporation rate (butylacetate=1)	:	No data available
Melting point	:	No data available
Freezing point	:	-38,87 °C (-37.97 F)
Boiling point	:	No data available
Flash point	:	Not applicable
Self ignition temperature	:	Not applicable
Decomposition temperature	:	No data available
Flammability (solid, gas)	:	No data available
Vapour pressure	:	0,002 mm Hg at 25°C
Relative vapor density at 20 °C	:	6,9 (Air = 1)
Relative density	:	No data available
Relative density of saturated gas/air mixture	:	13,6
Solubility	:	No data available
Log Pow	:	No data available
Log Kow	:	No data available
Viscosity, kinematic	:	No data available
Viscosity, dynamic	:	No data available
Explosive properties	:	No data available
Oxidizing properties	:	No data available
Explosive limits	:	Not applicable

9.2. Other information

No additional information available

SECTION 10: Stability and reactivity

10.1. Reactivity

Stable. Reacts with (some) metals. Mercury can react with metals to form amalgams.

10.2. Chemical stability

Not established.

10.3. Possibility of hazardous reactions

Not established. Hazardous polymerization will not occur.

10.4. Conditions to avoid

Direct sunlight. Extremely high or low temperatures.

10.5. Incompatible materials

Acetylene and acetylene derivatives, amines, ammonia, 3-bromopropyne, boron diiodophosphide, methyl azide, sodium carbide, heated sulfuric acid, methylsilane/oxygen mixtures, nitric acid/alcohol mixtures, tetracarbonylnickel/oxygen mixtures, alkyne/silver perchlorate mixtures, halogens and strong oxidizers. Mercury can attack copper alloys. Mercury can react with many metals (i.e. calcium, lithium, potassium, sodium, rubidium, aluminum) to form amalgams.

10.6. Hazardous decomposition products

If this product is exposed to extremely high temperature in the presence of oxygen or air, toxic vapor of mercury and mercury oxides will be generated.

SECTION 11: Toxicological information

11.1. Information on toxicological effects

Acute toxicity	:	Fatal if inhaled.
Skin corrosion/irritation	:	Not classified
		pH: Not applicable
Serious eye damage/irritation	:	Not classified
		pH: Not applicable
Respiratory or skin sensitisation	:	Not classified
Germ cell mutagenicity	:	Not classified
		Based on available data, the classification criteria are not met
Carcinogenicity	:	Not classified

MERCURY
Safety Data Sheet
according to the federal final rule of hazard communication revised on 2012 (HazCom 2012)

Mercury (7439-97-6)	
IARC group	3

Reproductive toxicity	: May damage fertility or the unborn child.
	Based on available data, the classification criteria are not met
Specific target organ toxicity (single exposure)	: Not classified
Specific target organ toxicity (repeated exposure)	: Causes damage to organs through prolonged or repeated exposure.
	Based on available data, the classification criteria are not met Causes damage to organs through prolonged or repeated exposure
Aspiration hazard	: Not classified
	Based on available data, the classification criteria are not met
Potential adverse human health effects and symptoms	: Based on available data, the classification criteria are not met. Fatal if inhaled.
Symptoms/injuries after inhalation	: Short-term over-exposures to high concentrations of mercury vapors can lead to breathing difficulty, coughing, acute,chemical pneumonia, and pulmonary edema (a potentially fatal accumulation of fluid in the lungs) . Depending on the concentration of over-exposure, cardiac abnormalities, damage to the kidney, liver or nerves and effects on the brain may occur. Long-term inhalation over-exposures can lead to the development of a wide variety of symptoms, including the following: excessive salivation, gingivitis, anorexia, chills, fever, cardiac abnormalities, anemia, digestive problems, abdominal pains, frequent urination, an inability to urinate, diarrhea, peripheral neuropathy (numbness, weakness, or burning sensations in the hands or feet), tremors (especially in the hands, fingers, eyelids, lips, cheeks, tongue, or legs), alteration of tendon reflexes, slurred speech, visual disturbances, and deafness. Allergic reactions (i.e. breathing difficulty) may also occur in sensitive individuals.
Symptoms/injuries after skin contact	: Symptoms of skin exposure can include redness, dry skin, and pain. Prolonged contact may lead to ulceration of the skin. Allergic reactions (i.e. rashes, welts) may occur in sensitive individuals. Dermatitis (redness and inflammation of the skin) may occur after repeated skin exposures.
Symptoms/injuries after eye contact	: Symptoms of eye exposure can include redness, pain, and watery eyes. A symptom of Mercury exposure is discoloration of the lens of the eyes.
Symptoms/injuries after ingestion	: If Mercury is swallowed, symptoms of such over-exposure can include metallic taste in mouth, nausea, vomiting, central nervous system effects, and damage to the kidneys. Metallic mercury is not usually absorbed sufficiently from the gastrointestinal tract to induce an acute, toxic response. Damage to the tissues of the mouth, throat, esophagus, and other tissues of the digestive system may occur. Ingestion may be fatal, due to effects on gastrointestinal system and kidneys.
Chronic symptoms	: Long-term over-exposure can lead to a wide range of adverse health effects. Anyone using Mercury must pay attention to personality changes, weight loss, skin or gum discolorations, stomach pains, and other signs of Mercury over-exposure. Gradually developing syndromes ("Erethism" and "Acrodynia") are indicative of potentially severe health problems. Mercury can cause the development of allergic reactions (i.e. dermatitis, rashes, breathing difficulty) upon prolonged or repeated exposures. Refer to Section 11 (Toxicology Information) for additional data.

SECTION 12: Ecological information

12.1.   Toxicity

Ecology - water	: Very toxic to aquatic life. Toxic to aquatic life with long lasting effects.

Mercury (7439-97-6)	
LC50 fishes 1	0,5 mg/l (Exposure time: 96 h - Species: Cyprinus carpio)
EC50 Daphnia 1	5,0 µg/l (Exposure time: 96 h - Species: water flea)
LC50 fish 2	0,16 mg/l (Exposure time: 96 h - Species: Cyprinus carpio [semi-static])

12.2.   Persistence and degradability

MERCURY (7439-97-6)	
Persistence and degradability	May cause long-term adverse effects in the environment.

12.3.   Bioaccumulative potential

MERCURY (7439-97-6)	
Bioaccumulative potential	Not established.

12.4.   Mobility in soil

No additional information available

12.5.   Other adverse effects

Other information	: Avoid release to the environment.

SECTION 13: Disposal considerations

13.1. Waste treatment methods

Waste disposal recommendations	: Dispose in a safe manner in accordance with local/national regulations. Waste disposal must be in accordance with appropriate federal, state, and local regulations. This product, if unaltered by use, should be recycled. If altered by use, recycling may be possible. Consult Bethlehem Apparatus Company for information. If Mercury must be disposed of as hazardous waste, it must be handled at a permitted facility or as advised by your local hazardous waste regulatory authority.
Ecology - waste materials	: Hazardous waste due to toxicity. Avoid release to the environment.

SECTION 14: Transport information

In accordance with DOT

14.1. UN number

UN-No.(DOT)	: 2809
DOT NA no.	UN2809

14.2. UN proper shipping name

DOT Proper Shipping Name	: Mercury
Department of Transportation (DOT) Hazard Classes	: 8 - Class 8 - Corrosive material 49 CFR 173.136
Hazard labels (DOT)	: 8 - Corrosive substances 6.1 - Toxic substances

DOT Symbols	: A - Material is regulated as a hazardous material only when be transported by air, W - Material is regulated as a hazardous material only when be transported by water
Packing group (DOT)	: III - Minor Danger
DOT Packaging Exceptions (49 CFR 173.xxx)	: 164
DOT Packaging Non Bulk (49 CFR 173.xxx)	: 164
DOT Packaging Bulk (49 CFR 173.xxx)	: 240

14.3. Additional information

Other information	: No supplementary information available.

Overland transport

No additional information available

Transport by sea

DOT Vessel Stowage Location	: B - (i) The material may be stowed "on deck" or "under deck" on a cargo vessel and on a passenger vessel carrying a number of passengers limited to not more than the larger of 25 passengers, or one passenger per each 3 m of overall vessel length; and (ii) "On deck only" on passenger vessels in which the number of passengers specified in paragraph (k)(2)(i) of this section is exceeded.
DOT Vessel Stowage Other	: 40 - Stow "clear of living quarters",97 - Stow "away from" azides

Air transport

DOT Quantity Limitations Passenger aircraft/rail (49 CFR 173.27)	: 35 kg
DOT Quantity Limitations Cargo aircraft only (49 CFR 175.75)	: 35 kg

SECTION 15: Regulatory information

15.1. US Federal regulations

Mercury (7439-97-6)	
Listed on the United States TSCA (Toxic Substances Control Act) inventory Listed on SARA Section 313 (Specific toxic chemical listings)	
EPA TSCA Regulatory Flag	S - S - indicates a substance that is identified in a proposed or final Significant New Uses Rule.
SARA Section 313 - Emission Reporting	1,0 %

15.2. International regulations

CANADA

MERCURY
Safety Data Sheet
according to the federal final rule of hazard communication revised on 2012 (HazCom 2012)

Mercury (7439-97-6)	
Listed on the Canadian DSL (Domestic Sustances List) inventory.	
WHMIS Classification	Class D Division 1 Subdivision A - Very toxic material causing immediate and serious toxic effects Class D Division 2 Subdivision A - Very toxic material causing other toxic effects Class E - Corrosive Material

EU-Regulations

Mercury (7439-97-6)
Listed on the EEC inventory EINECS (European Inventory of Existing Commercial Chemical Substances) substances.

Classification according to Regulation (EC) No. 1272/2008 [CLP]

Classification according to Directive 67/548/EEC or 1999/45/EC
Not classified

15.2.2.   National regulations

Mercury (7439-97-6)
Listed on the AICS (the Australian Inventory of Chemical Substances) Listed on Inventory of Existing Chemical Substances (IECSC) Listed on the Korean ECL (Existing Chemical List) inventory. Listed on New Zealand - Inventory of Chemicals (NZIoC) Listed on Inventory of Chemicals and Chemical Substances (PICCS) Poisonous and Deleterious Substances Control Law Pollutant Release and Transfer Register Law (PRTR Law) Listed on the Canadian Ingredient Disclosure List

15.3. US State regulations

Mercury (7439-97-6)				
U.S. - California - Proposition 65 - Carcinogens List	U.S. - California - Proposition 65 - Developmental Toxicity	U.S. - California - Proposition 65 - Reproductive Toxicity - Female	U.S. - California - Proposition 65 - Reproductive Toxicity - Male	No significance risk level (NSRL)
	Yes			

SECTION 16: Other information

Other information   : None.

Full text of H-phrases: see section 16:

Acute Tox. 1 (Inhalation:dust,mist)	Acute toxicity (inhalation:dust,mist) Category 1
Acute Tox. 2 (Inhalation)	Acute toxicity (inhalation) Category 2
Aquatic Acute 1	Hazardous to the aquatic environment — AcuteHazard, Category 1
Aquatic Chronic 1	Hazardous to the aquatic environment — Chronic Hazard, Category 1
Repr. 1B	Reproductive toxicity Category 1B
STOT RE 1	Specific target organ toxicity (repeated exposure) Category 1
H330	Fatal if inhaled
H360	May damage fertility or the unborn child
H372	Causes damage to organs through prolonged or repeated exposure
H400	Very toxic to aquatic life
H410	Very toxic to aquatic life with long lasting effects

NFPA health hazard   : 3 - Short exposure could cause serious temporary or residual injury even though prompt medical attention was given.

NFPA fire hazard   : 0 - Materials that will not burn.

NFPA reactivity   : 0 - Normally stable, even under fire exposure conditions, and are not reactive with water.

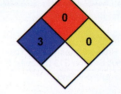

SDS US (GHS HazCom 2012)

This information is based on our current knowledge and is intended to describe the product for the purposes of health, safety and environmental requirements only. It should not therefore be construed as guaranteeing any specific property of the product

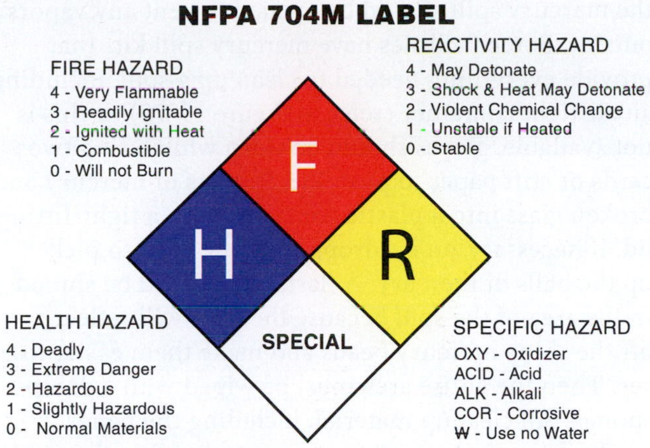

NFPA 704M LABEL

FIRE HAZARD
4 - Very Flammable
3 - Readily Ignitable
2 - Ignited with Heat
1 - Combustible
0 - Will not Burn

REACTIVITY HAZARD
4 - May Detonate
3 - Shock & Heat May Detonate
2 - Violent Chemical Change
1 - Unstable if Heated
0 - Stable

F
H R
SPECIAL

HEALTH HAZARD
4 - Deadly
3 - Extreme Danger
2 - Hazardous
1 - Slightly Hazardous
0 - Normal Materials

SPECIFIC HAZARD
OXY - Oxidizer
ACID - Acid
ALK - Alkali
COR - Corrosive
W̶ - Use no Water

FIGURE 14–4 The NFPA label identifies specific hazards of chemicals.

The Occupational Exposure to Hazardous Chemicals Standard also mandates that all employers train employees to follow the proper procedures or policies with regard to:

- Identifying the types and locations of all chemicals or hazards

- Locating and using the SDS manual containing all of the safety data sheets; SDSs must be readily accessible for all hazardous chemicals used

- Reading and interpreting chemical labels and hazard signs

- Using personal protective equipment (PPE) such as masks, gowns, gloves, and goggles

- Locating cleaning equipment and following the correct methods for managing spills and disposal of chemicals

- Reporting accidents or exposures and documenting any incidents that occur

BLOODBORNE PATHOGEN STANDARD

The **Bloodborne Pathogen Standard** has mandates to protect health care providers from diseases caused by exposure to body fluids. The Centers for Disease Control and Prevention (CDC) recommends the use of standard precautions for all patients because of possible exposure to body fluids. Examples of body fluids include blood and blood components, urine, stool, semen, vaginal secretions, cerebrospinal fluid, saliva, mucus, and other similar fluids. Three diseases that can be contracted by exposure to body fluids include hepatitis B, caused by the hepatitis B virus; hepatitis C, caused by the hepatitis C virus; and acquired immune deficiency syndrome (AIDS), caused by the human immunodeficiency virus (HIV). The mandates of this standard are discussed in detail in Section 15:4. Isolation precautions required while caring for patients who have communicable disease are found under *transmission-based precautions* in Section 15:9 of this text.

ENVIRONMENTAL SAFETY

Ergonomics is an applied science used to promote the safety and well-being of a person by adapting to the environment and using techniques to prevent injuries. Ergonomics includes correctly placing furniture and equipment, training in required muscle movements, avoiding repetitive motions, and being aware of the environment to prevent injuries. The prevention of accidents and injury centers around people and the immediate environment. The health care provider must be conscious of personal and patient/resident safety at all times. In addition, every health care provider must be alert to unsafe situations and report them immediately. Examples include burned-out lightbulbs, frayed electrical cords, scalding water in a sink or bath area, missing floor tiles or torn carpet, and other similar hazards.

Environmental hazards in health care facilities can also endanger patients, health care personnel, other individuals, and the environment.

Radiation exposure is a major concern in radiology departments and dental offices. In dental offices, a lead apron should be used to cover the patient before dental radiographs are taken. In addition, the dental provider taking the radiographs usually stands outside the room to activate the machine and obtain the radiograph. In radiology departments, all machines that emit radiation waves must be checked frequently to make sure they are operating correctly and not leaking radiation. Radiographers should stand behind a protective shield when activating the machines. To ensure that the level of exposure is safe, personnel in these departments wear dosimeter badges that measure exposure to radiation. Another substance that can cause radiation exposure is *radioactive iodine*. This substance is used to diagnose thyroid problems and treat thyroid diseases. After it has been given to a patient, small amounts of radiation are present in the neck area for several days. This is a beneficial treatment for the patient, but precautions must be taken to protect the patient's family and friends. Contact must be limited, especially with children and pregnant women. No eating utensils or food should be shared. Other radioactive substances used to treat cancer present the same problems. An example is radioactive seeds that are used to treat prostate cancer in men. At times, patients are even kept in isolation for several days to prevent radiation exposure to others. In addition, the tests and treatments result in radioactive waste. Most health care facilities dispose of radioactive wastes by placing them in a sealed container and sending them to a radioactive disposal site for treatment and disposal. The wastes are stored for a minimum of 10 half-lives and then monitored to determine the amount of residual radioactivity. When the level of radioactivity is safe, the wastes can be discarded in a secure government-approved location.

Medications and gases can be an environmental hazard. Antineoplastic drugs used to treat different cancers can be hazardous to health care personnel and pregnant individuals and must be handled with care. In operating rooms and dental offices, nitrous oxide, a gas used as an anesthetic, may cause spontaneous abortions in pregnant women.

In the same way, individuals and the environment can be harmed by improper disposal of biohazard wastes such as needles and syringes. Contaminated wastes containing body fluids, such as blood, can spread disease if they are not destroyed properly. Body parts, such as tissues or tumors that have been removed surgically, must also be disposed of correctly. All health care providers are responsible for identifying the specific hazards that present a danger to themselves, others in society, and the environment, and for taking proper precautions to deal with those hazards and follow the approved method of disposal.

Another example of biohazard waste is mercury. Mercury is a heavy silver element that is liquid at room temperature. Mercury is used in dental offices, older sphygmomanometers, and glass thermometers and can present a danger to people and the environment if it is not disposed of correctly. To avoid the chance of mercury contamination, the Occupational Health and Safety Administration (OSHA), the Environment Protection Agency (EPA), and the American Medical Association (AMA) recommend the use of mercury-free liquid clinical thermometers or digital thermometers and the use of aneroid or automated sphygmomanometers. If mercury is released by improper handling in a dental area or by breaking a clinical thermometer or sphygmomanometer, the mercury can evaporate and create a toxic vapor that can harm both humans and the environment. Mercury poisoning attacks the central nervous system in humans. Children, especially those under the age of six, are very susceptible. Mercury can contaminate water supplies and build up in the tissues of fish and animals. Therefore, proper cleanup of a mercury spill is essential. Only authorized individuals should clean up a mercury spill. A vacuum cleaner or broom should *never* be used to clean up mercury because this will break up the beads of mercury and allow them to vaporize more quickly. Mercury should *never* be poured down a drain or discarded in a toilet because this causes contamination of the water supply. If a mercury spill occurs, doors to other indoor areas should be closed and the windows in the room with

the mercury spill should be opened to vent any vapors outside. Some facilities have mercury spill kits that provide everything needed to clean up a spill, including an air tight container (refer to Figure 19-72). If this is not available, gloves should be worn while using two cards or stiff paper to push the droplets of mercury and broken glass into a plastic container with a tight-fitting lid. If necessary, an eyedropper can be used to pick up the balls of mercury. A flashlight should be shined in the area of the spill because the light will reflect off the shiny mercury beads and make them easier to see. Then the entire area must be wiped with a damp sponge. All cleanup material, including the paper, eyedropper, gloves, and sponge, are placed in the plastic container and labeled as "Mercury for Recycling." The lid is sealed tightly and the container is then sent to a mercury recycling center. Most waste disposal companies will accept mercury for recycling. Unbroken mercury thermometers, older sphygmomanometers, or unused dental mercury can be placed in a plastic container with a tight-fitting lid, labeled, and sent to a mercury recycling center. Dental offices also have other specific mercury exposures and handling procedures. Further dental information can be found in Section 19:14.

Legal

In addition, every health care provider must accept the responsibility to use good judgment in all situations, ask questions when in doubt, and follow approved policies and procedures to create a safe environment. Always remember that a health care provider has a legal responsibility to protect the patient from harm and injury.

Equipment and Solutions Safety

Basic rules that must be followed when working with equipment and solutions include:

- Do *not* operate or use any equipment until you have been instructed on how to use it.

- Read and follow the operating instructions for all major pieces of equipment. If you do not understand the instructions, ask for assistance.

- Do *not* operate any equipment if your instructor/immediate supervisor is not in the room.

- Report any damaged or malfunctioning equipment immediately. Make no attempt to use it. Some facilities use a lockout tag system for damaged electrical or mechanical equipment. A locking device is placed on the equipment to prevent the equipment from being used (**Figure 14–5**).

- Do not use frayed or damaged electrical cords. Do not use a plug if the third prong for grounding has been broken off. Never use excessive force to insert a plug into an outlet.

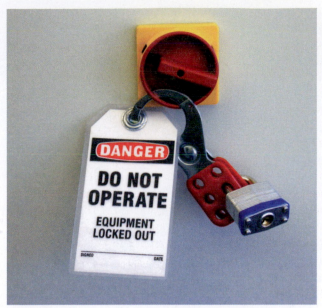

FIGURE 14–5 Some facilities use a lockout tag system for damaged equipment to prevent anyone from using the equipment. ©iStock.com/Brandon Clark

- Never handle any electrical equipment with wet hands or around water.

- Store all equipment in its proper place. Unused equipment should not be left in a patient's room, a hallway, or a doorway.

- When handling any equipment, observe all safety precautions that have been taught.

- Read SDSs before using any hazardous chemical solutions.

- Check the NFPA code on a chemical to determine the specific hazards associated with the chemical.

- Never use solutions from bottles that are not labeled.

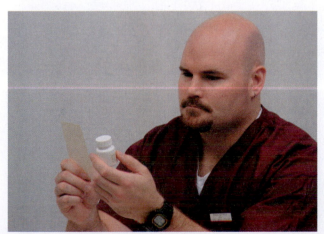

FIGURE 14–6 Read the label on a solution bottle at least three times to be sure you have the correct solution.

- Read the labels of solution bottles at least three times during use to be sure you have the correct solution (**Figure 14–6**).

- Do *not* mix any solutions together unless instructed to do so by your instructor/immediate supervisor or you can verify that they are compatible.

- Some solutions can be injurious or poisonous. Avoid contact with your eyes and skin. Avoid inhaling any fumes emitted by a solution. Use only as directed. Store all chemical solutions in a locked cabinet or closet following the manufacturer's recommendations. For example, some solutions must be kept at room temperature, while others must be stored in a cool area.

- Dispose of chemical solutions according to the instructions provided on the SDS for the solution.

- If any equipment is broken or any solutions spilled, immediately report the incident to an instructor/immediate supervisor. They will advise how to dispose of the equipment or how to remove the spilled solution (**Figure 14–7**).

Patient/Resident Safety

Basic rules that must be followed to protect a patient or resident include:

- Do *not* perform any procedure on patients unless you have been instructed to do so. Make sure you have the proper authorization. Follow instructions carefully. Ask questions if you do not understand. Use correct or approved methods while performing any procedure. Avoid shortcuts or incorrect techniques.

- Provide privacy for all patients. Knock on the door before entering any room (**Figure 14–8A**). Speak to the patient and identify yourself. Ask for permission to enter before going behind closed privacy curtains. Close the door and draw curtains for privacy before beginning a procedure on a patient (**Figure 14–8B**).

- Always identify your patient. Be absolutely positive that you have the correct patient. Check the identification wristband, if present. Ask the patient to state his or her name. Repeat the patient's name at least twice. Check the name on the patient's bed and on the patient's record.

- Always explain the procedure so the patient knows what you are going to do (**Figure 14–8C**). Answer any questions and make sure you have the patient's consent before performing any procedure. Never perform a procedure if a patient refuses to allow you to do so.

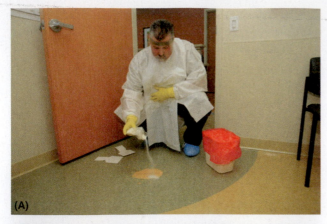

(A)

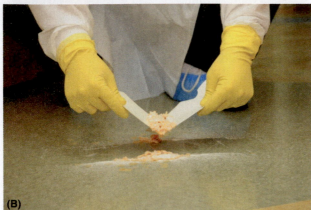

(B)

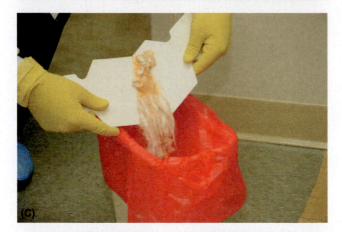

(C)

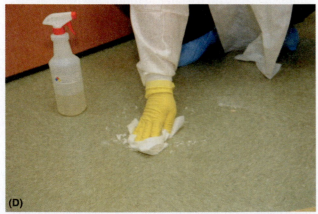

(D)

FIGURE 14–7 To clean a spill: (A) Pour coagulating powder on the spill. (B) When the material has been absorbed, pick up the residue and (C) place it in a biohazard container. (D) Clean the area thoroughly with a disinfecting solution.

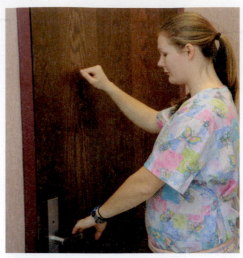

FIGURE 14–8A Always knock on the door or speak before entering a patient's room.

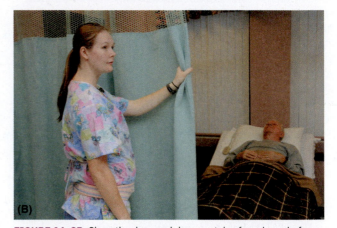

(B)

FIGURE 14–8B Close the door and draw curtains for privacy before beginning a procedure.

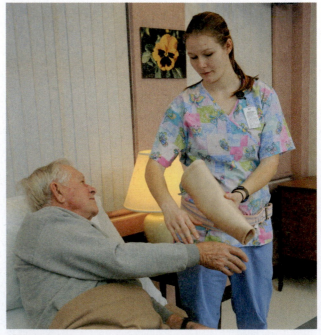

FIGURE 14–8C Explain the procedure and answer any questions to make sure you have the patient's consent.

- Observe the patient closely during any procedure. If you notice any change, immediately report this. Be alert to the patient's condition at all times.

- Frequently check the patient area, waiting room, office rooms, bed areas, or home environment for safety hazards. Report all unsafe situations immediately to the proper person or correct the safety hazard.

- Before leaving a patient/resident in a bed, observe all safety checkpoints. Make sure the patient is in a comfortable position. Check the bed to be sure that the side rails are elevated, if indicated; that the bed is at the lowest level to the floor; and that the wheels on the bed are locked to prevent movement of the bed. Place the call signal (a bell can be used in a home situation) and other supplies such as the telephone, television remote control, fresh water, and tissues within easy reach of the patient/resident (**Figure 14–9A**). Open the privacy curtains if they were closed. Leave the area neat and clean, and make sure no safety hazards are present. Wash your

hands thoroughly (**Figure 14–9B**). If your hands are not visibly dirty or contaminated with blood or body fluids, they can be cleaned with a waterless hand cleaner (**Figure 14–9C**).

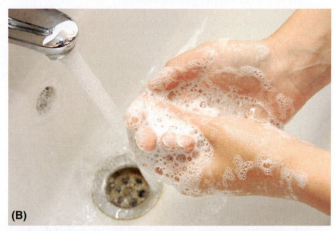

(B)

FIGURE 14–9B Wash your hands before and after any procedure, and any time they become contaminated during a procedure. © Voronin76/Shutterstock.com

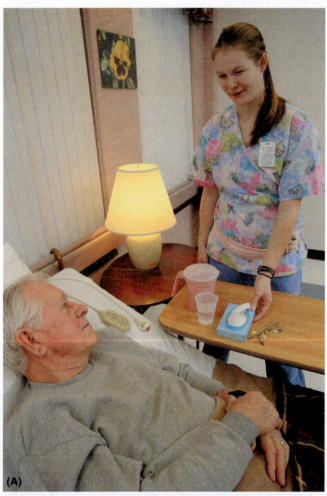

(A)

FIGURE 14–9A Lower the bed and place the call signal and other supplies within easy reach of the patient before leaving a patient.

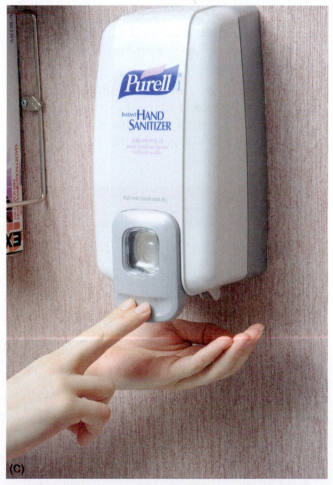

(C)

FIGURE 14–9C If your hands are not visibly dirty or contaminated with blood or body fluids, they can be cleaned with a waterless hand cleaner.

Personal Safety

Basic rules that must be followed to protect yourself and others include:

- Remember, it is your responsibility to protect yourself and others from injury.

- Use correct body mechanics while performing any procedure.

- Wear the required personal protective equipment (PPE) as discussed in Section 15:4. This may include a gown, mask, gloves, and protective eyewear.

- Walk—do *not* run—in the laboratory area or clinical area, in hallways, and especially on stairs. Keep to the right and watch carefully at intersections to avoid collisions. Use handrails on stairways.

- Promptly report any personal injury or accident, no matter how minor, to your instructor/immediate supervisor.

- If you see an unsafe situation or a violation of a safety practice, report it to your instructor/immediate supervisor promptly.

- Keep all areas clean and neat with all equipment and supplies in their proper locations at all times.

- Wash your hands frequently. Hands should always be washed before and after any procedure, and any time they become contaminated during a procedure (refer to Figure 14–9B).

- Keep your hands away from your face, eyes, mouth, and hair.

- Dry your hands thoroughly before handling any electrical equipment.

- Wear safety glasses when instructed to do so and in any situations that might result in possible eye injury.

- While working with your partner in patient simulations, observe all safety precautions taught in caring for a patient. Review the role each of you will have before you begin practicing a procedure so each person knows his or her responsibilities. Avoid horseplay and practical jokes; they cause accidents.

- If any solutions come in contact with your skin or eyes, immediately flush the area with cool water. Inform your instructor/immediate supervisor.

- If a particle gets in your eye, inform your instructor/immediate supervisor. Do *not* try to remove the particle or rub your eye.

checkpoint

1. What does SDS stand for? Why is it used?
2. What is the NFPA? Why is it important for health care providers?

PRACTICE: Go to the workbook and complete the assignment sheet for 14:2, Preventing Accidents and Injuries. Then return and continue with the procedure.

Procedure 14:2

Preventing Accidents and Injuries

Equipment and Supplies

Information section on Preventing Accidents and Injuries, several bottles of solutions, laboratory area with equipment

Procedure

1. Assemble equipment.
2. Review the safety standards in the information section for Preventing Accidents and Injuries. Note standards that are not clear and ask your instructor for an explanation.
3. Examine several bottles of solutions. Read the labels carefully. Read the safety or danger warnings on the bottles. Read SDSs provided with hazardous chemicals. Check the NFPA label and note specific hazards.
4. Practice reading the label three times to be sure you have the correct solution. Read the label before taking the bottle off the shelf, before pouring from the bottle, and after you have poured from the bottle.
5. Look at major pieces of equipment in the laboratory. Read the operating instructions for the equipment. Do *not* operate the equipment until you are taught how to do it correctly.
6. Role-play the following situations by using another student as a patient.
   - Show ways to provide privacy for the patient.
   - Identify the patient.

- Explain a procedure to the patient.

- Observe the patient during a procedure. List points you should observe to note a change in the patient's condition.

7. Check various patient areas in the laboratory. Note any safety hazards that may be present. Discuss how you can correct the problems. Report your findings to your instructor.

8. Discuss the following situations with another student and decide how you would handle them:

   - You see an unsafe situation or a violation of a safety practice

   - You see a wet area on the laboratory counter

   - You get a small cut on your hand while using a glass slide

   - A solution splashes on your arm

   - A particle gets in your eye

- A piece of equipment is not working correctly

- A bottle of solution does not have a label

- You break a glass beaker

9. Observe and practice all of the safety regulations as you work in the laboratory.

10. Study the regulations in preparation for the safety examination. You must pass the safety examination.

11. Replace all equipment used.

PRACTICE: Use the evaluation sheet for 14:2, Preventing Accidents and Injuries, to practice this procedure. When you believe you have mastered this skill, sign the sheet and give it to your instructor for further action.

 FINAL EVALUATION: Using the criteria listed on the evaluation sheet, your instructor will grade your performance.

Check

14:3 OBSERVING FIRE SAFETY

OBRA

Health care providers must know three basic facts about fires: how they start, how to prevent them, and how to respond when they occur.

Fires need three things in order to start (**Figure 14–10**):

- **Oxygen**: present in the air

- **Fuel**: any material that will burn

- **Heat**: sparks, matches, flames

The major cause of fires is unattended cooking fires. Other causes include misuse of electricity (overloaded circuits, frayed electrical wires, improperly grounded plugs), defects in heating systems and portable heaters, smoking and matches, candles, spontaneous ignition, improper rubbish disposal, children playing with matches and lighters, and arson.

FIRE EXTINGUISHERS

Fire extinguishers are classified and labeled according to the kind of fire they extinguish. The main classes are:

- **Class A**: used on fires involving combustibles such as paper, cloth, plastic, and wood

- **Class B**: used on fires involving flammable or combustible liquids such as gasoline, oil, paint, grease, and cooking fat

- **Class C**: used on electrical fires such as fuse boxes, appliances, wiring, and electrical outlets; the C stands for nonconductive; if possible, the electricity should be turned off before using an extinguisher on an electrical fire

- **Class D**: used on burning or combustible metals; often specific for the type of metal being used and not used on any other types of fires

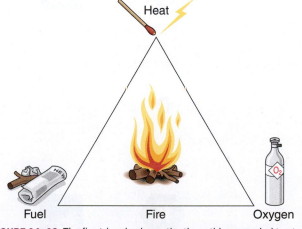

FIGURE 14–10 The fire triangle shows the three things needed to start a fire.

- **Class K**: used on burning cooking materials (fats, grease, and oils) and appliances in commercial cooking sites such as restaurants; uses a process call saponification by applying an alkaline mixture that creates a soapy foam to hold in the vapors and steam and extinguish the fire

Many different types of fire extinguishers are available. The main types include:

- **Water**: contains pressurized water and should only be used on Class A fires
- **Carbon dioxide**: contains carbon dioxide gas that provides a smothering action on the fire by forming a cloud of cool ice or snow that displaces the air and oxygen; leaves a powdery, snow-like residue that irritates the skin and eyes and can be dangerous if inhaled; most effective on Class B or C fires
- **Dry chemical**: contains a chemical that acts to smother a fire; type BC extinguishers contain potassium bicarbonate or sodium bicarbonate, which leaves a mildly corrosive residue that must be cleaned up as soon as possible; type ABC extinguishers contain monoammonium phosphate, a yellow powder that leaves a sticky residue that can damage electrical appliances such as computers; type K uses potassium acetate, potassium citrate, or potassium carbonate, which leaves a soapy foam that can damage appliances; all of the residues can irritate the skin and eyes; used on Class A, B, C, or K fires depending on the type of extinguisher
- **Halon**: contains a gas that interferes with the chemical reaction that occurs when fuels burn; used on electrical equipment because it does not leave a residue and will not damage appliances such as computers; most effective on Class C fires

Most fire extinguishers are labeled with a diagram and/or a letter showing the type of fire for which they are effective (**Figure 14–11**). Many extinguishers are used on different types of fires and will be labeled with more than one diagram or letter. In addition, some extinguishers put all of the diagrams on the label; however, a diagonal red

CLASSES OF FIRE EXTINGUISHERS

  CLASS A
Used for fires of ordinary combustibles such as wood, paper, cloth, and plastics

  CLASS B
Used for fires of flammable liquids and gases such as paint, gasoline, oil, grease, and cooking fires

  CLASS C
Used for electrical fires such as fuse boxes, electrical outlets, and appliances; if possible, turn off the electricity before using an extinguisher on this type of fire

  CLASS D
Used on burning or combustible metals such as magnesium, titanium, and sodium; specific for the type of metal; not used on other types of fires

  CLASS K
Used on burning cooking material such as fats, grease, and oils in commercial cooking sites

FIGURE 14–11 Fire extinguishers contain diagrams and/or letters to show the type of fire on which they should be used.

line is drawn through any diagram that depicts a fire for which the extinguisher should not be used. For example, if a diagonal red line is drawn through the diagram for electrical fires, it means the extinguisher should not be used on any electrical fire. Health care providers must become familiar with the types and locations of fire extinguishers in their place of employment so they are prepared to act when a fire occurs.

In case of fire, the main rule is to remain calm. If your personal safety is endangered, evacuate the area according to the stated method and sound the alarm. If the fire is small, confined to one area, and your safety is not endangered, determine what type of fire it is and use the proper extinguisher.

FIRE EMERGENCY PLAN

While working in a health care facility, know and follow the fire emergency plan established by the facility. The plan usually states that all patients and personnel in immediate danger should be moved from the area. The alarm should be activated as quickly as possible (**Figure 14–12**). All doors and windows should be closed, if possible, to prevent drafts, which cause fire to spread more rapidly. Electrical equipment and oxygen should be shut off. Elevators should never be used

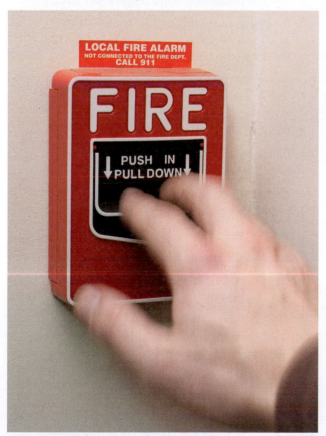

FIGURE 14–12 When a fire occurs, the fire alarm should be activated as quickly as possible. © Andre Blais/Shutterstock.com

during a fire. The acronym *RACE* is frequently used to remember the important steps. *RACE* stands for:

- **R** = Rescue anyone in immediate danger. Move patients to a safe area. If the patient can walk, escort them to a safe area. At times it may be necessary to move a patient in a bed or use the bed sheets as lift sheets to carry a patient to a safe area.

- **A** = Activate the alarm. Sound the alarm and give the location and type of fire.

- **C** = Contain the fire. Close windows and doors to prevent drafts. Shut off electrical equipment and oxygen if your safety is not endangered.

- **E** = Extinguish the fire or evacuate the area. If the fire is small and contained, and you are not in danger, locate the correct fire extinguisher to extinguish the fire. If the fire is large or spreading rapidly, or if you or a patient/resident are in danger, evacuate the area.

By following the fire emergency plan, knowing the location of fire extinguishers and exit doors, and remaining calm, the health care provider can help prevent loss of life or serious injury during a fire.

Safety

Preventing fires is everyone's job. Constantly be alert to potential causes of fires, and correct all situations that can lead to fires. Some rules for preventing fires are:

- Obey all "No Smoking" signs. Most health care facilities are "smoke-free" environments and do not permit smoking anywhere on the premises.

- Extinguish matches, cigarettes, and any other flammable items completely. Do not empty ashtrays into trash cans or plastic bags that can burn. Always empty ashtrays into separate metal cans or containers partially filled with sand or water.

- Dispose of all waste materials in proper containers.

- Before using electrical equipment, check for damaged cords or improper grounding. Avoid overloading electrical outlets.

- Store flammable materials such as kerosene or gasoline in proper containers and in a safe area. If you spill a flammable liquid, wipe it up immediately.

- Do not allow clutter to accumulate in rooms, closets, doorways, or traffic areas. Make sure no equipment or supplies block any fire exits.

- When oxygen is in use, observe special precautions. Post a "No Smoking—Oxygen in Use" sign. Remove all smoking materials, candles, lighters, and matches from the room. Avoid the use of electrically operated equipment whenever possible. Do not use flammable liquids such as alcohol, nail polish, and oils. Avoid static electricity by using cotton blankets, sheets, and gowns.

DISASTER PLANS

Legal

In addition to fires, other types of disasters may occur. Examples include tornadoes, hurricanes, earthquakes, floods, bomb threats, and active shooters. If an active shooter situation occurs in your facility, run and escape if possible, hide in a safe location out of sight of the shooter if escape is not possible, try to protect patients or residents by moving them to a secure location if this does not endanger you or the patient, silence any electronic devices and text 911 or put a sign in the window, and stay in place until law enforcement arrives. Always follow the facility's protocol regarding actions that should be taken and how to contact emergency personnel. In any type of disaster, stay calm, follow the most current policy of the health care facility, and provide for the safety of yourself and the patient. It is important to note that health care providers are legally responsible for familiarizing themselves with disaster policies so appropriate action can be taken when a disaster strikes.

checkpoint

| **1.** What does the acronym RACE stand for?

PRACTICE: Go to the workbook and complete the assignment sheet for 14:3, Observing Fire Safety. Then return and continue with the procedure.

Procedure 14:3

Observing Fire Safety

Equipment and Supplies

Fire alarm box, fire extinguishers

Procedure

1. Read the information section on Observing Fire Safety.

2. Learn the five classes of fire extinguishers and know for which kind of fire each type is used.

3. Locate the nearest fire alarm box. Read the instructions on how to operate the alarm. Be sure you could set off the alarm in case of a fire.

4. Locate any fire extinguishers in the laboratory or clinical area. Look for extinguishers in both the room and surrounding building. Identify each extinguisher and the kind of fire for which it is meant to be used.

5. Learn how to operate a fire extinguisher. Read the manufacturer's operating instructions carefully. Work with a practice extinguisher or do a mock demonstration.

    CAUTION: Do *not* discharge a real extinguisher in the laboratory or clinical area.

   Safety

   a. Check the extinguisher type to be sure it is the proper one to use for the mock fire (**Figure 14–13A**).

   b. Locate the lock or pin at the top handle. Release the lock following the manufacturer's instructions (**Figure 14–13B**).

   NOTE: During a mock demonstration, only pretend to release the lock.

   c. Grasp the handle to hold the extinguisher firmly in an upright position.

   d. Stand approximately 6–10 feet from the near edge of the fire.

   e. Aim the nozzle at the fire (**Figure 14–13C**).

   f. Discharge the extinguisher. Use a side-to-side motion. Spray toward the near edge of the fire at the bottom of the fire.

    CAUTION: Do not spray into the center or top of the fire, because this will cause the fire to spread in an outward direction.

   Safety

   g. Continue with the same side-to-side motion until the fire is extinguished.

   NOTE: The word PASS can help you remember the correct steps:

   P = Pull the pin.

   A = Aim the extinguisher at the near edge and bottom of the fire.

   S = Squeeze the handle to discharge the extinguisher.

   S = Sweep the extinguisher from side to side at the base of the fire.

   h. At all times, stay a safe distance from the fire to avoid personal injury.

    CAUTION: Avoid contact with residues from chemical extinguishers.

   Safety

i. After an extinguisher has been used, it must be recharged or replaced. Another usable extinguisher must be put in position when the extinguisher is removed.

6. Check the policy in your area for evacuating the laboratory or clinical area during a fire. Practice the method and know the locations of all exits.

NOTE: Remember to remain calm and avoid panic.

7. Replace all equipment used.

PRACTICE: Use the evaluation sheet for 14:3, Observing Fire Safety, to practice this procedure. When you believe you have mastered this skill, sign the sheet and give it to your instructor for further action.

 FINAL EVALUATION: Using the criteria listed on the evaluation sheet, your instructor will grade your performance.

PRACTICE: Study the safety regulations throughout Chapter 14 in preparation for the safety examination.

 FINAL EVALUATION: Take the safety examination and obtain a passing grade to demonstrate your knowledge of safety.

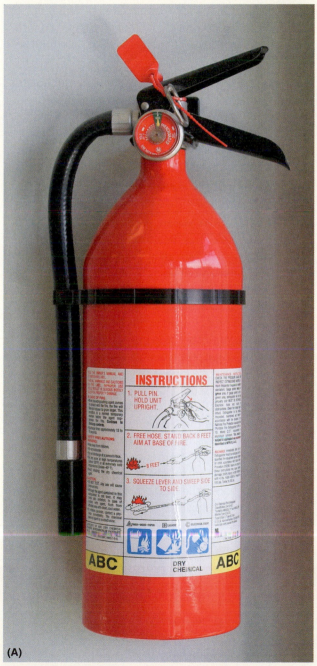

(A)

FIGURE 14–13A Check the extinguisher type to make sure it is the correct one to use. © Rob Byron/Shutterstock.com

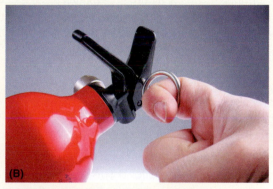

(B)

FIGURE 14–13B Release the pin on the fire extinguisher. © iStock.com/ Alessandro D'Alessandro

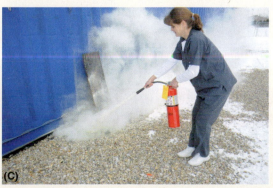

(C)

FIGURE 14–13C Aim the nozzle at the near edge of the fire, and push the handle to discharge the extinguisher.

Active Shooter in a Health Care Facility

An active shooter is defined as an individual who is actively engaged in killing or attempting to kill people in a facility or on a facility campus. According to the U.S. Department of Homeland Security, usually active shooters use a firearm and display no pattern or method for selection of their victims.

Most health care facilities are open to the public and have unusual hours, making it relatively easy for a shooter to gain access. Active shooter events in a health care setting present unique challenges: a vulnerable patient population, biohazard materials, and locked units.

Health care providers may be faced with decisions about leaving patients. They may not be able to evacuate due to age, injury, illness, or a medical procedure in progress. Some people who are able to avoid the incident will choose to remain in dangerous areas.

During an active shooter situation, the natural human reaction is to be startled, feel fear and anxiety, and even experience disbelief. There is usually a great deal of noise from alarms, gunfire and explosions, and people shouting and screaming. Training provides the means to regain your composure, recall what you have learned, and commit to action. A trained individual will more likely respond according to the training received, while the untrained will more likely not respond appropriately and can become part of the problem.

Hospitals, health centers, and schools represent a distinctive set of challenges for active shooter planning. The limitations as a result of size, location, critical care versus acute care, the presence of students, whether you have security, law enforcement availability, and response times are just a few of the many challenges when developing a response to an active shooter. There are several sets of planning guidance that have been developed for active shooter incidents for organizations such as schools, government, and business office settings. Most include the following:

- Exit if there is an accessible escape route. Leave your belongings behind and try to help others escape. Keep your hands visible so law enforcement can see that you are unarmed. If you can't get out, find a place to hide. Block entry to your hiding place if possible, for example, by pushing furniture against the door. Silence your cell phone or pager, and turn off any other sources of noise, such as a computer or television.

- As a last resort, and only if your life is in immediate danger, try to incapacitate the shooter. Find a makeshift weapon and act aggressively: yell and throw items. Try to remain calm, particularly if you are with patients or students at the time. When law enforcement or security arrives, follow their orders, knowing that they may shout commands and use pepper spray or tear gas.

Active shooter situations are unpredictable and evolve quickly. Because of this, health care providers must be prepared to deal with an active shooter situation before law enforcement personnel arrive on the scene. "Stop the Bleed" is a national awareness campaign; it is intended to encourage bystanders to become trained, equipped, and empowered to help in a bleeding emergency before other help arrives. In a Stop the Bleed course, three techniques are taught to help save a life before someone bleeds out: (1) correct use of hands to apply pressure to a wound; (2) how to pack a wound to control bleeding; (3) how to correctly apply a tourniquet. These three techniques will empower health care providers to assist in an emergency and potentially save a life. There is no single method to respond to an incident, but prior planning will allow providers to choose the best option during an active shooter situation, maximizing lives saved.

Case Study Investigation Conclusion

Sylvia needs to think of patient safety, equipment safety, environmental safety as well as her personal safety. What two techniques did Sylvia use to keep the patient safe? What personal protective equipment did she use to keep herself safe? Did you list moving the bed's power cord as one way she addressed environmental safety? The way Sylvia disposed of the used insulin needle showed her concern for equipment safety. Did your answer include all of these areas?

CHAPTER 14 SUMMARY

- Safety is the responsibility of every health care provider. It is essential that established safety standards be observed by everyone. This protects the provider, the employer, and the patient.

- One important aspect of safety is the correct use of body mechanics. Body mechanics refer to the way the body moves and maintains balance while making the most efficient use of all of its parts. Practicing basic principles of good body mechanics prevents strain and maintains muscle strength.

In addition, correct body mechanics make lifting, pulling, and pushing easier.

- Knowing and following basic safety standards is also important.

- An awareness of the causes and prevention of fires is essential. Following the fire emergency plan or other disaster plan, knowing the location of fire extinguishers and exit doors, and remaining calm, allows the health care provider to help prevent loss of life or serious injury during a fire or a disaster.

REVIEW QUESTIONS

1. List four reasons why it is important to use good body mechanics.

2. List three principles of good body mechanics that are important to follow in both lab and clinical areas while performing area tasks and procedures.

3. You are using an electrical microhematocrit centrifuge to spin blood. You see smoke coming from the back of the machine. What should you do?

4. List four (4) safety precautions that must be followed while using solutions.

5. Identify three (3) things that must be done before performing any procedure on a patient.

6. State five (5) checkpoints that must be observed before leaving a patient/resident in bed.

7. Identify the three (3) things fires need in order to start.

8. List five (5) rules that must be followed while oxygen is in use.

9. What does the acronym *PASS* stand for?

10. Describe the active shooter plan for your classroom according to school policy.

CRITICAL THINKING

1. Create a chart showing the five main types of fire extinguishers and the type of fire for which each is effective. Include examples of each in a health care setting.

2. Think about the tasks that a lab team member does each day. List the safety regulations that lab team member must be aware of as they accomplish their assignments for the day.

3. Take a picture of the fire alarm nearest your classroom. Research and describe the operation of that specific alarm.

ACTIVITIES

1. In a group of four, create a skill check off list to demonstrate safely using an extinguisher and putting out a fire. To practice: two people are partners that go in to put out the fire, one "scribe" observes and completes the check off list, and one person assists the scribe in spotting procedure specifics.

2. In a small group, develop a skit that demonstrates observation of OSHA standards in the event of a chemical spill such as mercury.

3. With a partner, research and create a safety training video or report to educate new health care students about the Bloodborne Pathogen Standard.
   a. Summarize your findings and design a brochure.
   b. Produce a short skit illustrating a typical situation encountered in health care.

Case Study Investigation

Ryan and Andrea worked at University Hospital during the Covid-19 pandemic. They worked in the Emergency Room and needed to be aware of how this virus was transmitted in order to use the proper personal protective equipment. After they went through training, they understood that this disease was highly contagious and potentially deadly. Ryan and Andrea knew that patients would sometimes have to remain in the ER for extended periods of time waiting on test results and they would have to use correct precautions when interacting with those patients. At the end of this chapter, you will be asked what PPE they needed to use and why.

■ LEARNING OBJECTIVES

After completing this chapter, you should be able to:

- Identify six classes of microorganisms by describing the characteristics of each class.
- List the six components of the chain of infection.
- Differentiate between antisepsis, disinfection, and sterilization.
- Define bioterrorism and identify at least four ways to prepare for a bioterrorism attack.
- Wash hands following aseptic technique.
- Observe standard precautions while working in the laboratory or clinical area.
- Wash, wrap, and autoclave instruments, linen, and equipment.
- Operate an autoclave with accuracy and safety.
- Follow basic principles of chemical disinfection.
- Clean instruments with an ultrasonic unit.
- Open sterile packages with no contamination.
- Don sterile gloves with no contamination.
- Prepare a sterile dressing tray with no contamination.
- Change a sterile dressing with no contamination.
- Don and remove a transmission-based isolation mask, gloves, and gown.
- Relate specific basic tasks to the care of a patient in a transmission-based isolation unit.
- Define, pronounce, and spell all key terms.

■ KEY TERMS

acquired immune deficiency
  syndrome (AIDS)

aerobic

airborne precautions

anaerobic

antisepsis (ant"-ih-sep'-sis)

asepsis (a-sep'-sis)

autoclave

bacteria

bioterrorism

cavitation (kav'-ih-tay'-shun)

chain of infection

chemical disinfection

clean

communicable disease

contact precautions

contaminated

disinfection

droplet precautions

Ebola

endogenous

epidemic

exogenous

fomites

fungi (fun'-guy)

health care–associated
  infection (HAI)

helminths

hepatitis B

hepatitis C

infectious agent

microorganism (my-crow-or'-
  gan-izm)

mode of transmission

nonpathogens

opportunistic

pandemic

parasite

pathogens (path'-oh-jenz')

personal protective equipment
  (PPE)

portal of entry

portal of exit

protective (reverse) isolation

protozoa (pro-toe-zo'-ah)

reservoir

rickettsiae (rik-et'-z-ah)

standard precautions

sterile

sterile field

sterilization

susceptible host

transmission-based
  precautions

ultrasonic units

viruses

15:1 UNDERSTANDING THE PRINCIPLES OF INFECTION CONTROL

Science   **OBRA**

Understanding the basic principles of infection control is essential for any health care provider in any field of health care. The principles described in this unit provide a basic knowledge of how disease is transmitted and the main ways to prevent disease transmission.

A **microorganism**, or microbe, is a small, living organism that is not visible to the naked eye. It must be viewed under a microscope. Microorganisms are found everywhere in the environment, including on and in the human body. Many microorganisms are part of the normal flora (plant life adapted for living in a specific environment) of the body and are beneficial in maintaining certain body processes. These are called **nonpathogens**. Other microorganisms cause infection and disease and are called **pathogens**, or germs. At times, a microorganism that is beneficial in one body system can become pathogenic when it is present in another body system. For example, a bacterium called

Escherichia coli (*E. coli*) is part of the natural flora of the large intestine. If *E. coli* enters the urinary system, however, it causes an infection.

A **parasite** is an organism that lives in or on an organism of another species (its host) and benefits by getting nutrients at the host's expense. Parasitic infections can be spread through contaminated water, food, waste, soil, and blood. Some parasites are spread by insects that act as a vector, or carrier, of the disease. Diseases caused by parasites include: body lice, Chagas Disease, cryptosporidiosis, foodborne illness, Giardia infections, and malaria. Medication is available to treat parasitic infections.

To grow and reproduce, microorganisms need certain things. Most microorganisms prefer a warm environment, and body temperature is ideal. Darkness is also preferred by most microorganisms, and many are killed quickly by sunlight. In addition, a source of food and moisture is needed. Some microorganisms, called **aerobic** organisms, require oxygen to live. Others, called **anaerobic** organisms, live and reproduce in the absence of oxygen. The human body is the ideal supplier of all the requirements of microorganisms.

CLASSES OF MICROORGANISMS

There are many different classes of microorganisms. In each class, some microorganisms are pathogenic to humans. The main classes include bacteria, protozoa, fungi, rickettsia, viruses, and helminths.

Bacteria

Bacteria are simple, one-celled organisms that multiply rapidly. They are classified by shape and arrangement. *Cocci* are round or spherical in shape (**Figure 15–1**). If cocci occur

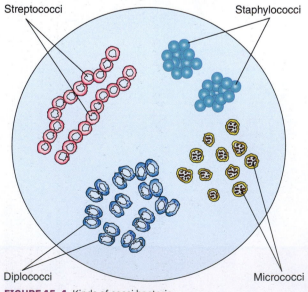

Streptococci

Staphylococci

Diplococci

Micrococci

FIGURE 15–1 Kinds of cocci bacteria.

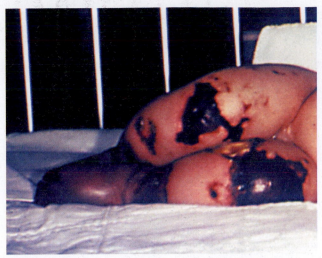

FIGURE 15–2 *Streptococcus pyogenes*, also called *Strep A* or flesh-eating strep, causes necrotizing fasciitis that destroys tissues and can result in amputation or death if not treated immediately. Courtesy of the CDC.

in pairs, they are diplococci. Diplococci bacteria cause diseases such as gonorrhea, meningitis, and pneumonia. If cocci occur in chains, they are streptococci. A common streptococcus causes a severe sore throat (strep throat) and rheumatic fever. *Streptococcus pyogenes*, also called *Strep A* or flesh-eating strep, causes necrotizing fasciitis that destroys tissues and can result in amputation or death (**Figure 15–2**). If cocci occur in clusters or groups, they are staphylococci. These are the most common pyogenic (pus-producing) microorganisms. Staphylococci cause infections such as boils, urinary tract infections, wound infections, and toxic shock. Rod-shaped bacteria are called *bacilli* (**Figure 15–3**). They can occur singly, in pairs, or in chains. Many bacilli contain flagella, which are thread-like

projections that are similar to tails and allow the organisms to move. Bacilli also have the ability to form spores, or thick-walled capsules, when conditions for growth are poor. In the spore form, bacilli are extremely difficult to kill. Diseases caused by different types of bacilli include tuberculosis, tetanus, pertussis (whooping cough), botulism, diphtheria, and typhoid. Listeria (Listeriosis) is a serious infection usually caused by eating food contaminated with the bacillus bacterium *Listeria monocytogenes*. Bacteria that are spiral or corkscrew in shape are called *spirilla* (**Figure 15–4**). These include the comma-shaped vibrio and the corkscrew-shaped spirochete. Diseases caused by spirilla include syphilis and cholera.

Antibiotics are used to kill bacteria. However, due to the overuse and misuse of antibiotics, some strains of bacteria have become antibiotic-resistant, which means that the antibiotic is no longer effective against the bacteria. If a bacterium becomes resistant to several drugs, it is called multidrug resistant, or a "superbug." Methicillin-resistant *Staphylococcus aureas* (MRSA) is an example. It causes a severe staph infection that is difficult to treat because it is resistant to many different antibiotics. Vancomycin-resistant enterococcus (VRE) is a bacterium that is resistant to vancomycin and several other drugs. Because no single antibiotic can eliminate VRE, drug combinations are often used to treat it. *Extended spectrum beta lactamase* (ESBL)-producing bacterium developed from an increased use of beta lactam antibiotics such as penicillin and ampicillin. ESBL is resistant to many antibiotics. Multidrug-resistant *Acinetobacter baumannii* (MRAB) is an example of a bloodstream infection that is difficult to treat due to drug resistance. In some cases, *A. baumannii* has been resistant to all drugs tested.

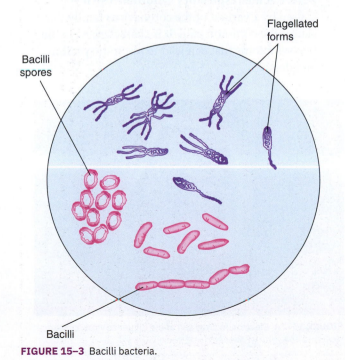

FIGURE 15–3 Bacilli bacteria.

FIGURE 15–4 Spirilla bacteria.

Carbapenem-resistant enterobacteriaceae (CRE) are resistant to most antibiotics and can cause pneumonia, kidney and bladder disease, and septicemia (pathogenic organisms in the bloodstream). All antibiotic-resistant bacterium are a major concern because they are difficult to treat, they cause increased hospital stays, and they increase the cost of health care. A major campaign has been launched to push for less antibiotic use, unless specifically indicated, to help prevent drug resistance.

Protozoa

Protozoa are one-celled animal-like organisms often found in decayed materials, animal or bird feces, insect bites, and contaminated water (**Figure 15–5**). Many contain flagella, which allow them to move freely. Some protozoa are pathogenic and cause diseases such as malaria, amebic dysentery (intestinal infection), trichomonas, and African sleeping sickness.

Fungi

Fungi are simple, plant-like organisms that live on dead organic matter. Yeasts and molds are two common forms that can be pathogenic. They cause diseases such as ringworm, athlete's foot, histoplasmosis, yeast vaginitis, and thrush (**Figure 15–6**). Antibiotics do not kill fungi. Antifungal medications are available for many of the pathogenic fungi, but they are expensive, must be taken internally for a long period, and may cause liver damage.

Rickettsiae

Rickettsiae are parasitic microorganisms, which means they cannot live outside the cells of another living organism. They are commonly found in fleas, lice, ticks, and mites, and are transmitted to humans by the bites of these insects. Rickettsiae cause diseases such as typhus fever and Rocky Mountain spotted fever. Antibiotics are effective against many different rickettsiae.

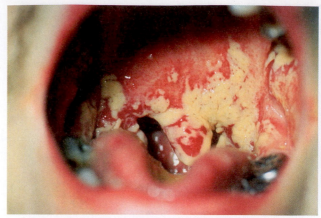

FIGURE 15–6 The yeast (fungus) called *thrush* causes these characteristic white patches on the tongue and in the mouth. Courtesy CDC.

Viruses

Viruses are the smallest microorganisms, visible only using an electron microscope (**Figures 15–7A to C**). They cannot reproduce unless they are inside another living cell. They are spread from human to human by blood and other body secretions. It is important to note that viruses are more difficult to kill because they are resistant to many disinfectants and are not affected by antibiotics. Viruses cause many diseases including the common cold, measles, mumps, chicken pox, herpes, warts, influenza, and polio. New and different viruses emerge constantly because viruses are prone to mutating and changing genetic information. In addition, viruses that infect animals can mutate to infect humans, often with lethal results.

There are many examples of these viruses:

- **Severe acute respiratory syndrome (SARS)** is caused by a variant of the coronavirus family that causes the common cold. It is characterized by flu-like symptoms that can lead to respiratory failure and death.

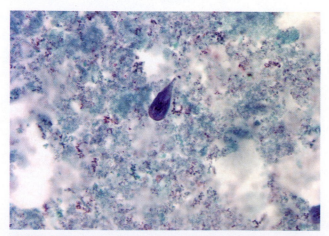

FIGURE 15–5 An intestinal protozoan, *Giardia intestinalis*, is the blue stained mass in the center of the photo. Courtesy CDC/DPDx-Melanie Moser.

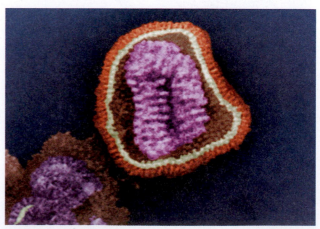

FIGURE 15–7A Electron micrograph of the influenza virus. Courtesy CDC/Erskine L. Palmer, Ph.D.; M.L. Martin. Photo credit: Frederick Murphy.

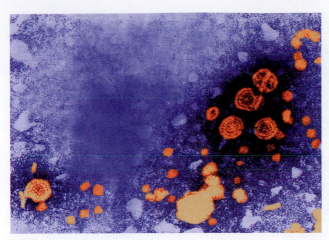

FIGURE 15–7B Electron micrograph of the hepatitis B virus. Courtesy CDC/Dr. Erskine Palmer.

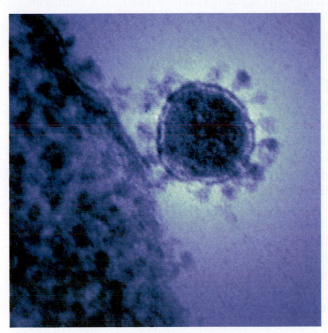

FIGURE 15–7C Electron micrograph of a coronavirus.

- **West Nile virus (WNV)** is a mosquito-borne flavivirus that first infected birds but now infects humans. In some individuals, it causes only a mild febrile illness. In other individuals who are older or have poor immune systems, it can cause severe neurologic illnesses such as encephalitis or meningitis, which can lead to death.

- **Monkeypox**, a hantavirus that affects monkeys, other primates, and rodents, mutated and spread to humans. Infection usually occurs after contacting the body secretions or excretions (urine and stool) of infected animals or ingesting food that has been contaminated by fluids from infected animals. A major outbreak occurred in the American Southwest when infected prairie dogs contaminated food with fecal material. Monkeypox is similar to smallpox. It causes severe flu-like symptoms, lymphadenopathy (disease of the lymph nodes), and pustules that cause severe scarring of the skin. If the eyes are infected, blindness can occur. It can be prevented and treated with a smallpox vaccination.

- Filoviruses such as **Ebola** and *Marburg* first affected primates and then spread to humans. These viruses cause hemorrhagic fever, a disease that begins with flu-like symptoms, fever, chills, headache, myalgia (muscle pain), and a skin rash. It quickly progresses to jaundice, pancreatitis, liver failure, massive hemorrhaging throughout the body, delirium, shock, and death. Most outbreaks of hemorrhagic fever have occurred in Africa, but isolated cases have appeared in other parts of the world when individuals were in contact with infected primates. A major epidemic of Ebola occurred in West Africa in 2014. It is discussed in detail in Section 1:2 of this text under *Pandemics*.

- The *H5N1* virus that causes avian or bird flu has devastated bird flocks in many countries. The infection has appeared in humans, but most cases have resulted from contact with infected poultry or contaminated surfaces. The spread from one person to another has been reported only rarely. However, because the death rate for bird flu is between 50 and 60 percent, a major concern is that the *H5N1* virus will mutate and spread more readily.

- *H1N1*, or swine flu, was declared a global pandemic in 2009. The virus spreads quickly and causes flu-like symptoms. In severe cases, it results in pneumonia, respiratory distress or failure, and, in some cases, death. As with the bird flu, it rarely spreads from one person to another. Most cases result from contact with infected hogs.

- The Coronavirus (COVID-19) pandemic is the result of a new virus that started in animals and mutated to infect humans. Highly contagious, many people have not developed antibodies against this virus allowing an unprecedented spread of infection and a high mortality rate. A COVID-19 infection causes flu-like symptoms and shortness of breath that may quickly advance to respiratory failure requiring a ventilator. It is discussed in Section 1:2 in this text under *Pandemics*.

In addition to these viruses, there are three other viral diseases of major concern to the health care provider: hepatitis B, hepatitis C, and acquired immune deficiency syndrome (AIDS).

Hepatitis B, or serum hepatitis, is caused by the HBV virus and is transmitted by blood, serum, and other body secretions. It affects the liver and can lead to the destruction and scarring of liver cells. A vaccine has been developed to protect individuals from this disease, but this vaccine is expensive and involves a series of three injections. Under federal law, employers must provide the vaccination at no cost to any health care team member with occupational exposure to blood or other body secretions that may carry the HBV virus. An individual does have the right to refuse the vaccination, but a written record must be kept proving that the vaccine was offered.

Hepatitis C is caused by the hepatitis C virus, or HCV, and is transmitted by blood and blood-containing body fluids. Many individuals who contract the disease are asymptomatic (display no symptoms); others have mild symptoms that are often diagnosed as influenza or flu. In either case, HCV can cause serious liver damage that may result in death. New direct acting antiviral drugs that are 90 to 99 percent effective have been approved by the FDA to treat HCV in the past several years. However, the drugs are extremely expensive and can cost as much as $1,000 per pill. At present, there is no preventive immunization, but a vaccine is being developed. Both HBV and HCV are extremely difficult to destroy. These viruses can even remain active for several days in dried blood. Health care providers must take every precaution to protect themselves from hepatitis viruses.

Acquired immune deficiency syndrome (AIDS) is caused by the human immunodeficiency virus (HIV) and suppresses the immune system (refer to Section 7:9 for detailed information). An individual with AIDS cannot fight off many cancers and infections that would not affect a healthy person. Presently, there is no cure, and no vaccine is available, so it is important for the health care provider to take precautions to prevent the spread of this disease.

Helminths

Helminths are multicellular parasitic organisms commonly called *worms* or *flukes*. They are transmitted to humans when humans ingest the eggs or larvae in contaminated food, ingest meat contaminated with the worms, or get bitten by infected insects. Some worms can also penetrate the skin to enter the body. Examples of helminths include hookworms, which attach to the small intestine and can infect the heart and lungs (**Figure 15–8**); ascariasis, which live in the small intestine and can cause an obstruction of the intestine; trichinella spiralis, which causes trichinosis and is contracted by eating raw or inadequately cooked pork products; enterobiasis, which is commonly called *pinworm* and

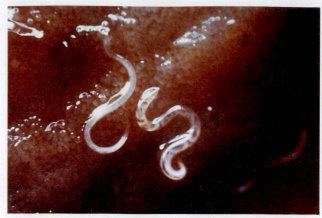

FIGURE 15–8 Hookworms attached to the mucosal lining of the intestine are one type of helminth. Courtesy CDC.

mainly affects young children; and taenia solium or the pork tapeworm, which is contracted by eating inadequately cooked pork.

TYPES OF INFECTION

Pathogenic microorganisms cause infection and disease in different ways. Some pathogens produce poisons, called *toxins*, which harm the body. An example is the bacillus that causes tetanus, which produces toxins that damage the central nervous system. Some pathogens cause an allergic reaction in the body, resulting in a runny nose, watery eyes, and sneezing. Other pathogens attack and destroy the living cells they invade. An example is the protozoan that causes malaria; it invades red blood cells and causes them to rupture.

Infections and diseases are also classified as endogenous, exogenous, health care–associated, or opportunistic. **Endogenous** means the infection or disease originates within the body. These include metabolic disorders, congenital abnormalities, tumors, and infections caused by microorganisms within the body. **Exogenous** means the infection or disease originates outside the body. Examples include pathogenic organisms that invade the body, radiation, chemical agents, trauma, electric shock, and temperature extremes. A **health care–associated infection (HAI)** (formerly referred to as *nosocomial or hospital-acquired*) is an infection acquired by an individual in a health care facility such as a hospital or long-term care facility. Health care–associated infections are usually present in the facility and transmitted by health care team members to the patient. Many of the pathogens transmitted in this manner are antibiotic-resistant and can cause serious and even life-threatening infections in patients. Common examples are staphylococcus, pseudomonas, and enterococci. Infection-control programs are used in health care facilities to prevent and deal with HAIs. The infection control professionals that run these programs are called *infection preventionists*, according to the Association for Professionals in Infection Control and Epidemiology (APIC). Their job is to reduce the incidence of HAIs. **Opportunistic** infections are those that occur when the body's defenses are weak. These diseases do not usually occur in individuals with intact immune systems. Examples include the development of a yeast infection called *candidiasis*, Kaposi's sarcoma (a rare type of cancer), or *Pneumocystis carinii* pneumonia in individuals who have AIDS.

Vaccines are used whenever available to prevent disease. A vaccine stimulates the immune system to produce antibodies, similar to the antibodies made by the body after exposure to a disease. They are made from very small amounts of weak or dead germs that can cause diseases. After getting vaccinated, an individual develops immunity to that disease without having to get the disease first. Vaccinations protect both the individual getting them and the community from the disease. Germs can travel quickly through a community and cause a major outbreak of a disease. If enough people are vaccinated against a certain disease, the germs can't travel as easily from person to person and the entire community is less likely to get the disease. This idea is called community immunity.

CHAIN OF INFECTION

For disease to occur and spread from one individual to another, certain conditions must be met. These conditions are commonly called the **chain of infection** (**Figure 15–9**). The parts of the chain include:

- **Infectious agent**: a pathogen, such as a bacterium or virus that can cause a disease

- **Reservoir**: an area where the infectious agent can live; some common reservoirs include the human body, animals, the environment, and **fomites**, or objects contaminated with infectious material that contains the pathogens. Common fomites include doorknobs, bedpans, urinals, linens, instruments, and specimen containers.

- **Portal of exit**: a way for the infectious agent to escape from the reservoir in which it has been growing. In the human body, pathogens can leave the body through urine, feces, saliva, blood, tears, mucous discharge, sexual secretions, and draining wounds.

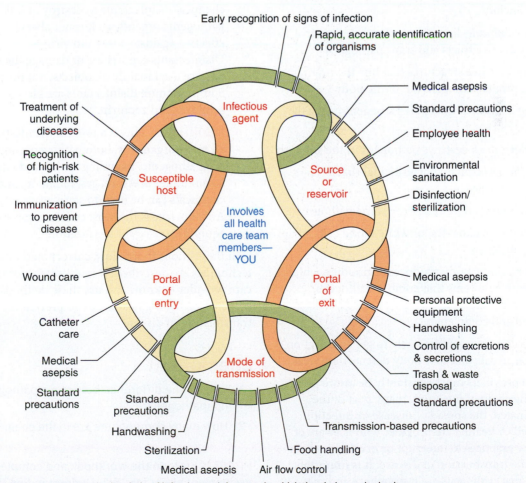

FIGURE 15–9 Note the components in the chain of infection and the ways in which the chain can be broken.

- **Mode of transmission**: a way that the infectious agent can be transmitted to another reservoir or host where it can live. The pathogen can be transmitted in different ways. One way is by *direct contact*, which includes person-to-person contact (physical or sexual contact) or contact with a body secretion containing the pathogen. Contaminated hands are one of the most common sources of direct contact transmission. Another way is by *indirect contact*, when the pathogen is transmitted from contaminated substances such as food, air, soil, insects, feces, clothing, instruments, and equipment. Examples include touching contaminated equipment and spreading the pathogen on the hands, breathing in droplets carrying airborne infections, and contacting *vectors* (insects, rodents, or small animals), such as being bitten by an insect carrying a pathogen.

- **Portal of entry**: a way for the infectious agent to enter a new reservoir or host. Some ways pathogens can enter the body are through breaks in the skin, breaks in the mucous membrane, the respiratory tract, the digestive tract, the genitourinary tract, and the circulatory system. If the defense mechanisms of the body are intact and the immune system is functioning, a human can frequently fight off the infectious agent and not contract the disease. Body defenses include:

  Mucous membrane: lines the respiratory, digestive, and reproductive tracts and traps pathogens

  Cilia: tiny, hair-like structures that line the respiratory tract and propel pathogens out of the body

  Coughing and sneezing: expels pathogens out of the body

  Hydrochloric acid: destroys pathogens in the stomach

  Tears in the eye: contain bacteriocidal (bacteria-killing) chemicals

  Fever: high temperatures destroy some pathogens

  Inflammation: leukocytes, or white blood cells, destroy pathogens

  Immune response: body produces antibodies, which are protective proteins that combat pathogens, and protective chemicals secreted by cells, such as interferon and complement

- **Susceptible host**: a person likely to get an infection or disease, usually because body defenses are weak.

Health care providers must constantly be aware of the parts in the chain of infection. If any part of the chain is eliminated, the spread of disease or infection will be stopped. A health care provider who is aware of this can follow practices to interrupt or break this chain and prevent the transmission of disease. It is important to remember that pathogens are everywhere and that preventing their transmission is a continuous process.

ASEPTIC TECHNIQUES

A major way to break the chain of infection is to use aseptic techniques while providing health care. **Asepsis** is defined as the absence of disease-producing microorganisms, or pathogens.

Sterile means free from all organisms, both pathogenic and nonpathogenic, including spores and viruses. **Contaminated** means that organisms and pathogens are present. Any object or area that may contain pathogens is considered to be contaminated. Aseptic techniques are directed toward maintaining cleanliness and eliminating or preventing contamination. Common aseptic techniques include handwashing, good personal hygiene, use of disposable gloves when contacting body secretions or contaminated objects, proper cleaning of instruments and equipment, and thorough cleaning of the environment.

Various levels of aseptic control are possible. These include:

- **Antisepsis**: Antiseptics prevent or inhibit growth of pathogenic organisms but are not effective against spores and viruses. They can usually be used on the skin. Common examples include alcohol and betadine.

- **Disinfection**: This is a process that uses chemical disinfectants to destroy or kill pathogenic organisms. It is not always effective against spores and viruses. Disinfectants can irritate or damage the skin and are used mainly on objects, not people. Some common disinfectants are bleach solutions and zephirin.

- **Sterilization**: This is a process that destroys all microorganisms, both pathogenic and nonpathogenic, including spores and viruses. Steam under pressure, gas, radiation, and chemicals can be used to sterilize objects. An autoclave is the most common piece of equipment used for sterilization.

In the sections that follow, correct methods of aseptic techniques are described. It is important for the health care provider to know and use these methods in every aspect of providing health care to prevent the spread and transmission of disease.

checkpoint

1. What is the difference between a pathogen and a nonpathogen?
2. How many components are in the chain of infection?

PRACTICE: Go to the workbook and complete the assignment sheet for 15:1, Understanding the Principles of Infection Control.

INTRODUCTION

Bioterrorism is the use of microorganisms, or biologic agents, as weapons to infect humans, animals, or plants. Throughout history, microorganisms have been used in biologic warfare. Some examples include:

- The Tartar army throwing bodies of dead plague victims over the walls of a city called Caffa in 1346, causing an epidemic of plague in the city

- The British army providing Delaware Indians with blankets and handkerchiefs contaminated with smallpox in 1763, resulting in a major outbreak of smallpox among the Indian population

- The Germans using a variety of animal and human pathogens in World War I

- The Japanese military using prisoners of war to experiment with many different pathogens in World War II

- The United States, Canada, the Soviet Union, and the United Kingdom developing biologic weapons programs until the late 1960s

- The release of sarin gas in Tokyo in 1995

- An unknown individual or individuals sending anthrax through the mail in the United States in 2001

Today, there is a major concern that these biologic agents will be used not only in wars but also against unsuspecting civilians.

BIOLOGIC AGENTS

Many different microorganisms can cause diseases in humans, animals, and plants. However, only a limited number are considered to be ideal for bioterrorism. Six characteristics of the "ideal" microorganism include:

- Inexpensive and readily available or easy to produce

- Spread through the air by winds or ventilation systems and inhaled into the lungs of potential victims, or spread by ingesting contaminated food or water

- Survives sunlight, drying, and heat

- Causes death or severe disability and public panic

- Easily transmitted from person to person

- Difficult to prevent or has no effective treatment

The Centers for Disease Control and Prevention (CDC) has identified and classified major bioterrorism agents. High-priority agents that have been identified include:

- **Smallpox**: Smallpox is a highly contagious infectious disease that is caused by a variola virus (**Figure 15–10**). A smallpox vaccination can provide protection against

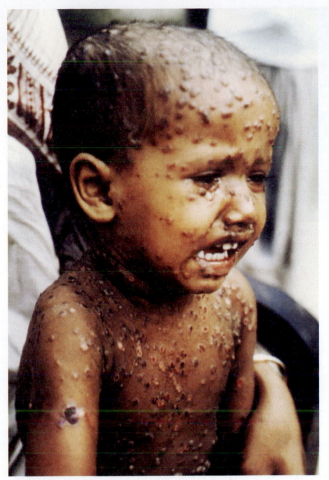

FIGURE 15–10 Smallpox is a highly contagious infectious disease caused by a variola virus. Courtesy CDC/Dr. Michael Schwartz.

some types of smallpox, but one type, hemorrhagic smallpox, is usually fatal. Until the 1970s, people were vaccinated against smallpox. However, after many years with no reported cases, the vaccinations were no longer required. Now, with the threat of a smallpox bioterrorism attack, the U.S. government has started a new vaccination program. The program encourages first responders, police, fire department, and health care personnel to be vaccinated.

- **Anthrax**: Anthrax is an infectious disease caused by the spores of bacteria called *Bacillus anthracis*. The spores are highly resistant to destruction and can live in soil for years. Grazing animals such as cattle, sheep, and goats eat the contaminated soil and become infected. Humans develop anthrax by exposure through the skin (cutaneous) (**Figure 15–11**), by eating undercooked or raw infected meat (gastrointestinal), or by inhaling the spores (pulmonary). Cutaneous and gastrointestinal anthrax are usually treated successfully with antibiotics, but some victims die. Inhalation anthrax causes death in more than 80 percent of its victims. An anthrax vaccine is available for prevention, and the military has an active vaccination program.

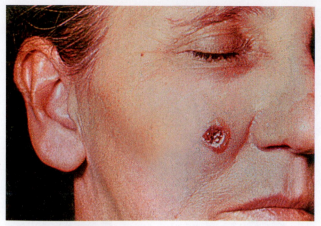

FIGURE 15–11 Cutaneous (skin) anthrax is usually treated successfully with antibiotics. Courtesy CDC.

- **Plague**: This is an infectious disease that is caused by bacteria called *Yersinia pestis*. Usually plague is transmitted by the bites of infected fleas. In some cases, the organism enters the body through a break in the skin or by contact with the tissue of an infected animal (bubonic plague). Rats, rock squirrels, prairie dogs, and chipmunks are the most common sources of plague in the United States. If the disease is not treated immediately with antibiotics, the infection spreads to the blood (septicemic plague) and lungs (pneumonic plague), and causes death. No vaccine for plague is available in the United States.

- **Botulism**: Botulism is a paralytic illness caused by a nerve toxin produced by bacteria called *Clostridium botulinum*. Three main types of botulism exist. One type is caused by eating foods that contain the toxin. A second type is caused by the presence of the toxin in a wound or injury to the skin. A third type occurs in infants who eat the spores that then grow in the intestine and release the toxin. The toxin rapidly causes muscle paralysis. If it is not treated with an antitoxin, the paralysis spreads to the respiratory muscles and causes death.

- **Tularemia**: This is an infectious disease caused by bacteria called *Francisella tularensis*. This bacteria is commonly found in animals such as rats, rabbits, and insects (ticks and deerflies). Humans get the disease through the bite of an infected animal or insect, by eating contaminated food, by drinking contaminated water, or by breathing in the bacteria. The disease causes death if it is not treated with appropriate antibiotics. Currently, the Food and Drug Administration (FDA) is reviewing a vaccine, but it is not available in the United States.

- **Hemorrhagic fever**: This is an infectious disease caused by a filovirus. Two filoviruses have been identified: the Ebola virus and the Marburg virus. The source of these viruses is still being researched,

but the common belief is that the viruses are transmitted from animals such as bats, monkeys, and chimpanzees. Once the viruses affect a human, the disease is spread rapidly from person to person by contact with body fluids. Treatment is supportive care with fluid and electrolyte replacement, respiratory support, and management of symptoms. Several experimental antiviral therapies were used during the 2014 outbreak of Ebola in West Africa, but none have proven to be effective in humans. In the 2014 outbreak, it is estimated that more than 70 percent of the infected people died.

Many other pathogenic microorganisms can be used in a bioterrorism attack. In fact, any pathogenic organism could be used in a bioterrorism attack. For this reason, health care providers must be constantly alert to the threat of infection with a biologic agent.

PREPARING FOR BIOTERRORISM

A bioterrorism attack could cause an epidemic and public health emergency. Large numbers of infected people would place a major stress on health care facilities. Fear and panic could lead to riots, social disorder, and disregard for authority. For these reasons, the Bioterrorism Act of 2002 was passed by Congress and signed into law in June 2002. This act requires the development of a comprehensive plan against bioterrorism to increase the security of the United States.

Preparing for bioterrorism will involve government at all levels—local, regional, state, and national (**Figure 15–12**). Some of the major aspects of preparation include:

- Community-based surveillance to detect early indications of a bioterrorism attack

- Notification of the public when a high-risk situation is detected

- Strict infection-control measures and public education about the measures

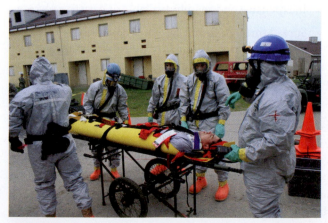

FIGURE 15–12 Response to a bioterrorism attack involves preparing and training emergency personnel at all government levels—local, regional, state, and federal. Courtesy U.S. Army/Photo by Lt. Col. Richard Goldenberg.

- Funding for studying pathogenic organisms, developing vaccines, researching treatments, and determining preventive actions

- Strict guidelines and restrictions for purchasing and transporting pathologic microorganisms

- Mass immunization, especially for military, first responders, police, fire department, and health care personnel

- Increased protection of food and water supplies

- Training personnel to properly diagnose and treat infectious diseases

- Establishing emergency management policies

- Criminal investigation of possible threats

- Improving the ability of health care facilities to deal with an attack by increasing emergency department space, preparing decontamination areas, and establishing isolation facilities

- Improving communications so information about bioterrorism is transmitted quickly and efficiently

Every health care provider must constantly be alert to the threat of bioterrorism. In today's world, it is likely that an attack will occur. Careful preparation and thorough training can limit the effect of the attack and save the lives of many people.

checkpoint

| **1.** List five (5) high priority bioterrorism agents.

PRACTICE: Go to the workbook and complete the assignment sheet for 15:2, Bioterrorism.

15:3 WASHING HANDS

Precaution   OBRA

Handwashing is a basic task required in any health care occupation. The method described in this unit has been developed to ensure that a thorough cleansing occurs. An aseptic technique is a method followed to prevent the spread of germs or pathogens. *Handwashing is the single most important method used to practice aseptic technique* (**Figure 15–13**). Handwashing is also the most effective way to prevent the spread of infection.

The hands are a perfect medium for the spread of pathogens. Thoroughly washing the hands helps prevent and control the spread of pathogens from one person to another. It also helps protect the health care provider from disease and illness.

The Centers for Disease Control and Prevention (CDC) publishes the results of handwashing research

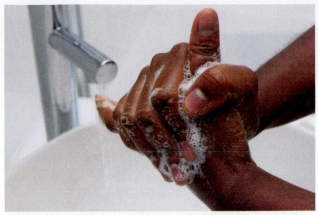

FIGURE 15–13 Handwashing is the most important method used to practice aseptic technique. © iStock.com/Jo Unruh.

and provides recommendations for hand hygiene. The recommendations call for regular handwashing using plain soap and water, antiseptic handwashing using an antimicrobial soap and water, and antiseptic hand rubs (waterless handwashing) using alcohol-based hand cleaners containing at least 60 to 90 percent alcohol. Regular handwashing is recommended for routine cleansing of the hands when the hands are visibly dirty or soiled with blood or other body fluids. Antiseptic handwashing is recommended before invasive procedures, in critical care units, while caring for patients on specific organism transmission-based precautions, and in specific circumstances defined by the infection-control program of the health care facility. Antiseptic hand rubs are recommended if the hands are not visibly dirty or are not soiled with blood or body fluids.

Handwashing should be performed frequently. The World Health Organization (WHO) has developed guidelines for handwashing called *My 5 Moments for Hand Hygiene*. The five essential times for handwashing include:

- Before touching a patient

- Before a clean or aseptic procedure

- After body fluid exposure or risk of exposure

- After touching a patient

- After touching the patient's surroundings

In addition, handwashing should be done:

- When you arrive at the facility and immediately before leaving the facility

- After contact with a patient's intact skin (for example, after taking a blood pressure)

- Before moving from a contaminated body site to a clean body site during patient care (for example, before washing the patient's hands after removing a bedpan)

- Any time the hands become contaminated during a procedure

- Before applying and immediately after removing gloves
- Any time gloves are torn or punctured
- Before and after handling any specimen
- After contact with any soiled or contaminated item
- After picking up any item off the floor
- After personal use of the bathroom
- After you cough, sneeze, or use a tissue
- Before and after any contact with your mouth or mucous membranes, such as eating, drinking, smoking, applying lip balm, or inserting or removing contact lenses

The recommended method for handwashing is based on the following principles; they should be observed whenever hands are washed:

- Soap is used as a cleansing agent because it aids in the removal of germs through its sudsy action and alkali content. Pathogens are trapped in the soapsuds and rinsed away. Liquid soap from a dispenser should be used whenever possible because bar soap can contain microorganisms.
- Warm water should be used. This is less damaging to the skin than hot water. It also creates a better lather with soap than does cold water.
- Friction must be used in addition to soap and water. This action helps rub off pathogens from the surface of the skin.
- All surfaces on the hands must be cleaned. This includes the palms, the backs/tops of the hands, and the areas between the fingers.
- Fingertips must be pointed downward. The downward direction prevents water from getting on the forearms and then running down to contaminate the clean hands.
- Dry paper towels must be used to turn the faucet on and off. This action prevents contamination of the hands from pathogens on the faucet. A dry towel must be used because pathogens can travel more readily through a wet towel.

Nails also harbor dirt and pathogens, and must be cleaned during the handwashing process. An orange/cuticle stick can be used. Care must be taken to use the blunt end of the stick because the pointed end can injure the nailbeds. A brush can also be used to clean the nails. If a brush or orange stick is not available or the nails are not visibly dirty, the nails can be rubbed against the palm of the opposite hand to get soap under the nails. Most health care facilities prohibit the use of artificial nails or extenders and require that nails be kept short, usually less than ¼-inch long. Artificial or long nails can harbor organisms and increase the risk for infection for both the patient and health care provider. In addition, long nails can puncture or tear gloves.

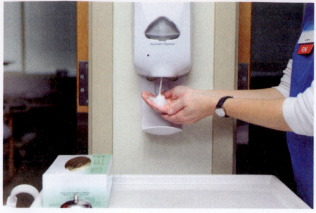

FIGURE 15–14 Waterless handwashing using an alcohol-based hand cleaner is an effective way to clean hands that are not visibly soiled.
© iStock.com/Nancy Louie.

Waterless hand cleaning with an alcohol-based gel, lotion, or foam has been proved safe for use during routine patient care. Its use is recommended when the hands are not visibly dirty and are not contaminated with blood or body fluids (**Figure 15–14**). Most waterless hand cleaning products contain at least 60 to 90 percent alcohol to provide antisepsis and a moisturizer to prevent drying of the skin. It is important to read the manufacturer's instructions before using any product. Usually, a small amount of the alcohol-based cleaner is applied to the palm of the hands. The hands are then rubbed vigorously so the solution is applied to all surfaces of the hands, fingers, nails, and wrists. The hands should be rubbed until they are dry, usually at least 20 to 30 seconds. Most manufacturers recommend that the hands be washed with soap and water after 6–10 cleanings with the alcohol-based product. In addition, if the hands are visibly soiled, or if there has been contact with blood or body fluid, the hands must be washed with soap and water.

Many facilities conduct handwashing audits. Staff are evaluated by trained observers during the WHO's five moments for hand hygiene to ensure that hand-washing is done correctly and at the appropriate times. In addition, an ultraviolet black light and special lotion can be used to test how clean hands are. Any germs that remain will glow under the light.

Every health care facility has written policies for hand hygiene as a part of their standard precautions manual. Health care team members must become familiar with and follow these policies to prevent the spread of infection.

checkpoint

1. What item is used to turn the water faucet on and off?
2. What is the single most important method used to practice aseptic technique?

PRACTICE: Go to the workbook and complete the assignment sheet for 15:3, Washing Hands. Then return and continue with the procedure.

Washing Hands

Equipment and Supplies

Paper towels, running water, waste container, hand brush or orange/cuticle stick, soap

Procedure

1. Assemble all equipment. Stand back slightly from the sink so you do not contaminate your uniform or clothing. Avoid touching the inside of the sink with your hands as it is considered contaminated. Remove any rings and push your wristwatch up above your wrist.

2. Turn the faucet on by holding a paper towel between your hand and the faucet (**Figure 15–15A**). Regulate the temperature of the water and let water flow over your hands. Discard the towel in the waste container.

   NOTE: Water should be warm.

   ⚠️ **Safety** **CAUTION:** Hot water will burn your hands.

3. With your fingertips pointing downward, wet your hands.

   NOTE: Washing in a downward direction prevents water from getting on your forearms and then running back down to contaminate your hands.

4. Use soap to create a lather on your hands.

5. Put the palms of your hands together and rub them using friction and a circular motion for at least 20 seconds.

6. Put the palm of one hand on the back of the other hand. Rub together several times. Repeat this after reversing the position of your hands (**Figure 15–15B**).

7. Interlace the fingers on both hands and rub them back and forth (**Figure 15–15C**).

8. Encircle your wrist with the palm and fingers of the opposite hand. Use a circular motion to clean the front, back, and sides of the wrist. Repeat for the opposite wrist.

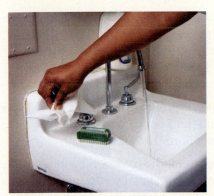

FIGURE 15–15A Use a dry towel to turn the faucet on.

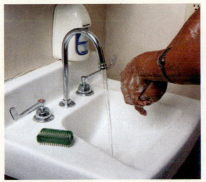

FIGURE 15–15B Point the fingertips downward and use the palm of one hand to clean the back of the other hand.

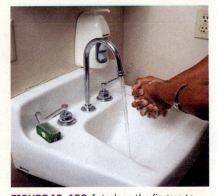

FIGURE 15–15C Interlace the fingers to clean between the fingers.

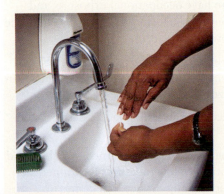

FIGURE 15–15D The blunt end of an orange stick can be used to clean the nails.

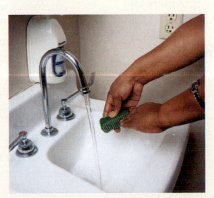

FIGURE 15–15E A hand brush can also be used to clean the nails.

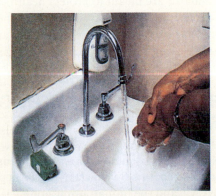

FIGURE 15–15F With the fingertips pointing downward, rinse the hands thoroughly.

(continues)

9. Clean the nails with an orange/cuticle stick or hand brush if they are visibly dirty or if this is the first hand cleaning of the day (**Figures 15–15D and E**). If the nails are not visibly dirty, they can be cleaned by rubbing them against the palm of the opposite hand.

 CAUTION: Use the blunt end of orange/cuticle stick to avoid injury.

NOTE: Steps 3 through 9 ensure that all parts of both hands are clean.

NOTE: Many health care facilities require washing the hands for 40–60 seconds (WHO recommendation is 40–60 seconds when visibly soiled). This is equivalent to singing the "Happy Birthday" song twice.

10. Rinse your hands from the forearms down to the fingertips, keeping fingertips pointed downward (**Figure 15–15F**).

11. Use a clean paper towel to dry hands thoroughly, from tips of fingers to wrist. Discard the towel in the waste container.

12. Use another dry paper towel to turn off the faucet.

 CAUTION: Wet towels allow passage of pathogens.

13. Discard all used towels in the waste container. Leave the area neat and clean.

14. Apply a water-based hand lotion if desired.

PRACTICE: Go to the workbook and use the evaluation sheet for 15:3, Washing Hands, to practice this procedure. When you believe you have mastered this skill, sign the sheet and give it to your instructor for further action.

✅ **FINAL EVALUATION:** Using the criteria listed on the evaluation sheet, your instructor will grade your performance.

15:4 OBSERVING STANDARD PRECAUTIONS

Precaution   OBRA

To prevent the spread of pathogens and disease, the chain of infection must be broken. In 1985, the Centers for Disease Control and Prevention (CDC) developed a set of common sense practices called standard precautions to prevent the spread of infection. The standards have been updated frequently. These standards are meant to protect health care providers and patients from disease transmission. The standard precautions discussed in this unit are an important way health care providers can break this chain.

BLOODBORNE PATHOGENS STANDARD

One of the main ways that pathogens are spread is by blood and body fluids. Three pathogens of major concern are the hepatitis B virus (HBV), the hepatitis C virus (HCV), and the human immunodeficiency virus (HIV), which causes AIDS. Consequently, extreme care must be taken at all times when an area, an object, or a person is contaminated with blood or body fluids. In 1991, the Occupational Safety and Health Administration (OSHA)

established *Bloodborne Pathogen Standards* that must be followed by all health care facilities. The employer faces civil penalties if the regulations are not implemented by the employer and followed by the employees. These regulations require all health care facility employers to:

- Develop a written exposure control plan, and update it annually, to minimize or eliminate employee exposure to bloodborne pathogens.

- Identify all employees who have occupational exposure to blood or potentially infectious materials such as semen, vaginal secretions, and other body fluids.

- Provide hepatitis B vaccine free of charge to all employees who have occupational exposure, and obtain a written release form signed by any employee who does not want the vaccine.

- Provide **personal protective equipment (PPE)** such as gloves, gowns, lab coats, masks, and face shields in appropriate sizes and in accessible locations.

- Provide adequate handwashing facilities and supplies.

- Ensure that the worksite is maintained in a clean and sanitary condition, follow measures for immediate decontamination of any surface that comes in contact with blood or infectious materials, and dispose of infectious waste correctly.

- Enforce rules of no eating, drinking, smoking, applying cosmetics or lip balm, handling contact lenses, and mouth pipetting or suctioning in any area that can be potentially contaminated by blood or other body fluids.

- Provide appropriate containers that are color coded (fluorescent orange or orange-red) and labeled for contaminated sharps (needles, scalpels) and other infectious or biohazard wastes.

- Post signs at the entrance to work areas where there is occupational exposure to biohazardous materials. Label any item that is biohazardous with the red biohazard symbol (**Figure 15–16**). The label must show both the symbol and the word "biohazard."

- Provide a confidential medical evaluation and follow-up for any employee who has an exposure incident. Examples might include an accidental needlestick or the splashing of blood or body fluids on the skin, eyes, or mucous membranes.

- Provide training about the regulations and all potential biohazards to all employees at no cost during working hours, and provide additional education as needed when procedures or working conditions are changed or modified.

In 2014, the CDC established more stringent precautions because of an outbreak of Ebola in West Africa. These requirements are discussed in detail in Section 15:9 of this text.

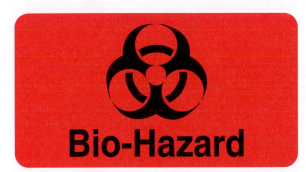

FIGURE 15–16 The universal biohazard symbol indicates a potential source of infection.

NEEDLESTICK SAFETY ACT

In 2001, OSHA revised its Bloodborne Pathogen Standards in response to Congress passing the *Needlestick Safety and Prevention Act* in November 2000. This act was passed after the Centers for Disease Control and Prevention (CDC) estimated that 600,000 to 800,000 needlesticks occur each year, exposing health care workers to bloodborne pathogens. Employers are required to:

- **Identify and use effective and safer medical devices**. OSHA defines safer devices as sharps with engineered injury protections, and includes,

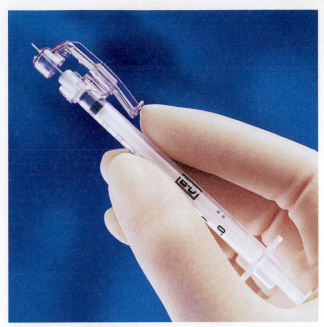

FIGURE 15–17 The Safety-Glide syringe is one example of a safer device to prevent needlesticks. Photo reprinted courtesy of BD [Becton, Dickinson and Company].

but is not limited to, devices such as syringes with a sliding sheath that shields the needle after use, needles that retract into a syringe after use, shielded or retracting catheters that can be used to administer intravenous medications or fluids, and intravenous systems that administer medication or fluids through a catheter port or connector site using a needle housed in a protective covering (**Figure 15–17**). OSHA also encourages the use of needleless systems, which include, but are not limited to, intravenous medication delivery systems that administer medication or fluids through a catheter port or connector site using a blunt cannula or other non-needle connection, and jet injection systems that deliver subcutaneous or intramuscular injections through the skin without using a needle.

- **Incorporate changes in annual updates of the exposure control plan**. Employers must include changes in technology that eliminate or reduce exposure to bloodborne pathogens in the annual update and document the implementation of any safer medical devices.

- **Solicit input from nonmanagerial employees who are responsible for direct patient care**. Employees who provide patient care and are exposed to injuries from contaminated sharps must be included in a multidisciplinary team that identifies, evaluates, and selects safer medical devices, and determines safer work practice controls.

- **Maintain a sharps injury log**. Employers with more than 11 employees must maintain a sharps injury log to help identify high-risk areas and evaluate ways to decrease injuries. Each injury recorded must protect the confidentiality of the injured employee but must state the type and brand of device involved in the incident, the work area or department where the exposure injury occurred, and a description of how the incident occurred.

STANDARD PRECAUTIONS

Employers are also required to make sure that every employee uses standard precautions at all times to prevent contact with blood or other potentially infectious materials. **Standard precautions** (**Figure 15–18**) are rules developed by the CDC to prevent the spread of infection.

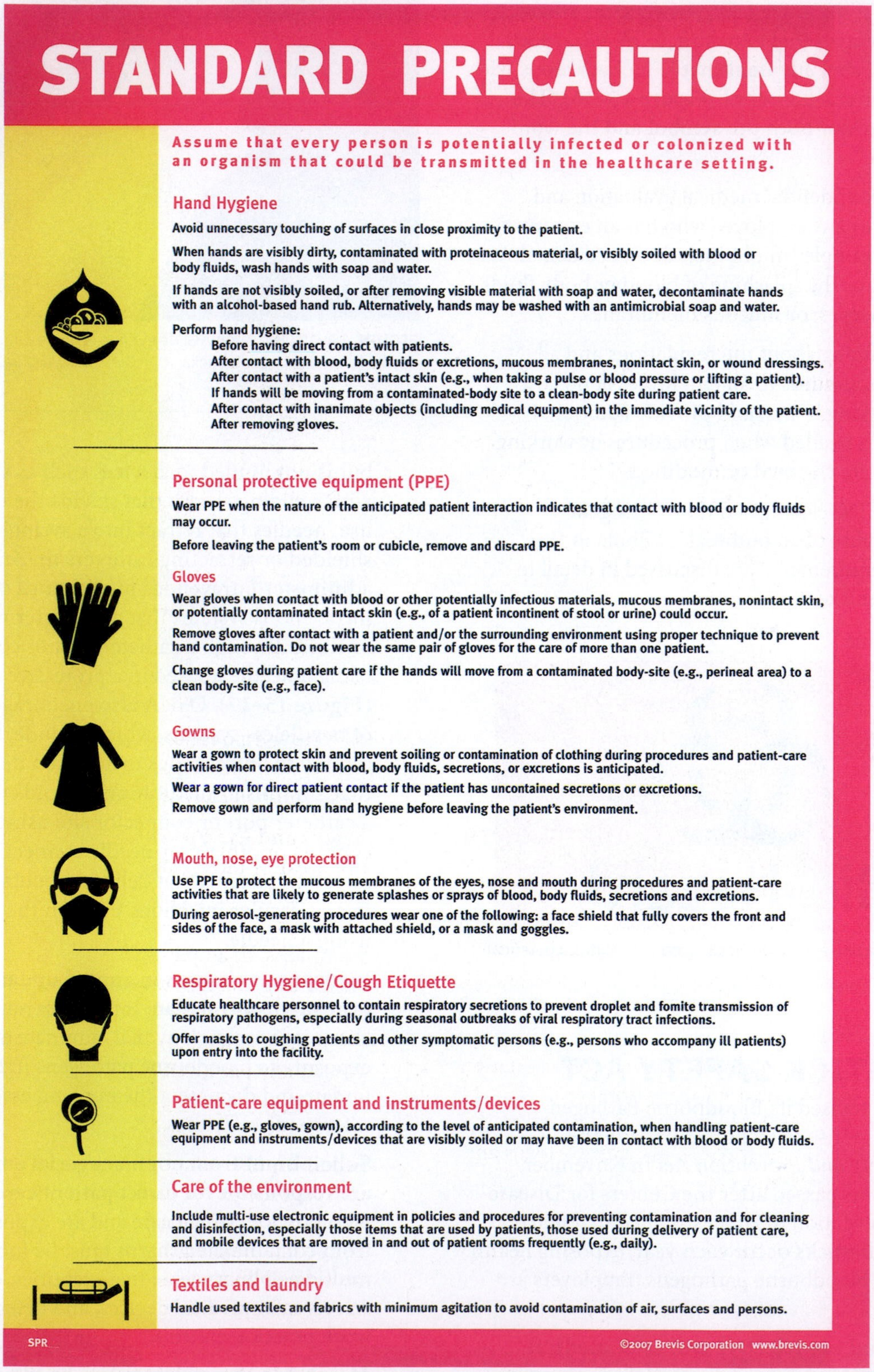

STANDARD PRECAUTIONS

Assume that every person is potentially infected or colonized with an organism that could be transmitted in the healthcare setting.

Hand Hygiene

Avoid unnecessary touching of surfaces in close proximity to the patient.

When hands are visibly dirty, contaminated with proteinaceous material, or visibly soiled with blood or body fluids, wash hands with soap and water.

If hands are not visibly soiled, or after removing visible material with soap and water, decontaminate hands with an alcohol-based hand rub. Alternatively, hands may be washed with an antimicrobial soap and water.

Perform hand hygiene:
    Before having direct contact with patients.
    After contact with blood, body fluids or excretions, mucous membranes, nonintact skin, or wound dressings.
    After contact with a patient's intact skin (e.g., when taking a pulse or blood pressure or lifting a patient).
    If hands will be moving from a contaminated-body site to a clean-body site during patient care.
    After contact with inanimate objects (including medical equipment) in the immediate vicinity of the patient.
    After removing gloves.

Personal protective equipment (PPE)

Wear PPE when the nature of the anticipated patient interaction indicates that contact with blood or body fluids may occur.

Before leaving the patient's room or cubicle, remove and discard PPE.

Gloves

Wear gloves when contact with blood or other potentially infectious materials, mucous membranes, nonintact skin, or potentially contaminated intact skin (e.g., of a patient incontinent of stool or urine) could occur.

Remove gloves after contact with a patient and/or the surrounding environment using proper technique to prevent hand contamination. Do not wear the same pair of gloves for the care of more than one patient.

Change gloves during patient care if the hands will move from a contaminated body-site (e.g., perineal area) to a clean body-site (e.g., face).

Gowns

Wear a gown to protect skin and prevent soiling or contamination of clothing during procedures and patient-care activities when contact with blood, body fluids, secretions, or excretions is anticipated.

Wear a gown for direct patient contact if the patient has uncontained secretions or excretions.

Remove gown and perform hand hygiene before leaving the patient's environment.

Mouth, nose, eye protection

Use PPE to protect the mucous membranes of the eyes, nose and mouth during procedures and patient-care activities that are likely to generate splashes or sprays of blood, body fluids, secretions and excretions.

During aerosol-generating procedures wear one of the following: a face shield that fully covers the front and sides of the face, a mask with attached shield, or a mask and goggles.

Respiratory Hygiene/Cough Etiquette

Educate healthcare personnel to contain respiratory secretions to prevent droplet and fomite transmission of respiratory pathogens, especially during seasonal outbreaks of viral respiratory tract infections.

Offer masks to coughing patients and other symptomatic persons (e.g., persons who accompany ill patients) upon entry into the facility.

Patient-care equipment and instruments/devices

Wear PPE (e.g., gloves, gown), according to the level of anticipated contamination, when handling patient-care equipment and instruments/devices that are visibly soiled or may have been in contact with blood or body fluids.

Care of the environment

Include multi-use electronic equipment in policies and procedures for preventing contamination and for cleaning and disinfection, especially those items that are used by patients, those used during delivery of patient care, and mobile devices that are moved in and out of patient rooms frequently (e.g., daily).

Textiles and laundry

Handle used textiles and fabrics with minimum agitation to avoid contamination of air, surfaces and persons.

SPR

©2007 Brevis Corporation www.brevis.com

FIGURE 15–18 Standard precautions must be observed while working with all patients. Reprinted with Permission from Brevis Corporation [www.brevis.com].

According to standard precautions, every body fluid must be considered a potentially infectious material, and all patients must be considered potential sources of infection, regardless of their disease or diagnosis.

Standard precautions must be used in any situation where health care providers may contact:

- Blood or any fluid that may contain blood
- Body fluids, secretions, and excretions, such as mucus, sputum, saliva, cerebrospinal fluid, urine, feces, vomitus, amniotic fluid (surrounding a fetus), synovial (joint) fluid, pleural (lung) fluid, pericardial (heart) fluid, peritoneal (abdominal cavity) fluid, semen, and vaginal secretions
- Mucous membranes
- Nonintact skin
- Tissue or cell specimens

The basic rules of standard precautions include:

- **Handwashing**: Hands must be washed before and after contact with any patient. If hands or other skin surfaces are contaminated with blood, body fluids, secretions, or excretions, they must be washed immediately and thoroughly with soap and water. If hands are not visibly soiled, an alcohol-based hand cleaner can be used. Hands must always be washed immediately before donning and immediately after removing gloves.

- **Gloves**: Gloves (**Figure 15–19**) must be worn whenever contact with blood, body fluids, secretions, excretions, mucous membranes, tissue specimens, or nonintact skin is possible; when handling or cleaning any contaminated items or surfaces; when performing any invasive (entering the body) procedure; and when performing venipuncture or blood tests. Rings must be removed before putting on gloves to avoid puncturing the gloves. Gloves must be changed after contact with each patient and even between tasks or procedures on the same patient if there is any chance the gloves are contaminated. Gloves should not be worn out of patient rooms or care areas. Hands must be washed immediately after gloves are removed. Care must be taken while removing gloves to avoid contamination of the skin. Gloves must *not* be washed or disinfected for reuse because washing may allow penetration of liquids through undetected holes and disinfecting agents may cause deterioration of the gloves.

- **Gowns**: Gowns must be worn during any procedure that may cause splashing or spraying of blood, body fluids, secretions, or excretions. This helps prevent contamination of clothing or uniforms. Contaminated gowns must be handled according to agency policy and local and state laws. Gowns should

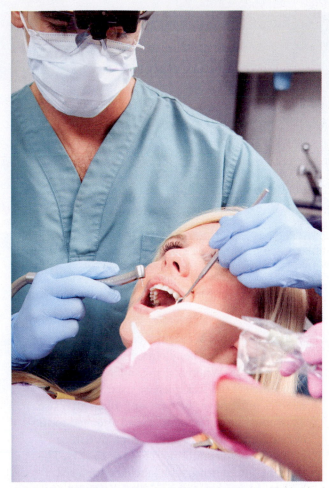

FIGURE 15–19 Gloves must be worn whenever contact with blood, body fluids, secretions, excretions, mucous membranes, or nonintact skin is possible. © Tyler Olson/Shutterstock.com.

only be worn once and then discarded. Gowns should not be worn out of patient rooms or care areas. Wash hands immediately after removing a gown.

- **Masks and Eye Protection**: Masks and protective eye-wear or face shields (**Figure 15–20**) must be worn during procedures that may produce splashes or sprays of blood, body fluids, secretions, or excretions. Examples include irrigation of wounds, suctioning, dental procedures, delivery of a baby, and surgical procedures. This prevents exposure of the mucous membranes of the mouth, nose, and eyes to any pathogens.

Masks must be used once and then discarded. In addition, masks should be changed anytime they become moist or wet. They should be removed by grasping the ties or elastic strap. Mask should not be worn out of patient rooms or care areas and should not be left dangling around the neck. Hands must be washed immediately after the mask is removed. Protective eyewear or face shields should provide protection for the front, top, bottom, and sides of the eyes. If eyewear is not disposable, it must be cleaned and disinfected before it is reused.

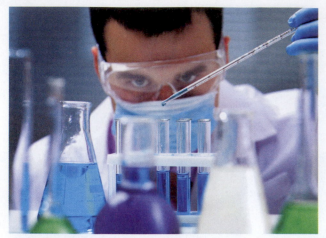

FIGURE 15–20 Gloves, a gown, a mask, and protective eyewear must be worn during any procedure that may produce droplets or cause splashing of blood, body fluids, secretions, or excretions. © YanLev/Shutterstock.com

- **Sharps**: To avoid accidental cuts or punctures, extreme care must be taken while handling sharp objects. Whenever possible, safe needles or needleless devices must be used. Disposable needles must never be bent or broken after use. They must be left uncapped and attached to the syringe and placed in a leakproof, puncture-resistant sharps container (**Figure 15–21**). The sharps container must be labeled with a red biohazard symbol. Surgical blades, razors, and other sharp objects must also be discarded in the sharps container.

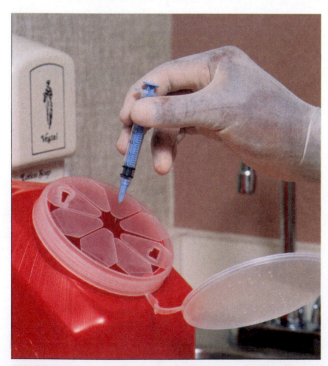

FIGURE 15–21 All needles and sharp objects must be discarded immediately in a leakproof, puncture-resistant sharps container.

Legal

The sharps containers must *not* be emptied or reused. Federal, state, and local laws establish regulations for the disposal of sharps containers.

- **Spills or Splashes**: Spills or splashes of blood, body fluids, secretions, or excretions must be wiped up immediately. Gloves must be worn while wiping up the area with disposable cleaning cloths. The area must then be cleaned with a disinfectant solution such as a 10 percent bleach solution. Furniture or equipment contaminated by the spill or splash must be cleaned and disinfected immediately. For large spills, an absorbent powder may be used to soak up the fluid. After the fluid is absorbed, the powder is swept up and placed in an infectious waste container (**Figure 15–22**).

- **Resuscitation Devices**: Mouthpieces or resuscitation devices should be used to avoid mouth-to-mouth resuscitation. These devices should be placed in convenient locations and be readily accessible for use. If these devices are not disposable, they must be disinfected between patient use.

- **Waste and Linen Disposal**: Health care providers must wear gloves and follow the agency policy

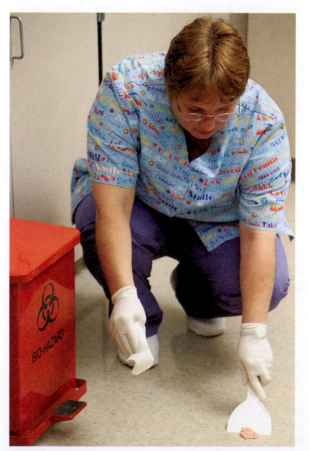

FIGURE 15–22 An absorbent powder may be used to soak up a spill of blood, body fluids, secretions, or excretions. Gloves must be worn while picking up the solidified spill.

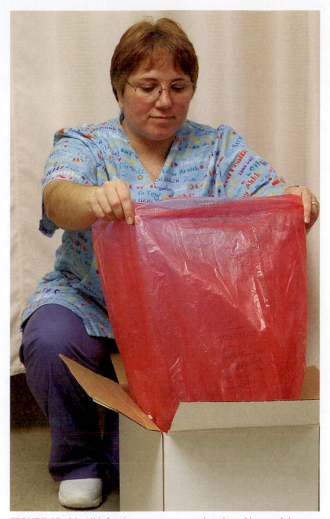

FIGURE 15–23 All infectious wastes must be placed in special infectious waste or biohazardous material bags.

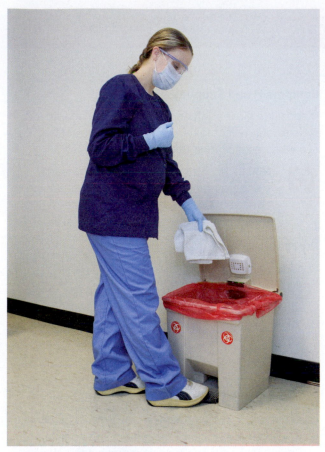

FIGURE 15–24 The health care worker must know the requirements for disposal of waste materials and dispose of wastes in the proper containers.

developed according to law to dispose of waste and soiled linen. Infectious wastes such as contaminated dressings; gloves; urinary drainage bags; incontinence pads; vaginal pads; disposable emesis basins, bedpans, and urinals; and body tissues must be placed in special infectious waste or biohazardous material bags (**Figure 15–23**) according to law. Other trash is frequently placed in plastic bags and incinerated. The health care team member must dispose of waste in the proper container (**Figure 15–24**) and know the requirements for disposal. Soiled linen should be placed in laundry bags to prevent any contamination. Linen soiled with blood, body fluids, or excretions is placed in a special bag for contaminated linen and is usually soaked in a disinfectant before being laundered. Gloves must be worn while handling any contaminated linen, and any bag containing contaminated linen must be clearly labeled and color coded.

- **Injuries**: Any cut, injury, needlestick, or splashing of blood or body fluids must be reported immediately. Agency policy must be followed to deal with the

injury or contamination. Every health care facility must have a policy stating actions that must be taken immediately when exposure or injury occurs, including reporting any injury, documenting any exposure incident, recording the care given, noting follow-up to the exposure incident, and identifying ways to prevent a similar incident.

Standard precautions must be followed at all times by all health care team members. By observing these precautions, health care providers can help break the chain of infection and protect themselves, their patients, and all other individuals.

checkpoint

1. What are the three (3) pathogens of major concern that the Bloodborne Pathogens Standard addresses?

2. What government agency developed the standard precautions rules?

PRACTICE: Go to the workbook and complete the assignment sheet for 15:4, Observing Standard Precautions. Then return and continue with the procedure.

Observing Standard Precautions

Equipment and Supplies

Disposable gloves, infectious waste bags, needle and syringe, sharps container, gown, masks, protective eyewear, resuscitation devices

Precaution

NOTE: This procedure will help you learn standard precautions. It is important for you to observe these precautions at all times while working in the laboratory or clinical area.

Procedure

1. Assemble equipment.

2. Review the precautions in the information section for Observing Standard Precautions. Note points that are not clear, and ask your instructor for an explanation.

3. Practice handwashing according to Procedure 15:3. Identify at least six times that hands must be washed according to standard precautions.

4. Name four instances when gloves must be worn to observe standard precautions. Put on a pair of disposable gloves. Practice removing the gloves without contaminating the skin. With a gloved hand, grasp the cuff of the glove on the opposite hand, handling only the outside of the glove (**Figure 15–25A**). Pull the glove down and turn it inside out while removing it (**Figure 15–25B**). Take care not to touch the skin with the gloved hand. Grasp the contaminated glove in the palm of the gloved hand (**Figure 15–25C**). Using the ungloved hand, slip the fingers under the cuff of the glove on the opposite hand (**Figure 15–25D**). Touching only the inside of the glove and taking care not to touch the skin, pull the glove down and turn it inside out while removing it (**Figure 15–25E**). Place the gloves in an infectious waste container (**Figure 15–25F**). Wash your hands immediately.

5. Practice putting on a gown. State when a gown is to be worn. To remove the gown, touch only the inside. Fold the contaminated gown so the outside is folded inward. Roll it into a bundle and place it in an infectious waste container if it is disposable, or in a bag for contaminated linen if it is not disposable.

Safety

CAUTION: If a gown is contaminated, gloves should be worn while removing the gown.

NOTE: Folding the gown and rolling it prevents transmission of pathogens.

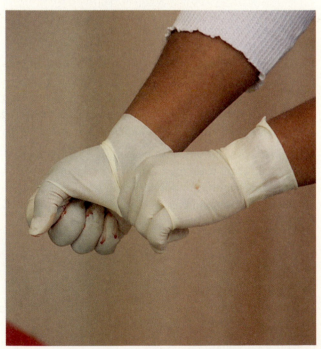

FIGURE 15–25A To remove the first glove, use a gloved hand to grasp the outside of the glove on the opposite hand.

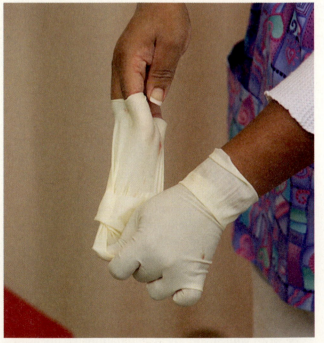

FIGURE 15–25B Pull the glove down and turn it inside out while removing it.

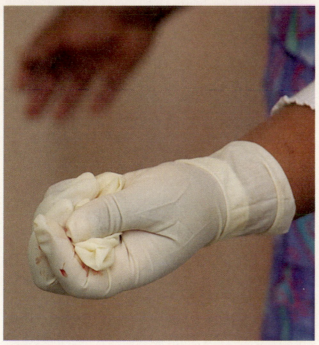

FIGURE 15–25C Grasp the contaminated glove in the palm of the gloved hand.

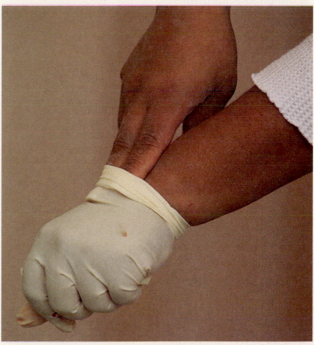

FIGURE 15–25D To remove the second glove, slip the fingers of the ungloved hand inside the cuff of the glove.

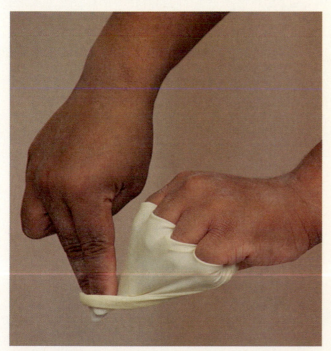

FIGURE 15–25E Touch only the inside of the glove while pulling it down and turning it inside out.

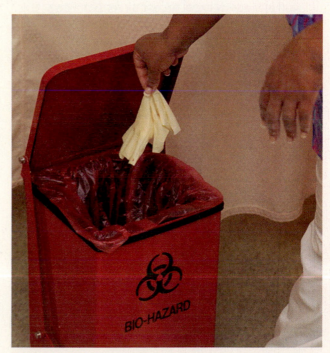

FIGURE 15–25F Place the gloves in an infectious waste container and wash your hands immediately.

(continues)

6. Practice putting on a mask and protective eyewear. To remove the mask, handle it by the ties only. Clean and disinfect protective eyewear after use if it is not disposable.

7. Practice proper disposal of sharps. Uncap a needle attached to a syringe, taking care not to stick yourself with the needle. Place the entire needle and syringe in a sharps container. Never recap a needle. State the rules regarding disposal of the sharps container.

8. Spill a small amount of water on a counter. Pretend that it is blood. Put on gloves and use disposable cloths or gauze to wipe up the spill. Put the contaminated cloths or gauze in an infectious waste bag. Use clean disposable cloths or gauze to wipe the area thoroughly with a disinfectant agent (**Figure 15–26**). Put the cloths or gauze in the infectious waste bag, remove your gloves, and wash your hands.

9. Practice handling an infectious waste bag. Fold down the top edge of the bag to form a cuff at the top of the bag. Wear gloves to close the bag after contaminated wastes have been placed in it. Put your hands under the folded cuff and gently expel excess air from the bag. Twist the top of the bag shut and fold down the top edges to seal the bag. Secure the fold with tape or a tie according to agency policy (**Figure 15–27**).

10. Examine mouthpieces and resuscitation devices that are used for resuscitation. You will

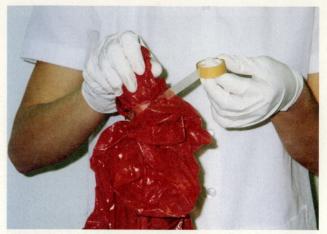

FIGURE 15–27 After folding down the top edge of the infectious waste bag, tie or tape it securely.

be taught to use these devices when you learn cardiopulmonary resuscitation (CPR).

11. Discuss the following situations with another student and determine which standard precautions should be observed:

- A patient has an open sore on the skin and pus is seeping from the area. You are going to bathe the patient.

- You are cleaning a tray of instruments that contains a disposable surgical blade and a needle with syringe.

- A tube of blood drops to the floor and breaks, spilling the blood on the floor.

- Drainage from dressings on an infected wound has soiled the linen on the bed you are changing.

- You work in a dental office and are assisting a dentist while a tooth is being extracted (removed).

12. Replace all equipment used. Wash hands.

PRACTICE: Go to the workbook and use the evaluation sheet for 15:4, Observing Standard Precautions. When you believe you have mastered this skill, sign the sheet and give it to your instructor for further action.

 FINAL EVALUATION: Using the criteria listed on the evaluation sheet, your instructor will grade your performance.

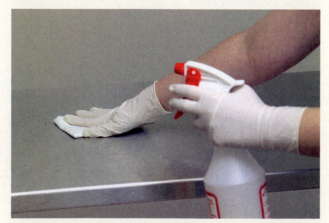

FIGURE 15–26 Wear gloves to spray the contaminated counter with a disinfectant. Then wipe the counter clean with a disposable cloth or gauze.

15:5 STERILIZING WITH AN AUTOCLAVE

Sterilization of instruments and equipment is essential in preventing the spread of infection. In any of the health care fields, you may be responsible for proper sterilization. The following basic principles relate to sterilization methods. The autoclave is the safest, most efficient sterilization method.

An **autoclave** is a piece of equipment that uses steam under pressure or gas to sterilize equipment and supplies (**Figure 15–28**). It is the most efficient method of sterilizing most articles, and it will destroy all microorganisms, both pathogenic and nonpathogenic, including spores and viruses.

Autoclaves are available in various sizes and types. Offices and health clinics usually have smaller units, and hospitals or surgical areas have large floor models. A pressure cooker can be used in home situations.

Before any equipment or supplies are sterilized in an autoclave, they must be prepared properly. All items must be washed thoroughly and then rinsed. Oily substances can often be removed with alcohol or ether. Any residue left on articles will tend to bake and stick to the article during the autoclaving process.

Items that are to remain sterile must be wrapped before they are autoclaved. A wide variety of wraps are available. The wrap must be a material that will allow for the penetration of steam during the autoclaving process. Samples of wraps include muslin, autoclave paper, special plastic or paper bags, and autoclave containers (**Figure 15–29**).

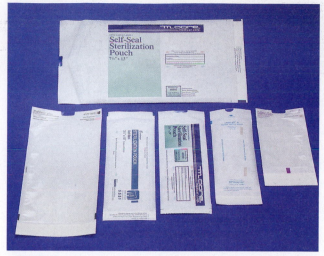

FIGURE 15–29 Special plastic or paper autoclave bags can be used to sterilize instruments.

Autoclave indicators are used to ensure that articles have been sterilized (**Figure 15–30A and B**). Examples of indicators include autoclave tape, sensitivity marks on bags or wraps, and indicator capsules. The indicator is usually placed on or near the article when the article is put into the autoclave. Indicators can also be placed in the center of a package, such as a tray of instruments, to show that sterilization of the entire package has occurred. The indicator will change appearance during the autoclaving process because of the length of time and the temperature, which lead to sterilization. Learn how to recognize that an article is sterile by reading the directions provided with indicators.

The autoclave must be loaded correctly for all parts of an article to be sterilized. Steam builds at the top of the chamber and moves downward. As it moves down, it pushes cool, dry air out of the bottom of the chamber. Therefore, materials must be placed so the steam can penetrate along the natural planes between the packages of articles in the autoclave. Place the articles in such a way that there is space between all pieces. Packages should be placed on the sides, not flat. Jars, basins, and cans should be placed on their sides, not flat, so that steam can enter and air can flow out. No articles should come in contact with the sides, top, or door of the autoclave.

The length of time and amount of pressure required to sterilize different items varies (**Figure 15–31**). *It is important to check the directions that come with the autoclave.* Because different types of articles require different times and pressures, it is important to separate loads so that all articles sterilized at one time require the same time and pressure. For example, rubber tubings usually require a relatively short time and can be damaged by long exposure. Certain instruments and needles

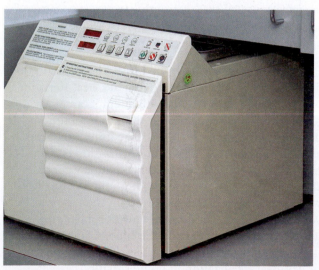

FIGURE 15–28 An autoclave uses steam under pressure to sterilize items.

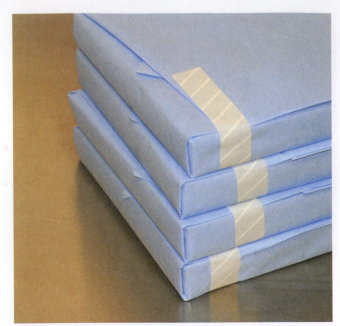

FIGURE 15–30A Autoclave indicators change color to show that sterilization has occurred. This photo shows before sterilization. Courtesy, SPSmedical Supply Corp.

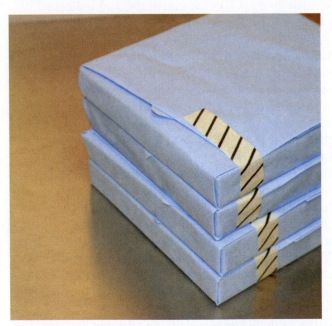

FIGURE 15–30B This photo shows after sterilization. Courtesy, SPSmedical Supply Corp.

Articles	Time at 250° to 254°F (121° to 123°C)
Glassware: empty, inverted	15 minutes
Instruments: metal in covered or open, padded or unpadded tray	
Needles, unwrapped	
Syringes: unassembled, unwrapped	
Instruments, metal combined with other materials in covered and/or padded tray	
Instruments wrapped in double-thickness muslin	20 minutes
Flasked solutions, 75–250 mL	
Rubber products: gloves, catheters, and tubings	
Syringes: unassembled, individually packed in muslin or paper	30 minutes
Needles, individually packaged in glass tubes or paper	
Dressings wrapped in paper or muslin (small packs only)	
Flasked solutions, 500–1,000 mL	
Sutures: silk, cotton, or nylon; wrapped in paper or muslin	
Treatment trays wrapped in muslin or paper	

FIGURE 15–31 The length of time required to sterilize different items varies.

require a longer time to ensure sterilization; therefore, items of this type should not be sterilized in the same load as rubber tubings.

Wet surfaces permit rapid infiltration of organisms, so it is important that all items are thoroughly dry before being removed from the autoclave. The length of drying time varies. Follow the manufacturer's instructions.

Sterilized items must be stored in clean, dustproof areas. Items usually remain sterile for 30 days after autoclaving. However, if the wraps loosen or tear, if they become wet, or if any chance of contamination occurs, the items should be rewrapped and autoclaved again.

NOTE: *At the end of the 30-day sterile period—providing that the wrap has not loosened, been torn, or gotten wet—remove the old autoclave tape from the package, replace with a new, dated tape, and resterilize according to correct procedure.*

Some autoclaves are equipped with a special door that allows the autoclave to be used as a dry-heat sterilizer. Dry heat involves the use of a high temperature for a long period. The temperature is usually a minimum of 320°F–350°F (160°C–177°C). The minimum time is usually 60 minutes. Dry-heat sterilization is a good method for sterilizing instruments that may corrode, such as knife blades, or items that would be destroyed by the moisture in steam sterilization, such as powders. Dry heat should never be used on soft rubber goods because the heat will destroy the rubber. Some types of plastic will also melt in dry heat. An oven can be used for dry-heat sterilization in home situations.

Procedures 15:5A and 15:5B describe wrapping articles for autoclaving and autoclaving techniques. These procedures may vary in different agencies and areas, but the same principles apply. In some facilities, many supplies are purchased as sterile, disposable items; needles and syringes are purchased in sterilized wraps, used once, and then destroyed. In other facilities, however, special treatment trays are sterilized and used more than once.

It is important that you follow the directions specific to the autoclave with which you are working as well as the agency policy for sterile supplies. Careless autoclaving permits the transmission of disease-producing organisms. Infection control is everyone's responsibility.

checkpoint

1. What are autoclave tape, sensitivity marks on bags, and indicator capsules used to indicate?

2. How long is a sterilized item to be stored?

PRACTICE: Go to the workbook and complete the assignment sheet for 15:5, Sterilizing with an Autoclave. Then return and continue with the procedures.

Procedure 15:5A

Wrapping Items for Autoclaving

Equipment and Supplies

Items to wrap: instrument, towel, bowl; autoclave wrap: paper, muslin, plastic or paper bag; autoclave tape or indicator; disposable or utility gloves; pen or autoclave marker; masking tape (if autoclave tape is not used)

Procedure

1. Assemble equipment.

2. Wash hands. Put on gloves.

   CAUTION: If the items to be autoclaved may be contaminated with blood, body fluids, or tissues, gloves must be worn while cleaning the items.

3. Sanitize the items to be sterilized. Instruments, bowls, and similar items should be cleaned thoroughly in soapy water (**Figure 15–32**). Rinse the items well in cool water to remove any soapy residue. Then rinse well with hot water. Dry the items with a towel. After the items are sanitized and dry, remove the gloves and wash hands.

   NOTE: If stubborn stains are present, it may be necessary to soak the items.

   NOTE: Check the teeth on serrated (notched like a saw) instruments. Scrub with a brush as necessary.

4. To prepare linen for wrapping, check first to make sure it is clean and dry. Fold the linen in half lengthwise. If it is very wide, fold lengthwise again. Fanfold or accordion pleat the linen from end to end until a compact package is formed (**Figure 15–33A**). All folds should be the same size. Fold back one corner on the top fold (**Figure 15–33B**). This provides a piece to grab when opening the linen.

   NOTE: Fanfolding linens allows for easy handling after sterilization.

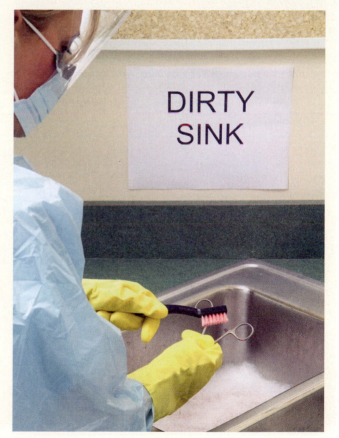

FIGURE 15–32 Wear gloves to scrub instruments thoroughly with soapy water.

5. Select the correct wrap for the item. Make sure the wrap is large enough to enclose the item to be wrapped.

   NOTE: Double-thickness muslin, disposable paper wraps, and plastic or paper bags are the most common wraps.

(continues)

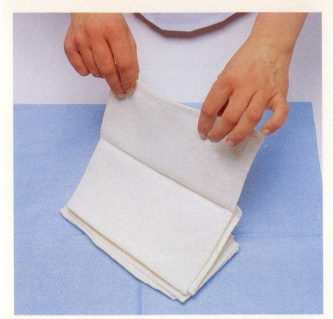

FIGURE 15–33A Fanfold clean, dry linen so all the folds are the same size.

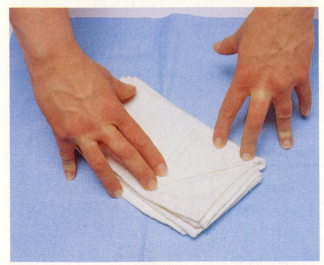

FIGURE 15–33B Fold back one corner on the top fold of the linen.

6. With the wrap positioned at a diagonal angle and one corner pointing toward you, place the item to be sterilized in the center of the wrap (**Figure 15–34A**)

   NOTE: Make sure that hinged instruments are open so the steam can sterilize all edges.

7. Fold up the bottom corner to the center (**Figure 15–34B**). Double back a small corner (**Figure 15–34C**).

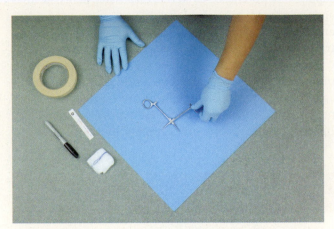

FIGURE 15–34A Place the instrument in the center of the wrap.

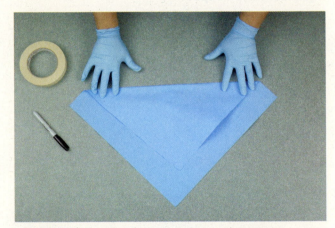

FIGURE 15–34B Fold up the bottom corner to the center.

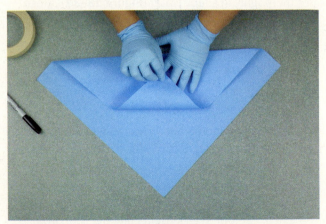

FIGURE 15–34C Turn a small corner back to form a tab.

8. Fold a side corner over to the center. Make sure the edges are sealed and that there are no air pockets. Bring back a small corner (**Figure 15–34D**).

    CAUTION: Any open areas at corners will allow pathogens to enter.
   Safety

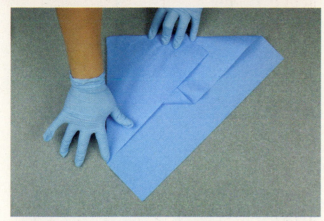

FIGURE 15–34D Fold in one side to the center.

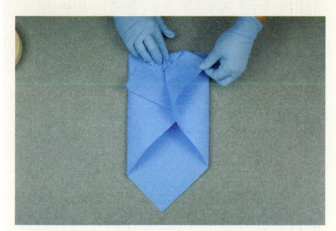

FIGURE 15–34E Fold in the opposite side and fold back a tab.

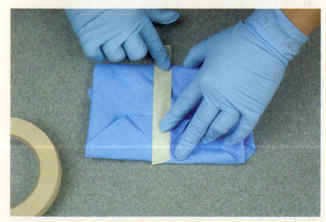

FIGURE 15–34F Secure the package with pressure-sensitive autoclave tape.

9. Fold in the other side corner. Again, watch for and avoid open edges. Bring back a small corner (**Figure 15–34E**).

10. Bring the final corner up and over the top of the package. Check the two edges to be sure they are sealed and tight. Tuck this under the pocket created by the previous folds. Leave a small corner exposed so it can be used when unwrapping the package.

   NOTE: This is frequently called an "envelope" wrap, because the final corner is tucked into the wrap similar to the way the flap is tucked into an envelope.

11. Secure with autoclave or pressure-sensitive indicator tape (**Figure 15–34F**).

   NOTE: If regular masking tape is used, attach an autoclave indicator to reflect when contents are sterilized.

12. Label the package by marking the tape with the date and contents. Some health care agencies may require you to initial the label.

   NOTE: For certain items, the type or size of item should be noted, for example, curved hemostat or mosquito hemostat, hand towel or bath towel, small bowl or large bowl.

   NOTE: Contents will not be sterile after 30 days, so the date of sterilization must be noted on the package.

13. Check the package. It should be firm enough for handling but loose enough for proper circulation of steam.

14. To use a plastic or paper autoclave bag (refer to Figure 15–29), select or cut the correct size for the item to be sterilized. Place the clean item inside the bag. Double fold the open end(s) and tape or secure with autoclave tape. Check the package to make sure it is secure.

   NOTE: In some agencies, the ends are sealed with heat before autoclaving.

   NOTE: If the bag has an autoclave indicator, regular masking tape can be used to seal the ends.

15. Replace all equipment used.

16. Wash hands.

PRACTICE: Go to the workbook and use the evaluation sheet for 15:5A, Wrapping Items for Autoclaving, to practice this procedure. When you believe you have mastered this skill, sign the sheet and give it to your instructor for further action.

FINAL EVALUATION: Using the criteria listed on the evaluation sheet, your instructor will grade your performance.

Loading and Operating an Autoclave

NOTE: Follow the operating instructions for your autoclave. The basic principles of loading apply to all autoclaves.

Equipment and Supplies

Autoclave, distilled water, small pitcher or measuring cup, items wrapped or prepared for autoclaving, time chart for autoclave, 15:5 information section

Procedure

Review the information section for 15:5, Sterilizing with an Autoclave. Then proceed with the following activities. You should read through the procedure first, checking against the diagram. Then practice with an autoclave.

1. Assemble equipment.

2. Wash and dry hands thoroughly.

3. Check the three-prong plug and the electrical cord. If either is damaged or prongs are missing, do not use the autoclave. If no problems are present, plug the cord into a wall outlet.

4. Use distilled water to fill the reservoir to within 2½ inches below the opening or to the level indicated on the autoclave.

    NOTE: Distilled water prevents the collection of mineral deposits and prolongs the life and effectiveness of the autoclave.

5. Check the pressure gauge to make sure it is at zero.

     CAUTION: Never open the door unless the pressure is zero.

6. Open the safety door by following the manufacturer's instructions. Some door handles require an upward and inward pressure; others require a side-pressure technique.

7. Load the autoclave. Make sure all articles have been prepared correctly. Check for autoclave indicators, secure wraps, and correct labels. Separate loads so all items require the same time, temperature, and pressure. Place packages on their sides. Place bowls or basins on their sides so air and steam can flow in and out of the containers (**Figure 15–35**). Make sure there is space between the packages so the steam can circulate.

    NOTE: Check to make sure no large packages block the steam flow to smaller packages. Place large packages on the bottom.

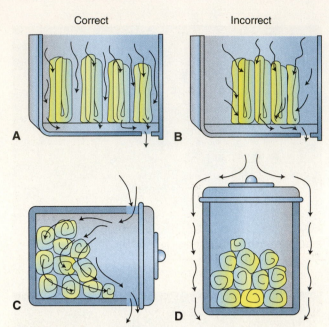

FIGURE 15–35 Packages should be placed on their sides and separated to allow steam to penetrate all sides of the packages: (A) correct placement; (B) incorrect placement. Bowls or basins should be placed on their sides so steam can flow in and out of the containers: (C) correct placement; (D) incorrect placement. Courtesy of STERIS Corporation.

 CAUTION: Make sure no item comes in contact with the sides, top, or door of the autoclave chamber.

8. Follow the instructions for filling the chamber with the correct amount of water. Most autoclaves have a "Fill" setting on the control. Allow water to enter the chamber until the water covers the fill plate inside the chamber.

9. When the correct amount of water is in the chamber, follow the instructions for stopping the flow of water. In many autoclaves, turning the control valve to "Sterilize" stops the flow of water from the reservoir.

10. Check the load in the chamber to be sure it is properly spaced. The chamber can also be loaded at this point, if this has not been done previously.

11. Close and lock the door.

     CAUTION: Be sure the door is securely locked; check by pulling slightly.

12. Read the time chart for the specific time and temperature required to sterilize the items that were placed in the autoclave.

13. After referring to the chart provided with the autoclave or reviewing Figure 15–31, set the control valves to allow the temperature and pressure to increase in the autoclave.

14. When the desired temperature (usually 250°F–254°F or 121°C–123°C) and pressure (usually 15 pounds) have been reached, set the controls to maintain the desired temperature during the sterilization process. Follow the manufacturer's instructions.

15. Based on the information in the time chart, set the timer to the correct time.

    NOTE: Many autoclaves require you to rotate the timer past 10 (minutes) before setting the time.

16. Check the pressure and temperature gauges at intervals to make sure they remain as originally set.

    NOTE: Most autoclaves automatically shut off when pressure reaches 35 pounds.

17. When the required time has passed, set the controls so the autoclave will vent the steam from the chamber.

18. Put on safety glasses.

     CAUTION: Never open the door without glasses. The escaping steam can burn the eyes.

19. Check the pressure and temperature gauges. When the pressure gauge is at zero, and the temperature gauge is at or below 212°F, open the door about ½ to 1 inch to permit thorough drying of the contents.

 CAUTION: Do not open the door until pressure is zero.

NOTE: Most autoclaves have a safety lock on the door that does not release until the pressure is at zero.

20. After the autoclaved items are completely dry, remove and store them in a dry, dust-free area.

     CAUTION: Handle supplies and equipment carefully. They may be hot.

21. If there are additional loads to run, leave the main valve in the vent position. This will keep the autoclave ready for immediate use.

22. If this is the final load, turn the autoclave off. Unplug the cord from the wall outlet; do not pull on the cord.

    NOTE: The autoclave must be cleaned on a regular basis. Follow manufacturer's instructions.

23. Replace all equipment used.

24. Wash hands.

PRACTICE: Go to the workbook and use the evaluation sheet for 15:5B, Loading and Operating an Autoclave, to practice this procedure. When you believe you have mastered this skill, sign the sheet and give it to your instructor for further action.

 FINAL EVALUATION: Using the criteria listed on the evaluation sheet, your instructor will grade your performance.

15:6 USING CHEMICALS FOR DISINFECTION

Many health care fields require the use of chemicals for aseptic control. Certain points that must be observed while using the chemicals are discussed in the following section.

Chemicals are frequently used for aseptic control. Many chemicals do not kill spores and viruses; therefore, chemicals are not a method of sterilization. Because sterilization does not occur, **chemical disinfection** is the appropriate term (rather than *cold sterilization*, a term sometimes used). A few chemicals will kill spores and viruses, but these chemicals frequently require that instruments be submerged in the chemical for 10 or more hours. It is essential to read the entire label to determine the effectiveness of a product before using any chemical.

Chemicals are used to disinfect instruments that do not penetrate body tissue. Many dental instruments, percussion hammers, scissors, and similar items are examples. In addition, chemicals are used to disinfect thermometers and other items that would be destroyed by the high heat used in the autoclave.

Proper cleaning of all instruments or articles is essential. Particles or debris on items may contaminate the chemicals and reduce their effectiveness. In addition, all items must be rinsed thoroughly because the presence of soap can also reduce the effectiveness of chemicals. The articles must be dry before being placed in the disinfectant to keep the chemical at its most effective strength.

Some chemical solutions used as disinfectants are 90 percent isopropyl alcohol, formaldehyde–alcohol, 2 percent phenolic germicide, 10 percent bleach (sodium hypochlorite) solution, glutaraldehyde, iodophor, Lysol, Cidex, and benzalkonium (Zephiran).

The manufacturer's directions should be read completely before using any solution. Some solutions must be diluted or mixed before use. The directions will also specify the recommended time for the most thorough disinfection.

Chemical solutions can cause rust to form on certain instruments, so antirust tablets or solutions are frequently added to the chemicals. Again, it is important to read the directions provided with the tablets or solution. If improperly used, antirust substances may cause a chemical reaction with a solution and reduce the effectiveness of the chemical disinfectant.

The container used for chemical disinfection must be large enough to accommodate the items. In addition, the items should be separate so each one will come in contact with the chemical. A tight-fitting lid must be placed on the container while the articles are in the solution to prevent evaporation, which could affect the strength of the solution. The lid also decreases the chance of dust or airborne particles falling into the solution.

The chemical disinfectant must completely cover the article. This is the only way to be sure that all parts of the article will be disinfected.

Before removing items from solutions, health care providers must wash their hands. Sterile gloves or sterile pick-ups or transfer forceps may be used to remove the instruments from the solution. The items should be rinsed with sterile water to remove any remaining chemical solution. After rinsing, the instruments are placed on a sterile or clean towel to dry, and then stored in a drawer or dust-free closet.

Solutions must be changed frequently. Some solutions can be used more than once, but others must be discarded after one use. Follow the manufacturer's instructions. However, if any time contamination occurs or dirt is present in the solution, discard it. A fresh solution must be used.

checkpoint

1. What kind of instruments are disinfected using chemicals?

PRACTICE: Go to the Workbook and complete the assignment sheet for 15:6, Using Chemicals for Disinfection. Then return and continue with the procedure.

Procedure 15:6

Using Chemicals for Disinfection

Equipment and Supplies

Chemicals, container with tight-fitting lid, basin, soap, water, instruments, brush, sterile pick-ups or transfer forceps, sterile towel, sterile gloves, eye protection, disposable gloves

Procedure

1. Assemble equipment.

2. Wash hands. Put on disposable or heavy-duty utility gloves and eye protection.

Precaution

NOTE: Wear gloves if any of the instruments or equipment may be contaminated with blood or body fluids. Wear eye protection if there is any chance splashing will occur.

3. Wash all instruments or equipment thoroughly. Use warm soapy water. Use the brush on serrated edges of instruments.

NOTE: All tissue and debris must be removed from the item or it will not be disinfected.

4. Rinse the item in cool water to remove soapy residue. Then rinse well with hot water. Dry all instruments or equipment thoroughly.

NOTE: Water on the instruments or equipment will dilute the chemical disinfectant.

5. Check the container. Make sure the lid fits securely.

NOTE: A loose cover will permit entrance of pathogens and/or evaporation of the chemical solution.

6. Place instruments in the container. Make sure there is a space between instruments. Leave hinged edges open so the solution can flow between the surfaces.

7. Carefully read label instructions about the chemical solution. Some solutions must be diluted. Check the manufacturer's recommended soaking time.

Safety

CAUTION: Reread instructions to be sure the solution is safe to use on instruments.

NOTE: An antirust substance must be added to some solutions.

8. Pour the solution into the container slowly to avoid splashing. Make sure that all instruments are covered (**Figure 15–36**). Close the lid of the container.

NOTE: Read label three times: before pouring, while pouring, and after pouring.

Safety

CAUTION: Avoid splashing the chemical on your skin. Improper handling of chemicals may cause burns or injuries.

9. Remove gloves. Wash hands.

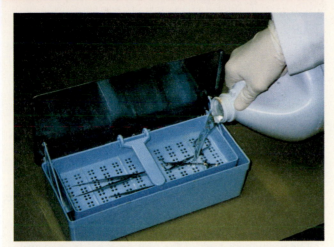

FIGURE 15–36 Pour the chemical disinfectant into the container until all instruments are covered with the solution.

10. Leave the instruments in the solution for the length of time recommended by the manufacturer.

    NOTE: The usual soaking time is 20–30 minutes.

    NOTE: If the solution requires a long period (for example, 10–12 hours) for disinfecting, label the container with the date and time the process began, ending date and time, and your initials.

11. When instruments have soaked the correct amount of time, use sterile gloves or sterile pick-ups or transfer forceps to remove the instruments from the solution. Hold the instruments over a sink or

basin and pour sterile water over them to rinse them thoroughly. Place them on a sterile towel to dry. A second sterile towel is sometimes used to dry the instruments or to cover the instruments while they are drying. Store the instruments in special drawers, containers, or dust-free closets.

NOTE: Some contamination occurs when instruments are exposed to the air. In some cases, such as with external instruments, this minimal contamination will not affect usage.

12. Replace all equipment used.

     CAUTION: If the disinfectant solution can be used again, label the container with the name of the disinfectant, date, and number of days it can be used according to manufacturer's instructions. When solutions cannot be reused, dispose of the solution according to the manufacturer's instructions.

13. Remove gloves. Wash hands.

PRACTICE: Go to the workbook and use the evaluation sheet for 15:6, Using Chemicals for Disinfection, to practice this procedure. When you believe you have mastered this skill, sign the sheet and give it to your instructor for further action.

 FINAL EVALUATION: Using the criteria listed on the evaluation sheet, your instructor will grade your performance.

15:7 CLEANING WITH AN ULTRASONIC UNIT

Ultrasonic units are used in many dental and medical offices and in other health agencies to remove dirt, debris, blood, saliva, and tissue from a large variety of instruments before sterilizing them. Ultrasonic cleaning uses sound waves to clean. When the ultrasonic unit is turned on, the sound waves produce millions of microscopic bubbles in a cleaning solution. When the bubbles strike the items being cleaned, they explode, a process known as **cavitation**, and drive the cleaning solution onto the article. Accumulated dirt and residue are easily and gently removed from the article.

Ultrasonic cleaning is not sterilization because spores and viruses remain on the articles. If sterilization is desired, other methods must be used after the ultrasonic cleaning.

Only ultrasonic solutions should be used in the unit. Different solutions are available for different materials. A general, all-purpose cleaning solution is usually used in the permanent tank and to clean many items. There are other specific solutions for alginate, plaster and stone removal, and tartar removal. The solution chart provided with the ultrasonic unit will state which solution should be used. It is important to read labels carefully before using any solutions. Some solutions must be diluted before use, and some can be used only on specific materials. All solutions are toxic. They can also cause skin irritation, so contact with the skin and eyes should be avoided. Solutions should be discarded when they become cloudy or contaminated, or if cleaning results are poor.

The permanent tank of the ultrasonic unit (**Figure 15–37**) must contain a solution at all times. A general, all-purpose cleaning solution is used most of the time. Glass beakers or auxiliary pans or baskets can then be placed in the permanent tank. The items to be cleaned and the proper cleaning solution are then put in

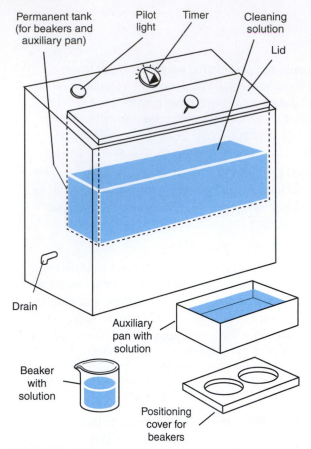

Permanent tank
(for beakers and
auxiliary pan)

Pilot
light

Timer

Cleaning
solution

Lid

Drain

Auxiliary
pan with
solution

Beaker
with
solution

Positioning
cover for
beakers

FIGURE 15–37 Parts of an ultrasonic cleaning unit.

the beakers or pans. The bottoms of the beakers or pans must always be positioned below the level of the solution present in the permanent tank. In this way, cavitation can be transmitted from the main tank and through the solution to the items being cleaned in the beakers or pans. The ultrasonic unit should never be operated without solutions in both containers. In addition, the items being cleaned must be submerged in the cleaning solution.

Many different items can be cleaned in an ultrasonic unit. Examples include instruments, dental impression trays, glass products, and most jewelry. The ultrasonic unit should not be used on jewelry with pearls or pasted stones. The sound waves can destroy the pearls or the paste holding the stones. Before cleaning, most of the dirt or particles should be brushed off the items being cleaned. It is better to clean a few articles at a time and avoid overloading the unit. If items are close together, the cavitation is poor because the bubbles cannot strike all parts of the items being cleaned.

The glass beakers used in the ultrasonic unit are made of a type of glass that allows the passage of sound waves. After continual use, the sound waves etch the bottom of the beakers. A white, opaque coating forms. The beakers must be discarded and replaced when this occurs. After each use, the beakers should be washed with soap and water and rinsed thoroughly to remove any soapy residue. They must be dry before being filled with solution because water in the beaker can dilute the solution.

The permanent tank of the unit must be drained and cleaned at intervals based on tank use or the appearance of the solution in the tank. A drain valve on the side of the tank is opened to allow the solution to drain. The tank is then wiped with a damp cloth or disinfectant. Another damp cloth or disinfectant is used to wipe off the outside of the unit. The unit should never be submerged in water to clean it. After cleaning, a fresh solution should be placed in the permanent tank.

The manufacturer's instructions must be read carefully before using any ultrasonic unit. Most manufacturers provide cleaning charts that state the type of solution and time required for a variety of cleaning problems. Each time an item is cleaned in an ultrasonic unit, the chart should be used to determine the correct cleaning solution and time required.

checkpoint

| **1.** What is cavitation?

PRACTICE: Go to the workbook and complete the assignment sheet for 15:7, Cleaning with an Ultrasonic Unit. Then return and continue with the procedure.

Procedure 15:7

Cleaning with an Ultrasonic Unit

Equipment and Supplies

Ultrasonic unit, permanent tank with solution, beakers, auxiliary pan or basket with covers, beaker bands, cleaning solutions, transfer forceps or pick-ups, paper towels, gloves, brush, soap, water for rinsing, articles for cleaning, solution chart

Procedure

1. Assemble all equipment.

2. 🔴 Precaution — Wash hands. Put on gloves if any items may be contaminated with blood, body fluids, secretions, or excretions.

NOTE: Use heavy-duty utility gloves if instruments are sharp.

3. Use a brush and soap and water to remove any large particles of dirt from articles to be cleaned. Rinse articles thoroughly. Dry items.

NOTE: Rinsing is important because soap may interact with the cleaning solution.

4. Check the permanent tank to be sure it has enough cleaning solution. An all-purpose cleaning solution is usually used in this tank.

    CAUTION: Never run the unit without solution in the permanent tank.

   NOTE: Many solutions must be diluted before use; if new solution is needed, read the instructions on the bottle.

5. Pour the proper cleaning solution into the auxiliary pan or beakers.

   NOTE: Use the cleaning chart to determine which solution to use.

    CAUTION: Read label before using.

    CAUTION: Handle solutions carefully. Avoid contact with skin and eyes.

6. Place the beakers, basket, or auxiliary pan into the permanent tank (**Figures 15–38A and B**). Use beaker positioning covers and beaker bands. Beaker bands are large bands that circle the beakers to hold them in position and keep them from hitting the bottom of the permanent tank.

7. Check to be sure that the bottoms of the beakers, basket, or pan are below the level of solution in the permanent tank.

   NOTE: For sonic waves to flow through solutions in the beakers, basket, or pan, the two solution levels must overlap.

8. Place articles to be cleaned in the beakers, basket, or pan. Be sure the solution completely covers the articles. Do not get solution on your hands.

   NOTE: Remember that pearls or pasted stones cannot be cleaned in an ultrasonic unit.

9. Turn the timer past 5 (minutes) and then set the proper cleaning time. Use the cleaning chart to determine the correct amount of time required for the items. Most articles are cleaned in 2–5 minutes.

10. Check that the unit is working. You should see a series of bubbles in both solutions. This is called *cavitation.*

     CAUTION: Do not get too close. Solution can spray into your face and eyes. Use beaker lids to prevent spray.

11. When the timer stops, cleaning is complete. Use transfer forceps or pick-ups to lift articles from the basket, pan, or beakers. Place the articles on paper towels. Then rinse the articles thoroughly under running water.

     CAUTION: Avoid contact with skin. Some solutions are toxic.

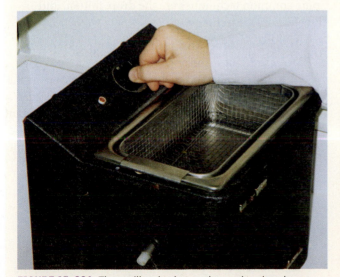

FIGURE 15–38A The auxiliary basket can be used to clean larger items in an ultrasonic unit.

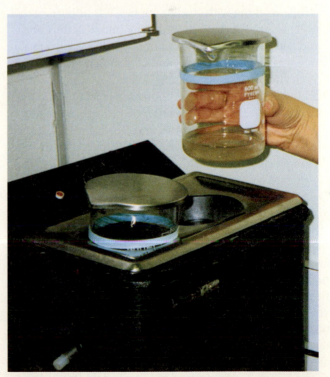

FIGURE 15–38B Glass beakers can be used to clean smaller items in an ultrasonic unit.

(continues)

12. Allow articles to air-dry or dry them with paper towels. Inspect the articles for cleanliness. If they are not clean, repeat the process.

13. Periodically change solutions in the permanent tank and auxiliary containers. Do this when solutions become cloudy or cleaning has not been effective. To clean the permanent tank, place a container under the side drain to collect the solution. Then open the valve and drain the solution from the tank. Wash the inside with a damp cloth or disinfectant. To clean the auxiliary pans or beakers, discard the solution. (It can be poured down the sink, but allow water to run for a time after disposing of the solution.) Then wash the containers and rinse thoroughly.

NOTE: If the bottoms of beakers are etched and white, the beakers must be discarded and replaced.

14. Clean and replace all equipment used. Make sure all beakers are covered with lids.

15. Wash hands.

PRACTICE: Go to the workbook and use the evaluation sheet for 15:7, Cleaning with an Ultrasonic Unit, to practice this procedure. When you believe you have mastered this skill, sign the sheet and give it to your instructor for further action.

 FINAL EVALUATION: Using the criteria listed on the evaluation sheet, your instructor will grade your performance.

15:8 USING STERILE TECHNIQUES

Many procedures require the use of sterile techniques to protect the patient from further infection. *Surgical asepsis* refers to procedures that keep an object or area free from living organisms. The main facts are presented here.

While working with sterile supplies, it is important that correct techniques be followed to maintain sterility and avoid contamination. It is also important that you are able to recognize sterile surfaces and contaminated surfaces.

A clean, uncluttered working area is required when working with sterile supplies. A sterile object must never touch a nonsterile object. If other objects are in the way, it is easy to contaminate sterile articles. If sterile articles touch the skin or any part of your clothing, they are no longer sterile. Because any area below the waist is considered contaminated, sterile articles must be held away from and in front of the body and above the waist.

Once a **sterile field** has been set up (for example, a sterile towel has been placed on a tray), never reach across the top of the field. Microorganisms can drop from your arm or clothing and contaminate the field. Always reach in from either side to place additional articles on the field. Keep the sterile field in constant view. Never turn your back to a sterile field. Avoid coughing, sneezing, or talking over the sterile field because airborne particles can fall on the field and contaminate it. A person must remain alert and honest to properly maintain a sterile field.

The 2-inch border around the sterile field (towel-covered tray) is considered contaminated. Therefore, 2 inches around the outside of the field must not be used when sterile articles are placed on the sterile field.

All sterile items must be checked carefully before they are used. If the item was autoclaved and dated, most health care facilities believe the date should not be more than 30 days from autoclaving. Follow agency guidelines for time limits. If tears or stains are present on the package, the item should *not* be used because it could be contaminated. If there are any signs of moisture on the package, it has been contaminated and should *not* be used.

Organisms and pathogens travel quickly through a wet surface, so the sterile field must be kept dry. If a sterile towel or article gets wet, contamination has occurred. It is very important to use care when pouring solutions into sterile bowls or using solutions around a sterile field.

Various techniques can be used to remove articles from sterile wraps, depending on the article being unwrapped. Some common techniques are the drop, mitten, and transfer-forceps techniques:

- **Drop technique:** This technique is used for gauze pads, dressings, and small items. The wrapper is partially opened and then held upside down over the sterile field. The item drops out of the wrapper and onto the sterile field (**Figure 15–39A**). It is important to keep fingers back so the article does not touch the skin as it falls out of the wrapper. It is also important to avoid touching the inside of the wrapper.

- **Mitten technique:** This technique is used for bowls, drapes, linen, and other similar items. The wrapper is opened and its loose ends are grasped around the wrist with the opposite hand (**Figure 15–39B**). In this way, a mitten is formed around the hand that is still holding the item (for example, a bowl). With the mitten hand, the item can be placed on the sterile tray.

- **Transfer forceps:** These are used for cotton balls, small items, or articles that cannot be removed by

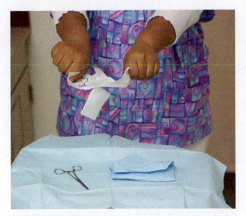

FIGURE 15–39A Sterile items can be dropped from the wrapper onto the sterile field.

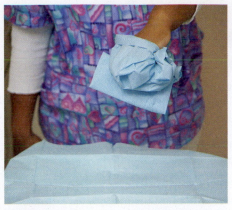

FIGURE 15–39B By using the wrap as a mitten, sterile supplies can be placed on a sterile field.

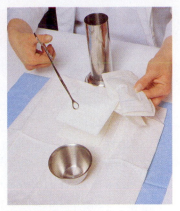

FIGURE 15–39C Sterile transfer forceps or pick-ups can be used to grasp sterile items and place them on a sterile field.

the drop or mitten techniques. Either sterile gloves or sterile transfer forceps (pick-ups) are used. Sterile transfer forceps or pick-ups are removed from their container of disinfectant solution and used to grasp the article from the opened package. The item is removed from the opened, sterile wrap and placed on the sterile field (**Figure 15–39C**). The transfer forceps must be pointed in a downward direction. If they are pointed upward, the solution will flow back to the handle, become contaminated, and return to contaminate the sterile tips when they are being used to pick up items. In addition, care must be taken not to touch the sides or rim of the forceps container while removing or inserting the transfer forceps. Also, the transfer forceps must be shaken gently to get rid of excess disinfectant solution before they are used.

Make sure the sterile tray is open and you are ready to do the sterile procedure *before* putting the sterile gloves on your hands. Sterile gloves are considered sterile on the outside and contaminated on the inside (side against the skin). Once they have been placed on the hands, it

is important to hold the hands away from the body and above the waist to avoid contamination. Handle only sterile objects while wearing sterile gloves.

Precaution *If at any time during a procedure there is any suspicion that you have contaminated any article, start over. Never take a chance on using contaminated equipment or supplies.*

A wide variety of commercially prepared sterile supplies is available. Packaged units are often set up for special procedures, such as changing dressings. Many agencies use these units instead of setting up special trays. Observe all sterile principles while using these units and read any directions provided with the units.

checkpoint

1. Around a sterile field, how wide of a border is considered contaminated?

PRACTICE: Go to the workbook and complete the assignment sheet for 15:8, Using Sterile Techniques. Then return and continue with the procedures.

Procedure 15:8A

Opening Sterile Packages

Equipment and Supplies

Sterile package of equipment or supplies, a table or other flat surface, sterile field (tray with sterile towel)

Procedure

1. Assemble equipment.

2. Wash hands.

3. Take equipment to the area where it will be used. Check the autoclave indicator and date

on the package. Check the package for stains, tears, moisture, or evidence of contamination. Do *not* use the package if there is any evidence of contamination.

NOTE: Contents are not considered sterile if 30 days have elapsed since autoclaving.

4. Pick up the package with the tab or sealed edge pointing toward you. If the item is small, it can be held in the hand while being unwrapped. If it is large, place it on a table or other flat surface.

(continues)

5. Loosen the wrapper fastener (usually tape).

6. Check to be sure the package is away from your body. If it is on a table, make sure it is not close to other objects.

   NOTE: Avoid possible contamination by keeping sterile supplies away from other objects.

7. Open the distal (furthest) flap of the wrapper by grasping the outside of the wrapper and pulling it away from you (**Figure 15–40A**).

    CAUTION: Do not reach across the top of the package. Reach around the package to open it.

8. With one hand, raise a side flap and pull laterally (sideways) away from the package (**Figure 15–40B**).

   CAUTION: Do not touch the inside of the wrapper at any time.

9. With the opposite hand, open the other side flap by pulling the tab to the side (**Figure 15–40C**).

   NOTE: Always reach in from the side. Never reach across the top of the sterile field or across any opened edges.

10. Open the proximal (closest) flap by lifting the flap up and toward you. Then drop it over the front of your hand (or the table) (**Figure 15–40D**).

    CAUTION: Be careful not to touch the inside of the package or the contents of the package.

11. Transfer the contents of the sterile package using one of the following techniques:

    a. **Drop**: Separate the ends of the wrap and pull apart gently. Avoid touching the inside of the wrap. Secure the loose ends of the wrap and hold the package upside down over the sterile field. Allow the contents to drop onto the sterile tray (**Figure 15–40E**).

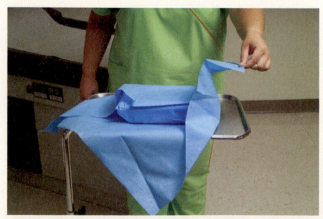

FIGURE 15–40A To open a sterile package, open the top flap away from you, handling only the outside of the wrap.

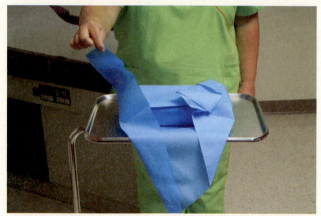

FIGURE 15–40B Open one side by pulling the wrap out to the side.

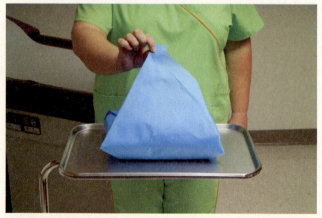

FIGURE 15–40C Open the opposite side by pulling the wrap out to the opposite side.

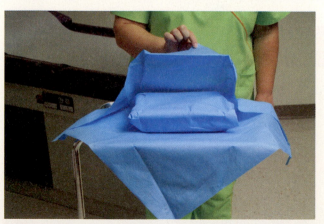

FIGURE 15–40D Open the side nearest to you by pulling back on the wrap.

b. **Mitten**: Grasp the contents securely by holding on to the outside of the wrapper as you unwrap it. With your free hand, gather the loose edges of the wrapper together and hold them securely around your wrist. This can be compared to making a mitten of the wrapper (with the sterile equipment on the outside of the mitten). Place the item on the sterile tray or hand it to someone who is wearing sterile gloves (refer to Figure 15–39B).

c. **Transfer forceps**: Remove forceps from their sterile container, taking care not to touch the side or rim of the container with the forceps. Hold the forceps pointed downward. Shake them gently to remove excess disinfectant solution. Take care not to touch anything with the forceps. Use the forceps to grasp the item in the package and then place the item on the sterile tray (**Figures 15–40F and G**).

NOTE: The method of transfer depends on the sterile item being transferred.

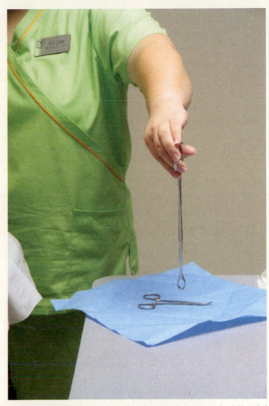

FIGURE 15–40F Hold the forceps pointed downward while picking up the sterile instrument that needs to be transferred.

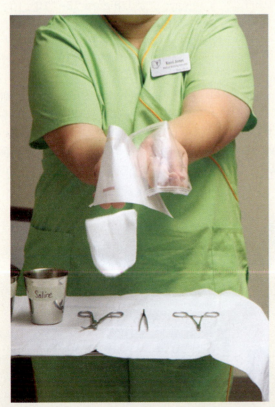

FIGURE 15–40E Separate the ends of the wrap and hold the package upside down to allow the contents to drop onto the sterile tray.

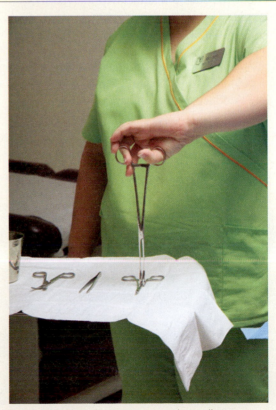

FIGURE 15–40G Place the instrument on the sterile tray.

(continues)

CAUTION: If at any time during the procedure there is any suspicion that you have contaminated any article, start over. Never take a chance on using equipment for a sterile procedure if there is any possibility that the equipment is contaminated.

12. Replace all equipment used.

13. Wash hands.

PRACTICE: Go to the workbook and use the evaluation sheet for 15:8A, Opening Sterile Packages, to practice this procedure. When you believe you have mastered this skill, sign the sheet and give it to your instructor for further action.

✅ **FINAL EVALUATION:** Using the criteria listed on the evaluation sheet, your instructor will grade your performance.

Procedure 15:8B

Preparing a Sterile Dressing Tray

Equipment and Supplies

Tray or Mayo stand, sterile towels, sterile basin, sterile cotton balls or gauze sponges, sterile dressings (different sizes), antiseptic solution, forceps in disinfectant solution

Procedure

1. Assemble all equipment.

2. Wash hands.

3. Check the date and autoclave indicator for sterility. If more than 30 days have elapsed, use another package with a more recent date. Put the unsterile package aside for resterilization. Check the package for stains, tears, moisture, or evidence of contamination. Do not use the package if there is any evidence of contamination.

4. Place the tray on a flat surface or a Mayo stand.

NOTE: Make sure the work area is clean and dry, and there is sufficient room to work.

5. Open the package that contains the sterile towel. Be sure it is held away from your body. Place the wrapper on a surface away from the tray or work area. Touch only the outside of the towel. Pick up the towel at its outer edge. Allow it to open by releasing the fanfolds (**Figure 15–41A**). Place the towel with the outer side (side you have touched) on the tray or Mayo stand (**Figure 15–41B**). The untouched, or sterile, side will be facing up to create a sterile field. Holding the outside edges of the towel, fanfold the back of the towel so the towel can be used later to cover the supplies.

 CAUTION: Do not reach across the top of the sterile field. Reach in from either side.

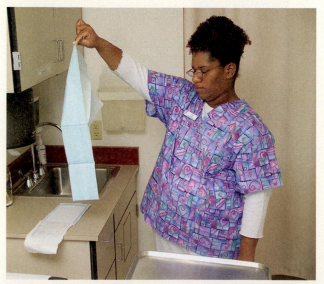

FIGURE 15–41A Pick up the sterile towel at its outer edge and allow it to open by releasing the fanfolds.

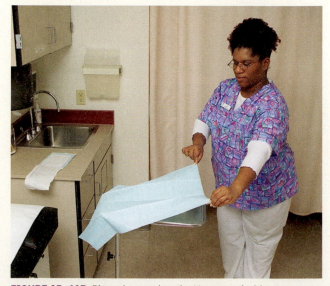

FIGURE 15–41B Place the towel on the Mayo stand without reaching across the top of the towel.

NOTE: If you are setting up a relatively large work area, one towel may not be large enough when fanfolded to cover the supplies. In such a case, you will need a second sterile towel (later) to cover your sterile field.

 CAUTION: At all times, make sure that you do not touch the sterile side of the towel. Avoid letting the towel come in contact with your uniform, other objects, or contaminated areas.

6. Correctly unwrap the package containing the sterile basin. Place the basin on the sterile field. Do not place it close to the edge.

    NOTE: A 2-inch border around the outside edges of the sterile field is considered to be contaminated. No equipment should come in contact with this border.

     CAUTION: Make sure that the wrapper does not touch the towel while placing the basin in position.

7. Unwrap the package containing the sterile cotton balls or gauze sponges. Use a dropping motion to place them in the basin. Do not touch the basin with the wrapper.

8. Unwrap the package containing the larger dressing. Use the sterile forceps to remove the dressing from the package and place it on the sterile field. Make sure the dressing is not too close to the edge of the sterile field.

    NOTE: The larger, outside dressing is placed on the sterile field first (before other dressings). In this way, the supplies will be in the order of use. For example, gauze dressings placed directly on the skin will be on top of the pile, and a thick abdominal pad used on top of the gauze pads will be on the bottom of the pile.

    NOTE: The forceps must be lifted straight up out of the container and must *not* touch the side or rim of the container. Keep the tips pointed down and above the waist at all times. Shake off excess disinfectant solution.

9. Unwrap the inner dressings correctly. Use the sterile forceps to place them on top of the other dressings on the sterile field, or use a drop technique.

    NOTE: Dressings are now in a pile; the dressing that will be used first is on the top of the pile.

    NOTE: The number and type of dressings needed is determined by checking the patient being treated.

10. Open the bottle containing the correct antiseptic solution. Place the cap on the table, with the inside of the cap facing up. Pour a small amount of the solution into the sink to clean the lip of the bottle. Then hold the bottle over the basin and pour a sufficient amount of the solution into the basin (**Figure 15–41C**).

     CAUTION: Make sure that no part of the bottle touches the basin or the sterile field. Pour carefully to avoid splashing. If the sterile field gets wet, the entire tray will be contaminated, and you must begin again.

11. Check the tray to make sure all needed equipment is on it.

12. Pick up the fanfolded edge of the towel by placing one hand on each side edge of the towel on the underside, or contaminated side. Do not touch the sterile side. Keep your hands and arms to the side of the tray, and bring the towel forward to cover the supplies.

    NOTE: A second sterile towel may be used to cover the supplies if the sterile field is too large to be covered by the one fanfolded towel (**Figure 15–41D**).

    CAUTION: Never reach across the top of the sterile tray.

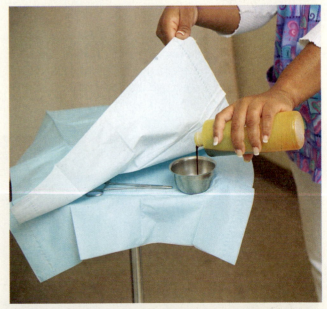

FIGURE 15–41C Avoid splashing the solution onto the sterile field while pouring it into the basin.

(continues)

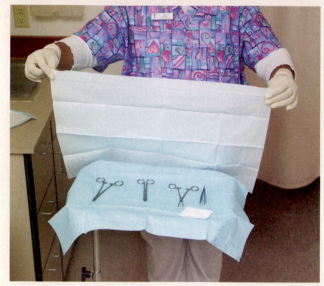

FIGURE 15–41D Use a second sterile towel to cover the first sterile towel and protect the sterile field, taking care not to reach across the field.

13. Once the sterile tray is ready, never allow it out of your sight. Take it to the patient area and use it immediately. If you need more equipment, you must take the tray with you. This is the only way to be completely positive that the tray does not become contaminated.

14. Replace equipment.

15. Wash hands.

PRACTICE: Go to the workbook and use the evaluation sheet for 15:8B, Preparing a Sterile Dressing Tray, to practice this procedure. When you believe you have mastered this skill, sign the sheet and give it to your instructor for further action.

 FINAL EVALUATION: Using the criteria listed on the evaluation sheet, your instructor will grade your performance.

Procedure 15:8C

Donning and Removing Sterile Gloves

Equipment and Supplies

Sterile gloves

Procedure

1. Obtain a package of sterile gloves and take it to the area where it is to be used. Check the package for stains, tears, moisture, or evidence of contamination. Do *not* use the package if there is any evidence of contamination.

2. Remove rings. Wash hands. Dry hands thoroughly.

3. Open the package of gloves, taking care not to touch the inside of the inner wrapper. The inner wrapper contains the gloves. Reach in from the sides to open the inner package and expose the sterile gloves (**Figure 15–42A**). The folded cuffs will be nearest to you.

 CAUTION: If you touch the *inside* of the package (where the gloves are), get a new package and start again.

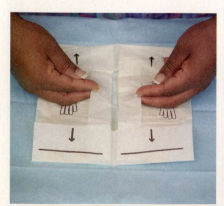

FIGURE 15–42A Reach in from the sides to open the inner package and expose the sterile gloves.

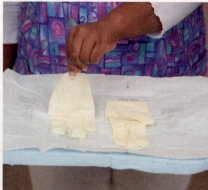

FIGURE 15–42B Pick up the first glove by grasping the glove on the top edge of the folded-down cuff.

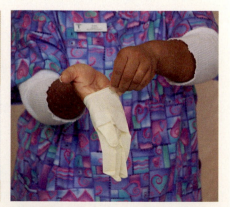

FIGURE 15–42C Hold the glove securely by the cuff and slip the opposite hand into the glove.

4. The glove for the right hand will be on the right side and the glove for the left hand will be on the left side of the package. With the thumb and forefinger of the nondominant hand, pick up the top edge of the folded-down cuff (inside of glove) of the glove for the dominant hand. Remove the glove carefully (**Figure 15–42B**).

 CAUTION: Do *not* touch the outside of the glove. This is sterile. Only the part that will be next to the skin can be touched. Remember, unsterile touches unsterile and sterile touches sterile.

5. Hold the glove by the inside cuff and slip the fingers and thumb of your other hand into the glove. Pull it on carefully (**Figure 15–42C**).

   NOTE: Hold the glove away from the body. Pull gently to avoid tearing the glove.

6. Insert your gloved hand under the cuff (outside) of the other glove and lift the glove from the package (**Figure 15–42D**). Do not touch any other area with your gloved hand while removing the glove from the package.

    CAUTION: If contamination occurs, discard the gloves and start again.

7. Holding your gloved hand under the cuff of the glove, insert your other hand into the glove (**Figure 15–42E**). Keep the thumb of your gloved hand tucked in to avoid possible contamination.

8. Turn the cuffs up by manipulating only the sterile surface of the gloves (sterile touches sterile). Go up under the folded cuffs, pull out slightly, and turn cuffs over and up (**Figure 15–42F**). Do not touch the inside of the gloves or the skin with your gloved hand.

9. Interlace the fingers to position the gloves correctly, taking care not to touch the skin with the gloved hands (**Figure 15–42G**).

    CAUTION: If contamination occurs, start again with a new pair of gloves.

10. Do not touch anything that is not sterile once the gloves are in place. Gloves are applied for the purpose of performing procedures requiring sterile technique. During the procedure, they will become contaminated with organisms related to the patient's condition, for example, wound drainage, blood, or other body discharges. Even a clean, dry wound may contaminate gloves.

    NOTE: Gloved hands should remain in position above the waist. Do *not* allow them to fall below waist.

11. After the procedure requiring sterile gloves is completed, dispose of all contaminated supplies before removing the gloves.

    NOTE: This reduces the danger of cross-infection caused by handling contaminated supplies without glove protection.

12. To remove the gloves, use one gloved hand to grasp the other glove by the outside of the cuff (**Figure 15–42H**). Taking care not to touch the skin, remove the glove by pulling it down over the hand (**Figure 15–42I**). It will be wrong side out when removed.

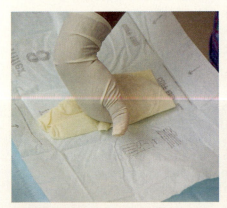

FIGURE 15–42D Slip the gloved fingers under the cuff of the second glove to lift it from the package.

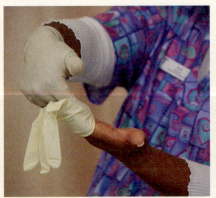

FIGURE 15–42E Hold the gloved hand under the cuff while inserting the other hand into the glove.

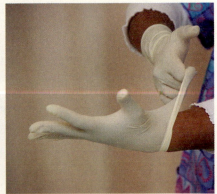

FIGURE 15–42F Insert the gloved fingers under the cuff, pull out slightly, and turn the cuffs over and up without touching the inside of the gloves or the skin.

(continues)

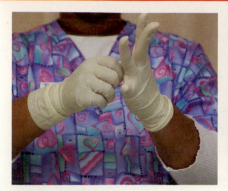

FIGURE 15–42G Interlace the fingers to position the gloves correctly, taking care not to touch the skin with the gloved hands.

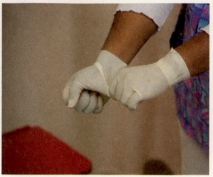

FIGURE 15–42H Use a gloved hand to grasp the other glove by the outside of the cuff.

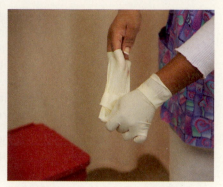

FIGURE 15–42I Remove the glove by pulling it down over the hand and turning it inside out.

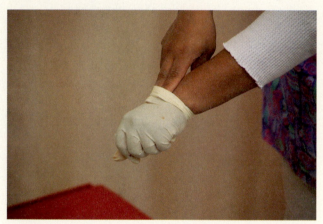

FIGURE 15–42J Insert your bare fingers inside the top of the second glove.

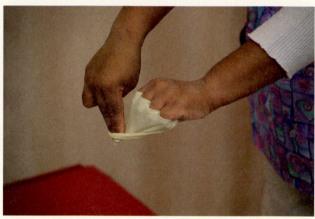

FIGURE 15–42K Pull the glove down gently, taking care to not touch the outside of the glove with your fingers.

NOTE: This prevents contamination of your hands by organisms picked up during performance of the procedure. Now you must consider the outside of the gloves contaminated, and the area inside, next to your skin, clean.

13. Insert your bare fingers inside the second glove (**Figure 15–42J**). Remove the glove by pulling it down gently, taking care not to touch the outside of the glove with your bare fingers (**Figure 15–42K**). It will be wrong side out when removed.

CAUTION: Avoid touching your uniform or any other object with the contaminated gloves.

14. Put the contaminated gloves in an infectious waste container immediately after removal.

15. Wash your hands immediately and thoroughly after removing gloves.

16. Once the gloves have been removed, do not handle any contaminated equipment or supplies such as soiled dressings or drainage basins. Protect yourself.

17. Replace equipment if necessary.

18. Wash hands thoroughly.

PRACTICE: Go to the workbook and use the evaluation sheet for 15:8C, Donning and Removing Sterile Gloves, to practice this procedure. When you believe you have mastered this skill, sign the sheet and give it to your instructor for further action.

FINAL EVALUATION: Using the criteria listed on the evaluation sheet, your instructor will grade your performance.

Changing a Sterile Dressing

Equipment and Supplies

Sterile tray with basin, solution, gauze sponges and pads (or a prepared sterile dressing package); sterile gloves; adhesive or nonallergic tape; disposable gloves; infectious waste bag; pen or computer

Procedure

1. Check doctor's written orders or obtain orders from immediate supervisor.

   NOTE: Dressings should *not* be changed without orders.

   NOTE: The policy of your agency will determine how you obtain orders for procedures.

2. Assemble equipment. Check autoclave indicator and date on all equipment. If more than 30 days have elapsed, use another package with a more recent date. Put the unsterile package aside for resterilization.

3. Wash hands thoroughly.

4. Prepare a sterile tray as previously taught in Procedure 15:8B or obtain a commercially prepared sterile dressing package.

   NOTE: Prepared packages are used by some agencies.

    CAUTION: Never let the tray out of your sight after it has been prepared.

5. Take all necessary equipment to the patient area. Place it where it will be convenient for use yet free from possible contamination by other equipment.

6. Introduce yourself. Identify the patient. Explain the procedure. Close the door and/or windows to avoid drafts and flow of organisms into the room.

7. Make sure the door is closed or draw curtains to provide privacy for the patient. If the patient is in a bed, elevate the bed to a comfortable working height and lower the siderail if it is elevated. Expose the body area needing the dressing change. Use sheets or drapes as necessary to prevent unnecessary exposure of the patient.

8. Fold down a 2- to 3-inch cuff on the top of the infectious waste bag. Position it in a convenient location. Tear off the tape you will need later to secure the clean dressing. Place it in an area where it will be available for easy access.

9. Put on disposable, nonsterile gloves. Gently but firmly remove the tape from the soiled dressing. Discard it in the infectious waste bag. Hold the skin taut and then lift the dressing carefully, taking care not to pull on any surgical drains. Note the type, color, and amount of drainage on the dressing. Discard dressing in the infectious waste bag.

   NOTE: Surgical drains are placed in some surgical incisions to aid in the removal of secretions. Care must be taken to avoid moving the drains when the dressing is removed.

10. Check the incision site. Observe the type and amount of remaining drainage, color of drainage, and degree of healing.

     CAUTION: Report any unusual observations immediately to your supervisor. Examples are bright red blood, pus, swelling, abnormal discharges at the wound site, or patient complaints of pain or dizziness.

11. Remove disposable gloves and place in infectious waste bag. Immediately wash your hands.

     CAUTION: Nonsterile disposable gloves should be worn while removing dressings to avoid contamination of the hands or skin by blood or body discharge.

12. Fanfold the top cover back to uncover the sterile field.

    CAUTION: Handle only the contaminated side (outside) of the towel. The side in contact with the tray's contents is the sterile side.

    NOTE: If a prepared package is used, open it at this time.

13. Don sterile gloves as previously taught in Procedure 15:8C.

14. Using thumb and forefinger or dressing forceps, pick up a gauze sponge from the basin. Squeeze it slightly to remove any excess solution. Warn the patient that the solution may be cool.

15. Cleanse the wound using a circular motion (**Figure 15–43A**).

    NOTE: Begin near the center of the wound and move outward or away from the wound. Make an ever-widening circle. Discard the wet gauze sponge after use. Never go back over the same area with the same gauze sponge. Repeat this procedure until the area is clean, using a new gauze sponge each time.

(continues)

16. Do not cleanse directly over the wound unless there is a great deal of drainage or it is specifically ordered by the physician. If this is to be done, use sterile gauze and wipe with a single stroke from the top to the bottom. Discard the soiled gauze. Repeat as necessary, using a new sterile gauze sponge each time.

17. The wound is now ready for clean dressings. Lift the sterile dressings from the tray and place them lightly on the wound (**Figure 15–43B**). Make sure they are centered over the wound.

    NOTE: The inner dressing is usually made up of 4-by-4-inch gauze sponges.

18. Apply outer dressings until the wound is sufficiently protected (**Figure 15–43C**).

    NOTE: Heavier dressings such as abdominal pads are usually used.

    NOTE: The number and size of dressings needed will depend on the amount of drainage and the size of the wound.

19. Place the precut tape over the dressing at the proper angle. Check to make sure that the dressing is secure and the ends are closed.

    NOTE: Tape should be applied so it runs opposite from body action or movement (**Figure 15–43D**). It should be the correct width for the dressing. It should be long enough to support the dressing, but it should not be too long because it may irritate the patient's skin.

20. Remove the sterile gloves as previously taught. Discard them in the infectious waste bag. Immediately wash your hands.

21. Check to be sure the patient is comfortable and that safety precautions have been observed before leaving the area.

22. Put on disposable, nonsterile gloves. Clean and replace all equipment used. Tie or tape the infectious waste bag securely. Dispose of it according to agency policy.

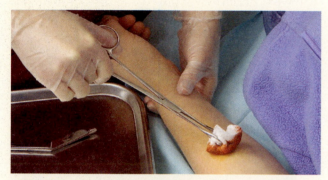

FIGURE 15–43A Use a circular motion to clean the wound, starting at the center of the wound and moving in an outward direction.

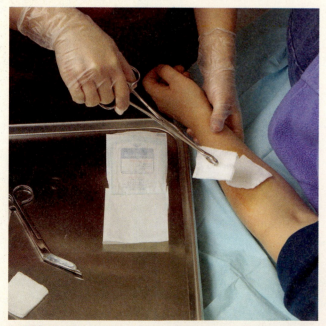

FIGURE 15–43B Position the inner sterile dressings so they are centered over the wound.

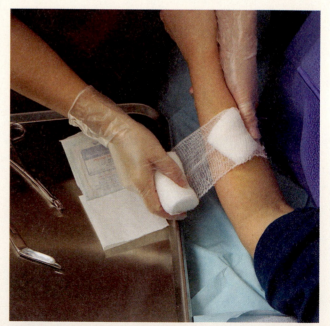

FIGURE 15–43C Apply the outer dressings until the wound is sufficiently protected.

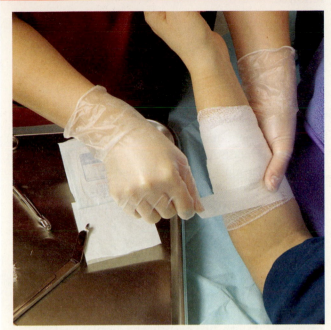

FIGURE 15–43D Tape should be applied so that it runs opposite to body action or movement.

CAUTION: Disposable, nonsterile gloves should be worn to provide a protective barrier while cleaning equipment or supplies that may be contaminated by blood or body fluids.

Safety

23. Remove disposable gloves. Wash hands thoroughly. Protect yourself from possible contamination.

24. Record the following information on the patient's chart or enter it into the computer: date, time, dressing change, amount and type of drainage, and any other pertinent information, or tell this information to your immediate supervisor.

Comm

EXAMPLE: 1/8/—, 9:00 A.M. Dressing changed on right abdominal area. Small amount of thick, light yellow discharge noted on dressings. No swelling or inflammation apparent at incision site. Sterile dressing applied. Your signature and title.

NOTE: Report any unusual observations immediately.

 NOTE: In health care agencies using electronic health records (EHRs), also known as electronic medical records (EMRs), the information is entered directly into the patient's record on a computer.

EHR

PRACTICE: Go to the workbook and use the evaluation sheet for 15:8D, Changing a Sterile Dressing, to practice this procedure. When you believe you have mastered this skill, sign the sheet and give it to your instructor for further action.

 FINAL EVLUATION: Using the criteria listed on the evaluation sheet, your instructor will grade your performance.

Check

15:9 MAINTAINING TRANSMISSION-BASED PRECAUTIONS

INTRODUCTION

OBRA In a health care career, you will deal with many different diseases/disorders. Some diseases are communicable and require isolation. A **communicable disease** is caused by a pathogenic organism that can be easily transmitted to others. An **epidemic** occurs when the communicable disease spreads rapidly from person to person and affects a large number of people at the same time. A **pandemic** exists when the outbreak of disease occurs over a wide geographic area and affects a high proportion of the population. Because individuals can travel readily throughout the world, a major concern is that worldwide pandemics will become more and more frequent.

Precaution **Transmission-based precautions** are a method or technique of caring for patients who have communicable diseases. Examples of communicable diseases are tuberculosis, wound infections, and pertussis (whooping cough). Standard precautions, discussed in information Section 15:4, Observing Standard Precautions, do not eliminate the need for specific transmission-based precautions. Standard precautions are used on all patients. Transmission-based precautions are used to provide extra protection against specific diseases or pathogens to prevent their spread.

Communicable diseases are spread in many ways. Some examples include direct contact with the patient; contact with dirty linen, equipment, and/or supplies; and contact with blood, body fluids, secretions, and excretions such as urine, feces, droplets (from sneezing, coughing, or spitting), and discharges from wounds. Transmission-based precautions are used to limit contact with pathogenic organisms. These techniques help prevent the spread of the disease to other people and protect patients, their families, and health care providers.

The type of transmission-based precautions used depends on the causative organism of the disease, the way the organism is transmitted, and whether the pathogen is antibiotic resistant (not affected by antibiotics). Personal protective equipment (PPE) is used to provide protection from the pathogen. Some transmission-based precautions require the use of gowns, gloves, face shields, and masks (**Figure 15–44**), while others require the use of only a mask.

Two terms are extensively used in transmission-based precautions: *contaminated* and *clean*. These words refer to the presence of organisms on objects.

- **Contaminated**, or dirty, means that objects contain disease-producing organisms. These objects must not be touched unless the health care provider is protected by gloves, gown, and other required items.

  NOTE: *The outside and waist ties of the gown, protective gloves, and mask are considered contaminated.*

- **Clean** means that objects or parts of objects do *not* contain disease-producing organisms and therefore have minimal chance of spreading the disease. Every effort must be made to prevent contamination of these objects or parts of objects.

  NOTE: *The insides of the gloves and gown are clean, as are the neckband, its ties, and the mask ties.*

The Centers for Disease Control and Prevention (CDC) in conjunction with the National Center for Infectious Diseases (NCID) and the Hospital Infection Control Practices Advisory Committee (HICPAC) has recommended four main classifications of precautions that must be followed: standard, airborne, droplet, and contact. Health care facilities are provided with a list of infections/conditions that shows the type and duration of precautions needed for each specific disease. In this way, facilities can follow the guidelines to determine

the type of transmission-based isolation that should be used along with the specific precautions that must be followed.

STANDARD PRECAUTIONS

Standard precautions (discussed in information Section 15:4, Observing Standard Precautions) are used on all patients. In addition, a patient must be placed in a private room if the patient contaminates the environment or does not (or cannot be expected to) assist in maintaining appropriate hygiene. Every health care provider must be well informed about standard precautions and must follow the recommendations for the use of gloves, gowns, and face masks when conditions indicate their use.

AIRBORNE PRECAUTIONS

Airborne precautions (**Figure 15–45**) are used for patients known or suspected to be infected with pathogens transmitted by airborne droplet nuclei. These are small particles of evaporated droplets that contain microorganisms and remain suspended in the air or on dust particles. Examples of diseases requiring these isolation precautions are rubella (measles), varicella (chicken pox), tuberculosis, coronavirus, and severe acute respiratory syndrome (SARS). Standard precautions are used at all times. In addition, the following precautions must be taken:

- The patient must be placed in an airborne infection isolation room (AIRR), and the door should be kept closed.

- Air in the room must be discharged to outdoor air or filtered before being circulated to other areas.

- Each person who enters the room must wear respiratory protection in the form of an N95, P100, or more powerful filtering mask such as a high-efficiency particulate air (HEPA) mask (**Figures 15–46A and B**). These masks contain special filters to prevent the entrance of the small airborne pathogens. The masks must be fit tested to make sure they create a tight seal each time they are worn by a health care provider. Men with facial hair cannot wear a standard filtering mask because a beard prevents an airtight seal. Men with facial hair can use a special HEPA-filtered hood.

- People susceptible to measles or chicken pox should not enter the room.

- If at all possible, the patient should not be moved from the room. If transport is essential, however, the patient must wear a surgical mask during transport to minimize the release of droplets into the air.

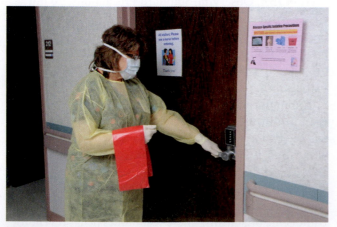

FIGURE 15–44 Some transmission-based precautions require the use of gowns, gloves, and a mask, while others require the use of only a mask.

AIRBORNE PRECAUTIONS
(in addition to Standard Precautions)
PRECAUCIONES CONTRA LA DISEMINACIÓN POR EL AIRE
(Además de las Precauciones Estándar)

Assume that every person is potentially infected or colonized with a transmissible pathogen

VISITORS STOP!
REPORT TO NURSE BEFORE ENTERING

¡VISITANTES ALTO!
INFORMAR A LA ENFERMERA ANTES DE INGRESAR

PATIENT PLACEMENT
in an **AIIR** (Airborne Infection Isolation Room). **Monitor air pressure** daily with visual indicators (e.g., flutter strips).

Keep door closed except for entry and exit.

In ambulatory settings instruct patients with a known or suspected airborne infection to wear a surgical mask and observe Respiratory Hygiene/Cough Etiquette. Once in an AIIR, the mask may be removed.

PATIENT TRANSPORT
Limit transport and movement of patients to **medically necessary purposes.**

If transport or movement outside an AIIR is necessary, instruct patients to **wear a surgical mask**, if possible, and observe Respiratory Hygiene/Cough Etiquette.

HAND HYGIENE
When hands are visibly dirty, or soiled with blood or body fluids, wash hands with soap and water.

If hands are not visibly soiled, decontaminate with an alcohol hand sanitizer or wash hands with soap & water.

PERSONAL PROTECTIVE EQUIPMENT
Wear a fit-tested NIOSH-approved **N95** or higher level respirator for respiratory protection when entering the room of a patient when the following diseases are suspected or confirmed: Listed on back.

UBICACIÓN DEL PACIENTE
Ubique al paciente en una Habitación de **Aislamiento de Infecciones Diseminadas por el Aire** (AIIR, por sus siglas en inglés). **Controle la presión del aire** diariamente con indicadores visuales (por ejemplo, cintas sensibles al flujo del aire).

Mantenga la puerta cerrada, excepto para la entrada y salida.

En entornos ambulatorios, indique o los pacientes que se sepa o sospeche que presentan una infección diseminada por el aire que usen una mascarilla quirúrgica y que se sigan las normas de Etiqueta para la Higiene Respiratoria/Tos. Una vez que hayan ingresado en la AIIR, pueden quitarse la mascarilla.

TRASLADO DEL PACIENTE
Limite el traslado y el movimiento de los pacientes solamente con fines **médicamente necesarios.**

Si es necesario trasladar o mover al paciente fuera de un AIIR, indíquele que **use una mascarilla quirúrgica**, si es posible, y que sigan las normas de Etiqueta para la Higiene Respiratoria/Tos.

HIGIENE DE MANOS
Cuando las manos estén visiblemente sucias o manchadas de sangre o fluidos corporales, lávese las manos con agua y jabón.

Si las manos no están visiblemente sucias, descontamínelas con un desinfectante de manos a base de alcohol o lávese las manos con agua y jabón.

EQUIPO DE PROTECCIÓN PERSONAL
Use un respirador **N95** o de nivel superior aprobado por NIOSH comprobando adecuadamente su ajuste para la protección respiratoria cuando ingrese a la habitación de un paciente y cuando se sospeche o confirme las siguientes enfermedades: Enumeradas al dorso

APR20.ES · ©2020 Brevis Corporation · www.brevis.com

FIGURE 15–45 Airborne precautions. Reprinted with Permission from Brevis Corporation [www.brevis.com].

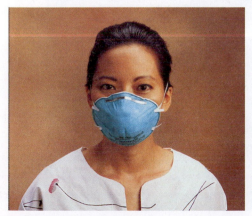

FIGURE 15–46A The N95 respirator mask. Courtesy of 3M Company, St. Paul, MN.

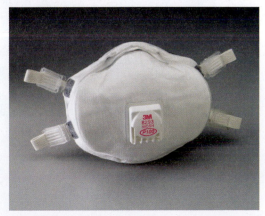

FIGURE 15–46B The P100 respirator mask. Courtesy of 3M Company, St. Paul, MN.

DROPLET PRECAUTIONS

Droplet precautions (**Figure 15–47**) must be followed for a patient known or suspected to be infected with pathogens transmitted by large-particle droplets expelled during coughing, sneezing, talking, or laughing. Examples of diseases requiring these isolation precautions include *Haemophilus influenzae* meningitis and pneumonia; *Neisseria* meningitis and pneumonia; multidrug-resistant *Streptococcus* meningitis, pneumonia, sinusitis, and otitis media; diphtheria; *Mycoplasma* pneumonia; pertussis; adenovirus; mumps; and severe viral influenza.

Standard precautions are used at all times. In addition, the following precautions must be taken:

- The patient should be placed in a private room. If a private room is not available and the patient cannot be placed in a room with a patient who has the same infection, a distance of at least 3 feet should separate the infected patient and other patients or visitors.

- Masks must be worn when entering the room.

- If transport or movement of the patient is essential, the patient must wear a surgical mask.

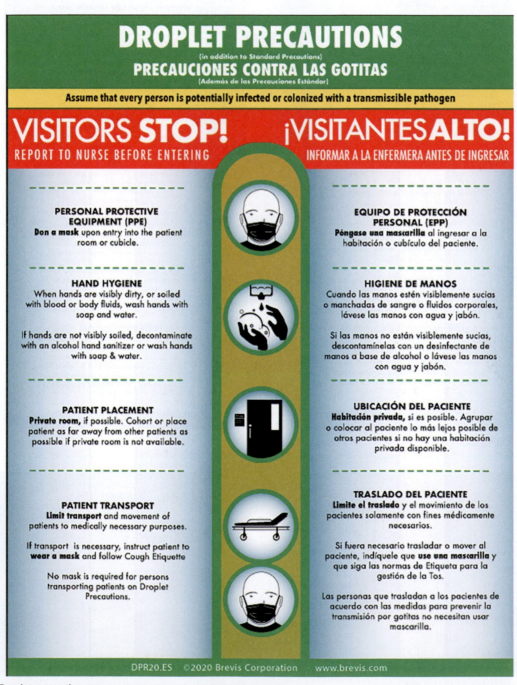

FIGURE 15–47 Droplet precautions. Reprinted with Permission from Brevis Corporation [www.brevis.com].

CONTACT PRECAUTIONS

Contact precautions (**Figure 15–48**) must be followed for any patients known or suspected to be infected with *epidemiological* (capable of spreading rapidly from person to person, an epidemic) microorganisms that can be transmitted by either direct or indirect contact. Examples of diseases requiring these precautions include any gastrointestinal, respiratory, skin, or wound infections caused by multidrug-resistant organisms; diapered or incontinent patients with enterohemorrhagic *E. coli*, *Shigella*, hepatitis A, or rotavirus; viral or hemorrhagic conjunctivitis or fevers; and any skin infections that are highly contagious or that may occur on dry skin, such as diphtheria, herpes simplex virus, impetigo, pediculosis (head or body lice), scabies, and staphylococcal infections. Standard precautions are used at all times. In addition, the following precautions must be taken:

- The patient should be placed in a private room or, if a private room is not available, in a room with a patient who has an active infection caused by the same organism.

- Gloves must be worn when entering the room.

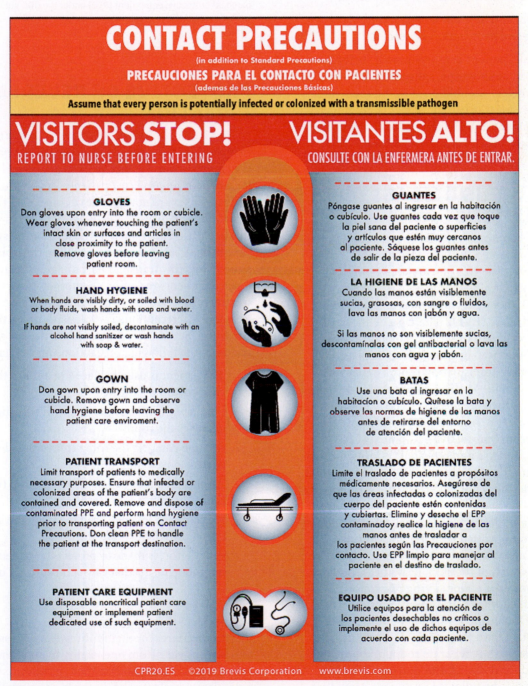

FIGURE 15–48 Contact precautions. Reprinted with Permission from Brevis Corporation [www.brevis.com].

- Gloves must be changed after having contact with any material that may contain high concentrations of the microorganism, such as wound drainage or fecal material.

- Gloves must be removed before leaving the room, and the hands must be washed with an antimicrobial agent.

- A gown must be worn in the room. The gown must be removed before leaving the room and care must be taken to ensure that clothing is not contaminated after gown removal.

- Movement and transport of the patient from the room should be for essential purposes only.

- The room and items in it must receive daily cleaning and disinfection as needed.

- If possible, patient-care equipment (bedside commode, stethoscope, sphygmomanometer, thermometer) should be left in the room and used only for this patient. If this is not possible, all equipment must be cleaned and disinfected before being used on another patient.

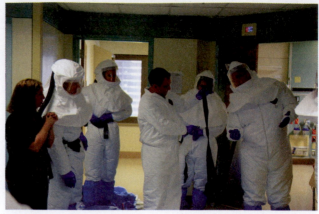

FIGURE 15–49 Intense and repeated training is required for donning personal protective equipment (PPE) under the CDC guidelines for Ebola virus disease (EVD) precautions. Courtesy of the CDC/U.S. DoD, Army Sgt. 1st Class Tyrone C. Marshall, Jr.

EBOLA VIRUS DISEASE (EVD) PRECAUTIONS

The first Ebola outbreak to reach epidemic proportions occurred in West Africa in 2014. In October of 2014, the CDC formulated more stringent infection control guidelines to be used when caring for patients with confirmed or suspected Ebola virus disease (EVD). These guidelines call for strict enforcement of standard, contact, and droplet precautions. The patient is to be placed in an airborne infection isolation room (AIIR) with restricted visitation. Medical equipment is dedicated to the patient whenever possible. The use of needles and blood draws are limited to necessity only. In addition, personal protective equipment (PPE) is a high priority. Intense and repeated training must be done to ensure that the correct PPE is used and that it is put on (donned) and taken off (doffed) properly (**Figure 15–49**). The proper order and procedure for donning and doffing is essential. The guidelines require a second trained staff member to supervise the donning and doffing of the PPE at all times. The PPE must cover all of the skin, head, neck, body, and feet. A powered air-purifying respirator (PAPR) or a N95 respirator (at a minimum) must be worn at all times. Double gloves should be worn when in direct contact with the patient. Diligent hand hygiene is essential. A separate room or area should be designated for donning and doffing of the PPE. All precautions must be followed by anyone providing care to an infected or suspected patient who has EVD.

PROTECTIVE OR REVERSE ISOLATION

Protective or reverse isolation refers to methods used to protect certain patients from organisms present in the environment. Protective isolation is used mainly for *immunocompromised* patients, or those whose body defenses are not capable of protecting them from infections and disease. Examples of patients who require this protection are patients whose immune systems have been depressed before receiving transplants (such as bone marrow transplants), patients who are severely burned, patients receiving chemotherapy or radiation treatments for cancer, or patients whose immune systems have failed. Precautions vary depending on the patient's condition. Standard precautions are used at all times. In addition, the following precautions may be taken:

- The patient is usually placed in a room that has been cleaned and disinfected

- Frequent disinfection occurs while the patient occupies the room

- Anyone entering the room must wear clean or sterile gowns, gloves, and masks

- All equipment or supplies brought into the room are clean, disinfected, or sterile

- Special filters may be used to purify the air that enters the room

- Every effort is made to protect the patient from microorganisms that cause infection or disease

SUMMARY

Exact procedures for maintaining transmission-based precautions vary from one facility to another. The procedures used depend on the type of units provided for isolation patients and on the kind of supplies or special isolation equipment available. Most facilities convert a regular patient room into an isolation room, but some facilities use special, two-room isolation units. Most facilities use disposable supplies such as gloves, gowns, and treatment packages. Therefore, it is essential that you learn the isolation procedure followed by your agency. However, the basic principles for maintaining transmission-based isolation are the same regardless of the facility. Therefore, if you know these basic principles, you will be able to adjust to any setting.

checkpoint

| **1.** What is reverse isolation?

PRACTICE: Go to the workbook and complete the assignment sheet for 15:9, Maintaining Transmission-Based Precautions. Then return and continue with the procedures.

Procedure 15:9A

Donning and Removing Transmission-Based Isolation Garments

OBRA

NOTE: The following procedure deals with contact transmission-based precautions. For other types of transmission-based precautions, follow only the steps that apply.

Equipment and Supplies

Isolation gown, surgical mask, gloves, googles and/or a face shield, small plastic bag, linen cart or container, infectious waste container, paper towels, sink with running water

Procedure

1. Assemble equipment.

   NOTE: In many agencies, clean isolation garments and supplies are kept available on a cart outside the isolation unit or in the outer room of a two-room unit. A waste container should be positioned just inside the door.

2. Wash hands.

3. Remove rings and place them in your pocket or pin them to your uniform.

4. Remove your watch and place it in a small plastic bag or centered on a clean paper towel. If placed on a towel, handle only the bottom part of the towel; do not touch the top.

   NOTE: The watch will be taken into the room and placed on the bedside stand for taking vital signs. Because it cannot be sterilized, it must be kept clean.

   NOTE: In some agencies, a plastic-covered watch is left in the isolation room or the room has a clock with a second hand.

5. If uniform sleeves are long, roll them up above the elbows before putting on the gown.

6. Lift the gown by placing your hands inside the shoulders.

NOTE: The inside of the gown and the ties at the neck are considered clean.

NOTE: Most agencies use disposable gowns that are discarded after use.

NOTE: In some agencies, a mask is applied before donning the gown. Either order is satisfactory.

7. Work your arms into the sleeves of the gown by gently twisting (**Figure 15–50A**). Take care not to touch your face with the sleeves of the gown.

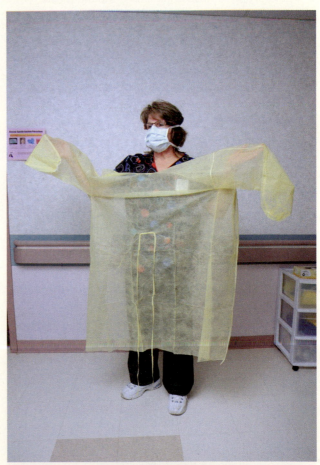

FIGURE 15–50A Put on the gown by placing your hands inside the shoulders to ease your arms into the sleeves.

(continues)

8. Place your hands *inside* the neckband, adjust until it is in position, and then tie the bands at the back of your neck (**Figure 15–50B**).

9. Reach behind and fold the edges of the gown over so that the uniform is completely covered. Tie the waistbands (**Figure 15–50C**). Some waistbands are long enough to wrap around your body before tying.

10. Put on the mask. Secure it under your chin. Make sure to cover your mouth and nose. Handle the mask as little as possible. Tie the mask securely behind your head and neck. Tie the top ties first and the bottom ties second .

    NOTE: The tie bands on the mask are considered clean. The mask is considered contaminated.

    ⊕ **Precaution** **CAUTION:** The mask is considered to be contaminated anytime it gets wet. If the mask gets wet, you must wash your hands, and remove and discard the old mask. Then wash your hands again, and put on a clean mask.

    NOTE: The policy in some facilities calls for the mask to be put into position before the gown. The CDC states that procedures will vary. Follow your agency policy regarding the order of donning the equipment.

11. If goggles or a face shield are to be worn, place the goggles or face shield over the face and eyes and adjust them to fit properly.

12. If gloves are to be worn, put them on. Make sure that the cuff of each glove comes over the top of the cuff of the gown (**Figure 15–50D**). In this way, there are no open areas for organisms to enter.

13. You are now ready to enter the isolation room. Double-check to be sure you have all equipment and supplies that you will need for patient care before you enter the room.

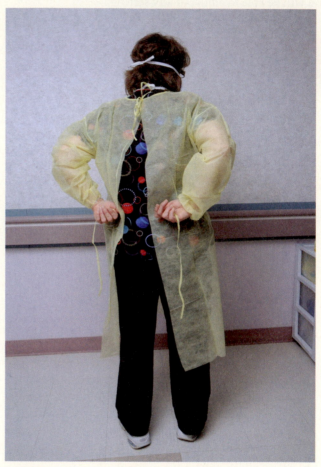

FIGURE 15–50C Tie the waist ties and make sure the back edges of the gown overlap to cover your uniform.

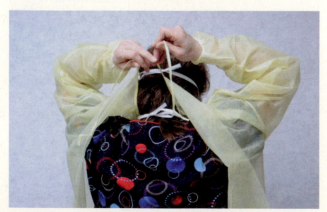

FIGURE 15–50B Slip your fingers inside the neckband to tie the gown at the neck.

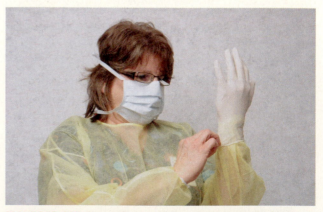

FIGURE 15–50D Put on gloves, making sure that the cuff of each glove is over the top of the cuff on the gown.

14. When patient care is complete, you will be ready to remove isolation garments. In a two-room isolation unit, go to the outer room. In a one-room unit, remove garments while you are standing close to the inside of the door. Take care to avoid touching the room's contaminated articles.

15. Untie the waist ties (**Figure 15–51A**), and loosen the gown at the waist.

    NOTE: The waist ties are considered contaminated.

16. If gloves are worn, remove the first glove by grasping the outside of the cuff with the opposite gloved hand. Pull the glove over the hand so that the glove is inside out (**Figure 15–51B**). Remove the second glove by placing the bare hand inside the cuff. Pull the glove off so it is inside out. Place the disposable gloves in the infectious waste container.

17. If goggles or a face shield are worn, remove the goggles or face shield from the back by lifting the head band or strap. Avoid touching the outside of either device. If they are disposable, place them in an infectious waste can. If they are reusable, place them in the proper container for disinfecting.

    ⚠️ **Safety** **CAUTION:** If you touch the contaminated outside of the goggles or face shield, wash your hands or use an alcohol-based hand cleaner.

18. Untie the neck ties (**Figure 15–51C**). Loosen the gown at the shoulders, handling only the inside of the gown.

    NOTE: The neck ties are considered clean.

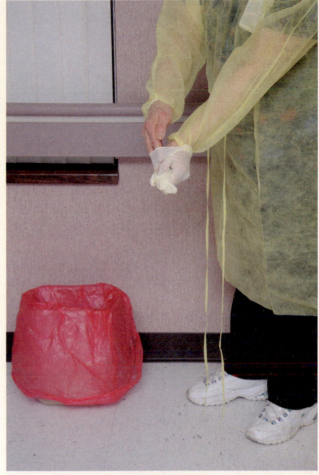

FIGURE 15–51B To remove the gloves, pull them over the hand so the glove is inside out.

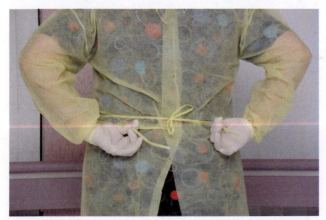

FIGURE 15–51A Untie the waist ties of the gown before removing the gloves.

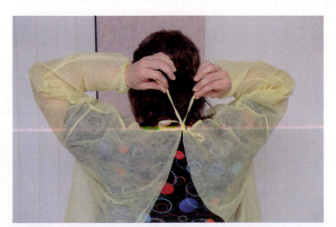

FIGURE 15–51C Untie the neck ties but avoid touching the outside of the gown.

(continues)

19. Slip the fingers of one hand inside the opposite cuff. Do *not* touch the outside. Pull the sleeve down over the hand (**Figure 15–51D**).

     CAUTION: The outside of the gown is considered contaminated and should not be touched.

    Safety

20. Using the gown-covered hand, pull the sleeve down over the opposite hand (**Figure 15–51E**).

21. Ease your arms and hands out of the gown. Keep the gown in front of your body and keep your hands away from the outside of the gown. Use as gentle a motion as possible.

    NOTE: Excessive flapping of the gown will spread organisms.

22. With your hands inside the gown at the shoulders, bring the shoulders together and turn the gown so that it is inside out (**Figure 15–51F**). In this manner, the outside of the contaminated gown is on the inside. Fold the gown in half and then roll it together. Place it in the infectious waste container (**Figure 15–51G**).

    NOTE: Avoid excess motion during this procedure because motion causes the spread of organisms.

23. Remove the mask next. Untie the bottom ties of the mask first followed by the top ties. Holding the mask by the top ties only, drop it into the infectious waste container

    NOTE: The ties of the mask are considered clean. Do not touch any other part of the mask, because it is considered contaminated.

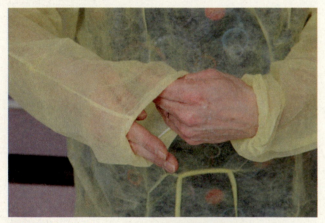

FIGURE 15–51D To remove the gown, slip the fingers of one hand under the cuff of the opposite arm to pull the gown down over the opposite hand.

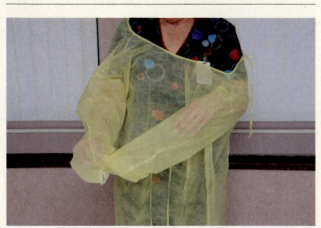

FIGURE 15–51E Using the gown-covered hand, grasp the outside of the gown on the opposite arm and pull the gown down over the hand.

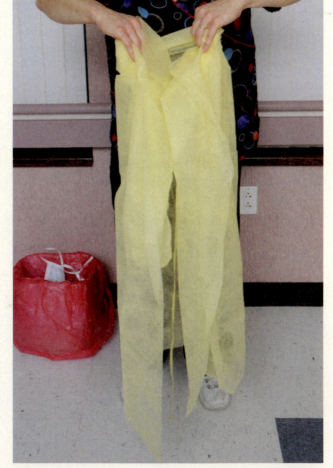

FIGURE 15–51F With your hands inside the gown at the shoulders, bring the shoulders together and turn the gown so it is inside out, with the contaminated side on the inside.

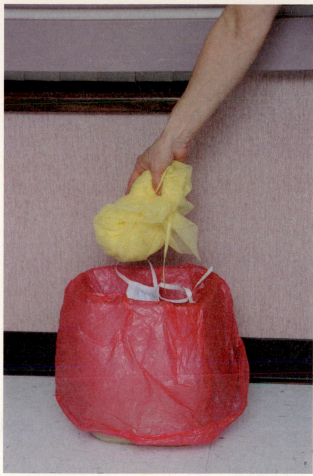

FIGURE 15–51G After folding the gown, discard it in an infectious waste container.

24. To avoid unnecessary transmission of organisms, use paper towels to turn on the water faucet. Wash and dry your hands thoroughly. Use dry, clean paper towels to turn off the water faucet.

25. Touch only the inside of the plastic bag to remove your watch. Discard the bag in the waste container. If the watch is on a paper towel, handle only the "clean," top portion (if necessary). Discard the towel in the infectious waste container.

26. Use a clean paper towel to open the door. Discard the towel in the waste container before leaving the room.

 CAUTION: The inside of the door is considered contaminated.

NOTE: The waste container should be positioned just inside the door of the room.

27. After leaving the isolation room, wash hands thoroughly. This will help prevent the spread of the disease. It also protects you from the illness.

PRACTICE: Go to the workbook and use the evaluation sheet for 15:9A, Donning and Removing Transmission-Based Isolation Garments, to practice this procedure. When you believe you have mastered this skill, sign the sheet and give it to your instructor for further action.

 FINAL EVALUATION: Using the criteria listed on the evaluation sheet, your instructor will grade your performance.

Working in a Hospital Transmission-Based Isolation Unit

OBRA

NOTE: The following procedure describes some basic methods of working in an isolation room. These will vary from facility to facility. *It is essential for you to learn and follow your agency's policies.*

Equipment and Supplies

Clothes hamper, two laundry bags, two trays, dishes, cups, bowls, waste container lined with a plastic bag, infectious waste bags, bags, tape, pencil, pen, paper

Procedure

1. Assemble all equipment.

   NOTE: Any equipment or supplies to be used in the isolation room must be assembled before entering the room.

2. Wash hands.

3. Put on appropriate isolation garments as previously instructed.

4. Tape paper to the outside of the isolation door. This will be used to record vital signs.

5. Enter the isolation room. Take all needed equipment into the room.

6. **Comm** Introduce yourself. Greet and identify patient. Provide patient care as needed.

   NOTE: All care is provided in a routine manner. However, transmission-based isolation garments must be worn as ordered.

7. To record vital signs:

   a. Take vital signs using the watch in the plastic bag. (If the watch is not in a plastic bag, hold it with the bottom part of a paper towel.) Use other equipment in the room as needed.

   b. Open the door touching only the inside, or contaminated side.

   c. Using a pencil, record the vital signs on the paper taped to the door. Do not touch the outside of the door at any time.

   NOTE: The pencil remains in the room because it is contaminated.

8. To transfer food into the isolation unit:

   a. The transfer of food requires two people; one person must stay outside the unit and one inside.

   b. The person inside the isolation unit picks up the empty tray in the room and opens the door, touching only the inside of the door.

   c. The person outside holds the tray while the dishes are being transferred (**Figure 15–52**).

   d. When transferring food, the two people should handle the opposite sides of the dishes. In this manner, one person will not touch the other person.

   e. Glasses should be held near the top by the transfer person on the outside. The transfer person on the inside should receive the glasses by holding them on the bottom.

9. To dispose of leftover food or waste:

   a. Liquids can be poured down the sink or flushed down the toilet.

   b. Soft foods such as mashed potatoes or cooked vegetables can be flushed down the toilet.

   c. Hard particles of food, such as bone, should be placed in the plastic-lined trash container.

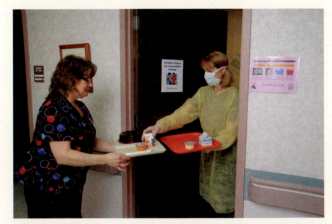

FIGURE 15–52 To transfer food into an isolation unit, a health worker holds the tray so the worker in isolation can transfer the food onto the tray kept inside the unit.

d. Disposable utensils or dishes should be placed in the plastic-lined trash container.

e. Metal utensils should be washed and kept in the isolation room to be used as needed for other meals. These utensils, however, are contaminated. When they are removed from the isolation room, they must be disinfected or double bagged and labeled before being sent for decontamination and reprocessing.

10. To transfer soiled linen from the unit, two people are required:

a. All dirty linen should be folded and rolled.

b. Place linen in the isolation linen bag.

c. The person outside the unit should cuff the top of a clean infectious waste laundry bag and hold it. Hands should be kept on the inside of the bag's cuff to avoid contamination.

d. The person in isolation should seal the isolation linen bag. The bag is then placed inside the outer bag, which is being held by the person outside (**Figure 15–53**).

e. The outer bag should be folded over at the top and taped by the person outside. The bag should be labeled as "BIOHAZARDOUS LINEN."

f. At all times, no direct contact should occur between the two people transferring linen.

NOTE: Many agencies use special isolation linen bags. Hot water dissolves the bags during the washing process. Therefore, no other personnel handle the contaminated linen after it leaves the isolation unit.

11. To transfer trash from the isolation unit, two people are required:

a. Any trash in the isolation room should be in plastic bags. Any trash or disposable items contaminated with blood, body fluids, secretions, or excretions should be placed in infectious waste bags.

b. When the bag is full, expel excess air by pushing gently on the bag.

c. Tie a knot at the top of the bag to seal it or fold the top edge twice and tape it securely.

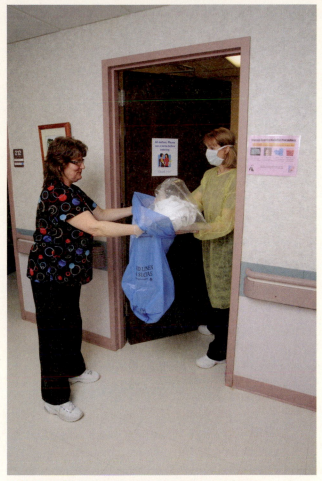

FIGURE 15–53 To transfer linen from an isolation unit, the worker in the unit places the sealed bag containing the infectious linen inside a second bag held by a "clean" worker outside the unit.

d. Place this bag inside a cuffed biohazardous waste bag held by a "clean" person outside the unit.

e. The outside person then ties the outer bag securely or tapes the outer bag shut.

f. The double-bagged trash should then be burned. Double-bagged infectious waste is autoclaved before incineration or disposal as infectious waste according to legal requirements.

g. At all times, direct contact between the two people transferring trash must be avoided.

(continues)

12. To transfer equipment from the isolation unit, two people are required:

    a. Thoroughly clean and disinfect all equipment in the unit.

    b. After cleaning, place equipment in a plastic bag or special isolation bag. Label the bag with the contents and the word "ISOLATION."

    c. After folding the bag down twice at the top, tape the bag shut.

    d. A second person outside the isolation room should hold a second, cuffed infectious waste bag.

    e. The person in isolation places the sealed, contaminated bag inside the bag being held outside the unit. The person in isolation should have no direct contact with the clean bag.

    f. The person outside the unit turns down the top of the infectious waste bag twice and securely tapes the bag. The outside person then labels the bag with the contents, for example, "ISOLATION DISHES."

    g. The double-bagged material is then sent to Central Supply or another designated area for sterilization and/or decontamination.

13. The transmission-based isolation unit must be kept clean and neat at all times. Equipment no longer needed should be transferred out of the unit using the appropriate isolation technique.

14. Before leaving an isolation room, ask the patient whether a urinal or bedpan is needed. This will save time and energy by reducing the need to return to provide additional patient care shortly after leaving. Also, before leaving, check all safety and comfort points to make sure patient care is complete.

15. Remove isolation garments as previously instructed in Procedure 15:9A.

16. Wash hands thoroughly.

PRACTICE: Go to the workbook and use the evaluation sheet for 15:9B, Working in a Hospital Transmission-Based Isolation Unit, to practice this procedure. When you believe you have mastered this skill, sign the sheet and give it to your instructor for further action.

FINAL EVALUATION: Using the criteria listed on the evaluation sheet, your instructor will grade your performance.

Paint Away Those Germs?

Health care–associated infections (HAIs) are a major problem for health care providers. The Centers for Disease Control and Prevention (CDC) estimates that one out of every 31 patients receiving health care may acquire an HAI. In addition, the CDC estimates that HAIs in hospitals alone result in 10 billion dollars of excess medical costs every year. Methicillin-resistant *Staphylococcus aureus*, commonly called MRSA, is one of the most common HAIs. MRSA is a bacterium that causes severe infections in humans. It is difficult to treat because it is resistant to many antibiotics, which means the antibiotics will not eliminate the organism.

Now, thanks to biotechnology researchers at the Rensselaer Polytechnic Institute, it is possible to use paint to kill MRSA germs. The researchers studied a naturally occurring enzyme, lysostaphin, that is used by nonpathogenic (non-disease producing) strains of staphylococcus bacteria to defend themselves against *Staphylococcus aureus*. Lysostaphin is harmless to humans and toxic only to MRSA. It is not an antibiotic to which bacteria could become resistant, and it does not leach chemicals into the environment. Lysostaphin kills MRSA bacteria by slicing open the cell wall, causing the MRSA cell to literally explode and die.

One problem encountered during the research was that the lysostaphin was not stable and would not remain in other substances for long periods. The researchers solved this problem by packing the lysostaphin in carbon nanotubes, tiny structures that lock the enzyme in place. The nanotubes containing the enzyme were then put in a can of ordinary house paint, which was used to paint a wall. Studies showed that 100 percent of MRSA organisms were destroyed when they came in contact with the paint. The paint remained effective even after repeated washings. Recently, the Environmental Protection Agency (EPA) registered a microbicidal paint that kills greater than 99 percent of MRSA (methicillin-resistant *Staphylococcus aureus*), E. coli (*Escherichia coli*), and VRE (Vancomycin-resistant *Enterococcus faecalis*) pathogens within 2 hours of exposure on painted surfaces. Within several years, this initial research could provide many benefits for both health care and other commercial products. By creating coatings containing nanotubes of lysostaphin, commercial products could be developed for walls, furniture, medical equipment, food-processing equipment, and even items such as shoes, masks, or hospital gowns. If this happens, a simple, inexpensive, naturally occurring substance could prevent HAI infections, save lives, and decrease medical costs.

Case Study Investigation Conclusion

What PPE would allow Andrea and Ryan to work safely in the Emergency Department in the middle of COVID-19? As health care team members became ill, Andrea and Ryan had to cross-train in other areas of the hospital, for example, transport and ICU. Would these new duties affect the type of PPE and isolation techniques they would need to use?

CHAPTER 15 SUMMARY

- Understanding the basic principles of infection control is essential for any health care provider in any health care field. Disease is caused by a wide variety of pathogens. An understanding of the types of pathogens, methods of transmission, and the chain of infection allows health care providers to take precautions to prevent the spread of disease.

- Bioterrorism is the use of microorganisms as weapons to infect humans, animals, or plants. Careful preparation of a comprehensive plan against bioterrorism and thorough training of all individuals can limit the effect of the attack and save the lives of many people.

- Asepsis is defined as "the absence of disease-producing microorganisms, or pathogens." Antisepsis refers to methods that prevent or inhibit the growth of pathogenic organisms.

- Disinfection is a process that uses chemical disinfectants to destroy or kill pathogenic organisms, but it is not always effective against spores and viruses.

- Sterilization is a process that destroys all microorganisms, including spores and viruses.

- Following the standard precautions established by the CDC helps prevent the spread of pathogens by way of blood, body fluids, secretions, and excretions. The standard precautions provide guidelines for handwashing; wearing gloves; using gowns, masks, and protective eyewear when splashing is likely; proper handling and disposal of contaminated sharp objects; proper disposal of contaminated waste; and proper methods to wipe up spills of blood, body fluids, secretions, and excretions.

- Sterile techniques are used in specific procedures, such as changing dressings. Health care providers must learn and follow sterile techniques when they are required to perform these procedures.

- Transmission-based precautions are used for patients who have communicable diseases. An awareness of the major types of transmission-based precautions presented in this unit will help the health care provider prevent the transmission of communicable diseases.

- Infection control must be followed when performing every health care procedure. By learning and following the principles discussed in this unit, health care providers will protect themselves, patients, and others from disease.

REVIEW QUESTIONS

1. Differentiate between antisepsis, disinfection, and sterilization.

2. List the five (5) essential times for handwashing as identified by the World health Organization (WHO).

3. Name the different types of personal protective equipment (PPE) and state when each type must be worn to meet the requirements of standard precautions.

4. What level of infection control is achieved by an ultrasonic cleaner? Chemicals? An autoclave?

5. Name three (3) methods that can be used to place sterile items on a sterile field. Identify the types of items that can be transferred by each method.

6. Which side of sterile gloves is considered contaminated?

7. List the three (3) main types of transmission-based precautions and the basic principles that must be followed for each type.

8. What special precautions for personal protective equipment (PPE) must be followed under the CDC guidelines for Ebola virus disease (EVD)?

CRITICAL THINKING

1. List the six (6) classifications of microorganisms and describe the characteristics of each. What is the treatment for each type of microorganism?

2. Develop a plan showing at least four (4) ways you can protect yourself and your family from a bioterrorism attack.

3. When completing a sterile dressing change, why do you use nonsterile gloves when removing the old dressing?

ACTIVITIES

1. With a partner, research the effects of practices of sanitation and disinfection on health and wellness. Include the implications for public health during the COVID-19 pandemic. Present your findings to the class, citing evidence from your investigation.

2. In a small group, pick a disease from the list below. Create a flow chart that lists the six (6) components of the chain of infection as applied to this disease and strategies to break each part of the chain.

- COVID-19
- tuberculosis
- dysentery
- pneumonia
- Ebola
- herpes
- MRSA infection (from wound drainage)
- AIDS

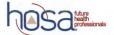 | **CONNECTION**

Competitive Event: Epidemiology

Event Summary: Epidemiology provides members with the opportunity to gain knowledge in regard to health and disease in populations. This competitive event consists of a written examination of concepts related to the study of epidemiology. Competitors are expected to recognize, identify, define, interpret, and apply these concepts in a multiple choice test.

This event aims to inspire members to be proactive future health professionals and improve their scientific literacy as well as provide insights into public health careers.

Details on this competition can be found at

www.hosa.org/guidelines

Case Study Investigation

DeShawn is a 32-year-old man who was a former football player and is now working construction. He is married with two children and just got laid off last month. He is 6'4" tall and weighs 280 lbs. DeShawn hasn't been to the doctor in 3 years but goes to Dr. Elliott after experiencing a persistent headache and dizziness. Suspecting hypertension, Dr. Elliott asks him to stop by the office every afternoon for two weeks to have his blood pressure monitored. At the end of this chapter, you will be asked why this is a good plan for DeShawn.

◾ LEARNING OBJECTIVES

After completing this chapter, you should be able to:

- List the five main vital signs.
- Read a clinical thermometer to the nearest two-tenths of a degree.
- Measure and record oral temperature accurately.
- Measure and record rectal temperature accurately.
- Measure and record axillary temperature accurately.
- Measure and record tympanic (aural) temperature accurately.
- Measure and record temporal temperature accurately.
- Measure and record radial pulse to an accuracy within ±2 beats per minute.
- Count and record respirations to an accuracy within ±1 respiration per minute.
- Measure and record apical pulse to an accuracy within ±2 beats per minute.
- Measure and record blood pressure to an accuracy within ±2 mm of actual reading.
- State the normal range for oral, axillary, and rectal temperature; pulse; respirations; and systolic and diastolic pressure.
- Define, pronounce, and spell all key terms.

■ KEY TERMS

apical pulse *(ape'-ih-kal)*

apnea *(ap'-nee"-ah)*

arrhythmia *(ah-rith'-me-ah)*

aural temperature

axillary temperature

blood pressure

bradycardia *(bray'-dee-car'-dee-ah)*

bradypnea *(brad"-ip-nee'-ah)*

character

Cheyne-Stokes *(chain'-stokes")*

clinical thermometers

cyanosis

diastolic *(die"-ah-stall'-ik)*

dyspnea *(dis(p)'-nee"-ah)*

electronic thermometers

fever

homeostasis *(home"-ee-oh-stay'-sis)*

hypertension

hyperthermia *(high-pur-therm'-ee-ah)*

hypotension

hypothermia *(high-po-therm'-ee-ah)*

noncontact infrared thermometer

oral temperature

orthopnea *(of"-thop-nee'-ah)*

pain

pulse

pulse deficit

pulse oximeter

pulse pressure

pyrexia

rales (rawls)

rate

rectal temperature

respirations

rhythm

sphygmomanometer *(sfig"-moh-ma-nam'-eh-ter)*

stethoscope *(steth'-uh-scope)*

systolic *(sis"-tall'-ik)*

tachycardia *(tack"-eh-car'-dee-ah)*

tachypnea *(tack"-ip-nee'-ah)*

temperature

temporal scanning thermometers

temporal temperature

tympanic thermometers

vital signs

volume

wheezing

LEGAL ALERT

Legal Before performing any procedures in this chapter, know and follow the standards and regulations established by the scope of practice; federal laws and agencies; state laws; state or national licensing, registration, or certification boards; professional organizations; professional standards; and agency policies.

It is your responsibility to learn exactly what you are legally permitted to do and to perform only procedures for which you have been trained.

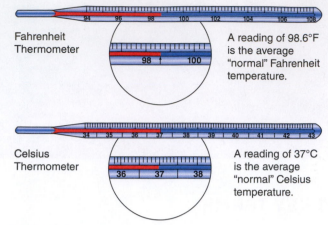

Fahrenheit Thermometer

A reading of 98.6°F is the average "normal" Fahrenheit temperature.

Celsius Thermometer

A reading of 37°C is the average "normal" Celsius temperature.

FIGURE 16–1 Normal oral body temperature on Fahrenheit and Celsius thermometers.

16:1 MEASURING AND RECORDING VITAL SIGNS

Vital signs are defined as various determinations that provide information about the basic body conditions of the patient. The five main vital signs are temperature, pulse, respirations, blood pressure, and pain. Other important vital signs that provide information about the patient's condition include a measurement of the percentage of oxygen in the blood, the color of the skin, the size of the pupils in the eyes and their reaction to light, the level of consciousness, and the patient's response to stimuli. As a health care provider, it will be your responsibility to measure and record the vital signs of patients. It is essential that vital signs be accurate. They are often the first indication of a disease or abnormality in the patient.

Temperature is a measurement of the balance between heat lost and heat produced by the body. Temperature can be measured in the mouth (oral), rectum (rectal), armpit (axillary), ear (aural), by the temporal artery in the forehead (temporal), or on surface of the skin with a noncontact thermometer. A low or high reading can indicate disease. Most temperatures are measured in degrees on a thermometer that has a Fahrenheit scale. However, some health care facilities are now measuring temperature in degrees on a Celsius (centigrade) scale. A comparison of the two scales is shown in **Figure 16–1** and in Appendix C. At times, it may be necessary to convert Fahrenheit temperatures to Celsius, or Celsius to Fahrenheit. The formulas for the conversion are discussed in detail in Section 13:6 of this text.

Pulse is the pressure of the blood felt against the wall of an artery as the heart contracts and relaxes, or beats. The rate, rhythm, and volume are recorded. **Rate** refers to the number of beats per minute, **rhythm** refers to regularity, and **volume** refers to strength, force, or quality. The pulse

is usually taken over the radial artery, although it may be felt over any superficial artery that has a bone behind it. Any abnormality can indicate disease.

Respirations reflect the breathing rate of the patient. In addition to the respiration count, the rhythm (regularity) and character (type) of respirations are noted. Abnormal respirations usually indicate that a health problem or disease is present.

Blood pressure is the force exerted by the blood against the arterial walls when the heart contracts or relaxes. Two readings (systolic and diastolic) are noted to show the greatest pressure and the least pressure. Both are very important. Abnormal blood pressure is often the first indication of disease.

Pain is an unpleasant sensation that is perceived in the nervous system when illness or injury occurs. Pain can be acute or chronic. Acute pain lasts for a short amount of time, as with post-operative pain or pain from a physical injury. Chronic pain is long term, as with cancer pain, arthritis, or other on-going illness. When assessing pain, it is important to remember that pain is what the person says it is. Only they can describe what they are feeling. Pain is a very individual experience and everyone tolerates it differently. Some people have a high pain tolerance and complain very little, even when they are in severe pain. Others with a low tolerance may cry and yell out with the slightest amount of pain. Pain can be measured using a scale of 0 to 10, with 0 being no pain, 1 being very mild pain, and 10 being the worst pain imaginable. The patient states what number they perceive the pain to be, and pain control can be administered accordingly. After the patient has received treatment, the health care provider should ask again what they perceive the pain to be to assess how effective the treatment was. If the patient is unable to rate their pain with a number, a series of faces ranging from happy to very sad can be shown to describe how they are feeling (**Figure 16–2**). A patient must be assessed for pain frequently because it is often the first sign of a problem.

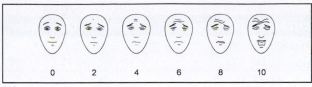

(A)

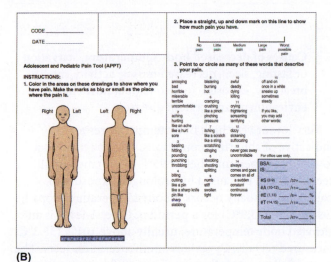

(B)

FIGURE 16–2 (A) Pain can be measured by asking the patient to rate the level of pain on a scale of 0 to 10. (B) For children, a special scale tool can be used that will allow a child to color an area of the body where they have pain or to circle words that can help describe what they are feeling. Top image, Hicks CL, von Baeyer CL, Spafford P, van Korlaar I, Goodenough B. Faces Pain-Scale-Revised: Toward a Common Metric in Pediatric Pain Measurement. PAIN 2001; 93: 173-183. With the instructions and translations as found on the website www.iasp-pain.org/FPSR; Bottom image, From Savedra, M., Tesller, M., Holzemer, W., & Ward, J. (1992). University of California, San Francisco, School of Nursing, San Francisco, CA 94143-0606. Copyright © 1989, 1992. Used with permission.

Another vital sign is the apical pulse. This pulse is taken with a stethoscope at the apex of the heart. The actual heartbeat is heard and counted. At times, because of illness, hardening of the arteries, a weak or very rapid radial pulse, or doctor's orders, you will be required to take an apical pulse. Also, because infants and small children have a very rapid radial pulse that is difficult to count, apical pulses are usually taken.

Comm
If you note any abnormality or change in any vital sign, it is your responsibility to report this immediately to your supervisor. If you have difficulty obtaining a correct reading, ask another individual to check the patient. Never guess or report an inaccurate reading.

checkpoint

1. What are the five (5) areas where temperature can be measured?

PRACTICE: Go to the workbook and complete the assignment sheet for 16:1, Measuring and Recording Vital Signs.

16:2 MEASURING AND RECORDING TEMPERATURE

OBRA

Legal
Body temperature is one of the main vital signs. Guidelines for measuring and recording temperature will vary depending on state laws and policies of health care agencies. It is your legal responsibility to know and follow the guidelines for your state and agency.

Science
Temperature is defined as "the balance between heat lost and heat produced by the body." Heat is lost through perspiration, respiration, and excretion (urine and feces). Heat is produced by the metabolism of food and by muscle and gland activity. A constant state of fluid balance, known as **homeostasis**, is the ideal health state in the human body. The rates of chemical reactions in the body are regulated by body temperature. Therefore, if body temperature is too high or too low, the body's fluid balance and homeostatic state is affected.

VARIATIONS IN BODY TEMPERATURE

The normal range for body temperature is 97°–100° Fahrenheit, or 36.1°–37.8° Celsius (sometimes called centigrade). However, variations in body temperature can occur. Some reasons for variations include:

- **Individual differences**: some people have accelerated body processes and usually have higher temperatures; others have slower body processes and usually have lower temperatures

- **Time of day**: body temperature is usually lower in the morning, after the body has rested, and higher in the evening, after muscular activity and daily food intake have taken place

- **Body sites**: parts of the body where temperatures are taken lead to variations; temperature variations by body site are shown in **Table 16–1**.

Oral temperatures are taken in the mouth. This is usually the most common, convenient, and comfortable method of obtaining a temperature. Eating, drinking hot or cold liquids, and/or smoking can alter the temperature in the mouth. It is important to make sure the patient has *not* had anything to eat or drink or has *not* smoked for at least 15 minutes prior to taking the patient's oral temperature. If the patient has done any of these things, explain why you cannot take the temperature and that you will return to do so.

TABLE 16–1 Average Temperature Variations by Body Site

	Oral and/or Tympanic	Rectal, Aural, and/or Temporal	Axillary and/or Groin
Average Temperature	98.6°F (37°C)	99.6°F (37.6°C)	97.6°F (36.4°C)
Normal Range of Temperature	97.6°F–99.6°F (36.5°C–37.5°C)	98.6°F–100.6°F (37°C–38.1°C)	96.6°F–98.6°F (36°C–37°C)

Rectal temperatures are taken in the rectum. This is an internal measurement and is the most accurate of all methods. Rectal temperatures are frequently taken on infants and small children and on patients with hypothermia (below-normal body temperature).

Axillary temperatures are taken in the armpit, under the upper arm. The arm is held close to the body, and the thermometer is inserted between the two folds of skin. A *groin* temperature is taken between the two folds of skin formed by the inner part of the thigh and the lower abdomen. Both axillary and groin are external temperatures and, thus, less accurate.

Science

Aural temperatures are taken with a special tympanic thermometer that is placed in the ear or auditory canal. The thermometer detects and measures the thermal, infrared energy radiating from blood vessels in the tympanic membrane, or eardrum. Because this provides a measurement of body core temperature, the range is similar to rectal or internal body temperature. Most tympanic thermometers record temperature in less than 2 seconds; so, this is a fast and convenient method for obtaining temperature. However, a drawback to using tympanic thermometers is that inaccurate results will be obtained if the thermometer is not inserted into the ear correctly or if an ear infection or a wax buildup is present.

Temporal temperatures are taken with a special temporal scanning thermometer that is passed in a straight line across the forehead, midway between the eyebrows and upper hairline. The thermometer measures the temperature in the temporal artery to provide an accurate measurement of blood temperature. A normal temporal temperature is similar to a rectal temperature because it measures the temperature inside the body or bloodstream. Because a temporal scanning thermometer is easy to use and usually produces accurate results, it is a common way to record body temperature. However, if the forehead has a wig or covering on it, is lying on a pillow, or has profuse perspiration on it, an inaccurate result may be obtained.

Body temperatures can be above or below the normal range for a variety of reasons:

- **Causes of increased body temperature**: illness, infection, exercise, excitement, and high temperatures in the environment

- **Causes of decreased body temperature**: starvation or fasting, sleep, decreased muscle activity, mouth breathing, exposure to cold temperatures in the environment, and certain diseases

Very low or very high body temperatures are indicative of abnormal conditions. **Hypothermia** is a low body temperature, below 95°F (35°C) measured rectally. It can be caused by prolonged exposure to cold. Death usually occurs if body temperature drops below 93°F (33.9°C) for a period of time. A **fever** is an elevated body temperature, usually above 101°F (38.3°C) measured rectally. **Pyrexia** is another term for fever. The term *febrile* means a fever is present; *afebrile* means no fever is present or the temperature is within the normal range. Fevers are usually caused by infection or injury. **Hyperthermia** occurs when the body temperature exceeds 104°F (40°C) measured rectally. It can be caused by prolonged exposure to hot temperatures, brain damage, and serious infections. Immediate actions must be taken to lower body temperature because temperatures above 106°F (41.1°C) can quickly lead to convulsions, brain damage, and death.

TYPES OF THERMOMETERS

Clinical thermometers may be used to record temperatures, but very few health care agencies use them. A clinical thermometer consists of a slender glass tube containing mercury or a heat-reactive mercury-free liquid such as alcohol, which expands when exposed to heat. Thermometers containing mercury are banned in many states. This is supported by the World Health Organization (WHO), the National Institutes of Health (NIH), the U.S. Environmental Protection Agency (EPA), and the American Hospital Association.

There are different types of clinical thermometers (**Figure 16–3**). The glass oral thermometer has a long, slender bulb or a blue tip. A security oral thermometer has a shorter, rounder bulb and is usually marked with a blue tip. A rectal thermometer has a short, stubby, rounded bulb and may be marked with a red tip. Disposable plastic sheaths may be used to cover the thermometer when it is used on a patient.

Electronic thermometers are used in most health care facilities. This type of thermometer uses a heat sensor to record temperature and displays the temperature

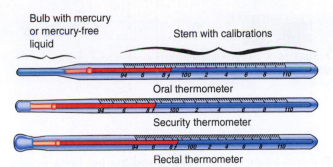

Bulb with mercury or mercury-free liquid

Stem with calibrations

Oral thermometer

Security thermometer

Rectal thermometer

FIGURE 16–3 Types of clinical thermometers.

on a viewer in a few seconds (**Figure 16–4**). Electronic thermometers can be used to take oral, rectal, axillary, and/or groin temperatures. Most facilities have electronic thermometers with blue probes for oral or axillary use and red probes for rectal use. To prevent cross-contamination, a disposable cover is placed over the thermometer probe before the temperature is taken. By changing the

disposable cover after each use, one unit can be used on many patients. Electronic digital thermometers are excellent for home use because they eliminate the hazard of a mercury spill that occurs when a clinical thermometer containing mercury is broken (**Figure 16–5**). The small battery-operated unit usually will register the temperature in about 60 seconds on a digital display screen. Disposable probe covers prevent contamination of the probe.

Tympanic thermometers are specialized electronic thermometers that use an infrared ray to record the aural temperature in the ear (**Figure 16–6**). A disposable plastic cover is placed on the ear probe. By inserting the probe into the auditory canal and pushing a scan button, the temperature is recorded on the screen within 1–2 seconds. It is important to read and follow instructions while using this thermometer to obtain an accurate reading.

Temporal scanning thermometers are specialized electronic thermometers that use an infrared scanner to measure the temperature in the temporal artery of the forehead (**Figure 16–7**). The

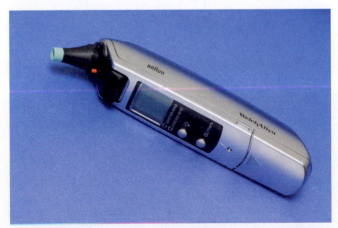

Oral Probe

Disposable probe cover

Rectal probe

FIGURE 16–4 An electronic thermometer registers the temperature in easy-to-read numbers on a viewer.

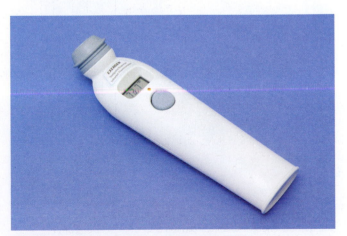

FIGURE 16–5 Electronic digital thermometers are excellent for home use.

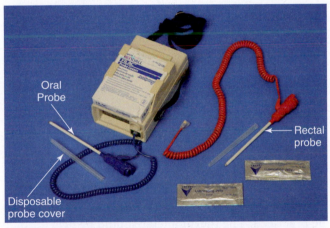

FIGURE 16–6 Tympanic thermometers record the aural temperature in the ear.

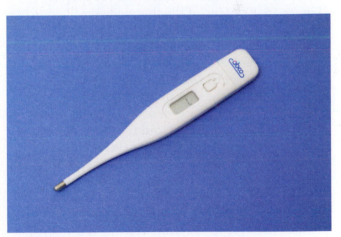

FIGURE 16–7 Temporal scanning thermometers measure the temperature in the temporal artery of the forehead.

thermometer probe is placed on the forehead and passed in a straight line across the forehead, midway between the eyebrows and upper hairline. In this area, the temporal artery is less than 2 millimeters (mm) below the skin surface and easy to find. The temperature registers on the screen in 1–2 seconds. This thermometer provides an accurate measurement of internal body temperature, is easy to use, and is noninvasive. It is important to make sure that the area of forehead scanned is not covered by hair, a wig, or a hat. If the person's head is lying on a pillow, the side of the forehead by the pillow should not be used for the measurement. Any type of head covering or a pillow prevents heat from dissipating and causes the reading to be falsely high. In addition, if the forehead has profuse perspiration, a cooling of the skin could cause falsely low readings.

Noncontact infrared thermometers (NCITs) use light wavelength technology to measure the thermal energy radiating from the skin without requiring any physical contact with the person (**Figure 16–8**). Many of the thermometers resemble the shape of a gun so they can be easily pointed at a person and held steady for an accurate temperature measurement. Some of the thermometers use a laser light that can be positioned on the skin to see where the temperature is being recorded. The thermometers are easy to use, and they record the temperature in a matter of seconds. Most models require holding a trigger down until a laser appears or the unit indicates it has been activated. While holding the trigger down, the thermometer is pointed toward the person and held as steady as possible until the temperature reading is displayed

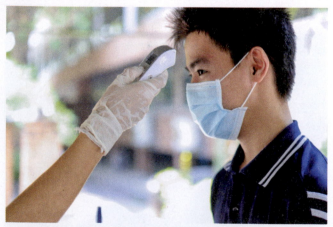

FIGURE 16–8 Non-contact infrared thermometers can measure the thermal energy radiating from the skin without having any physical contact with the individual whose temperature is being measured.

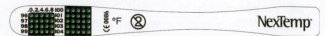

FIGURE 16–9 Plastic disposable thermometers have chemical dots that change color to register body temperature. Courtesy Medical Indicators, Inc.

on the screen. It is important to make sure that the area being checked is dry and has not been covered with clothing. Since these thermometers measure the surface temperature rather than internal temperature, normal range usually is comparable to axillary or groin temperatures. This type of thermometer was used widely during the COVID-19 pandemic and is ideal for screening the temperatures of many individuals quickly and accurately with no contamination of the thermometer.

Plastic or paper disposable thermometers are used in some health care facilities and in homes (**Figure 16–9**). These thermometers contain special chemical dots or strips that change color when exposed to specific temperatures. Some types are placed on the forehead and skin temperature is recorded. Other types are used orally. Both types are used once and discarded.

READING AND RECORDING TEMPERATURE

Electronic, tympanic, temporal, and noncontact infrared thermometers are easy to read because they have digital displays. Reading a glass clinical thermometer is a procedure that must be practiced. The thermometer should be held at eye level and rotated slowly to find the solid column of mercury or mercury-free liquid (**Figure 16–10**). The thermometer is read at the point where the liquid line ends. Each long line on a thermometer is read as 1 degree. An exception to this is the long line for 98.6°F (37°C), which is the normal oral body temperature. Each short line represents 0.2 (two-tenths) of a degree. Temperature is always recorded to the next nearest two-tenths of a degree. In **Figure 16–11**, the line ends at 98.6°F (the inset explains the markings for each line).

 To record the temperature, write 98[6] instead of 98.6. This reduces the possibility of making

Comm an error in reading. For example, a temperature of 100.2 could easily be read as 102. By writing 100[2], the chance of error decreases. If a temperature is taken orally, it is not necessary to indicate that it is an oral reading.

If it is taken rectally, place an (R) beside the recording; if in the axillary area, use an (Ax); if in the eardrum or tympanically (aurally), use an (A) or (T) or (Tym); and if over the temporal artery, or temporally, use a (TA). For example:

- 98⁶ is an oral reading
- 99⁶ (R) is a rectal reading
- 97⁶ (Ax) is an axillary reading
- 98⁶ (A) is an aural reading
- 99⁶ (TA) is a temporal artery reading

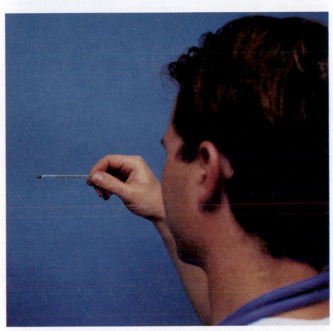

FIGURE 16–10 A clinical thermometer must be held at eye level to find the solid column of mercury or mercury-free liquid.

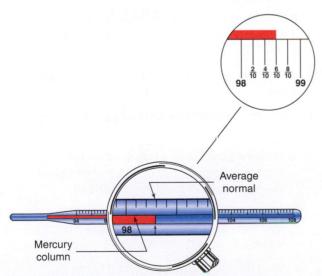

Average normal

Mercury column

FIGURE 16–11 Each line on a thermometer equals two-tenths of a degree, so the thermometer shown reads 98.6°F.

CLEANING THERMOMETERS

Thermometers must be cleaned thoroughly after use. The procedure used varies with different agencies and types of thermometers. In some agencies, the glass clinical thermometer is washed and rinsed. Cool water is used to prevent breakage and to avoid destroying the column of liquid. The thermometer is then soaked in a disinfectant solution (frequently 70 percent alcohol) for a minimum of 30 minutes before it is used again. Other agencies cover the clinical thermometer with a plastic sheath that is discarded after use (**Figure 16–12**).

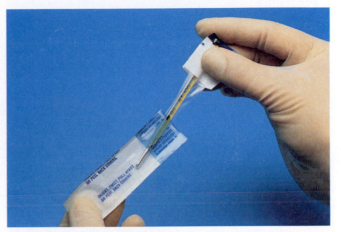

FIGURE 16–12 A clinical thermometer can be covered with a plastic sheath that is discarded after each use.

The probe on electronic thermometers is covered with a plastic sheath that is discarded after each use. These covers prevent the thermometers from coming into contact with each patient's mouth or skin and prevent transmission of germs. Electronic thermometers all use disposable probes so contamination of the thermometer is limited. Some health care facilities do use disinfectants to wipe the outside of electronic thermometers to prevent the spread of infection between patients. In most cases, it is best to follow the recommendations of the manufacturer for cleaning and proper care of electronic thermometers. Every health care provider should learn and follow the agency's policy for cleaning and care of thermometers.

checkpoint

1. What are three (3) reasons for variation in body temperature?

PRACTICE: Go to the workbook and complete the assignment sheet for 16:2, Measuring and Recording Temperature. Then return and continue with the procedures.

Measuring and Recording Oral Temperature with a Clinical Thermometer

Equipment and Supplies

Oral thermometer, plastic sheath (if used), holder with disinfectant solution, tissues or dry cotton balls, container for used tissues, watch with second hand, soapy cotton balls, disposable gloves, notepaper, pen and/or computer

Procedure

1. Assemble equipment.

2. Wash hands and put on gloves.

    CAUTION: Follow standard precautions for contact with saliva or the mucous membrane of the mouth.

   Precaution

3. Introduce yourself. Identify the patient. Explain the procedure.

   Comm

4. Position the patient comfortably. Ask the patient if they have eaten, have had hot or cold fluids, or have smoked in the past 15 minutes.

   NOTE: Eating, drinking liquids, or smoking can affect the temperature in the mouth. Wait at least 15 minutes if the patient says "yes" to your question.

5. Remove the clean thermometer by the upper end. Use a clean tissue or dry cotton ball to wipe the thermometer from stem to bulb.

   NOTE: If the thermometer was soaking in a disinfectant, rinse first in cool water.

    CAUTION: Hold the thermometer securely to avoid breaking.

   Safety

6. Read the thermometer to be sure it reads 96°F (35.6°C) or lower. Check carefully for chips or breaks.

    CAUTION: Never use a cracked thermometer because it may injure the patient.

   Safety

7. If a plastic sheath is used, place it on the thermometer.

8. Insert the bulb under the patient's tongue, toward the side of the mouth (**Figure 16–13**). Ask the patient to hold it in place with the lips, and caution against biting it.

   NOTE: Check to be sure patient's mouth is closed.

9. Leave the thermometer in place for 3–5 minutes.

   NOTE: Some agencies require that a clinical thermometer be left in place for 5–8 minutes. Follow your agency's policy.

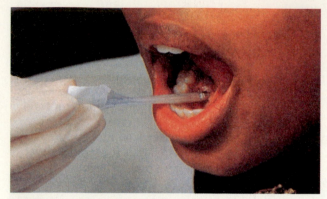

FIGURE 16–13 Insert the bulb of the thermometer under the patient's tongue (sublingually).

10. Remove the thermometer. Hold it by the stem and use a tissue or cotton ball to wipe toward the bulb.

    NOTE: If a plastic sheath was used to cover the thermometer, there is no need to wipe the thermometer. Simply remove the sheath, taking care not to touch the part that was in the patient's mouth.

    CAUTION: Do **not** hold the bulb end. This could alter the reading because of the warmth of your hand.

    Safety

11. Read the thermometer. Record the reading on notepaper.

    NOTE: Recheck the reading and your notation for accuracy.

    NOTE: If the reading is less than 97°F, reinsert the thermometer in the patient's mouth for 1–2 minutes.

12. Check the patient for comfort and safety before leaving.

13. Clean the thermometer following agency policy. General guidelines include:

    a. Wearing gloves, use a soapy cotton ball to wipe the thermometer once from the top to the tip or bulb. Discard the cotton ball.

    b. With the bulb pointed downward, hold the thermometer by the stem and rinse it in cool water.

    c. Hold the thermometer securely between your thumb and index finger. Use a snapping motion of the wrist to shake the thermometer down to 96°F (35.6°C) or lower.

    (continues)

d. Place the thermometer in a small basin or container filled with a disinfectant solution. Make sure the thermometer is completely covered by the solution (**Figure 16–14**).

e. Allow the thermometer to soak for the recommended time, usually 30 minutes.

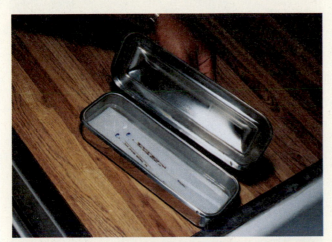

FIGURE 16–14 Soak the thermometer in a disinfectant solution for a minimum of 30 minutes.

14. Replace all equipment.

15. Remove gloves and discard in infectious waste container. Wash hands.

16. Record all required information on the patient's chart or enter it into the computer. For example: date and time, T 98⁶, and your signature and title. Report any abnormal reading to your supervisor immediately.

NOTE: In health care agencies using electronic health records (EHRs), the information is entered directly into the patient's record on a computer.

PRACTICE: Go to the workbook and use the evaluation sheet for 16:2A, Measuring and Recording Oral Temperature with a Clinical Thermometer, to practice this procedure. When you believe you have mastered this skill, sign the sheet and give it to your instructor for further action.

 FINAL EVALUATION: Using the criteria listed on the evaluation sheet, your instructor will grade your performance.

Procedure 16:2B

Measuring Oral Temperature with an Electronic Thermometer

Equipment and Supplies

Electronic thermometer with blue probe, sheath (probe cover) gloves, paper, pen and/or computer, container for soiled sheath

Procedure

1. Assemble equipment.

    NOTE: Read the operating instructions for the electronic thermometer so you understand how the particular model operates.

2. Wash hands. Put on gloves if needed.

    CAUTION: Follow standard precautions.

   NOTE: Some health care facilities do not require gloves for an oral temperature taken with an electronic thermometer because there is usually no contact with oral fluids. Follow agency policy.

3. Introduce yourself. Identify the patient. Explain the procedure.

4. Position the patient comfortably. Ask the patient if they have eaten, have had hot or cold fluids, or have smoked in the past 15 minutes. Wait at least 15 minutes if the patient answers "yes."

5. If the blue probe has to be connected to the thermometer unit, insert the probe into the correct receptacle. If the thermometer has an "on" or "activate" button, push the button to turn on the thermometer.

6. Cover the probe with the sheath or probe cover (**Figure 16–15A**).

7. Insert the covered probe under the patient's tongue toward the side of the mouth. Ask the patient to close their mouth but to avoid biting down on the thermometer. Most probes are heavy, so it is usually necessary to hold the probe in position (**Figure 16–15B**).

(continues)

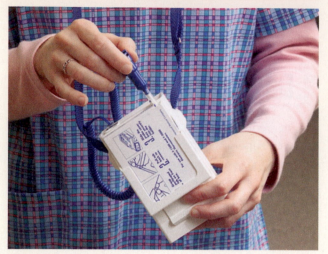

FIGURE 16–15A Install a probe cover on the thermometer.

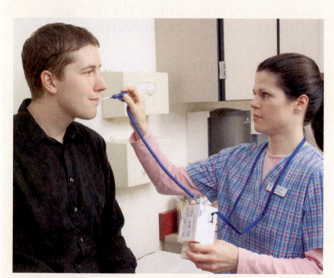

FIGURE 16–15B While taking a temperature, hold the probe of the electronic thermometer in place.

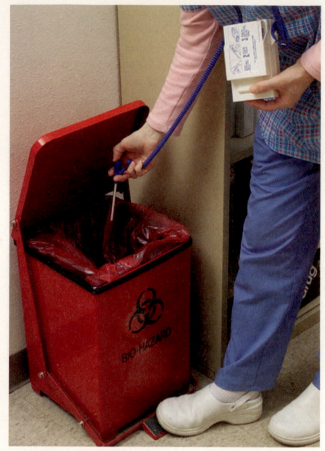

FIGURE 16–15C Discard the probe cover in an infectious waste container without touching the cover.

8. When the unit signals that the temperature has been recorded, remove the probe.

   NOTE: Many electronic thermometers have an audible "beep." Others indicate that temperature has been recorded when the numbers stop flashing and become stationary.

    CAUTION: Do not touch the probe cover. It is contaminated with the patient's saliva.

   Precaution

9. Read and record the temperature. Recheck your reading for accuracy.

10. Without touching the sheath or probe cover, discard the sheath in an infectious waste container (**Figure 16–15C**). Most thermometers have an eject button that is pushed to remove the sheath.

11. Observe all safety checkpoints before leaving the patient.

12. Return the probe to the correct storage position in the thermometer unit. Turn off the unit if this is necessary. Place the unit in the charging stand if the model has a charging unit.

13. Replace all equipment.

14. Remove gloves if worn and discard in an infectious waste container. Wash hands.

15.   Record all required information on the patient's chart or enter it into the electronic health record (EHR). For example: date and time, T 98⁸, and your signature and title. Report any abnormal reading immediately to your supervisor.

   Comm   EHR

(continues)

PRACTICE: Go to the workbook and use the evaluation sheet for 16:2B, Measuring Oral Temperature with an Electronic Thermometer, to practice this procedure. When you believe you have mastered this skill, sign the sheet and give it to your instructor for further action.

 FINAL EVALUATION: Using the criteria listed on the evaluation sheet, your instructor will grade your performance.

Procedure 16:2C

Measuring and Recording Rectal Temperature

Equipment and Supplies

Electronic thermometer with red probe or rectal thermometer, plastic sheath or probe cover, lubricant, tissues/cotton balls, waste bag or container, watch with second hand, paper, pen and/or computer, disposable gloves

NOTE: A manikin is frequently used to practice this procedure.

Procedure

1. Assemble equipment.

2. Wash hands and put on gloves.

    CAUTION: Follow standard precautions if contact with rectal discharge is possible.

3. Introduce yourself. Identify the patient. Explain the procedure. Screen unit, draw curtains, and/or close door to provide privacy for the patient.

4. Prepare the thermometer.

   a. Insert the red probe on the electronic thermometer. Cover the probe with a disposable sheath or probe cover. Turn the thermometer on.

   b. If a clinical thermometer is being used, remove it from its container. If the thermometer was soaking in a disinfectant, hold it by the stem end and rinse in cool water. Use a dry tissue/cotton ball to wipe from stem to bulb. Check that the thermometer reads 96°F (35.6°C) or lower. Check condition of thermometer. If a plastic sheath is used, position it on the thermometer.

    CAUTION: Breaks in a thermometer can injure the patient. Never use a cracked thermometer.

5. Place a small amount of lubricant on the tissue. Roll the tip of the probe or the bulb end of the thermometer in the lubricant to coat it. Leave the lubricated thermometer on the tissue until the patient is properly positioned.

6. Turn the patient on their side. If possible, use Sims' position (lying on left side with right leg bent up near the abdomen). Infants are usually placed on their backs, with legs raised and held securely, or on their abdomens (**Figure 16–16**).

7. Fold back covers just enough to expose the anal area.

   NOTE: Avoid exposing the patient unnecessarily.

8. With one hand, raise the upper buttock gently. With the other hand, insert the lubricated thermometer approximately 1–1½ inches (½–1 inch for an infant) into the rectum. Tell the patient what you are doing.

   NOTE: At times, rotating the thermometer slightly will make it easier to insert.

    CAUTION: Never force the thermometer. It can break. If you are unable to insert it, obtain assistance.

9. Fold the bedcovers back over your hand and the patient to provide privacy for the patient. Keep your hand on the thermometer the entire time it is in place.

    CAUTION: *Never* let go of the thermometer. It could slide further into the rectum or break.

(continues)

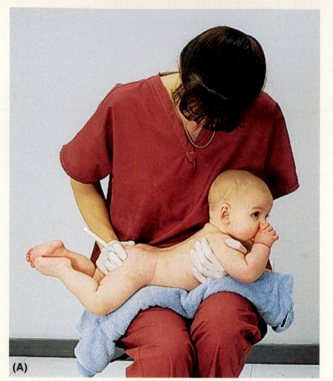
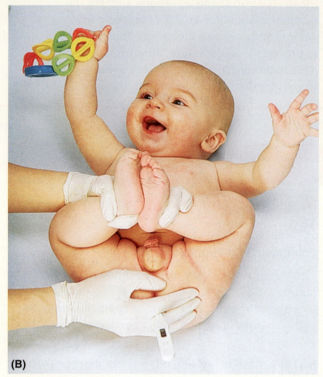

FIGURE 16–16 The infant can be positioned on the (A) abdomen or (B) back for a rectal temperature.

10. Hold the thermometer in place for 3–5 minutes for a clinical thermometer, or until the electronic thermometer beeps or signals that the temperature has registered.

11. Remove the thermometer gently. Tell the patient what you are doing.

12. Eject the probe cover of the electronic thermometer into an infectious waste container. If a clinical thermometer was used, use a tissue to remove excess lubricant from the thermometer. Wipe it from stem to bulb while holding it by the stem area only. Discard the tissue into an infectious waste container.

13. Read and record. Recheck your reading for accuracy. Remember to place an (R) next to the recording to indicate a rectal temperature was taken.

14. Reposition the patient. Observe all safety checkpoints before leaving the patient.

15. Clean the thermometer following agency policy.

16. Replace all equipment.

17. Remove gloves and discard in infectious waste container. Wash hands.

18. Comm · EHR Record all required information on the patient's chart or enter it into the electronic health record (EHR). For example: date and time, T 99⁶ (R), and your signature and title. Report any abnormal reading immediately to your supervisor.

PRACTICE: Go to the workbook and use the evaluation sheet for 16:2C, Measuring and Recording Rectal Temperature, to practice this procedure. When you believe you have mastered this skill, sign the sheet and give it to your instructor for further action.

 FINAL EVALUATION: Using the criteria listed on the evaluation sheet, your instructor will grade your performance.

Measuring and Recording Axillary Temperature

Equipment and Supplies

Electronic thermometer with blue probe or oral thermometer, probe cover or sheath, disposable gloves (if needed), tissues/towel, waste container, watch with second hand, paper, pen and/or computer

Procedure

1. Assemble equipment.

2. Wash hands. Put on gloves if necessary.

    CAUTION: Follow standard precautions if contact with open sores or body fluids is possible.
   Precaution

3. Introduce yourself. Identify the patient. Explain the procedure.
   Comm

4. Prepare the thermometer.

   a. Insert the blue probe on the electronic thermometer. Cover the probe with a disposable sheath or probe cover. Turn the thermometer on.

   b. If a clinical thermometer is being used, remove it from its container. Use a tissue to wipe from stem to bulb. Check the thermometer for damaged areas. Read the thermometer to be sure it reads below 96°F (36.5°C). Place a plastic sheath on the thermometer, if used.

5. Expose the axilla and use a towel to pat the armpit dry.

   NOTE: Moisture can alter a temperature reading. Do not rub area hard because this too can alter the reading.

6. Raise the patient's arm and place the tip or bulb end of the thermometer in the hollow of the axilla (**Figure 16–17**). Bring the arm over the chest or abdomen.

7. Leave the thermometer in place for 10 minutes for a clinical thermometer, or until the electronic thermometer beeps or signals that the temperature has registered.

8. Remove the thermometer. Eject the probe cover of the electronic thermometer into an infectious waste container. If a clinical thermometer was used, use a tissue to wipe from stem to bulb to remove moisture. Hold by the stem end only.

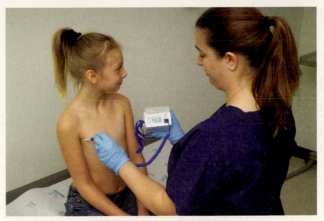

FIGURE 16–17 To take an axillary temperature, insert the thermometer in the hollow of the axilla, or armpit.

 CAUTION: Holding the bulb end will change the reading.
Safety

9. Read and record. Check your reading for accuracy. Remember to mark (Ax) by the recording to indicate axillary temperature.

10. Reposition the patient. Be sure to check for safety and comfort before leaving.

11. Clean the thermometer following agency policy.

12. Replace all equipment used.

13. Remove gloves if worn and discard in an infectious waste container. Wash hands.

14. Record all required information on the patient's chart or enter it into the electronic health record
    Comm   EHR
    (EHR). For example: date and time, T 97⁶ (Ax), and your signature and title. Report any abnormal reading immediately to your supervisor.

PRACTICE: Go to the workbook and use the evaluation sheet for 16:2D, Measuring and Recording Axillary Temperature, to practice this procedure. When you believe you have mastered this skill, sign the sheet and give it to your instructor for further action.

 FINAL EVALUATION: Using the criteria listed on the evaluation sheet, your instructor will grade your performance.
Check

Measuring and Recording Tympanic (Aural) Temperature

Equipment and Supplies

Tympanic thermometer, probe cover, disposable gloves, paper, pencil/pen and/or computer, container for soiled probe cover

Procedure

1. Assemble equipment.

    NOTE: Read the operating instructions so you understand exactly how the thermometer must be used.

2. Wash hands. Put on gloves if needed.

    CAUTION: Follow standard precautions if contact with open sores or body fluids is possible.

3. Introduce yourself. Identify the patient. Explain the procedure.

4. Remove the thermometer from its base and turn it on. A *ready* or series of lines will usually appear on the screen.

5. Install a probe cover according to instructions (**Figure 16–18A**). This will usually activate the thermometer.

6. Position the patient. Infants under 1 year of age should be positioned lying flat with the head turned for easy access to the ear. Small children can be held on the parent's lap, with the head held against the parent's chest for support. Adults who can cooperate and hold the head steady can either sit or lie flat. Patients in bed should have the head turned to the side, and stabilized against the pillow.

7. Hold the thermometer in your right hand to take a temperature in the right ear, and in your left hand to take a temperature in the left ear. With your other hand, pull the ear pinna (external lobe) up and back on any child over 1 year of age and on adults (**Figure 16–18B**). Pull the ear pinna straight back for infants under 1 year of age.

   NOTE: Pulling the pinna correctly straightens the auditory canal so the probe tip will point directly at the tympanic membrane.

8. Insert the covered probe into the ear canal as far as possible to seal the canal. Do not apply pressure.

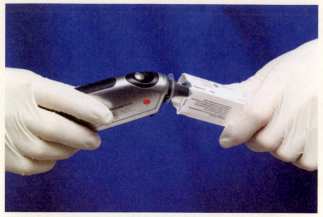

FIGURE 16–18A Install a disposable probe cover on the tympanic thermometer.

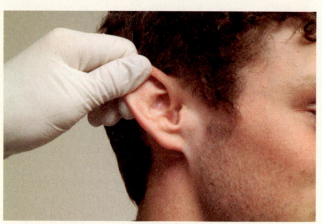

FIGURE 16–18B Before inserting the tympanic thermometer, pull the pinna up and back on adults and children older than 1 year.

9. Rotate the thermometer handle slightly until it is aligned with the patient's jaw. Hold the thermometer steady and press the scan or activation button (**Figure 16–18C**). Hold it for the required amount of time, usually 1–2 seconds, until the reading is displayed on the screen.

10. Remove the thermometer from the patient's ear. Read and record the temperature. Place an (A), (T), or (Tym) by the recording to indicate tympanic temperature.

    NOTE: The temperature will remain on the screen until the probe cover is removed.

     CAUTION: If the temperature reading is low or does not appear to be accurate, change the probe cover and repeat the procedure. The opposite ear can be used for comparison.

(continues)

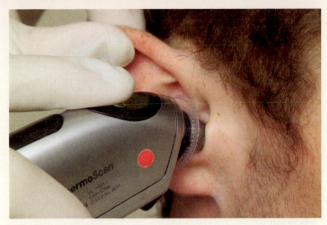

FIGURE 16–18C After inserting the covered probe of the tympanic thermometer into the ear canal, press the scan or activation button and hold the thermometer steady until the temperature reading is displayed.

11. Press the eject button on the thermometer to discard the probe cover into a waste container.

12. Return the thermometer to its base.

13. Reposition the patient. Observe all safety checkpoints before leaving the patient.

14. Remove gloves if worn and discard in an infectious waste container. Wash hands.

15.   Record all required information on the patient's chart or enter it into the electronic health record (EHR). For example: date and time, T 98⁸ (A), and your signature and title. Report any abnormal reading immediately to your supervisor.

PRACTICE: Go to the workbook and use the evaluation sheet for 16:2E, Measuring and Recording Tympanic (Aural) Temperature, to practice this procedure. When you believe you have mastered this skill, sign the sheet and give it to your instructor for further action.

 FINAL EVALUATION: Using the criteria listed on the evaluation sheet, your instructor will grade your performance.

Procedure 16:2F
OBRA

Measuring and Recording Temporal Temperature

Equipment and Supplies

Temporal scanning thermometer, disinfectant wipe or probe cover, paper, pen and/or computer

Procedure

1. Assemble equipment.

     NOTE: Read the operating instructions for the temporal scanning thermometer so you understand how the particular model works.

2. Wash hands.

3. Introduce yourself. Identify the patient. Explain the procedure.

4. Remove the protective cap on the lens of the thermometer. Hold the thermometer upside down to clean the lens with a disinfectant wipe and allow it to dry. Check the lens for cleanliness after it has dried.

    NOTE: Holding the thermometer upside down prevents excess moisture from entering the sensor area. The moisture will not harm the sensor, but a temperature cannot be taken until the sensor lens is dry.

    NOTE: Some temporal thermometers use disposable probe covers. If a probe cover is used, the probe does not have to be cleaned with a disinfectant.

5. Position the patient comfortably. Adults who can cooperate and hold the head steady can either sit or lie flat. Infants younger than 1 year should be positioned lying flat on the back. Small children can be held on the parent's lap, with the head held against the parent's chest for support, or lying flat.

6. Check the forehead to make sure there is no sign of perspiration. If perspiration is present, use a towel to pat the forehead dry. Make sure no covering, such as a hat, wig, or hair, is on the forehead. If the patient was lying on a pillow, do not use the side of the forehead that was on the pillow.

     CAUTION: Head coverings or a pillow prevent heat from dissipating from the forehead and cause a falsely high temperature reading.

7. Gently position the probe flat on the center of the forehead, midway between the eyebrow and hairline. Press and hold the scan button.

(continues)

8. Slide the thermometer across the forehead lightly and slowly (**Figure 16–19**). Keep the sensor flat and in contact with the skin until you reach the hairline on the side of the face.

   NOTE: The thermometer will emit a beeping sound and a red light will blink to indicate that a measurement is taking place.

9. Release the scan button and remove the thermometer from the head.

    NOTE: If sweating is profuse and you are not able to dry the forehead completely, use a different method to obtain the temperature.

   Safety

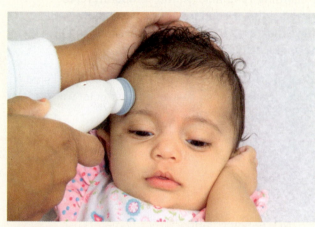

FIGURE 16–19 To take a temporal temperature, hold the scan button while lightly sliding the thermometer across the forehead midway between the eyebrow and hairline.

10. Read and record the temperature that is displayed on the thermometer. Double-check your reading.

11. Press and release the activation button quickly to turn off the thermometer. If a probe cover was used, remove and discard the cover. Wipe the lens with a disinfectant wipe and let it air dry. Put the protective cap on the lens to protect the lens.

    NOTE: Most thermometers will turn off automatically after 30 seconds to 1 minute.

12. Reposition the patient. Observe all safety checkpoints before leaving the patient.

13. Replace all equipment.

14. Wash hands.

15. Record all required information on the patient's chart or enter it into the electronic health record (EHR). For example: date and time, T 99⁸ (TA), your signature and title. Report any abnormal reading immediately to your supervisor.

    Comm   EHR

PRACTICE: Go to the workbook and use the evaluation sheet for 16:2F, Measuring and Recording Temporal Temperature, to practice this procedure. When you believe you have mastered this skill, sign the sheet and give it to your instructor for further action.

 FINAL EVALUATION: Using the criteria listed on the evaluation sheet, your instructor will grade your performance.

Check

16:3 MEASURING AND RECORDING PULSE

 Pulse is a vital sign that you will be required to take. There are certain facts you must know when you take this measurement.

OBRA

 Pulse refers to the pressure of the blood pushing against the wall of an artery as the heart beats and rests. In other words, it is a throbbing of the arteries that is caused by the contractions of the heart. The pulse is more easily felt in arteries that lie fairly close to the skin and can be pressed against a bone by the fingers.

Science

The pulse can be felt at different arterial sites on the body. Some of the major sites are shown in **Figure 16–20** and include:

- **Temporal:** on either side of the forehead
- **Carotid:** at the neck on either side of the trachea
- **Brachial:** inner aspect of forearm at the antecubital space (crease of the elbow)
- **Radial:** at the inner aspect of the wrist, above the thumb
- **Femoral:** at the inner aspect of the upper thigh where the thigh joins with the trunk of the body
- **Popliteal:** behind the knee
- **Dorsalis pedis or pedal:** at the top of the foot arch
- **Posterior tibial:** just below and behind the medial malleolus (the bony part of the ankle that sticks out on the inner, or big toe side, of the leg)

NOTE: *Pulse is usually taken over the radial artery.*

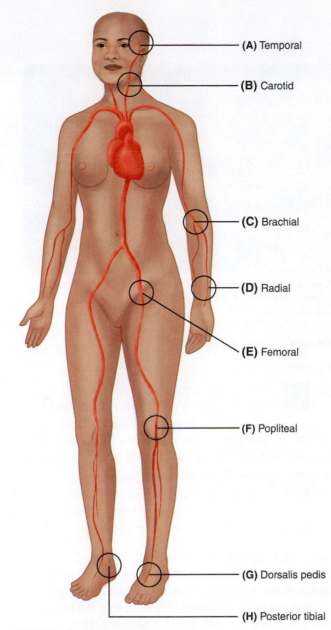

(A) Temporal

(B) Carotid

(C) Brachial

(D) Radial

(E) Femoral

(F) Popliteal

(G) Dorsalis pedis

(H) Posterior tibial

FIGURE 16–20 Major pulse sites.

Each time a pulse is measured, three different facts must be noted: the rate, the rhythm, and the volume of the pulse. These facts are important to provide complete information about the pulse. For example, a pulse of 82, strong and regular, is much different than a pulse of 82, weak and very irregular.

The rate of the pulse is measured as the number of beats per minute. Pulse rates vary among individuals, depending on age, sex, and body size:

- **Adults**: general range of 60–100 beats per minute
- **Adult men**: 60–70 beats per minute
- **Adult women**: 65–80 beats per minute
- **Children aged over 7**: 70–100 beats per minute
- **Children aged 1–7**: range of 80–110 beats per minute
- **Infants**: 100–160 beats per minute

- **Bradycardia**: a pulse rate under 60 beats per minute
- **Tachycardia**: a pulse rate over 100 beats per minute (except in children)

Comm

NOTE: *Any variations or extremes in pulse rates should be reported immediately.*

Rhythm of the pulse is also noted. Rhythm refers to the regularity of the pulse, or the spacing of the beats. It is described as *regular* or *irregular*. An **arrhythmia** is an irregular or abnormal rhythm, usually caused by a defect in the electrical conduction pattern of the heart.

Volume, or the strength, force, quality, or intensity of the pulse, is also noted. It is described by words such as *bounding*, *strong*, *weak*, or *thready*.

Various factors will change pulse rate. Increased, or accelerated, rates can be caused by exercise, stimulant drugs, excitement, fever, dehydration, shock, nervous tension, and other similar factors. Decreased, or slower, rates can be caused by sleep, depressant drugs, heart disease, coma, physical training, and other similar factors.

Another measurement that is frequently taken in addition to pulse is the oxygen level of the blood. **Pulse oximeters** are simple clip-like devices that are used to obtain this measurement (**Figure 16–21**). The oximeter is placed on a finger, toe, or ear lobe. When it is in place, the oximeter uses light to determine the percentage of oxygen in the blood and displays the result on the screen. In addition, many oximeters also measure pulse rate. A normal range of blood oxygen saturation level is 95 to 100 percent. Levels below 90 are considered to be hypoxia, a deficiency of oxygen reaching the tissues, and may indicate the need for supplemental oxygen.

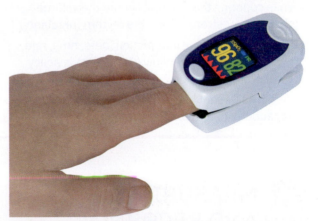

FIGURE 16–21 A pulse oximeter measures the percentage of oxygen in the blood. Many oximeters also measure the pulse rate per minute.

checkpoint

| **1.** What artery site is usually used to obtain a pulse?

PRACTICE: Go to the workbook and complete the assignment sheet for 16:3, Measuring and Recording Pulse. Then return and continue with the procedure.

Measuring and Recording Radial Pulse

Equipment and Supplies

Watch with second hand, paper, pen and/or computer

Procedure

1. Assemble equipment.

2. Wash hands.

3. Introduce yourself. Identify the patient. Explain the procedure.

4. Place the patient in a comfortable position, with the arm supported and the palm of the hand turned downward.

   NOTE: If the forearm rests on the chest, it will be easier to count respirations after taking the pulse.

5. With the tips of your first two or three fingers, locate the pulse on the thumb side of the patient's wrist (**Figure 16–22**).

   NOTE: Do not use your thumb; use your fingers. The thumb contains a pulse that you may confuse with the patient's pulse.

6. When the pulse is felt, exert slight pressure and start counting. Use the second hand of the watch and count for 1 full minute.

   NOTE: In some agencies, the pulse is counted for 30 seconds and the final number multiplied by 2. To detect irregularities, it is better to count for 1 full minute.

7. While counting the pulse, also note the volume (character or strength) and the rhythm (regularity).

8. Record the following information: date, time, rate, rhythm, and volume. Follow your agency's policy for recording.

9. Check the patient before leaving. Observe all safety precautions to protect the patient.

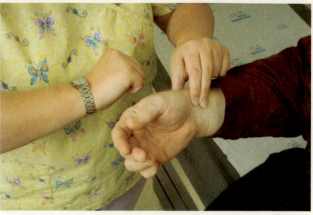

FIGURE 16–22 To count a radial pulse, put the tips of two or three fingers on the thumb side of the patient's wrist.

10. Replace all equipment used.

11. Wash hands.

12. Record all required information on the patient's chart or enter it into the computer. For example: date, time, P 82 strong and regular, and your signature and title. Report any unusual observations immediately to your supervisor.

     NOTE: In health care agencies using electronic health records (EHRs), the information is entered directly into the patient's record on a computer.

PRACTICE: Go to the workbook and use the evaluation sheet for 16:3, Measuring and Recording Radial Pulse, to practice this procedure. When you believe you have mastered this skill, sign the sheet and give it to your instructor for further action.

 FINAL EVALUATION: Using the criteria listed on the evaluation sheet, your instructor will grade your performance.

16:4 MEASURING AND RECORDING RESPIRATIONS

 Respirations are another vital sign that you must observe, count, and record correctly. This section provides the main points you must note when counting and recording the quality of respirations.

 Respiration is the process of taking in oxygen (O_2) and expelling carbon dioxide (CO_2) from the lungs and respiratory tract. One respiration consists of one inspiration (breathing in) and one expiration (breathing out).

Each time respiration is measured, three different facts must be noted: the rate, the character, and the rhythm of respirations. These three facts provide complete information about how the patient is breathing. For example, a respiration measurement of 18, deep and regular, is much different than a measurement of 18, very shallow and irregular.

Rate of respirations counts the numbers of breaths per minute. The normal rate for respirations in adults is a range of 12–20 breaths per minute. In children, respirations are slightly faster than those for adults and average 16–30 per minute. In infants, the rate may be 30–50 per minute.

In addition to rate, the character and rhythm of respirations should be noted. **Character** refers to the depth and quality of respirations. Words used to describe character include *deep, shallow, labored, difficult, stertorous* (abnormal sounds like snoring), and *moist*. Rhythm refers to the regularity of respirations, or equal spacing between breaths. It is described as *regular* or *irregular*.

The following terminology is used to describe abnormal respirations:

- **Dyspnea**: difficult or labored breathing
- **Apnea**: absence of respirations, usually a temporary period of no respirations
- **Tachypnea**: rapid, shallow respiratory rate above 25 respirations per minute
- **Bradypnea**: slow respiratory rate, usually below 10 respirations per minute
- **Orthopnea**: severe dyspnea in which breathing is very difficult in any position other than sitting erect or standing
- **Cheyne-Stokes**: abnormal breathing pattern characterized by periods of dyspnea followed by periods of apnea; frequently noted in the dying patient

- **Rales**: bubbling, crackling, or noisy sounds caused by fluids or mucus in the air passages
- **Wheezing**: difficult breathing with a high-pitched whistling or sighing sound during expiration; caused by a narrowing of bronchioles (as seen in asthma) and/or an obstruction or mucus accumulation in the bronchi
- **Cyanosis**: a dusky, bluish discoloration of the skin, lips, and/or nail beds as a result of decreased oxygen and increased carbon dioxide in the bloodstream

Respirations must be counted in such a way that the patient is unaware of the procedure. Because respirations are partially under voluntary control, patients may breathe more quickly or more slowly when they become aware of the fact that respirations are being counted. Do not tell the patient you are counting respirations. Also, leave your hand on the pulse site while counting respirations. The patient will think you are still counting pulse and will not be likely to alter the respiratory rate.

checkpoint

1. What three (3) facts provide complete information about respirations?

PRACTICE: Go to the workbook and complete the assignment sheet for 16:4, Measuring and Recording Respirations. Then return and continue with the procedure.

Procedure 16:4

Measuring and Recording Respirations

Equipment and Supplies

Watch with second hand, paper, pen and/or computer

Procedure

1. Assemble equipment.

2. Wash hands.

3. Introduce yourself. Identify the patient.

4. After the pulse rate has been counted, leave your hand in position on the pulse site and count the number of times the chest rises and falls during 1 minute (**Figure 16–23**).

   NOTE: This is done so the patient is not aware that respirations are being counted. If patients are aware, they can alter their rate of breathing.

5. Count each expiration and inspiration as one respiration.

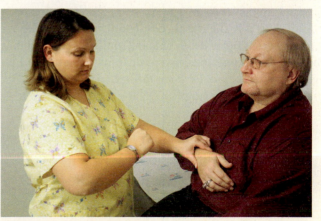

FIGURE 16–23 Positioning the patient's hand on his chest makes it easier to count pulse and respiration.

6. Note the depth (character) and rhythm (regularity) of the respirations.

7. Record the following information: date, time, rate, character, and rhythm.

(continues)

8. Check the patient before leaving the area. Observe all safety precautions to protect the patient.

9. Replace all equipment.

10. Wash hands.

11. Record all required information on the patient's chart or enter it into the computer. For example: date, time, R 16 deep and regular (or even), and your signature and title. Report any unusual observations immediately to your supervisor.

 NOTE: In health care agencies using electronic health records (EHRs), the information is entered directly into the patient's record on a computer.

PRACTICE: Go to the workbook and use the evaluation sheet for 16:4, Measuring and Recording Respirations, to practice this procedure. When you believe you have mastered this skill, sign the sheet and give it to your instructor for further action.

 FINAL EVALUATION: Using the criteria listed on the evaluation sheet, your instructor will grade your performance.

16:5 GRAPHING TPR

 In some agencies, you may be required to chart temperature, pulse, and respirations (TPR) on graphic records. This section provides basic information about these records.

Graphic sheets are special records used for recording temperature, pulse, and respirations. The forms vary in different health care facilities, but all contain the same basic information. The graphic chart presents a visual diagram of variations in a patient's vital signs. The progress is easier to follow than a list of numbers that give the same information. Graphic charts are used most often in hospitals and long-term-care facilities. However, similar records may be kept in medical offices or other health care facilities. Patients are sometimes taught how to maintain these records.

Some charts make use of color coding. For example, temperature is recorded in blue ink, pulse is recorded in red ink, and respirations are recorded in green ink. Other agencies use blue ink for 7 AM to 7 PM (days) and red ink for 7 PM to 7 AM (nights). Follow the policy of your institution.

Factors that affect vital signs are often included on the graph. Examples include surgery, medications that lower temperature (such as aspirin), and antibiotics.

  Computer software programs may also be used to create a graphic chart for vital signs. After vital signs have been entered into the computer, the software program records the entries on a graphic chart. The chart can be printed and used as a patient record or kept in a patient's electronic health record (EHR).

 The graph is a medical record, so it must be neat, legible, and accurate. Double-check all information recorded on the graph. If an error occurs, it should be crossed out carefully with red ink and initialed. Correct information should then be inserted on the graph.

checkpoint

1. How can a health care provider apply data from graphs to provide information or solutions to health related issues?

PRACTICE: Read the complete procedure for 16:5, Graphing TPR. Then go back and start doing the procedure. Your assignment will follow the procedure.

Procedure 16:5

Graphing TPR

Equipment and Supplies

Blank TPR graphic sheets in the workbook, TPR sample graph, assignment sheets on graphing in the workbook, pen, ruler, or computer with graphic program

Procedure

1. Assemble equipment.

2. Examine the sample graphic sheet (**Figure 16–24**). This will vary, depending on the agency. However, most graphic sheets contain time blocks across the top and number blocks for TPRs on the side. Note areas for recording temperature, pulse, and respirations. Refer to the example while completing the procedure steps.

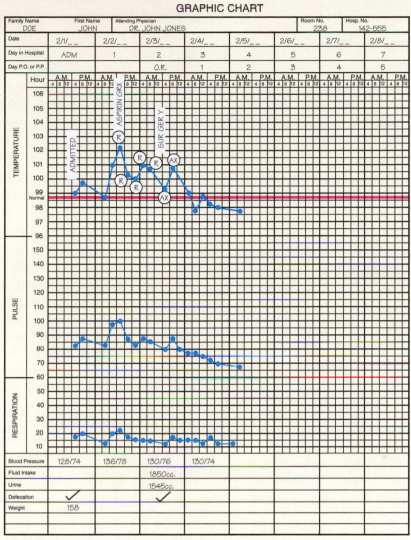

FIGURE 16–24 A sample graphic sheet.

---

3. Using a blank graphic sheet, fill in patient information in the spaces provided at the top. Write last name first in most cases. Be sure patient identification, hospital, and room number are accurate.

NOTE: Forms vary. Follow directions as they apply to your form.

4. Fill in the dates in the spaces provided after DATE.

NOTE: A graphic chart provides a day-to-day visual representation of the variations in a patient's TPRs.

5. If your chart calls for DAY IN HOSPITAL below the dates, enter *Adm* under the first date. This stands for day of admission. The second date would then be day 1, or first full day in the hospital. The third date would be day 2, and so forth.

6. Some graphs contain a third line, DAYS PO or PP, which means days post-op (after surgery) or postpartum (after delivery of a baby). The day of surgery would be shown as *OR* or *Surgery*. The next day would be day 1, or first day after surgery. The day of delivery of a baby is shown as *Del*, with the next day as day 1, or first day after delivery. Numbers continue in sequence for each following day.

7. Go to the Assignment Sheet #1. Note the TPRs. On the graphic sheet, find the correct *Date and Time* column. Move down the column until the correct temperature number is found on the side of the chart. Mark this with a dot (•) in the box. Do the same for pulse and respirations.

(continues)

CAUTION: Double-check your notations. Be sure they are accurate.

CHECKPOINT: Your instructor will check your notations.

8. Repeat step 7 for the next TPR. Check to be sure you are in the correct time column. Mark the dots clearly under the time column and at the correct temperature measurement, pulse rate, or respiration rate.

9. Use a straight paper edge or ruler to connect the dots for temperature. Do the same with the dots for pulse and, finally, with the dots for respiration.

   NOTE: A ruler makes the line straight and neat, and the readings are more legible.

10. Continue to graph the remaining TPRs from Assignment Sheet #1. Double-check all entries for accuracy. Use a ruler to connect all dots for each of the vital signs.

11. Any drug that might alter or change temperature or other vital sign is usually noted on the graph in the time column closest to the time when the drug was first given. Turn the paper sideways and write the name of the drug in the correct time column. Aspirin is often recorded in this column because it lowers temperature. A rapid drop in body temperature would be readily explained by the word *aspirin* in the time column. Antibiotics and medications that alter heart rate are also noted in many cases.

12. Other events in a patient's hospitalization are also recorded in the time column. Examples include surgery and discharge. In some hospitals, if the patient is placed in isolation, this is also noted on the graph.

13. Blood pressure, weight, height, defecation (bowel movements), and other similar kinds of information are often recorded in special areas at the bottom of the graphic record. Record any information required in the correct areas on your form.

14. Recheck your graph for neatness, accuracy, and completeness of information.

PRACTICE: Go to the workbook and complete Assignment Sheet #1 for Graphing TPR. Give it to your instructor for grading. Note all changes. Then complete Assignment Sheet #2 for Graphing TPR in the workbook. Repeat this process by completing Graphing TPR Assignment Sheets #3 to #5 until you have mastered graphic records.

FINAL EVALUATION: Your instructor will grade your performance on this skill according to the accuracy of the completed assignments.

16:6 MEASURING AND RECORDING APICAL PULSE

An **apical pulse** is a pulse count taken with a stethoscope at the apex of the heart. The actual heartbeat is heard and counted. A **stethoscope** is an instrument used to listen to internal body sounds. The stethoscope amplifies the sounds so they are easier to hear. Parts of the stethoscope include the earpieces, tubing, and bell or thin, flexible disk called a *diaphragm* (**Figure 16–25**). The tips of the earpieces should be bent forward when they are placed in the ears. The earpieces should fit snugly but should not cause pain or discomfort. To prevent the spread of microorganisms, the earpieces and bell/diaphragm of the stethoscope should be cleaned with a disinfectant before and after every use.

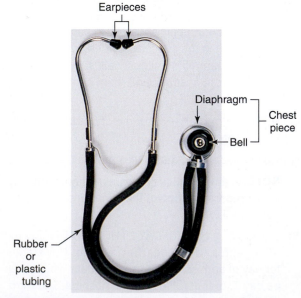

FIGURE 16–25 Parts of a stethoscope.

Usually, a physician orders an apical pulse. It is frequently ordered for patients with irregular heartbeats, hardening of the arteries, or weak or rapid radial pulses. Because children and infants have very rapid radial pulse counts, apical pulse counts are usually taken (**Figure 16–26**). It is generally easier to count a rapid pulse while listening to it through a stethoscope than by feeling it with your fingers.

It is important that you protect the patient's privacy when counting an apical pulse. Avoid exposing the patient during this procedure.

Science Two separate heart sounds are heard while listening to the heartbeat. The sounds resemble a "lubb-dupp." Each lubb-dupp counts as one heartbeat. The sounds are caused by the closing of the heart valves as blood flows through the chambers of the heart. Any abnormal sounds or beats should be reported immediately to your supervisor.

Math A **pulse deficit** is a condition that occurs with some heart conditions. In some cases, the heart is weak and does not pump enough blood to produce a pulse. In other cases, the heart beats too fast (tachycardia), and there is not enough time for the heart to fill with blood; therefore, the heart does not produce a pulse during each beat. In such cases, the apical pulse rate is higher than the pulse rate at other pulse sites on the body. For the most accurate determination of a pulse deficit, one person should check the apical pulse while a second person checks another pulse site, usually the radial pulse (**Figure 16–27**). If this is not possible, one person should first check the apical pulse and then immediately check the radial pulse. Then, subtract the rate of the radial pulse from the rate of the apical pulse. The difference is the pulse deficit. For example, if the apical pulse is 130 and the radial pulse is 92, the pulse deficit would be 38 (130 − 92 = 38).

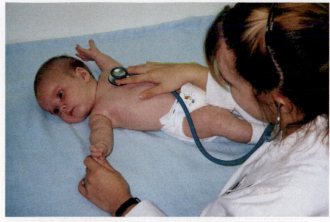
FIGURE 16–26 An apical pulse is frequently taken on infants and small children because their pulses are more rapid.

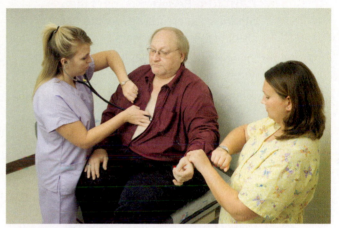
FIGURE 16–27 To determine a pulse deficit, one person should count an apical pulse while another person is counting a radial pulse.

checkpoint

| **1.** What are the three (3) parts of a stethoscope?

PRACTICE: Go to the workbook and complete the assignment sheet for 16:6, Measuring and Recording Apical Pulse. Then return and continue with the procedure.

Procedure 16:6

Measuring and Recording Apical Pulse

Equipment and Supplies

Stethoscope, watch with second hand, paper, pen and/or computer, disinfectant wipe

Procedure

1. Assemble equipment. Use a disinfectant to wipe the ear-pieces and the bell/diaphragm of the stethoscope.

2. Wash hands.

3. **Comm** Introduce yourself. Identify the patient and explain the procedure. If the patient is an infant or child, explain the procedure to the parent(s).

   NOTE: It is usually best to say, "I am going to listen to your heartbeat." Some patients do not know what an apical pulse is.

4. Close the door to the room. Screen the unit or draw curtains around the bed to provide privacy.

(continues)

5. Uncover the left side of the patient's chest. The stethoscope must be placed directly against the skin.

   NOTE: If the diaphragm of the stethoscope is cold, warm it by placing it in the palm of your hand before placing it on the patient's chest.

6. Place the stethoscope tips in your ears. Locate the apex of the heart, 2–3 inches to the left of the breastbone. Use your index finger to locate the fifth intercostal (between the ribs) space at the midclavicular (collarbone) line (**Figure 16–28**). Place the bell/diaphragm over the apical region and listen for heart sounds.

    CAUTION: Be sure the tips of the stethoscope are facing forward before placing them in your ears.
   Safety

7. Count the apical pulse for 1 full minute. Note the rate, rhythm, and volume.

   NOTE: Remember to count each lubb-dupp as one beat.

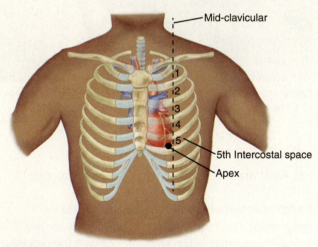

FIGURE 16–28 Locate the apex of the heart at the fifth intercostal (between the ribs) space by the midclavicular (middle of the collarbone) line.

8. If you doubt your count, recheck your count for another minute.

9. Record your reading. Note date, time, rate, rhythm, and volume. Chart according to the agency policy. Some use an A and others use an AP to denote apical pulse.

    NOTE: If both a radial and apical pulse are taken, it may be recorded as A82/R82. If a pulse deficit exists, it should be noted.
   Math
   For example, with A80/R64, there is a pulse deficit of 16 (that is, 80 − 64 = 16). This would be recorded as A80/R64 pulse deficit: 16.

10. Check all safety and comfort points before leaving the patient.

11. Use a disinfectant wipe to clean the earpieces and the bell/diaphragm of the stethoscope. If the tubing contacted the patient's skin, wipe the tubing with a disinfectant. Replace all equipment.

12. Wash hands.

13. Record all required information on the patient's chart or enter it into the computer.
    Comm
    For example: date, time, AP 86 strong and regular, and your signature and title. If any abnormalities or changes were observed, note and report these immediately.

     NOTE: In health care agencies using electronic health records (EHRs), the information is entered directly into the patient's record on a computer.
    EHR

PRACTICE: Go to the workbook and use the evaluation sheet for 16:6, Measuring and Recording Apical Pulse, to practice this procedure. When you believe you have mastered this skill, sign the sheet and give it to your instructor for further action.

 FINAL EVALUATION: Using the criteria listed on the evaluation sheet, your instructor will grade your performance.
Check

16:7 MEASURING AND RECORDING BLOOD PRESSURE

 Blood pressure (BP) is one of the vital signs you will be required to take. It is important that your recording be accurate and that you understand what the blood pressure reading means.
OBRA

 Blood pressure is a measurement of the pressure that the blood exerts on the walls of the arteries during the various stages of heart activity. Blood pressure is read in millimeters (mm) of mercury (Hg) on an instrument known as a *sphygmomanometer*.
Science

There are two types of blood pressure measurements: systolic and diastolic. **Systolic** pressure occurs in the walls of the arteries when the left ventricle of the heart is contracting and pushing blood into the arteries. **Diastolic** pressure is the constant pressure in the walls of the arteries when the left ventricle of the heart is at rest,

TABLE 16-2 Classifications of Blood Pressure in Adults

Category	Blood Pressure Level in Millimeters of Mercury (mm Hg)		
	Systolic		Diastolic
Normal blood pressure	<120	and	<80
Elevated	120–129	and	<80
Stage 1	130–139	or	80–89
Stage 2	>140	or	>90
Hypertensive Crisis	>180	and/or	>120

Legend: < less than; > greater than

or between contractions. Blood has moved forward into the capillaries and veins, so the volume of blood in the arteries has decreased.

Normal values and classifications for diastolic and systolic pressure are shown in **Table 16–2**.

Blood pressure is recorded as a fraction. The systolic reading is the top number, or numerator. The diastolic reading is the bottom number, or denominator. For example, a systolic reading of 120 and a diastolic reading of 80 is recorded as 120/80.

Math

Pulse pressure is the difference between systolic and diastolic pressure. The pulse pressure is an important indicator of the health and tone of arterial walls. A normal range for pulse pressure in adults is 30–50 mm Hg. For example, if the systolic pressure is 120 mm Hg and the diastolic pressure is 80 mm Hg, the pulse pressure is 40 mm Hg (120 − 80 = 40). The pulse pressure should be approximately one-third of the systolic reading. A high pulse pressure can be caused by an increase in blood volume or heart rate, or a decrease in the ability of the arteries to expand.

Elevated blood pressure is when systolic blood pressure is between 120 and 129 mm Hg *and* diastolic is less than 80 mm Hg. Elevated blood pressure is a warning that high blood pressure will develop unless steps are taken to prevent it. Research has proven the elevated blood pressure can harden arteries, dislodge plaque, and block vessels that nourish the heart. Proper nutrition and a regular exercise program are the main treatments for elevated blood pressure.

Health care providers must realize when obtaining accurate blood pressure measurements it is important to take in consideration socioeconomic status and psychological factors. Stress triggers the body to produce a surge of hormones that temporarily increase the blood pressure by causing the heart to beat faster and the blood vessels to narrow. Recognizing "white-coat" hypertension (when blood pressure readings are higher at the doctors' office than in other settings) is important.

Socioeconomic status appears to also be a contributing factor to hypertension. Whether it is less access to healthy food, higher BMI, or the stress of economic pressure, health care providers must keep patient status in mind when treating for this disease.

Hypertension, or high blood pressure, is indicated when pressures are greater than 130 mm Hg systolic and 80 mm Hg diastolic. *Stage 1 hypertension* is defined as a systolic between 130 and 139 mm Hg *or* a diastolic between 80 and 89 mm Hg. People in this category only take medication if they have had a heart attack or stroke or have an underlying condition. Lifestyle changes, for example, a low sodium diet and exercise, are suggested as treatment. *Stage 2 hypertension* occurs when blood pressure is a systolic of more than 140 mm Hg *or* a diastolic of more than 90 mm Hg. This level of hypertension is addressed not only with lifestyle changes, but medication is added to the treatment regimen. A *hypertensive crisis* occurs when blood pressure is measured at a systolic over 180 mm Hg and/or a diastolic over 120 mm Hg. This level of pressure can damage blood vessels and cause a cardiovascular accident (CVA) or stroke. Immediate medication changes are indicated and possible immediate hospitalization if there are signs of organ damage. Common causes include stress, anxiety, obesity, high salt intake, aging, kidney disease, thyroid deficiency, and vascular conditions such as arteriosclerosis. Hypertension is often called a "silent killer" because most individuals do not have any signs or symptoms of the disease. If hypertension is not treated, it can lead to stroke, kidney disease, and/or heart disease.

Hypotension, or low blood pressure, is indicated when pressures are less than 90 mm Hg systolic and 60 mm Hg diastolic. Hypotension may occur with heart failure, dehydration, depression, severe burns, hemorrhage, and shock. *Orthostatic*, or postural, hypotension occurs when there is a sudden drop in both systolic and diastolic pressure when an individual moves from a lying to a sitting or standing position. It is caused by the inability of blood vessels to compensate quickly to the change in position. The individual becomes light-headed and dizzy, and may experience blurred vision. The symptoms last a few seconds until the blood vessels compensate and more blood is pushed to the brain.

Many factors can influence blood pressure readings. These factors can cause blood pressure to be high or low. Some examples include:

- **Factors causing changes in readings**: force of the heartbeat, resistance of the arterial system, elasticity of the arteries, volume of blood in the arteries, and position of the patient (lying down, sitting, or standing)

- **Factors that may increase blood pressure**: excitement, anxiety, nervous tension, exercise, eating, pain, obesity, smoking, and/or stimulant drugs

- **Factors that may decrease blood pressure**: rest or sleep, depressant drugs, shock, dehydration, hemorrhage (excessive loss of blood), and fasting (not eating)

A **sphygmomanometer** is an instrument used to measure blood pressure in millimeters of mercury (mm Hg). There are three main types of sphygmomanometers: mercury, aneroid, and electronic. The mercury sphygmomanometer has a long column of mercury (**Figure 16–29**). Each mark on the gauge represents 2 mm Hg. The mercury sphygmomanometer must always be placed on a flat, level surface or mounted on a wall. If it is calibrated correctly, the level of mercury should be at zero when viewed at eye level. Even though the mercury sphygmomanometer has proven to be the most accurate instrument for measuring blood pressure, the Occupational Health and Safety Administration (OSHA) discourages its use because of the possibility of a mercury spill and contamination. Because of this, very few health care facilities use a mercury sphygmomanometer. The aneroid sphygmomanometer does not have a mercury column (**Figure 16–30A**). However, it is calibrated in mm Hg. Each line represents 2 mm Hg pressure. When the cuff is deflated, the needle must be on zero (**Figure 16–30B**).

If the needle is not on zero, the sphygmomanometer should not be used until it is recalibrated. Electronic sphygmomanometers are used in many health care facilities. Blood pressure and pulse readings are shown on a digital display after a cuff is placed on the patient. Automatic sphygmomanometers are also available for use (**Figure 16–31**). They register the blood pressure after a cuff is positioned on the arm and a start button is activated. They are frequently used by patients who monitor their blood pressure at home. It is important to read and follow the instructions provided with the sphygmomanometer to obtain accurate readings.

In order to obtain accurate blood pressure readings, it is important to observe several factors. The American Heart Association (AHA) recommends that the patient sit quietly for at least 5 minutes before blood pressure is taken. The AHA also recommends that two separate readings be taken and averaged, with a minimum wait of 30 seconds between readings.

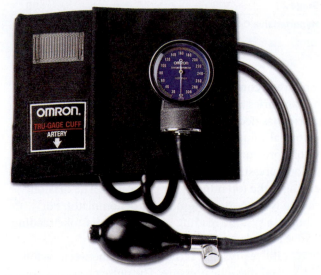

FIGURE 16–30A The gauge on an aneroid sphygmomanometer does not contain a column of mercury. Courtesy, Omron Healthcare, Inc.

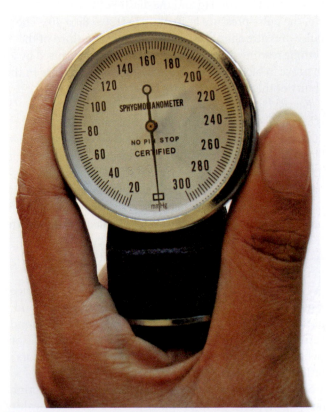

FIGURE 16–30B If the needle is not on zero when the aneroid cuff is deflated, the sphygmomanometer should not be used until it is recalibrated. ©iStock.com/Tiburon Studios.

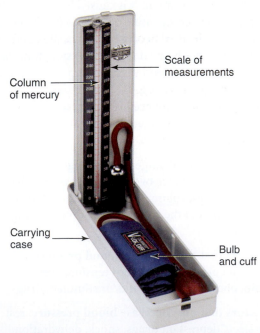

Scale of measurements

Column of mercury

Carrying case

Bulb and cuff

FIGURE 16–29 The gauge on a mercury sphygmomanometer has a long column of mercury. Courtesy, W.A. Baum Co., Inc.

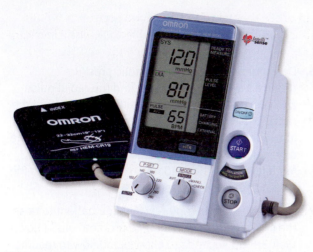

FIGURE 16–31 Automatic sphygmomanometers provide a digital display of blood pressure and pulse readings. Courtesy, Omron Healthcare, Inc.

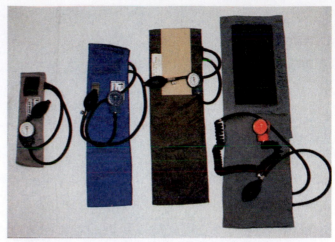

FIGURE 16–32 It is important to use the correct size cuff because cuffs that are too wide or too narrow will result in inaccurate readings.

The size and placement of the sphygmomanometer cuff is also important (**Figure 16–32**). The cuff contains a rubber bladder that fills with air to apply pressure to the arteries. Cuffs that are too wide or too narrow give inaccurate readings. A cuff that is too small will give an artificially high reading; if it is too large, it will give an artificially low reading. To ensure the greatest degree of accuracy, the width of the cuff should be approximately 40 percent of the circumference (distance around) of the patient's upper arm. The length of the bladder should be approximately 80 percent of the circumference of the patient's upper arm. The patient should be seated or lying comfortably and have the forearm supported on a flat surface. The area of the arm covered by the cuff should be at heart level. The arm must be free of any constrictive clothing. The fully deflated cuff should be placed on the arm with the center of the bladder in the cuff directly over the brachial artery, and the lower edge of the cuff 1–1½ inches above the antecubital area (bend of the elbow). Disposable cuffs are available for use when strict infection control is needed. They are available in a variety of sizes and help prevent the transmission of disease. If a nondisposable cuff is used, it can be wiped down with a disinfectant wipe between patients.

A final point relating to accuracy is placement of the stethoscope bell/diaphragm. The bell/diaphragm should be placed directly over the brachial artery at the antecubital area and held securely but with as little pressure as possible.

Comm For a health care provider, a major responsibility is accuracy in taking and recording blood pressure. If you have difficulty obtaining an accurate reading, ask another individual to check the reading. If you note any abnormalities, report these to your supervisor immediately. A physician, physician's assistant, certified nurse practitioner, or other authorized individual will determine whether an abnormal blood pressure is an indication for treatment.

checkpoint

1. Blood pressure is read in millimeters of _____.
2. What artery is used to obtain a blood pressure reading?

PRACTICE: Go to the workbook and complete the assignment sheets for 16:7, Measuring and Recording Blood Pressure, Reading a Mercury Sphygmomanometer, and Reading an Aneroid Sphygmomanometer. Then return and continue with the procedure.

Procedure 16:7
OBRA

Measuring and Recording Blood Pressure

Equipment and Supplies

Stethoscope, sphygmomanometer, disinfectant wipe, paper, pen and/or computer

Procedure

1. Assemble equipment. Use disinfectant wipe to clean the earpieces and bell/diaphragm of the stethoscope.
2. Wash hands.

(continues)

3. Introduce yourself. Identify the patient. Explain the procedure.

    Comm

    NOTE: If possible, allow the patient to sit quietly for 5 minutes before taking the blood pressure.

    NOTE: Reassure the patient as needed. Nervous tension and excitement can alter or elevate blood pressure.

4. Roll up the patient's sleeve to approximately 5 inches above the elbow. Position the arm so that it is supported, comfortable, and close to the level of the heart. The palm should be up.

    NOTE: If the sleeve constricts the arm, remove the garment. The arm must be bare and unconstricted for an accurate reading.

5. Wrap the deflated cuff around the upper arm 1–2 inches above the elbow and over the brachial artery. The center of the bladder inside the cuff should be over the brachial artery.

    ⚠️ **CAUTION:** Do not pull the cuff too tight. The cuff should be smooth and even.

    Safety

6. Determine the palpatory systolic pressure (**Figure 16–33A**). To do this, find the radial pulse and keep your fingers on it. Inflate the cuff until the radial pulse disappears. Inflate the cuff 30 mm Hg above this point. Slowly release the pressure on the cuff while watching the gauge. When the pulse is felt again, note the reading on the gauge. This is the palpatory systolic pressure.

7. Deflate the cuff completely. Ask the patient to raise the arm and flex the fingers to promote blood flow. Wait 30–60 seconds to allow blood flow to resume completely.

8. Use your fingertips to locate the brachial artery (**Figure 16–33B**). The brachial artery is located on the inner part of the arm at the antecubital space (area where the elbow bends). Place the stethoscope over the artery (**Figure 16–33C**). Put the earpieces in your ears.

    NOTE: Earpieces should be pointed forward.

9. Check to make sure the tubings are separate and not tangled together.

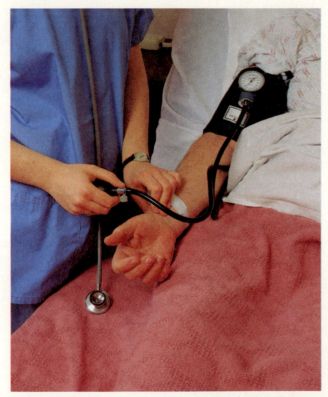

FIGURE 16–33A Determine the palpatory systolic pressure by checking the radial pulse as you inflate the cuff.

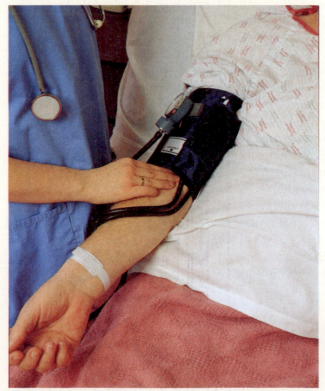

FIGURE 16–33B Locate the brachial artery on the inner part of the arm at the antecubital space.

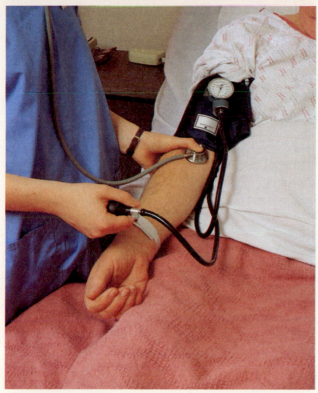

FIGURE 16–33C Place the stethoscope over the brachial artery as you listen for the blood pressure sounds.

10. Gently close the valve on the rubber bulb by turning it in a clockwise direction. Inflate the cuff to 30 mm Hg above the palpatory systolic pressure.

    NOTE: Make sure the sphygmomanometer gauge is at eye level.

11. Open the bulb valve slowly and let the air escape gradually at a rate of 2–3 mm Hg per second (or per heartbeat if the heart rate is very slow).

    NOTE: Deflating the cuff too rapidly will cause an inaccurate reading.

12. When the first sound is heard, note the reading on the manometer. This is the systolic pressure.

13. Continue to release the air until there is an abrupt change of the sound, usually soft or muffled. Note the reading on the manometer. Continue to release the air until the sound changes again, becoming first faint and then no longer heard. Note the reading on the manometer. The point at which the first change in sound occurs is the diastolic pressure in children.

The diastolic pressure in adults is the point at which the sound becomes very faint or stops.

NOTE: If you still hear the sound after it becomes faint, continue until the sound stops or to the zero mark. Record all readings (the reading when the sound became very faint and the reading when the sound stopped or the zero reading). For a systolic of 122 and a diastolic change to a faint sound at 78 with a final stoppage of sound at 32, this can be written as 122/78/32.

14. Continue to listen for sounds for 10–20 mm Hg below the last sound. If no further sounds are heard, rapidly deflate the cuff.

15. If you need to repeat the procedure to recheck your reading, completely deflate the cuff, wait 1 minute, and repeat the procedure. Ask the patient to raise the arm and flex the fingers to promote blood flow.

     CAUTION: If you cannot obtain a reading, report to your supervisor promptly.

16. Record the time and your reading. The reading is written as a fraction, with systolic over diastolic. For example, BP 124/72 (or 124/80/72 if the change in sound is noted).

17. Remove the cuff. Expel any remaining air by squeezing the cuff. Use a disinfectant wipe to clean the stethoscope earpieces and diaphragm/bell. Replace all equipment.

18. Check patient for safety and comfort before leaving.

19. Wash hands.

20. Record all required information on the patient's chart or enter it into the computer. For example: date, time, BP 126/74, and your signature and title. Report any abnormal readings immediately to your supervisor.

     NOTE: In health care agencies using electronic health records (EHRs), the information is entered directly into the patient's record on a computer.

PRACTICE: Go to the workbook and use the evaluation sheet for 16:7, Measuring and Recording Blood Pressure, to practice this procedure. When you believe you have mastered this skill, sign the sheet and give it to your instructor for further action.

 FINAL EVALUATION: Using the criteria listed on the evaluation sheet, your instructor will grade your performance.

An Artificial Heart That Eliminates the Need for Heart Transplants?

Artificial hearts have been in use for many years. They are used to keep a patient alive until a heart transplant can be found. The first artificial heart that sustained life for more than a matter of hours was used on Barney Clark, a Seattle dentist, in 1982. It was implanted by Dr. William DeVries. This heart, the Jarvik-7, was connected to an electrical generator the size of a refrigerator. Wires connected the heart with the generator. Barney Clark lived for 112 days connected to this device.

Now, researchers have developed a new type of artificial heart. By using miniaturized electronics and high-capacity lithium batteries, scientists have created a heart that allows a patient to wear a battery pack on their waist. Electrical energy passes through the patient's skin to power the implanted heart. This allows the patient to resume many normal daily activities. The patient is no longer attached by wires to a power source. Patients have lived for many months with this type of heart while waiting for a suitable transplant.

One artificial heart that received FDA approval in 2010 is the Thoratec Heart-Mate II. This device was approved for patients who are waiting for a transplant and to extend the life of patients who are not candidates for a transplant. Another artificial heart that received FDA approval in 2011 is the Berlin Heart, and it was approved for use in pediatric patients who are waiting for a transplant. Many other artificial heart devices are going through clinical studies for FDA approval.

Most of these devices are called ventricular-assist devices (VADs) because they work with the patient's diseased heart to maintain circulation in the body. Researchers are now working on an artificial heart that will work in place of a patient's damaged heart. Currently, one total artificial heart (TAH) made by SynCardia is available in the United States. It consists of two ventricles and four valves that allow blood to be pumped through the body. It has a preset rate of 125 beats per minute. It works efficiently, but it is still meant to be a temporary replacement while a patient waits for a heart transplant. It requires a person to carry a backpack containing an external air compressor that pumps the implanted heart from the outside. The compressor can be powered with batteries or plugged into an electrical source. Research now is directed toward creating a TAH with an internal compressor and/or electrical source. This total artificial heart will have computerized intelligence to understand when additional blood is needed by the body. It will be able to respond to the demands of the body and increase or decrease the heart rate as needed. It will be created from materials that will not cause a rejection reaction in the body. And finally, it will last for many years.

Case Study Investigation Conclusion

What were possible reasons for monitoring DeShawn's blood pressure for two weeks? What psychological reasons may be impacting his blood pressure? What other possible factors do you think Dr. Elliott may have considered when having DeShawn monitored before prescribing medication?

CHAPTER 16 SUMMARY

- Vital signs are important indicators of health states of the body. The five main vital signs are temperature, pulse, respiration, blood pressure, and pain.
- Temperature is a measurement of the balance between heat lost and heat produced by the body. It can be measured orally, rectally, aurally (by way of the ear), temporally, and between folds of skin, such as the axillary or groin area.
- Pulse is the pressure of the blood felt against the wall of an artery as the heart contracts or beats. Pulse can be measured at various body sites, but the most common site is the radial pulse, which is at the wrist.
- An apical pulse is taken at the apex of the heart by listening to the heart with a stethoscope.

- Blood oxygen levels can be measured with pulse oximeters.
- Respiration refers to the breathing process. Each respiration consists of an inspiration (breathing in) and an expiration (breathing out).
- Blood pressure is the force exerted by the blood against the arterial walls when the heart contracts or relaxes. Two measurements are noted: systolic and diastolic.
- Pain is an unpleasant sensation that is perceived by the nervous system when illness or injury occurs. Pain can be acute or chronic and must be assessed frequently.
- Vital signs are major indications of body function. A thorough understanding of vital signs will allow the health care team member to report abnormalities to the correct individual.

REVIEW QUESTIONS

1. What increment of measurement does each short line on a clinical thermometer represent?
2. What is pain and how can it be assessed?
3. State the normal value or range for an adult for each of the following:
   a. oral or tympanic temperature
   b. rectal or temporal temperature
   c. axillary or groin temperature
   d. pulse
   e. respiration
4. What three (3) factors must be noted about every pulse?
5. Why is an apical pulse taken?

6. What is the pulse deficit if an apical pulse is 112 and the radial pulse is 88?
7. Define each of the following:
   a. Bradycardia   d. Tachypnea
   b. Arrhythmia   e. Rales
   c. Dyspnea
8. How does systolic pressure differ from diastolic pressure? What are the normal ranges for each?
9. If the systolic blood pressure is 132 and the diastolic pressure is 88, what is the pulse pressure?
10. Differentiate between hypertension and hypotension, and list the basic causes of each.

CRITICAL THINKING

1. List the five (5) main vital signs. Describe why the assessment of vital signs is important.
2. When counting respirations, why is it necessary to leave your hand on the pulse site?
3. Why does shock or dehydration decrease blood pressure?

ACTIVITIES

1. With a partner, create a spreadsheet listing the adult normal range for oral, axillary, and rectal temperature; pulse; respirations; and systolic and diastolic blood pressure.
2. On a piece of paper, write all of your classmates' names, leaving space to record their vital signs. Obtain the correct equipment and take accurate measurements of temperature, pulse, and respiration on each of your classmates. Create a spreadsheet that shows the range of temperature, pulse, and respirations for all of your classmates.

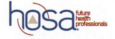 | CONNECTION

Competitive Event: Emergency Medical Technician

Event Summary: Emergency Medical Technician provides HOSA members with the opportunity to gain knowledge and skills required for emergency medical care. This competitive event consists of 2 rounds and each team consists of 2 people. Round One is a written, multiple choice test and the top scoring teams will advance to Round Two for the skills assessment. This event aims to inspire members to be proactive future health professionals and be equipped with resilience, physical strength and problem-solving skills to provide immediate treatment in emergencies.

Details on this competitive event may be found at www.hosa.org/guidelines

Case Study Investigation

Jamal and Miguel were certified in first aid during their health science class last year. They were playing soccer in the park with friends on a beautiful fall day, and they were winning! Suddenly, two players, Sean and Tran, ran into each other; Sean was knocked down and got right up, but Tran stayed down and complained of left leg pain. At the end of this chapter, you will be asked what Jamal and Miguel should do for their teammates until help arrives.

■ LEARNING OBJECTIVES

After completing this chapter, you should be able to:

- Demonstrate cardiopulmonary resuscitation for one-person rescue, two-person rescue, infants, children, and obstructed-airway victims.
- Describe first aid for:
  - Bleeding and wounds
  - Shock
  - Poisoning
  - Burns
  - Heat exposure
  - Cold exposure
  - Bone and joint injuries, including fractures
  - Specific injuries to the eyes, head, nose, ears, chest, abdomen, and genital organs
  - Sudden illness including heart attack, stroke, fainting, convulsions, and diabetic reactions
- Apply dressings and bandages, observing all safety precautions and using the circular, spiral, figure-eight, and recurrent, or finger, wrap.
- Define, pronounce, and spell all key terms.

■ KEY TERMS

abrasion *(ah"-bray'-shun)*

amputation

avulsion *(ay"-vul'-shun)*

bandages

burn

cardiopulmonary resuscitation *(car'-dee-oh-pull'-meh-nahree re"-suh-sih-tay'-shun)*

cerebrovascular accident *(seh-ree'-bro-vass"-kulehr ax'-ih-dent)*

convulsion

diabetic coma

diaphoresis *(dy"-ah-feh-ree'-sis)*

dislocation

dressing

fainting

first aid

fracture

frostbite

heart attack

heat cramps

heat exhaustion

heat stroke

hemorrhage

hypothermia

incision

infection

insulin shock

laceration

poisoning

puncture

shock

sprain

strain

stroke

triage *(tree'-ahj)*

wound

17:1 PROVIDING FIRST AID

INTRODUCTION

In every health care career, you may have experiences that require a knowledge of first aid. This section provides basic guidelines for all the first aid topics discussed in the remaining sections of this unit. *All students are strongly encouraged to take the First Aid Certification Course through their local Red Cross divisions to become proficient in providing first aid.*

First aid is not full and complete treatment. Rather, **first aid** is best defined as "immediate care that is given to the victim of an injury or illness to minimize the effect of the injury or illness until experts can take over." Application of correct first aid can often mean the difference between life and death, or recovery versus permanent disability. In addition, by knowing the proper first-aid measures, you can help yourself and others in a time of emergency.

BASIC PRINCIPLES OF FIRST AID

Comm

In any situation where first-aid treatment is necessary, it is essential that you remain calm. Avoid panic. Evaluate the situation thoroughly. Always have a reason for anything you do.

The treatment you provide will vary depending on the type of injury or illness, the environment, others present, equipment or supplies on hand, and the availability of medical help. Therefore, it is important for you to think about all these factors and determine what action is necessary.

The first step of first aid is to recognize that an emergency exists. Many senses can alert you to an emergency. Listen for unusual sounds, such as screams, calls for help, breaking glass, screeching tires, or changes in machinery or equipment noises. Look for unusual sights, such as an empty medicine container, damaged electrical wires, a stalled car, smoke or fire, a person lying motionless, blood, or spilled chemicals. Note any unusual, unfamiliar, or strange odors, such as those of chemicals, natural gas, or pungent fumes. Watch for unusual appearances or behaviors in others, such as difficulty in breathing, clutching of the chest or throat, abnormal skin colors, slurred or confused speech, unexplained confusion or drowsiness, excessive perspiration, signs of pain, and any symptoms of distress. Sometimes, signs of an emergency are clearly evident. An example is an automobile accident with victims in cars or on the street. Other times, signs are less obvious and require an alert individual to note that something is different or wrong. An empty medicine container and a small child with slurred speech, for example, are less obvious signs.

Safety

After determining that an emergency exists, the next step is to take appropriate action to help the victim or victims. Check the scene and make sure it is safe to approach (**Figure 17–1**). A quick glance at the area can provide information on what has occurred, dangers present, number of people involved, and other important factors. If live electrical wires are lying on the ground around an accident victim, for example, a rescuer could be electrocuted while trying to assist the victim. An infant thrown from a car during an automobile accident may be overlooked. A rescuer who pauses briefly to assess the situation will avoid such dangerous pitfalls and provide more efficient care. If the scene is not safe, call for medical help. Do not endanger your own life or the lives of

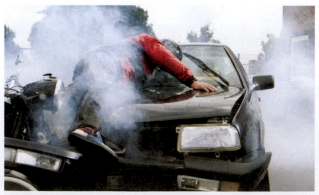

FIGURE 17–1 Check the scene and make sure it is safe to approach before checking any accident victim. © corepics/www.Shutterstock.com

other bystanders. Allow professionals to handle fires, dangerous chemicals, damaged electrical wires, and other life-threatening situations.

If the scene appears safe, approach the victim. Determine whether the victim is conscious. If the victim shows no sign of consciousness, tap them gently and call to them. If the victim shows signs of consciousness, try to find out what happened and what is wrong. Never move an injured victim unless the victim is in a dangerous area, such as an area filled with fire and/or smoke, flood waters, or carbon monoxide or poisonous fumes, or one with dangerous traffic, where vehicles cannot be stopped. If it is necessary to move the victim, do so as quickly and as carefully as possible. Victims have been injured more severely by improper movement at the scenes of accidents, so avoid any unnecessary movement.

 In an emergency, it is essential to call the emergency medical services (EMS) as soon as possible (**Figure 17–2**). The time factor is critical. Early access to the EMS system and advanced medical care increases the victim's chance of survival. Dial 911 on a telephone or cellular phone to contact any of the emergency medical services. Sometimes, it may be necessary to instruct others to contact EMS while you are giving first aid. Make sure that complete, accurate information is given to EMS. Describe the situation, actions taken, exact location, telephone number from which you are calling, assistance required, number of people involved, and the condition of the victim(s). Do not hang up the receiver until EMS has all the necessary information. If you are alone, call EMS immediately before providing any care to:

Comm

- An unconscious adult

- An unconscious child who has reached puberty

- An unconscious infant or child with a high risk for heart problems

- Any victim for whom you witness a sudden cardiac arrest

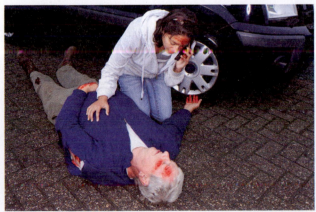

FIGURE 17–2 Call for emergency medical services (EMS) as soon as possible. © iStockphoto/Studio-Annika

If you are alone, shout for help and start cardiopulmonary resuscitation (CPR) if needed for:

- An unconscious infant or child from 1 year of age to puberty

- Any victim of submersion or near drowning

- Any victim with cardiac arrest caused by a drug overdose or trauma

If no one arrives to call EMS, continue providing care by giving five cycles of CPR (approximately 2 minutes). Then go to the nearest telephone, call for EMS, and return immediately to the victim.

 After calling for help, provide care to the victim. If possible, obtain the victim's permission before providing any care. Introduce yourself and ask if you can help. If the victim can respond, they should give you permission before you provide care. If the victim is a child or minor, and a parent is present, obtain permission from the parent. If the victim is unconscious, confused, or seriously ill and unable to consent to care, and no other relative is available to give permission, you can assume that you have permission. It is important to remember that every individual has the right to refuse care. If a person refuses to give consent for care, do not proceed. If possible, have someone witness the refusal of care. If a life-threatening emergency exists, call EMS, alert them to the situation, and allow the professionals to take over.

HIPAA

At times, it may be necessary to **triage** the situation. Triage is a method of prioritizing treatment. If a victim has more than one injury or illness, the most severe injury or illness must be treated first. If two or more people are involved, triage also determines which person is treated first. Life-threatening emergencies must be treated first. Examples include:

- No pulse

- No breathing or difficulty in breathing

- Severe bleeding

- Persistent pain in the chest or abdomen

- Vomiting or passing blood

- Poisoning

- Head, neck, or spine injuries

- Open chest or abdominal wounds

- Shock

- Severe partial-thickness and all full-thickness burns

Proper care for these emergencies is described in the sections that follow. If the victim is conscious, breathing, and able to talk, reassure the victim and try to determine what has happened. Examine the victim thoroughly. Always have a sound reason for anything you do. Examples include:

- Ask the victim about pain or discomfort

- Check the victim for other types of injuries, such as fractures (broken bones), burns, shock, and specific injuries

- Note any abnormal signs or symptoms
- Check vital signs
- Note the temperature, color, and moistness of the skin
- Check and compare the pupils of the eyes
- Look for fluids or blood draining from the mouth, nose, or ears
- Gently examine the body for cuts, bruises, swelling, and painful areas

Report any abnormalities noted to emergency medical services when they arrive at the scene.

Obtain as much information regarding the accident, injury, or illness as possible. This information can then be given to the correct authorities. Information can be obtained from the victim, other persons present, or by examination of items present at the scene. Emergency medical identification contained in a bracelet, necklace, medical card, or Vial-of-Life is an important source of information. Empty medicine containers, bottles of chemicals or solutions, or similar items also can reveal important information. Be alert to all such sources of information. Use this information to determine how you may help the victim.

SUMMARY

Some general principles of care should be observed whenever first aid is necessary. Some of these principles are:

- Obtain qualified assistance as soon as possible. Report all information obtained, observations noted, treatment given, and other important facts to the correct authorities. It may sometimes be necessary to send someone at the scene to obtain help.
- Avoid any unnecessary movement of the victim. Keep the victim in a position that will allow for providing the best care for the type of injury or illness.
- Reassure the victim. A confident, calm attitude will help relieve the victim's anxiety.
- If the victim is unconscious or vomiting, do not give them anything to eat or drink. It is best to avoid giving a victim anything to eat or drink while providing first-aid treatment, unless the specific treatment requires that fluids or food be given.
- Protect the victim from cold or chilling, but avoid overheating the victim.
- Work quickly, but in an organized and efficient manner.

Do *not* make a diagnosis or discuss the victim's condition with observers at the scene. It is essential to maintain confidentiality and protect the victim's right to privacy while providing treatment.

HIPAA

- Make every attempt to avoid further injury.

CAUTION: *Provide only the treatment that you are qualified to provide.*

Legal

checkpoint

| 1. What is the definition for first aid?

PRACTICE: Go to the workbook and complete the assignment sheet for 17:1, Providing First Aid.

17:2 PERFORMING CARDIOPULMONARY RESUSCITATION

INTRODUCTION

At some time in your life, you may find an unconscious victim who has no pulse and/or is not breathing. This is an emergency situation.

Legal

Correct action can save a life. Students are strongly encouraged to take certification courses in cardiopulmonary resuscitation (CPR) offered by the American Red Cross and the American Heart Association. This section provides the basic facts about CPR for health care providers according to American Heart Association standards. *The information provided is not intended to take the place of an approved certification course.*

The word parts of **cardiopulmonary resuscitation** provide a fairly clear description of the procedure: cardio (the heart) plus pulmonary

Science

(the lungs) plus resuscitation (to remove from apparent death or unconsciousness). When you administer CPR, you breathe for the person *and* circulate the blood. The purpose is to keep oxygenated blood flowing to the brain and other vital body organs until the heart and lungs start working again, or until medical help is available.

Clinical death occurs when the heart stops beating and the victim stops breathing. *Biological death* refers to the death of the body cells. Biological death occurs 4–6 minutes after clinical death and can result in permanent brain damage, as well as damage to other vital organs. If CPR can be started immediately after clinical death occurs, the victim may be revived.

COMPONENTS OF CPR

Cardiopulmonary resuscitation is a life-saving technique used for people who have no pulse and have stopped breathing. The American Heart Association uses a CPR sequence of *CABD* (circulation, airway, breathing, defibrillation), with a major emphasis on chest compressions. The goal is to start compressions within 10 seconds of recognizing cardiac arrest. This sequence is used for adults, children, and infants and includes:

- **C stands for circulation**. By applying pressure to a certain area of the sternum (breastbone), the heart is compressed between the sternum and vertebral column. Blood is squeezed out of the heart and into the blood vessels. In this way, oxygen is supplied to body cells.

- **A stands for airway**. To open the victim's airway, use the *head-tilt/chin-lift* method (**Figure 17–3**). Put one hand on the victim's forehead and put the fingertips of the other hand under the bony part of the jaw, near the chin. Tilt the head back without closing the victim's mouth. This action prevents the tongue from falling back and blocking the air passage. If the victim has a suspected neck or upper spinal cord injury, try

to open the airway by lifting the chin without tilting the head back. If it is difficult to keep the jaw lifted with one hand, use a *jaw-thrust maneuver* to open the airway. Assume a position at the victim's head and rest your elbows on the surface on which the victim is lying. Grasp the angles of the victim's lower jaw by positioning one hand on each side. Lift with both hands to move the lower jaw forward, making every attempt to avoid excessive backward tilting or side-to-side movement of the head.

- **B stands for breathing**. Breathing means that, while using a barrier device, you breathe into the victim's mouth or nose to supply needed oxygen or provide ventilations. Each breath should take about 1 second and the chest should rise. Rapid or forceful breaths should be avoided because they can force air into the esophagus and stomach, causing gastric distension (expansion of the stomach when air enters it). This can cause serious complications, such as vomiting, aspiration of fluids into the lungs, and even pneumonia.

 CAUTION: *OSHA requires health care providers to use standard precautions in the workplace. This requires a barrier device for CPR. Use a CPR pocket face mask with a one-way valve to provide a barrier and prevent the transmission of disease (**Figure 17–4**). Special training is required for the use of this mask. Other protective barrier face shields are also available.*

Precaution

- **D stands for defibrillation**. One of the most common causes of cardiac arrest is ventricular fibrillation, which is an arrhythmia, or abnormal electrical conduction pattern in the heart. When the heart is fibrillating, it does not pump blood effectively. A defibrillator is a machine that delivers an electric shock to the heart to try to restore the normal electrical pattern and rhythm.

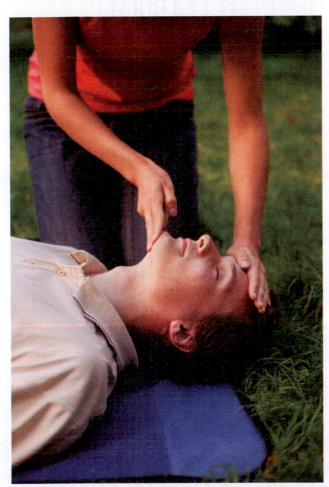

FIGURE 17–3 Open the airway by using the head-tilt/chin-lift method.
© iStockphoto/JanekWD

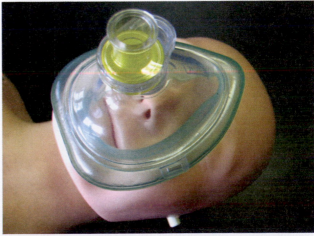

FIGURE 17–4 Use a CPR barrier mask to prevent transmission of disease while giving respirations. © Barbara J. Petrick/www.Shutterstock.com

Automated external defibrillators (AEDs) are now available for use by trained emergency medical responders, emergency medical technicians, and even citizens (**Figure 17–5**). After electrode pads are positioned on the victim's chest (follow the placement diagrams shown on the AED or the pads), the AED determines the heart rhythm, recognizes abnormal rhythms that may respond to defibrillation, and sounds an audible or a visual warning telling the operator to push a "shock" button. Some AEDs are fully automatic and even administer the shock. Anytime a shock is administered with an AED, it is essential to make sure no one is touching the victim. The rescuer should state, "Clear the victim," and look carefully to make sure no one is in contact with the victim before pushing the shock button. Serious injuries, such as cardiac arrest, could occur in other rescuers if they are shocked by the AED.

Newer models of AEDs allow the rescuer to deliver either adult or child defibrillator shocks. By using smaller pediatric electrodes and/or a switch on the AED, the rescuer can deliver a smaller electrical shock. The pediatric dose is recommended for any child from 1 to 8 years of age. The adult defibrillator dose and adult electrodes should be used for any child 8 years or older. In addition, if an AED does not have the option of a pediatric dosage, the adult dosage and electrodes should be used on the child. For infants younger than 1 year, a manual defibrillator is preferred, but an AED with pediatric dosage can be used. Studies have shown that the sooner the defibrillation is provided, the greater the chances of survival are from a cardiac arrest caused by an arrhythmia. However, it is essential to remember that CPR is used until an AED is available. CPR will circulate the blood and prevent biological death.

It is important to know and follow the *CABD*s in proper sequence while administering CPR.

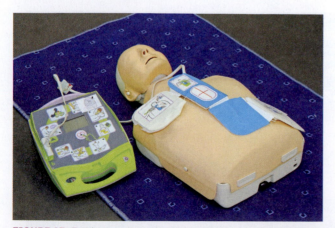

FIGURE 17–5 When cardiac arrest occurs, an automated external defibrillator (AED) can be used to analyze the electrical rhythm of the heart and to apply a shock to try to restore the normal heart rhythm. © Baloncici/www.Shutterstock.com

BASIC PRINCIPLES OF CPR

Extreme care must be taken to evaluate the victim's condition before CPR is started. The victim should be assessed for responsiveness first. To determine if a victim is conscious, tap the victim gently and ask, "Are you OK?" If you know the victim, call the victim by name and speak loudly. If there is no response and the victim is unconscious, call for help. The American Heart Association and the American Red Cross recommend a *"call first, call fast"* priority. If you are alone, *call first* before providing any care to:

- An unconscious adult
- An unconscious child who has reached puberty as defined by the presence of secondary sex characteristics
- An unconscious infant or child with a high risk for heart problems
- Any victim for whom you witness a sudden cardiac arrest

If you are alone, shout for help, and start CPR if needed for:

- An unconscious infant or child from 1 year of age to puberty
- Any victim of submersion or near drowning
- Any victim with cardiac arrest caused by a drug overdose or trauma; in a victim with an opioid-related cardiac arrest, starting CPR is a higher priority than administering naloxone (Narcan)

If no help arrives to call EMS, administer five cycles of CPR (about 2 minutes), and then *call fast* for EMS. Return to the victim immediately to continue providing care until EMS arrives. If you have a cell phone, you can put it on speaker mode and call EMS while providing CPR.

Check the pulse and breathing simultaneously. Check the carotid pulse in the neck to determine whether cardiac compression is needed. At the same time, check breathing by watching for the chest to rise and fall. If you do not feel a pulse within 5–10 seconds, or you are not sure if you feel a pulse, start compressions.

Position the victim on their back. If you must turn the victim, support the victim's head and neck, and keep the victim's body in as straight a line as possible.

 CAUTION: *Cardiac compressions are not given if the pulse can be felt. If a person has stopped breathing or is not breathing normally (gasping), but still has a pulse, it may be necessary to give only pulmonary respiration.*

Safety

Correct hand placement is essential before performing chest compressions. For adults, the hand is placed on the lower half of the sternum between the nipples. While kneeling alongside the victim, find the correct position by using the middle finger of your hand that is closest to the victim's feet to follow the ribs up to where the ribs meet the sternum, at the substernal notch (**Figure 17–6A**). Keep the middle finger on the notch and position the index finger above it so two fingers are on the sternum. Then place the heel of your opposite hand (the hand closest to the victim's head) on the sternum, next to the index finger (**Figure 17–6B**). Measuring in this manner minimizes the danger of applying pressure to the tip of the sternum, called the xiphoid process.

CAUTION: *The xiphoid process can be broken off quite easily and therefore should not be pressed.*

Safety

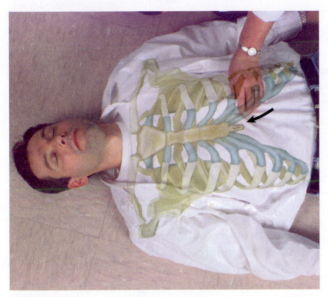

FIGURE 17–6A To position hands correctly for chest compressions, first use a finger to follow the ribs up to where they meet the sternum at the substernal notch.

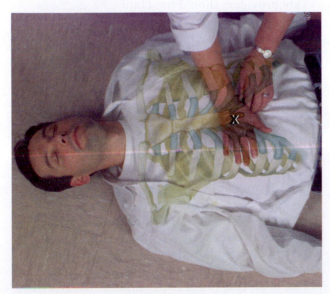

FIGURE 17–6B Place the heel of your opposite hand two-fingers' width above the substernal notch. This should place the hand on the lower half of the sternum between the nipples.

After positioning your hands on the sternum, straighten your arms and align your shoulders directly over your hands. To give compressions, push straight down on the victim's sternum with a hard, fast motion. On an adult, the sternum should be compressed at least 2 inches. After each compression, allow the chest to recoil completely. Deliver compressions at a rate of at least 100–120 compressions per minute and minimize interruptions in compressions. Proper administration of compressions will produce adequate blood flow and improve the victim's chances of survival.

Once 30 chest compressions are delivered, open the airway by using the head-tilt/chin-lift method or, if a neck or spinal cord injury is suspected, the jaw-thrust maneuver. This step will sometimes start the victim breathing. If the victim is not breathing, or not breathing normally (gasping), use a barrier device and give two breaths, each breath lasting approximately 1 second. Make sure the breaths are effective by watching for the victim's chest to rise. Do not give breaths too quickly or with too much force because this can cause gastric distension (stomach expansion due to air accumulation). Pause very briefly between breaths to allow air flow back out of the lungs. In addition, take a breath between the two breaths to increase the oxygen content of the rescue breath. After giving two breaths, immediately return to compressions.

CPR FOR ADULTS, INFANTS, AND CHILDREN

Cardiopulmonary resuscitation can be performed on adults, children, and infants. In addition, it can be done by one person or two persons. Rates of ventilations and compressions vary according to the number of persons giving CPR and the age of the victim.

- **One-person adult rescue**: For adults, a lone rescuer should provide 30 compressions followed by 2 ventilations, for a cycle ratio of 30:2. Compressions should be hard, fast, and deep, and given at the rate of at least 100–120 per minute. Five 30:2 cycles should be completed every 2 minutes. The hands should be positioned correctly on the sternum. The two hands should be interlaced and only the heel of the palm should rest on the sternum. Pressure should be applied straight down to compress the sternum at least 2 inches or 5 centimeters (cm) but not more than 2.4 inches or 6 cm.

- **Two-person adult rescue**: Two people performing a rescue on an adult victim allows one person to give breaths while the second person provides compressions (**Figure 17–7**). During the rescue, the person giving breaths can check the effectiveness of the compressions by feeling for a carotid pulse while chest compressions are administered.

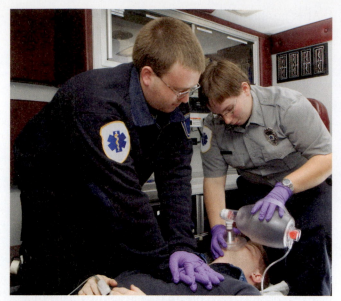

FIGURE 17-7 In a two-person rescue, one person gives breaths while the second person provides compressions. © iStockphoto/Nancy Louie

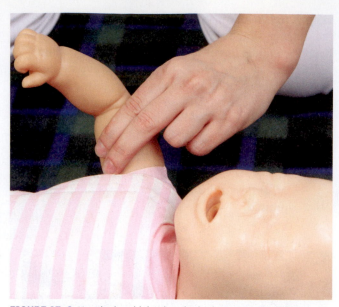

FIGURE 17-8 Use the brachial pulse site in the arm to check for a pulse in an infant. © pryzmat/www.Shutterstock.com.

One rescuer applies the compressions at the rate of at least 100–120 per minute. After every 30 compressions, the second rescuer provides 2 ventilations. Thus, there is a 30:2 ratio. The two rescuers should switch duties every 5 cycles, or about every 2 minutes. Switching should take less than 5 seconds.

- **Infants**: Cardiopulmonary resuscitation is given to any infant from birth to 1 year of age. It is different than that for an adult because of the infant's size. The brachial pulse site in the arm is used to check pulse (**Figure 17–8**). Compressions are given by placing two fingers on the lower half of the sternum just below an imaginary line drawn between the nipples. The sternum should be compressed at least ⅓ the depth of the chest, approximately 1½ inches (4cm). Compressions are given at a rate of at least 100–120 per minute. Once 30 compressions have been given, open the airway using the head-tilt/chin-lift method. The infant's head should not be tilted as far back as an adult's because this can obstruct the infant's airway. Ventilations are given by using a barrier device and covering both the infant's nose and mouth. Breaths are given until the infant's chest visibly rises. Extreme care must be taken to avoid overinflating the lungs and/or forcing air into the stomach. A lone rescuer gives 30 compressions followed by 2 ventilations for a 30:2 ratio. The infant's back must be supported at all times when giving compressions. If two rescuers are available to perform CPR on an infant, a two-thumb technique can be used by one rescuer to perform compressions while the second

rescuer gives breaths. The rescuer providing compressions stands at the infant's feet and places their thumbs next to each other on the lower half of the sternum just below the nipple line. The rescuer then wraps their hands around the infant to support the infant's back with the fingers. A ratio of 15 compressions to 2 ventilations is used by the two rescuers. If an infant has a pulse and is receiving rescue breathing, a ventilation rate of 30 per minute (1 breath every 2 seconds) is recommended.

- **Children**: Cardiopulmonary resuscitation for children depends on the size of the child. Health care providers should use child CPR methods for any child from 1 year of age to puberty (approximately 12 years of age). If a child shows signs of puberty, as evidenced by secondary sex characteristics, adult CPR methods should be used. The initial steps of CPR for a child are the same steps used in adult CPR, except that the head is not tilted as far back when the airway is opened. The main differences relate to compressions. The heel of one hand (or two hands) is placed on the lower half of the sternum in the same position used for adult compressions. If only one hand is used, the other hand remains on the forehead to keep the airway open. The sternum is compressed at least ⅓ the depth of the chest, approximately 2 inches (5 cm). Compressions are given at a rate of at least 100–120 per minute. After each set of 30 compressions, 2 breaths are given until the chest visibly rises. This provides a 30:2 ratio. Approximately five cycles of CPR should be completed every 2 minutes. For two-rescuer child CPR, a ratio of 15:2 is used. If a child has a pulse and is receiving rescue breathing, a ventilation rate of 25 per minute (1 breath every 2 to 3 seconds) is recommended.

CHOKING VICTIMS

 OBRA A choking victim has an obstructed airway (an object blocking the airway). Special measures must be taken to clear this obstruction.

- If an adult victim is conscious, coughing, talking or making noise, and/or able to breathe, the airway is not completely obstructed. Remain calm and encourage the victim to remain calm. Encourage the victim to cough hard. Coughing is the most effective method of expelling the object from the airway.

- If the adult victim is conscious but not able to talk, make noise, breathe, or cough, the airway is completely obstructed. The victim usually grasps their throat and appears cyanotic (blue discoloration of the skin) (**Figure 17–9**). Immediate action must be taken to clear the airway. Abdominal thrusts, as described in Procedure 17:2E, are given to provide a force of air to push the object out of the airway.

- If the adult victim has an obstructed airway and becomes unresponsive, administer adult CPR. Start with compressions (do not check for a pulse). Every time the airway is opened to give breaths, the rescuer should look in the victim's mouth for the object. If the object is visible, the rescuer should use a C-shaped or hooking motion to remove the object. If the object is not seen, the rescuer should try to administer breaths and then continue with chest compressions.

- If the adult victim is pregnant or obese, or you cannot reach around the victim to give abdominal thrusts, perform chest thrusts.

- If an infant (birth to 1 year old) has an obstructed airway, a different sequence of steps is used to remove the obstruction. The sequence includes five back blows, five chest thrusts, and a finger sweep of the mouth if the object is seen. The sequence, described in detail in Procedure 17:2F, is repeated until the object is expelled, the infant loses consciousness, or other qualified medical help arrives. If the infant becomes unresponsive, start infant CPR.

- If a child aged 1 to puberty (approximately age 12) has an obstructed airway, the same sequence of steps used for an adult is followed. A finger sweep of the mouth is *not* performed unless the object can be seen in the mouth.

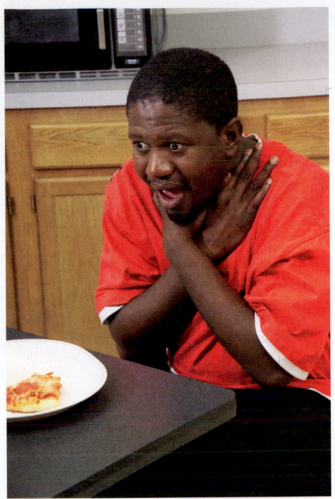

FIGURE 17–9 A choking victim usually grasps his throat and appears cyanotic.

Once CPR is started, it must be continued unless one of the following situations occur:

- The victim recovers and starts to breathe.

- Other qualified medical help arrives and takes over.

- A physician or other legally qualified person orders you to discontinue the attempt.

- The rescuer is so physically exhausted that CPR can no longer be continued.

- The scene suddenly becomes unsafe.

- You are given a legally valid do not resuscitate (DNR) order.

checkpoint

| **1.** What does the acronym *CABD* stand for?

PRACTICE: Go to the workbook and complete the assignment sheet for 17:2, Performing Cardiopulmonary Resuscitation. Then return and continue with the procedures.

Performing CPR—One-Person Adult Rescue

Equipment and Supplies

CPR manikin, barrier device, alcohol or disinfecting solution, gauze sponges

Procedure

⚠️ **Safety** **CAUTION:** Only a CPR training manikin (**Figure 17–10**) should be used to practice this procedure. *Never* practice CPR on another person.

1. Assemble equipment. Position the manikin on a firm surface, usually the floor.

2. *Check for consciousness.* Shake the "victim" by tapping the shoulder. Ask, "Are you OK?" If the victim does not respond, activate EMS immediately. Follow the "call first, call fast" priority. Get an AED if available.

3. *Palpate the carotid pulse.* Kneeling at the victim's side, place the fingertips of your hand on the victim's voice box. Then, slide the fingers toward you and into the groove at the side of the victim's neck, where you should find the carotid pulse. Take at least 5 seconds but not more than 10 seconds to feel for the pulse (**Figure 17–11A**). At the same time, watch for breathing by looking to see if the chest is rising and falling.

   NOTE: The pulse may be weak, so check carefully.

4. *If the victim has a pulse but is not breathing, provide rescue breaths.* Give one breath every 5–6 seconds. Count, "One, one thousand; two, one thousand; three, one thousand; four, one thousand; and breathe," to obtain the correct timing. Recheck the pulse every 2 minutes to make sure the heart is still beating.

5. *If the victim does not have a pulse, or you are not sure if they have a pulse, administer chest compressions* as follows:

   a. Locate the correct place on the sternum. While kneeling alongside the victim, use the middle finger of your hand that is closest to the victim's feet to follow the ribs up to where the ribs meet

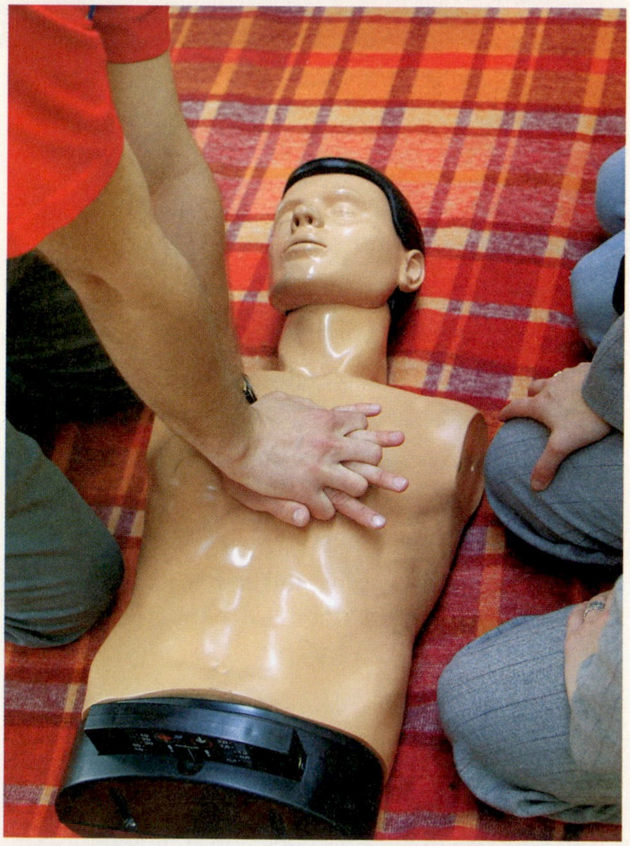

FIGURE 17–10 Use only training manikins while practicing CPR.
© prism68/www.Shutterstock.com

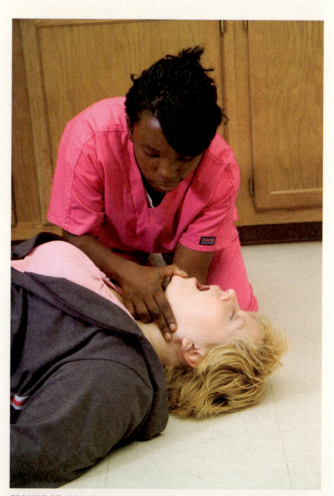

FIGURE 17–11A Palpate the carotid pulse for at least 5 but not more than 10 seconds to determine whether the heart is beating.

the sternum, at the substernal notch. Keep the middle finger on the notch and position the index finger above it so two fingers are on the sternum. Then, place the heel of the opposite hand (the one closest to the victim's head) on the sternum, next to the index finger.

 CAUTION: The heel of your hand should be in the center of the chest on the lower half of the sternum at the nipple line.

b. Place your other hand on top of the hand that is correctly positioned. Keep your fingers off the victim's chest. It may help to interlock your fingers.

c. Rise up on your knees so that your shoulders are directly over the victim's sternum. Lock your elbows and keep your arms straight.

NOTE: This position will allow you to push straight down on the sternum and compress the heart, which lies between the sternum and vertebral column.

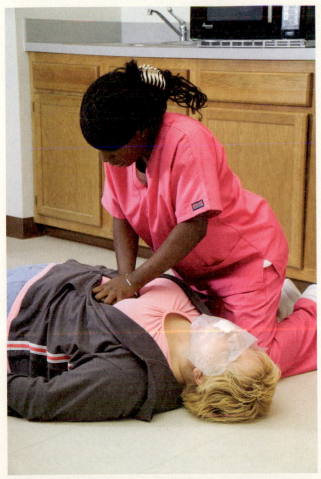

FIGURE 17–11B Use hard and fast motions to compress the chest straight down while giving 30 compressions.

d. Push down hard and fast to compress the chest at least 2 inches or 5 centimeters but not more than 2.4 inches or 6 centimeters **(Figure 17–11B)**. Use a smooth, even motion.

e. Administer 30 compressions at the rate of at least 100–120 per minute. Count, "One, two, three," and so forth, to obtain the correct rate.

f. Allow the chest to recoil or re-expand completely after each compression. Keep your hands on the sternum during the upstroke (chest relaxation period).

NOTE: When the chest recoils or re-expands completely, this allows more blood to refill the heart between compressions.

g. Administer 30 fast, deep chest compressions.

NOTE: Make every effort to minimize any interruptions to chest compressions. There is no blood flow to the brain and heart when compressions are not being performed.

6. *Open the airway.* Use the head-tilt/chin-lift method. Place one hand on the victim's forehead. Place the fingertips of the other hand under the bony part of the victim's jaw, near the chin. Tilt the head without closing the victim's mouth. Check for breathing by watching for chest movement as you open the airway.

NOTE: This action moves the tongue away from the back of the throat and prevents the tongue from blocking the airway.

 CAUTION: If the victim has a suspected neck or upper spinal cord injury, use a jaw-thrust maneuver to open the airway. Assume a position on either side of the patient's head. Grasp the angles of the victim's lower jaw by positioning one hand on each side. Lift with both hands to move the lower jaw forward, making every attempt to avoid excessive backward tilting or side-to-side movement of the head.

7. *If the victim is breathing,* keep the airway open and obtain medical help. *If the victim is not breathing,* administer mouth-to-mouth resuscitation as follows:

a. Keep the airway open.

b. Place the barrier mask on the face with the narrow section on the bridge of the nose. Using the thumb and index finger, make a "C" on the side of the mask and press down on the face to create a seal.

(continues)

c. Position your mouth on the barrier mask.

d. Give two breaths, each lasting approximately 1 second until the chest visibly rises (**Figure 17–11C**). Pause slightly between breaths. This allows air to flow out and provides you with a chance to take a breath and increase the oxygen level for the second rescue breath.

e. Watch the chest for movement to be sure the air is entering the victim's lungs. Avoid overinflating the lungs and/or forcing air into the stomach.

Precaution

CAUTION: Follow standard precautions. Use a CPR pocket face mask with a one-way valve to provide a barrier and prevent the transmission of disease.

Safety

CAUTION: Giving breaths too quickly or with too much force can cause gastric distention (bloating of the stomach when air enters it). This can lead to serious

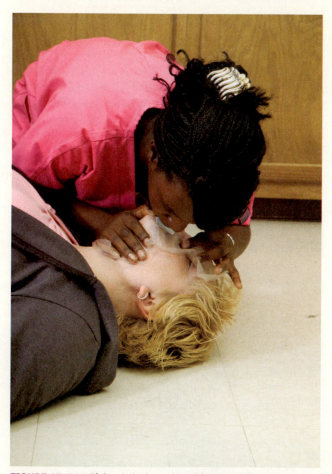

FIGURE 17–11C If the victim is not breathing, open the airway and use a barrier device to give two breaths. Watch for the chest to visibly rise.

complications, such as vomiting, aspiration (foreign material entering the lungs), and pneumonia.

8. Continue the cycles of 30 compressions followed by 2 ventilations until EMS providers take over, an AED arrives, or the victim recovers.

9. If an AED is available, give five cycles of CPR and then use the AED. Even though AEDs have different manufacturers and models, they all operate in basically the same way.

a. Position the AED at the victim's side next to the rescuer who is using it. If another person arrives to help, the second person can activate EMS (if this has not already been done) and then administer cycles of CPR on the victim's other side.

b. Open the case on the AED and turn on the power control.

NOTE: Some AEDs power on automatically when the case is opened.

c. Expose the victim's chest and attach the chest electrodes to bare skin. If the chest is covered with sweat or water, quickly wipe it dry. Choose the correct size electrode pad. Use adult size pads for any victim 8 years and older. Peel the backing off of the electrode pad. Place one pad on the upper right side of the chest, below the clavicle (collarbone) and to the right of the sternum (breastbone). Place the second electrode pad on the left side of the chest to the left of the nipple and a few inches below the axilla (armpit). Most AEDs have a diagram showing correct placement. If the victim has an implanted device such as a pacemaker, try to avoid putting the pads directly over the device. If possible, do not place the pads directly on a medication patch. If it does not delay shock, remove the patch and quickly wipe the area clean.

d. If necessary, attach the connecting cables of the electrodes to the electrode pad and AED. Some types of electrodes are preconnected.

e. Clearly state, "Clear the victim." Look carefully to make sure no one is touching the victim. Push the analyze control to allow the AED to evaluate the heart rhythm (**Figure 17–12**). The analysis may take 5–15 seconds.

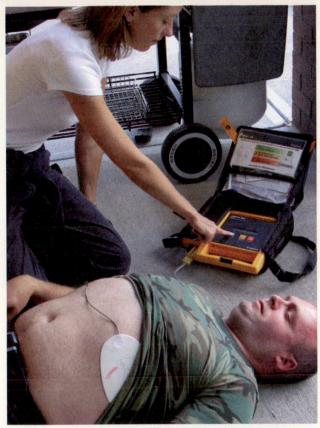

FIGURE 17–12 "Clear" the victim before pushing the control to allow the automated external defibrillator (AED) to analyze the victim's heart rhythm.

If the chest is very hairy and the AED is unable to analyze, press down firmly on the pads. If it still fails to analyze, pull the pads off and place new pads where the hair was pulled off by the previous pads.

f. Follow the recommendations of the AED. If the AED says NO SHOCK, resume CPR by giving 30 compressions followed by 2 ventilations.

g. If the AED says SHOCK, make sure the victim is clear. Loudly state, "Clear victim," and look to make sure no one is touching the victim. Push the shock button.

CAUTION: If another rescuer is touching the victim, the rescuer will also receive the shock. This can cause a serious injury and/or a cardiac arrest.

Safety

h. Begin cycles of CPR by starting with chest compressions immediately after the shock is delivered to the victim. After 2 minutes of CPR, most AEDs will prompt you to reanalyze the rhythm and deliver additional shocks if necessary.

10. After you begin CPR, do not stop unless:

a. The victim recovers

b. Qualified medical help arrives to take over and give CPR and/or apply an AED

c. A physician or other legally qualified person orders you to discontinue the attempt

d. You are so physically exhausted that you cannot continue

e. The scene suddenly becomes unsafe

f. You are given a legally valid do not resuscitate (DNR) order

11. After the practice session, use a gauze pad saturated with 70-percent alcohol or a 10-percent bleach disinfecting solution to clean the manikin. Wipe the face and clean inside the mouth thoroughly. Saturate a clean gauze pad with the solution and lay it on the mouth area for at least 30 seconds. Use another gauze pad to wipe the area dry. Follow manufacturer's instructions for any additional cleaning required.

NOTE: A 10-percent bleach solution is more effective than alcohol. Some manikins have disposable mouthpieces that are discarded after use. If the mouthpiece is discarded, the remainder of the face should still be disinfected.

12. Replace all equipment used. Wash hands.

PRACTICE: Go to the workbook and use the evaluation sheet for 17:2A, Performing CPR—One-Person Adult Rescue, to practice this procedure. When you believe you have mastered this skill, sign the sheet and give it to your instructor for further action.

FINAL EVALUATION: Using the criteria listed on the evaluation sheet, your instructor will grade your performance.

Check

Performing CPR—Two-Person Adult Rescue

Equipment and Supplies

CPR manikin, barrier device, alcohol or disinfecting solution, gauze sponges

Procedure

CAUTION: Only a CPR training manikin should be used to practice this procedure. *Never* practice CPR on another person.

Safety

1. Assemble equipment. Position the manikin on a firm surface, usually the floor.

2. Check for consciousness. Gently shake the victim and ask, "Are you OK?" If the victim does not respond, activate EMS immediately. Follow the "call first, call fast" priority. Get an AED if available.

3. If the victim is unconscious, the first rescuer starts CPR. The second rescuer activates EMS and obtains an AED if available.

4. Feel for the carotid pulse for at least 5 seconds and not more than 10 seconds. At the same time, check for breathing by watching the chest rise and fall.

5. If there is no pulse, or you are not sure if there is a pulse, give chest compressions. Locate the correct hand position on the sternum. Give 30 hard, fast, and deep compressions at a rate of at least 100–120 per minute.

6. Open the victim's airway using the head-tilt/chin-lift method. Place one hand on the victim's forehead. Place the fingertips of the other hand under the bony part of the victim's jaw, near the chin. Tilt the victim's head back without closing the victim's mouth. Check for breathing by watching for the chest to rise as you open the airway.

7. If the *victim is not breathing*, or not breathing normally (gasping), use a barrier device and give two breaths, each lasting approximately 1 second. Watch the chest for movement to be sure air is entering the victim's lungs. Avoid overinflating the lungs and/or forcing air into the stomach. Until the second rescuer returns, provide compressions and respirations as in a one-person rescue. Give 30 compressions for every 2 breaths.

CAUTION: Follow standard precautions. Use a CPR pocket face mask with a one-way valve to provide a barrier and prevent the transmission of disease.

Precaution

8. When the second rescuer returns after calling for help, the first rescuer should complete the cycle of 30 compressions and 2 respirations.

9. The second rescuer should get into position for compressions and locate the correct hand placement while the first rescuer is giving the two breaths. The second rescuer should begin compressions at the rate of at least 100–120 per minute (**Figure 17–13**). The second rescuer should count out loud, "One, two, three, four, five . . ." After each set of 30 compressions, the second rescuer should pause very briefly to allow the first rescuer to give 2 breaths. Rescue then continues with 2 breaths after each 30 compressions.

10. After every five cycles of CPR (approximately 2 minutes) the rescuers should change positions. The person giving compressions can provide a clear signal to change positions, such as, "Change, two, three, four. ..." The compressor should complete a cycle of 30 compressions. The ventilator should give 2 breaths at the end of the 30 compressions. The ventilator should then move to the chest and locate the correct hand placement for compressions. The compressor should move to the head and open the airway. The new compressor

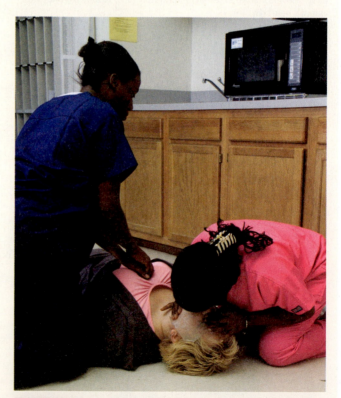

FIGURE 17–13 In a two-person rescue, two breaths are given after every 30 compressions.

should then give 30 hard, fast, and deep compressions at the rate of at least 100–120 per minute. The rescue should continue with 2 ventilations after each 30 compressions.

11. If an AED is available, one rescuer should set up the AED while the other rescuer is giving cycles of CPR. When the AED is ready to analyze the heart rhythm, the rescuer operating the AED must make sure the other rescuer is clear of the victim. The steps for using the AED are discussed in detail in step 9 of Procedure 17:2A.

12. The rescuers should continue CPR until qualified medical help arrives, the victim recovers, a physician or other legally qualified person orders CPR discontinued, the scene suddenly becomes unsafe, or they are presented with a legally valid do not resuscitate (DNR) order.

13. After the practice session, use a gauze pad saturated with 70-percent alcohol or a 10-percent bleach disinfecting solution to clean the manikin. Wipe the face and clean inside the mouth

thoroughly. Saturate a clean gauze pad with the solution and lay it on the mouth area for at least 30 seconds. Use another gauze pad to wipe the area dry. Follow manufacturer's instructions for any additional cleaning required.

NOTE: A 10-percent bleach solution is more effective than alcohol. Some manikins have disposable mouthpieces that are discarded after use. If the mouthpiece is discarded, the remainder of the face should still be disinfected.

14. Replace all equipment used. Wash hands.

PRACTICE: Go to the workbook and use the evaluation sheet for 17:2B, Performing CPR—Two-Person Adult Rescue, to practice this procedure. When you believe you have mastered this skill, sign the sheet and give it to your instructor for further action.

 FINAL EVALUATION: Using the criteria listed on the evaluation sheet, your instructor will grade your performance.

Performing CPR on Infants

Equipment and Supplies

CPR infant manikin, barrier device, alcohol or disinfecting solution, gauze pads

Procedure

 CAUTION: Only a CPR training manikin should be used to practice this procedure. *Never* practice CPR on a human infant.

1. Assemble equipment.

2. Check for responsiveness. Gently shake the infant or tap the infant's foot (for reflex action) to determine consciousness. Call to the infant.

   NOTE: For CPR techniques, infants are usually considered to be under 1 year old.

3. If the infant is unconscious call aloud for help, and begin the steps of CPR. If no one arrives to activate EMS, stop CPR after five cycles (approximately 2 minutes) to activate EMS. Resume CPR as quickly as possible.

   NOTE: If the infant is known to have a high risk for heart problems or a sudden collapse was witnessed, activate EMS and then begin CPR.

4. Check the pulse over the brachial artery. Place your fingertips on the inside of the upper arm and halfway between the elbow and shoulder (refer to Figure 17–8). Put your thumb on the posterior (outside) of the arm. Squeeze your fingers gently toward your thumb. Feel for the pulse for at least 5 but not more than 10 seconds. At the same time, check for breathing by watching to see if the chest rises and falls.

5. *If a pulse is present, but the infant is not breathing,* provide ventilations by giving the infant 1 ventilation every 2 seconds (approximately 30 breaths per minute). Recheck the pulse every 2 minutes.

6. *If no pulse is present or if the heart rate is below 60 beats per minute with signs of poor circulation such as cyanosis,* administer cardiac compressions. Locate the correct position for compressions by drawing an imaginary line between the nipples. Place two fingers on the sternum just below this imaginary line. Give compressions at the rate of at least 100–120 per minute (**Figure 17–14A**). Make sure the infant is on a firm surface, or use one hand to support the

(continues)

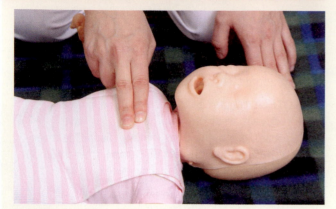

FIGURE 17–14A Use two fingers to give hard and fast compressions to the infant, at a rate of at least 100 – 120 compressions per minute.
© pryzmat/www.Shutterstock.com

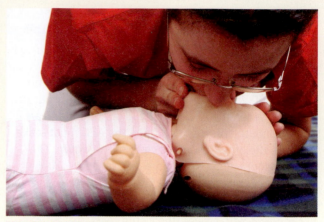

FIGURE 17–14B If the infant is not breathing, give 2 breaths.
© pryzmat/www.Shutterstock.com

infant's back while administering compressions. Press hard, fast, and deep enough to compress the infant's chest at least ⅓ the depth of the chest, approximately 1½ inches (4 cm). Give 30 compressions at the rate of at least 100–120 per minute. Allow the chest to recoil or re-expand completely between compressions.

7. Once 30 compressions are delivered, use the head-tilt/chin-lift method to open the infant's airway. Tip the head back gently, taking care not to tip it as far back as you would an adult's head.

 CAUTION: Tipping the head too far will cause an obstruction of the infant's airway.
Safety

8. *If there is no breathing,* give 2 breaths, each breath lasting approximately 1 second (**Figure 17–14B**). Using a barrier device, cover the infant's nose and mouth with your mouth. Breathe until the chest rises visibly during each ventilation. Allow for chest deflation after each breath.

 CAUTION: Follow standard precautions. Use a CPR pocket face mask with a one-way valve to provide a barrier and prevent the transmission of disease.
Precaution

9. After 2 breaths are given, administer 30 chest compressions.

10. Continue the cycle of 30 compressions followed by 2 ventilations. To establish the correct rate, count, "One, two, three, four, five … "

11. If a second rescuer arrives to assist, the second rescuer should activate EMS if this has not been done. Then both rescuers can perform CPR on the infant.

   a. The first rescuer should finish a cycle of 30 compressions followed by 2 respirations.

   b. The second rescuer should stand at the infant's feet and place their thumbs next to each other on the lower half of the sternum just below the nipple line. The rescuer then wraps their hands around the infant to support the infant's back with the fingers, and uses the thumbs to administer 15 compressions.

   c. After 15 compressions, the person giving compressions pauses very briefly so the other rescuer can give 2 ventilations.

   NOTE: The ratio of compressions to ventilations is 15:2 for a two-person rescue on an infant.

   d. The rescuers should switch positions after every six to eight cycles (approximately 2 minutes) of CPR.

12. The rescuers should continue the cycles of CPR until qualified medical help arrives, the infant recovers, a physician or other legally qualified person orders CPR discontinued, or they are presented with a legally valid do not resuscitate (DNR) order (very rare for infants).

13. After the practice session, use a gauze pad saturated with 70-percent alcohol or a 10-percent bleach disinfecting solution to clean the manikin. Wipe the face and clean inside the mouth thoroughly. Saturate a clean gauze pad with the solution and lay it on the mouth area for at least 30 seconds. Use another gauze pad to wipe the area dry. Follow manufacturer's instructions for specific cleaning.

   NOTE: The 10-percent bleach solution is more effective than alcohol. Some manikins have disposable mouthpieces that are discarded after use. If the mouthpiece is discarded, the remainder of the face should still be disinfected.

14. Replace all equipment used. Wash hands.

PRACTICE: Go to the workbook and use the evaluation sheet for 17:2C, Performing CPR on Infants, to practice this procedure. When you believe you have mastered this skill, sign the sheet and give it to your instructor for further action.

 FINAL EVALUATION: Using the criteria listed on the evaluation sheet, your instructor will grade your performance.

Check

Procedure 17:2D

Performing CPR on Children

Equipment and Supplies

CPR child manikin, barrier device, alcohol or disinfecting solution, gauze pads

Procedure

 CAUTION: Only a CPR training manikin should be used to practice this procedure. *Never* practice CPR on a human child.

Safety

1. Assemble equipment.

2. Check for responsiveness. Gently shake the child to determine consciousness. Call to the child.

   NOTE: Health care providers should use child CPR techniques on any child from 1 year of age to puberty (approximately age 12) as evidenced by the development of secondary sex characteristics.

3. If the child is unconscious call aloud for help, and begin the steps of CPR. If no one arrives to call EMS, stop CPR after five cycles (approximately 2 minutes) to activate EMS and obtain an AED if available. Resume CPR as quickly as possible.

   NOTE: If the child is known to have a high risk for heart problems or a sudden collapse was witnessed, activate EMS first and then begin CPR.

4. Check the pulse at the carotid pulse site. Feel for the pulse for at least 5 but not more than 10 seconds. At the same time, check breathing by watching to see if the chest rises and falls.

5. *If a pulse is present, but the child is not breathing,* provide ventilations by giving the child 1 ventilation every 2–3 seconds (approximately 20–30 breaths per minute). Recheck the pulse every 2 minutes.

6. *If no pulse is present or if the heart rate is below 60 beats per minute with signs of poor circulation such as cyanosis,* administer cardiac compressions. Place the heel of one hand on the lower half of the sternum just below a line drawn between the nipples or in the same position used for adult CPR.

Keep the other hand on the child's forehead. If the child is larger, two hands can be positioned on the chest for compressions. Give compressions at the rate of at least 100–120 per minute. Make sure the child is on a firm surface, or use one hand to support the child's back while administering compressions. Press hard, fast, and deep enough to compress the child's chest at least ⅓ the depth of the chest, approximately 2 inches (5 cm). Give 30 compressions at the rate of at least 100–120 per minute. Allow the chest to recoil or re-expand completely between compressions.

7. Once 30 compressions are done, use the head-tilt/chin-lift method to open the child's airway. Tip the head back gently, taking care not to tip it as far back as you would an adult's head.

8. *If there is no breathing,* give 2 breaths, each breath lasting approximately 1 second (**Figure 17–15**). Using a barrier device, cover the child's nose and mouth with your mouth, or pinch the child's nose and cover the child's mouth with your mouth. Breathe until the chest rises visibly during each ventilation. Allow for chest deflation after each breath.

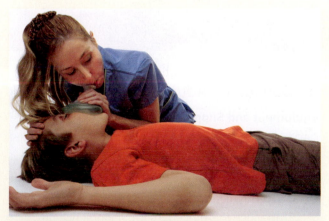

FIGURE 17–15 Using a barrier device, give 2 breaths. © iStockphoto/Leah-Anne Thompson

(continues)

CAUTION: Follow standard precautions. Use a CPR pocket face mask with a one-way valve to provide a barrier and prevent the transmission of disease.

9. Once 2 breaths are given, administer 30 compressions.

10. Continue the cycle of 30 compressions followed by 2 ventilations. To establish the correct rate, count, "One, two, three, four, five ..."

11. If a second rescuer arrives to assist, the second rescuer should activate EMS if this has not been done. Then both rescuers can perform CPR on the child.

   a. The first rescuer should finish a cycle of 30 compressions followed by 2 respirations.

   b. The second rescuer should locate the proper position on the sternum for compressions. As soon as the first rescuer delivers the 2 respirations, the second rescuer should administer 15 compressions.

   c. After 15 compressions, the person giving compressions pauses very briefly so the other rescuer can give 2 ventilations.

   NOTE: The ratio of compressions to ventilations is 15:2 for a two-person rescue on a child.

   d. The rescuers should switch positions after every six to eight cycles (approximately 2 minutes) of CPR.

12. If an AED is available, one rescuer should set up the AED while the other rescuer is giving cycles of CPR. When the AED is ready to analyze the heart rhythm, the rescuer operating the AED must make sure the other rescuer is clear of the victim. The steps for using the AED are discussed in detail in step 9 of Procedure 17:2A.

CAUTION: Adult electrode pads should be used on any child 8 years or older. Child or pediatric electrodes are used only on children from 1 to 8 years of age. In addition, if an AED does not have the option of a pediatric dosage, the adult dosage and electrodes should be used on the child.

13. The rescuers should continue the cycles of CPR until qualified medical help arrives, the child recovers, a physician or other legally qualified person orders CPR discontinued, or they are presented with a legally valid do not resuscitate (DNR) order.

14. After the practice session, use a gauze pad saturated with 70-percent alcohol or a 10-percent bleach disinfecting solution to clean the manikin. Wipe the face and clean inside the mouth thoroughly. Saturate a clean gauze pad with the solution and lay it on the mouth area for at least 30 seconds. Use another gauze pad to wipe the area dry. Follow manufacturer's instructions for specific cleaning.

   NOTE: The 10-percent bleach solution is more effective than alcohol. Some manikins have disposable mouthpieces that are discarded after use. If the mouthpiece is discarded, the remainder of the face should still be disinfected.

15. Replace all equipment used. Wash hands.

PRACTICE: Go to the workbook and use the evaluation sheet for 17:2D, Performing CPR on Children, to practice this procedure. When you believe you have mastered this skill, sign the sheet and give it to your instructor for further action.

FINAL EVALUATION: Using the criteria listed on the evaluation sheet, your instructor will grade your performance.

Procedure 17:2E

Performing CPR—Obstructed Airway on Conscious Adult or Child

Equipment and Supplies

CPR manikin or choking manikin, barrier device, alcohol or disinfecting solution, gauze sponges

Procedure

CAUTION: Only a manikin should be used to practice this procedure. Do not practice on another person. Hand placement can be tried on another person, but the actual abdominal thrust should *never* be performed unless the person is choking.

1. Assemble equipment. Position the manikin in an upright position sitting on a chair.

2. Determine whether the victim has an airway obstruction. Ask, "Are you choking?" Check to see whether the victim can cough or speak.

CAUTION: If the victim is coughing forcefully, the airway is not completely obstructed. Encourage the victim to remain calm and cough hard. Coughing is usually very effective for removing an obstruction.

3. If the victim cannot cough, talk, make noise, or breathe, activate EMS.

4. Perform abdominal thrusts to try to remove the obstruction. Follow these steps:

   a. Stand behind the victim.

   b. Wrap both arms around the victim's waist.

   c. Make a fist of one hand (**Figure 17–16A**). Place the thumb side of the fist in the middle of the victim's abdomen, slightly above the navel (umbilicus) but well below the xiphoid process at the end of the sternum.

   d. Grasp the fist with your other hand.

   e. Use quick, upward thrusts to press into the victim's abdomen (**Figure 17–16B**).

   NOTE: The thrusts should be delivered hard enough to cause a force of air to push the obstruction out of the airway.

    CAUTION: Make sure that your forearms do not press against the victim's rib cage while the thrusts are being performed.

   f. If you cannot reach around the victim to give abdominal thrusts or if a victim is in the later stages of pregnancy, give chest thrusts. Stand behind the victim. Wrap your arms under the victim's axillae (armpits) and around to the center of the chest. Make a fist with one hand and place the thumb side of the fist against the center of the sternum but well above the xiphoid process. Grab your fist with your other hand and thrust inward.

   g. Repeat the thrusts until the object is expelled or until the victim becomes unconscious.

5. If the victim loses consciousness, begin CPR. Activate EMS if this has not already been done. Then start the cycle of CPR. Start with compressions—do not check for a pulse. Every time you open the airway you should look in the mouth before giving breaths (**Figure 17–17**). If you see an object, use a C-shaped or hooking motion to remove the object. To perform CPR:

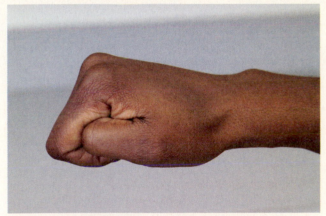

FIGURE 17–16A Make a fist of one hand.

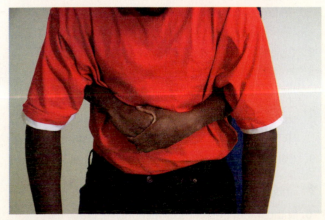

FIGURE 17–16B Place the thumb side of the fist above the umbilicus but well below the xiphoid process at the end of the sternum. Grasp the fist with your other hand and use quick, upward thrusts to press into the victim's abdomen.

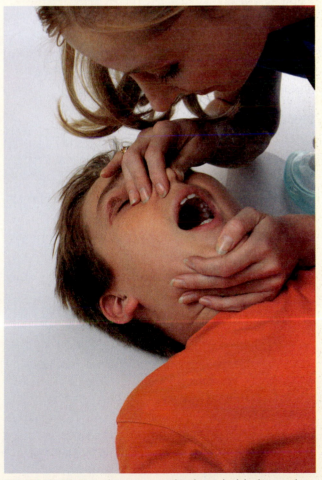

FIGURE 17–17 Every time you open the airway, look in the mouth before giving breaths. © iStockphoto/Leah-Anne Thompson

(continues)

a. Give 30 fast, deep chest compressions.

b. Open the airway.

c. Check the mouth for a foreign body. If you are able to see an object, use a hooking motion with your finger to try to remove it.

d. Using a barrier device, try to give 2 breaths.

e. Give 30 compressions and continue the cycle.

6. Do *not* stop CPR unless the victim recovers, qualified medical help arrives to take over, a physician or other legally qualified person orders you to discontinue the attempt, you are so physically exhausted you cannot continue, or the scene suddenly becomes unsafe.

7. Make every effort to obtain medical help for the victim as soon as possible.

8. After the practice session, replace all equipment used. Wash hands.

PRACTICE: Go to the workbook and use the evaluation sheet for 17:2E, Performing CPR—Obstructed Airway on Conscious Adult or Child, to practice this procedure. When you believe you have mastered this skill, sign the sheet and give it to your instructor for further action.

 FINAL EVALUATION: Using the criteria listed on the evaluation sheet, your instructor will grade your performance.

Check

Procedure 17:2F

Performing CPR—Obstructed Airway on Conscious Infant

Equipment and Supplies

CPR infant manikin, barrier device, alcohol or disinfecting solution, gauze sponges

Procedure

 CAUTION: Only an infant manikin should be used to practice this procedure. Do *not* practice on a real infant.

Safety

1. Assemble equipment. Kneel or sit with the infant in your lap.

   NOTE: An infant is any baby to 1 year of age. Health care providers should use the adult choking sequence for any child older than 1 year.

2. Check for responsiveness. Gently shake the infant or tap the infant's foot (for reflex action) to determine consciousness. Call to the infant.

3. If the infant is conscious and coughing forcefully, allow the infant to cough. The airway is not completely obstructed, and the coughing may expel the object.

4. If the infant cannot cry, make any sounds, is making a high-pitched noise while inhaling or no noise at all, is turning cyanotic, and does not appear to be breathing, the airway is completely obstructed. Activate EMS immediately.

5. Quickly bare the infant's chest to expose the sternum (breastbone).

6. Give five back blows. Hold the infant face down, with your arm supporting the infant's body and your hand supporting the infant's head and jaw. Position the head lower than the chest (**Figure 17–18A**). Use the heel of your other hand to give five firm back blows between the infant's shoulder blades.

    CAUTION: When performing back blows on an infant, do not use excessive force.

   Safety

7. Support the infant's head and neck to turn the infant face up. Hold the infant with your forearm resting on your thigh. Keep the infant's head lower than the chest.

8. Give five chest thrusts. Position two to three fingers on the sternum just below an imaginary line drawn between the nipples. Press straight down five times (**Figure 17–18B**), each time with the intention of creating enough force to dislodge the obstruction.

9. Continue the cycle of five back blows followed by five chest thrusts until EMS arrives or the infant becomes unresponsive.

10. If the infant becomes unresponsive, place the infant on a firm surface. Open the airway and look for an object. If an object is visible, use a C-shaped or hooking motion to remove it. Then perform CPR

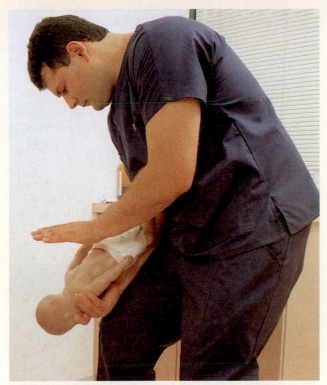

FIGURE 17–18A To give an infant five back blows, position the infant face down, with the head lower than the chest.

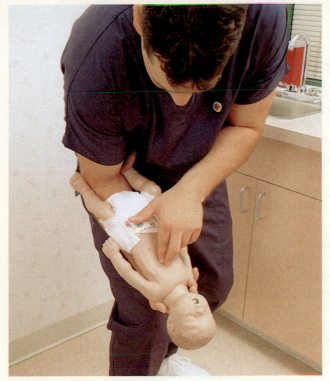

FIGURE 17–18B Give the infant five chest thrusts, keeping the head lower than the chest.

starting with compressions—do not check for a pulse. Follow the normal procedure for an infant, except look in the mouth every time you are ready to give breaths.

   a. Give 30 fast, deep chest compressions.

   b. Open the airway.

   c. Check the mouth for a foreign body. If you are able to see an object, use a hooking motion with your finger to try to remove it.

   d. Using a barrier device, try to give 2 breaths.

   e. Give 30 compressions and continue the cycle.

11. Do *not* stop CPR unless the infant recovers, qualified medical help arrives to take over, a physician or other legally qualified person orders you to discontinue the attempt, you are so physically exhausted you cannot continue, or the scene suddenly becomes unsafe.

12. Make every effort to obtain medical help for the infant as soon as possible.

13. After the practice session, use a gauze pad saturated with 70-percent alcohol or a 10-percent bleach disinfecting solution to clean the manikin. Wipe the face and clean inside the mouth thoroughly. Saturate a clean gauze pad with the solution and lay it on the mouth area for at least 30 seconds. Use another gauze pad to wipe the area dry. Follow manufacturer's recommendations for specific cleaning or care.

NOTE: A 10-percent bleach solution is more effective than alcohol. Some manikins have disposable mouthpieces that are discarded after use. If the mouthpiece is discarded, the remainder of the face should still be disinfected.

14. Replace all equipment used. Wash hands.

PRACTICE: Go to the workbook and use the evaluation sheet for 17:2F, Performing CPR—Obstructed Airway on Conscious Infant, to practice this procedure. When you believe you have mastered this skill, sign the sheet and give it to your instructor for further action.

Check

FINAL EVALUATION: Using the criteria listed on the evaluation sheet, your instructor will grade your performance.

PROVIDING FIRST AID FOR BLEEDING AND WOUNDS

INTRODUCTION

In any health care career, as well as in your personal life, you may need to provide first aid to control bleeding or care for wounds. A **wound** involves injury to the soft tissues. Wounds are usually classified as open or closed. With an open wound, there is a break in the skin or mucous membrane. With a closed wound, there is no break in the skin or mucous membrane but injury occurs to the underlying tissues. An example of a closed wound is a bruise or hematoma. Wounds can result in bleeding, infection, and/or tetanus (lockjaw, a serious infection caused by bacteria). First aid care must be directed toward controlling bleeding before the bleeding leads to death, and toward either preventing or obtaining treatment for infection.

TYPES OF OPEN WOUNDS

Open wounds are classified into types according to the injuries that occur. Some main types are abrasion, incision, laceration, puncture, avulsion, and amputation.

- **Abrasion:** With this type of wound, the skin is scraped off. Bleeding is usually limited, but infection must be prevented because dirt and contaminants often enter the wound.

- **Incision:** This is a cut or injury caused by a sharp object, such as a knife, scissors, or razor blade. The edges of the wound are smooth and regular. If the cut is deep, bleeding can be heavy and can lead to excessive blood loss. In addition, damage to muscles, nerves, and other tissues can occur (**Figure 17–19A**).

- **Laceration:** This type of wound involves tearing of the tissues by way of excessive force. The wound often has jagged, irregular edges (**Figure 17–19B**). Bleeding may be heavy. If the wound is deep, contamination may lead to infection.

- **Puncture:** This type of wound is caused by a sharp object, such as a pin, nail, or pointed instrument. Gunshot wounds can also cause puncture wounds that are extremely dangerous because the damage is hidden under the skin and not visible. With all puncture wounds, external bleeding is usually limited, but internal bleeding can occur. In addition, the chance for infection is increased, and tetanus may develop if tetanus bacteria enter the wound.

- **Avulsion:** This type of wound occurs when tissue is torn or separated from the victim's body. It can result in a piece of torn tissue hanging from the ear, nose, hand, or other body part. Bleeding is heavy and usually extensive. It is important to preserve the body part while caring for this type of wound because a surgeon may be able to reattach it.

- **Amputation:** This type of injury occurs when a body part is cut off and separated from the body. Loss of a finger, toe, hand, or other body part can occur. Bleeding can be heavy and extensive. Care must be taken to preserve the amputated part because a surgeon may be able to reattach it. The part should be wrapped in a cool, moist dressing (use sterile water or normal saline, if possible) and placed in a plastic bag. The plastic bag should be kept cool or placed in ice water and transported with the victim. The body part should never be placed directly on ice because ice can freeze the tissue.

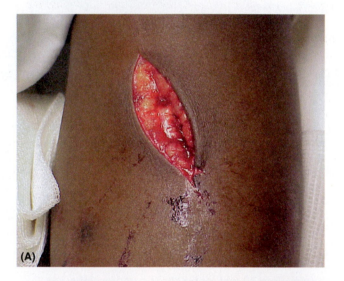
(A)

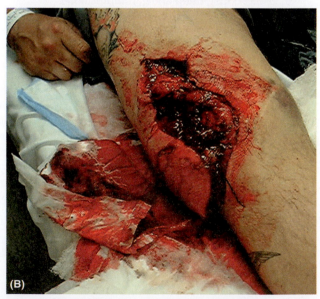
(B)

FIGURE 17–19 Open wounds include (A) an incision that has smooth, regular edges and (B) a laceration that has jagged irregular edges.
Courtesy of Ronald Stram, MD, Albany Medical Center, Albany, NY. Courtesy of Dr. Deborah Funk, Albany Medical Center

CONTROLLING BLEEDING

Controlling bleeding is the first priority in caring for wounds because it is possible for a victim to bleed to death in a short period of time. Bleeding can come from arteries, veins, and capillaries. *Arterial blood* usually spurts from a wound, results in heavy blood loss, and is bright red. Arterial bleeding is life-threatening and must be controlled quickly. *Venous blood* is slower, steadier, and dark red or maroon. Venous bleeding is constant and can lead to a large blood loss, but it is easier to control. *Capillary blood* "oozes" from the wound slowly, is less red than arterial blood, and clots easily. The four main methods for controlling bleeding are listed in the order in which they should be used: direct pressure, elevation, pressure bandage, and a tourniquet in extreme emergencies.

CAUTION: *If possible, use some type of protective barrier, such as gloves or plastic wrap, while controlling bleeding. If this is not possible in an emergency, use thick layers of dressings and try to avoid contact of blood with your skin. Wash your hands thoroughly and as soon as possible after giving first aid to a bleeding victim.*

Precaution

- **Direct pressure**: Using your gloved hand over a thick dressing or sterile gauze, apply pressure directly to the wound (**Figure 17–20A**). If no dressing is available, use a clean cloth or linen-type towel. In an emergency, it may be necessary to use a piece of clothing or another material from the environment. Continue to apply pressure for 5–10 minutes or until the bleeding stops. If blood soaks through the dressing, apply a second dressing over the first and continue to apply direct pressure. Do *not* disturb blood clots once they have formed. Direct pressure will usually stop most bleeding.

- **Elevation**: Whenever possible, if the injury is on an arm or a leg raise the injured part above the level of the victim's heart to allow gravity to aid in stopping the blood flow from the wound. Continue applying direct pressure while elevating the injured part (**Figure 17–20B**).

CAUTION: *If fractures (broken bones) are present or suspected, the part should not be elevated.*

Safety

- **Pressure bandage**: Apply a pressure bandage to hold the dressings in place. Maintain direct pressure and elevation while applying the pressure bandage. The procedure for applying a pressure bandage is described in step 4 of Procedure 17:3.

- **Tourniquet**: A tourniquet should *not* be used unless all other methods to control bleeding have not been effective, it is a life-threatening situation, medical help will be delayed, and you have been instructed on how to how to apply it. Commercial tourniquets are available in many first-aid kits. Follow the directions

provided with it. If a commercial tourniquet is not available, a strip of material or 2–4 inch-wide bandage can be used to create a tourniquet. The procedure for applying a tourniquet is described in step 5 of Procedure 17:3. It is always essential to note the time the tourniquet is applied so this information can be given to the medical responders.

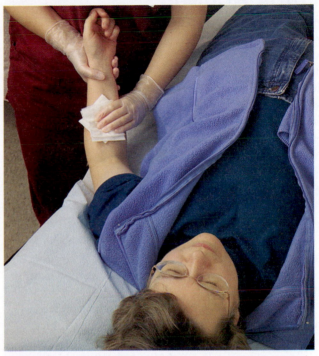

FIGURE 17–20A If possible, use some type of protective barrier, such as gloves or plastic wrap, while applying direct pressure to control bleeding.

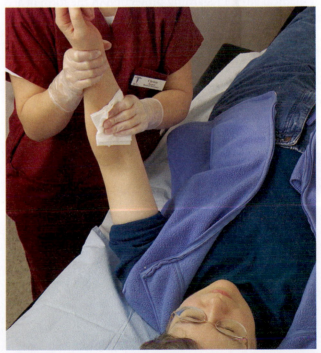

FIGURE 17–20B Whenever possible, if the injury is on an arm or a leg, continue to apply direct pressure while elevating the injured limb above the level of the heart.

After severe bleeding has been controlled, obtain medical help for the victim. Do not disturb any blood clots or remove the dressings that were used to control the bleeding because this may result in additional bleeding. Make no attempt to clean the wound because this too is likely to result in additional bleeding.

MINOR WOUNDS

In treating minor wounds that do not involve severe bleeding, prevention of infection is the first priority. Wash your hands thoroughly before treating the wound. Put on gloves to avoid contamination from blood or fluid draining from the wound. Use soap and water and sterile gauze, if possible, to wash the wound. Wipe in an outward direction, away from the wound. Discard the wipe after each use. Rinse the wound thoroughly with cool water. Use sterile gauze to gently blot the wound dry. Apply a sterile dressing or bandage. Watch for any signs of infection. Be sure to tell the victim to obtain medical help if any signs of infection appear.

Infection can develop in any wound. It is important to recognize the signs of infection and to seek medical help if they appear. Some signs and symptoms are swelling, heat, redness, pain, fever, pus, and red streaks leading from the wound. Prompt medical care is needed if any of these symptoms occur.

Tetanus bacteria can enter an open wound and lead to serious illness and death. Tetanus infection is most common in puncture wounds and wounds that involve damage to tissue underneath the skin. When this type of wound occurs, it is important to obtain information from the patient regarding their last tetanus shot and to get medical advice regarding protection in the form of a tetanus shot or booster.

With some wounds, objects can remain in the tissues or become embedded in the wound. Examples of such objects include splinters, small pieces of glass, small stones, and other similar objects. If the object is at the surface of the skin, remove it gently with sterile tweezers or tweezers wiped clean with alcohol or a disinfectant. Any objects embedded in the tissues should be left in the skin and removed by a physician.

CLOSED WOUNDS

Closed wounds (those not involving breaks in the skin) can occur anywhere in the body as a result of injury. If the wound is a bruise, cold applications can be applied to reduce swelling. Other closed wounds can be extremely serious and cause internal bleeding that may lead to death. Signs and symptoms may include pain, tenderness, swelling, deformity, cold and clammy skin, rapid and weak pulse, a drop in blood pressure, uncontrolled restlessness, excessive thirst, vomited blood, or blood in the urine or feces. Get medical help for the victim as soon as possible. Check breathing, treat for shock, avoid unnecessary movement, and avoid giving any fluids or food to the victim.

SUMMARY

While caring for any victim with severe bleeding or wounds, always be alert for the signs of shock (see Section 17:4). Be prepared to treat shock while providing care to control bleeding and prevent infection in the wound.

 At all times, remain calm while providing first aid. Reassure the victim. Obtain appropriate assistance or medical care as soon as possible in every case requiring additional care.

Comm

checkpoint

1. List four (4) types of wounds.
2. If a finger is amputated, how would you handle the severed part?

PRACTICE: Go to the workbook and complete the assignment sheet for 17:3, Providing First Aid for Bleeding and Wounds. Then return and continue with the procedure.

Procedure 17:3

Providing First Aid for Bleeding and Wounds

Equipment and Supplies

Sterile dressings and bandages, disposable gloves

Procedure
Severe Wounds

1. Follow the steps of priority care, if indicated:

   a. Check the scene. Move the victim only if absolutely necessary.

   b. Check the victim for consciousness, a pulse, and breathing.

   c. Call emergency medical services (EMS).

   d. Provide care to the victim.

2. To control severe bleeding, proceed as follows:

   a. 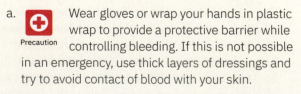 Wear gloves or wrap your hands in plastic wrap to provide a protective barrier while controlling bleeding. If this is not possible in an emergency, use thick layers of dressings and try to avoid contact of blood with your skin.

   Precaution

b. Using your hand over a thick dressing or sterile gauze, apply pressure directly to the wound.

c. Continue to apply pressure to the wound for approximately 5–10 minutes. Do *not* release the pressure to check whether the bleeding has stopped.

d. If blood soaks through the first dressing, apply a second dressing on top of the first dressing, and continue to apply direct pressure.

NOTE: If sterile gauze is not available, use clean material or a bare hand.

 CAUTION: Do *not* disturb blood clots once they have formed. This will cause the bleeding to start again.

3. Whenever possible, and the wound is on an arm or leg, elevate the injured part above the level of the victim's heart.

NOTE: This allows gravity to help stop the blood flow to the area.

 CAUTION: Do *not* move the injured part if a fractured bone is suspected.

NOTE: Direct pressure and elevation are used together. Do *not* stop direct pressure while elevating the injured part.

4. To hold the dressings in place, apply a pressure bandage. Maintain direct pressure while applying the pressure bandage. To apply a pressure bandage, proceed as follows:

a. Apply additional dressings over the dressings already on the wound.

b. Use a roller bandage to hold the dressings in place by wrapping the roller bandage around the dressings. Use overlapping turns to cover the dressings and to hold them securely in place.

c. Tie off the ends of the bandage by placing the tie directly over the dressings (**Figure 17–21**).

d. Make sure the pressure bandage is secure. Check a pulse site below the pressure bandage to make sure the bandage is not too tight. A pulse should be present, and there should be no discoloration of the skin to indicate impaired circulation. If any signs of impaired circulation are present, loosen and replace the pressure bandage.

5. If the bleeding continues and it becomes life-threatening and medical help is delayed, it may be necessary to apply a tourniquet. Do *not* apply a tourniquet if you have not been taught how to apply it. To apply a tourniquet, proceed as follows:

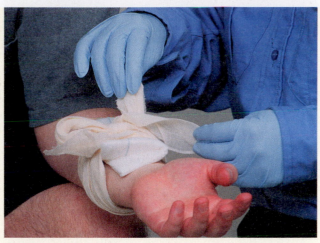

FIGURE 17–21 Tie the ends of the bandage directly over the dressings to secure a pressure bandage.

a. Commercial tourniquets are available in many first-aid kits. Follow the directions provided to apply it.

b. If a commercial tourniquet is not available, use a strip of material or 2–4 inch-wide bandage and wrap it around the limb about 2–3 inches above the bleeding wound.

c. Tie a knot in the bandage and position a stick or stiff rod on top of the knot. Tie another knot to hold the stick in place. Twist the stick only until the bandage is tight enough to stop the bleeding and then secure the stick in place.

NOTE: A tourniquet prevents blood flow to the extremity below it and can result in severe and irreversible nerve and muscle damage.

d. Note the time the tourniquet is applied so this information can be given to the medical responders.

6. Obtain medical help for the victim as soon as possible. Severe bleeding is a life-threatening emergency.

7. While caring for any victim experiencing severe bleeding, be alert for the signs and symptoms of shock. Treat the victim for shock if any signs or symptoms are noted.

8. During treatment, constantly reassure the victim. Encourage the victim to remain calm by remaining calm yourself.

9. After controlling the bleeding, wash your hands as thoroughly and quickly as possible to avoid possible contamination from the blood. Wear gloves and use a disinfectant solution to wipe up any blood spills. Always wash your hands thoroughly after removing gloves.

(continues)

Procedure
Minor Wounds

1. Wash hands thoroughly with soap and water. Put on gloves.

2. Use sterile gauze, soap, and water to wash the wound. Start at the center and wash in an outward direction. Discard the gauze after each pass.

3. Rinse the wound thoroughly with cool water to remove all of the soap.

4. Use sterile gauze to dry the wound. Blot it gently.

5. Apply a sterile dressing to the wound.

6. Caution the victim to look for signs of infection. Tell the victim to obtain medical care if any signs of infection appear.

7. If tetanus infection is possible (for example, in cases involving puncture wounds), tell the victim to contact a physician regarding a tetanus shot.

CAUTION: Do *not* use any antiseptic solutions to clean the wound and do not apply any substances to the wound unless specifically instructed to do so by a physician or your immediate supervisor.

8. Obtain medical help as soon as possible for any victim requiring additional care. Any victim who has particles embedded in a wound, risk for tetanus, severe bleeding, or other complications must be referred for medical care.

9. When care is complete, remove gloves and wash hands thoroughly.

PRACTICE: Go to the workbook and use the evaluation sheet for 17:3, Providing First Aid for Bleeding and Wounds, to practice these procedures. When you believe you have mastered these skills, sign the sheet and give it to your instructor for further action.

FINAL EVALUATION: Using the criteria listed on the evaluation sheet, your instructor will grade your performance.

17:4 PROVIDING FIRST AID FOR SHOCK

INTRODUCTION

Shock is a state that can exist with any injury or illness requiring first aid. It is important that you are able to recognize it and provide treatment.

Shock, also called *hypoperfusion*, can be defined as "a clinical set of signs and symptoms associated with an inadequate supply of blood to body organs, especially the brain and heart." If it is not treated, shock can lead to death, even when a victim's injuries or illness might not themselves be fatal. After just 4–6 minutes of hypoperfusion, brain cells are damaged irreversibly.

CAUSES OF SHOCK

Many different things can cause the victim to experience shock: **hemorrhage** (excessive loss of blood); excessive pain; infection; heart attack; stroke; poisoning by chemicals, drugs, or gases; lack of oxygen; psychological trauma; and dehydration (loss of body fluids) from burns, vomiting, or diarrhea. The nine main types of shock are shown in **Table 17–1**. All types of shock impair circulation and decrease the supply of oxygen to body cells, tissues, and organs.

SIGNS AND SYMPTOMS

When shock occurs, the body attempts to increase blood flow to the brain, heart, and vital organs by reducing blood flow to other body parts. This can lead to the following signs and symptoms that indicate shock:

- Skin is pale or cyanotic (bluish) in color. Check the nail beds and the mucous membrane around the mouth.

- Skin is cool to the touch.

- **Diaphoresis**, or excessive perspiration, may result in a wet, clammy feeling when the skin is touched.

- Pulse is rapid, weak, and difficult to feel. Check the pulse at one of the carotid arteries in the neck.

- Respirations are rapid, shallow, and may be irregular.

- Blood pressure is very low or below normal, and may not be obtainable.

- Victim experiences general weakness. As shock progresses, the victim becomes listless and confused. Eventually, the victim loses consciousness.

- Victim experiences anxiety and extreme restlessness.

- Victim may experience excessive thirst, nausea, and/or vomiting.

- Victim may complain of blurred vision. As shock progresses, the victim's eyes may appear sunken and have a vacant or confused expression. The pupils may dilate or become large.

TABLE 17-1 Types of Shock

Type of Shock	Cause	Description
Anaphylactic	Hypersensitive or allergic reaction to a substance, such as food, medications, insect stings or bites, or snake bites	Body releases histamine causing vasodilation (blood vessels get larger) Blood pressure drops and less blood goes to body cells Urticaria (hives) and respiratory distress may occur
Cardiogenic	Damage to heart muscle from heart attack or cardiac arrest	Heart cannot effectively pump blood to body cells
Hemorrhagic	Severe bleeding or loss of blood plasma	Decrease in blood volume causes blood pressure to drop Decreased blood flow to body cells
Hypovolemic	Excessive loss of body fluids due to bleeding, prolonged diarrhea, excessive vomiting, protracted diaphoresis, and severe burns	Loss of body fluids affects homeostatic balance and organs to not get enough blood or oxygen Causes weakness, fainting, and dizziness Can lead to organ failure
Metabolic	Loss of body fluid from severe vomiting, diarrhea, or a heat illness Disruption in acid-base balance as occurs in diabetes	Decreased amount of fluid causes dehydration and disruption in normal acid-base balance of body Blood pressure drops and less blood circulates to body cells
Neurogenic	Injury and trauma to brain and/or spinal cord	Nervous system loses ability to control the size of blood vessels Blood vessels dilate and blood pressure drops Decreased blood flow to body cells
Psychogenic	Emotional distress, such as anger, fear, or grief	Emotional response causes sudden dilation of blood vessels Blood pools in areas away from the brain Some individuals faint
Respiratory	Trauma to respiratory tract Respiratory distress or arrest (chronic disease, choking)	Interferes with exchange of oxygen and carbon dioxide between lungs and bloodstream Insufficient oxygen supply for body cells
Septic	Acute infection (toxic shock syndrome)	Poisons or toxins in blood cause vasodilation Blood pressure drops Less oxygen supply to body cells

TREATMENT FOR SHOCK

It is essential to get medical help for the victim as soon as possible because shock is a life-threatening condition. Treatment for shock is directed toward (1) eliminating the cause of shock; (2) improving circulation, especially to the brain and heart; (3) providing an adequate oxygen supply; and (4) maintaining body temperature. Some of the basic principles for treatment include:

- Reduce the effects of or eliminate the cause of shock: control bleeding, provide oxygen if available, ease pain through position change, and/or provide emotional support.

CAUTION: *If neck or spine injuries are suspected, the victim should not be moved unless it is necessary to remove them from danger.*

Safety

- The position for treating shock must be based on the victim's injuries.

    The best position for treating shock is usually to keep the victim lying flat on the back because this improves circulation. Raising the feet and legs approximately 12 inches can also provide additional blood for the heart and brain. However, if the victim is vomiting or has bleeding and injuries of the jaw or mouth, the victim should be positioned on the side to prevent them from choking on blood and/or vomitus, or vomited material. If a victim is experiencing breathing problems, it may be necessary to raise the victim's head and shoulders to make breathing easier. If the victim has a head (not neck) injury and has difficulty breathing, the victim should be positioned lying flat or with the head raised slightly. It is important to position the victim based on the injury or illness involved.

- Cover the patient with blankets or additional clothing to prevent chilling or exposure to the cold. Blankets may also be placed between the ground and the victim. However, it is important to avoid overheating the victim. If the skin is very warm to the touch and perspiration is noted, remove some of the blankets or coverings.

- Avoid giving the victim anything to eat or drink. If the victim complains of excessive thirst, a wet cloth can be used to provide some comfort by moistening the lips and mouth.

Remember that it is important to look for signs of shock while providing first aid for any injury or illness. Provide care that will reduce the effect of shock. Obtain medical help for the victim as soon as possible.

1. List three (3) causes of shock.

PRACTICE: Go to the workbook and complete the assignment sheet for 17:4, Providing First Aid for Shock. Then return and continue with the procedure.

Procedure 17:4

Providing First Aid for Shock

Equipment and Supplies

Blankets, watch with second hand (optional), disposable gloves

Procedure

1. Follow the steps of priority care, if indicated:

a. Check the scene. Move the victim only if absolutely necessary.

b. Check the victim for consciousness, a pulse, and breathing.

c. Call emergency medical services (EMS).

d. Provide care to the victim.

e. Control severe bleeding.

> **CAUTION:** Wear gloves or use a protective barrier while controlling bleeding.
> *Precaution*

2. Obtain medical help for the victim as soon as possible. Call or send someone to obtain help.

3. Observe the victim for any signs of shock. Look for a pale or cyanotic (bluish) color to the skin. Touch the skin and note if it is cool, moist, or clammy to the touch. Note diaphoresis, or excessive perspiration. Check the pulse to see if it is rapid, weak, or irregular. If you are unable to feel a radial pulse, check the carotid pulse. Check the respirations to see if they are rapid, weak, irregular, shallow, or labored. If equipment is available, check blood pressure to see if it is low. Observe the victim for signs of weakness, apathy, confusion, or consciousness. Note if the victim is nauseated or vomiting, complaining of excessive thirst, restless or anxious, or complaining of blurred vision. Examine the eyes for a sunken, vacant, or confused appearance, and dilated pupils.

4. Try to reduce the effects or eliminate the cause of shock.

a. Control bleeding by applying pressure at the site.

b. Provide oxygen, if possible.

c. Attempt to ease pain through position changes and comfort measures.

d. Give emotional support.

5. Position the victim based on the injuries or illness present.

a. If an injury of the neck or spine is present or suspected, do *not* move the victim.

b. If the victim has bleeding and injuries to the jaw or mouth, or is vomiting, position the victim's body on either side. This allows fluids, vomitus, and/or blood to drain and prevents the airway from becoming blocked by these fluids.

c. If the victim is having difficulty breathing, position the victim on the back, but raise the head and shoulders slightly to aid breathing.

d. If the victim has a head injury, position the victim lying flat or with the head raised slightly.

NOTE: Never allow the head to be positioned lower than the rest of the body.

e. If none of these conditions exist, position the victim lying flat on the back. To improve circulation, raise the feet and legs approximately 12 inches (**Figure 17–22**). If raising the legs causes pain or leads to difficult breathing, lower the legs to the flat position.

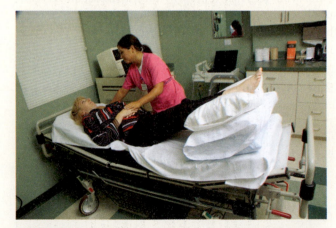

FIGURE 17–22 Position a shock victim flat on the back and elevate the feet and legs approximately 12 inches. Do *not* use this position if the victim has a neck, spinal, head, or jaw injury, or if the victim is having difficulty breathing.

CAUTION: Do not raise the legs if the victim has head, neck, or back injuries, or if there are possible fractures of the hips or legs.

Safety

f. If in doubt on how to position a victim according to the injuries involved, keep the victim lying down flat or in the position in which you found them. Avoid any unnecessary movement.

6. Place enough blankets or coverings on the victim to prevent chilling. Sometimes, a blanket can be placed between the victim and the ground. Avoid overheating the victim.

7. Do not give the victim anything to eat or drink. If the victim complains of excessive thirst, use a moist cloth to wet the lips, tongue, and inside of the mouth.

8. Constantly reassure the victim. Encourage the victim to remain calm by remaining calm yourself.

Comm

9. Observe and provide care to the victim until medical help is obtained.

10. Replace all equipment used. Wash hands.

PRACTICE: Go to the workbook and use the evaluation sheet for 17:4, Providing First Aid for Shock, to practice this procedure. When you believe you have mastered this skill, sign the sheet and give it to your instructor for further action.

✓ **FINAL EVALUATION:** Using the criteria listed on the evaluation sheet, your instructor will grade your performance.

Check

17:5 PROVIDING FIRST AID FOR POISONING

INTRODUCTION

Poisoning can occur anywhere, anytime—not only in health care settings, but also in your personal life. **Poisoning** is a condition that occurs when contact is made with any chemical substance that causes injury, illness, or death. It can be caused by ingesting (swallowing) various substances, inhaling poisonous gases, injecting substances, or contacting the skin with poison. Any substance that causes a harmful reaction when applied or ingested can be called a poison. *Anaphylactic shock* is a common reaction to poisoning (refer to Table 17–1). Immediate action is necessary for any poisoning victim. Treatment varies depending on the type of poison, the injury involved, and the method of contact.

If the poisoning victim is unconscious, check for pulse and breathing. Provide CPR if there is no pulse and/or artificial respiration if the victim is not breathing. Obtain medical help as soon as possible. If the unconscious victim is breathing, position the victim on their side so fluids can drain from the mouth. Obtain medical help quickly.

INGESTION POISONING

 If a poison has been swallowed, immediate care must be provided before the poison can be absorbed into the body. Basic steps of first aid include:

Comm

- Call a poison control center (PCC) or a physician immediately. If you cannot contact a PCC, call emergency medical services (EMS). Most areas have poison control centers that provide information on specific antidotes and treatment. Information can also be obtained at the American Association of Poison Control Centers at *www.aapcc.org*, or by calling 1-800-222-1222.

- Save the label or container of the substance taken so this information can be given to the PCC or physician.

- Calculate or estimate how much was taken and the time at which the poisoning occurred.

- If the victim vomits, save a sample of the vomitus.

- If the PCC tells you to induce vomiting, get the victim to vomit. To induce vomiting, tickle the back of the victim's throat or give the victim warm saltwater to drink.

 CAUTION: *Vomiting must not be induced in unconscious victims, victims who swallowed an acid or alkali, victims who swallowed petroleum products, victims who are convulsing, or victims who have burns on the lips and mouth.*

Safety

- Activated charcoal may be recommended by the PCC to bind to the poison so it is not absorbed into the body. Activated charcoal should only be given to victims who are conscious and able to swallow. It is available in most drug stores. The directions on the bottle should be followed to determine the correct dosage.

INHALATION POISONING

 If poisoning is caused by inhalation of dangerous gases, the victim must be removed immediately from the area before being treated. A commonly inhaled poison is carbon monoxide. It is odorless, colorless, and very difficult to detect. If excessive amounts of gas or fumes are present, and the scene is not safe, do not enter the area. Wait for EMS to arrive. If a quick rescue can be achieved without inhaling the gases, the basic steps of first aid include:

- Before entering the danger area, take a deep breath of fresh air and do not breathe the gas while you are removing the victim from the area.
- After rescuing the victim, immediately check for pulse and breathing.
- Provide CPR and/or artificial respiration if needed.
- Obtain medical help immediately; death may occur very quickly with this type of poisoning.

CONTACT POISONING

If poisoning is caused by chemicals or poisons coming in contact with the victim's skin, care for the victim includes:

- Use large amounts of water to wash the skin for at least 15–20 minutes to dilute the substance and remove it from the skin.
- Remove any clothing and jewelry that contain the substance.
- Call a PCC or physician for additional information.
- Obtain medical help as soon as possible for burns or injuries that may result from contact with the poison.

Contact with a poisonous plant, such as poison ivy, oak, or sumac, can cause a serious skin reaction if not treated immediately. Basic steps of first aid include:

- Wash the area thoroughly with soap and water.
- Apply a corticosteroid cream the first few days to decrease inflammation.
- If a rash or weeping sores develop after 2–3 days, lotions, such as calamine or Caladryl®, or a paste

made from baking soda and water may help relieve the discomfort.

- If the condition is severe and affects large areas of the body or face, obtain medical help.

INJECTION POISONING

Injection poisoning occurs when an insect or spider stings or a snake bites an individual. If an arm or a leg is affected, place the limb in a gravity-neutral position, close to heart level.

For an *insect sting*, first-aid treatment includes:

- Remove any embedded stinger by scraping the stinger away from the skin with the edge of a rigid card, such as a credit card, or a tongue depressor. Do not use tweezers because tweezers can puncture the venom sac attached to the stinger, injecting more poison into body tissues.
- Wash the area well with soap and water.
- Apply a sterile dressing and a cold pack to reduce swelling.

If a *tick* is embedded in the skin, first-aid treatment includes:

- Use tweezers to slowly pull the tick out of the skin.
- Wash the area thoroughly with soap and water.
- Apply an antiseptic.
- Watch for signs of infection.
- Obtain medical help if needed.

Ticks can cause Rocky Mountain spotted fever or Lyme disease, dangerous diseases if untreated.

For a *snakebite* or *spider bite*, first-aid treatment includes:

- Wash the wound.
- Immobilize the injured area, place the limb in a gravity-neutral position, close to heart level.
- Do not cut the wound or apply a tourniquet.
- Monitor the breathing of the victim and give artificial respiration if necessary.
- Obtain medical help for the victim as soon as possible.
- If possible, try to obtain a description of the snake so it can be identified and the correct anti-snake venom can be given to the victim.

For any type of injection poisoning, watch for allergic reaction in all victims (**Figure 17–23**). Signs and symptoms of allergic reaction include redness and swelling at the site, itching, hives, pain, swelling of the throat, difficult or labored breathing, dizziness, and a change in the level of consciousness. Maintain respirations and obtain medical help as quickly as possible for the victim who experiences an allergic reaction.

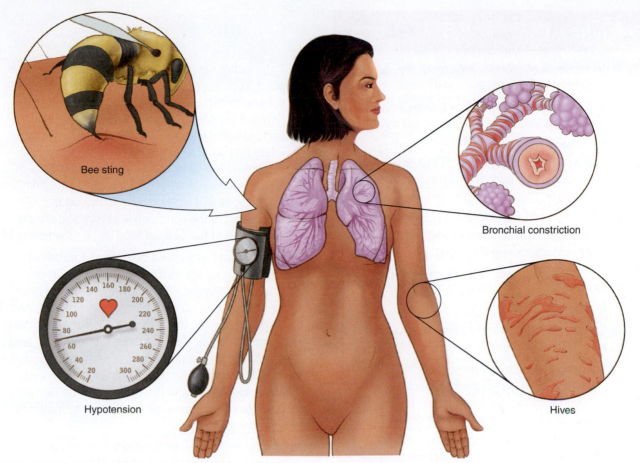

Bee sting

Bronchial constriction

Hypotension

Hives

FIGURE 17–23 Watch for allergic reactions in injection poisoning victims.

SUMMARY

Comm

In all poisoning victims, observe for signs of anaphylactic shock. Treat the victim for shock, if necessary. Try to remain calm and confident while providing first aid for poisoning victims. Reassure the victim as needed. Act quickly and in an organized, efficient manner.

checkpoint

1. What are three (3) ways to be poisoned?
2. What agency do you contact when poisoned?

PRACTICE: Go to the workbook and complete the assignment sheet for 17:5, Providing First Aid for Poisoning. Then return and continue with the procedure.

Procedure 17:5

Providing First Aid for Poisoning

Equipment and Supplies

Telephone, disposable gloves

Procedure

1. Follow the steps of priority care, if indicated:
   a. Check the scene. Move the victim only if absolutely necessary.
   b. Check the victim for consciousness, a pulse, and breathing.
   c. Call emergency medical services (EMS).
   d. Provide care to the victim.
   e. Control severe bleeding.

   Precaution

   CAUTION: Wear gloves or use a protective barrier while controlling bleeding.

2. Check the victim for signs of poisoning. Signs may include burns on the lips or mouth, odor, a container of poison, or presence of the poisonous substance on the victim or in the victim's mouth. Information may also be obtained from the victim or from an observer.

   (continues)

3. If the victim is conscious, not convulsing, and has swallowed a poison:

   a. Try to determine the type of poison, how much was taken, and when the poison was taken. Look for the container near the victim.

   b. Call a poison control center (PCC) or physician immediately for specific information on how to treat the poisoning victim. Provide as much information as possible.

   c. Follow the instructions received from the PCC. Obtain medical help if needed.

   d. If the victim vomits, save a sample of the vomitus.

4. If the PCC tells you to get the victim to vomit, induce vomiting. Give the victim warm saltwater or tickle the back of the victim's throat.

    CAUTION: Do *not* induce vomiting if the victim is unconscious or convulsing, has burns on the lips or mouth, or has swallowed an acid, alkali, or petroleum product.

   Safety

5. If the PCC tells you to give the victim activated charcoal, follow the directions on the container. Make sure the victim is conscious and able to swallow before giving the charcoal.

   NOTE: Activated charcoal binds to the poison so it is not absorbed into the body.

6. If the victim is unconscious:

   a. Check for a pulse and breathing. If the victim does not have a pulse, give CPR. If the victim is not breathing, give artificial respiration.

   b. If the victim is breathing, position the victim on their side to allow fluids to drain from the mouth.

   c. Call a PCC or physician for specific treatment. Obtain medical help immediately.

   d. If possible, save the poison container and a sample of any vomitus. Check with any observers to find out what was taken, how much was taken, and when the poison was taken.

7. If chemicals or poisons have splashed on the victim's skin, wash the area thoroughly with large amounts of water. Remove any clothing and jewelry containing the substance. If a large area of the body is affected, a shower, tub, or garden hose may be used to rinse the skin. Obtain medical help immediately for burns or injuries caused by the poison.

8. If the victim has come in contact with a poisonous plant, such as poison ivy, oak, or sumac, wash the area of contact thoroughly with soap and water. Remove any contaminated clothing. Initially, corticosteroid creams can be applied to decrease inflammation. If a rash or weeping sores develop in the next few days after exposure, lotions, such as calamine or Caladryl®, or a paste made from baking soda and water may help relieve the discomfort. If the condition is severe and affects large areas of the body or face, obtain medical help.

9. If the victim has inhaled poisonous gas, do not endanger your life by trying to treat the victim in the area of the gas. If excessive amounts of gas or fumes are present, and the scene is not safe, wait for EMS to arrive. If it is safe to enter the area, take a deep breath of fresh air before entering the area and hold your breath while you remove the victim from the area. When the victim is in a safe area, check for a pulse and breathing. Provide CPR and/or artificial respiration as needed. Obtain medical help immediately.

10. If poisoning is caused by injection from an insect bite or sting or a snakebite, proceed as follows:

    a. If an arm or a leg is affected, place the limb in a gravity-neutral position, close to heart level.

    b. For an *insect sting*, remove any embedded stinger by scraping it off with an object like a credit card. Wash the area well with soap and water. Apply a sterile dressing and a cold pack to reduce swelling.

    c. If a *tick* is embedded in the skin, use tweezers to gently pull the tick out of the skin. Wash the area thoroughly with soap and water, and apply an antiseptic. Obtain medical help if needed.

    d. For a *snakebite* or *spider bite*, wash the wound. Immobilize the injured area, positioning it lower than the heart if possible. Monitor the breathing of the victim and give artificial respiration if necessary. Obtain medical help for the victim as soon as possible.

    e. Watch for the signs and symptoms of allergic reaction in all victims. Signs and symptoms of allergic reaction include redness and swelling at the site, itching, hives (**Figure 17–24**), pain, swelling of the throat, difficult or labored breathing, dizziness, and a change in the level of

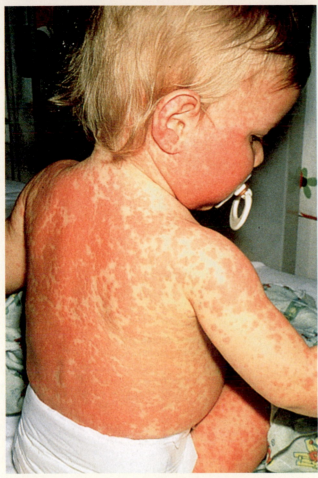

FIGURE 17–24 Hives are a common sign of an allergic reaction. Courtesy of Robert A. Silverman, M.D., Clinical Associate Professor, Department of Pediatrics, Georgetown University

consciousness. Maintain respirations and obtain medical help as quickly as possible for the victim experiencing an allergic reaction.

11. Observe for signs of anaphylactic shock while treating any poisoning victim. Treat for shock as necessary.

12. Remain calm while treating the victim. Reassure the victim.

13. Always obtain medical help for any poisoning victim. Some poisons may have delayed reactions. Always keep the telephone numbers of a PCC and other sources of medical assistance in a convenient location so you will be prepared to provide first aid for poisoning.

14. Wash hands thoroughly after providing care.

PRACTICE: Go to the workbook and use the evaluation sheet for 17:5, Providing First Aid for Poisoning, to practice this procedure. When you believe you have mastered this skill, sign the sheet and give it to your instructor for further action.

✅ **FINAL EVALUATION:** Using the criteria listed on the evaluation sheet, your instructor will grade your performance.

17:6 PROVIDING FIRST AID FOR BURNS

TYPES OF BURNS

A **burn** is an injury that can be caused by fire, heat, chemical agents, radiation, and/or electricity. Burns are classified as either superficial, partial thickness, or full thickness (**Figure 17–25**). Characteristics of each type of burn are as follows:

- **Superficial, or first-degree, burn**: This is the least severe type of burn. It involves only the top layer of skin, the epidermis, and usually heals in 5–6 days without permanent scarring. The skin is usually reddened or discolored. There may be some mild swelling, and the victim feels pain. Three common causes are overexposure to the sun (sunburn), brief contact with hot objects or steam, and exposure of the skin to a weak acid or alkali.

- **Partial-thickness, or second-degree, burn**: This type of burn involves injury to the top layers of skin, including both the epidermis and dermis. A blister or vesicle forms. The skin is red or has a mottled (blotchy with many shades of color) appearance. Swelling usually occurs, and the surface of the skin frequently appears to be wet. This is a painful burn and may take 3–4 weeks to heal. Frequent causes include excessive exposure to the sun, a sunlamp, or artificial radiation; contact with hot or boiling liquids; and contact with fire.

- **Full-thickness, or third-degree, burn**: This is the most severe type of burn and involves injury to all layers of the skin plus the underlying tissue. The

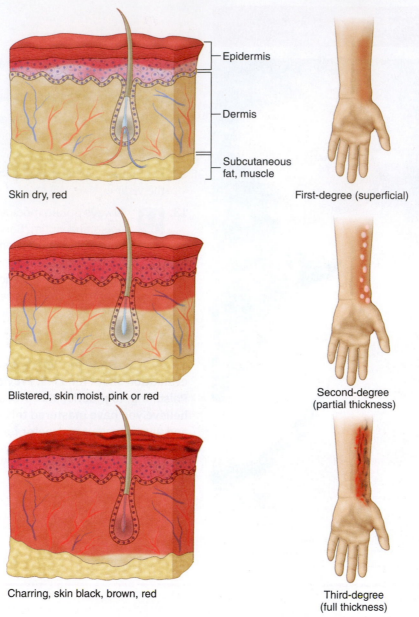

Epidermis

Dermis

Subcutaneous
fat, muscle

Skin dry, red

First-degree (superficial)

Blistered, skin moist, pink or red

Second-degree
(partial thickness)

Charring, skin black, brown, red

Third-degree
(full thickness)

FIGURE 17–25 Types of burns.

area involved has a white or charred appearance. This type of burn can be either extremely painful or, if nerve endings are destroyed, relatively painless. Third-degree burns can be life threatening because of fluid loss, infection, and shock. Frequent causes include exposure to fire or flames, prolonged contact with hot objects, contact with electricity, and immersion in hot or boiling liquids.

TREATMENT

First-aid treatment for burns is directed toward removing the source of heat, cooling the affected skin area, covering the burn, relieving pain, observing and treating for shock, and preventing infection. Medical treatment is not usually required for superficial and mild partial-thickness burns. However, medical care should be obtained if more than 15 percent of the surface of an adult's body is burned (10 percent in a child).

The rule of nines is used to calculate the percentage of body surface burned (**Figure 17–26**). For example, if an adult has burns on both legs, this would equal 18 percent of the body surface, and medical treatment should be obtained. Medical care should also be obtained if the burns affect the face or respiratory tract; if the victim has difficulty breathing; if burns cover more than one body part; if the victim has a partial-thickness burn and is under 5 or over 60 years of age; or if the burns resulted from chemicals, explosions, or electricity. All victims with full-thickness burns should receive medical care.

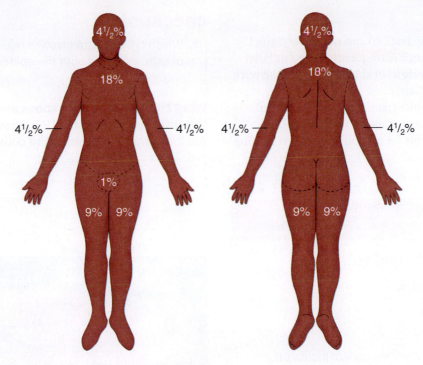

FIGURE 17–26 The *rule of nines* is used to calculate the percentage of body surface burned.

Superficial and Mild Partial-Thickness Burns

The main treatment for superficial and mild partial-thickness burns is to cool the area by flushing it with large amounts of cool water. Do *not* use ice or ice water on burns because doing so causes the body to lose heat. After the pain subsides, use dry, sterile gauze to blot the area dry. Apply a dry, sterile dressing to prevent infection. If nonadhesive dressings are available, it is best to use them because they will not stick to the injured area. If possible, elevate the affected part to reduce swelling caused by inflammation. If necessary, obtain medical help.

 CAUTION: *Do not apply cotton, tissues, ointment, powders, oils, grease, butter, or any other substances to the burned area unless you are instructed to do so by a physician or your immediate supervisor. Do not break or open any blisters that form on burns because doing so will just cause an open wound that is prone to infection.*

Safety

Severe Partial-Thickness and Full-Thickness Burns

Call for medical help immediately if the victim has severe partial-thickness or full-thickness burns. Cover the burned areas with thick, sterile dressings. Elevate the hands or feet if they are burned. If the feet or legs

are burned, do *not* allow the victim to walk. If particles of clothing are attached to the burned areas, do *not* attempt to remove these particles. Watch the victim closely for signs of respiratory distress and/or shock. Provide artificial respiration and treatment for shock, as necessary. Watch the victim closely until medical help arrives.

Chemical Burns

For burns caused by chemicals splashing on the skin, use large amounts of water to flush the affected areas for 15–30 minutes or until medical help arrives. Gently remove any clothing, socks and shoes, or jewelry that contains the chemical to minimize the area injured. Continue flushing the skin with cool water and watch the victim for signs of shock until medical help can be obtained.

If the eyes have been burned by chemicals or irritating gases, flush the eyes with large amounts of water for at least 15–30 minutes or until medical help arrives. If only one eye is injured, be sure to tilt the victim's head in the direction of the injury so the injured eye can be properly flushed. Start at the inner corner of the eye and allow the water to run over the surface of the eye and to the outside. Continue flushing the eye with cool water and watch the victim for signs of shock until medical help can be obtained.

 CAUTION: *Make sure that the water (or remaining chemical) does not enter the unin-jured eye.*

Safety

SUMMARY

Loss of body fluids (dehydration) can occur very quickly with severe burns, so shock is frequently noted in burn victims. Be alert for any signs of shock and treat the burn victim for shock immediately.

Comm

Remain calm while treating the burn victim. Reassure the victim. Obtain medical help as quickly as possible for any burn victim requiring medical assistance.

checkpoint

1. Which type of burn involves injury to the top layer of skin, including both the epidermis and dermis?

PRACTICE: Go to the workbook and complete the assignment sheet for 17:6, Providing First Aid for Burns. Then return and continue with the procedure.

Procedure 17:6

Providing First Aid for Burns

Equipment and Supplies

Water, sterile dressings, disposable gloves

Procedure

1. Follow the steps of priority care, if indicated:

   a. Check the scene. Move the victim only if absolutely necessary.

   b. Check the victim for consciousness, a pulse, and breathing.

   c. Call emergency medical services (EMS) if necessary.

   d. Provide care to the victim.

   e. Check for bleeding. Control severe bleeding.

   Precaution

   CAUTION: Wear gloves or use a protective barrier while controlling bleeding.

2. Check the burned area carefully to determine the type of burn. A reddened or discolored area is usually a superficial, or first-degree, burn. If the skin is wet, red, swollen, painful, and blistered, the burn is usually a partial-thickness, or second-degree, burn (**Figure 17–27A**). If the skin is white or charred and there is destruction of tissue, the burn is a full-thickness, or third-degree, burn (**Figure 17–27B**).

   NOTE: Victims can have more than one type of burn at one time. Treat for the most severe type of burn present.

3. For a superficial or mild partial-thickness burn:

   a. Cool the burn by flushing it with large amounts of cool water. If this is not possible, apply clean or sterile cloths that are cold and wet. Continue applying cold water until the pain subsides.

   b. Use sterile gauze to gently blot the injured area dry.

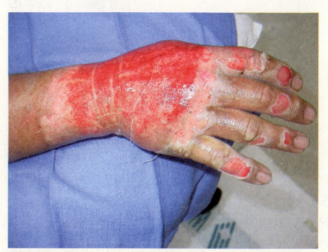

FIGURE 17–27A The skin is wet, red, swollen, painful, and blistered when a partial-thickness burn is present. The Victorian Adult Burns Service, Alfred Hospital, Melbourne, Australia

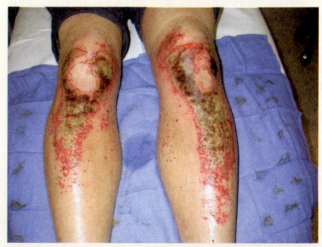

FIGURE 17–27B A full-thickness burn destroys or affects all layers of the skin plus fat, muscle, bone, and nerve tissue. The skin is white or charred in appearance. The Victorian Adult Burns Service, Alfred Hospital, Melbourne, Australia

   c. Apply dry, sterile dressings to the burned area. If possible, use nonadhesive (nonstick) dressings because they will not stick to the burn.

   d. If blisters are present, do *not* break or open them.

e. If possible, elevate the burned area to reduce swelling caused by inflammation.

f. Obtain medical help for burns to the face, or if burns cover more than 15 percent of the surface of an adult's body or 10 percent of the surface of a child's body. If the victim is having difficulty breathing, or any other distress is noted, obtain medical help.

g. Do *not* apply any cotton, ointment, powders, grease, butter, or similar substances to the burned area.

   NOTE: These substances may increase the possibility of infection.

4. For a severe partial-thickness or any full-thickness burn:

   a. Call for medical help immediately.

   b. Use thick, sterile dressings to cover the injured areas.

   c. Do *not* attempt to remove any particles of clothing that have stuck to the burned areas.

   d. If the hands and arms or legs and feet are affected, elevate these areas.

   e. If the victim has burns on the face or is experiencing difficulty in breathing, elevate the head.

   f. Watch the victim closely for signs of shock and provide care if necessary.

5. For a burn caused by a chemical splashing on the skin:

   a. Using large amounts of water, immediately flush the area for 15–30 minutes or until medical help arrives.

   b. Remove any articles of clothing, socks and shoes, or jewelry contaminated by the substance.

   c. Continue flushing the area with large amounts of cool water.

   d. Obtain medical help immediately.

6. If the eye has been burned by chemicals or irritating gases:

   a. If the victim is wearing contact lenses or glasses, ask them to remove them quickly.

   b. Tilt the victim's head toward the injured side.

   c. Hold the eyelid of the injured eye open. Pour cool water from the inner part of the eye (the part closest to the nose) toward the outer part (**Figure 17–28**).

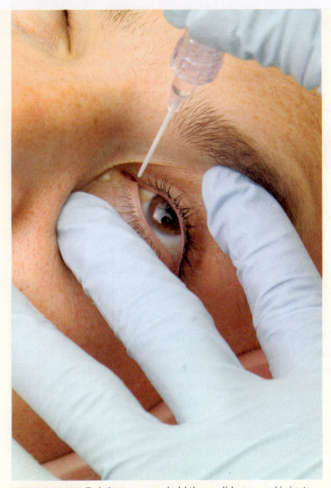

FIGURE 17–28 To irrigate an eye, hold the eyelid open and irrigate from the inner part of the eye toward the outer part.

   d. Use cool water to irrigate the eye for 15–30 minutes or until medical help arrives.

   ⚠ **Safety** **CAUTION:** Take care that the water or chemicals do not enter the uninjured eye.

   e. Obtain medical help immediately.

7. Observe for the signs of shock in all burn victims. Treat for shock as necessary.

8. **Comm** Reassure the victim as you are providing treatment. Remain calm and encourage the victim to remain calm.

9. Obtain medical help immediately for any burn victim with extensive burns, full-thickness burns, burns to the face, signs of shock, respiratory distress, eye burns, and/or chemical burns to the skin.

10. Wash hands thoroughly after providing care.

(continues)

17:7 PROVIDING FIRST AID FOR HEAT EXPOSURE

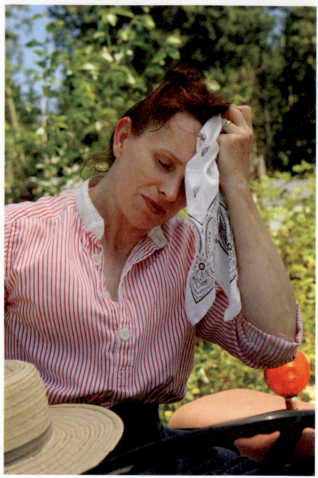

FIGURE 17–29 Excessive exposure to heat or high external temperatures can lead to a life-threatening emergency. © iStockphoto/Mike Rodriguez

Excessive exposure to heat or high external temperatures can lead to a life-threatening emergency (**Figure 17–29**). Overexposure to heat can cause a chemical imbalance in the body that can eventually lead to death. Harmful reactions can occur when fluids such as water or electrolytes such as salt are lost through perspiration or when the body cannot eliminate excess heat.

Heat cramps are caused by exposure to heat. They are muscle pains and spasms that result from the loss of fluids and electrolytes through perspiration. Firm pressure applied to the cramped muscle will provide relief from the discomfort. The victim should rest and move to a cooler area. In addition, small sips of water or an electrolyte solution, such as sport drinks, can be given to the victim.

Heat exhaustion occurs when a victim is exposed to heat and experiences a loss of fluids through sweating. Signs and symptoms include pale and clammy skin, profuse perspiration (diaphoresis), fatigue or tiredness, weakness, headache, muscle cramps, nausea and/or vomiting, and dizziness and/or fainting. Body temperature is about normal or just slightly elevated. It is important to treat heat exhaustion as quickly as possible. If it is not treated, it can develop into heat stroke. Treatment methods include moving the victim to a cooler area whenever possible; loosening or removing excessive clothing; applying cool, wet cloths; laying the victim down and elevating the victim's feet 12 inches; and giving the victim small sips of cool water, approximately 4 ounces every 15 minutes if the victim is alert and conscious. If the victim vomits, develops shock, or experiences respiratory distress, medical help should be obtained immediately.

Heat stroke is caused by prolonged exposure to high temperatures. It is a medical emergency. The body is unable to eliminate the excess heat, and internal body temperature rises to 105°F (40.6°C) or higher. Normal body defenses such as the sweating mechanism no longer function. Signs and symptoms in addition to the high body temperature include red, hot, and dry skin. The pulse is usually rapid, but may remain strong. The victim may lose consciousness.

Treatment is geared primarily toward ways of cooling the body quickly because a high body temperature can cause convulsions and/or death in a very short period of time. The victim can be placed in a tub of cool water, or the skin can be sponged with cool water. Ice or cold packs can be placed on the victim's wrists, ankles, in each axillary (armpit) area, and in the groin. Be alert for signs of shock at all times. Obtain medical help immediately.

 After victims have recovered from any condition caused by heat exposure, they must be warned to avoid abnormally warm or hot temperatures for several days. They should also be encouraged to drink sufficient amounts of water and/or electrolyte solutions.

Comm

checkpoint

1. List the three (3) main conditions that can occur from heat-related exposure?

PRACTICE: Go to the workbook and complete the assignment sheet for 17:7, Providing First Aid for Heat Exposure. Then return and continue with the procedure.

Procedure 17:7

Providing First Aid for Heat Exposure

Equipment and Supplies

Water, wash cloths or small towels

Procedure

1. Follow the steps of priority care, if indicated:
   a. Check the scene. Move the victim only if absolutely necessary.
   b. Check the victim for consciousness, a pulse, and breathing.
   c. Call emergency medical services (EMS) if necessary.
   d. Provide care to the victim.
   e. Check for bleeding. Control severe bleeding.

   CAUTION: Wear gloves or use a protective barrier while controlling bleeding.
   Precaution

2. Observe the victim closely for signs and symptoms of heat exposure. Information may also be obtained directly from the victim or from observers. If the victim has been exposed to heat or has been exercising strenuously, and is complaining of muscular pain or spasm, they are probably experiencing heat cramps. If the victim has close-to-normal body temperature but has pale and clammy skin, is perspiring excessively, and complains of nausea, headache, weakness, dizziness, or fatigue, they are probably experiencing heat exhaustion. If body temperature is high (105°F or 40.6°C or higher), skin is red, dry, and hot, and the victim is weak or unconscious, they are experiencing heat stroke.

3. If the victim has heat cramps:
   a. Use your hand to apply firm pressure to the cramped muscle(s). This helps relieve the spasms.
   b. Encourage relaxation. Allow the victim to lie down in a cool area, if possible.
   c. If the victim is alert and conscious and is not nauseated or vomiting, give them small sips of cool water or an electrolyte solution such as a sport drink. Encourage the victim to drink approximately 4 ounces every 15 minutes.
   d. If the heat cramps continue or get worse, obtain medical help.

4. If the victim has heat exhaustion:
   a. Move the victim to a cool area, if possible. An air-conditioned room is ideal, but a fan can also help circulate air and cool the victim.
   b. Help the victim lie down flat on the back. Elevate the victim's feet and legs 12 inches.
   c. Loosen any tight clothing. Remove excessive clothing such as jackets and sweaters.
   d. Apply cool, wet cloths to the victim's face.
   e. If the victim is conscious and is not nauseated or vomiting, give them small sips of cool water or an electrolyte solution such as a sport drink. Encourage the victim to drink approximately 4 ounces every 15 minutes.
   f. If the victim complains of nausea and/or vomits, discontinue the water. Obtain medical help.

5. If the victim has heat stroke:
   a. Immediately move the victim to a cool area, if at all possible.
   b. Remove excessive clothing.
   c. Sponge the bare skin with cool water, or place ice or cold packs on the victim's wrists, ankles, and in the axillary and groin areas. The victim can also be placed in a tub of cool water to lower body temperature.

   CAUTION: Watch that the victim's head is not submerged in water. If the victim is unconscious, you may need assistance to place them in the tub.
   Safety

   d. If vomiting occurs, position the victim on their side. Watch for signs of difficulty in breathing and provide care as indicated.
   e. Obtain medical help immediately. This is a life-threatening emergency.

6. Shock can develop quickly in all victims of heat exposure. Be alert for the signs of shock and treat as necessary.

   CAUTION: Obtain medical help for heat cramps that do not subside, heat exhaustion with signs of shock or vomiting, and all heat stroke victims as soon as possible.
   Safety

(continues)

7. Reassure the victim as you are providing treatment. Remain calm.

   Comm

8. Wash hands thoroughly after providing care.

PRACTICE: Go to the workbook and use the evaluation sheet for 17:7, Providing First Aid for

Heat Exposure, to practice this procedure. When you believe you have mastered this skill, sign the sheet and give it to your instructor for further action.

✅ **FINAL EVALUATION:** Using the criteria listed on the evaluation sheet, your instructor will grade your performance.

Check

17:8 PROVIDING FIRST AID FOR COLD EXPOSURE

Exposure to cold external temperatures can cause body tissues to freeze and body processes to slow. If treatment is not provided immediately, the victim can die. Factors such as wind velocity, amount of humidity, and length of exposure all affect the degree of injury.

Prolonged exposure to the cold can result in **hypothermia**, a condition in which the body temperature is less than 95°F (35°C). Elderly individuals are more susceptible to hypothermia than are younger individuals (**Figure 17–30**). Signs and symptoms include shivering, numbness, weakness or drowsiness, low body temperature, poor coordination, confusion, and loss of consciousness. If prolonged exposure continues, body processes will slow down and death can occur. Treatment consists of getting the victim to a warm area; removing wet clothing; slowly warming the victim by wrapping in blankets or putting on dry clothing; covering the head with a warm cap to retain body heat; and, if the victim is fully conscious, giving warm nonalcoholic, noncaffeinated liquids by mouth. Avoid warming the victim too quickly because rapid warming can cause dangerous heart arrhythmias.

Frostbite is actual freezing of tissue fluids accompanied by damage to the skin and underlying tissues (**Figure 17–31**). It is caused by exposure to freezing or below-freezing temperatures. Early signs and symptoms include redness and tingling. As frostbite progresses, signs and symptoms include pale, glossy skin that is white or grayish yellow in color; blisters; skin that is cold to the touch; numbness; and sometimes, pain that gradually subsides until the victim does not feel any pain. If exposure continues, the victim may become confused, lethargic, and incoherent. Shock may develop followed by unconsciousness and death. First aid for frostbite is directed at maintaining respirations, treating for shock, warming the affected parts, and preventing further injury. Frequently, small areas of the body are affected by frostbite. Common sites include the fingers, toes, ears, nose, and cheeks. Extreme care must be taken to avoid further injury to areas damaged by frostbite. Because the victim usually does not feel pain, the part must be warmed carefully, taking care not to burn the injured tissue. The parts affected may be immersed in warm water at 100°F–104°F (37.8°C–40°C) until normal color returns to the skin and/or feeling returns.

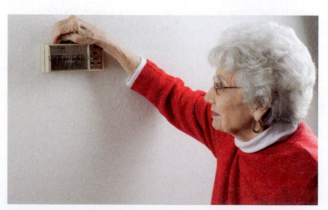

FIGURE 17–30 Elderly individuals are more susceptible to hypothermia than are younger individuals. © iStockphoto/David Sucsy

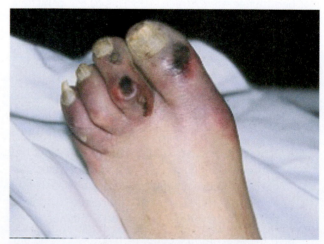

FIGURE 17–31 Frostbite is actual freezing of tissue fluids accompanied by damage to skin and underlying tissues. Courtesy of Dr. Deborah Funk, Albany Medical Center

CAUTION: *Heat lamps, hot water above 104°F (40°C), or heat from a stove or oven should not be* **Safety** *used. Furthermore, the parts should not be rubbed or massaged because this may cause gangrene (death of the tissue). Avoid opening or breaking any blisters that form because doing so will create an open wound. Do not allow the victim to walk or stand if the feet, legs, or toes are affected. Dry, sterile dressings can be placed between toes or fingers to prevent them from rubbing and causing further injury. Medical help should be obtained as quickly as possible.*

Shock is frequently noted in victims exposed to the cold. Be alert for all signs of shock and treat for shock as necessary.

check**point**

| **1.** What does the term *hypothermia* mean?

PRACTICE: Go to the workbook and complete the assignment sheet for 17:8, Providing First Aid for Cold Exposure. Then return and continue with the procedure.

Procedure 17:8

Providing First Aid for Cold Exposure

Equipment and Supplies

Blankets, warm water, thermometer, sterile gauze

Procedure

1. Follow the steps of priority care, if indicated:

   a. Check the scene. Move the victim only if absolutely necessary.

   b. Check the victim for consciousness, a pulse, and breathing.

   c. Call emergency medical services (EMS) if necessary.

   d. Provide care to the victim.

   e. Check for bleeding. Control severe bleeding.

    CAUTION: Wear gloves or use a protective barrier while controlling **Precaution** bleeding.

2. Observe the victim closely for signs and symptoms of cold exposure. Information may also be obtained directly from the victim or observers. Note shivering, numbness, weakness or drowsiness, confusion, low body temperature, and lethargy. Check the skin, particularly on the toes, fingers, ears, nose, and cheeks. Suspect frostbite if any areas are pale, glossy, white or grayish yellow, and cold to the touch, and if the victim complains of any part of the body feeling numb or painless.

3. Move the victim to a warm area as soon as possible.

4. Immediately remove any wet or frozen clothing. Loosen any tight clothing that decreases circulation.

5. Slowly warm the victim by wrapping the victim in blankets or dressing the victim in dry, warm clothing. Put a cap on the victim's head to prevent loss of body heat. If a body part is affected by frostbite, immerse the part in warm water measuring 100°F–104°F (37.8°C–40°C).

 CAUTION: Warm a victim of hypothermia slowly. Rapid warming can cause heart **Safety** problems or increase circulation to the surface of the body, which causes additional cooling of vital organs.

 CAUTION: Do *not* use heat lamps, hot water above the stated temperatures, or **Safety** heat from stoves or ovens. Excessive heat can burn the victim.

6. After the body part affected by frostbite has been thawed and the skin becomes flushed, discontinue warming the area because swelling may develop rapidly. Dry the part by blotting gently with a towel or soft cloth. Gently wrap the part in clean or sterile cloths. Use sterile gauze to separate the fingers and/or toes to prevent them from rubbing together.

 CAUTION: *Never* rub or massage the frostbitten area because doing so can **Safety** cause gangrene.

7. Help the victim lie down. Do not allow the victim to walk or stand if the legs, feet, or toes are injured. Elevate any injured areas.

8. Observe the victim for signs of shock. Treat for shock as necessary.

9. If the victim is conscious and is not nauseated or vomiting, give warm liquids to drink.

 CAUTION: Do *not* give beverages containing alcohol or caffeine. Give the **Safety** victim warm broth, water, or milk.

10. Reassure the victim while providing treatment. Remain calm and encourage the **Comm** victim to remain calm.

11. Obtain medical help as soon as possible.

12. Wash hands thoroughly after providing care.

(continues)

PRACTICE: Go to the workbook and use the evaluation sheet for 17:8, Providing First Aid for Cold Exposure, to practice this procedure. When you believe you have mastered this skill, sign the sheet and give it to your instructor for further action.

FINAL EVALUATION: Using the criteria listed on the evaluation sheet, your instructor will grade your performance.

Check

17:9 PROVIDING FIRST AID FOR BONE AND JOINT INJURIES

Injuries to bones and joints are common in accidents and falls. A variety of injuries can occur to bones and joints. Such injuries sometimes occur together; other times, these injuries occur by themselves. Examples of injuries to bones and joints are fractures, dislocations, sprains, and strains.

FRACTURES

A **fracture** is a break in a bone. A closed, or simple, fracture is a bone break that is not accompanied by an external or open wound on the skin. A compound, or open, fracture is a bone break that is accompanied by an open wound on the skin. The types of fractures are discussed in Section 7:4 (also refer to Figure 17–25).

Signs and symptoms of fractures can vary. Not all signs and symptoms will be present in every victim. Common signs and symptoms include:

- Deformity
- Limited motion or loss of motion
- Pain and tenderness at the fracture site
- Swelling and discoloration
- The protrusion of bone ends through the skin
- The victim heard a bone break or snap or felt a grating sensation (crepitation)
- Abnormal movements within a part of the body

Basic principles of treatment for fractures include:

- Maintain respirations
- Treat for shock
- Keep the broken bone from moving
- Prevent further injury
- Use devices such as splints and slings to prevent movement of the injured part
- Obtain medical help whenever a fracture is evident or suspected

DISLOCATIONS

A **dislocation** is when the end of a bone is either displaced from a joint or moved out of its normal position within a joint. This injury is frequently accompanied by a tearing or stretching of ligaments, muscles, and other soft tissue.

Signs and symptoms that may occur include:

- Deformity
- Limited or abnormal movement
- Swelling
- Discoloration
- Pain and tenderness
- A shortening or lengthening of the affected arm or leg

First aid for dislocations is basically the same as that for fractures. No attempt should be made to reduce the dislocation (that is, replace the bone in the joint). The affected part must be immobilized in the position in which it was found. Immobilization is accomplished by using splints and/or slings. Movement of the injured part can lead to additional injury to nerves, blood vessels, and other tissue in the area. Obtain medical help immediately.

SPRAINS

A **sprain** is an injury to the tissues surrounding a joint; it usually occurs when the part is forced beyond its normal range of movement. Ligaments, tendons, and other tissues are stretched or torn. Common sites for sprains include the ankles and wrists.

Signs and symptoms of a sprain include swelling, pain, discoloration, and sometimes, impaired motion. Frequently, sprains resemble fractures or dislocations. If in doubt, treat the injury as a fracture.

First aid for a sprain includes:

- Apply a cold application to decrease swelling and pain; place a barrier, for example a thin towel between the cold container and the skin
- Elevate the affected part
- Encourage the victim to rest the affected part

- Apply an elastic bandage to provide support for the affected area but avoid stretching the bandage too tightly

- An easy acronym to remember this treatment is *RICE*: rest, ice, compression, and elevation

- Obtain medical help if swelling is severe or if there is any question of a fracture.

STRAINS

A **strain** is the overstretching of a muscle; it is caused by overexertion or lifting. A frequent site for strains is the back. Signs and symptoms of a strain include sudden pain, swelling, and/or bruising.

Basic principles of first-aid treatment for a strain include:

- Encourage the victim to rest the affected muscle while providing support.

- Recommend bed rest with a backboard under the mattress for a strained back.

- Apply cold applications to reduce the swelling; place a barrier, for example a thin towel, between the cold container and the skin.

- After the swelling decreases, apply warm, wet applications because warmth relaxes the muscles; different types of cold and heat packs are available (**Figure 17–32**).

- Obtain medical help for severe strains and all back injuries.

SPLINTS

Splints are devices that can be used to immobilize injured parts when fractures, dislocations, and other similar injuries are present or suspected. Many commercial splints are available, including inflatable, or air, splints; padded boards; and traction splints. Splints can also be made from cardboard, newspapers, blankets, pillows, boards, and other similar materials.

Some basic principles regarding the use of splints are as follows:

- Splints should be long enough to immobilize the joint above and the joint below the injured area (**Figure 17–33**). By preventing movement in these joints, the injured bone or area is held in position and further injury is prevented.

- Splints should be padded, especially at bony areas and over the site of injury. Cloths, thick dressings, towels, and similar materials can be used as padding.

- Strips of cloth, roller gauze, triangular bandages folded into bands or strips, and similar materials can be used to tie splints in place.

- Splints must be applied so that they do not put pressure directly over the site of injury.

- If an open wound is present, use a sterile dressing to apply pressure and control bleeding.

 CAUTION: *Wear gloves or use a protective barrier while controlling bleeding to avoid contamination from the blood.*

Precaution

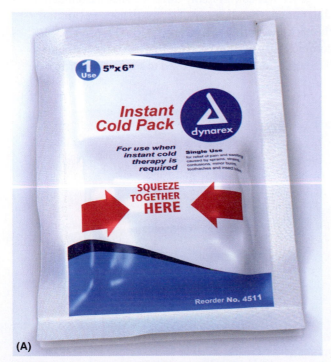

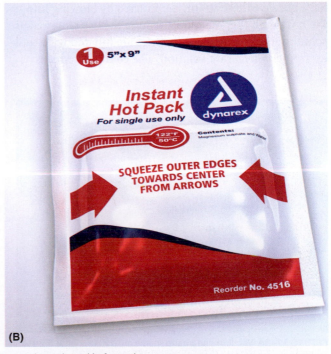

FIGURE 17–32 Disposable (A) cold and (B) heat packs contain chemicals that must be activated before using. Courtesy, Dynarex

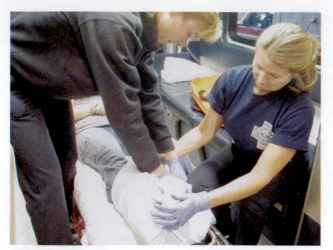

FIGURE 17–33 A pillow can be used to splint an ankle injury to immobilize the joint above and below the injured area. Courtesy of Larry Torrey, RN, EMT-P

 CAUTION: *Leave the dressing in place, and apply the splint in such a way that it does not put pressure on the wound.*

Safety

- *Never* make any attempt to replace broken bones or reduce a fracture or dislocation. Do *not* move the victim. Splint wherever you find the victim.

- *Pneumatic* splints are available in various sizes and shapes for different parts of the arms and legs. Care must be taken to avoid any unnecessary movement while the splint is being positioned. There are two main types of pneumatic splints: air (inflatable) and vacuum (deflatable).

If an *air splint* is positioned over a fracture site, air pressure is used to inflate the splint. Some air splints have nozzles; these splints are inflated by blowing into the nozzles. Other air splints require the use of a pressure solution in a can, while still others are inflated with cool air from a refrigerant solution. The coldness reduces

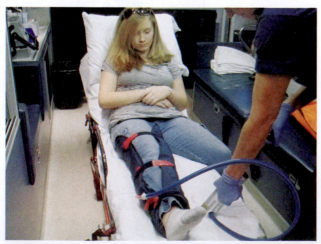

FIGURE 17–34 Vacuum pneumatic splints are deflated until the splint molds to the fracture site to provide support. Courtesy of Larry Torrey, RN, EMT-P

swelling. Care must be taken to avoid overinflating air splints. To test whether the splint is properly inflated, use a thumb to apply slight pressure to the splint; an indentation mark should result.

Vacuum pneumatic splints are deflated after being positioned over a fracture site. Air is removed from the splint with a hand pump or suction pump until the splint molds to the fracture site to provide support (**Figure 17–34**). Care must be taken to avoid overdeflation of the splint. A pulse site below the splint should be checked to make sure the splint is not applying too much pressure and cutting off circulation.

- Traction splints are special devices that provide a pulling or traction effect on the injured bone. They are frequently used for fractures of the femur, or thigh bone.

 CAUTION: *Only persons specifically trained in the application of traction splints should apply them.*

Legal

- After a splint is applied, it is essential to note the circulation and the effects on the nerve endings of the skin below the splint to make sure the splint is not too tight. Check skin temperature (it should be warm to the touch), skin color (pale or blue indicates poor circulation), swelling or edema, numbness or tingling, and pulse, if possible.

 CAUTION: *If any signs of impaired circulation or impaired neurological status are present, immediately loosen the ties holding the splint.*

Safety

SLINGS

Slings are available in many different forms. Commercial slings usually have a series of straps that extend around the neck and/or thoracic (chest) region (**Figure 17–35**). A common type of sling used for first aid is the triangular bandage. Slings are usually used to support the arm, hand,

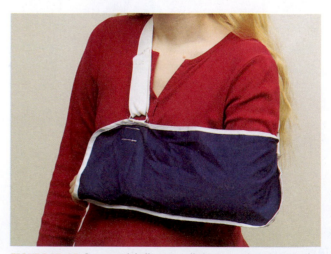

FIGURE 17–35 Commercial slings usually have a series of straps that extend around the neck and/or thoracic region.

forearm, and shoulder. They may be used when casts are in place. In addition, they are also used to provide immobility if a fracture of the arm, collarbone, or shoulder is suspected. Basic principles to observe with slings include:

- When a sling is applied to an arm, the sling should be positioned in such a way that the hand is higher than the elbow. The purpose of elevating the hand is to promote circulation, prevent swelling (edema), and decrease pain.

- Circulation in the limb and nerve supply to the limb must be checked frequently. Specifically, check for skin temperature (should be warm if circulation is good), skin color (blue or very pale indicates poor circulation), swelling (edema), amount of pain, and tingling or numbness. Nail beds can also be used to check circulation. When the nail beds are pressed slightly, they blanch (turn white). If circulation is good, the pink color should return to the nail beds immediately after the pressure is released (refer to **Figures 17–46A and B**).

- If a sling is being applied because of a suspected fracture to the bone, extreme care must be taken to move the injured limb as little as possible while the sling is being applied. The victim can sometimes help by holding the injured limb in position while the sling is slipped into place.

- If a triangular bandage is used, care must be taken so that the knot tied at the neck does not press against a bone. The knot should be tied to either side of the spinal column. Place gauze or padding under the knot of the sling to protect the skin.

- When shoulder injuries are suspected, it may be necessary to keep the arm next to the body. After a sling has been applied, another bandage can be placed around the thoracic region to hold the arm against the body.

NECK AND SPINE INJURIES

Injuries to the neck or spine are the most dangerous types of injuries to bones and joints.

 CAUTION: *If a victim who has such injuries is moved, permanent damage resulting in paralysis can occur. If at all possible, avoid any movement of a victim with neck or spinal injuries. Wait until a backboard, cervical collar, and adequate help for transfer is available.*

Safety

SUMMARY

Victims with injuries to bones and/or joints also experience shock. Always be alert for signs of shock and treat as needed.

 Injuries to bones and/or joints usually involve a great deal of anxiety, pain, and discomfort, so constantly reassure the victim. Encourage the victim to relax, and position the victim as comfortably as possible. Advise the victim that medical help is on the way. First-aid measures are directed toward relieving the pain as much as possible.

Comm

Obtain medical help for all victims of bone or joint injuries. The only definite diagnosis of a closed fracture is an X-ray of the area. Whenever a fracture and/or dislocation is suspected, treat the victim as though one of these injuries has occurred.

checkpoint

| **1.** What might a blue skin color indicate?

PRACTICE: Go to the workbook and complete the assignment sheet for 17:9, Providing First Aid for Bone and Joint Injuries. Then return and continue with the procedure.

Procedure 17:9

Providing First Aid for Bone and Joint Injuries

Equipment and Supplies

Blankets, splints of various sizes, air or inflatable splints, triangular bandages, strips of cloth or roller gauze, disposable gloves

Procedure

1. Follow the steps of priority care, if indicated:

   a. Check the scene. Move the victim only if absolutely necessary. If the victim must be moved from a dangerous area, pull in the direction of the long axis of the body (that is, from the head or feet). If at all possible, tie an injured leg to the other leg or secure an injured arm to the body before movement.

    CAUTION: If neck or spinal injuries are suspected, avoid any movement of the victim unless movement is necessary to save the victim's life.

   Safety

   b. Check the victim for consciousness, a pulse, and breathing.

   c. Call emergency medical services (EMS) if necessary.

   (continues)

d. Provide care to the victim.

e. Control severe bleeding. If an open wound accompanies a fracture, take care not to push broken bone ends into the wound.

CAUTION: Wear gloves or use a protective barrier while controlling bleeding.

2. Observe for signs and symptoms of a fracture, dislocation, or joint injury. Note deformities, such as a shortening or lengthening of an extremity, limited motion or loss of motion, pain, tenderness, swelling, discoloration, and bone fragments protruding through the skin. Also, the victim may state that they heard a bone snap or crack, or may complain of a grating sensation.

3. Immobilize the injured part to prevent movement.

CAUTION: Do *not* attempt to straighten a deformity, replace broken bone ends, or reduce a dislocation. Avoid any unnecessary movement of the injured part. If a bone injury is suspected, treat the victim as though a fracture or dislocation has occurred. Use splints or slings to immobilize the injury.

4. To apply splints:

a. Obtain commercial splints or improvise splints by using blankets, pillows, newspapers, boards, cardboard, or similar supportive materials.

b. Make sure that the splints are long enough to immobilize the joint both above and below the injury.

c. Position the splints, making sure that they do *not* apply pressure directly at the site of injury. Two splints are usually used. However, if a pillow, blanket, or similar item is used, one such item can be rolled around the area to provide support on all sides.

d. Use thick dressings, cloths, towels, or other similar materials to pad the splints. Make sure bony areas are protected. Avoid direct contact between the splint material and the skin.

NOTE: Many commercial splints are already padded. However, additional padding is often needed to protect the bony areas.

e. Use strips of cloth, triangular bandages folded into strips, roller gauze, or other similar material to tie or anchor the splints in place. The use of elastic bandage is discouraged because the bandage may cut off or interfere with circulation. If splints are long, three to five ties may be required. Tie the strips above and below the upper joint and above and below the lower joint. An additional tie should be placed in the center region of the splint.

f. Avoid any unnecessary movement of the injured area while splints are being applied. If possible, have another individual support the area while you are applying the splints.

5. To apply air (inflatable) splints:

a. Obtain the correct splint for the injured part.

NOTE: Most air splints are available for full arm, lower arm, wrist, full leg, lower leg, and ankle/foot.

b. Some air splints have zippers for easier application, but others must be slipped into position on the victim. If the splint has a zipper, position the open splint on the injured area, taking care to avoid any movement of the affected part. Use your hand to support the injured area. Close the zipper. If the splint must be slipped into position, slide the splint onto your arm first. Then, hold the injured leg or arm and slide the splint from your arm to the victim's injured extremity. This technique prevents unnecessary movement.

c. Inflate the splint. Many splints are inflated by blowing into the nozzle. Others require the use of a pressure solution in a can. Follow instructions provided by the manufacturer of the splint.

d. Check to make sure that the splint is not overinflated. Use your thumb to press a section of the splint. Your thumb should leave a slight indentation if the splint is inflated correctly.

6. To apply a sling, follow the manufacturer's instructions for commercial slings. To use a triangular bandage for a sling (**Figure 17–36**), proceed as follows:

a. If possible, obtain the help of another individual to support the injured arm while the sling is being applied. Sometimes, the victim can hold the injured arm in place.

b. Place the long straight edge of the triangular bandage on the uninjured side. Allow one end to extend over the shoulder of the uninjured arm. The other end should hang down in front of the victim's chest. The short edge of the triangle should extend back and under the elbow of the injured arm.

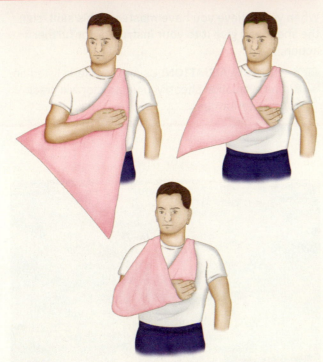

FIGURE 17–36 Steps for applying a triangular bandage as a sling.

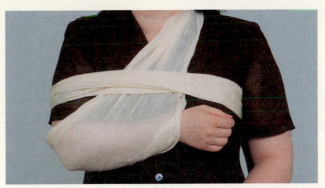

FIGURE 17–37 If a shoulder injury is suspected, use a long bandage to secure the arm against the body to stabilize the shoulder joint.

 CAUTION: Avoid excessive movement of the injured limb while positioning the sling.

c. Bring the long end of the bandage up and over the shoulder of the injured arm.

d. Use a square knot to tie the two ends together near the neck. Make sure the knot is not over a bone. Tie it to either side of the spinal column. Place gauze or padding between the knot and the skin. Make sure the hand is elevated 5–6 inches above the elbow.

e. The point of the bandage is now near the elbow. Bring the point forward, fold it, and pin it to the front of the sling. If no pin is available, coil the end and tie it in a knot.

 CAUTION: If you use a pin, put your hand between the pin and the victim's skin while inserting the pin.

f. Check the position of the sling. The fingers of the injured hand should extend beyond the edge of the triangular bandage. In addition, the hand should be slightly elevated to prevent swelling (edema).

g. If a shoulder injury is suspected, it may be necessary to secure the arm close to the body. Apply a large bandage around the thoracic region to stabilize the shoulder joint (**Figure 17–37**).

7. After splints and/or slings have been applied, check for signs of impaired circulation. Skin color should be pink. A pale or cyanotic (bluish) color is a sign of poor circulation. The skin should be warm to the touch. Swelling can indicate poor circulation. If the victim complains of pain or pressure from the splints and/or slings, or of numbness or tingling in the area below the splints/sling, circulation may be impaired. Slightly press the nail beds on the foot or hand so they temporarily turn white. If circulation is good, the pink color will return to the nail beds immediately after pressure is released. If you note any signs of impaired circulation, loosen the splints and/or sling immediately.

8. Watch for signs of shock in any victim with a bone and/or joint injury. Remember, inadequate blood flow is the main cause of shock. Watch for signs of impaired circulation, such as a cyanotic (bluish) tinge around the lips or nail beds. Treat for shock, as necessary.

9. If medical help is delayed, cold applications, such as cold compresses or an ice bag, can be used on the injured area to decrease swelling.

 CAUTION: To prevent injury to the skin, make sure that the ice bag is covered with a towel or other material.

10. Place the victim in a comfortable position, but avoid any unnecessary movement.

 CAUTION: Avoid *any* movement if a neck or spinal injury is suspected.

11. Reassure the victim while providing first aid. Try to relieve the pain by carefully positioning the injured part, avoiding unnecessary movement, and applying cold.

(continues)

12. Obtain medical help as quickly as possible.

13. Wash hands thoroughly after providing care.

PRACTICE: Go to the workbook and use the evaluation sheet for 17:9, Providing First Aid for Bone and Joint Injuries, to practice this procedure.

When you believe you have mastered this skill, sign the sheet and give it to your instructor for further action.

 FINAL EVALUATION: Using the criteria listed on the evaluation sheet, your instructor will grade your performance.

Check

17:10 PROVIDING FIRST AID FOR SPECIFIC INJURIES

Although treatment for burns, bleeding, wounds, poisoning, and fractures is basically the same for all regions of the body, injuries to specific body parts require special care. Examples of these parts are the eyes, ears, nose, brain, chest, abdomen, and genital organs.

EYE INJURIES

Any eye injury always involves the danger of vision loss, especially if treated incorrectly. In most cases involving serious injury to the eyes, it is best *not* to provide major treatment. Obtaining medical help, preferably from an eye specialist, is a top priority of first-aid care.

- **Foreign objects** such as dust, dirt, and similar small particles frequently enter the eye. These objects cause irritation and can scratch the eye or become embedded in the eye tissue. Signs and symptoms include redness, a burning sensation, pain, watering or tearing of the eye, and/or the presence of visible objects in the eye. If the foreign body is floating freely, prevent the victim from rubbing the eye, wash your hands thoroughly, and gently draw the upper lid down over the lower lid. This stimulates the formation of tears. The proximity of the lids also creates a wiping action, which may remove the particle. If this does not remove the foreign body, use your thumb and forefinger to grasp the eyelashes and gently raise the upper eyelid. Tell the victim to look down and tilt their head toward the injured side. Use water to gently flush the eye or use the corner of a piece of sterile gauze to gently remove the object.

   CAUTION: *If this does not remove the object or if the object is embedded, make no attempt to remove it.*
  Safety

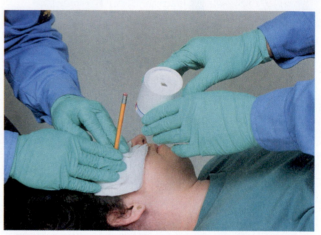

FIGURE 17–38 A cup can be used to stabilize an object impaled in the eye and to prevent it from moving.

Apply a dry, sterile dressing and obtain medical help for the victim. Serious injury can occur if any attempt is made to remove an object embedded in the eye tissue.

- **Blows to the eye** from a fist, an accident, or an explosion may cause contusions or black eyes as a result of internal bleeding and torn tissues inside the eye. Because this can lead to loss of vision, the victim should be examined as soon as possible by an eye specialist. Apply sterile dressings or an eye shield, keep the victim lying flat, and obtain medical help. It is sometimes best to cover both eyes to prevent involuntary movement of the injured eye.

- **Penetrating injuries** that cut the eye tissue are extremely dangerous.

  ⚠ **CAUTION:** *If an object is protruding from the eye, make no attempt to remove the object. Rather, support it by loosely applying dressings. A paper cup with a hole cut in the bottom can also be used to stabilize the object and prevent it from moving (**Figure 17–38**).*
  Safety

Apply dressings to both eyes to prevent involuntary movement of the injured eye. Avoid applying pressure to the eye while applying the dressings. Keep the victim lying flat on their back to prevent fluids from draining out of the eye. Obtain medical help immediately.

EAR INJURIES

Injuries to the ear can result in rupture or perforation of the eardrum. These injuries also require medical care. Treatment for specific types of ear injuries is as follows:

- Wounds of the ear frequently result in torn or detached tissue. Apply sterile dressings with light pressure to control bleeding.

CAUTION: *If possible, wear gloves or use a protective barrier while controlling bleeding.*

Save any torn tissue and wrap it in gauze moistened with cool sterile water or sterile normal saline solution. Put the gauze-wrapped tissue in a plastic bag to keep it cool and moist. Send the torn tissue to the medical facility along with the victim.

NOTE: *If sterile water is not available, use cool, clean water.*

- Keep the victim lying flat, but raise their head (if no other conditions prohibit raising the head).

- If the eardrum is ruptured or perforated, place sterile gauze loosely in the outer ear canal. Do *not* allow the victim to hit the side of the head in an attempt to restore hearing. Do *not* put any liquids into the ear. Obtain medical help for the victim.

- Clear or blood-tinged fluid draining from the ear can be a sign of a skull or brain injury. Allow the fluid to flow from the ear. Keep the victim lying down. If possible, turn the victim on their injured side and elevate the head and shoulders slightly to allow the fluid to drain. Obtain medical help immediately and report the presence and description of the fluid.

CAUTION: *Wear gloves or use a protective barrier to avoid skin contact with fluid draining from the ear.*

HEAD OR SKULL INJURIES

Wounds or blows to the head or skull can result in injury to the brain. Again, it is important to obtain medical help as quickly as possible for the victim.

- Signs and symptoms of brain injury include clear or blood-tinged cerebrospinal fluid draining from the nose or ears, loss of consciousness, headache, visual disturbances, eye pupils unequal in size, muscle paralysis, speech disturbances, convulsions, and nausea and vomiting.

- Keep the victim lying flat and treat for shock. If there is no evidence of neck or spinal injury, raise the victim's head slightly by supporting the head and shoulders on a small pillow or a rolled blanket or coat.

- Watch closely for signs of respiratory distress and provide artificial respiration as needed.

- Make *no* attempt to stop the flow of fluid from the nose or ears. Loose dressings can be positioned to absorb the flow.

CAUTION: *Wear gloves or use a protective barrier to avoid contamination from the cerebrospinal fluid.*

- Do *not* give the victim any liquids. If the victim complains of excessive thirst, use a clean, cool, wet cloth to moisten the lips, tongue, and inside of the mouth.

- If the victim loses consciousness, note how long the victim is unconscious and report this to the emergency rescue personnel.

- Monitor the pulse and breathing of the unconscious victim in case CPR and/or artificial respiration becomes necessary.

NOSE INJURIES

Injuries to the nose frequently cause a nosebleed, also called an *epistaxis*. Nosebleeds are usually more frightening than they are serious. Nosebleeds can also be caused by change in altitude, strenuous activity, high blood pressure, and rupture of small blood vessels after a cold. Treatment for a nosebleed includes:

- Keep the victim quiet and remain calm.

- If possible, place the victim in a sitting position with the head leaning slightly forward.

- Apply pressure to control bleeding by pressing the bleeding nostril toward the midline. If both nostrils are bleeding, press both nostrils toward the midline.

NOTE: *If both nostrils are blocked, tell the victim to breathe through the mouth.*

CAUTION: *Wear gloves or use a protective barrier to avoid contamination from blood.*

- If application of pressure against the midline or septum does not stop the bleeding, insert a small piece of gauze in the nostril and then apply pressure on the outer surface of the nostril. Be sure to leave a portion of the gauze extending out of the nostril so that the packing can be removed later.

CAUTION: *Do not use cotton balls because the fibers will shed and stick.*

- Apply a cold compress to the bridge of the nose. A covered ice pack or a cold, wet cloth can be used.

- If the bleeding does not stop or a fracture of the nose is suspected, obtain medical assistance. If a person has repeated nosebleeds, a referral for medical attention should be made. Nosebleeds can indicate an underlying condition, such as high blood pressure, that requires medical care and treatment.

CHEST INJURIES

Injuries to the chest are usually medical emergencies because the heart, lungs, and major blood vessels may be involved. Chest injuries include sucking chest wounds, penetrating wounds, and crushing injuries. In all cases, obtain medical help immediately.

- **Sucking chest wound**: This is a deep, open chest wound that allows air to flow directly in and out with breathing. The partial vacuum that is usually present in the pleura (sacs surrounding the lungs) is destroyed, causing the lung on the injured side to collapse. Immediate medical help must be obtained. Leave the open chest wound exposed to air without a dressing. If a nonocclusive dressing (a dressing like a gauze pad that allows liquids and gases to pass through) is used for active bleeding, care must be taken to ensure that the dressing doesn't lead to occlusion. Maintain an open airway (through the nose or mouth) and provide artificial respiration as needed. If possible, position the victim on their injured side and elevate the head and chest slightly. This allows the uninjured lung to expand more freely and prevents pressure on the uninjured lung from blood and damaged tissue.

- **Penetrating injuries to the chest**: These injuries can result in sucking chest wounds or damage to the heart and blood vessels. If an object (for example, a knife) is protruding from the chest, do *not* attempt to remove the object. If possible, immobilize the object by placing dressings around it and taping the dressings in position (**Figure 17–39**). Place the victim in a comfortable position, maintain respirations, and obtain medical help immediately.

- **Crushing chest injuries**: These injuries are caused in vehicular accidents or when heavy objects strike the chest. Fractured ribs and damage to the lungs and/or heart can occur. Place the victim in a comfortable position and, if possible, elevate the head and shoulders to aid breathing. If an injury to the neck or spine is suspected, avoid moving the victim. Obtain medical help immediately.

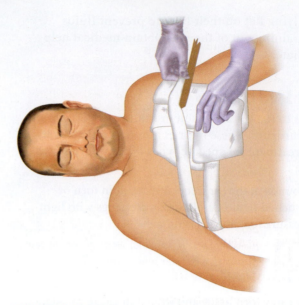

FIGURE 17–39 Immobilize an object protruding from the chest by placing dressings around the object and taping the dressings in place.

ABDOMINAL INJURIES

Abdominal injuries can damage internal organs and cause bleeding in major blood vessels. The intestines and other abdominal organs may protrude from an open wound. Medical help must be obtained immediately; bleeding, shock, and organ damage can lead to death in a short period of time.

- Signs and symptoms include severe abdominal pain or tenderness, protruding organs, open wounds, nausea and vomiting (particularly of blood), abdominal muscle rigidity, and symptoms of shock.

- Position the victim flat on their back. Place a pillow or rolled blanket under the knees to bend the knees slightly. This helps relax the abdominal muscles. Elevate the head and shoulders slightly to aid breathing.

 CAUTION: *If an injury to the neck or spine is suspected, avoid moving the victim.*
Safety

- Remove clothing from around the wound or protruding organs. Use a large sterile dressing moistened with sterile water or normal saline solution to cover the area. If sterile water or normal saline is not available, use warm tap water to moisten the dressings. Cover the dressings with plastic wrap, if available, to keep the dressings moist. Then, cover the dressings with aluminum foil or a folded towel to keep the area warm.

 CAUTION: *Make no attempt to reposition protruding organs.*
Safety

- Avoid giving the victim any fluids or food. If the victim complains of excessive thirst, use a cool, wet cloth to moisten the lips, tongue, and inside of the mouth.

INJURIES TO GENITAL ORGANS

Injuries to genital organs can result from falls, blows, or explosions. Zippers catching on genitals and other accidents sometimes bruise the genitals. Because injuries to the genitals may cause severe pain, bleeding, and shock, medical help is required. Basic principles of first aid include the following:

- Control severe bleeding by using a sterile (or clean) dressing to apply direct pressure to the area.

Precaution

CAUTION: *Wear gloves or use a protective barrier to prevent contamination from the blood.*

- Treat the victim for shock.

- Do not remove any penetrating or inserted objects.

- Save any torn tissue and wrap it in gauze moistened with cool sterile water or sterile normal saline. Put the gauze-wrapped tissue in a plastic bag to keep it cool and moist. Send the torn tissue to the medical facility along with the victim.

- Use a covered ice pack or other cold applications to decrease bleeding and relieve pain.

- Obtain medical help.

SUMMARY

Shock frequently occurs in victims with specific injuries to the eyes, ears, chest, abdomen, or other vital organs. Be alert for the signs of shock and immediately treat all victims.

Comm

Most of the specific injuries discussed in this section result in extreme pain for the victim. It is essential that you reassure the victim constantly and encourage the victim to relax as much as possible. Direct first-aid care toward providing as much relief from pain as possible.

checkpoint

| **1.** Define *epistaxis*.

PRACTICE: Go to the workbook and complete the assignment sheet for 17:10, Providing First Aid for Specific Injuries. Then return and continue with the procedure.

Procedure 17:10

Providing First Aid for Specific Injuries

Equipment and Supplies

Blankets, pillows, dressings, bandages, tape, aluminum foil or plastic wrap, eye shields or sterile dressings, sterile water, disposable gloves

Procedure

1. Follow the steps of priority care, if indicated:
   a. Check the scene. Move the victim only if absolutely necessary.
   b. Check the victim for consciousness, a pulse, and breathing.
   c. Call emergency medical services (EMS), if necessary.
   d. Provide care to the victim.
   e. Check for bleeding. Control severe bleeding.

   Precaution

   CAUTION: Wear gloves or use a protective barrier while controlling bleeding.

2. Observe the victim closely for signs and symptoms of specific injuries. Do a systematic examination of the victim. Always have a reason for everything you do. Explain what you are doing to the victim and/or observers.

   Comm

3. If the victim has an eye injury, proceed as follows:
   a. If the victim has a free-floating particle or foreign body in the eye, warn the victim *not* to rub the eye. Wash your hands thoroughly to prevent infection. Gently grasp the upper eyelid and draw it down over the lower eyelid. If this does not remove the object, use your thumb and forefinger to grasp the eyelashes and gently raise the upper eyelid. Tell the victim to look down and tilt their head slightly to the injured side. Use water to gently flush the eye or use the corner of a piece of sterile gauze to gently remove the object. If this does not remove the object or if the object is embedded, proceed to step b.
   b. If an object is embedded in the eye, make *no* attempt to remove it. Rather, apply a dry, sterile dressing to loosely cover the eye. Obtain medical help.
   c. If an eye injury has caused a contusion, a black eye, internal bleeding, and/or torn tissue in the eye, apply sterile dressings or eye shields to both eyes. Keep the victim lying flat. Obtain medical help.

   NOTE: Both eyes are covered to prevent involuntary movement of the injured eye.

(continues)

d. If an object is protruding from the eye, make *no* attempt to remove the object. If possible, support the object in position by loosely placing dressings around it. A paper cup with the bottom removed can also be used to surround and prevent any movement of the object. Apply dressings to the uninjured eye to prevent movement of the injured eye. Keep the victim lying flat. Obtain medical help immediately.

4. If the victim has an ear injury:

a. Control severe bleeding from an ear wound by using a sterile dressing to apply light pressure.

 CAUTION: Wear gloves or use a protective barrier to prevent contamination from the blood.
Precaution

b. If any tissue has been torn from the ear, preserve the tissue by placing it in gauze moistened with cool, sterile water or normal saline solution. Place the gauze-wrapped tissue in a plastic bag. Send the torn tissue to the medical facility along with the victim.

NOTE: If sterile water is not available, use cool, clean water.

c. If a rupture or perforation of the eardrum is suspected or evident, place sterile gauze loosely in the outer ear canal. Caution the victim against hitting the side of the head to restore hearing. Obtain medical help.

d. If cerebrospinal fluid is draining from the ear, make no attempt to stop the flow of the fluid. If no neck or spinal injury is suspected, turn the victim on their injured side and slightly elevate the head and shoulders to allow the fluid to drain. A dressing may be positioned to absorb the flow. Obtain medical help immediately.

 CAUTION: Wear gloves or use a protective barrier to prevent contamination from the cerebrospinal fluid.
Precaution

5. If the victim has a brain injury:

a. Keep the victim lying flat. Treat for shock. If there is no evidence of a neck or spinal injury, place a small pillow or a rolled blanket or coat under the victim's head and shoulders to elevate the head slightly.

 CAUTION: Never position the victim's head lower than the rest of the body.
Safety

b. Watch closely for signs of respiratory distress. Provide artificial respiration if needed.

NOTE: Remove the pillow if artificial respiration is given.

c. If cerebrospinal fluid is draining from the ears, nose, and/or mouth, make no attempt to stop the flow. Position dressings to absorb the flow.

 CAUTION: Wear gloves or use a protective barrier to prevent contamination from the cerebrospinal fluid.
Precaution

d. Avoid giving the victim any fluids by mouth. If the victim complains of excessive thirst, use a cool, wet cloth to moisten the lips, tongue, and inside of the mouth.

e. If the victim is unconscious, note for how long and report this information to the emergency rescue personnel.

f. Constantly monitor the pulse and breathing of the unconscious victim and provide CPR and/or artificial respiration if needed.

g. Obtain medical help as quickly as possible.

6. If the victim has a nosebleed:

a. Try to keep the victim calm. Remain calm yourself.

b. Position the victim in a sitting position, if possible. Lean the head forward slightly. If the victim cannot sit up, slightly elevate the head.

c. Apply pressure by pressing the nostril(s) toward the midline. Continue applying pressure for at least 5 minutes and longer, if necessary, to control the bleeding.

 NOTE: If both nostrils are bleeding and must be pressed toward the midline, tell the victim to breathe through the mouth.
Comm

 CAUTION: Wear gloves or use a protective barrier to prevent contamination from the blood.
Precaution

d. If application of pressure does not control the bleeding, insert gauze into the bleeding nostril, taking care to allow some of the gauze to hang out. Then, apply pressure again by pushing the nostril toward the midline.

e. Apply cold compresses to the bridge of the nose. Use a cold, wet cloth or a covered ice bag.

f. If the bleeding does not stop, if a fracture is suspected, or if the victim has repeated nosebleeds, obtain medical help.

   NOTE: Nosebleeds can indicate a serious underlying condition, such as high blood pressure, that requires medical attention.

7. If the victim has a chest injury:

   a. If the wound is a sucking chest wound, leave the wound open or apply a nonocclusive dressing. Make sure the dressing does not prevent the movement of air.

   b. Maintain an open airway. Constantly be alert for signs of respiratory distress. Provide artificial respiration as needed.

   c. If there is no evidence of a neck or spinal injury, position the victim with their injured side down. Slightly elevate the head and chest by placing small pillows or blankets under the victim.

   d. If an object is protruding from the chest, make *no* attempt to remove it. If possible, immobilize the object with dressings, and tape around it.

   e. Obtain medical help immediately for all chest injuries.

8. If the victim has an abdominal injury:

   a. Position the victim flat on the back. Place a small pillow or a rolled blanket or coat under the victim's knees to flex them slightly. Elevate the head and shoulders to aid breathing. If movement of the legs causes pain, leave the victim lying flat.

   b. If abdominal organs are protruding from the wound, make *no* attempt to reposition the organs. Remove clothing from around the wound or protruding organs. Use a sterile dressing that has been moistened with sterile water or normal saline solution to cover the area. If sterile water or normal saline is not available, use warm tap water to moisten the dressings.

   c. Cover the dressing with plastic wrap, if available, to keep the dressing moist. Then,

apply a folded towel or aluminum foil to keep the area warm.

   d. Avoid giving the victim any fluids or food. If the victim complains of excessive thirst, use a cool, wet cloth to moisten the lips, tongue, and inside of the mouth.

   e. Obtain medical help immediately.

9. If the victim has an injury to the genital organs:

   a. Control severe bleeding by using a sterile dressing to apply direct pressure.

   Precaution   **CAUTION:** Wear gloves or use a protective barrier to prevent contamination from the blood.

   b. Position the victim flat on the back. Separate the legs to prevent pressure on the genital area.

   c. If any tissue is torn from the area, preserve the tissue by wrapping it in gauze moistened with cool, sterile water or normal saline solution. Put the gauze-wrapped tissue in a plastic bag and send it to the medical facility along with the victim.

   d. Apply cold compresses such as covered ice bags to the area to relieve pain and reduce swelling.

   e. Obtain medical help for the victim.

10. Be alert for the signs of shock in all victims. Treat for shock immediately.

11.
    Comm   Constantly reassure all victims while providing care. Remain calm. Encourage the victim to relax as much as possible.

12. Always obtain medical help as quickly as possible. Shock, pain, and injuries to vital organs can cause death in a very short period of time.

13. Wash hands thoroughly after providing care.

PRACTICE: Go to the workbook and use the evaluation sheet for 17:10, Providing First Aid for Specific Injuries, to practice this procedure. When you believe you have mastered this skill, sign the sheet and give it to your instructor for further action.

✅ **FINAL EVALUATION:** Using the criteria listed on the evaluation sheet, your instructor will grade your performance.
Check

17:11 PROVIDING FIRST AID FOR SUDDEN ILLNESS

The victim of a sudden illness requires first aid until medical help can be obtained. Sudden illness can occur in any individual. At times, it is difficult to determine the exact illness being experienced by the victim. However, by knowing the signs and symptoms of some major disorders, you should be able to provide appropriate first-aid care. Information regarding a specific condition or illness may also be obtained from the victim, medical alert bracelets or necklaces, or medical information cards. Be alert to all of these factors while caring for the victim of a sudden illness.

HEART ATTACK

A **heart attack** is also called a *coronary thrombosis, coronary occlusion,* or *myocardial infarction*. It may occur when one of the coronary arteries supplying blood to the heart is blocked. If the attack is severe, the victim may die. If the heart stops beating, cardiopulmonary resuscitation (CPR) must be started. Main facts regarding heart attacks are as follows:

- Signs and symptoms of a heart attack may vary depending on the amount of heart damage. Severe, painful pressure under the breastbone (sternum) with pain radiating to the shoulders, arms, neck, and jaw is a common symptom (**Figure 17–40**). The victim usually experiences intense shortness of breath. The skin, especially near the lips and nail beds, becomes pale or cyanotic (bluish). The victim feels very weak but is also anxious and apprehensive. Nausea, vomiting, diaphoresis (excessive perspiration), and loss of consciousness may occur. The signs and symptoms of a heart attack in females are often more subtle. They may experience unusual fatigue and sleep disturbances for weeks prior to the attack. Cold sweats are common, as is pain in other areas than the chest, such as the arms, back, stomach, neck, and/or jaw. Heart attacks are often misdiagnosed in females.

- First aid for a heart attack is directed toward encouraging the victim to relax, placing the victim in a comfortable position to relieve pain and assist breathing, and obtaining medical help. Shock frequently occurs, so provide treatment for shock. Prevent any unnecessary stress and avoid excessive movement because any activity places additional strain on the heart. Reassure the victim constantly, and obtain appropriate medical assistance as soon as possible.

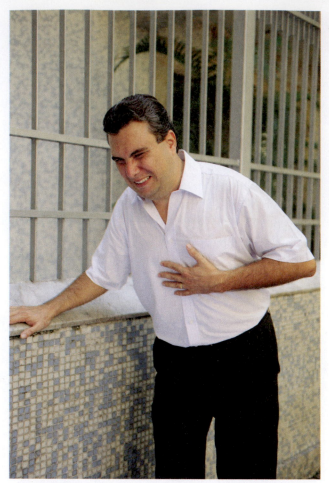

FIGURE 17–40 Severe pressure under the sternum with pain radiating to the shoulders, arms, neck, and jaw is a common symptom of a heart attack. © mangostock/www.Shutterstock.com

- Legal After calling EMS, the American Heart Association recommends that patients who can should take an aspirin. Aspirin keeps platelets in the blood from sticking together to cause a clot. However, there are legal restrictions as to which health care providers can administer medications. Only qualified individuals should give the victim aspirin.

CEREBROVASCULAR ACCIDENT OR STROKE

A **stroke** is also called a **cerebrovascular accident** (CVA), apoplexy, or cerebral thrombosis. It is caused by either the presence of a clot in a cerebral artery that provides blood to the brain or hemorrhage from a blood vessel in the brain.

- Signs and symptoms of a stroke vary depending on the part of the brain affected. Some common signs and symptoms are numbness (especially on one side of the body), paralysis (especially on one side of the body), eye pupils unequal in size, mental confusion, sudden severe headache, loss of balance or coordination, slurred speech, nausea, vomiting, difficulty breathing and swallowing, and loss of consciousness.

- A quick and easy way to remember the signs and symptoms of stroke is to think *FAST*:

  F = Face: ask the person to smile. If one side of the face appears to be drooping or crooked, it may be a sign of stroke.

  A = Arms: ask the person to raise both of their arms. If they have difficulty lifting one, or keeping one raised, it may be a sign of stroke.

  S = Speech: ask the person to speak. If the words are slurred or they have difficulty speaking, it may be a sign of stroke.

  T = Time: if they have any of these symptoms, call 911 immediately.

- First aid for a stroke victim is directed toward maintaining respirations, lying the victim flat on the back with the head slightly elevated or on the side to allow secretions to drain from the mouth, and avoiding any fluids by mouth. Reassure the victim, prevent any unnecessary stress, and avoid any unnecessary movement.

  Comm

  NOTE: *Always remember that although the victim may be unable to speak or may appear to be unconscious, they may be able to hear and understand what is going on.*

- It is very important to know exactly when the symptoms started and to obtain medical help as quickly as possible. Immediate care during the first 3 hours can help prevent brain damage. If the CVA is caused by a blood clot, treatment with thrombolytic or "clot busting" drugs such as TPA (tissue plasminogen activator) or angioplasty of the cerebral arteries can dissolve a blood clot and restore blood flow to the brain. If the CVA is caused by a hemorrhage, thrombolytic therapy is not an option. In this case, treatment will depend on the cause of the bleed (hypertension, use of anticoagulants, trauma, etc.). In some cases, surgery can be done to stop the bleeding.

FAINTING

Fainting occurs when there is a temporary reduction in the supply of blood to the brain. It may result in partial or complete loss of consciousness. The victim usually regains consciousness after being in a supine position (that is, lying flat on the back).

- Early signs of fainting include dizziness, extreme pallor, diaphoresis, coldness of the skin, nausea, and a numbness and tingling of the hands and feet.

- If early symptoms are noted, help the victim to lie down or to sit in a chair and position their head at the level of the knees.

- If the victim loses consciousness, try to prevent injury. Provide first aid by keeping the victim in a supine position. If no neck or spine injuries are suspected, use a pillow or blankets to elevate the victim's legs and feet 12 inches. Loosen any tight clothing and maintain an open airway. Use cool water to gently bathe the victim's face. Check for any injuries that may have been caused by the fall. Permit the victim to remain flat and quiet until color improves and the victim has recovered. Then, allow the victim to get up gradually. If recovery is not prompt, if other injuries occur or are suspected, or if fainting occurs again, obtain medical help. Fainting can be a sign of a serious illness or condition that requires medical attention.

CONVULSION

A **convulsion**, which is a type of *seizure*, is a strong, involuntary contraction of muscles. Convulsions may occur in conjunction with high body temperatures, head injuries, brain disease, and brain disorders such as epilepsy.

- Convulsions cause a rigidity of body muscles followed by jerking movements. During a convulsion, a person may stop breathing, bite the tongue, lose bladder and bowel control, and injure body parts. The face and lips may develop a cyanotic (bluish) color. The victim may lose consciousness. After regaining consciousness at the end of the convulsion, the victim may be confused and disoriented, and complain of a headache.

- First aid is directed toward preventing self-injury. Removing dangerous objects from the area, providing a pillow or cushion under the victim's head, and providing artificial respiration, as necessary are all ways to assist the victim.

- Do *not* try to place anything between the victim's teeth. This can cause severe injury to your fingers, and/or damage to the victim's teeth or gums.

- Do *not* use force to restrain or stop the muscle movements; this only causes the contractions to become more severe.

- When the convulsion is over, watch the victim closely. If fluid, such as saliva or vomitus, is in the victim's mouth, position the victim on their side to allow the fluid to drain from the mouth. Allow the victim to sleep or rest.

- Obtain medical help if the seizure lasts more than a few minutes, if the victim has repeated seizures, if other severe injuries are apparent, if the victim does not have a history of seizures, or if the victim does not regain consciousness.

DIABETIC REACTIONS

Diabetes mellitus is a metabolic disorder caused by an insufficient production of insulin (a hormone produced by the pancreas). Insulin helps the body transport glucose, a form of sugar, from the bloodstream into body cells where the glucose is used to produce energy. When there is a lack of insulin, sugar builds up in the bloodstream. Insulin injections can reduce and control the level of sugar in the blood. Individuals with diabetes are in danger of developing two conditions that require first aid: diabetic coma and insulin shock (**Figure 17–41**).

- **Diabetic coma** or *hyperglycemia* is caused by an increase in the level of glucose in the bloodstream. The condition may result from an excess intake of sugar, failure to take insulin, or insufficient production of insulin. Signs and symptoms include confusion; weakness or dizziness; nausea and/or vomiting; rapid, deep respirations; dry, flushed skin; and a sweet or fruity odor to the breath. The victim will eventually lose consciousness and die unless the condition is treated. Medical assistance must be obtained as quickly as possible.

- **Insulin shock** or *hypoglycemia* is caused by an excess amount of insulin (and a low level of glucose) in the bloodstream. It may result from failure to eat the recommended amounts, vomiting after taking insulin, or taking excessive amounts of insulin. Signs and symptoms include muscle weakness; mental confusion; restlessness or anxiety; diaphoresis; pale, moist skin; hunger pangs; and/or palpitations (rapid, irregular heartbeats).

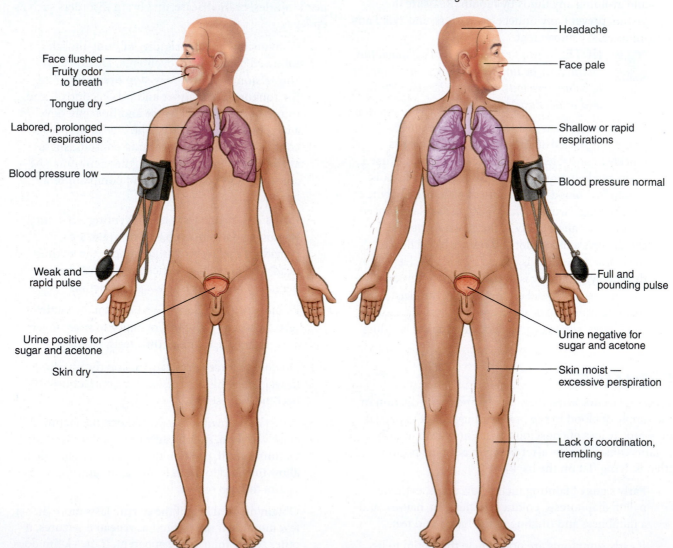

Diabetic coma (Hyperglycemia)
- Appears to be in stupor or coma
- High blood glucose levels

Face flushed
Fruity odor to breath
Tongue dry
Labored, prolonged respirations
Blood pressure low
Weak and rapid pulse
Urine positive for sugar and acetone
Skin dry

Insulin shock (Hypoglycemia)
- Excited, nervous, dizziness, confused, irritable, inappropriate responses
- Low blood glucose levels

Headache
Face pale
Shallow or rapid respirations
Blood pressure normal
Full and pounding pulse
Urine negative for sugar and acetone
Skin moist — excessive perspiration
Lack of coordination, trembling

FIGURE 17–41 Diabetic coma (hyperglycemia) versus insulin shock (hypoglycemia).

The victim may lapse into a coma and develop convulsions. The onset of insulin shock is sudden, and the victim's condition can deteriorate quickly; therefore, immediate first-aid care is required. If the victim is conscious, give them a drink containing sugar, such as sweetened orange juice. A cube or teaspoon of granulated sugar can also be placed in the victim's mouth. If the victim is confused, avoid giving hard candy. Unconsciousness could occur, and the victim could choke on the hard candy. Many individuals with diabetes use tubes of glucose that they carry with them (**Figure 17–42**). If the victim is conscious and can swallow and a glucose tube is available, it can be given to the victim.

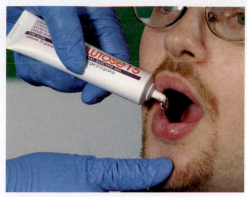

FIGURE 17–42 A victim experiencing insulin shock needs glucose or some form of sugar as quickly as possible.

The intake of sugar should quickly control the reaction. If the victim loses consciousness or convulsions start, provide care for the convulsions and obtain medical assistance immediately.

 By observing symptoms carefully and obtaining as much information as possible from the victim, you can usually determine whether the condition is diabetic coma or insulin shock. Ask the victim, "Have you eaten today?" and "Have you taken your insulin?" If the victim has taken insulin but has not eaten, insulin shock is developing because there is too much insulin in the body. If the victim has eaten but has not taken insulin, diabetic coma is developing. In cases when you know that the victim is diabetic but the victim is unconscious and there are no definite symptoms of either condition, you may not be able to determine whether the condition is diabetic coma or insulin shock. In such cases, the recommendation is to put granulated sugar under the victim's tongue and activate emergency medical services (EMS). This is the lesser of two evils. If the patient is in diabetic coma, the blood sugar level can be lowered as needed when the victim is transported for medical care. If the victim is in

insulin shock, however, brain damage can occur if the blood-sugar level is not raised immediately. Medical care cannot correct brain damage.

SUMMARY

 In all cases of sudden illness, constantly reassure the victim and make every attempt to encourage the victim to relax and avoid further stress. Be alert for the signs of shock and provide treatment for shock to all victims. The pain, anxiety, and fear associated with sudden illness can contribute to shock.

checkpoint

1. What is a myocardial infarction?
2. When evaluating stroke, what does the acronym FAST stand for?

PRACTICE: Go to the workbook and complete the assignment sheet for 17:11, Providing First Aid for Sudden Illness. Then return and continue with the procedure.

Procedure 17:11

Providing First Aid for Sudden Illness

Equipment and Supplies

Blankets, pillows, sugar, clean cloth, cool water, disposable gloves

Procedure

1. Follow the steps of priority care, if indicated.
   a. Check the scene. Move the victim only if absolutely necessary.
   b. Check the victim for consciousness, a pulse, and breathing.
   c. Call emergency medical services (EMS), if necessary.
   d. Provide care to the victim.
   e. Check for bleeding. Control severe bleeding.

    CAUTION: Wear gloves or use a protective barrier while controlling bleeding.

2. Closely observe the victim for specific signs and symptoms. If the victim is conscious, obtain information about the history of the illness, type and amount of

(continues)

pain, and other pertinent details. If the victim is unconscious, check for a medical bracelet or necklace or a medical information card. Always have a reason for everything you do. Explain your actions to any observers, especially if it is necessary to check the victim's wallet for a medical card.

3. If you suspect the victim is having a heart attack, provide first aid as follows:

a. Place the victim in the most comfortable position possible, but avoid unnecessary movement. Some victims will want to lie flat, but others will want to be in a partial or complete sitting position. If the victim is having difficulty breathing, use pillows or rolled blankets to elevate the head and shoulders.

b. Obtain medical help for the victim immediately. Advise EMS that oxygen may be necessary.

c. Encourage the victim to relax. Reassure the victim. Remain calm and encourage others to remain calm.

d. Watch for signs of shock and treat for shock as necessary. Avoid overheating the victim.

e. If the victim complains of excessive thirst, use a wet cloth to moisten the lips, tongue, and inside of the mouth. Small sips of water can also be given to the victim, but avoid giving large amounts of fluid.

⚠ CAUTION: Do *not* give the victim ice water or very cold water because the cold can intensify shock.
Safety

4. If you suspect that the victim has had a stroke:

a. Place the victim in a comfortable position. Keep the victim lying flat or slightly elevate the victim's head and shoulders to aid breathing. If the victim has difficulty swallowing, turn the victim on their side to allow secretions to drain from the mouth and prevent choking on the secretions.

b. Reassure the victim. Encourage the victim to relax.

c. Avoid giving the victim any fluids or food by mouth. If the victim complains of excessive thirst, use a cool, wet cloth to moisten the lips, tongue, and inside of the mouth.

d. Attempt to determine the exact time the symptoms started and obtain medical help for the victim as quickly as possible.

5. If the victim has fainted:

a. Keep the victim in a supine position (that is, lying flat on the back). Raise the legs and feet 12 inches.

b. Check for a pulse and breathing. Provide CPR and/or artificial respiration, if necessary.

c. Loosen any tight clothing.

d. Use cool water to gently bathe the face.

e. Check for any other injuries.

f. Encourage the victim to continue lying down until their skin color improves.

g. If no other injuries are suspected, allow the victim to get up slowly. First, elevate the head and shoulders. Then place the victim in a sitting position. Allow the victim to stand slowly. If any signs of dizziness, weakness, or pallor are noted, return the victim to the supine position.

h. If the victim does not recover quickly, or if any other injuries occur, obtain medical care. If fainting has occurred frequently, refer the victim for medical care.

NOTE: Fainting can be a sign of a serious illness or condition.

6. If the victim is having a convulsion, provide first aid as follows:

a. Remove any dangerous objects from the area. If the victim is near heavy furniture or machinery that cannot be moved, move the victim to a safe area.

b. Place soft material such as a blanket, small pillow, rolled jacket, or other similar material under the victim's head to prevent injury.

c. Closely observe respirations at all times. During the convulsion, there will be short periods of apnea (cessation of breathing).

NOTE: If breathing does not resume quickly, artificial respiration may be necessary.

d. Do *not* try to place anything between the victim's teeth. This can cause injury to the teeth and/or gums.

e. Do *not* attempt to restrain the muscle contractions. This only makes the contractions more severe.

f. Note how long the convulsion lasts and what parts of the body are involved. Be sure to report this information to the EMS personnel.

g. After the convulsion ends, closely watch the victim. Encourage the victim to rest.

h. Obtain medical assistance if the convulsion lasts more than a few minutes, if the victim has repeated convulsions, if other severe injuries are apparent, if the victim does not have a history of convulsions, or if the victim does not regain consciousness.

7. If the victim is in diabetic coma:

a. Place the victim in a comfortable position. If the victim is unconscious, position them on either side to allow secretions to drain from the mouth.

b. Frequently check pulse and respirations. Provide CPR and/or artificial respiration as needed.

c. Obtain medical help immediately so the victim can be transported to a medical facility.

8. If the victim is in insulin shock:

a. If the victim is conscious and can swallow, offer a drink containing sugar or oral glucose if a tube is available.

b. If the victim is unconscious, place a small amount of granulated sugar under the victim's tongue.

c. Place the victim in a comfortable position. Position an unconscious victim on either side to allow secretions to drain from the mouth.

d. If the victim is unconscious, monitor the pulse and breathing. Provide CPR and/or artificial respiration as needed.

e. If recovery is not prompt, obtain medical help immediately.

9. Observe all victims of sudden illness for signs of shock. Treat for shock as necessary.

10. Constantly reassure any victim of sudden illness. Encourage relaxation to decrease stress.

    Comm

11. Wash hands thoroughly after providing care.

PRACTICE: Go to the workbook and use the evaluation sheet for 17:11, Providing First Aid for Sudden Illness, to practice this procedure. When you believe you have mastered this skill, sign the sheet and give it to your instructor for further action.

✅ **FINAL EVALUATION:** Using the criteria listed on the evaluation sheet, your instructor will grade your performance.

Check

17:12 APPLYING DRESSINGS AND BANDAGES

In many cases requiring first aid, it will be necessary for you to apply dressings and bandages. This section provides basic information on types of bandages and dressings and on application methods.

A **dressing** is a sterile covering placed over a wound or an injured part. It is used to control bleeding, absorb blood and secretions, prevent infection, and ease pain. Materials that may be used as dressings include gauze pads in a variety of sizes and compresses of thick, absorbent material (**Figure 17–43**). Fluff cotton should *not* be used as a dressing because the loose cotton fibers may contaminate the wound. In an emergency when no dressings are available, a clean handkerchief or pillowcase may be used. The dressing is held in place with tape or a bandage.

Bandages are materials used to hold dressings in place, to secure splints, and to support and protect body parts. Bandages should be applied snugly enough to control bleeding and prevent movement of the dressing, but

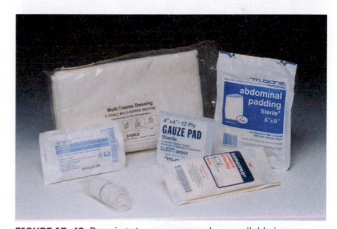

FIGURE 17–43 Dressings to cover a wound are available in many different sizes.

not so tightly that they interfere with circulation. Types of bandages include roller gauze bandages, triangular bandages, and elastic bandages (**Figure 17–44**).

- **Roller gauze bandages** come in a variety of widths, most commonly 1-, 2-, and 3-inch widths. They can be used to hold dressings in place on almost any part of the body.

- **Triangular bandages** can be used to secure dressings on the head/scalp or as slings. A triangular bandage is sometimes used as a covering for a large body part such as a hand, foot, or shoulder. By folding the triangular bandage into a band of cloth called a *cravat* (**Figure 17–45**), the bandage can be used to secure splints or dressings on body parts.

- **Elastic bandages** are easy to apply because they readily conform, or mold, to the injured part. However, they can be quite hazardous; if they are applied too tightly or are stretched during application, they can cut off or constrict circulation. Elastic bandages are sometimes used to provide support and stimulate circulation.

Several methods are used to wrap bandages. The method used depends on the body part involved. Some common wraps include the spiral wrap, the figure-eight wrap for joints, and the finger, or recurrent, wrap. The wraps are described in Procedure 17:12, immediately following this information section.

After any bandage has been applied, it is important to check the body part below the bandage to make sure the bandage is not so tight as to interfere with blood circulation. Signs that indicate poor circulation include swelling, a pale or blue (cyanotic) color to the skin, coldness to the touch, and numbness or tingling. If the bandage has been applied to the hand, arm, leg, or foot, press lightly on the nail beds to blanch them, that is, make them turn white (**Figure 17–46A**). The pink color should return to the nail beds immediately after pressure is released (**Figure 17–46B**). If the pink color does not return or returns slowly, this is an indication of poor or impaired circulation. If any signs of impaired circulation are noted, loosen the bandages immediately.

checkpoint

| **1.** List three (3) types of bandages.

PRACTICE: Go to the workbook and complete the assignment sheet for 17:12, Applying Dressings and Bandages. Then return and continue with the procedure.

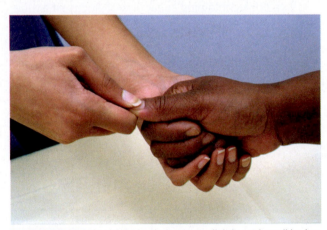

FIGURE 17–46A To check circulation, press lightly on the nail bed to blanch it or make it turn white.

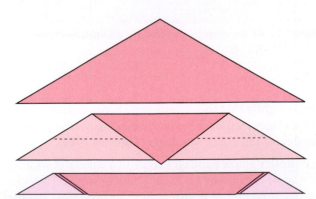

FIGURE 17–44 Roller gauze and elastic bandages can be used to hold dressings in place.

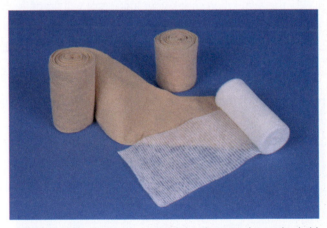

FIGURE 17–45 Folding a cravat bandage from a triangular bandage.

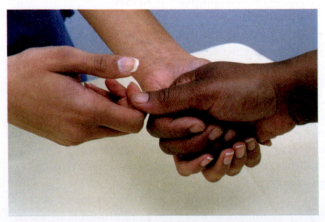

FIGURE 17–46B If the nail bed does not turn to pink immediately after pressure is released, circulation may be impaired.

Applying Dressings and Bandages

Equipment and Supplies

Sterile gauze pads, triangular bandage, roller gauze bandage, elastic bandage, tape, disposable gloves

Procedure

1. Assemble equipment.

2. **Precaution** Wash hands. Put on gloves if there is any chance of contact with blood or body fluids.

3. Apply a dressing to a wound as follows:

   a. Obtain the correct size dressing. The dressing should be large enough to extend at least 1 inch beyond the edges of the wound.

   b. Open the sterile dressing package, taking care not to touch or handle the sterile dressing with your fingers.

   c. Use a pinching action to pick up the sterile dressing so you handle only one part of the outside of the dressing. The ideal situation would involve the use of sterile transfer forceps or sterile gloves to handle the dressing. However, these items are usually not available in emergency situations.

   d. Place the dressing on the wound. The untouched (sterile) side of the dressing should be placed on the wound. Do *not* slide the dressing into position. Instead, hold the dressing directly over the wound and then lower the dressing onto the wound.

   e. Secure the dressing in place with tape or with one of the bandage wraps.

   ⚠️ **Safety** **CAUTION:** If tape is used, do not wrap it completely around the part. This can lead to impaired circulation.

4. Apply a triangular bandage to the head or scalp (**Figure 17–47**):

   a. Fold a 2-inch hem on the base (longest side) of the triangular bandage.

   b. Position and secure a sterile dressing in place over the wound.

   c. Keeping the hem on the outside, position the middle of the base of the bandage on the forehead, just above the eyebrows.

   d. Bring the point of the bandage down over the back of the head.

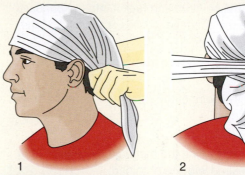
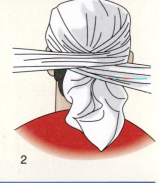

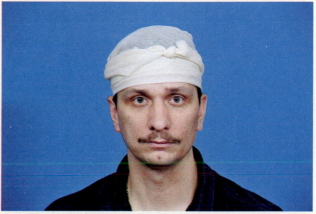

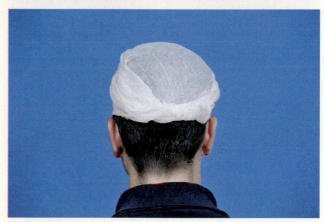

FIGURE 17–47 Steps for applying a triangular bandage to the head or scalp.

   e. Bring the two ends of the base of the bandage around the head and above the ears. Cross the ends when they meet at the back of the head. Bring them around to the forehead.

   f. Use a square knot to tie the ends in the center of the forehead.

   g. Use one hand to support the head. Use the other hand to gently but firmly pull down on the point of the bandage at the back of the head until the bandage is snug against the head.

(continues)

h. Bring the point up and tuck it into the bandage where the bandage crosses at the back of the head.

5. Make a cravat bandage from a triangular bandage (review Figure 17–45):

   a. Bring the point of the triangular bandage down to the middle of the base (the long end of the bandage).

   b. Continue folding the bandage lengthwise until the desired width is obtained.

6. Apply a circular bandage with the cravat bandage (**Figure 17–48**):

   a. Place a sterile dressing on the wound.

   b. Place the center of the cravat bandage over the sterile dressing.

   c. Bring the ends of the cravat around the body part and cross them when they meet.

   d. Bring the ends back to the starting point.

   e. Use a square knot to tie the ends of the cravat over the dressing.

    CAUTION: Avoid tying or wrapping the bandage too tightly. This could impair circulation.

NOTE: Roller gauze bandage can also be used.

 CAUTION: This type of wrap is *never* used around the neck because it could strangle the victim.

7. Apply a spiral wrap using roller gauze bandage or elastic bandage:

   a. Place a sterile dressing over the wound.

   b. Hold the roller gauze or elastic bandage so that the loose end is hanging off the bottom of the roll.

   c. Start at the farthest end (the bottom of the limb) and move in an upward direction.

   d. Anchor the bandage by placing it on an angle at the starting point. To do this, encircle the limb once, leaving a corner of the bandage uncovered. Turn down this free corner and then encircle the part again with the bandage (**Figure 17–49A**).

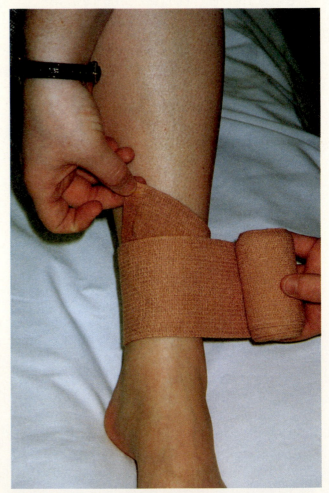

FIGURE 17–49A Anchor the bandage by leaving a corner exposed. This corner is then folded down and covered when the bandage is circled around the limb.

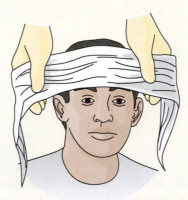

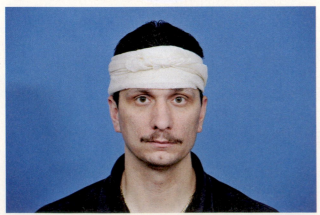

FIGURE 17–48 Applying a circular bandage with a cravat bandage.

e. Continue encircling the limb. Use a spiral type motion to move up the limb. Overlap each new turn approximately half the width of the bandage.

f. Use one or two circular turns to finish the wrap at the end point.

g. Secure the end by taping, pinning, or tying. To avoid injury when pins are used, place your hand under the double layer of bandage and between the pin and the skin before inserting the pin (**Figure 17–49B**). The end of the bandage can also be cut in half and the two halves brought around opposite sides and tied into place.

8. Use roller gauze bandage or elastic bandage to apply a figure-eight ankle wrap:

a. Position a dressing over the wound.

b. Anchor the bandage at the instep of the foot.

c. Make one or two circular turns around the instep and foot (**Figure 17–50A**).

d. Bring the bandage up over the foot in a diagonal direction. Bring it around the back of the ankle and then down over the top of the foot. Circle it under the instep. This creates the figure-eight pattern.

e. Repeat the figure-eight pattern. With each successive turn, move downward and backward toward the heel (**Figure 17–50B**). Overlap the previous turn by one-half to two-thirds the width of the bandage.

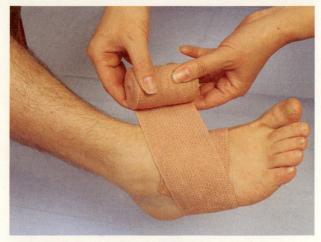

FIGURE 17–50A Bring the bandage over the foot in a diagonal direction for the start of the figure-eight pattern.

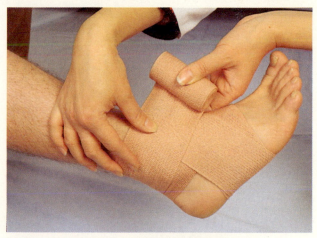

FIGURE 17–50B Keep repeating the figure-eight pattern by moving downward and backward toward the heel with each turn.

 NOTE: Hold the bandage firmly, but do not pull it too tightly. If you are using elastic bandage, avoid stretching the material during the application.

f. Near completion, use one or two final circular wraps to circle the ankle.

g. Secure the bandage in place by taping, pinning, or tying the ends, as described in step 7g.

 CAUTION: To avoid injury to the victim when pins are used, place your hand between the bandage and the victim's skin.

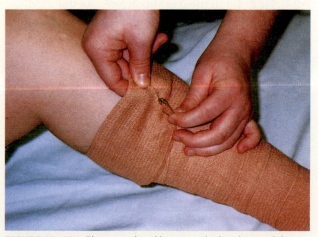

FIGURE 17–49B Place your hand between the bandage and the victim's skin while inserting a pin.

(continues)

9. Use roller gauze bandage to apply a recurrent wrap to the fingers (**Figure 17–51**).

   a. Place a sterile dressing over the wound.

   b. Hold the roller gauze bandage so that the loose end is hanging off the bottom of the roll.

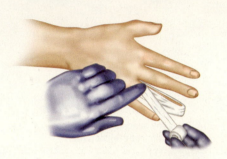

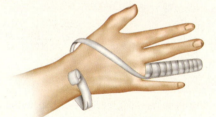

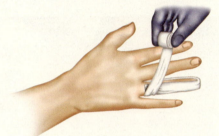

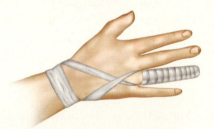

FIGURE 17–51 Recurrent wrap for the finger.

   c. Place the end of the bandage on the bottom of the finger. Then, bring the bandage up to the tip of the finger and down to the bottom of the opposite side of the finger. With overlapping wraps, fold the bandage backward and forward over the finger three or four times.

   d. Start at the bottom of the finger and use a spiral wrap up and down the finger to hold the recurrent wraps in position.

   e. Complete the bandage by using a figure-eight wrap around the wrist. Bring the bandage in a diagonal direction across the back of the hand. Circle the wrist at least two times. Bring the bandage back over the top of the hand and circle the bandaged finger. Repeat this figure-eight motion at least twice.

   f. Secure the bandage by circling the wrist once or twice. Tie the bandage at the wrist.

10. After any bandage has been applied, check the circulation below the bandage at frequent intervals. If possible, check for a pulse at a site below the bandage. Note any signs of impaired circulation, including swelling, coldness, numbness or tingling, pallor or cyanosis, and poor return of pink color after nail beds are blanched by lightly pressing on them.

 CAUTION: If any signs of poor circulation are noted, loosen the bandages immediately.
Safety

11. Obtain medical help for any victim who may need additional care.

12. Remove gloves and wash hands.

PRACTICE: Go to the workbook and use the evaluation sheet for 17:12, Applying Dressings and Bandages, to practice this procedure. When you believe you have mastered this skill, sign the sheet and give it to your instructor for further action.

 FINAL EVALUATION: Using the criteria listed on the evaluation sheet, your instructor will grade your performance.
Check

A SkinGun to Treat Burns?

Burns are a very common injury. Their intensity can range from a superficial burn, such as mild sunburn, to a partial-thickness burn that damages the top layers of skin, to a full-thickness burn that damages all layers of the skin and underlying tissue. Superficial burns usually heal by themselves in 5–6 days. For more severe burns, the major treatment is a skin graft, which involves taking skin from other parts of a patient's body or using sheets of artificial skin to cover the burn. The grafts can take weeks and even months to heal and are prone to infections. Frequently, the grafted skin causes scars and disfigurement.

Now, Dr. Jörg Gerlach and a team of researchers at the University of Pittsburgh's McGowan Institute for Regenerative Medicine have developed a SkinGun that is similar to a paint spray gun or airbrush. The process begins with surgeons using a dermatome, a special knife that can remove a very thin layer of the patient's healthy skin. Skin stem cells are isolated from this layer of skin and put into a water solution for approximately 90 minutes. Then, this mixture of cells and water is put into syringes and inserted into the nozzle of the gun. The gun is attached to a processor-controlled pneumatic (air) device that produces an even flow of solution. The skin cells are then sprayed directly onto the burn. The sprayed wound is covered with a specially created dressing that contains tubes connected to a source of nutrients and antibiotics that provide nourishment for the cells and help prevent infections. The entire process takes less than two hours for most patients. In clinical trials, the burns heal in just days instead of the weeks for skin grafts. In addition, there is less scarring of the tissue. At the present time, the SkinGun can only be used on partial-thickness burns, but research continues to improve the method so it can be used to treat full-thickness burns. In addition, researchers are working on finding a way to restore full pigmentation on patients with darker skin pigmentation.

The SkinGun has had successful clinical trials. All patients treated were able to grow new skin with minimal or no scarring in a short period of time without the complications that occur with skin grafts. It is currently in the process of obtaining FDA approval.

A second similar device called a ReCell uses almost an identical procedure to treat burns. It is approved for use in Europe, Australia, and China and is in the process of obtaining FDA approval for use in the United States.

When these devices are approved, treatment of burn patients will be more efficient and effective in the future. In addition, researchers are hopeful that they will be able to treat other types of skin damage or scarring, such as acne scarring and wounds and surgical incisions that fail to heal with traditional treatments.

Case Study Investigation Conclusion

What did you decide Miguel and Jamal should do? If Tran is bleeding because of his injury, what should they do? Do they need to check Sean for injury? Who is responsible for calling EMS? What items could they use to improvise if they don't have medical supplies?

CHAPTER 17 SUMMARY

- First aid is defined as "the immediate care given to the victim of an injury or illness to minimize the effect of the injury or illness until experts can take over."

- The basic principles of first aid were presented in this unit. Methods of cardiopulmonary resuscitation (CPR) for infants, children, adults, and choking victims were described. Proper first aid for bleeding, shock, poisoning, burns, heat and cold exposure, bone and joint injuries, specific injuries, and sudden illness were covered. Instructions were given for the application of common dressings and bandages.

- By learning and following the suggested methods, the health care provider can administer correct first-aid treatment in emergency situations until the help of experts can be obtained.

REVIEW QUESTIONS

1. What is the first step in administering CPR?

2. What are the first five (5) steps of priority care in any sudden illness procedure?

   Review the following case histories. List the correct first-aid care, in proper order of use, that should be used to treat each victim.

3. You are slicing carrots and cut off the end of your finger.
   a. How do you handle the finger? Why?
   b. What other condition would you assess for when your patient has a large blood loss?
   c. How would you treat the condition in 3b?

4. You find your 2-year-old brother in the bathroom. An empty bottle of aspirin tablets is on the floor. His mouth is covered with a white powdery residue.
   a. What do you do with the bottle found on the floor? Why?
   b. What is anaphylactic shock?

5. Liliana is a certified nursing assistant (CNA) assigned to the Alzheimer's unit in Green Pastures Veteran Retirement Home. One of her residents, Bob, loves to be outside enjoying sunny days as much as possible. Bob went outside right after lunch and fell asleep on a lawn chair. Liliana got busy with a new admission and finally woke Bob up 4½ hours later. Bob was suffering from a first-degree burn on his arms and shoulders and a second-degree burn on his forehead and nose.
   a. When the nurse used the "rule of nines" when evaluating Bob's burn, what was being calculated?
   b. What are four (4) causes of a burn injury?

6. Mark was playing tennis on a hot summer day with his friend Justin. Suddenly Justin collapses on the tennis court. When Mark gets to Justin, his skin is hot, red, and dry. He is breathing, but he is unconscious.
   a. Why should Mark not pour water in Justin's mouth?
   b. List the three (3) types of heat exposures in their order of severity.

7. Juliana went on her first ski trip during the Winter Break holiday. She didn't have the correct cold weather gear. When Juliana came inside after her first day on the slopes, her feet were pale, and her skin was glossy with a white or grayish yellow color; her toes were a little painful.
   a. What does hypothermia mean?
   b. Why is rubbing or massaging Juliana's feet contraindicated?

8. Ryan brought his two sons, Luke and Joseph, to the construction site where he works. As they were leaving, 2-year-old Joseph was running to catch up with his dad and big brother and fell, catching himself with his arm before he hit his head. He started screaming and crying, holding his left arm. When Ryan looked at it, it was oddly shaped.
   a. Why do you want to immobilize the area involved?
   b. What materials might Ryan use from the construction site to splint Joseph's arm?

9. You are on the couch watching television with your parents. Suddenly your father complains of severe pain in his chest and left arm. He is very short of breath and his lips appear cyanotic.
   a. If you suspect he is having a heart attack, what is the first thing you would do?
   b. If he needs CPR, why would you move him off of the couch and onto the floor?

REVIEW QUESTIONS (continued)

10. You are working in the chemistry lab. Suddenly an experiment boils over, explodes, and shards of material splash into your lab partner's face and eyes. She starts screaming with pain.
    a. Why is it inappropriate to rub or try to wipe the shards of material out of your lab partner's eyes?

11. You are driving and the car ahead of you loses control, goes off the road, and hits a tree. When you get to the car, the driver is slumped over the wheel. His arm is twisted at an odd angle. You notice a small fire at the rear of the car. In the back seat, a small child in a car seat is crying.
    a. What problems in this situation need to be addressed?
    b. In what order of priority would you triage these problems?

CRITICAL THINKING

1. When holding pressure on a wound, why do you reinforce and not remove bloody dressing?

2. When only one eye is injured, why do you cover both eyes?

ACTIVITIES

1. With a partner, pick one (1) of the first aid skills. Create a scenario and skill checklist that would utilize one or more of those skills.

2. Turn in the checklist to your instructor. Each team will go outside of the room. The rest of the class gets the skill checklist and sets up the classroom for the skill. The instructor will hand the team a scenario. They will have 3 minutes to read it and plan what they need to do. Then, they come into the room and complete the first-aid skill. The class will complete the checklist to provide feedback.

3. Practice applying dressings and bandages, observing all safety precautions and using the circular, spiral, figure-eight, and finger wrap. Schedule a time for the class to wrap ankles and bandage the athletic class. Teach the athletes how to take care of their ankle wraps.

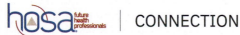 | CONNECTION

Competitive Event: CPR/First Aid

Event Summary: CPR/First Aid provides members with the opportunity to gain knowledge and skills required for team first aid and basic life support. This competitive event consists of 2 rounds and each team consists of 2 people. Round One is a written, multiple choice test and the top scoring teams will advance to Round Two for the skills assessment. This event aims to inspire members to be proactive future health professionals and be equipped with the skills to provide immediate, lifesaving actions in the absence of emergency services.

Details on this competitive event can be found at:

www.hosa.org/guidelines

Case Study Investigation

Jasmine Patel has just finished Respiratory Therapy school and is applying for her first job at Community Hospital. She has interned there for the last 10 months. Jasmine wants to be prepared for her interview. She will have her résumé and references ready but is worried about doing and saying the right thing during the actual interview. At the end of this chapter, you will be asked how Jasmine can optimize her chances of landing this job and starting her career.

■ LEARNING OBJECTIVES

After completing this chapter, you should be able to:

- Identify at least five skills that employers consider to be essential for job retention.
- Write a cover letter or letter of introduction containing all required information and using correct form for letters.
- Prepare a résumé containing all necessary information and meeting professional standards.
- Demonstrate how to complete a job application form that meets standards of neatness and accuracy.
- Demonstrate how to participate in a job interview meeting professional standards.
- Determine gross and net income.
- Calculate an accurate budget for a one-month period, accounting for fixed expenses and variable expenses without exceeding net monthly income.
- Define, pronounce, and spell all key terms.

■ KEY TERMS

application forms
budget
cover letter
deductions
externships

fixed expenses
gross income
income
internships
job interview

letter of introduction
net income
résumé *(rez'-ah-may)*
variable expenses

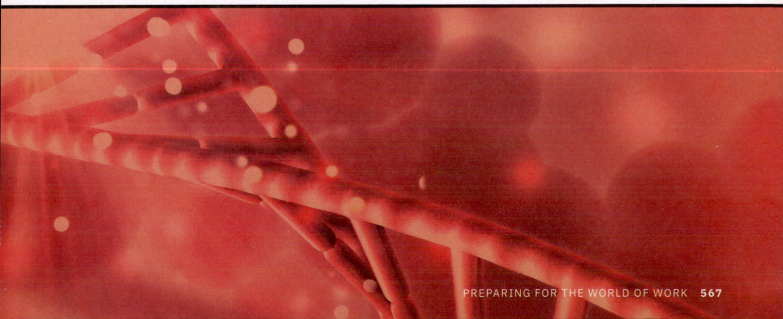

DEVELOPING
JOB-KEEPING SKILLS

PREPARING FOR A JOB

When you have completed your health science education, you will be ready to obtain a position in health care. Two things that may help you prepare for a health care position are internships and externships, which are work experiences that offer you the opportunity to gain experience in your chosen field.

Externships are often required as a part of a health science education program and are generally set up by your instructor. An externship is usually unpaid, but it will allow you to go to a health care facility to observe and/or perform the skills you have learned. It is important that you make every effort to work to the best of your ability during your externships because employers frequently select future employees from externs.

Internships usually come toward the end of a health science program and can serve as a "bridge" between the training program and professional life. An internship may be paid, unpaid, or partially paid. An intern is supervised, but the intern is usually allowed to apply the knowledge and skills learned in an actual work situation. Again, employers often hire the best interns after their internships are completed.

When looking for a job, make sure you do all of the following:

- Assess your strengths and weaknesses to help determine the type of job for which you would be best suited. If you have completed an externship or internship, use those experiences to help determine the positions that allow you to excel.

- Determine the type of job you would like, hours you are available to work, location or area where you would like to work, potential health care agency employers, and positions you are qualified to hold.

- Develop a positive attitude—be proud of what you have accomplished, and be prepared to discuss your achievements.

- Do a job search, prepare a letter of introduction and résumé, complete all information for your portfolio, and prepare for a job interview. All of these topics will be discussed in more detail later in this chapter.

CHARACTERISTICS OF A GOOD EMPLOYEE

To obtain and keep a job you must develop certain characteristics to be a good employee. A recent survey of employers asked for information on the deficiencies of high school graduates. The most frequent complaints included poor grammar, spelling, speech, communication, and math skills. Other complaints included lack of respect for work, lack of self-initiative, poor personal appearance, not accepting responsibility, excessive tardiness, poor attendance, and inability to accept criticism. Any of these defects would be detrimental to a health care provider.

Employers envision new employees improving over time. Employees must always strive toward personal development and meeting employer expectations. Some of those expectations include being loyal, flexible, and having integrity. Employers also expect every employee to understand the organizational structure (refer to Section 2:4 in this text) and follow this chain of command. Questions and problems can be resolved in a quick and efficient manner if the correct person is consulted. Effective decision making is the mark of a well-educated, experienced, and valued employee.

It is essential that you develop good job-keeping skills to be successful in a health care career. Being aware of and striving to achieve the qualities needed for employment are as important as acquiring the knowledge and skills required in your chosen health care profession.

Job-keeping skills include:

- **Use correct grammar at all times.** This includes both the written and spoken word. Patients often judge ability on how well a person speaks or writes information. While at work, do not use texting speech or writing. Also, the use of words like *ain't* indicates a lack of education and does not create a favorable or professional impression. You must constantly strive to use correct grammar. Listen to how other health care professionals speak and review basic concepts of correct grammar. It may even be necessary to take a communications course to learn to speak correctly. Because you will be completing legal written records for health care, the use of correct spelling, punctuation, and sentence structure is also essential. Use a dictionary to check spelling, or use the spell-check tool on a computer system. Refer to standard English books or grammar manuals for information on sentence structure and punctuation. Constantly strive to improve both oral and written communication skills.

- **Report to work on time and when scheduled.** Because many health care facilities provide care 7 days a week, 365 days per year, and often 24 hours per day, an employee who is frequently late or absent can cause a major disruption in schedule and contribute to an insufficiency of personnel to provide patient care. Most health care facilities have strict rules regarding absenteeism, and a series of absences can result in job loss.

Comm

- **Be prepared to work when you arrive at work.** An employer does not pay workers to socialize, text friends and family, check their social media, make personal telephone calls, consult others about personal or family problems, bring their children to work, shop online, play games, or work in a sloppy and inefficient manner. Develop a good work ethic. Observe all legal and ethical responsibilities. Follow the policies and procedures of your health care facility. Recognize your limitations and seek help when you need it. Be willing to learn new procedures and techniques. Watch efficient and knowledgeable staff members and learn by their examples. Constantly strive to do the best job possible. A worker who has self-initiative, who sees a job that needs to be done and does it, is a valuable employee who is likely to be recognized and rewarded.

- **Practice teamwork.** Because health care typically involves a team of different professionals working together to provide patient care, it is important to be willing to work with others. If you are willing to help others when they need help, they will likely be willing to help you. Two or three people working together can lift a heavy patient much more readily than one can.

- **Promote a positive attitude.** By being positive, you create a good impression and encourage the same attitude in others. Too often, employees concentrate only on the negative aspects of their jobs. Every job has some bad points that are easy to criticize. It is also easy to criticize the bad points in others with whom you work. However, this leads to a negative attitude and helps create poor morale in everyone. By concentrating on the good aspects of a job and the rewards it can provide, work will seem much more pleasant, and employees will obtain more satisfaction from their efforts.

- **Accept responsibility for your actions.** Most individuals are more than willing to take credit for the good things they have done. In the same manner, it is essential to take responsibility for mistakes. If you make a mistake, report it to your supervisor and make every effort to correct the error. Every human being will do something wrong at some time. Recognizing an error, taking responsibility for it, and making every effort to correct it or prevent it from happening again is a sign of a competent employee. Honesty is essential in health care. Not accepting responsibility for your actions is dishonest. It is often a reason for dismissal and can prevent you from obtaining another position.

- **Be willing to learn.** Health care changes constantly because of advances in technology and research. Every health care provider must be willing to learn new things and adapt to change. Participating in staff development programs (**Figure 18–1**); taking courses at technical schools, colleges, or online; attending special seminars or meetings; reading professional journals; and asking questions of other qualified individuals are all ways to improve your knowledge and skills. Employers recognize these efforts. Ambition is often rewarded with a higher salary and/or job advancement.

Without good job-keeping skills, no amount of knowledge will help you keep a job. Therefore, it is essential for you to strive to develop the qualities that employers need in their employees. Be courteous, responsible, enthusiastic, cooperative, reliable, punctual, and efficient. Strive hard to be the best you can be. If you do this, you will not only be likely to retain your job, but you will probably be rewarded with job advancement, increased salary, and personal satisfaction.

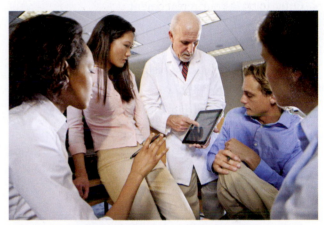

FIGURE 18–1 Participating in staff development programs is one way to improve your own knowledge and skills. © Golden Pixels LLC/Shutterstock.com.

RESIGNING FROM A JOB

As you progress through your career, there will most likely come a time when you will need to resign from your current position. There are many reasons for needing to resign, and these include:

- A job offer with better hours, more pay, better benefits, more educational and advancement opportunities, or better job security

- A job offer that allows you to use more of your education and skills or is in a specialized area in which you are interested, such as pediatrics or obstetrics

- Personal reasons, such as marriage, moving, illness, or pregnancy

It is always best to have a new position before resigning from a current position. If you do not, make sure you have adequate funds to live on until you have a new position. Handle your resignation in a professional manner. Make sure you treat your current employer well, because you may need to rely on them for a reference.

When resigning:

- Always give notice—usually at least one pay period or a minimum of 2 weeks. If you can give more notice, do so.

- Make sure the first person you tell is your supervisor or the person in charge—it is not a good idea to let them hear the news from your other team members.

- Be positive about your reasons for leaving, and emphasize how your current position has benefited you. Let them know you are grateful for the experience.

- Work to the best of your ability until your resignation date. Make sure you complete all open assignments and leave detailed progress reports for your supervisor and team members.

- Offer to train your replacement.

- Ask for a letter of recommendation to put in your portfolio.

When resigning, a letter of resignation must be submitted and must include:

- Date you are submitting your resignation letter

- Addressed correctly to your supervisor or the person in charge of your department; copies should be given to any other people who should be notified in your health care facility

- Date resignation is effective

- Reason for leaving—keep this brief and positive

- Thank them for giving you the opportunity to work at their health care facility, and be sure to end the letter on a positive note

- Signature

In the event that you are fired or laid off:

- Stay positive, no matter how difficult.

- Do not blame others—look for the reason within yourself and learn from experience. In future interviews, you can tell potential employers how you learned from your error. Accept responsibility for whatever caused you to be fired.

- Do not criticize the health care facility to others. Do not make any statements or express any opinions that you may later regret.

- Ask the employer if a letter of resignation would be accepted instead of being fired. It looks better to future employers if you resigned instead of being fired. If the employer agrees, be sure to thank them.

Before you leave, make sure you have contact information for key supervisors and other team members who you want to keep as part of your network of contacts. Be sure to thank them for having had the opportunity

to work with them. Throughout your health care career, you may need to call on former colleagues and employers for consultations, recommendations, advice, and help. The health care world is very interconnected, so it is important you make your career decisions with respect and dignity.

checkpoint

1. List five (5) job-keeping skills.

2. When you are resigning your position, who is the first person you should tell?

PRACTICE: Go to the workbook and complete the assignment sheet for 18:1, Developing Job-Keeping Skills.

18:2 WRITING A COVER LETTER AND PREPARING A RÉSUMÉ

INTRODUCTION

Before you look for a job, evaluate your interests and abilities. Decide what type of job you would like. Make sure you obtain the education needed to perform the job. Then, look at different job sources to try to find a position you will like. There are many different sources for finding job openings. Some of them include:

- Internet job search sites such as *www.monster.com*, *www.careerbuilder.com*, *www.indeed.com*, *www.healthecareers.com*, *www.ziprecruiter.com*, or *www.careervitals.com*

- Job listings posted by health care facilities on their websites

- Job fairs sponsored by schools, employment agencies, or health care facilities

- Recommendations from practicum shadowing clinical sites, externships, and internships

- Personal networking: supervisors, mentors, acquaintances

- Joining professional social networking sites such as *www.linkedin.com*. These sites allow you to search for available jobs as well as network with other health care professionals. You are also able to "follow" healthcare agencies you are interested in to see when they have new job openings available.

- Advertisements in newspapers

- Recommendations from friends and relatives

- School counselors or bulletin boards
- Employment agencies
- Professional organizations: check their Internet sites or contact the local organizations

Once you have identified possible places of employment, prepare to apply for the position. In most cases, this involves writing a cover letter, or letter of introduction, and a résumé.

COVER LETTER OR LETTER OF INTRODUCTION

The purpose of a **cover letter** or **letter of introduction** is to obtain an interview. You must create a good impression in the letter so that the employer will be interested in hiring you. In many cases, you will be responding to a job advertised either on the Internet, or through other sources. However, a résumé may be sent to potential employers even though they have not advertised a job opportunity. A cover letter or letter of introduction should accompany all résumés.

The letter should be completed on a computer and printed on good quality paper that is white or light in color. It must be neat, complete, and written according to correct form for letters. The correct form for composing business letters is discussed in detail in Section 24:5 in this text. Care must be taken to ensure that spelling and punctuation are correct. Remember, this letter is the employer's first impression of you.

Comm

If possible, the letter should be addressed to the correct individual. If you know the name of the agency or company, call to obtain this information or try to locate it on their website. Be sure you obtain the correct spelling of the person's name as well as the person's correct title. If you are responding to a box number, follow the instructions in the advertisement or posting. Another possibility is to address the letter to the director of human resources or the head of a particular department.

The letter usually contains three to four paragraphs. The contents of each paragraph are described as follows:

- **Paragraph one:** State your purpose for writing and express interest in the position for which you are applying. If you are responding to an advertisement or posting, state the name and date of the publication or posting site. If you were referred by another individual, give this person's name and title.

- **Paragraph two:** State why you believe you are qualified for the position. It may also state why you want to work for this particular employer. Information should be brief because most of the information will be included on your résumé.

- **Paragraph three:** State that a résumé is included, or attached if you are submitting your cover letter

and résumé online. You may also want to draw the employer's attention to one or two important features on your résumé. If you are not including a résumé, state that one is available on request. Whenever possible, it is best to include a résumé.

- **Paragraph four:** Close the letter with a request for an interview. Be sure you clearly state how the employer can contact you for additional information. Include a telephone number, e-mail address, and the times you will be available to respond to a telephone call. When including an e-mail address, it is very important that you create a professional e-mail account name that has your first name, last name, and no nicknames or slang. Yahoo! and Google offer free e-mail accounts. Finally, include a "thank you" to the potential employer for considering your application.

Figure 18–2 is a sample cover letter to serve as a guide to writing a good letter. However, remember this is only one guide. Letters must be varied to suit each circumstance.

RÉSUMÉ

A **résumé** is a record of information about an individual. It is a thorough yet concise summary of an individual's education, skills, accomplishments, and work experience. It is used to provide an employer with basic information that details your qualifications as an employee. At the same time, a good résumé will help you clarify your job objective and be better prepared for a job interview.

A résumé should be prepared on a computer using a word-processing program so that it can be easily changed or updated, and it should be attractive in appearance. Like a cover letter, a résumé creates an impression on the employer. Information should be presented in an organized fashion. At the same time, the résumé should be concise and pertinent. Good-quality paper that is white or light in color; correct spelling and punctuation; straight, even margins; and an attractive style are essential. It is also a good idea to prepare a digital copy of your résumé so it can be attached to an e-mail without changing its formatting or design.

Résumé format can vary. Review sample sources and find a style that you feel best presents your information. A one-page résumé is usually sufficient.

Parts of a résumé can also vary. Some of the most important parts that should be included are shown in **Figures 18–3A and 18–3B** and are described as follows:

- **Personal identification:** This includes your name, address, telephone number including area code, and e-mail address.

- **Employment objective, job desired, or career goal:** Briefly state the title of the position for which you are applying.

18 Hireme Lane
Job City, Ohio 44444
June 3, 20--

Mr. Prospective Employer
Director of Human Resources
Health Care Facility
12 Nursing Lane
Dental City, Ohio 44833

Dear Mr. Employer:

In response to your advertisement in the _____
on _____, 20 _____, I would like to apply for the position
of _____.

I recently graduated from _____. I majored in
_____ and feel I am well qualified for this position. I enjoy
working with people and have a sincere interest in additional training
in _____.

My résumé is enclosed. I have also enclosed a specific list of skills that I mastered
during my school experience. I feel that previous positions noted on the résumé
have provided me with a good basis for meeting your job requirements.

Thank you for considering my application. I would appreciate a personal interview
at your earliest convenience to discuss my qualifications. Please contact me at the
above address, via e-mail at iamjobhunting@yahoo.com, or by telephone at
589-1111 after 2:00 PM any day.

Sincerely,

Iamjob Hunting

FIGURE 18–2 A sample cover letter.

- **Educational background:** List the name and address of your high school. Be sure to include special courses or majors if they relate to the job position. If you have taken additional courses or special training, list them also. If you have completed college or technical school, this information should be placed first. If you have an A to B average in school, include this information. If your average is lower than a B, do *not* include this information.

- **Work or employment experience:** This includes previous positions of employment. Always start with the most recent position and work backward. Each entry should include the name and address of the employer, dates employed, your job title, and a brief description of duties. Avoid use of the word *I*. For example, instead of stating, "I sterilized supplies," state, "sterilized supplies," using action verbs to describe duties.

- **Skills:** List special knowledge, computer, technology, and work skills you have that can be used in the job you are seeking. The list of skills should be specific and indicate your qualifications and ability

Florence Nurse
22 South Main Street
Nursing, Ohio 33303
(400) 589-1111
florence.nurse@gmail.com

Employment Objective: Nursing Assistant Position

Skills

Recording Vital Signs	Making Beds
Moving and Transferring Patients	Observing Infection Control
Administering CPR and First Aid	Providing Personal Hygiene
Understanding Medical Terminology	Collecting Specimens
Applying Heat or Cold Applications	Ambulating Patients

Education

Career High School	Graduation: June 5, 2021
5 Diamond Street	Major: Health Science Careers
Nursing, Ohio 33303	Grade Average: As and Bs

Certification: State Approved Nurse Assistant

Work Experience

Summer 2020 to Present	Country King Fried Chicken 5 Southern Lane Mansfield, Ohio 33302
Fast Food Worker	Operate register Record orders Promote customer relations
Summer of 2019 and 2020	Madison Ram Hospital 602 Esley Lane Mansfield, Ohio 33301
Volunteer Worker	Deliver mail and flowers Assist nurses with patients

Extracurricular Activities

School Marching Band	Member for 3 years
HOSA	Class treasurer for 2 years
Red Cross Club	Member for 3 years
Red Cross Blood Mobile	Volunteer worker for 3 years
March of Dimes Walkathon	Walker for 5 years
Church Youth Group	Member for 7 years

FIGURE 18–3A A sample résumé with information centered.

to perform the job duties. When work experience is limited, a list of skills is important to show an employer that you are qualified for the position.

- **Other activities:** These can include organizations of which you are a member, offices held, community service, special awards received, volunteer work, hobbies, special interests, and other similar facts. Keep this information brief, but do not hesitate to include facts that indicate school, church, and community involvement. This section can show an employer that you are a well-rounded person who participates in activities, assumes leadership roles, strives to achieve, and practices good citizenship. Write out the full names of organizations rather than the identifying letters.

- **Credentials:** If you have obtained any kind of credential, please note them. Examples include certified nursing assistant, licensed vocational nurse, pharmacy technician, certified dental assistant, and CPR certification.

THOMAS J. TOOTH

340 DENTAL LANE   **FLOSS, OHIO 44598**   **(524) 333-2435**   **TJTooth@yahoo.com**

CAREER GOAL: POSITION AS A DENTAL ASSISTANT IN GENERAL PRACTICE WITH A GOAL OF BECOMING A CERTIFIED DENTAL ASSISTANT

EDUCATION: OHIO TECHNICAL SCHOOL, OPPORTUNITY, OHIO 44597
GRADUATED IN JUNE 2021
MAJORED IN DENTAL ASSISTANT PROGRAM FOR TWO YEARS

SKILLS: IDENTIFICATION OF TEETH, CHARTING CONDITIONS OF THE TEETH, MIXING DENTAL CEMENTS AND BASES, POURING MODELS AND CUSTOM TRAYS, PREPARING ANESTHETIC SYRINGE, SETTING UP BASIC DENTAL TRAYS, STERILIZING OF INSTRUMENTS, DEVELOPING AND MOUNTING RADIOGRAPHS, TYPING BUSINESS LETTERS, COMPLETING INSURANCE FORMS

WORK EXPERIENCE: DENTAL LAB PRODUCTS, 55 MODEL STREET, FLOSS, OHIO 44598
EMPLOYED SEPTEMBER 2020 TO PRESENT AS DENTAL LAB ASSISTANT
PROFICIENT IN MODELS, CUSTOM TRAYS, PROSTHETIC DEVICES

DRUGGIST STORES, 890 PHARMACY LANE, OPPORTUNITY, OHIO 44597
EMPLOYED JUNE 2019 TO AUGUST 2020 AS SALESPERSON
EXPERIENCE IN CUSTOMER RELATIONS, INVENTORY, REGISTER, AND SALES PROMOTION

ACTIVITIES: HOSA TREASURER, FIRST PLACE STATE AWARD IN HOSA DENTAL ASSISTANT CONTEST, VOLUNTEER WORKER DURING DENTAL HEALTH WEEK, MEMBER OF SCHOOL PEP CLUB, HOBBIES INCLUDE FOOTBALL, SWIMMING, BASKETBALL, AND READING, VOLUNTEER FOR MEALS-ON-WHEELS

PERSONAL TRAITS: DEPENDABLE, CONSIDERATE OF OTHERS, WILLING TO LEARN, ADAPTABLE TO NEW SITUATIONS, RESPECTFUL AND HONEST, ADEPT AT DENTAL TERMINOLOGY, ABLE TO PERFORM A VARIETY OF DENTAL SKILLS

FIGURE 18–3B A sample résumé with left margin highlights.

- **References:** Most sources recommend not including references on a résumé. Even the statement "references will be furnished on request" is now usually omitted. However, at least three references should be printed on a separate sheet of paper. The paper should be the same paper used for the résumé and include the same heading showing your name, address, telephone number, and e-mail address. The reference sheet can be given to an employer during the job interview. For a high school student with limited experience, references can provide valuable additional information. Always be sure you have an individual's permission before using that person as a reference. List the full name, title, address, telephone number, and e-mail address of the reference. It is best not to use relatives or high school friends as references. Select professionals in your field, clergy, teachers, work supervisors, or other individuals with responsible positions.

Honesty is always the best policy, and this is particularly true regarding résumés. Never give information that you think will look good but is exaggerated or only partly true. Inaccurate or false information can cost you a job.

Before preparing your résumé, it is important to list all of the information you wish to include. Then, select the format that best presents this information. The two sample résumés shown in **Figures 18–3A** and **18–3B** are meant to serve as guidelines only. Do not hesitate to evaluate other formats and present your information in the best possible way.

The envelope should be the correct size for your letter of introduction and résumé. Do *not* fold the letter into small sections and put it in an undersized envelope. This creates a sloppy impression. When possible, it is best to buy standard business envelopes that match your paper. A 9 × 12 envelope eliminates the need to fold the cover letter and résumé and helps create a more professional appearance. Be sure the envelope is addressed correctly and neatly. It should also be computer printed. If you respond online, upload your cover letter first and then your résumé so the employer will open your information in the correct order.

CAREER PASSPORT OR PORTFOLIO

A *career passport* or *portfolio* is a professional way to highlight your knowledge, abilities, and skills as you prepare for employment or extended education. It allows you to present yourself in an organized and efficient manner when you interview for schools or employment. Final content will vary for each individual, but most career passports or portfolios will contain the following types of information:

- **Introductory letter**: a brief synopsis of yourself including your background, education, and future goals

- **Résumé**: an organized record of information on education, employment experience, special skills, and activities

- **Skill list and competency level**: a list of skills you have mastered and the level of competency for each skill; some health science programs provide summaries of competency evaluations that can be used; if your program does not provide this, a list of skills and final competency grades can be compiled by using the evaluation sheets in the *Simmers DHO Health Science Workbook*

- **Letter(s) of recommendation**: letters of recommendation from your instructors, guidance counselors, supervisors at clinical areas or agencies where you perform volunteer work, respected members of the community, advisors of activities in which you participate, and presidents of organizations of which you are a member

- **Copies of work-based learning evaluations and documentation of hours**: copies of evaluations you receive at work-based learning sites, such as externships and internships, practicum shadowing clinical sites, volunteer activities, and/or paid work experiences; create a spreadsheet that tracks the hours at each paid or unpaid work-based learning or clinical shadowing site.

- **Credentials**: copies of a school transcript or a recent grade card and copies of any health care related certificates, such as CPR certification, first aid certification, OSHA safety certification, or certificates of completion for the National Health Science test offered by the National Consortium for Health Science Education (NCHSE)

- **Service projects**: documentation of service learning or community service and any associated credentials or recognition you may have been awarded for that effort; examples of service learning may be anything from organizing a food drive for dogs at the Humane Society to organizing the Tuesday evening activity at your local long-term care facility for a year. Record the progress of your project by taking pictures and documenting the hours of planning and implementation. Make sure to ask for letters of recommendation from the people you are working with.

- **Documentation of mastering job-keeping skills**: documentation—written in brief paragraphs—of how you have mastered job-keeping skills; the Partnership for 21st Century Skills is a national organization that has developed a framework that describes the skills, knowledge, and expertise students must master in order to succeed in work and life. This framework is based on the following:

    Core subjects and 21st century themes: The core subjects essential to student success include: English, language arts, world languages, arts, math, economics, science, geography, history, government, and civics. The 21st century themes that must be woven into academic content are global awareness; financial, economic, business, and entrepreneurial literacy; civic literacy; health literacy; and environmental literacy.

    Learning and innovation skills: These are the skills that separate students who are ready for the complexity of life and work in the 21st century from those who are not, and they include: creativity and innovation, critical thinking and problem solving, and communication and collaboration.

Information, media, and technology skills: In an increasingly technology-driven environment, these skills are critical to success and they include: information technology, media literacy, and information and communication technology literacy.

Life and career skills: Succeeding in the 21st century requires more than thinking skills and content knowledge, it is also essential to develop life and career skills that include: flexibility and adaptability, initiative and self-direction, social and cross-cultural skills, productivity and accountability, and leadership and responsibility.

Write brief paragraphs to document how you have mastered each of these skills and place them in your portfolio.

- **Leadership and organization abilities**: information that demonstrates leadership and organization abilities you have mastered; oral presentations (for example, conducting meetings or facilitating small group discussions) should be documented by written minutes or a short video. Participation in HOSA or SkillsUSA should be included.

NOTE: *If you are a member of a student organization for health science, such as HOSA or SkillsUSA, please check their websites for specific portfolio requirements.*

Organize the above information in a neat binder, portfolio, or computer file. Use tab dividers or electronic folders to separate it into organized sections. Make sure that you use correct grammar and punctuation on all written information. The effort you put into creating a professional portfolio or passport will be beneficial when you have this document ready to present during a school or job interview. It is also a good idea to keep an electronic version of your portfolio for easy updates, so you have a back-up of all the information in case anything happens to your portfolio, or in case an employer asks you to send your résumé and portfolio for them to review before your interview.

checkpoint

1. How many paragraphs should be included in a cover letter or letter of introduction?

PRACTICE: Go to the workbook and complete the assignment sheet for 18:2, Writing a Cover Letter and Preparing a Résumé. Then return and continue with the procedure.

Procedure 18:2

Writing a Cover Letter and Preparing a Résumé

Equipment and Supplies

Good-quality paper, inventory sheet for résumés (see workbook), computer with word-processing software, and a printer

Procedure

1. Assemble equipment.

2. Re-read the preceding information section on writing a cover letter or letter of introduction and résumé. Read the section on *Composing Business Letters* in Section 24:5 in this text.

3. Review the sample cover letter and résumés.

4. Go to the workbook and complete the inventory sheet for résumés. Check dates for accuracy. Be sure that names are spelled correctly. Use the telephone book or the internet to check addresses and zip codes.

5. Carefully evaluate all your information. Determine the best method of presenting your information. Try different ways of writing your material. Do not hesitate to show several different versions to your instructor or others and get their opinions on which way seems most effective.

6. Create a rough draft of a cover letter or letter of introduction. Follow the correct form for letters as shown in Section 24:5 in this text. Use correct spacing and margins. Check for correct spelling and punctuation.

7. Create a final cover letter. Be sure it contains the required information. Proofread the letter for spelling errors and other mistakes. If possible, ask someone else to proofread your letter and evaluate it.

8. Create a rough draft of your résumé. Format the information in an attractive manner. Be sure that spacing is standard throughout the résumé and margins are even on all sides.

9. Review your sample résumé. Reword any information, if necessary. Be sure all information is pertinent and concise. Ask your instructor or others for opinions regarding suggested changes.

10. Create your final résumé. Take care to avoid errors. Use the spell-check function of your word-processing program to check for misspelled words. Proofread the final copy, checking carefully for errors. If possible, ask someone else to proofread your résumé and evaluate it.

11. Replace all equipment.

PRACTICE: Go to the workbook and use the evaluation sheet for 18:2, Writing a Cover Letter and Preparing a Résumé, to practice this procedure. When you believe you have mastered this skill, sign the sheet and give it to your instructor for further action.

Give your instructor your cover letter and résumé along with the evaluation sheet.

 FINAL EVALUATION: Using the criteria listed on the evaluation sheet, your instructor will grade your cover letter and résumé.

Check

18:3 COMPLETING JOB APPLICATION FORMS

Even though you provide each potential employer with a résumé, most employers still require you to complete an application form. **Application forms** are used by employers to collect specific information. Forms vary from employer to employer, but most request similar information.

Before completing any application form, it is essential that you first read the entire form. Note areas where certain information is to be placed. Read instructions that state how the form is to be completed. Some forms request that the applicant complete the application in handwritten form, but most now provide the application in a computerized format to be completed on a computer and either printed out or submitted electronically by e-mail.

Some employers will send you the application form before your interview so you have time to fill it out and print it or submit it electronically (unless they require you to do it in handwritten form). If they do not send it to you in advance, make sure you have all the required information with you when you go for a job interview.

 Basic rules for completing a job application form include:

Comm

- Fill out each item neatly and completely.

- Do *not* leave any areas blank. Put "none" or "NA" (meaning "not applicable") when the item requested does not apply to you.

- Be sure addresses include zip codes and all other required information.

- Watch spelling and punctuation. Use spell-check when completing an application on a computer. Errors will not impress the potential employer.

- Complete the form in the manner requested (on a computer or handwritten).

- Use a black pen if handwritten.

- If the application is not available electronically, scan the application into a computer word program, key

in all information, check for accuracy, and then print the completed application form. Use spell-check. This method allows for easy correction of errors.

- Make sure all information is legible.

- Do *not* write in spaces that state "office use only" or "do not write below this line." Employers often judge how well you follow directions by your reaction to these sections.

- Be sure all information is correct and truthful. Remember, material can be checked and verified. A simple half-truth can cost you a job.

- Proofread your completed application. Check for completeness, spelling, proper answers to questions, and any errors.

- If references are requested, be sure to include all information, such as title, address, telephone number, and e-mail address. Before using anyone's name as a reference, it is best to obtain that person's permission. Be prepared to provide reference information when you go for a job interview. Most sources suggest listing at least three references on a separate sheet of the same type of paper used for the résumé.

Even though questions vary on different forms, some basic information is usually requested on all of them. In order to be sure you have this information, it is useful to take a "wallet card" with you. A sample card is included in the workbook (as 18:3 Assignment #2). You could also save all this information on your mobile device so you have easy access to it while filling out an application.

Remember that employers use application forms as a screening method. To avoid being eliminated from consideration for a position of employment, be sure your application creates a favorable impression.

check**point**

1. If you fill out an application on paper, what color ink should you use?

2. How many references should you have?

PRACTICE: Go to the workbook and complete the assignment sheets for 18:3, Completing Job Application Forms. Then return and continue with the procedure.

Completing Job Application Forms

Equipment and Supplies

Computer with word-processing software and scanner or pen, wallet card (sample in workbook) or mobile device with wallet card information saved on it, sample application forms (sample in workbook)

Procedure

1. Assemble equipment. If a scanner is available, scan the application form into the word-processing program of a computer. The application form can then be completed with the computer and printed on a printer.

2. Complete all information on the wallet card. A sample is included in the workbook (Section 18:3 Assignment #2). Check dates and be sure information is accurate. List full addresses, zip codes, e-mail addresses, and names.

3. Review the preceding information section on completing job application forms. Read additional references, as needed.

4. Read the entire sample application form (Section 18:3 Assignment #3) in the workbook. Be sure you understand the information requested for each part. Read all directions completely.

5. If a scanner is not available, use a black ink pen to print all information. If a scanner and computer are available, scan the application form into a word-processing program. After keying in all information, the completed application can be printed.

6. Complete all areas of the form. Use "none" or "NA" as a reply to items that do not apply to you.

7. Take care not to write in spaces labeled "office use only" or "do not write below this line." Leave these areas blank.

8. In the space labeled "signature," sign your name. Note any statement that may be printed by the signature line. Be sure you are aware of what you are signing and the permission you may be giving. Most employers request permission to contact previous employers and/or references, and a verification that the information is accurate.

9. Recheck the entire application. Be sure information is correct and complete. Note and correct any spelling errors. Be sure you have answered all of the questions.

10. Replace all equipment.

PRACTICE: Go to the workbook and use the evaluation sheet for 18:3, Completing Job Application Forms, to practice this procedure. Obtain sample job application forms from your instructor or other sources. When you believe you have mastered this skill, sign the sheet and give it to your instructor for further action. Give the instructor your printed application form along with the evaluation sheet.

Check

FINAL EVALUATION: Using the criteria listed on the evaluation sheet, your instructor will grade your job application form.

18:4 PARTICIPATING IN A JOB INTERVIEW

A job interview is what you are seeking when you send a cover letter or letter of introduction and a résumé. You must prepare for an interview just as hard as you did when composing your résumé. A poor interview can mean a lost job.

A **job interview** is usually the last step before getting or being denied a particular position of employment. Usually, you have been screened by the potential employer and have been selected for an interview as a result of your résumé and application form. Keep in mind that most employers now also check an applicant's social media accounts, such as Facebook, Instagram, Snapchat, and Twitter, in the prescreening process, so it is very important to make sure your social media accounts reflect a professional image. A potential employer will not be impressed by pictures of you drinking, smoking, or acting inappropriately. Make sure you clean up your social media accounts before applying for a job. To the employer, the interview serves at least two main purposes:

- Provides the opportunity to evaluate you in person, obtain additional information, and ascertain whether you meet the job qualifications

- Allows the employer to tell you about the position in more detail

Careful preparation is needed before going to an interview. Be sure you have all required information. Your "wallet card," résumé, and completed application form (if it was given to you in advance) must be ready. If you have completed a career passport or portfolio, be sure to take it to the interview. If possible, find out about the position and the agency offering the job. In this way, you will be more aware of the agency's needs.

Be sure of the scheduled date and time of the interview. Know the name of the individual you must contact and the exact place of the interview. Write this information down and take it with you, or save it on your mobile device for easy access.

Dress carefully. It is best to dress conservatively. Business suits or coats, or a dress shirt and slacks, and ties are still best for men. Business suits, dresses, skirts, or dress pants are best for women. Even though it shouldn't be the case, first impressions can affect the employer. All clothes should fit well and be clean and pressed, if needed. Avoid bright, flashy colors and very faddish styles.

Check your entire appearance. Hair should be clean and neatly styled. Nails should be clean. Women should avoid wearing bright nail polish, too much makeup, and perfume. Men should be clean shaven or have well-maintained facial hair. Be sure that your teeth are clean and your breath is fresh. Jewelry should not be excessive. And last but not least, use a good antiperspirant. When you are nervous, you may perspire.

It is best to arrive 5–10 minutes early for your interview. Late arrival could mean a lost job. Allow for traffic, trains blocking the road, and other complications that might interfere with your arriving on time. Do not bring any friends or relatives to the interview with you. Before your interview starts, turn off all mobile devices.

During the interview, observe all of the following points:

- Greet the interviewer by name when you are introduced. Introduce yourself and smile.

- Remain standing until the interviewer asks you to sit. Be aware of your posture and sit straight. Keep both feet flat on the floor or cross your legs at the ankles only.

- Use correct grammar. Avoid using slang words.

- Speak slowly and clearly. Do not mumble.

- Be polite. Practice good manners.

- **Comm** Maintain eye contact (**Figure 18–4**). Avoid looking at the floor, ceiling, or away from the interviewer. Looking at the middle of the interviewer's forehead or at the tip of the interviewer's nose can sometimes help when you are nervous and experiencing difficulty with direct eye contact.

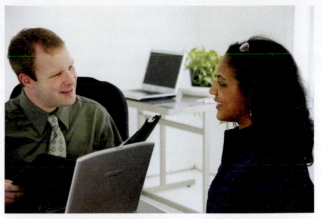

FIGURE 18–4 Sit straight and maintain eye contact during the interview. © Rob Marmion/www.Shutterstock.com.

- Listen closely to the interviewer. Do not interrupt in the middle of a sentence. Allow the interviewer to take the lead.

- Answer all questions thoroughly, but do not go into long, drawn-out explanations. Make sure your answers show how you are qualified for the job.

- Do *not* smoke, chew gum, or eat candy during the interview.

- Smile but avoid excessive laughter or giggling.

- Be yourself. Do not try to assume a different personality or different mannerisms; doing so will only increase your nervousness.

- Be enthusiastic. Display your positive attitude.

- Avoid awkward habits, such as swinging your legs, jingling change in your pocket, waving your hands or arms, or patting at your hair.

- Never discuss personal problems, finances, or other situations in an effort to get the job. This usually has a negative effect on the interviewer.

- Do not criticize former employers or degrade them in any way.

- Answer all questions truthfully to the best of your ability.

- Think before you respond. Try to organize the information you present.

- Be proud of yourself, to a degree. You have skills and are trained. Make sure the interviewer is aware of this. However, be sure to show a willingness to learn and to gain additional knowledge.

- Do not immediately question the employer about salary, fringe benefits, insurance, and other similar items. This information is usually mentioned before the end of the interview. If the employer asks whether you have any questions have one prepared. Ask about the job description or responsibilities, type of uniform required, potential for career growth, continuing education or in-service programs, and job orientation. These types of questions indicate a sincere interest in the job rather than a "What's in it for me?" attitude.

- Do not expect a definite answer at the end of the interview. The interviewer will usually tell you that they will contact you.

- Thank the interviewer for the interview as you leave. Smile, be polite, and exit with confidence.

- Never try to extend the interview if the interviewer indicates that they are ready to end it.

After the interview, it is best to send a follow-up note, letter, or e-mail to thank the employer for the interview. You may indicate that you are still interested in the position. You may also state that you are available for further questioning. When an employer is evaluating several applicants, a thank-you note is sometimes the deciding factor in who gets the job.

 Because you may be asked many different questions during an interview, it is impossible to prepare all answers ahead of time. However, it is wise to think about some potential questions and your responses to them. The following is a suggested list of questions to review. Additional questions may be found in any book on job interviews.

- **Tell me a little about yourself**. (Note: Stick to job-related information.)

- **What are your strong points/weak points?** (Note: Be sure to turn a weakness into a positive point. For example, say, "One of my weaknesses is poor spelling, but I use a dictionary or spell-check to check spelling and try to learn to spell 10 new words each week.")

- **Why do you feel you are qualified for this position?**

- **What jobs have you held in the past? Why did you leave those jobs?** (Note: Avoid criticizing former employers.)

- **What school activities are you involved in?**

- **What kind of work interests you?**

- **Why do you want to work here?**

- **What skills do you have that would be of value?**

- **What is your attitude toward work?**

- **What do you want to know about this job opening?**

- **What were your favorite subjects in school and why?**

- **What does success mean to you?**

- **How do you manage your time?**

- **What is your image of the ideal job?**

- **How skilled are you with computers?**

- **What are the three most important things to you in a job?**

- **Do you prefer to work alone or with others? Why?**

- **How many days of school did you miss last year?**

- **What do you do in your spare time?**

- **Do you have any plans for further education?**

 Any questions that may reflect discrimination or bias do *not* have to be answered during a job interview. Federal law prohibits discrimination with regard to age, cultural or ethnic background, marital status, parenthood, disability, religion, race, and gender. Employers are aware that it is illegal to ask questions of this nature, and the large majority will not ask such questions. If an employer does ask a question of this nature, however, you have the right to refuse to answer. An example of this type of question might be, "I see you married recently. Do you plan to start having children in the next year or two?" Be polite but firm in your refusal. A statement such as "I prefer not to answer that question" or "Can I ask you how this would affect the job we are discussing?" is usually sufficient.

 At the end of the interview, you may be asked to provide proof of your eligibility to work. Under the Bureau of Immigration Reform Act of 1986, employers are now required by federal law to ask you to complete an Employment Eligibility Verification Form I-9. This form helps the employer verify that you are legally entitled to work in the United States. To complete this form, you must provide documents that indicate your identity. A birth certificate, passport, and/or immigration card can be used for this purpose. You must also have a photo identification, such as a driver's license, and a social security card. The employer must make copies of these documents and include them in your file. Having these forms readily available shows that you are prepared for a job.

checkpoint

1. What are two (2) documents that employers may ask for to confirm your eligibility to work?

2. How early should you arrive for an interview?

PRACTICE: Go to the workbook and complete the assignment sheet for 18:4, Participating in a Job Interview. Then return and continue with the procedure.

Participating in a Job Interview

Equipment and Supplies

Desk, two chairs, evaluation sheets, lists of questions

Procedure

1. Assemble equipment. Role-play a mock interview with four people. Arrange for two people to evaluate the interview, one person to be the interviewer, and you to be the interviewee.

2. Position the two evaluators in such a way that they can observe both the interviewer and the interviewee. Make sure they will not interfere with the interview.

3. The interviewer should be seated at the desk and have a list of possible questions to ask during the interview.

4. Play the role of the interviewee. Prepare for this role by doing the following:

   a. Be sure you have all necessary information. Prepare your wallet card or save your wallet card information in your mobile device, résumé, job application form, and/or career passport or portfolio.

   b. Dress appropriately for the interview (as outlined in the preceding information section).

   c. Arrive at least 5–10 minutes early for the interview.

   d. Turn off all your mobile devices.

5. When you are called for the interview, introduce yourself. Be sure to refer to the interviewer by name.

6. Sit in the chair indicated. Be aware of your posture, making sure to sit straight. Keep your feet flat on the floor or cross your legs at the ankles only.

7. Listen closely to the interviewer. Answer all questions thoroughly and completely. Think before you speak. Organize your information.

8. Maintain eye contact. Avoid distracting mannerisms.

9. Use correct grammar. Avoid slang expressions. Speak in complete sentences. Practice good manners.

10. When you are asked whether you have any questions, ask questions pertaining to the job responsibilities. Avoid a series of questions on salary, fringe benefits, vacation, time off, and so forth.

11. At the end of the interview, thank the interviewer for their time.

12. Check your performance by looking at the evaluation sheets completed by the two evaluators. Study suggested changes.

13. Replace all equipment.

PRACTICE: Go to the workbook and use the evaluation sheet for 18:4, Participating in a Job Interview, to practice this procedure. When you believe you have mastered this skill, sign the sheet and give it to your instructor for further action.

 FINAL EVALUATION: Using the criteria listed on the evaluation sheet, your instructor will grade your performance.

Check

18:5 DETERMINING NET INCOME

Math

Obtaining a job means, in part, that you will be earning your own money. This often means that you will be responsible for your own living expenses. To avoid debt and financial crisis, it is important that you learn about managing your money effectively, including understanding how to determine net income.

The term **income** usually means money that you earn or that is available to you. However, the amount you actually earn and the amount you receive to spend may vary. The following two terms explain the difference.

- **Gross income**: This is the total amount of money you earn for hours worked. It is the amount determined before any deductions have been taken out of your pay.

- **Net income**: This is commonly referred to as "take-home pay." It is the amount of money available to you after all payroll **deductions** have been taken out of your salary. Some common deductions are the Federal Insurance Contributions Act (FICA) that includes the Social Security tax and the Medicare tax, federal and state taxes, and city taxes. Other deductions may include payroll deductions such as those for a company-sponsored 401K savings plan, medical or life insurance, union dues, and other similar items.

To determine gross income, simply multiply your wage per hour times the number of hours worked. For example, if you earn $14.00 per hour and work a 40-hour week, 14 × 40 = $560.00. In this example, then, $560.00 would be your gross income.

To determine net income, you must first determine the amounts of the various deductions that will be taken out of your gross pay. Deduction percentages usually vary depending on your income level. You can usually determine approximate deduction percentages and, therefore, your approximate net income by referring to tax charts. Tax charts for federal taxes are available on the Internet at *www.irs.gov*. Tax charts for cities and states can usually be found on the treasurer's Internet site for the particular city or state. Never hesitate to ask your employer about deduction percentages. It is your responsibility to check your own paycheck for accuracy. Starting with the example of gross pay of $560.00, the following shows how net pay may be determined.

| Gross Pay | $560.00 |

- Deduction for federal tax in this income range is usually approximately 15 percent. Check tax tables for accuracy.

  15%, or 0.15, × 560 = $84.00   560.00
  $\underline{-84.00}$
  476.00

- Deduction for state tax is approximately 2 percent.

  2%, or 0.02, × 560 = $11.20   476.00
  $\underline{-11.20}$
  464.80

- Deduction for city tax is approximately 1 percent.

  1%, or 0.01, × 560 = $5.60   464.80
  $\underline{-5.60}$
  459.20

- Deduction for FICA includes 6.2 percent of the first $137,700 in income for the Social Security tax and a Medicare tax deduction of 1.45 percent of the total in income, for a total deduction of 7.65 percent.

  7.65%, or 0.0765, × 560 = $42.84   459.20
  $\underline{-42.84}$
  416.36

- Net income after taxes, then, would be $416.36. Therefore, before you even receive your paycheck, $143.64 will be deducted from it. Additional deductions for insurance, uniforms, union dues, savings plans, contributions to charity, and other items may also be taken out of your gross pay.

In order to manage your money effectively, it is essential that you be able to calculate your net income. Because this is the amount of money you will have to spend, it will to some extent determine your lifestyle.

checkpoint

| **1.** What is net income?

PRACTICE: Read and complete Procedure 18:5, Determining Net Income.

Procedure 18:5

Determining Net Income

Equipment and Supplies

Assignment sheet for 18:5, Determining Net Income; pen or pencil

Procedure

1. Assemble equipment. If a calculator is available, you may use it to complete this assignment.

2. Read the instructions on the assignment sheet in the workbook for 18:5, Determining Net Income. Use the assignment sheet with this procedure.

3. Determine your wage per hour by using your salary in a current job or an amount assigned by your instructor. Multiply this amount by the number of hours you work per week. This is your gross weekly pay.

4. If your instructor has federal tax tables, read the tax tables to determine the percentage, or amount of money, that will be withheld for federal tax. If tax tables are not available, look on the Internet at *www.irs.gov* or check with your employer to obtain this information.

   NOTE: The average withholding tax for an initial income bracket is usually approximately 15 percent. If you cannot find the exact amount or percentage, use this amount (0.15) for an approximate determination.

5. Multiply the percentage for federal tax by your gross weekly pay to determine the amount deducted for federal tax.

6. Determine the deduction for state tax by reading your state tax tables, checking the state treasurer's site on the Internet, or by consulting your employer.

   NOTE: An average state tax is 2 percent. If you cannot find the exact amount or percentage, use this amount (0.02) for an approximate determination.

7. Multiply the percentage for state tax by your gross weekly pay to determine the amount deducted for state tax.

8. Determine the deduction for any city or corporation tax by reading the city/corporation tax tables, checking the city/corporation treasurer's site on the Internet, or consulting your employer.

   NOTE: An average city/corporation tax is 1 percent. If you cannot find the exact amount or percentage, use this amount (0.01) for an approximate determination.

9. Multiply the percentage for city/corporation tax by your gross weekly pay to determine the amount deducted for city/corporation tax.

10. Check the current deduction for FICA, or Social Security tax and Medicare tax, by checking the Social Security website or asking your employer for this information. Determine the deduction for FICA by multiplying your gross weekly pay by this percentage.

NOTE: In 2020, the FICA rate was 6.2 percent of the first $137,700 in income for the Social Security tax and 1.45 percent of total income for the Medicare tax. Use this total of 7.65 percent, or 0.0765, if you cannot obtain another percentage.

11. List the amounts for any other deductions. Examples include insurance, 401K savings plans, charitable donations, union dues, and similar items.

12. Add the amounts determined for federal tax, state tax, city/corporation tax, FICA, and other deductions together.

13. Subtract the total amount for deductions from your gross weekly pay. The amount left is your net, or take-home, pay.

14. Recheck any figures, as needed.

15. Replace all equipment.

PRACTICE: Go to the workbook and use the evaluation sheet for 18:5, Determining Net Income. Practice determining net income according to the criteria listed on the evaluation sheet. When you believe you have mastered this skill, sign the sheet and give it to your instructor for further action.

Check
FINAL EVALUATION: Using the criteria listed on the evaluation sheet, your instructor will grade your performance.

18:6 CALCULATING A BUDGET

Math
In order to use your net income wisely, it is best to prepare a budget. A **budget** is an itemized list of living expenses. It must be realistic to be effective.

A budget usually consists of two main types of expenses: fixed expenses and variable expenses. **Fixed expenses** include items such as rent or house payments, utilities, food, car payments, student loan payments, and insurance payments. **Variable expenses** include items such as entertainment, clothing purchases, and donations.

The easiest way to prepare a budget is to simply list all anticipated expenses for a one-month period. Then determine your net monthly pay. Allow a fair percentage of the net monthly pay for each of the budget items listed.

Savings should be incorporated into every budget. If saving money is regarded as an obligation, it is easier to set aside money for this purpose. When an emergency occurs, money is then available to cover the unexpected expenditure.

Some payments are due once or twice a year. An example is insurance payments. To be realistic, a monthly amount should be budgeted for this purpose. To determine a monthly amount, divide the total yearly cost for the insurance by 12. Then budget this amount each month. In this way, when insurance payments are due, the money is available for payment, and one month's budget will not have to bear the full amount of the insurance payment.

Money Management International (MMI), a nonprofit consumer counseling organization, recommends that the following percentage ranges of total net income be used while preparing a realistic budget:

- **Housing:** 20–35 percent
- **Food:** 15–30 percent
- **Utilities:** 4–7 percent
- **Transportation (including car loan, insurance, gas, and maintenance):** 6–20 percent
- **Insurance (including health, life, and/or disability):** 4–6 percent
- **Health (including prescriptions, eye care, dental care):** 2–8 percent
- **Clothing:** 3–10 percent
- **Personal care (including soap, toothpaste, laundry detergent, cosmetics, etc.):** 2–4 percent
- **Miscellaneous (including travel, child care, entertainment, gifts, etc.):** 1–4 percent
- **Savings:** 5–9 percent

It is important to remember that these percentages and line items are just suggested guidelines. Each individual must determine their own needs and allocate monies accordingly. However, MMI does state that personal debt should not exceed 10–20 percent of net income. Financial difficulties usually occur when debt exceeds this limit.

It is important that budgeted expenses do not exceed net monthly income. It may sometimes be necessary to limit expenses that are not fixed. Entertainment, clothing purchases, and similar items are examples of expenses that can be limited.

The final step is to live by your budget and avoid any spending over the allotted amounts. This is one way to prevent financial problems and excessive debt. If your fixed expenses or net income increases, you will have to revise your budget. Remember, creating a budget leads to careful management of hard-earned money.

checkpoint

1. What percentage of income is recommended to be spent on housing? Clothing?

PRACTICE: Read Procedure 18:6, Calculating a Budget. Then go to the workbook and complete the corresponding assignment sheet.

Procedure 18:6 Math

Calculating a Budget

Equipment and Supplies

Workbook assignment sheet for 18:6, Calculating a Budget; pen or pencil

Procedure

1. Assemble equipment. If a calculator is available, you may use it to complete this procedure.
2. Go to the workbook and read the instructions on the assignment sheet for 18:6, Calculating a Budget.
3. Determine your fixed expenses for a one-month period. This includes amounts you must pay for rent, utilities, loans, credit card accounts, insurance, and similar items. List these expenses.
4. Determine your variable expenses for a one-month period. This includes amounts for clothing purchases, personal items, donations, entertainment, and similar items. List these expenses.
5. List any other items that must be included in your monthly budget. Be sure to list a reasonable amount for each item.
6. Determine a reasonable amount for savings. Many people prefer to set aside a certain percentage of their net monthly pay as savings.
7. Determine your net monthly pay. Double-check all figures for accuracy.
8. Add all of your monthly budget expenses together. The sum represents your total expenditures per month.
9. Compare your expense total to your net monthly income. If your expense total is higher than your net income, you will have to revise your budget and reduce any expenses that are not fixed. If your expense total is lower than your net income, you may increase the dollar amounts of your budget items. If the other figures in your budget are realistic, it may be wise to increase the dollar amount of savings.
10. When the expense total in your budget equals your monthly net income, you have a balanced budget. Live by this budget and avoid any expenditures not listed on the budget.
11. Replace all equipment.

PRACTICE: Go to the workbook and use the evaluation sheet for 18:6, Calculating a Budget, to practice this procedure. When you believe you have mastered this skill, sign the sheet and give it to your instructor for further action. Give your instructor a completed budget along with the evaluation sheet.

Check

FINAL EVALUATION: Using the criteria listed on the evaluation sheet, your instructor will grade your budget.

Today's Research   Tomorrow's Health Care

A Bravery Gene?

Anxiety and fear have been felt by every human being. However, some individuals are so anxious or fearful they are not able to function within society. For example, individuals with agoraphobia have an abnormal fear of being helpless in a situation from which they cannot escape, so they stay in an environment in which they feel secure. Many agoraphobic people never leave their homes; they avoid all public or open places. Scientists are not really certain how fear works in the brain, so conditions such as these are difficult to treat.

Many scientists are researching a genetic basis for fear. Some early research involved the Shumyatsky group at Rutgers University where they analyzed brain tissue to locate a gene in a tiny prune-shaped region of the brain called the *amygdala*, an area of the brain that is extremely active when animals or humans are afraid or anxious. This gene produces a protein called *stathmin*, which is highly concentrated in the amygdala but very hard to detect in other areas of the brain. Scientists removed this stathmin gene and bred a line of mice that were all missing this gene. Tests showed that this breed of mice was twice as willing to explore unknown territories as unaltered mice. In addition, if the mice were trained to expect a small electrical shock after being presented with a stimulus, such as a sound or sight, this group of mice did not seem as fearful when the sound or sight was given. Researchers theorized that stathmin helps form fearful memories in the amygdala of the brain, the area where unconscious fears seemed to be stored. If the production of stathmin could be halted or inhibited by medication, it is possible that fears would not be stored as unconscious memories. Recent research has shown that stathmin may also play a crucial role in epileptic seizures. Patients with temporal lobe epilepsy seizures frequently experience pain as an aura or warning that a seizure is going to occur. In addition, the Shumyatsky group is currently studying the role of other amygdala-enriched genes to determine their role in memory and learned fear.

Other researchers have identified two genes that may be associated with autism—glutamate receptor interacting protein 1 and 2, or GRIP1/2—that appear to be linked to problems with social interactions. Using mice genetically engineered to lack both normal and mutant GRIP1/2 proteins, the scientists noted that these mice interacted with other mice twice as much as mice with the GRIP1/2 proteins. Research continues on how these genes function to disrupt social interactions and create anxiety.

Several groups of researchers are studying a gene encoded as Lef1. It seems to function in the hypothalamus of the brain by disrupting the development of nerve cells that affect stress and anxiety. One group of researchers worked with brains of fish that were missing this gene and determined that more than 20 genes involved in mood disorders like depression and anxiety are affected by the loss of Lef1. The fish exhibited signs consistent with these disorders by being reluctant to explore the environment, remaining immobile at the bottom of the fish tank, and growing much slower than other fish. Although brain complexity varies greatly from fish to humans, the researchers have found that Lef1 appears to mediate anxiety in all species.

Statistics from the World Health Organization (WHO) show almost 300 million people worldwide suffer from anxiety disorders and depression. If researchers can identify genes or genetic defects that affect how fear is learned and experienced, it may lead to a future with more effective therapies and medications for conditions such as post-traumatic stress disorder, phobias, human anxiety disorders, depression, epilepsy, and autism.

How many ideas did you come up with that Jasmine could implement? Some things are readily available and some she will have to work toward.

Since she had interned for 10 months, what references might she call on?

■ CHAPTER 18 SUMMARY

- Even if an individual is proficient in many skills, it does not necessarily follow that the individual will obtain the "ideal" job. Just as it is important to learn the skills needed in your chosen health care career, it is important to learn the skills necessary to obtain a job.

- Job-keeping skills important to an employer include using correct grammar in both oral and written communications, reporting to work on time and when scheduled, being prepared to work, following correct policies and procedures, having a positive attitude, working well with others, taking responsibility for your actions, and being willing to learn.

- Without good job-keeping skills, no amount of knowledge will help you keep a job.

- It is important to prepare for an interview. Careful consideration should be given to dress and appearance. Answers should be prepared for common interview questions.

- Practice completing job application forms. A neat, correct, and thorough application form will also help you get a job.

- Everyone should be able to calculate gross and net income. In addition, everyone should be able to develop a budget based on needs and income. Having and following a budget makes it more likely that money earned will be spent wisely and minimizes the chance of debt.

■ REVIEW QUESTIONS

1. What is the main purpose of a cover letter or letter of introduction? When is it used?

2. List the main sections of a résumé and briefly describe the information that should be included in each section.

3. State six (6) basic principles that must be followed while completing a job application form.

4. You have obtained a job and will receive a wage of $15.20 per hour. Calculate the following:
   a. Gross pay for a 40-hour week
   b. Federal tax deduction of 15 percent
   c. State tax deduction of 3 percent
   d. City tax deduction of 0.5 percent
   e. FICA or Social Security and Medicare tax deduction of 7.65 percent
   f. Net pay after above deductibles

■ CRITICAL THINKING

1. Choose five (5) job-keeping skills that you believe you have mastered. Write a paragraph describing why you believe you have mastered these skills. Include examples. Set up your electronic Career Portfolio and include this document as part of your writing example.

2. Why is it important to be honest in composing your résumé?

3. Create answers for the following interview questions:
   a. Why do you believe you are qualified for this job?
   b. Why do you want to leave your current job?
   c. Tell me about two or three of your major accomplishments and why you feel they are important.

4. Calculate your monthly budget when you get a job as a Radiology Technician making $25.50 an hour, working a 40-hour week. List fixed and variable expenses. Do not exceed your net monthly income.

■ ACTIVITIES

1. Start your personal Career Portfolio by creating:
   a. Cover letter or letter of introduction
   b. Résumé

2. Get an application that your instructor has obtained from local health care facilities. Complete it meeting the standards of neatness and correctness.

3. With a partner, create a job interview scenario. Practice presenting this with the candidate completely prepared and then completely unprepared.

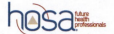 | CONNECTION

Competitive Event: Job Seeking Skills

Event Summary: Job Seeking Skills provides HOSA members with the opportunity to gain knowledge and skills required to apply for and obtain employment. This competitive event requires competitors to prepare a cover letter and résumé, and participate in a job interview with judge. This event aims to inspire members to learn more about applying for health-related positions.

Details on this competitive event can be found at

www.hosa.org/guidelines

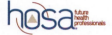 | CONNECTION

Leadership

Summary: The goal of the Academic Testing Center is to provide as many International Leadership Conference HOSA delegates as space permits with the opportunity to demonstrate their basic knowledge in preparation to become future health professionals.

The series of events in the Academic Testing Center are written tests based on items from the identified text specific to each event. Competitors will recognize, identify, define, interpret, and apply knowledge in a 50-item multiple choice test with a tie-breaker question. The written test will measure knowledge and understanding at the recall, application, and analysis levels. Higher-order thinking skills will be incorporated.

Details on this competitive event can be found at

www.hosa.org/guidelines

PART 2

SPECIAL HEALTH CARE SKILLS

> **LEGAL ALERT**
>
>
> Legal
>
> Before performing any procedures in this section, know and follow the standards and regulations established by the scope of practice; federal laws and agencies; state laws; state or national licensing, registration, or certification boards; professional organizations; and agency policies.
>
> *It is your responsibility to learn exactly what you are legally permitted to do and to perform only procedures for which you have been trained.*

Introduction

This part is divided into six major chapters. The topics are designed to provide you with the basic knowledge and skills required to perform a wide variety of procedures used in specific health care careers. Before you start a chapter, read the chapter objectives so you will know exactly what is expected of you. The objectives identify the competencies you should have mastered on completing the chapter.

For each procedure discussed in this part, you will find information and procedure sections in the textbook. In the workbook, you will find two types of sheets: assignment sheets and evaluation sheets. Following are brief explanations of these main components of the textbook and workbook.

1. *Information Sections (Textbook):* Each topic in the text begins with an information section to provide the basic knowledge you must have to perform the procedures. The sections explain why things are done, give necessary facts, and stress key points that should be observed. Each information section refers you to a specific assignment sheet in the workbook.

2. *Assignment Sheets (Workbook):* The assignment sheets provide a review of the main facts and related information about the procedures. After you have

read the information in the text, try to answer the questions on the assignment sheet. Then refer back to the text to see whether your answers are correct. Let your instructor grade your completed assignment sheet. Note and learn from any points that were incorrect. Be sure you understand all information before performing the procedure.

3. *Procedure Sections (Textbook):* The procedure sections provide step-by-step instructions on how to perform the procedures. Follow the steps while you practice the procedures. Each procedure lists the equipment and supplies you will need. Be sure you have all the necessary equipment and supplies before you begin.

   At times you will see one of three words within the procedure sections: *Note, Caution,* and *Checkpoint.* **NOTE** means to carefully read the comment following. These comments usually stress points of knowledge or explain why certain techniques are used. **CAUTION** means that a safety factor is involved and that you should proceed carefully while doing this step to avoid injury to yourself or the patient. **EVALUATION** means to ask your instructor to check you at this point in the procedure. Checkpoints are usually located at critical points in the procedures. Each procedure section in this part of the text refers you to a specific evaluation sheet in the workbook.

4. *Evaluation Sheets (Workbook):* Each evaluation sheet contains a list of the criteria on which you will be tested when you have demonstrated that you have mastered a particular procedure. Use these sheets as you practice the procedures. Make sure that your performance meets the established standards. When you believe you have mastered a particular procedure, sign the evaluation sheet and give it to your instructor. Your instructor will grade you by using the listed criteria and checking each step against your performance.

As was the case in Part 1, you will notice icons throughout this part of the textbook. The purpose of these icons is to accentuate particular factors or denote specific types of knowledge. The icons and their meanings are as follows:

 Observe Standard Precautions
Precaution

 Instructor's Check—Call Instructor at This Point
Check

 Safety—Proceed with Caution
Safety

 OBRA Requirement—Based on Federal Law for Nurse Assistant
OBRA

 Math Skill
Math

 Legal Responsibility
Legal

 Science Skill
Science

 Career Information
Career

 Communications Skill
Comm

 Technology
Technology

 Health Insurance Portability and Accountability Act
HIPAA

 Electronic Health Records
EHR

Case Study Investigation

Dr. Green is interviewing LaTonya for a dental assisting position in her clinic. What skills would she desire in a competent employee? What workplace experience might be beneficial? What personal characteristics would she expect LaTonya to have? What specific questions might Dr. Green ask? At the end of the chapter, you will be asked to compile a list of desirable traits, skills, and qualities for an ideal dental assisting candidate.

■ LEARNING OBJECTIVES

After completing this chapter, you should be able to:

- Name all the structures and tissues of a tooth.
- Identify deciduous and permanent teeth.
- Identify teeth by the Universal/National Numbering System and the FDI System.
- Identify surfaces of the teeth.
- Chart conditions of teeth.
- Operate and maintain dental equipment.
- Identify dental instruments and set up dental trays for oral examination, amalgam restoration, composite restoration, and surgical extraction.
- Position a patient in a dental chair.
- Demonstrate the Bass method of brushing.
- Demonstrate flossing technique.
- Prepare alginate and take an impression from dentures.
- Prepare polysulfide impression material and load a syringe.
- Pour plaster and stone models.
- Make a custom tray.
- Describe proper maintenance of anesthetic carpules and an aspirating syringe.
- Load an anesthetic aspirating syringe.
- Mix cements and bases for dental use.
- Mix composite for restorations.
- List the advantages of digital dental radiography.
- Define, pronounce, and spell all key terms.

KEY TERMS

air compressor

alginate *(ahl'-jih-nate")*

alveolar process *(al-vee'-o-lar)*

amalgam *(ah-mahl'-gam)*

anesthesia *(an-es-thee'-sha)*
   Note: th as in "thin"

anesthetic carpules (cartridges)

anterior

apex

apical foramen

aspirating syringes

assistant's carts

base

bicuspids

bite-wings

buccal *(buck'-kal)*

burs

carious lesions (caries) *(care'-ee"-us lee'-shunz)*

cavity

cement

cementum

cervix

composite *(kom-poz'-it)*

contra angle

crown

cuspids

custom trays

dental chair

dental lights

dentin

dentitions

distal

doctor's carts

enamel

Federation Dentaire International (FDI) System

gingiva *(jin'-jih"-vah)*

halitosis *(hal"-ih-toe'-sis)*

high-speed handpiece

high-velocity oral evacuator (HVE)

impression

incisal

incisors

labial *(lab'-ee"-ahl)*

line angles

liner

lingual *(lynn'-gwal)*

low-speed handpiece

mandibular

maxillary

mesial *(me'-ze-ahl)*

model

molars

occlusal *(oh-klew'-sal)*

occlusal films

odontology

oral-evacuation system

panoramic

pedodontic (child) films *(pee-doe-don'tick)*

periapical films *(per-ree-ape'ih-kal)*

periodontal ligament *(pear"-e-o-don'-till)*

periodontium

permanent (succedaneous) teeth *(suk'-se-dane"-ee-us)*

plaque *(plak')*

plaster

point angles

polysulfide

posterior

primary (deciduous) teeth *(de'-sid"-ju-wus)*

prophylaxis angle *(proh"-fill-ax'-sis an'-gull)*

pulp

quadrants

radiographs

radiolucent *(ray"-dee-oh-lew'-sent)*

radiopaque *(ray"-dee-oh-payk')*

restoration

rheostats *(ree"-oh-stats')*

root

saliva ejector

silicone

stone

temporary

tri-flow (air-water) syringe

Universal/National Numbering System

Dental assistants work under the supervision of doctors called dentists, and they are important members of the dental health care team. Educational requirements vary from state to state, but can include on-the-job training, one- or two-year health science education programs, and/or an associate's degree.

Legal Certification is available through the Dental Assisting National Board (DANB) after an individual has graduated from a Commission on Dental Accreditation (CODA)–accredited program of dental assisting or has met the requirements established in their state for completing a

- Presenting a professional appearance and attitude
- Obtaining knowledge regarding health care delivery systems, organizational structure, and teamwork
- Meeting all legal responsibilities
- Communicating effectively
- Being sensitive to and respecting cultural diversity
- Learning dental terminology
- Comprehending human anatomy, physiology, and pathophysiology with an emphasis on oral anatomy and physiology
- Observing all safety precautions
- Practicing all principles of infection control

specific number of hours of work experience in a period of two years of full-time or four years of part-time employment as a dental assistant. The duties of dental assistants vary depending on the size and type of practice, and on the dental practice laws of the state in which they work. Each state has a dental practice act that governs which duties dental assistants can perform under the scope of practice. It is the responsibility of the dental assistant to know and follow the state regulations. In addition to the knowledge and skills presented in this chapter, dental assistants must also learn and master skills such as:

- Taking and recording vital signs
- Administering first aid and cardio-pulmonary resuscitation
- Promoting good nutrition and a healthy lifestyle to maintain dental health
- Using computer and technology skills
- Performing administrative duties such as answering the telephone, scheduling appointments, preparing correspondence, completing insurance forms, maintaining accounts, recording dental histories, and maintaining patient records
- Ordering and maintaining supplies and materials

LEGAL ALERT

Legal Before performing any procedures in this chapter, know and follow the standards and regulations established by the scope of practice; federal laws and agencies; state laws; state or national licensing, registration, or certification boards; professional organizations; professional standards; and agency policies.

It is your responsibility to learn exactly what you are legally permitted to do and to perform only procedures for which you have been trained.

19:1 IDENTIFYING THE STRUCTURES AND TISSUES OF A TOOTH

Science An understanding of the basic structures and tissues of a tooth is essential for a dental assistant. **Odontology** is the study of the anatomy, growth, and diseases of the teeth. Teeth are accessory organs of the digestive tract that aid in the *mastication*, or

chewing, of food. Individuals have two **dentitions**, or sets, of teeth: a primary, or deciduous, dentition, and a permanent, or succedaneous, dentition (**Figure 19–1**). At birth, a newborn has approximately 44 teeth buds at various stages of development. When a child is approximately 6 months old, these teeth buds begin to erupt into the mouth to form the primary dentition. When a child is approximately 2–3 years old, all of the 20 primary teeth will have erupted. These teeth maintain proper spacing for the permanent, or succedaneous, teeth and are used for mastication and speech. Between the ages of 6 and 12 years, all of the primary teeth are lost and are replaced by the permanent dentition. These permanent teeth begin to erupt when a child is approximately 5–6 years old. They continue erupting and replacing primary teeth until the individual reaches approximately 17–20 years of age, when the third molars, or wisdom teeth, erupt. Most of the 32 teeth in the permanent dentition are in place by 12 years of age. A child 5–12 years old who has both primary and permanent teeth erupted in the mouth has a *mixed dentition*.

Every tooth in both the primary and permanent dentitions has four main sections, or divisions: the crown, the root, the cervix, and the apex (**Figure 19–2**):

- **Crown:** This is the section of the tooth that is visible in the mouth. It is protected on the outside by the tissue called *enamel*.

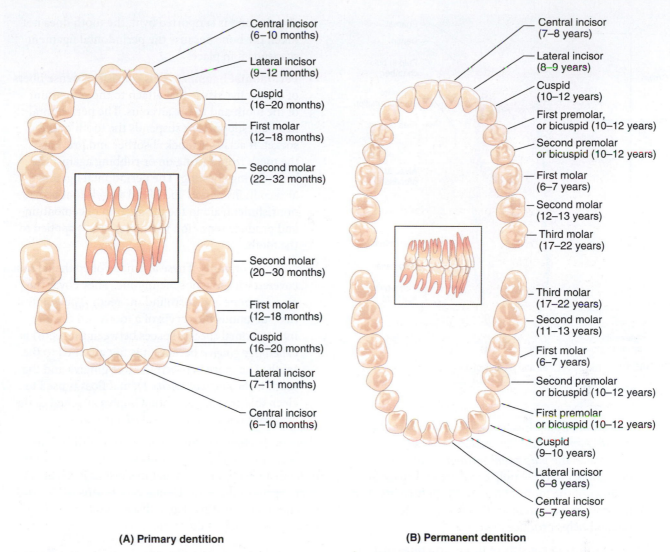

FIGURE 19–1 Eruption times of (A) primary (deciduous) and (B) permanent (succedaneous) teeth.

- **Root:** This is the section of the tooth below the gingiva, or gums. It is covered on the outside by the tissue called *cementum*. The root is normally not visible in the mouth; it helps anchor, or hold, the tooth in the bony socket of the jaw. A tooth may have a single root or multiple roots. If it has two roots, it is called *bifurcated*; if it has three roots, it is called *trifurcated*.

- **Cervix:** This is also called the *neck, cervical line,* or *cemento-enamel junction,* because it is the area where the enamel covering the crown meets the cementum covering the root. It is the narrow section where the crown joins with the root.

- **Apex:** This is the tip of the root of the tooth. It contains an opening called the **apical foramen,** through which nerves and blood vessels enter the tooth.

Each tooth is made of four main tissues: enamel, cementum, dentin, and pulp (refer to Figure 19–2):

- **Enamel:** This is the hardest tissue in the body and covers the outside of the crown. It is made up mainly

of calcium and phosphorus, and forms a protective layer for the tooth. Once a tooth is fully developed, the enamel cannot grow or repair itself.

- **Cementum:** This is the hard, bonelike tissue that covers the outside of the root. In addition to providing a thin layer of protection, it also helps hold the tooth in place. Cementum is formed throughout the life of the tooth.

- **Dentin:** This is the tissue that makes up the main bulk of the tooth. It lies under the enamel of the crown and under the cementum of the root. It is a bone-like substance that is softer than enamel but harder than cementum and bone. Although it has no nerves, it carries sensations of pain and temperature to the pulp. Dentin is a living tissue that is capable of limited repair and continued growth. The internal surface of dentin forms the wall of the pulp chamber.

- **Pulp:** This is the soft tissue located in the innermost area of the tooth. It is made up of blood vessels and nerves held in place by connective tissue.

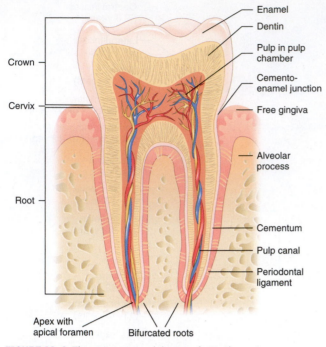

Enamel
Dentin
Pulp in pulp chamber
Cemento-enamel junction
Free gingiva
Crown
Cervix
Alveolar process
Root
Cementum
Pulp canal
Periodontal ligament
Apex with apical foramen
Bifurcated roots

FIGURE 19–2 The structures and tissues of a tooth.

The section of pulp located in the crown is called the *pulp chamber*, and the section located in the root is called the *pulp canal* (or *root canal*). The pulp chamber and the pulp canal create a space in the center of the tooth known as the *pulp cavity*. The pulp provides sensation and nourishment for the tooth and helps produce dentin.

The **periodontium** consists of those structures that surround and support the teeth, and includes the alveolar process, the periodontal ligament, and the gingiva:

- **Alveolar process** or ridge: This is the bone tissue of the maxilla (upper jawbone) and mandible (lower jawbone) that surrounds the roots of the teeth. It contains a series of sockets, or *alveoli*—one for each tooth. Although the root of the tooth sits in the alveolus and is supported by it, the tooth does not touch the bone because the periodontal ligament suspends it in place.

- **Periodontal ligament**: This consists of dense fibers of connective tissue that attach to the cementum of the tooth and to the alveolus. The periodontal ligament supports or suspends the tooth in the socket. It acts as a shock absorber and prevents the tooth from resting on or rubbing against the bone during chewing. The periodontal ligament also contains nerves and blood vessels that provide nourishment, aid in the production of cementum, and produce sensation when pressure is applied to the tooth.

- **Gingiva**, or gums: These are made of epithelial tissue covered with mucous membrane. They cover the alveolar bone and surround the teeth. The gingiva that surrounds the cervix of a tooth and fills the interproximal spaces (spaces between the teeth) is called *free gingiva* because it is not attached to the tooth. The space between the free gingiva and the tooth is the *gingival sulcus*. Dental floss is used to clean this area of the tooth. Gingiva attached to the alveolar bone is called *attached gingiva*.

The supporting structures and tissues of the teeth are meant to last a lifetime. However, disease can affect the teeth and supporting structures just as it can affect other organs of the body. Dental care is directed toward preventing and treating dental disease and preserving and prolonging the life of the teeth.

checkpoint

| **1.** What does odontology mean?

PRACTICE: Go to the workbook and complete the assignment sheet for 19:1, Identifying the Structures and Tissues of a Tooth. Then return and continue with the procedure.

Procedure 19:1

Identifying the Structures and Tissues of a Tooth

Equipment and Supplies

Anatomical model or chart of the structures and tissues of a tooth, paper, and pen or pencil

Procedure

1. Assemble equipment.

2. Wash hands.

3. Review Section 19:1, Identifying the Structures and Tissues of a Tooth, and then answer the following questions by writing the answers or discussing the information with a lab partner:

   a. Differentiate between primary (deciduous) and permanent (succedaneous) dentitions.

   b. State the ages when primary teeth begin to erupt in the mouth and when they finish erupting.

   c. What is the first primary tooth to erupt?

d. State the age when permanent teeth begin to erupt to replace the primary teeth.

e. What is the first permanent tooth to erupt?

f. What is the total number of primary teeth? Of permanent teeth?

g. What does the term *mixed dentition* mean? At what ages does it usually occur?

4. Use an anatomical model or chart of a tooth to identify and locate each of the following sections or divisions of a tooth:

a. crown

b. root

c. cervix

d. apex and apical foramen

5. Use an anatomical model or chart of a tooth to identify and describe the function of each of the following tissues of a tooth:

a. enamel

b. cementum

c. dentin

d. pulp

6. Use an anatomical model or chart of a tooth to identify and state the function of each of the following structures of the periodontium:

a. alveolar process

b. periodontal ligament

c. gingiva

7. Without looking at the model or chart, draw a tooth and label all of the divisions, tissues, and supporting structures. Then compare your drawing to the model or chart. Check it for accuracy and correct any errors.

NOTE: If you make any errors, return to Section 19:1 to review the material. Then correct your drawing.

8. Replace all equipment.

9. Wash hands.

PRACTICE: Go to the workbook and use the evaluation sheet for 19:1, Identifying the Structures and Tissues of a Tooth, to practice this procedure. When you believe you have mastered this skill, sign the sheet and give it to your instructor for further action.

 FINAL EVALUATION: Using the criteria listed on the evaluation sheet, your instructor will grade your performance.

Check

19:2 IDENTIFYING THE TEETH

Science

The four main types of teeth and their locations and characteristics are:

- **Incisors**
  Located in the front and center of the mouth
  Broad, sharp edge
  Used to cut or bite food
  Important for pronouncing *s*'s and *t*'s when speaking
  Central incisors are in the center
  Lateral incisors are on the sides of the centrals

- **Cuspids**
  Also called *canines*, or *eyeteeth*
  Located at angles of lips
  Used to tear food
  Longest teeth in the mouth

- **Bicuspids**
  Also called *premolars*
  Located before the molars, from front to back
  Not present in primary dentition
  Used to pulverize or grind food

- **Molars**
  Teeth in the back of the mouth
  Largest and strongest teeth
  Used to chew and grind food

Primary, or **deciduous**, **teeth**: This is the first set of teeth. Although they are also called "baby" teeth, this is an inappropriate term because it implies that the primary teeth have no permanent value and are unimportant. In reality, they serve the important function of maintaining correct spacing for permanent teeth. There are 20 primary teeth:

Ten maxillary (upper):
  Two central incisors
  Two lateral incisors
  Two cuspids (canines)
  Two 1st molars
  Two 2nd molars

Ten mandibular (lower):
  Two central incisors
  Two lateral incisors
  Two cuspids (canines)

Two 1st molars
Two 2nd molars

NOTE: *There are no bicuspids (premolars) in primary dentition.*

To name the primary teeth, the mouth is divided into **quadrants** or four sections: maxillary right, maxillary left, mandibular right, and mandibular left. A *transverse*, or horizontal, plane separates the mouth into an upper, or *maxillary*, and lower, or *mandibular*, arch or jaw. Each tooth is then labeled as either **maxillary** or **mandibular**. Teeth in the sockets, or alveoli, of the maxilla, or upper jawbone, are called *maxillary*. Teeth in the alveoli of the mandible, or lower jawbone, are called *mandibular*. A *midsagittal plane*, also called a *median* or *midline plane*, divides the mouth into a right and left half. Each tooth is then identified as *right* or *left*, depending on its location in the mouth. In **Figure 19–3A**, positions of the teeth are shown as though you were facing another person and looking into the mouth. This creates a mirror image and right and left are reversed.

NOTE: *Your left is the patient's right; your right is the patient's left.*

Each primary tooth has a specific name. For example, the central incisor in the maxillary right quadrant or arch is called the *maxillary right central incisor*. The central incisor in the maxillary left quadrant is called the *maxillary left central incisor*. The central incisor in the mandibular left quadrant is called the *mandibular left central incisor*. The central incisor in the mandibular right quadrant is called the *mandibular right central incisor*. The same pattern applies to all of the lateral incisors, cuspids, 1st molars, and 2nd molars.

Permanent, or **succedaneous**, **teeth**: This is the second set of teeth (**Figure 19–3B**). There are 32 permanent teeth:

Sixteen maxillary (upper):
Two central incisors
Two lateral incisors
Two cuspids (canines)
Two 1st bicuspids (premolars)

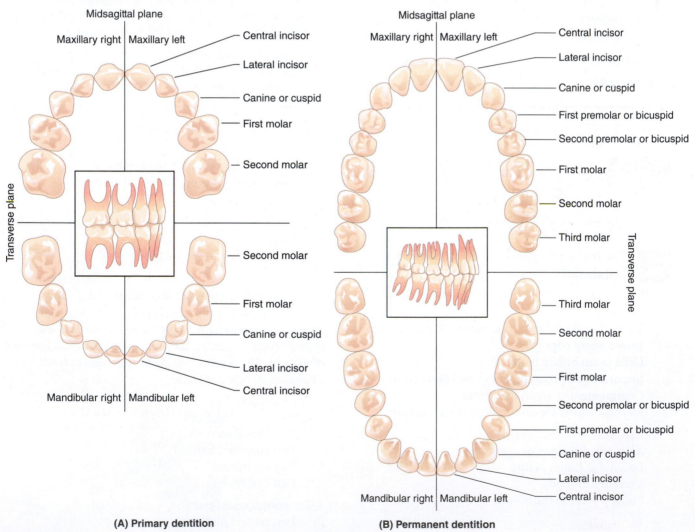

(A) Primary dentition

(B) Permanent dentition

FIGURE 19–3 (A) Primary (deciduous) teeth and (B) permanent (succedaneous) teeth.

Two 2nd bicuspids (premolars)
Two 1st molars
Two 2nd molars
Two 3rd molars (wisdom teeth)

Sixteen mandibular (lower):
Two central incisors
Two lateral incisors
Two cuspids (canines)
Two 1st bicuspids (premolars)
Two 2nd bicuspids (premolars)
Two 1st molars
Two 2nd molars
Two 3rd molars (wisdom teeth)

NOTE: *Each permanent tooth in Figure 19–3B has its own name, depending on the quadrant it is in. Each is labeled as* maxillary *or* mandibular *and* right *or* left, *following the same pattern used to name each primary tooth.*

checkpoint

1. What is the difference between deciduous and permanent teeth?

PRACTICE: Go to the workbook and complete the assignment sheet for 19:2, Identifying the Teeth. Then return and continue with the procedure.

Procedure 19:2

Identifying the Teeth

Equipment and Supplies

Model or unlabeled chart of primary or deciduous teeth, model or unlabeled chart of permanent or succedaneous teeth, paper, pen or pencil

Procedure

1. Assemble equipment.

2. Wash hands.

3. Use the model or unlabeled chart of primary (deciduous) teeth to practice the following:

   a. Point to all of the upper teeth and state the name *maxillary*. Write the word *maxillary* on paper. Check for correct spelling.

   b. Point to all of the lower teeth and state the name *mandibular*. Write the word *mandibular* on paper. Check for correct spelling.

   c. Imagine a line in the midsagittal (median or midline) plane that divides the mouth into right and left sides. Point to all the teeth on the right side of the mouth. Point to all the teeth on the left side of the mouth.

   NOTE: Remember, you are on the outside of the mouth looking in. Teeth on your right side are *left* teeth, and teeth on your left side are *right* teeth.

   d. Point to all four central incisors, lateral incisors, cuspids, 1st molars, and 2nd molars. State the names out loud.

   e. Name each tooth by its correct name. For example, say *maxillary right central incisor*, *maxillary right lateral incisor*, and continue until you have named all the teeth.

   f. Number your paper from 1 to 20. Write the names for all 20 primary teeth. Check the spelling of each name.

4. Use the model or unlabeled chart of the permanent (succedaneous) teeth to practice the following:

   a. Point to all the upper, or maxillary, teeth.

   b. Point to all the lower, or mandibular, teeth.

   c. Point to all the teeth on the right side of the mouth. Point to all the teeth on the left side of the mouth.

   d. Point to each of the central incisors, lateral incisors, cuspids, 1st bicuspids, 2nd bicuspids, 1st molars, 2nd molars, and 3rd molars.

   e. Name each tooth by its correct name. For example, state *maxillary right 3rd molar*, *maxillary right 2nd molar*, and continue until you have named all the teeth.

   f. Number your paper from 1 to 32. Write the names for all 32 permanent teeth. Check the spelling of each name.

5. Replace all equipment.

6. Wash hands.

PRACTICE: Go to the workbook and use the evaluation sheet for 19:2, Identifying the Teeth, to practice this procedure. When you believe you have mastered this skill, sign the sheet and give it to your instructor for further action.

 FINAL EVALUATION: Using the criteria listed on the evaluation sheet, your instructor will grade your performance.

19:3 IDENTIFYING TEETH USING THE UNIVERSAL/NATIONAL NUMBERING SYSTEM AND THE FEDERATION DENTAIRE INTERNATIONAL (FDI) SYSTEM

Several charting methods are used to identify the teeth. The most common method used in the United States is the Universal/National Numbering System. It was adopted by the American Dental Association in 1968 and is used on most dental insurance forms and dental charts.

The **Universal/National Numbering System** is an abbreviated form for identifying the teeth. Each tooth has a number or letter by which it is identified. It is much easier to call a permanent tooth *number 8* rather than to call it the *maxillary right central incisor*.

The Universal/National Numbering System for identifying primary, or deciduous, teeth is as follows:

- Teeth are identified by letters from *A* to *T*.
- Labeling takes place in a circular pattern.
- Starting at the maxillary right 2nd molar, which is *A*, and moving to the left side of the maxillary arch, each tooth is assigned a different letter. The maxillary left 2nd molar is *J*.
- Dropping down to the mandibular left 2nd molar, which is *K*, and moving from the left to the mandibular right teeth, continue lettering each mandibular tooth. The mandibular right 2nd molar is *T*.

- **Figure 19–4** demonstrates how primary or deciduous teeth are identified by the Universal/National Numbering System. Remember, this is a mirror image. The teeth on *your* right are the patient's left teeth, and teeth on *your* left are the patient's right teeth.

- In some areas, a lowercase *d* is used for primary or deciduous teeth. If this method is used, the maxillary right 2nd molar is *d-1*. Numbering continues across the maxillary arch until the maxillary left 2nd molar, which is *d-10*. Dropping down to the mandibular arch, the mandibular left 2nd molar is *d-11*. Numbering continues across the arch until the mandibular right 2nd molar, which is *d-20*.

The Universal/National Numbering System for identifying permanent, or succedaneous, teeth is as follows:

- Teeth are identified by numbers from 1 to 32.
- The mouth is encircled as each tooth is labeled.
- Starting at the maxillary right 3rd molar, which is *1*, and moving around the arch to the left side of the maxillary arch, each tooth is assigned a number. The maxillary left 3rd molar is number *16*.
- Dropping down to the mandibular left 3rd molar, which is number *17*, and moving from the left to the mandibular right teeth, continue numbering each tooth in the mandibular arch. The mandibular right 3rd molar is number *32*.
- Figure 19–4 demonstrates how permanent teeth are identified by the Universal/National Numbering System.

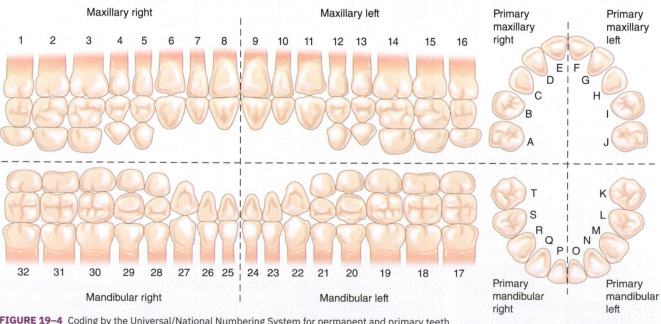

FIGURE 19–4 Coding by the Universal/National Numbering System for permanent and primary teeth.

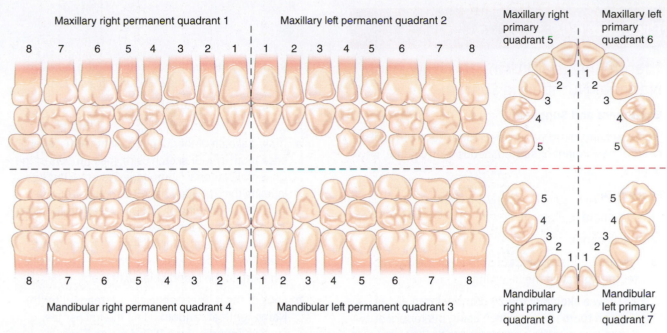

Maxillary right permanent quadrant 1 | Maxillary left permanent quadrant 2

Maxillary right primary quadrant 5 | Maxillary left primary quadrant 6

Mandibular right permanent quadrant 4 | Mandibular left permanent quadrant 3

Mandibular right primary quadrant 8 | Mandibular left primary quadrant 7

FIGURE 19–5 The Federation Dentaire International (FDI) system of coding for permanent and primary teeth.

The **Federation Dentaire International (FDI) System** is another method for numbering the teeth. It is used in some dental offices in the United States, and is the most widely used system in Canada and European countries. It uses a two-digit code that identifies the quadrant and the tooth. This makes it easy to use on a computerized system. The FDI system to identify primary or deciduous teeth is as follows:

- The mouth is divided into 4 quadrants.
- Code numbers are assigned to each quadrant: maxillary right is 5, maxillary left is 6, mandibular left is 7, and mandibular right is 8.
- Teeth in each quadrant are numbered from 1 to 5, starting with the central incisor and ending with the second molar.
- The number of the quadrant is used first, followed by the number of the tooth to code the tooth. For example, the maxillary right central incisor is tooth number 51. The 5 represents maxillary right and the 1 represents the central incisor.
- **Figure 19–5** demonstrates how primary teeth are identified by the FDI System.

The FDI System to identify permanent or succedaneous teeth is as follows:

- The mouth is divided into 4 quadrants.
- Code numbers are assigned to each quadrant: maxillary right is 1, maxillary left is 2, mandibular left is 3, and mandibular right is 4.
- Teeth in each quadrant are numbered from 1 to 8, starting with the central incisor and ending with the third molar.

- The number of the quadrant is used first, followed by the number of the tooth to code the tooth. For example, the mandibular left lateral incisor is tooth number 32. The 3 represents mandibular left and the 2 represents lateral incisor.
- Figure 19–5 demonstrates how permanent teeth are identified by the FDI System.

The FDI System can also be used to describe the oral cavity and/or the maxillary or mandibular arches:

- *00* refers to the entire oral cavity; for example: *panoramic X-ray 00*
- *01* refers to the entire maxillary arch; for example: *fluoride treatment 01*
- *02* refers to the entire mandibular arch; for example: *denture 02*

Dental assistants must use the method of numbering the dentist prefers. It is important to become familiar with the various systems to assist with charting conditions and completing insurance forms.

checkpoint

1. What are two methods used to identify teeth by using a number?

PRACTICE: Go to the workbook and complete the assignment sheet for 19:3, Identifying Teeth Using the Universal/National Numbering System and Federation Dentaire International (FDI) System. Then return and continue with the procedure.

Identifying Teeth Using the Universal/ National Numbering System

Equipment and Supplies

Model or chart of primary or deciduous teeth, model or chart of permanent or succedaneous teeth, paper, pen or pencil

Procedure

1. Assemble equipment.

2. Wash hands.

3. Use the model or chart of primary or deciduous teeth to practice the following:

   a. Draw a sketch of the 20 primary teeth. Label each tooth in your sketch using the letters of the Universal/National Numbering System. Start by labeling the maxillary right 2nd molar as *A*. Continue labeling all maxillary teeth from *A* to *J*, moving from the maxillary right teeth to the maxillary left teeth. Then, label the mandibular teeth from *K* to *T*, moving from the mandibular left teeth to the mandibular right teeth.

   b. Look at the model or chart of primary teeth. Name teeth at random using the full names, such as *maxillary right central incisor*. Then, determine the correct letter for each tooth. In the previous example, the letter would be *E*. Refer to your sketch as needed.

   c. Call out letters from *A* to *T* at random. Name the tooth that corresponds with each letter.

   d. Repeat the previous two steps until you feel confident about using the Universal/National Numbering System to identify primary teeth.

   e. Repeat naming each primary or deciduous tooth but use the letter *d* with a number from 1 to 20

to identify the teeth. For example, the *maxillary right central incisor* is *d-5* using this system.

4. Use the model or chart of permanent or succedaneous teeth to practice the following:

   a. Draw a sketch of the 32 permanent teeth. Label each tooth in your sketch using the numbers of the Universal/National Numbering System. Start by labeling the maxillary right 3rd molar as number *1*. Continue labeling all maxillary teeth from 1 to 16, moving from the maxillary right teeth to the maxillary left teeth. Then, label the mandibular teeth from 17 to 32, moving from the mandibular left teeth to the mandibular right teeth.

   b. Look at the model or chart of permanent teeth. Name teeth at random using the full names, such as *mandibular left 2nd molar*. Then, determine the correct number for each tooth. In the previous example, the number would be *18*. Refer to your sketch as needed.

   c. Call out numbers from 1 to 32 at random. Name the tooth that corresponds with each number.

   d. Repeat the previous two steps until you feel confident about using the Universal/National Numbering System to identify permanent teeth.

5. Replace all equipment.

6. Wash hands.

PRACTICE: Go to the workbook and use the evaluation sheet for 19:3A, Identifying Teeth Using the Universal/National Numbering System, to practice this procedure. When you believe you have mastered this skill, sign the sheet and give it to your instructor for further action.

 FINAL EVALUATION: Using the criteria listed on the evaluation sheet, your instructor will grade your performance.

Check

Identifying Teeth Using the Federation Dentaire International (FDI) Numbering System

Equipment and Supplies

Model or chart of primary teeth, model or chart of permanent teeth, paper, pen or pencil

Procedure

1. Assemble equipment.

2. Wash hands.

3. Use the model or chart of primary or deciduous teeth to practice the following:

   a. Draw a sketch of the 20 primary teeth. Divide the mouth into four quadrants. Draw a transverse line to separate the teeth into maxillary or upper and mandibular or lower teeth. Draw a midsagittal line to separate the mouth into right and left sides.

b. Label the maxillary right quadrant as *5*, the maxillary left quadrant as *6*, the mandibular left quadrant as *7*, and the mandibular right quadrant as *8*.

c. Label the teeth in each quadrant from 1 to 5. Begin with the central incisor as *1*, and end with the second molar as *5*.

d. Examine the model of primary teeth. Name teeth at random using correct names, such as *maxillary left central incisor*. Then, combine the number of the quadrant with the number of the tooth to determine the correct code for the tooth. In the previous example, the correct code for the tooth is number *61*. The *6* represents maxillary left, and the *1* represents central incisor.

e. Call out number codes at random. Name the tooth that corresponds with each number.

f. Repeat the previous two steps until you feel confident about using the FDI System to identify primary teeth.

4. Use the model or chart of permanent or succedaneous teeth to practice the following:

a. Draw a sketch of the 32 permanent teeth. Divide the mouth into four quadrants. Draw a transverse line to separate the teeth into maxillary or upper and mandibular or lower teeth. Draw a midsagittal line to separate the mouth into right and left sides.

b. Label the maxillary right quadrant as *1*, the maxillary left quadrant as *2*, the mandibular

left quadrant as *3*, and the mandibular right quadrant as *4*.

c. Label the teeth in each quadrant from 1 to 8. Begin with the central incisor as *1*, and end with the third molar as *8*.

d. Examine the model of permanent teeth. Name teeth at random using correct names, such as *mandibular left first bicuspid*. Then, combine the number of the quadrant with the number of the tooth to determine the correct code for the tooth. In the previous example, the correct code for the tooth is number *34*. The *3* represents mandibular left and the *4* represents first bicuspid.

e. Call out number codes at random. Name the tooth that corresponds with each number.

f. Repeat the previous two steps until you feel confident about using the FDI System to identify permanent teeth.

5. Replace all equipment.

6. Wash hands.

PRACTICE: Go to the workbook and use the evaluation sheet for 19:3B, Identifying Teeth Using the Federation Dentaire International (FDI) Numbering System, to practice this procedure. When you believe you have mastered this skill, sign the sheet and give it to your instructor for further action.

 FINAL EVALUATION: Using the criteria listed on the evaluation sheet, your instructor will grade your performance.

Check

19:4 IDENTIFYING THE SURFACES OF THE TEETH

Science

To chart conditions of the teeth, the dental assistant must be familiar with the crown surfaces of the teeth.

The first step is to differentiate between anterior and posterior teeth (**Figure 19–6**).

- **Anterior** means "toward the front." The central and lateral incisors and cuspids are anterior teeth.

- **Posterior** means "toward the back." The bicuspids and molars are posterior teeth.

Each tooth then is divided into two main sections: the crown and the root. The crown is the part that is visible in the mouth, or oral cavity. The root is the section that is located below the gingiva, or gums. The crown is divided into five sections, or surfaces.

Crown surfaces of the anterior teeth (**Figure 19–7**) are as follows:

- **Labial**: crown surface next to the lips; *facial* surface

- **Lingual**: crown surface next to the tongue

- **Incisal**: cutting or biting edge of the tooth

- **Mesial**: side surface closest to or facing toward the midline (the imaginary line dividing mouth into a right half and a left half)

- **Distal**: side surface away from the midline (that is, the side surface facing toward the back of the mouth)

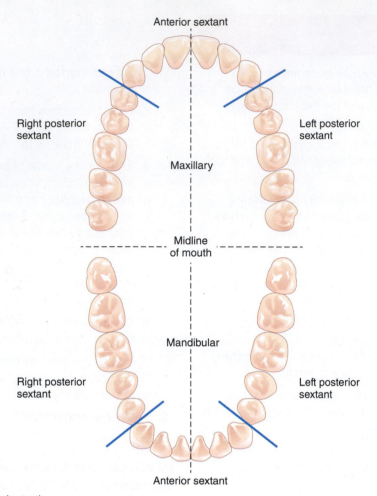

FIGURE 19–6 Anterior and posterior teeth.

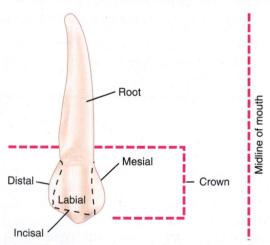

FIGURE 19–7 Crown surfaces on an anterior tooth. The lingual (tongue) surface is not seen on this diagram.

Crown surfaces of the posterior teeth (**Figure 19–8**) are as follows:

- **Buccal**: crown surface next to face or cheek; *facial* surface

- **Lingual**: crown surface next to the tongue

- **Occlusal**: chewing or grinding surface of the tooth

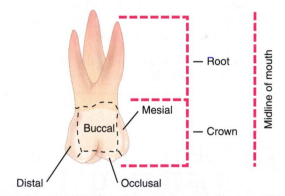

FIGURE 19–8 Crown surfaces on a posterior tooth. The lingual (tongue) surface is not seen on this diagram.

- **Mesial**: side surface toward the midline of the mouth

- **Distal**: side surface away from the midline of the mouth

Abbreviations used for the crown surfaces will depend on the doctor's preference. However, some commonly used abbreviations for the crown surfaces include:

Mesial	*M*
Distal	*D*
Labial	*La*
Lingual	*L* or *Li* or *Lin*

Incisal   *I*

Occlusal   *O*

Buccal   *B*

Line angles form where two crown surfaces meet. The name of each angle is formed by combining the names of the surfaces involved. Use the following guidelines when naming line angles:

- Drop the suffix *-al* of the *first* word and replace it with *o*.

- Whenever mesial or distal surfaces are involved, use *mesial* or *distal* as the first part of the word. For example, a line angle formed by the mesial and labial surfaces would be called a *mesiolabial* line angle.

- Use *incisal* or *occlusal* as the last part of the word. For example, a line angle formed by the lingual and occlusal surfaces would be called a *linguoocclusal* line angle.

Point angles form where three crown surfaces meet. The name of each point angle is formed by combining the names of the surfaces involved. Use the following guidelines when naming point angles:

- Drop the suffix *-al* of the first *two* words and replace with *o*.

- Use *mesial* or *distal* as the first part of the word. For example, a point angle formed by the distal, labial, and incisal surfaces would be called a *distolabioincisal* point angle.

- Use *incisal* or *occlusal* as the last part of the word. For example, a point angle formed by the mesial, lingual, and occlusal surfaces would be called a *mesiolinguoocclusal* point angle.

An anterior tooth has eight line angles and four point angles. The names of the angles and suggested list of abbreviations include:

Line Angles of Anterior Teeth

Linguoincisal	*LiI*
Labioincisal	*LaI*
Mesiolabial	*MLa*

Mesioincisal	*MI*
Mesiolingual	*MLi*
Distolingual	*DLi*
Distoincisal	*DI*
Distolabial	*DLa*

Point Angles of Anterior Teeth

Mesiolinguoincisal	*MLiI*
Mesiolabioincisal	*MLaI*
Distolabioincisal	*DLaI*
Distolinguoincisal	*DLiI*

A posterior tooth has eight line angles and four point angles. The names of the angles and suggested list of abbreviations include:

Line Angles of Posterior Teeth

Mesioocclusal	*MO*
Mesiolingual	*MLi*
Mesiobuccal	*MB*
Distoocclusal	*DO*
Distolingual	*DLi*
Distobuccal	*DB*
Linguoocclusal	*LiO*
Buccoocclusal	*BO*

Point Angles of Posterior Teeth

Mesiolinguoocclusal	*MLiO*
Mesiobuccoocclusal	*MBO*
Distobuccoocclusal	*DBO*
Distolinguoocclusal	*DLiO*

PRACTICE: Go to the workbook and complete the assignment sheet for 19:4, Identifying the Surfaces of the Teeth. Then return and continue with the procedure.

checkpoint

1. What is a point angle?

2. How many point angles does an anterior tooth possess?

Procedure 19:4

Identifying the Surfaces of the Teeth

Equipment and Supplies

Model of the teeth, paper, pen or pencil

Procedure

1. Assemble equipment.

2. Wash hands.

3. Use the model of the teeth to point out and identify the teeth and surfaces.

4. Identify the anterior teeth. Identify the posterior teeth.

5. Locate the following crown surfaces on the anterior teeth:

   a. labial

   b. incisal edge

   c. lingual

   d. mesial (draw an imaginary line to separate the mouth into a right and left side)

   e. distal

   (continues)

6. Locate the following crown surfaces on the posterior teeth:

   a. buccal
   b. occlusal
   c. lingual
   d. mesial
   e. distal

7. Locate the line angles on the anterior teeth. Write the correct names on paper. Remember, a line angle forms where two crown surfaces meet. There are a total of eight line angles.

8. Locate the line angles on the posterior teeth. Write the correct names on paper. There are a total of eight line angles.

9. Locate the point angles on the anterior teeth. Write the correct names on the paper. Remember, a point angle forms where three crown surfaces meet. There are a total of four point angles.

10. Locate the point angles on the posterior teeth. Write the correct names on the paper. There are a total of four point angles.

11. Practice steps 4–10 until you feel confident about identifying the surfaces on the teeth.

12. Replace all equipment.

13. Wash hands.

PRACTICE: Go to the workbook and use the evaluation sheet for 19:4, Identifying the Surfaces of the Teeth, to practice this procedure. When you believe you have mastered this skill, sign the sheet and give it to your instructor for further action.

FINAL EVALUATION: Using the criteria listed on the evaluation sheet, your instructor will grade your performance.

Check

19:5 CHARTING CONDITIONS OF THE TEETH

Comm

Legal

A dental assistant may be required to record conditions of the teeth on dental charts or insurance forms. Forms, symbols, and abbreviations vary from office to office. Dental charts are legal records. They must be complete, neat, and correct. Information must be current and should be updated each time a patient visits the office. The dental charts must be stored in a locked file cabinet to maintain confidentiality and to prevent loss. If the dental charts are electronic files, all safeguards must be used to prevent unauthorized access to the computer files.

A dental chart may contain the following sections:

- **Personal patient information**: full name of patient, birth date or age, address, telephone number, place of employment, physician's name and address, and insurance information

- **Medical history**: diseases or medical conditions patient has, special medical precautions, allergies, and other pertinent medical information (Section 24:4 in this textbook discusses a medical history in detail.)

- **Charting area**: anatomic or geometric diagrams of the teeth

- **Treatment section**: written record of treatment, services performed, and in some cases, fees and amounts paid

- **Radiographic history**: record of date and type of dental radiographs or X-rays

- **Remarks**: area for written notations by dentist or dental hygienist

In **Figure 19–9A**, permanent, or succedaneous, teeth are represented by the anatomic diagrams (diagrams containing images that look like the teeth). The teeth are numbered according to the Universal/National Numbering System. Maxillary teeth are above the transverse line, and mandibular teeth are below the line. In **Figure 19–9B**, both primary and permanent teeth are represented by the geometric diagrams (diagrams containing circles to represent teeth). Primary teeth are labeled with letters according to the Universal/National Numbering System. Permanent teeth are labeled with numbers.

Surfaces of the teeth are also shown in Figures 19–9A and 19–9B. The surfaces have been shaded to help familiarize you with chart representations. Note the examples for the following surfaces, the numbers of which refer to the Universal/National Numbering System:

- **Occlusal**: numbers 1 and 32
- **Incisal**: numbers 8 and 25
- **Buccal**: numbers 3 and 30
- **Labial**: numbers 9 and 24
- **Lingual**: numbers 5, 10, 23, and 28

- **Mesial**: numbers 6 and 27; not actually shown as a separate surface on the anatomic diagram but noted along the mesial edges of other surfaces
- **Distal**: numbers 12 and 21; not actually shown as a separate surface on the anatomic diagram but noted along the distal edges of other surfaces

NOTE: *Figures 19–9A and 19–9B are sample charts. Dental charts vary slightly. Never hesitate to ask questions about which surfaces are represented by different diagrams.*

Notation methods for dental charting vary. In some dental offices, a pencil is used so that if errors occur, they can be erased. In other offices, a pencil is initially used but charting is completed in ink. In most offices, colored pencils are used. Red indicates carious lesions (decay) or treatment needed. Blue indicates treatment completed, such as restorations or crowns. Many offices use electronic records and the software automatically enters the selected colors for treatment needed or treatment completed. Check with the doctor to determine which system is used and learn this system. Never hesitate to ask questions while you learn the preferred method.

Symbols used for anatomic diagrams can also vary. Again, check with the doctor to determine which symbols you should use.

Samples of symbols are shown on **Figures 19–10A** and **19–10B**. The numbers used in this figure refer to the Universal/National Numbering System:

○ *Carious lesion (decay):* Circle or outline any area involving a carious lesion or decay. In Figures 19–10A and 19–10B, carious lesions are shown on the following teeth and surfaces:

1. occlusal	6. distal
2. distoocclusal	7. incisal
3. mesioocclusodistal	8. lingual
4. buccal	9. labial
5. lingual	10. mesiolingual

● *Amalgam (silver filling material) restoration:* Use a circle filled in solid to indicate amalgam restoration (number 12, occlusal amalgam restoration)

☉ *Esthetic or composite (filling material colored to blend with tooth) restoration:* Use a circle with dot in the middle to indicate esthetic restoration such as composite or silicates (number 11, composite on labial surface)

X *Missing tooth:* Draw an X over the entire diagram of a missing tooth (number 13)

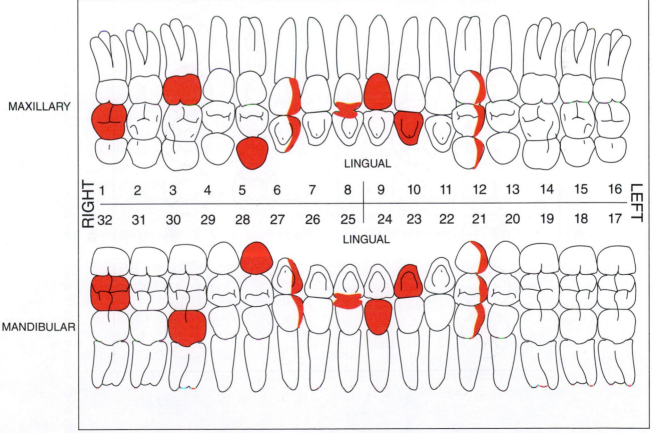

MAXILLARY

LINGUAL

RIGHT	1	2	3	4	5	6	7	8	9	10	11	12	13	14	15	16	LEFT
	32	31	30	29	28	27	26	25	24	23	22	21	20	19	18	17	

LINGUAL

MANDIBULAR

FIGURE 19–9A A sample anatomic diagram dental chart of permanent dentition with different crown surfaces shaded.

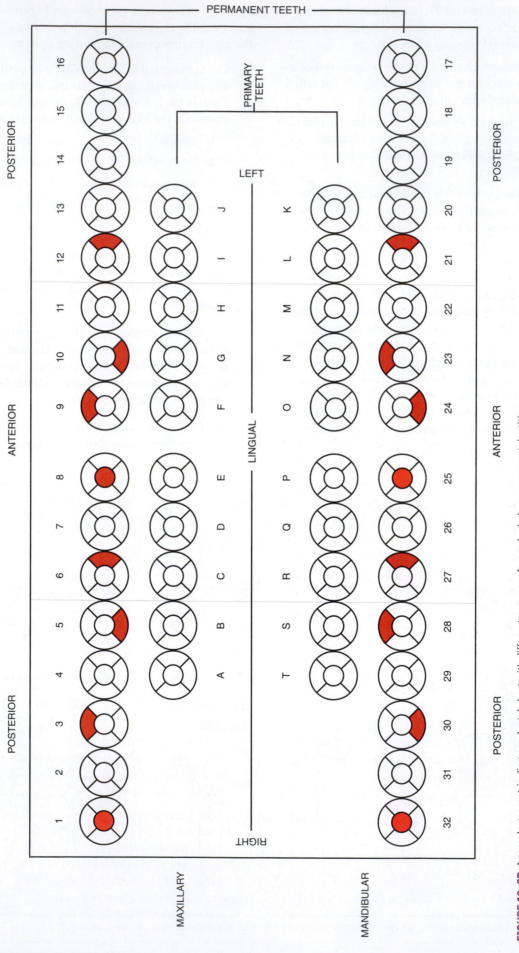

FIGURE 19–9B A sample geometric diagram dental chart with different crown surfaces shaded on permanent dentition.

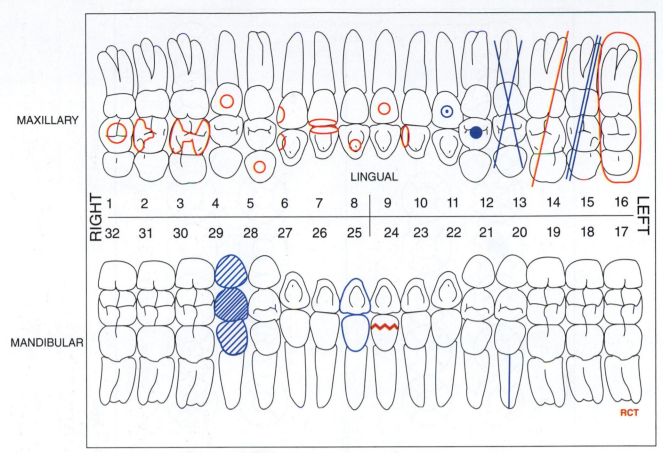

FIGURE 19–10A An anatomic diagram of permanent dentition with conditions noted by symbols.

/ *Tooth needs extraction:* Draw one line through the entire diagram of a tooth to be extracted (number 14)

// *Extracted tooth:* Draw two lines through the entire diagram of a tooth that has been extracted (number 15); some offices use an X in place of the two lines.

O *Impacted tooth:* Circle the entire diagram of an impacted tooth (tooth that is unable to erupt into its proper position) (number 16)

RCT or ENDO *Needs endodontic treatment:* Write under a tooth that needs endodontic (root canal) treatment (number 17)

| *Endodontic treatment:* Draw a heavy line in the pulp canal of a tooth with completed endodontic (root canal) treatment (number 20)

⋀⋁ *Fractured tooth:* Draw a saw line in the affected area of a fractured tooth (number 24)

O *Porcelain or esthetic crown:* Circle entire crown for a porcelain or esthetic crown (number 25)

⊜ *Gold crown:* Circle the entire crown and fill in with lines for a gold crown (number 29)

NOTE: *Remember, these are only one group of symbols. Many other symbols are in use. Learn the symbols you are required to use.*

Comm

In addition to using symbols in the anatomic diagram, all treatments or services rendered to the patient are also recorded on the dental chart. The following points should be noted:

- Only services performed are recorded in this section. Treatment performed by a previous dentist, the presence of carious lesions, or missing teeth are *not* noted here.

- Information must be recorded in ink.

- Information must be neat, correct, and complete.

- Abbreviations are used to denote teeth, surfaces, treatment completed, and base cements.

- Information recorded usually includes date, numbers of teeth treated, and services performed (for example, examination, radiographs, restorations, crowns, impressions).

- If treatment was not done to a *particular tooth* (for example, only full-mouth radiographs and examination were performed), the number column should be left blank for the Universal/National Numbering System. If the FDI system is used, the code *00* for the entire oral cavity, *01* for the entire maxillary arch, and *02* for the entire mandibular arch is entered on the chart.

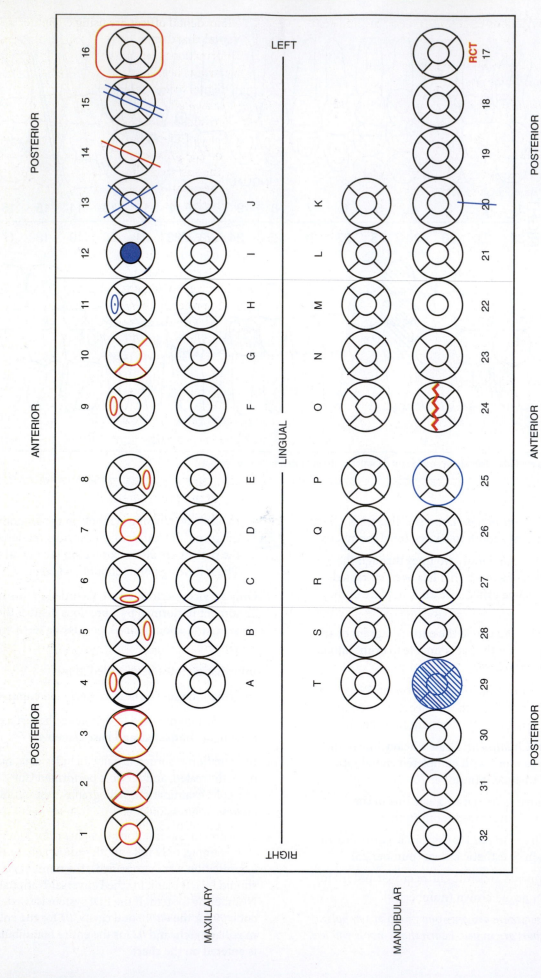

FIGURE 19–10B A geometric diagram with conditions noted by symbols on permanent dentition.

Common abbreviations used for services rendered are as follows:

NOTE: *This list varies from area to area. Use the abbreviations your doctor prefers.*

AM or *Amal*: amalgam restoration, silver filling

Anes: anesthetic

BWXR: bite-wing X-rays

Com or *Ant*: composite restoration, anterior restoration, or esthetic restoration

Cr or *CR*: crown; type may be included (*FGCr* for full gold crown, *PFMCr* for porcelain-fused-to-metal crown, and *PJCr* for porcelain jacket crown)

Ex. or *Clin. Ex.*: examination or clinical examination

Ext.: extraction

FMXR: full-mouth series of X-rays

Imp.: impression; type may be included (*Alg* for alginate, *RB* for rubber base)

Pro or *Prophy*: prophylaxis, cleaning teeth

RCT or *Endo*: root canal, or endodontic, treatment

Check your understanding of what treatment was completed in the following examples of charting by referring to the previous list of abbreviations.

2/10/—		Ex., Pro, FMXR
3/1/—	30	AM to MOD, Anes
5/6/—	8	Ant to MLa

EHR

Many dental offices are using computerized dental charting in place of manual charting. Information is entered directly into the patient's electronic health record (EHR), also called an electronic dental record (EDR). Many different types of software are available for dental charting. Some software are voice activated and totally automatic. Other software require the use of a keyboard or light pen to input the information. The software program places the correct symbol on the surface(s) indicated. Most software also color code the notation when the doctor or assistant indicates whether the tooth "needs treatment" or "treatment is complete." Dental charting software is easy to use once an individual becomes familiar with how it operates. However, the user must still know how to indicate tooth surface or work performed. In addition, the computer, keyboard, and/or light pen must be covered with protective barriers so they are not contaminated with the spray of saliva and body fluids during a dental procedure. The barriers must be changed between patients to prevent cross-contamination.

checkpoint

1. Are dental charts a legal record?

2. What does red coloring in a dental chart indicate?

PRACTICE: Read Procedure 19:5, Charting Conditions of the Teeth. Then go to the workbook and complete assignment sheet 19:5, Charting Conditions of the Teeth.

Procedure 19:5
Comm

Charting Conditions of the Teeth

Equipment and Supplies

Dental cards or charts; charting assignments in workbook; pen, pencil, or colored pencils

Procedure

1. Assemble equipment.

2. Wash hands.

3. Use the dental card or chart to complete Charting Assignment 1.

4. Use a pen, pencil, or colored pencils to complete all information. Your instructor will specify which to use.

5. Fill in the patient information area with name, address, and telephone number. You may place your name, address, and telephone number on the practice chart.

6. Chart each condition noted on the assignment. Check to be sure you are using the correct anatomic diagram. Refer to Section 19:5, Charting Conditions of the Teeth, to determine correct symbols.

7. On the anatomic diagrams of the teeth and in the services rendered area, chart all treatment completed. Use appropriate abbreviations for treatment completed. Refer to Section 19:5, Charting Conditions of the Teeth, to determine common abbreviations for services rendered.

8. Double-check all notations on the chart for accuracy. Make sure all notations are neat and legible.

9. When you have completed Charting Assignment 1, give it to your instructor. Your instructor will grade the assignment according to the criteria listed on the evaluation sheet.

10. Replace all equipment.

11. Wash hands.

(continues)

19:6 OPERATING AND MAINTAINING DENTAL EQUIPMENT

Correct use and maintenance of dental equipment may be one of the responsibilities of the dental assistant. Remember always to check the manufacturer's recommendations prior to using or maintaining any equipment. This section provides some basic facts about the various pieces of dental equipment. Note that the equipment discussed is used for four-handed dentistry. The term *four-handed dentistry* describes the dentist and dental assistant working together as a team while seated on either side of a patient who is lying in a supine position in the dental chair.

Precaution

Infection control is essential while operating and maintaining any piece of dental equipment. During dental procedures, equipment can be contaminated with blood, saliva, and body fluids. Standard precautions, described in Section 15:4, must be observed at all times. All personnel performing or assisting with any dental procedure must wear personal protective equipment (PPE) (**Figure 19–11**). This includes protective eyewear, a mask, gloves, and a gown or special clothing. The masks and gloves are disposable and are discarded after interaction with each patient. Protective eyewear should be cleaned and disinfected between patients. Some dental offices use disposable gowns that are impermeable to fluids. The gowns are discarded after each patient. Other dental offices use special uniforms, laboratory coats, or jackets. This type of protective clothing may not be worn outside the dental office. The Occupational Safety and Health Administration (OSHA) requires doctors to provide protective clothing that is laundered in the office or by a commercial laundry service. All office personnel assisting with dental procedures change into the protective clothing when they arrive at work. If they leave the office for any reason, they must remove the protective clothing and dress in their own clothes. When the protective clothing is removed, it must be folded inward to keep contaminated areas on the inside. In addition, the clothing must be changed at least daily, or immediately if it has been splashed with body fluids. These regulations were established by OSHA to protect dental personnel, their families, and the public from exposure to clothing that has been contaminated by the mist of body fluids that is expelled during every dental procedure.

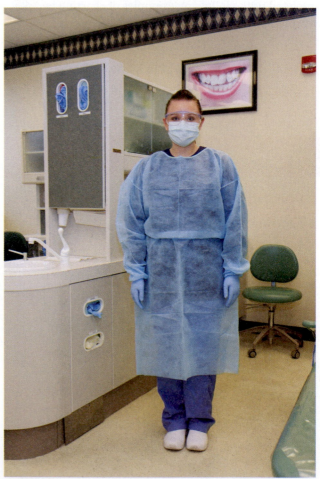

FIGURE 19–11 All personnel performing or assisting with any dental procedure must wear personal protective equipment (PPE).

Precaution

Standard precautions must also be followed while using any dental instruments, equipment, or supplies. Protective barriers must be placed on many parts of the equipment prior to use (**Figure 19–12**). Special covers can be purchased for the dental chair, handles and switches on the dental light, handpieces, air-water syringe, high-volume evacuator, tubing, and the X-ray tube head. Plastic wrap or aluminum foil can also be used to cover surfaces such as the handles and switches on the dental light. Clear plastic wrap can be used on the X-ray tube head. Plastic-backed paper or plastic wrap can be used on the headrest, armrest, and other parts of the dental chair, and to cover the tops of the dental carts. Some offices use clear plastic dry-cleaning bags to cover the dental chair. After the procedure is complete, the bag is removed from the chair, turned inside out, and used as a trash bag for the other barriers (**Figure 19–13**).

Precaution

After any dental procedure, standard precautions must be followed to clean and disinfect or sterilize any contaminated equipment. The assistant must wear gloves to remove the contaminated barriers. The areas must then be disinfected. All surfaces are sprayed with a disinfectant and wiped to remove any particles or debris. The areas are then sprayed a second time, and the solution is left in place for the period of time recommended by the manufacturer, usually 10 minutes (**Figures 19–14A** and **19–14B**). All surfaces are then wiped again, and the contaminated gloves removed. After the hands are washed thoroughly, clean protective barriers must be put in place before the next dental procedure. By observing standard precautions and proper disinfection/sterilization procedures, the transmission of disease by dental equipment can be prevented.

Most **dental lights** are mounted on the ceiling of the dental unit or attached to the dental chair. The light is used to illuminate the oral cavity, or mouth, while the doctor works. The light is positioned 30–50 inches from the oral cavity. Both the doctor and assistant should be able to adjust the position of the light. Most lights contain dimmer switches to adjust the intensity of the light. Prior to a procedure, protective barriers such as plastic wrap, aluminum foil, or commercial covers are placed on the handles and switches of the light. These must be removed and replaced with clean barriers after each patient. In

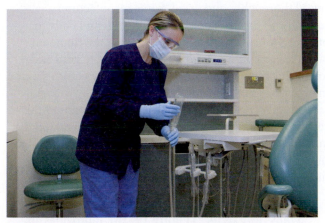

FIGURE 19–12 Protective barriers, such as plastic wrap or commercial covers, must be placed on many parts of the dental equipment prior to use.

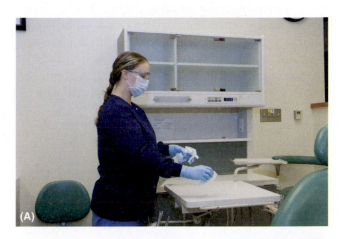

(A)

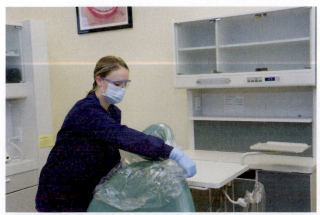

FIGURE 19–13 After a dental procedure is complete, the plastic bag used to cover the chair can be turned inside out and used as a trash bag for the other barriers.

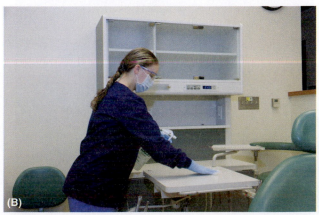

(B)

FIGURE 19–14 After a dental procedure is complete, contaminated surfaces are (A) sprayed with a disinfectant and then (B) wiped and sprayed a second time with a disinfectant.

addition, all parts that are touched must be disinfected after each patient. Most manufacturers recommend the use of a mild detergent and a soft cloth to clean the light shield. The soft cloth prevents the formation of scratches on the light shield. At least once a week, all moving parts on the light should be lubricated with a general, all-purpose oil.

The **dental chair** (**Figure 19–15**) is designed to position the patient comfortably while providing the doctor and the dental assistant with easy access to the oral cavity. Most chairs have thin, narrow headrests so the doctor and the dental assistant can position themselves close to the patient. The chair reclines to place the patient in a supine, or lying down, position. Most chairs contain controls on both sides and/or on the floor so they can be operated by the doctor or the dental assistant. The control to raise and lower the height of the chair is usually located on the chair base and is operated by foot. The control to recline or raise the chair is usually located on the side of the chair and near the headrest; it is operated by hand. Some chairs have foot controls to raise or lower the chair because this eliminates the need for protective barriers. Chairs also have foot controls to lock the chairs in position. This prevents movement of the chair while the patient is getting in or out of it. Some chairs have digital controls that regulate all movements. The control pad is usually attached to the cart. Cleaning the chair between patients is mandatory for infection control. The headrest, armrest, and any other contaminated area must be wiped clean with a disinfectant, then resprayed, left in place for the required time, and wiped again. The headrest and/ or the top of the chair is usually covered with a plastic disposable cover, which is discarded and replaced with a clean one after each patient. Most manufacturers recommend frequent, thorough cleaning with special upholstery cleaners or mild soap solutions.

The **air compressor** provides air pressure to operate the handpieces and air syringes on the dental units. It is usually located in a storage area or basement, and air lines are installed to carry the air pressure to the dental units.

The compressor is usually set to provide 100 pounds of pressure. The pressure gauge on the air compressor should be checked frequently. If pressure goes above 120 pounds, the doctor should be notified. Careful maintenance of the air compressor is essential. Many have filters that must be changed routinely. Manufacturer's recommendations must be read and followed.

The **oral-evacuation system**, also called a *central vacuum system*, uses water to provide the dental units with a suction action. It aids in removing particles, debris, and liquids from the oral cavity. Its action is similar to that of a vacuum cleaner. The system consists of a main pump with vacuum lines to the dental unit and is usually located in a storage area or utility closet. Electrical control switches to turn the pump on and off are usually located on or near the dental unit. Wastes and liquids drawn into the system are discharged into a sanitary sewer line. A solids collector trap or filter is located on the oral evacuation unit or in the dental unit. This trap catches large particles and must be cleaned daily. The particles should be emptied into a paper towel and placed in the correct waste container. The trap should be washed with a mild detergent, rinsed thoroughly, and dried. Some manufacturers recommend using a germicide spray or liquid daily to prevent the growth of organisms and the development of unpleasant odors. Again, it is important to read and follow the manufacturer's instructions on specific care and maintenance of the oral-evacuation system.

Assistant's carts vary from office to office, but most carts contain the same basic equipment. Drawers or areas for instrument storage are found on some carts. Other carts have sliding tops with storage areas under the tops. In addition, the following equipment is usually located on the cart:

- **Tri-flow**, or **air-water**, **syringe**: This is also called a *three-way syringe* (**Figure 19–16**). It provides air, water, or a combination of air and water for various dental procedures. Protective barrier covers are placed on the syringe handle and tubing prior to

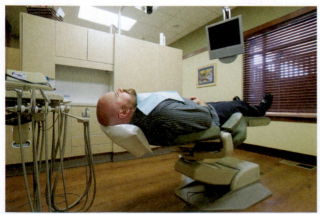

FIGURE 19–15 The dental chair allows the patient to be positioned comfortably while providing the doctor and the dental assistant easy access to the oral cavity.

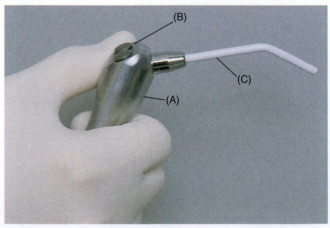

FIGURE 19–16 Parts of an air-water, or tri-flow, syringe: (A) handle; (B) air-water control; and (C) disposable tip.

each patient examination. After each use, the air-water syringe should be run for at least 30 seconds to flush out the unit. Plastic disposable tips are used in many offices. Other offices use a metal tip that is removable for sterilization in an autoclave. It must be changed and replaced with a sterile tip after each patient. The syringe and tubing must be wiped with a disinfectant after each patient.

- **Saliva ejector**: This provides constant, low-volume suction to remove saliva and other fluids from the mouth. Most ejectors contain screw-type knobs that are used to turn the suction on and off. The tips are disposable (**Figure 19–17**). They must be changed after each patient. The tip holder is covered with a protective barrier during use. The barrier is removed after each patient, the holder and tubing are disinfected, and a new barrier is put in place. At least once daily, the inside of the tip holder must be cleaned thoroughly with a brush. A germicide solution or spray can also be used to clean the inside of the tip holder. The tubing can be sanitized by turning the saliva ejector on and drawing a disinfecting and deodorizing solution into it.

- **High-velocity oral evacuator (HVE)**: This is also called a *high-volume* or *high-vacuum evacuator* (**Figure 19–18**). It is used to remove particles, debris, and large amounts of liquid from the oral cavity. Various tips can be used in the evacuator. Most offices use plastic disposable tips that are discarded after each patient. Metal tips and nondisposable, heavy plastic tips are cleaned and sterilized in an autoclave. The evacuator holder is covered with a protective barrier during the procedure. The barrier is removed after each patient, the holder and tubing are disinfected, and a new barrier is put in place. A disinfecting and deodorizing solution can be suctioned into the tubing to sanitize the interior of the unit. Most units contain filter screens to trap larger particles drawn into the evacuator. These screens must be changed or emptied and cleaned daily. In addition, a slide valve is usually attached to the unit. This is used to turn the unit on and off with ease. The valve should be removed daily for thorough cleaning. It should be lubricated with a silicone-type lubricant to prevent sticking.

Style and type of **doctors' carts** also vary from office to office. Many contain air-water syringes in addition to a variety of handpieces. Most carts also have **rheostats**, or foot controls used to operate the handpieces and control the speed. Basic handpieces found on a doctor's cart include the air-water syringe, high-velocity oral evacuator (HVE), and/or saliva ejector. Two other hand-pieces are as follows:

- **Low-speed handpiece**: This is also called a *conventional-speed handpiece* (**Figure 19–19**). It is used for dental caries (decay) removal and fine-finishing work. The lower speed of this handpiece allows the doctor maximum control. Different attachments can be used on this handpiece. Two of the most common are the contra angle and the prophylaxis angle.

(1) **Contra angle**: This is used for cutting and polishing during various dental procedures. Instruments called burs are inserted into the contra angle. **Burs** are rotary instruments used to cut, shape, finish, and polish teeth, restorations,

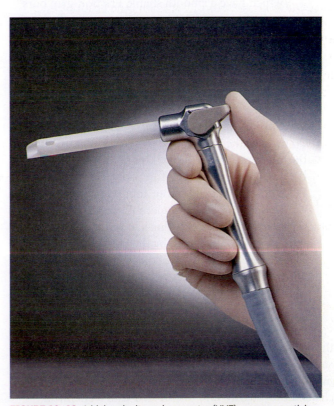

FIGURE 19–18 A high-velocity oral evacuator (HVE) removes particles, debris, and large amounts of liquid from the oral cavity. Courtesy, Hager Worldwide, Inc.

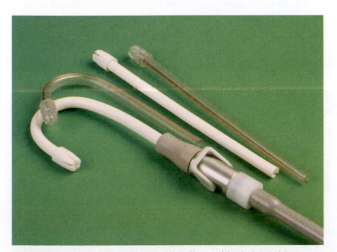

FIGURE 19–17 A saliva ejector with a disposable tip in position.
Courtesy, Practicon Inc.

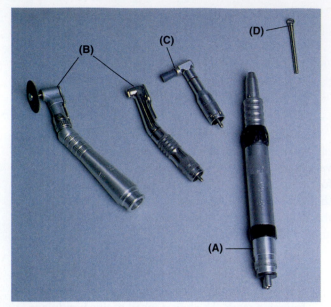

FIGURE 19–19 (A) A low-speed handpiece with (B) contra-angle heads with and without a disc, (C) a right angle or prophylaxis attachment, and (D) a round bur.

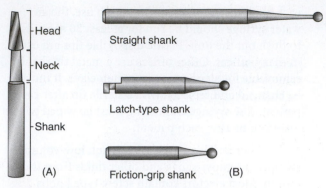

FIGURE 19–20 (A) Parts of a bur and (B) types of burs.

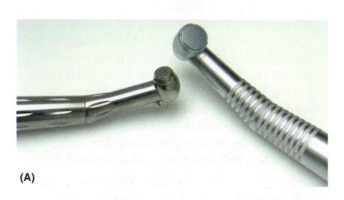

(A)

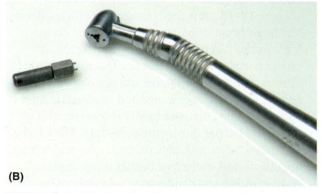

(B)

FIGURE 19–21 High-speed handpieces are used to do most of the cutting and preparation of the mouth during dental procedures. (A) A high-speed handpiece with a push button to insert and remove burs. (B) A high-speed handpiece with a bur tool to insert and remove burs.

and dental appliances. Burs have three parts: the *head* or cutting portion, the *shank* or part inserted in the handpiece, and the neck, which joins the head to the shank. Some contra angles use latch-type burs, which contain a groove at the shank. Others use friction-grip, or FG, burs, which have a smooth shank. Friction-grip burs are held in place by a friction chuck in the head of the contra angle (**Figure 19–20**).

(2) **Prophylaxis angle**: This attachment holds polishing cups, disks, and brushes that are used to clean the teeth or to polish restorations.

- **High-speed handpiece**: This is sometimes called an *ultraspeed handpiece* (**Figure 19–21**). It is used to do most of the cutting and preparation of the tooth during dental procedures. This handpiece contains a friction-grip chuck; therefore, only friction-grip, or FG, burs can be used. A bur tool/wrench or a button release lever on the handpiece is used to insert and remove the burs. When this handpiece is used, intense heat is generated by the friction action of the bur. This requires the handpiece to be water-cooled with a fine mist of water when it is used. An HVE or saliva ejector is used to suction the water that accumulates in the patient's mouth.

After each patient, handpieces must be scrubbed thoroughly to remove debris, rinsed, dried, and sterilized. If a handpiece cannot be sterilized according to manufacturer's instructions, it must be flushed with water, cleaned thoroughly, and disinfected with a chemical germicide. All tubings must be wiped with a disinfectant. The burs should be cleaned well with a bur brush and then sterilized. Manufacturer's recommendations must

be followed when sterilizing burs because different types of materials used in burs require different methods of sterilization. Both low-speed and high-speed handpieces require lubrication. It is important to follow the manufacturer's instructions regarding the type of lubrication and method of application.

 CAUTION: *Because of possible contamination from saliva, blood, or body fluids, standard precautions must be observed while handpieces are in use. Personal protective equipment (PPE) that includes a gown or protective clothing, gloves, masks, and protective eyewear must be worn at all times. Gloves and masks are discarded after each patient. In addition, masks must be changed any time they become moist or wet.*

Precaution

Protective eyewear must be disinfected, rinsed to remove the disinfectant, and dried before being used for another patient.

The dental assistant's responsibilities for the use and maintenance of dental equipment vary. It is your responsibility to learn exactly what maintenance is expected. Read specific manufacturer's instructions for the equipment you handle.

checkpoint

| 1. What does the term *"four-handed dentistry"* mean?

PRACTICE: Go to the workbook and complete the assignment sheet for 19:6, Operating and Maintaining Dental Equipment. Then return and continue with the procedure.

Procedure 19:6

Operating and Maintaining Dental Equipment

Equipment and Supplies

Dental light; dental chair; air compressor; oral-evacuation system; assistant's cart with equipment; doctor's cart with equipment; latch-type bur; friction-grip (FG) bur; bur tool; lubricants; cleaning brush; soft cloths; disinfecting solution; protective barriers; personal protective equipment (gloves, gown, face mask, and eye protection)

Procedure

1. Assemble equipment.

2. Wash hands. Put on personal protective equipment (PPE).

    CAUTION: Observe standard precautions at all times. Equipment may be contaminated with saliva, body fluids, and blood.
   Precaution

    CAUTION: Dry hands thoroughly. You will be working with electrical equipment.
   Safety

3. Practice operating the dental light:

   a. Locate the on/off switch. Turn the light on.

   b. Position the light so that it is above the dental chair. From a seated position, practice moving the light.

   NOTE: You will be sitting on a chair while assisting the doctor and will frequently reposition the light.

   c. Locate the dimmer switch. Turn the switch to adjust the intensity of the light.

   d. Practice applying protective barriers to the handles and/or switches of the light. Use commercial covers, plastic wrap, or aluminum foil to cover and protect the areas of the light that may be touched during a dental procedure.

    CAUTION: Remember to wear gloves while removing contaminated
   Precaution

protective barriers. After the covers are discarded, wipe the areas with a disinfectant. Then, respray the areas and leave the disinfectant in place for the amount of time recommended by the manufacturer. Then, rewipe all areas. Remove the gloves, and wash your hands. Put on clean gloves. Then, apply clean protective barriers.

   e. Use a mild detergent and a soft cloth to clean the shield of the light.

   f. Locate all moving parts on the light fixture. Use a general, all-purpose oil to lubricate these parts, if lubrication is needed.

4. Practice operating the dental chair:

   a. Locate the chair lock. It is usually on the base of the chair. Lock and unlock the chair.

    CAUTION: The chair must be locked when a patient is getting in or out of it.
   Safety

   b. Locate the elevation control, which raises and lowers the height of the chair. It is usually a foot control on the base of the chair. Raise and lower the chair.

    CAUTION: The chair must be in its lowest position when a patient is getting in or out of the chair.
   Safety

   NOTE: At least once each week, the chair should be elevated to its highest position and then lowered to its lowest position. This lubricates the hydraulic system.

   c. Locate the forward-backward control, which reclines or raises the back of the chair. It is usually located on the side of the chair and near the headrest or on a foot control. Put the chair in a reclining position. Raise the chair to a sitting position.

   NOTE: The chair must be in an upright position when a patient is getting in or out of it.

(continues)

d. Locate the reset button, found on many chairs. It is usually located near the forward-backward control. Operate the button. It automatically raises the back of the chair to an upright position and lowers the chair to its lowest position from the floor.

NOTE: Some chairs have digital controls located on a small pad that is usually attached to the dental cart. All movements of the chair are controlled by the different buttons on the pad.

e. Place a clean, disposable cover on the headrest and back of the chair. Some offices also drape the armrests and other parts of the chair with plastic-backed paper or plastic wrap. Wear gloves to remove contaminated protective barriers, wipe the areas with a disinfectant, respray the area and leave the solution in place for the correct amount of time, and then rewipe. Remove the gloves, and wash your hands before putting clean protective barriers in place.

f. Use a mild detergent and a soft cloth to wash the chair. Rinse and dry the chair.

NOTE: Some manufacturers recommend special upholstery cleaners.

5. Practice operating and maintaining the air compressor:

a. Read the manufacturer's instructions.

b. Turn the compressor on. Most compressors are operated by a switch in the operatory area. Others must be turned on manually by plugging in an electrical cord. Before inserting the plug into an electrical socket, always check the electrical cord for breaks or tears, and the plug for the third prong. Some air compressors operate immediately after being plugged into an electric wall socket; others have on/off switches.

c. Watch the pressure gauge on the compressor. If the pressure goes above 120 pounds, turn the compressor off, and notify your doctor immediately.

NOTE: Most air compressors are set to provide 100 pounds of pressure.

d. Turn the compressor off.

6. Practice operating and maintaining the oral-evacuation system:

a. Read the manufacturer's instructions.

b. Turn the system on. Some systems have on/off switches in the dental units; other smaller systems have switches on the evacuation units themselves.

c. Turn the system off.

d. Locate the solids collector trap (**Figure 19–22**). Empty any particles in the trap onto a paper towel. Place the towel and particles in the proper waste container. Wash the trap with a mild detergent, rinse, and dry. Replace the trap on the system.

 CAUTION: Always wear gloves when emptying the solids collector trap.

Precaution

NOTE: Many manufacturers recommend using a germicide spray or solution in the trap to prevent the growth of organisms and the development of unpleasant odors.

NOTE: Systems vary, so follow individual instructions on removing and replacing the trap.

7. Practice operating the tri-flow, or air-water, syringe. It is located on the assistant's cart and/or the doctor's cart.

a. Push the button to release air. It is usually marked with an *A* (for air).

b. Direct the tip of the syringe into a cup or sink. Push the button to release water. It is usually marked with a *W* (for water).

c. Continue to hold the tip over a cup or sink. Push both the air and water buttons. Water under air pressure will spray out of the syringe.

d. Remove and replace the syringe tip. The tip must be sterilized after each patient. Most offices use plastic tips that are disposable and discarded in an infectious-waste container after use.

e. Use a disinfectant solution to clean the tip holder and tubing.

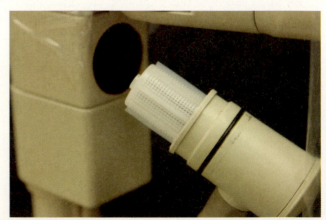

FIGURE 19–22 The oral evacuation system has a solids collector trap that must be emptied, or discarded if it is disposable.

8. Practice operating the saliva ejector:

   a. Insert a tip into the ejector.

   b. Locate the screw knob or control and turn the ejector on.

      NOTE: The oral-evacuation system must be on before the ejector will work.

   c. Turn the ejector off.

   d. Remove the tip. The tips are disposable and are placed in an infectious-waste container after being used on a patient.

   e. Use a brush to clean inside the ejector tip holder. Use a disinfectant solution to clean the tip holder and tubing.

   f. Turn the saliva ejector on. Place the end into a disinfecting and deodorizing solution to draw the solution into the ejector unit to sanitize it.

9. Practice operating the high-velocity oral evacuator (HVE).

   a. Insert a tip into the evacuator. Tips can be plastic or metal.

   b. Locate the slide valve. Move the valve to turn the HVE on. Move it in the opposite direction to turn it off.

   c. Remove the slide valve from the HVE. Scrub it with a brush. Rinse it thoroughly. Dry the valve. Place a silicone lubricant on the valve. Replace the valve in the HVE unit.

      NOTE: The lubricant prevents the slide valve from sticking.

   d. Locate the filter screen on the HVE unit. It is usually located under the cart or on the tubing. Empty the particles in the screen onto a paper towel. Place the towel and particles in an infectious-waste container. Scrub the screen gently with a brush. Rinse the screen and replace it in the HVE unit. Some screens are disposable. These are discarded in an infectious waste container and replaced with a new screen.

      NOTE: Follow specific instructions on removing and replacing the screen.

   e. Remove the tip. Place a disposable tip in an infectious-waste container. Scrub a metal tip, using a brush to clean the inside. Rinse the tip. Sterilize it correctly.

   f. Use a disinfectant solution to clean the tip holder and tubing.

   g. Turn the HVE on. Place the tip into a disinfecting and deodorizing solution to draw the solution into the tubing to sanitize it.

10. Practice maintaining the low-speed handpiece. It is located on the doctor's cart.

    a. Read the manufacturer's instructions.

    b. Insert a contra-angle head or attachment on the handpiece. Tighten the handpiece to hold the head in place.

       NOTE: The handpiece should be kept open when an attachment or head is not in place. If the handpiece is closed while empty, the units that hold the heads in place can be damaged.

    c. Check the contra angle to determine which type of bur is required. If a small latch is present on the back, latch-type burs are required. Obtain a bur that has a groove at the end and insert it in the contra angle. Close the latch to hold the bur in place. If no latch is present on the contra angle, friction-grip, or FG, burs are required. Obtain an FG bur. Use a bur tool to push the bur into position on the contra angle.

       NOTE: Some new handpieces have levers that are pushed to insert and remove burs. Bur tools are not used with these handpieces.

    d. Remove the bur from the contra angle by releasing the latch, pushing the bur out with the bur tool, or using the lever on the handpiece, if a lever is present.

    e. Remove the contra angle from the handpiece by loosening the top of the handpiece. Use a low-speed lubricant to lubricate the contra angle. Spray the lubricant into the hole at the end, where the contra angle attaches to the handpiece.

    f. Insert and remove a prophylaxis angle on the handpiece. Use a low-speed lubricant to moisten the hole at the end of the prophylaxis angle, where the angle attaches to the handpiece.

    g. Remove the handpiece from the unit. Scrub it thoroughly to remove debris, rinse and dry it, and then sterilize it. Use a disinfectant to clean the outside of the tubing. Follow manufacturer's instructions to sterilize the burs and the contra angle or prophylaxis angle.

(continues)

h. Follow manufacturer's instructions to lubricate the handpiece. Most handpieces unclip in the center. Spray low-speed lubricant into the lower end of the top section; the tubing looks like two *V*s in this area. Then, unscrew the handpiece from the base. The lower end of this section has four holes. Spray low-speed lubricant into the second largest hole only. Reassemble the handpiece. Push the rheostat, or foot control, on the cart to operate the handpiece and to remove excess oil. Turn it off and use a paper towel to wipe the handpiece dry. Then, clean the handpiece again with a disinfectant.

NOTE: Most manufacturers recommend daily lubrication.

11. Practice maintaining the high-speed handpiece:

a. Use a bur tool to insert and remove a friction-grip bur on the handpiece.

NOTE: Only friction-grip burs are used in this handpiece.

NOTE: Some new handpieces have levers that are pushed to insert and remove burs. Bur tools are not used with these handpieces.

b. Remove the handpiece from the unit. Scrub it thoroughly to remove debris, rinse and dry it, and then sterilize it. Use a disinfectant to clean the outside of the tubing.

c. Follow manufacturer's instructions to lubricate the handpiece. Most handpieces are unscrewed at the base. Spray high-speed lubricant into the large hole only. Reassemble the handpiece. Operate the handpiece to remove excess lubricant. Wipe the handpiece dry with a paper towel and then clean the handpiece again with a disinfectant.

12. Clean and replace all equipment.

13. Remove PPE. Wash hands.

PRACTICE: Go to the workbook and use the evaluation sheet for 19:6, Operating and Maintaining Dental Equipment, to practice this procedure. When you believe you have mastered this skill, sign the sheet and give it to your instructor for further action.

 Check

FINAL EVALUATION: Using the criteria listed on the evaluation sheet, your instructor will grade your performance.

19:7 IDENTIFYING DENTAL INSTRUMENTS AND PREPARING DENTAL TRAYS

Assisting with a variety of dental procedures may be one of the responsibilities of the dental assistant. Correct preparation includes setting up trays of instruments and supplies used in specific procedures. Therefore, a dental assistant must be familiar with dental instruments.

Various methods are used for setting up trays for specific dental procedures. In some settings, the trays are set up immediately before use. The dental assistant prepares the room, seats the patient, and then sets up a tray with supplies and sterilized instruments. The instruments and supplies are determined by the procedure that will be performed on the patient. In other settings, preset sterilized trays are used. Tray contents are determined by the doctor.

Trays are set up for oral examinations, amalgam restorations, composite restorations, surgical extractions, and other similar procedures. During an oral examination, the patient's teeth are cleaned and examined. Dental radiographs or X-rays may be taken. Amalgam and composite are the two main restorative materials used to repair carious lesions or tooth decay. The doctor removes the damaged tooth structure and creates an opening called a *cavity preparation*. Amalgam, the silver restorative material, or composite, an esthetic restorative material, is then placed in the cavity preparation. A surgical extraction is the removal of a damaged tooth. After determining the procedure that is to be performed, the dental assistant seats the patient and positions the correct tray containing the sterilized instruments. Additional instruments or supplies can be added if needed. In many settings, preset trays are color coded (for example, red for amalgam, blue for composite) and are sterilized as a unit.

Items on the trays should be organized and placed in proper sequence. Instruments are usually arranged in the order of use. After an instrument is used, it is returned to the same place on the tray, in case it is needed again. This makes it easier for the dental assistant to locate instruments and increases overall efficiency (**Figure 19–23**).

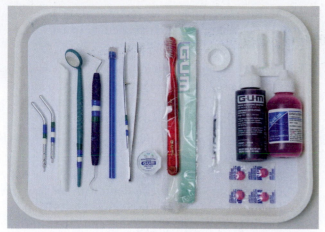

FIGURE 19–23 Instruments are arranged in order of use to make it easier for the dental assistant to locate them.

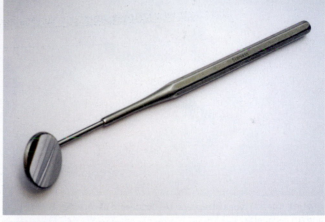

FIGURE 19–24 Mouth mirror. © iStock.com/andrewmedina

The main parts of a dental hand instrument are:

- **Blade, nib, or point**: A blade is the cutting portion of an instrument; a nib is the blunt, serrated, or smooth working end of a condensing (packing) instrument; a point is the sharp end used to explore and detect.

- **Shank**: The portion that connects the shaft, or handle, to the blade, nib, or point.

- **Shaft**: The handle of the instrument, usually hexagonal (six sides) to provide a better grip.

Some instruments are single ended, which means they have only one working end with a blade, nib, or point. Other instruments are double ended, which means they have a working edge on each end of the instrument. Some double-ended instruments have the same type of working surface at each end, but one end is larger than the other. Others have one working end for the right side of a preparation and the second end for the left side. In some cases, an instrument has ends with different functions, but both ends are used for the same procedure.

Instruments used vary from office to office. However, some instruments are standard and are used in all dental offices. The following list briefly describes some of the main instruments:

- **Mouth mirror**: Used to view areas of the oral cavity, reflect light on dark surfaces, and retract the lips for better visibility. It is used in every basic tray set up. Mirrors are available in various sizes and with plain or magnifying ends (**Figure 19–24**).

- **Explorer**: Used to examine the teeth, detect carious lesions, and note other oral conditions. Explorers are available in many shapes and sizes. They may be single or double ended (**Figure 19–25**).

- **Cotton pliers**: Used to carry objects such as cotton pellets or rolls to and from the mouth. Some lock, some do not. They are also called *operating pliers* or *college pliers* (**Figure 19–26**).

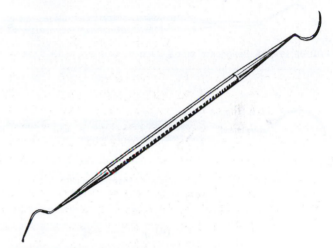

FIGURE 19–25 Double-ended explorer.

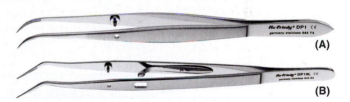

FIGURE 19–26 (A) Nonlocking cotton pliers. (B) Locking cotton pliers. Courtesy of Hu-Friedy Mfg., LLC.

- **Scalers**: Sharp instruments used to remove calculus (tartar) and debris from the teeth and subgingival pockets. Scalers are used mainly for prophylactic (cleaning) or periodontal (gum or gingiva) treatments. They are available in many types or shapes (**Figure 19–27**).

- **Periodontal probes**: Used to measure the depth of the gingival sulcus (the space between the tooth and the free gingiva). It has a round, tapered blade with a blunt tip that is marked in millimeters (mm) (**Figure 19–28A**). A combination double-ended instrument called an *expro* has an explorer at one end and a periodontal probe at the other end (**Figure 19–28B**).

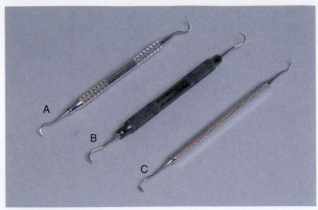

FIGURE 19–27 Types of scalers: (A) Sickle and Jacquette; (B) Sickle; and (C) Jacquette.

- **Excavators**: Used mainly for removal of caries and refinement of the internal opening in a cavity preparation.

  (1) **Spoon**: Used to remove soft decay from a cavity. It is also used to remove excess dental cement. It is a cutting instrument with a small curve or scoop at the working end (**Figure 19–29A**).

  (2) **Hoe**: Used primarily on anterior teeth to remove caries, smooth and shape a cavity preparation, and/or form line angles. A hoe has one or more angles to the shaft, with the last length forming the blade (**Figure 19–29B**). It is also used in scraping, planing, and direct-thrust cutting.

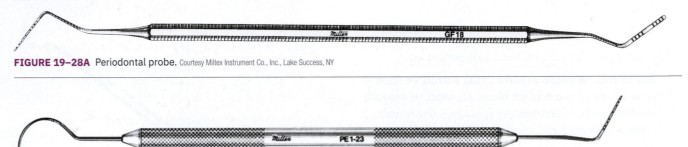

FIGURE 19–28A Periodontal probe. Courtesy Miltex Instrument Co., Inc., Lake Success, NY

(1)   **(2)**

FIGURE 19–28B An expro is a combination instrument with (1) an explorer at one end and (2) a periodontal probe at the other end. Courtesy Miltex Instrument Co., Inc., Lake Success, NY

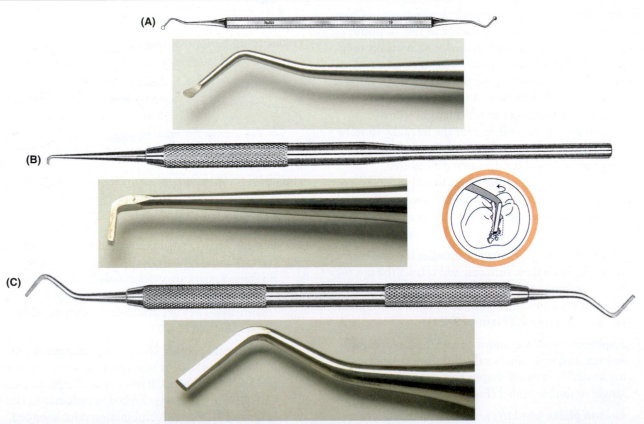

FIGURE 19–29 Types of excavators: (A) A spoon with a close-up view of the working end. (B) A hoe with a close-up view of the working end and a view of the instrument in a tooth. (C) A hatchet with a close-up view of the working end. Courtesy Miltex Instrument Co. Inc., Lake Success, NY Courtesy of Hu-Friedy Mfg., Co.,Inc., Courtesy of Hu-Friedy Mfg., Co.,Inc.

(3) **Hatchet**: Used to refine internal line angles, smooth and shape the sides of a cavity preparation, and remove hard-type caries. It is usually a double-ended right and left instrument (**Figure 19–29C**).

- **Chisels**: Used for cutting and shaping enamel. Instruments in this group include:

  (1) **Enamel hatchet**: Similar to other hatchets but the blade is larger, heavier, and beveled on only one side.

  (2) **Gingival margin trimmer**: Special chisel for placing bevels on gingival enamel margins of proximo occlusal cavity preparations. Most are double ended for either the distal or mesial side of the tooth. It has the chisel blade placed at an angle to the shaft, not straight across like a hatchet. In addition, the blade is curved, not flat like a hatchet (**Figure 19–30**).

- **Cleoid-discoid carver**: A double-ended cutting instrument. It is also available as a cleoid or discoid single-ended instrument. The cleoid has a claw-shaped cutting end, and the cutting edge surrounds the entire end. The discoid is disc shaped and also has the cutting edge around the blade. It is used as a carver for amalgam, but can also be used as an excavator (**Figure 19–31**).

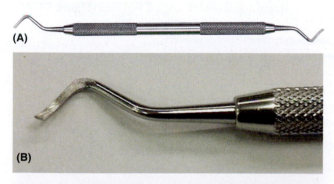

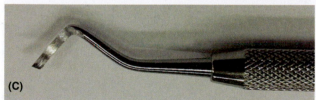

FIGURE 19–30 A gingival margin trimmer (GMT) (A) with a close-up of (B) a mesial working end and (C) a distal working end. Courtesy of Hu-Friedy Mfg., LLC

- **Plastic filling instrument (PFI)**: Used to shape and condense restorative material that is still malleable (capable of being shaped or formed). It is also used with cements before setting occurs. Most have a small condenser at one end and a paddle-like cutting blade at the other end (**Figure 19–32**).

- **Amalgam instruments**: Used mainly with amalgam restorations. Some examples are as follows:

  (1) **Amalgam carrier**: Used to carry small masses of freshly mixed amalgam to the cavity preparation (**Figure 19–33**).

  (2) **Amalgam carvers**: Used to carve or shape freshly placed amalgam and restore the tooth to natural anatomy. One example is the Hollenback carver (**Figure 19–34**).

  (3) **Condenser-plugger**: Used for condensing and packing amalgam into the prepared cavity. The ends may be serrated or plain (**Figure 19–35**).

  (4) **Matrix retainer and matrix band**: The matrix retainer is used to hold the matrix band in place (**Figure 19–36**). A matrix band is a short strip of steel or other metal that is not affected by mercury. It is used to form a wall around a cavity so amalgam can be packed into place.

NOTE: *Plastic matrix strips are used with composite restorative material.*

- **Burnisher**: Contains working points in the shapes of balls or "beavertails." Burnishers are used primarily to burnish (adapt) the margins of gold restorations to a better fit. Burnishers are also used to polish other metals (**Figure 19–37**).

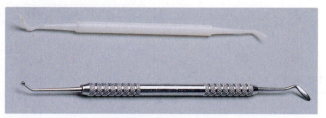

FIGURE 19–32 Plastic filling instruments (PFIs).

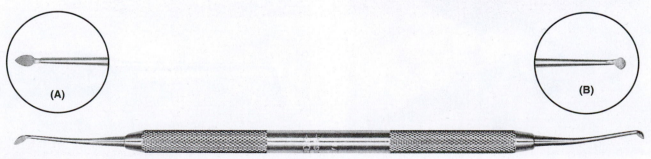

FIGURE 19–31 Carvers: (A) cleoid and (B) discoid. Courtesy of Hu-Friedy Mfg., Co.,Inc.

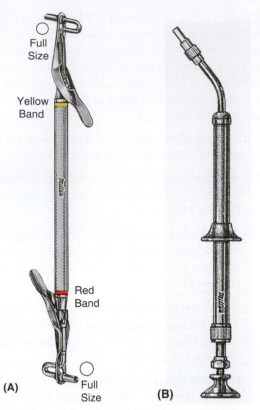

Full Size

Yellow Band

Red Band

Full Size

(A)   (B)

FIGURE 19–33 Amalgam carriers: (A) lever type and (B) plunger type. Courtesy Miltex Instrument Co., Inc., Lake Success, NY

- **Plastic composite instruments**: A set of plastic instruments used with composite restorations. Because metal instruments can discolor composite, doctors use plastic instruments.

- **Surgical instruments**: Instruments used depend on the type of oral surgery being performed. The main instruments used in extraction procedures are listed. Other specific instruments and supplies such as chisels, hemostats, needle holders, and suture materials might also be used.

  (1) **Surgical forceps**: Also called *extracting forceps*. These are used for extracting teeth. There are many different types, one for each type of tooth to be extracted (**Figure 19–38**).

  (2) **Periosteal elevators**: Used for lifting the mucous membrane and tissue covering the bone. It is a double-ended instrument with a blade at each end (**Figure 19–39**).

  (3) **Root (extraction) elevator**: Used to loosen the tooth out of its socket prior to being removed with forceps. There are various types, shapes, and sizes (**Figure 19–40**).

  (4) **Root-tip pick**: Used to remove small tips from a socket such as a root tip or piece of bone. There are straight and contra-angled versions (**Figure 19–41**).

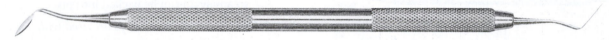

FIGURE 19–34 Hollenback carver. Courtesy of Hu-Friedy Mfg., Co.,Inc.

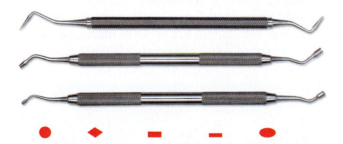

FIGURE 19–35 Types of condenser-pluggers with different shaped ends. Courtesy of Hu-Friedy Mfg., Co.,Inc.

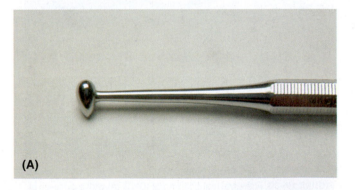

(A)

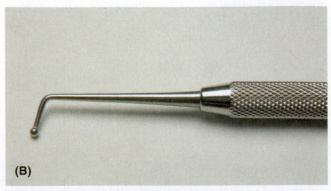

(B)

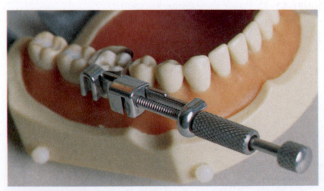

FIGURE 19–36 Matrix retainer and band.

FIGURE 19–37 (A) Oval burnisher. (B) Ball burnisher.

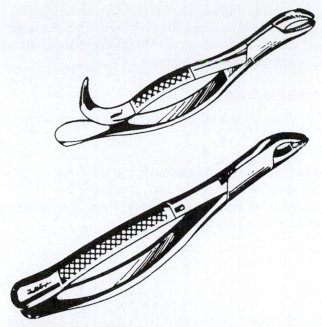

FIGURE 19–38 Surgical forceps. Courtesy Miltex Instrument Co., Inc., Lake Success, NY

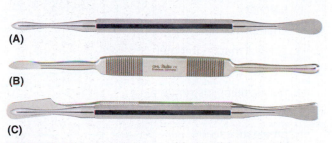

(A)

(B)

(C)

FIGURE 19–39 Periosteal elevators: (A) MOLT, (B) OHL, and (C) Pritchard elevator. Permission granted by Integra Miltex, a business of Integra Life-Sciences Corporation, Plainsboro, New Jersey, USA

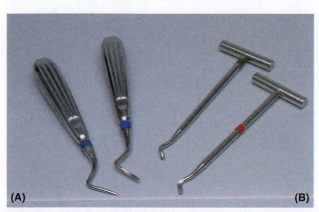

(A)   **(B)**

FIGURE 19–40 Root (extraction) elevators: (A) apical and (B) Potts or T-handled.

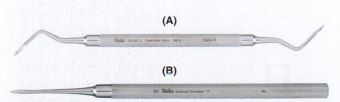

(A)

(B)

FIGURE 19–41 Root-tip picks (A) double ended and (B) straight. Permission granted by Integra Miltex, a business of Integra Life-Sciences Corporation, Plainsboro, New Jersey, USA

(5) **Rongeur forceps**: Used to trim or cut bone tissue. The tips of the forceps may be round or square with a tough sharp blade that extends around both sides and the end of the tips (**Figure 19–42**).

(6) **Lancet**: Used to lance and incise tissue. A lancet is similar to a scalpel and blade.

(7) **Bone or surgical chisels**: Used for cutting bone structure in oral surgery. Some are used by hand, others require the use of a surgical mallet (**Figure 19–43**).

When setting up trays for various procedures, it is important to remember to place only items that are usually needed. Setting the tray with instruments and supplies that are needed only occasionally can decrease efficiency and crowd all the items. Items usually kept in the cart or drawers include the drape and clips, dental bases and cements, restorative materials, extra cotton products or dressings, and instruments used for specific problems or procedures. Some instruments and supplies are placed on almost all trays. Examples include the mouth mirror, cotton pliers, explorer, cotton pellets, cotton rolls, and gauze sponges.

Trays can be set up for a variety of dental procedures. Four examples of tray setups include:

- **Prophylactic, or general examination, tray**: This type of tray is used for basic examination and cleaning of the teeth. Supplies and instruments placed on the tray include scalers; a periodontal probe for an adult; prophylactic cups, paste, and brushes; and fluoride treatment supplies.

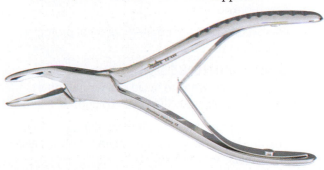

FIGURE 19–42 Rongeur forceps. Permission granted by Integra Miltex, a business of Integra Life-Sciences Corporation, Plainsboro, New Jersey, USA

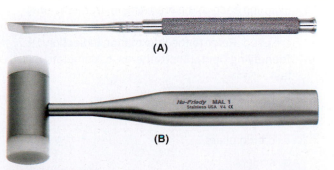

(A)

(B)

FIGURE 19–43 (A) Bone or surgical chisel and (B) mallet. Courtesy of Hu-Friedy Mfg., LLC

- **Amalgam restoration tray**: This type of tray is used for an amalgam restoration procedure. Instruments placed on the tray include amalgam carriers, condenser-pluggers, and carvers.

- **Composite, or esthetic, restoration tray**: This type of tray is used for the placement of a composite restoration. Special composite instruments such as a fine brush and plastic instruments are placed on this tray.

- **Surgical extraction tray**: This type of tray is used for extraction, or removal, of teeth. Instruments and supplies vary depending on the type of extraction. In most cases, however, surgical instruments such as extracting forceps, root elevators, root-tip picks, periosteal elevators, Rongeur forceps, lancets, bone chisels, and a needle holder with suture materials are placed on the tray.

checkpoint

1. What are four (4) items that are on almost all dental trays?

PRACTICE: Go to the workbook and complete the assignment sheet for 19:7, Identifying Dental Instruments and Preparing Dental Trays. Then return and continue with the procedure.

Procedure 19:7

Identifying Dental Instruments and Preparing Dental Trays

Equipment and Supplies

Patient records; radiographs (X-rays); variety of instruments; cotton pellets and rolls; tray for supplies and instruments; cements; mixing pads; drape and clips; carts with handpieces; assorted supplies and equipment for specific procedures; personal protective equipment (PPE) including gloves, gown, mask, and eye shield

Procedure

1. Assemble equipment.

2. Wash hands. Put on required personal protective equipment (PPE).

    CAUTION: Observe standard precautions at all times to avoid contamination by saliva, body fluids, and blood.

3. Read the information sections on dental instruments, amalgam, composite, cements, and anesthesia.

4. Place the dental tray in a convenient location. Make sure the tray is clean.

5. Examine each of the following instruments until you are able to identify them and state why they are used. Refer to the information in Section 19:7, Identifying Dental Instruments, to complete this task.

   a. mouth mirror

   b. explorers

   c. cotton pliers

   d. scalers

   e. periodontal probe

   f. spoons

   g. hoes

   h. hatchet

   i. enamel hatchet

   j. gingival margin trimmer

   k. cleoid-discoid carver

   l. plastic filling instrument

   m. amalgam carrier

   n. amalgam carvers

   o. condenser-plugger

   p. matrix retainer and band

   q. burnisher

   r. plastic composite instruments

   s. surgical forceps

   t. periosteal elevator

   u. root (extraction) elevator

   v. root-tip pick

   w. Rongeur forceps

   x. lancet

   y. bone or surgical chisel and mallet

6. Set up trays for the following procedures: prophylactic cleaning and oral examination, amalgam restoration, composite restoration, and surgical extraction. Perform the following steps for each procedure and tray.

   a. Lay out the general patient equipment, including records, radiographs (X-rays), drape, clips, and other similar items.

       NOTE: If electronic health records (EHRs) are used, open the patient's record on the computer so it is available for the doctor to review.

b. Review the parts of the carts. Think about which handpieces will be used. Make sure all are in good working condition.

c. Set the tray with the main instruments to be used. Place these instruments in the order of use. Refer to references and information sections to be sure you include all required instruments. Make sure that the basic instruments (mirror, explorer, cotton pliers) are on the trayd.

d. Have the correct dental cements or bases available for any procedure that might involve the use of these materials. Do not forget to have mixing pads and instruments ready for use.

e. Think about additional equipment that might be used. Add these to the tray. Such items might include prophy paste, fluoride trays, matrix bands, wooden wedges, finishing strips, and articulation paper.

f. Add additional equipment that might be necessary. Examples might include the amalgamator and special handpieces.

g. Add needed supplies. These might include cotton pellets, rolls, gauze, and other similar items.

7. Review all of the equipment and supplies you have prepared for each of the four procedures (**Figure 19–44**). Read the steps of each procedure and make sure that you have the equipment and materials the doctor will require for each.

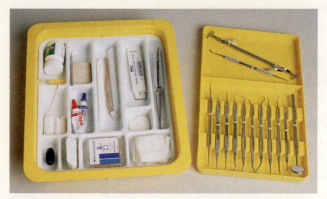

FIGURE 19–44 Always double-check to make sure all required instruments and supplies are on the tray before starting any dental procedure.

8. Remember that equipment, supplies, and instruments used vary from doctor to doctor. It is the dental assistant's responsibility to know the doctor's preferences and to prepare these things for use.

9. Replace all equipment.

10. Remove PPE. Wash hands.

PRACTICE: Go to the workbook and use the evaluation sheet for 19:7, Identifying Dental Instruments and Preparing Dental Trays, to practice this procedure. When you believe you have mastered this skill, sign the sheet and give it to your instructor for further action.

FINAL EVALUATION: Using the criteria listed on the evaluation sheet, your instructor will grade your performance.

Check

19:8 POSITIONING A PATIENT IN THE DENTAL CHAIR

Positioning a patient in the dental chair is one of the responsibilities of a dental assistant. Correct positioning of a patient in the dental chair allows the doctor to complete dental procedures efficiently. In four-handed dentistry, the patient is placed in a supine, or lying-down, position.

Safety

Before a patient gets in or out of the chair, the chair must be locked in the upright position. The patient could be injured if the chair moves. Always check the chair to be sure it is in a locked position before seating a patient or before assisting a patient out of the chair.

The patient's head rests on the upper, narrow headrest of the chair. Positioning the patient's head in this narrow section of the chair allows the doctor and the dental assistant closer access to the oral cavity. Short adults and children must be positioned in the chair starting with correct placement of the head first.

The chair must be elevated from the floor to the height that will allow both the doctor to be seated comfortably near the chair and the patient's head to be above the doctor's lap.

After a patient has been seated in the chair, it is best to recline the chair slowly. Lowering a patient to a supine position quickly can cause dizziness, discomfort, and fear in some patients. It is best to lower the chair part way, pause to allow the patient time to adjust to the change in position, and then finish lowering the chair. The chair should recline until the patient is lying almost flat. An imaginary line from the patient's chin to the patient's ankles should be parallel to the floor. The patient's nose and knees should be at about the same level.

Explain all chair movements to the patient. Inform the patient before elevating or lowering the chair, before reclining the back of the chair, and before returning the patient to a sitting position. Unexpected movements can frighten the patient.

Before any dental procedure is performed, a protective drape is placed over the patient's chest. This protects the patient's clothing during the procedure. Most drapes have a paper side and a plastic side. The plastic side is placed against the patient's clothing; the paper side is placed facing up. In this way, the paper absorbs moisture and the plastic keeps moisture from soaking through to the patient's clothing.

The patient should also be given safety glasses to wear during the procedure. This protects the patient's eyes from spray and fluids that might be present during a dental procedure. After the procedure is complete, the safety glasses must be cleaned and disinfected before being used on another patient.

After the patient is in the correct position, the light should be positioned 30–50 inches from the oral cavity, or mouth. Care must be taken to ensure that the light illuminates the mouth but does not shine in the patient's eyes.

When positioning a patient in the dental chair, it is important to show a friendly and pleasant attitude toward the patient. Make the patient feel welcome and allow the patient to talk about their interests. Knowledge about the patient allows the dental assistant to ask questions such as, "How was your vacation?" or "How did your basketball team do in the last game?" Displaying an interest in patients makes them more at ease and less apprehensive. When a procedure is complete, a comment such as, "It was good to see you again, Mrs. Brown" or, "I hope you enjoy your first year at college" is much better than, "You're done for today."

checkpoint

1. Before a patient gets in or out of the chair, it must be locked in what position?

PRACTICE: Go to the workbook and complete the assignment sheet for 19:8, Positioning a Patient in the Dental Chair. Then return and continue with the procedure.

Procedure 19:8

Positioning a Patient in the Dental Chair

Equipment and Supplies

Dental chair and light; headrest cover; drape; alligator clips; protective barriers for dental light; personal protective equipment (PPE) including gown, gloves, mask, and protective eyewear; protective eyewear for the patient; disinfectant solution; gauze sponges

Procedure

1. Wash hands.

2. Assemble equipment. Use a disposable plastic cover to cover the headrest and/or top of the chair. Use protective barriers, such as commercial covers, plastic wrap, or aluminum foil to cover the handles and/or switches of the dental light, the handpieces, and the tubings. Use plastic cloths to cover the tops of dental carts.

3. Introduce yourself. Identify the patient. Explain the procedure.

    NOTE: Patients are often apprehensive.

4. Lock the chair to prevent movement of the chair.

    CAUTION: Double-check the lock to prevent injury to the patient.

5. Assist the patient into the chair as needed.

6. Adjust the headrest for comfort and correct position.

7. Use the alligator clips to secure the drape around the patient's neck and shoulders. Place the plastic side of the drape against the patient's clothing (**Figure 19–45**).

   NOTE: The drape can also be applied later, when the patient is in a reclining position.

   NOTE: In some offices, the patient's health history is updated at this time.

8. Give the patient safety glasses to wear during the procedure.

9. Use the elevation control to raise the chair to the height desired by the doctor. This is usually about 8–12 inches above the seat of the doctor's chair.

    NOTE: Tell the patient you are raising the chair before doing so.

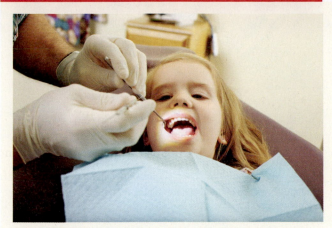

FIGURE 19–45 A protective drape is used to protect the patient's clothing during dental procedures. © iStock.com/eyecrave

10. Use the backward control to place the patient in the correct reclining position. Pause after reclining the patient halfway to allow the patient to adjust to the change in position. When the patient is fully reclined, the patient's nose and knees should be at about the same level.

NOTE: Inform the patient before performing any movement of the chair. Observe the patient closely for signs of respiratory distress.

11. Position the light 30–50 inches from the oral cavity. Leave the light off until the doctor is ready to work on the patient.

    NOTE: Make sure the light does *not* shine in the patient's eyes.

12. Put on gloves, a gown (if not wearing protective clothing), a mask, and protective eyewear before assisting the doctor with any dental procedure that may result in the splashing of saliva, blood, or body fluids.

CAUTION: Observe all standard precautions while assisting with dental procedures.

13. When the doctor is done, lock the chair. Check to be sure it does not move. Position the dental light out of the patient's way.

14. Warn the patient *not* to get out of the chair until it has stopped moving.

15. Use the reset button to lower the chair and to return it to an upright position. Remove the drape and place it in an infectious-waste container.

16. Help the patient out of the chair.

17. After the patient has left the area, remove the protective barriers from the light, dental chair, handpieces, tubing, and carts. Put the barriers in an infectious waste container. Use a disinfectant solution to wipe all contaminated areas. Then, respray all areas, leave the disinfectant in place for the required amount of time, and rewipe the areas.

18. Clean and prepare all instruments and handpieces for sterilization. Replace all equipment.

19. Remove personal protective equipment. Wash hands thoroughly.

PRACTICE: Go to the workbook and use the evaluation sheet for 19:8, Positioning a Patient in the Dental Chair, to practice this procedure. When you believe you have mastered this skill, sign the sheet and give it to your instructor for further action.

FINAL EVALUATION: Using the criteria listed on the evaluation sheet, your instructor will grade your performance.

19:9 DEMONSTRATING BRUSHING AND FLOSSING TECHNIQUES

Using correct brushing and flossing techniques is essential to prevent dental disease. Teaching the patient the correct methods to use is part of the responsibility of a dental assistant.

Correct brushing and flossing are important parts of prophylactic (preventive) care. Purposes include:

- Prevention of decay, or **carious lesions (caries)**
- Removal of plaque; **plaque** is a thin, tenacious, filmlike deposit that adheres to the teeth and can lead to decay; plaque contains microorganisms and a protein substance
- Prevention of **halitosis** (bad breath)

The importance of proper brushing and flossing techniques must be stressed to the patient. Demonstrations should be given to all patients.

Talk slowly and clearly. Repeat and stress important points. After the demonstration is complete, ask the patient to demonstrate the technique (**Figure 19–46**). This is a good method to determine whether the patient understands the main points.

The brushing technique taught will depend on the preference of the doctor. A common technique is the Bass method. The brush is placed at a 45-degree angle to the gumline, and then a vibrating motion is used.

Five surfaces on each tooth must be cleaned:

- **Chewing or biting surface**: the top surfaces of the teeth

- **Facial surface**: the tooth side that faces the inside of the lips and cheeks; facial surfaces are seen from the front, as in a smile

- **Lingual surface**: the tooth side nearest the tongue

- **Side, or interproximal, surfaces**: the surfaces located between the teeth; there are two on each tooth; floss is used to clean these surfaces because a brush cannot get between the teeth, and the bristles do not provide enough coverage

Toothbrushes vary in size, shape, and texture of the bristles. A soft-bristled brush is usually recommended. It will not injure the gum, or gingival tissue. The head of the brush should be the correct size and fit easily into the mouth. Brushes should be discarded when the bristles are frayed or worn. Many kinds of mechanical toothbrushes powered by electricity and/or batteries are also available. They are very effective in cleaning the teeth if used correctly. They can be beneficial for people with limited function of the hands and arms, such as people with arthritis.

Toothpastes or dentifrices are used to clean the teeth and provide a pleasant taste. Many doctors recommend toothpaste with fluoride. The American Dental Association supports the use of fluoride as an aid in preventing decay. Toothpastes with tartar control help prevent the hard deposits that accumulate on the teeth.

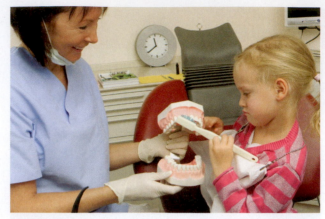

FIGURE 19–46 Asking the patient to demonstrate the brushing technique is a good method of determining that the main points have been understood. © iStock.com/Hightower_NRW

Toothpastes with whitening agents help remove stains from teeth. The type of toothpaste recommended to the patient depends on the needs of the patient and the doctor's preference.

Dental floss is used to remove plaque and bacteria from the side surfaces of the teeth. Floss is available in waxed and unwaxed types. The type suggested to the patient depends on the doctor's preference. Both types are effective if used correctly. Floss is also available in different colors and flavors. The colors and flavors do not improve the action of the floss, but they may motivate the patient to floss more frequently.

checkpoint

| **1.** What is halitosis?

PRACTICE: Go to the workbook and complete the assignment sheet for 19:9, Demonstrating Brushing and Flossing Techniques. Then return and continue with the procedures.

Procedure 19:9A

Demonstrating Brushing Technique

Equipment and Supplies

Soft-textured toothbrush; demonstration model of teeth; personal protective equipment (gloves, gown, face mask, and eye protection)

Procedure

1. Assemble equipment.

2. Wash hands. Put on personal protective equipment (PPE).

 CAUTION: Observe standard precautions at all times to avoid contamination by saliva, body fluids, and blood.

3. Introduce yourself. Identify the patient.

4. Explain the importance of correctly brushing the teeth. Stress that proper brushing helps prevent decay and removes plaque, a soft deposit leading to decay. Also stress that teeth should be brushed immediately after eating.

5. Suggest the use of a soft-textured brush to prevent gum damage.

   NOTE: If the doctor has recommended another type of toothbrush, follow the doctor's preference.

6. Use a toothbrush and demonstration model of teeth to show the patient how to brush the teeth.

7. Tell the patient to begin brushing in one area of the mouth and then to systematically brush each tooth. Suggest starting on the facial surfaces of the right, rear teeth.

8. Place the brush at a 45-degree angle to the gumline (**Figure 19–47A**).

9. Rotate the brush slightly and gently push the bristles between the teeth.

10. Use a very short, back-and-forth, light vibrating movement to clean the teeth.

11. Move the brush to the next group of teeth. Repeat steps 8–10. Continue until the facial surfaces of all the teeth are clean.

12. Repeat steps 8–10 on the lingual, or tongue, surfaces of the teeth. To brush the lingual surfaces of the front, or anterior, teeth, place the brush in a vertical position (**Figure 19–47B**).

13. Brush the biting surfaces of all teeth. Place the brush on the surfaces. Use a very short, vibrating motion (**Figure 19–47C**). Move the brush to the next area. Repeat until all biting surfaces are clean.

14. Stress to the patient that the areas between the teeth must be cleaned with floss.

15. Ask whether the patient has any questions. Make sure the patient understands the technique to use.

     NOTE: Asking the patient to demonstrate the technique is a good method of determining whether the main points have been understood.

    Comm

16. Clean and replace all equipment.

17. Remove PPE. Wash hands.

PRACTICE: Go to the workbook and use the evaluation sheet for 19:9A, Demonstrating Brushing Technique, to practice this procedure. When you believe you have mastered this skill, sign the sheet and give it to your instructor for further action.

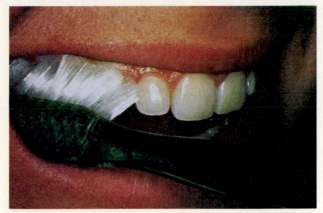

FIGURE 19–47A Place the brush at a 45-degree angle to the gumline.

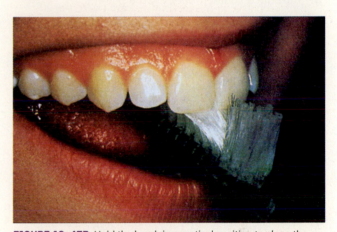

FIGURE 19–47B Hold the brush in a vertical position to clean the lingual, or tongue, surfaces of the anterior teeth.

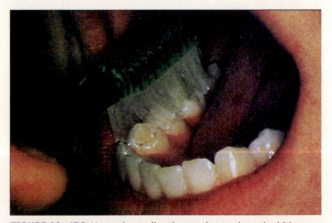

FIGURE 19–47C Use a short, vibrating motion to clean the biting surfaces of the teeth.

 FINAL EVALUATION: Using the criteria listed on the evaluation sheet, your instructor will grade your performance.

Check

Demonstrating Flossing Technique

Equipment and Supplies

Dental floss; demonstration model of teeth; personal protective equipment (gloves, gown, face mask, and eye protection)

Procedure

1. Assemble equipment.

2. Wash hands. Put on personal protective equipment (PPE).

   Precaution

   CAUTION: Observe standard precautions at all times to avoid contamination by saliva, body fluids, and blood.

3. Introduce yourself. Identify the patient.

4.
   Comm

   Explain the importance of flossing. Stress that flossing is the way to remove food and plaque from between the teeth. Mention that this is an area where decay often begins because brushing is not enough. A toothbrush cannot clean these areas.

5. Use dental floss and a demonstration model of the teeth to show the patient how to floss the teeth.

6. Remove 12–18 inches of floss from the spool.

   NOTE: Floss is waxed or unwaxed. The type recommended depends on the doctor's preference.

7. Wrap the floss around the middle fingers of both hands. This anchors the floss. As floss is used, unroll new floss from the middle finger of one hand and wrap used floss around the middle finger of the opposite hand.

8. To clean the maxillary (upper) teeth, wrap the floss around the index finger of one hand and the thumb of the other hand or the two thumbs (**Figure 19–48A**). To clean the mandibular (lower) teeth, use the index fingers of both hands.

   NOTE: Floss still remains anchored on middle fingers.

9. Keep the fingers and thumb approximately 1–2 inches apart. This is the length of floss to be used.

10. Gently insert the floss between the teeth. Do not snap the floss into the gums.

    Safety

    CAUTION: Snapping the floss into the gums can injure the gingival tissue.

11. Gently slide the floss into the space between the gum and tooth. Stop when you feel resistance. Curve the floss into a C-shape around the side of the tooth (**Figure 19–48B**).

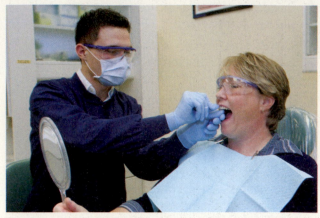

FIGURE 19–48A To floss maxillary teeth, wrap the floss around the index finger of one hand and the thumb of the other hand, or use both thumbs.

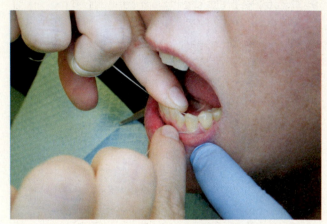

FIGURE 19–48B After curving the floss into a C-shape around the side of the tooth, use an up-and-down motion to clean the side.

12. Hold the floss tightly against the tooth and move the floss away from the gum by scraping the floss up and down against the side of the tooth to remove plaque and debris.

    Safety

    CAUTION: A side-to-side or front-to-back motion could cut the gums.

13. Repeat steps 10–12 until both sides of every tooth in the mouth have been flossed. Move the floss on the fingers as it becomes soiled or after finishing the side of a tooth. Use fresh floss at all times.

14. Warn the patient that some bleeding and soreness may occur the first few times teeth are flossed. If bleeding or soreness continues, flossing should be stopped and the doctor notified.

15. Make sure the patient understands the procedure.

    Comm

    NOTE: Asking the patient to demonstrate the technique is a good way to determine whether the main points have been understood.

16. Clean and replace all equipment.
17. Remove PPE. Wash hands.

PRACTICE: Go to the workbook and use the evaluation sheet for 19:9B, Demonstrating Flossing Technique, to practice this procedure. When you

believe you have mastered this skill, sign the sheet and give it to your instructor for further action.

Check

FINAL EVALUATION: Using the criteria listed on the evaluation sheet, your instructor will grade your performance.

19:10 TAKING IMPRESSIONS AND POURING MODELS

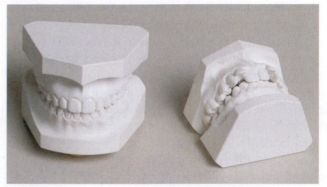

FIGURE 19–50 A model is a positive reproduction of the teeth that is used for the construction of dentures, partials, or other prosthetics.

INTRODUCTION

The dental assistant may prepare a wide variety of impression and model materials for the doctor. This section provides basic facts about the purposes and types of some of these materials.

An **impression** is a negative reproduction of a tooth, several teeth, or the dental arch (**Figure 19–49**). It is taken to form a model of the area for restorative treatment that will take place outside of the mouth. Common materials used to take impressions are alginate, polysulfide, and the silicones such as polysiloxane or polyvinylsiloxane.

A **model**, also called a *cast*, is a positive reproduction of the arches or teeth that is created from the negative impression (**Figure 19–50**). Common materials used for models are plaster or stone. A model serves as the basis for construction of dentures, partials, or other prosthetics

for the mouth. A model is also used for making orthodontic appliances, mouth guards, and custom trays used to take impressions of a patient's teeth.

ALGINATE

Alginate is an *irreversible hydrocolloid* impression material. It cannot be returned from a gel to its original state. Advantages include:

- It is simple and economical to use.
- Setting time can be controlled by the water temperature.
- It has adequate strength for an accurate impression.
- It yields an adequate basic reproduction of detail.
- It can be used for impressions of the teeth and/or tissue.
- It is easily removed from tissues and instruments during cleaning.

Disadvantages include:

- It is not good for final impressions of cavity preparations or small areas requiring fine detail, such as final impressions for crowns or bridges.
- It changes in dimension by shrinking as it loses water content and must be poured immediately for an accurate duplication.
- It tears or breaks easily when set.

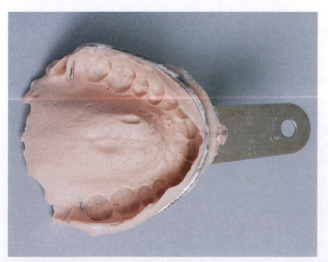

FIGURE 19–49 An impression is a negative reproduction of a tooth, several teeth, or a dental arch.

Alginate powder is supplied as a fast set (type I) or regular set (type II), flavored or unflavored, and/or regular or heavy-bodied material. Some alginates have an antimicrobial agent added to prevent the growth of microorganisms in the impression. Some are powder-free to reduce inhalation of the dry material.

Proper measuring techniques are essential to obtain the correct set. Always follow the manufacturer's directions. Some manufacturers require that the alginate powder be fluffed (shake the can lightly with the lid on) before being put in the powder scoop. Others require packing the powder into the scoop. It is also essential to measure the water carefully and to use the measuring container provided by the manufacturer. Inaccurate measurements of the powder and water can affect the setting time, strength, and accuracy of the final impression. Alginate material should be stored in a cool, dry place to avoid deterioration. The lid should be replaced immediately after the material is used to prevent moisture contamination.

A new form of premixed alginate with a dispensing unit may also be used. The premixed alginate is loaded into the dispensing unit (**Figure 19–51**). A disposable tip is attached to the end of the unit and the alginate is dispensed directly into the impression tray. This type of alginate is more expensive, so it is not used as frequently as powdered alginate.

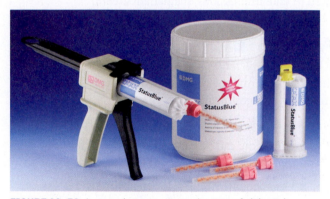

FIGURE 19–51 A newer but more expensive type of alginate is premixed and can be dispensed directly into the impression tray.
Courtesy, DMG America

POLYSULFIDE

Polysulfide, also called *rubber-base*, is an *elastomeric* impression material that is elastic and rubbery in nature. It is supplied in two tubes of paste: a base and a catalyst (accelerator). Usually the two are mixed manually using a mixing pad and spatula. There are special cartridges of rubber base material that can be placed in an extruder gun. The extruder gun mixes the base and catalyst together and dispenses it directly into a tray and/or syringe.

Four types are produced. One is a light-bodied material for use in a syringe. A regular- or medium-bodied material is available for use in both syringes and trays. Heavy-bodied and extra heavy-bodied materials are used in trays. Frequently, two types are used together. A syringe is used to place light-bodied material into the area of the impression. Then, a custom tray filled with heavy-bodied or extra heavy-bodied material is placed into the mouth and over the light-bodied material to complete the impression.

Polysulfide materials can be used for any dental procedure that requires an impression. They are particularly good for use in cavity preparations that require fine detail, such as an impression taken prior to the construction of a crown. Polysulfide materials are not subject to dimension changes as much as are alginates. However, polysulfide materials should be poured promptly if possible, preferably within 1–2 hours after they are made. Disadvantages of polysulfide materials are the sulfur-like odor, taste, long setting-time (approximately 10 minutes), and the fact that they cause permanent stains on cloth and other materials.

SILICONES

Silicone impression materials include polysiloxane or polyvinylsiloxane. They are available in light-bodied, regular (medium)-bodied, and heavy-bodied versions. Silicones can be supplied in two tubes, a base and an accelerator (catalyst), which are mixed together manually. The most common type of silicones for impressions are cartridges of the base and accelerator, which are placed in a special mixing device called an *extruder*, or *automix gun* (**Figure 19–52A**). A disposable mixing tip is placed on the end of this gun, and as the pastes are expelled into the mixing tip, the accelerator (catalyst) and base are automatically mixed. The mixed material can be extruded directly into the impression tray (**Figure 19–52B**). Syringe-tipped mixing tubes can also be used, and the material can be placed directly on the area of the impression as it is expelled from the gun. This provides for easy cleanup after use.

Polysiloxane or polyvinylsiloxane materials are not affected by fluids in the oral cavity. This allows these materials to spread evenly over the impression area, creating a highly accurate impression. This impression retains its shape and size for a long period. Another important advantage is that these materials are odor-free and have a pleasant taste. One disadvantage is that latex gloves may inhibit the setting of these materials; thus, vinyl gloves must be worn while taking impressions. A second disadvantage is that they are more expensive than rubber-base or polysulfide impression materials.

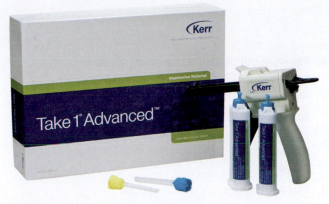

FIGURE 19–52A An extruder gun automatically mixes the cartridges of catalyst and base of polysiloxane or polyvinylsiloxane impression materials. *Courtesy of Kerr Corporation*

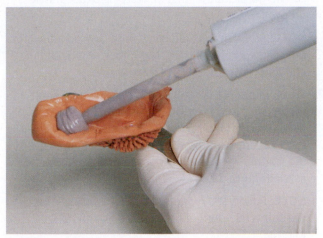

FIGURE 19–52B The mixed silicone can be extruded directly into the impression tray.

GYPSUM MATERIALS

There are two main gypsum products used to form models: plaster and stone. **Plaster** is the weaker of the two. It is used mainly where strength is not a critical factor, such as for study models and preliminary models. It is also a less expensive material. **Stone** is a more refined gypsum product than is plaster. It produces a stronger, more regular and uniform model. However, it is more expensive than plaster. Stone is used for making diagnostic models or casts and for any work requiring a high degree of strength and accuracy.

Basic principles for the use of plaster and stone include:

- Both products must be stored in a tightly closed container and in a cool, dry area. Moisture contamination of gypsum products leads to defective models or casts.

- Correct amounts of water and powder must be used. Usually, 50 milliliters (mL) of water is used

for 100 grams (g) of plaster; and 30 milliliters (mL) of water is used for 100 grams (g) of stone. If an insufficient amount of water is used, the mixture will be too thick and crumbly to flow into the impression. If too much water is used, the model will be weak, set slowly, and develop air bubbles that destroy the effectiveness of the model. It is important to read and follow the manufacturer's directions.

- Impressions should be clean and dry before the models or casts are poured. Drying by blotting is preferred. Drying with an air blast can cause dehydration or shrinkage of the impression material, especially of alginate.

- The use of cold water when mixing plaster provides the greatest amount of working time. When you are learning how to prepare the plaster mix, use the coldest water available to provide more time.

- Air bubbles in the mix can ruin a model. Stir and spatulate the mix in such a way that as little air as possible enters the mix. To remove as many air bubbles as possible, always place the bowl on a vibrator before pouring.

 Precaution Because contact with saliva, body fluids, and/or blood is very possible while taking impressions and pouring models, the Centers for Disease Control and Prevention (CDC) has established guidelines for infection control. Gloves, a gown (or protective clothing), face mask, and eye protection must be worn at all times. Hands must be washed immediately after removing gloves at the end of the procedure. All completed impressions must be rinsed gently for at least 30 seconds with room temperature tap water to remove any mouth debris. The impression must then be disinfected with a solution such as 10-percent sodium hypochlorite (household bleach), iodophor, glutaraldehyde, or phenylphenol. All mixing containers, spatulas, and impression trays must be disinfected or sterilized prior to being used for another patient. Standard precautions must be followed at all times while taking impressions and pouring models.

checkpoint

1. What is another word for a dental model?

2. What is an extruder?

PRACTICE: Go to the workbook and complete the assignment sheet for 19:10, Taking Impressions and Pouring Models. Then return and continue with the procedures.

Preparing Alginate

Equipment and Supplies

Alginate powder; large, rubber mixing bowl or disposable mixing bowl; spatula; powder scoop and water-measuring cup provided by the manufacturer; room-temperature water; denture; impression trays; disinfectant solution or spray; personal protective equipment (PPE)

Procedure

1. Assemble equipment. Select an impression tray to fit the denture.

   NOTE: If an impression is being made of the patient's mouth, the doctor usually measures and selects the impression tray to be used.

2. Wash hands. Put on personal protective equipment (PPE).

    CAUTION: The denture or the mouth will contain saliva, body fluids, and even blood at times. Standard precautions must be observed while taking an impression of the mouth.

   Precaution

3. Make sure all equipment, especially the bowl and spatula, are clean.

   NOTE: Some dental offices use disposable mixing bowls and spatulas. This eliminates the need to disinfect or sterilize the bowl and spatula after use.

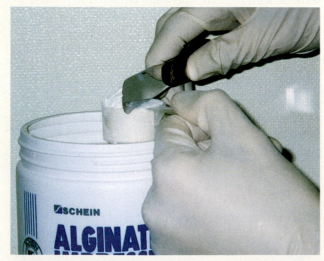

FIGURE 19–53A Use the spatula to level the scoop of alginate powder.

4. Measure out the correct amount of room-temperature (70°F or 21°C) water using the manufacturer's measuring vial.

   NOTE: Follow the manufacturer's directions for the correct amount of water. Usually, one measure of water is used with one scoop or envelope of powder.

5. Place the water in the mixing bowl.

6. Fluff the powder in the container by rolling the container from side to side several times if directed to do so by the manufacturer. Open the lid cautiously to avoid inhaling the powder, which can be hazardous if inhaled. Wearing a face mask reduces this risk.

   NOTE: Some brands of alginate are packed into the scoop and not fluffed. It is important to read and follow manufacturer's instructions.

7. Measure out the correct amount of powder using the powder scoop provided by the manufacturer. Fill the scoop with powder. Tap the top of the scoop lightly with the spatula to fill air voids. With the spatula, level the powder at the top of the scoop (**Figure 19–53A**).

   NOTE: Follow the manufacturer's instructions for the correct amount of powder. A basic guide is as follows:

   Three scoops: large maxillary impression

   Two scoops: medium maxillary or any mandibular impression

   One scoop: partial impression

8. Add the measured powder to the water in the bowl.

9. Use a circular motion to press the spatula against the side of the bowl and to mix all of the powder with the water.

10. Use a stropping (beating or pressing) action with the spatula to press the mix against the side of the bowl (**Figure 19–53B**). Rotate the bowl as you mix. This makes the mix creamy and smooth and removes air bubbles.

    NOTE: Mixing devices are available for mixing alginate. The powder and water are placed in the bowl on the device. The assistant uses slight pressure to hold a spatula against the side of the bowl and turns the device on. The device spins the bowl at approximately 300 times per minute to create a bubble-free mixture of alginate.

11. Mixing should be completed within 1 minute for regular-set and 30–45 seconds for fast-set alginate.

12. The impression tray can be sprayed with a special lubricant spray before being filled. This makes it easier to remove the alginate at the end of the procedure (**Figure 19–53C**). Some impression trays require the use of an adhesive. Follow manufacturer's instructions provided with the impression trays.

13. Fill the impression tray with the mix starting with the back of the tray and moving to the anterior portion of the tray (**Figure 19–53D**). Smooth the surface with a wet finger or wet spatula (**Figure 19–53E**). Remove any excess material from the back of the tray.

> **CAUTION:** Regular-set alginate mix sets in 2–4 minutes, and fast-set alginate sets in 1–2 minutes, so work quickly.
> *Safety*

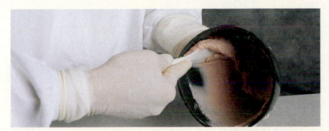

FIGURE 19–53B Use a stropping action to press the mix against the side of the bowl.

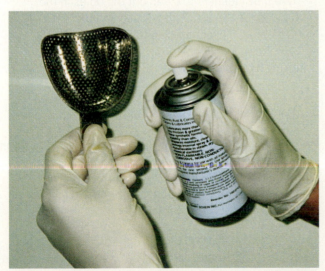

FIGURE 19–53C Before using the impression tray, spray it with lubricant to make it easier to remove the alginate material from the tray when the procedure is complete.

NOTE: Make sure the impression tray is the correct size.

14. Hand the filled impression tray to the doctor. Pass the tray handle first. The doctor will insert the tray into the patient's mouth and hold the tray in place until the alginate sets.

> **NOTE:** In some states, a dental assistant may be allowed to take a preliminary impression of a patient's dentition. Check the legal requirements for your state.
> *Safety*

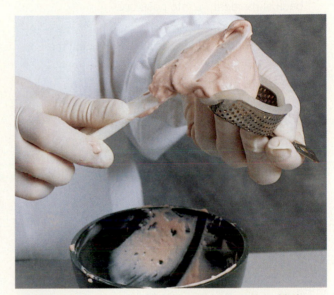

FIGURE 19–53D Place the alginate into the tray starting with the back of the tray and pushing the material to the front of the tray.

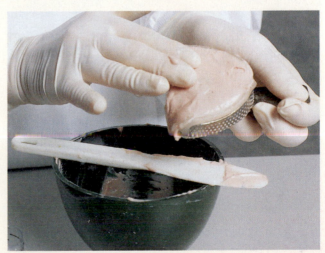

FIGURE 19–53E Smooth the surface of the alginate with a wet finger or spatula.

(continues)

15. To take an impression from a denture, soak the denture in water first.

NOTE: This allows the denture to more readily come out of the alginate.

Precaution **CAUTION:** Gloves should be worn while handling any denture to avoid contamination from saliva or fluids from the mouth.

16. Shake the excess water from the denture. Place it in position on the alginate. Press the anterior teeth of the denture into place. Then, press the back of the denture into position.

CAUTION: Do not press too hard or the denture will go completely through the alginate.
Safety

17. Use steady pressure with the index finger and the middle finger to hold the denture in place (**Figure 19–53F**). Hold for at least 1 minute.

18. After the alginate has set completely (usually in 2–4 minutes), check it for smoothness. If it is smooth and does *not* stick to your fingers, it is ready.

19. Gently remove the denture from the alginate.

NOTE: A very slight side-to-side motion often releases the denture.

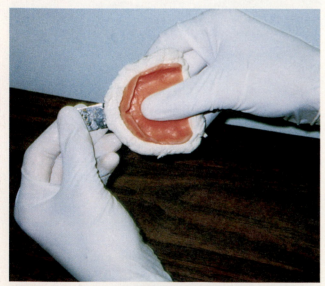

FIGURE 19–53F Use steady pressure to hold the denture in the alginate.

20. Use room-temperature tap water to gently rinse the impression for at least 30 seconds. Spray the impression with a disinfecting solution to prevent contamination from saliva, blood, or mouth fluids that may be present on the impression.

21. Pour the model as quickly as possible, preferably within 20 minutes. If you are unable to immediately pour the model, wrap the alginate impression in a wet paper towel. Place the towel-wrapped impression in a plastic bag or covered air-tight container to maintain 100 percent humidity. Soaking an impression in a bowl of water is not recommended. Label the bag or container with the patient's name and date.

CAUTION: The alginate will shrink almost immediately if left to air-dry, and this shrinkage leads to an inaccurate model.
Safety

22. Clean the bowl and spatula. Place all excess alginate in a trash container. *Never* pour alginate into the sink because it will clog the drain. The bowl and spatula must be disinfected or sterilized. Some offices use disposable bowls and spatulas. These are discarded in an infectious-waste container.

23. To clean the impression tray, remove the alginate. Discard all alginate in a trash container. Use pipe cleaners to clean out the holes in the tray. Scrub the tray with a brush and place it in the ultrasonic unit for cleaning. Sterilize the tray according to manufacturer's instructions prior to using it on another patient.

24. Replace all equipment.

25. Remove PPE. Wash hands thoroughly.

PRACTICE: Go to the workbook and use the evaluation sheet for 19:10A, Preparing Alginate, to practice this procedure. When you believe you have mastered this skill, sign the sheet and give it to your instructor for further action.

Check **FINAL EVALUATION:** Using the criteria listed on the evaluation sheet, your instructor will grade your performance.

Preparing Polysulfide

Equipment and Supplies

Tubes of accelerator and base polysulfide materials, paper mixing pad (coated), metal spatula, impression tray, adhesive, syringe, tip, paper to make funnel, cleaning brush, disinfecting solution or spray, personal protective equipment (PPE)

Procedure

1. Assemble equipment.

2. Wash hands. Put on personal protective equipment (PPE).

    CAUTION: The mouth will contain saliva, body fluids, and even blood at times. Standard precautions must be observed while taking an impression of the mouth.

3. Prepare tray and/or syringe, depending on which will be used. Use heavy-bodied polysulfide material for a tray and light-bodied polysulfide material for a syringe.

   a. To prepare the impression tray, apply adhesive over the entire surface of the tray if directed to do so by the manufacturer. Allow the adhesive to dry.

   b. To prepare the syringe, put a plastic tip on the end of the syringe (**Figure 19–54A**). Make a paper funnel to load the syringe: fold the paper in half; then, fold a bias fold with one end ¼ inch and one end 1 inch (**Figure 19–54B**).

4. Mark the mixing pad with the length of strip desired (**Figure 19–54C**). The amount is determined by the impression to be taken.

5. Dispense an even line of accelerator material. Wipe off excess accelerator from the end of the tube and close the cap immediately.

   NOTE: Strip of accelerator must be smooth and even for correct proportions.

6. Dispense a strip of base material that is the same length as the accelerator. Wipe off excess base material from the end of the tube and close the cap immediately.

   NOTE: Strip will be wider in diameter, but it is the same weight.

   NOTE: Keep the materials separate (**Figure 19–54D**). If either tube is contaminated by the contents of the other tube, polymerization will occur and cause the entire contents of the tube to set or harden.

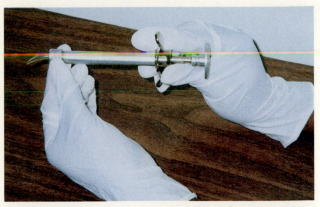

FIGURE 19–54A Put a plastic tip on the syringe before mixing the polysulfide material.

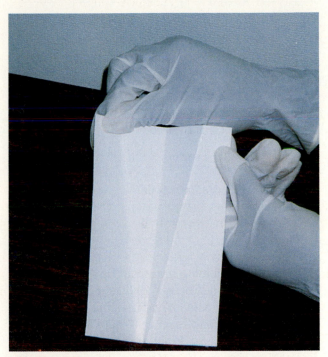

FIGURE 19–54B Fold a sheet of mixing-pad paper to make a paper funnel to load the polysulfide syringe.

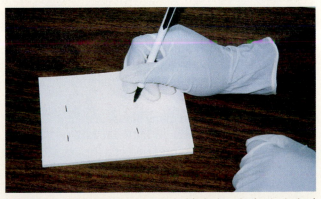

FIGURE 19–54C Mark the mixing pad with the length of strip desired.

(continues)

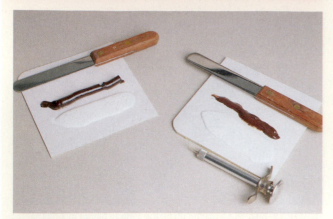

FIGURE 19–54D Keep the materials separate while dispensing equally long strips of the accelerator and base.

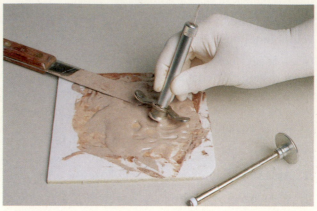

FIGURE 19–54E The syringe can also be filled by pushing the end of the barrel into the polysulfide material.

7. Use accelerator material to coat both sides of the metal spatula. Then, push the accelerator material into the base material.

8. Mix the accelerator and the base. Use smooth strokes and broad sweeps. Mix well until no strips or streaks of color are evident.

   NOTE: Mixing should be complete in 45–60 seconds.

9. Place the polysulfide mix in the prepared impression tray. If a syringe is to be used, first place the material in the paper funnel. Then, roll the funnel and squeeze the material into the syringe. Another way to fill the syringe with the polysulfide material is to remove the plastic tip and plunger. Use a repetitive stroking motion to push the end of the barrel into the material so that the material fills the inside of the syringe (**Figure 19–54E**). Replace the plastic tip and plunger so the syringe is ready to use.

10. If a syringe is used, pass this to the doctor first. The doctor uses the syringe to place the impression material directly in the area of the impression. The filled impression tray is then passed to the doctor for insertion into the patient's mouth. After insertion, the doctor or assistant must hold the tray in position for a minimum of six minutes until the material sets.

    CAUTION: In many states, a dental assistant is *not* permitted to take a polysulfide impression of a patient's dentition. The assistant's role is to prepare the material for the doctor.

    Legal

    NOTE: Work quickly before the impression sets. Curing time is usually 6–10 minutes.

11. After the impression tray is removed from the mouth, rinse it in room-temperature tap water for 30 seconds. Spray it with a disinfectant or soak it in a disinfecting solution.

     CAUTION: The impression may be contaminated with saliva, blood, and mouth fluids. Observe standard precautions.

    Precaution

12. A model can now be poured. It is best to pour a model as quickly as possible for the greatest degree of accuracy.

13. To clean the syringe, first squeeze out excess material. Then, soak the syringe in warm water for approximately 15 minutes. Soak the impression tray after the impression has been removed.

    NOTE: Soaking allows the material to set and makes it easy to peel off the tray, spatula, or syringe.

14. Use a brush to remove any material left on the spatula or tray or in the syringe. Clean the syringe, spatula, and tray in an ultrasonic unit. Follow manufacturer's instructions to sterilize the syringe, spatula, and tray.

    NOTE: The syringe tips are disposable and discarded after use. Disposable impression trays are sometimes used for polysulfide impressions.

15. Discard all excess polysulfide material and the mixing sheet in an infectious-waste container. Replace all equipment. Check to be sure the caps are closed tightly on both tubes of material.

16. Remove PPE. Wash hands thoroughly.

PRACTICE: Go to the workbook and use the evaluation sheet for 19:10B, Preparing Polysulfide, to practice this procedure. When you believe you have mastered this skill, sign the sheet and give it to your instructor for further action.

 Check

FINAL EVALUATION: Using the criteria listed on the evaluation sheet, your instructor will grade your performance.

Procedure 19:10C

Pouring a Plaster Model

Equipment and Supplies

Alginate or polysulfide impression; mixing bowl; hard spatula; plaster; metric graduate; scale; vibrator; glass slab or tile square; water; personal protective equipment (gloves, gown, face mask, and eye protection)

Procedure

1. Assemble equipment (**Figure 19–55A**).
2. Wash hands. Put on personal protective equipment (PPE).

    Precaution

   CAUTION: Observe standard precautions while working with an impression.

3. Prepare an alginate impression or use a polysulfide impression a doctor has prepared. Blot excess disinfecting solution from the impression.
4. Measure the water (**Figure 19–55B**). Use 50 milliliters (mL) or the amount recommended by the manufacturer. The water should be room temperature (70°F or 21°C) or cooler.

   NOTE: Colder water allows more working time.

5. Pour the water into the bowl.
6. Weigh the plaster powder. Use 100 grams (g).
7. Sift the powder into the bowl, allowing it to drop to the bottom of the bowl (**Figure 19–55C**). Allow the powder to absorb all of the water.
8. With the spatula, use a wiping and scraping motion to mix the powder and water.

   Safety **CAUTION:** Avoid using a whipping motion because this creates air bubbles.

9. Scrape the mix against the side of the bowl to remove any lumps.
10. Place the bowl on the vibrator platform. Hold the bowl in place to remove air bubbles from the mix (**Figure 19–55D**).
11. Test the mix by holding the bowl upside down. The mixture should not flow out of the bowl. Cut through the mixture with the spatula. The mix is the correct consistency if it does not run back together (**Figure 19–55E**).
12. Place a plastic bag over the vibrator. Place the impression on the covered vibrator platform.

    NOTE: The plastic cover protects the vibrator.

FIGURE 19–55A Equipment for pouring a plaster model.

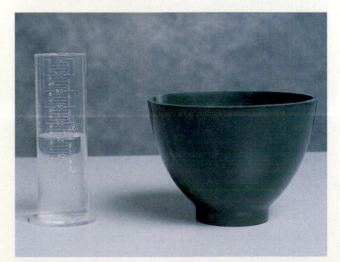

FIGURE 19–55B Measure 50 milliliters (mL) of water at 70°F (21°C) or cooler.

(continues)

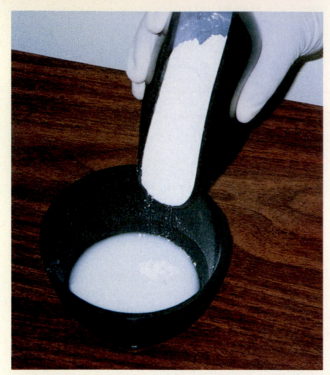

FIGURE 19–55C Allow the plaster to drop to the bottom of the bowl and absorb the water.

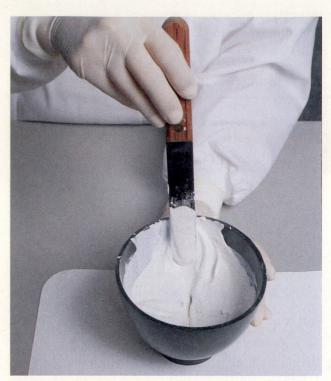

FIGURE 19–55E The consistency of the plaster mix is correct if the mix does not run back together after being cut with a spatula.

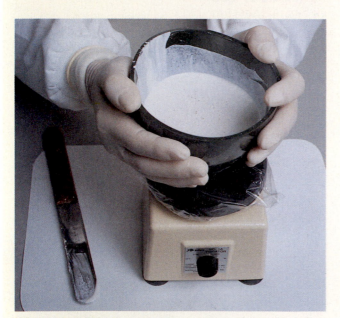

FIGURE 19–55D Use both hands to grasp the bowl of mix firmly on the vibrator platform to remove air bubbles from the plaster.

13. Use the spatula to place a small amount of plaster on the back, or heel, of the impression (**Figure 19–55F**). Vibrate the tray lightly so the mix flows into the impression, filling the "teeth."

 CAUTION: Use only a small amount of plaster at a time to ensure even filling and prevent air bubble formation.

14. Repeat step 13. Add the mix to the same area each time. Try to keep the flow as even as possible. Repeat until the impression is completely filled.

15. Form the base of the model by placing the remaining mix on a glass slab or tile (**Figure 19–55G**). The mix should be approximately 1 inch thick.

16. Very carefully invert the entire impression and place it on the base. Do not push down on the model.

    NOTE: Use a damp paper towel to create an arch on the mandibular model to keep the plaster mix out of this area.

    NOTE: In some dental settings, the remaining mix is simply placed on top of the model and built up to the correct thickness. In other settings, a base former is used. It is filled with plaster to form the base; the impression is then inverted on top.

17. Smooth the mix on the sides of the impression and base so the two areas join (**Figure 19–55H**). The model should be kept as level as possible.

18. Remove excess amounts of mix from the sides and top of the model. Keep the model basically smooth.

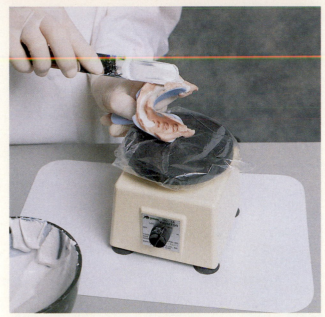

FIGURE 19–55F While holding the impression tray on the vibrator platform, place a small amount of plaster mix on the back, or heel, of the impression.

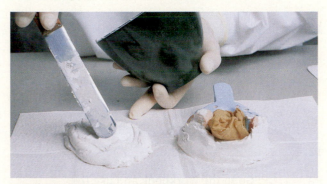

FIGURE 19–55G Form the base of the model by placing the rest of the plaster mix on a glass slab or tile. The impression is then inverted onto this base.

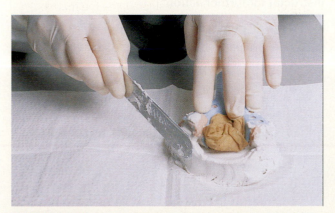

FIGURE 19–55H Smooth the mix on the sides of the model to join the base to the model.

19. Put the model in a safe place. Allow it to set. Do not disturb it for at least 1 hour.

NOTE: Setting time varies from 1 to 3 hours.

 NOTE: The model will get hot. As heat is produced, the water evaporates, and the model sets (becomes solid). This is called an *exothermic* reaction.

20. When the model is completely dry, remove it from the impression tray. Use a laboratory knife or spatula to gently scrape away any plaster material on the impression tray (**Figure 19–55I**). Use firm but steady pressure to lift the tray away from the model. Do *not* pull or twist the tray from side to side because this may break the model, separate it from the base, or break the teeth.

21. Clean and replace all equipment. Place all waste plaster in a trash container. Use large amounts of water to flush the sink. Scrub the bowls and other equipment thoroughly. If the impression tray is not disposable, it must be cleaned and sterilized prior to being used for another patient. Clean the counter top immediately.

22. Remove PPE. Wash hands.

PRACTICE: Go to the workbook and use the evaluation sheet for 19:10C, Pouring a Plaster Model, to practice this procedure. When you believe you have mastered this skill, sign the sheet and give it to your instructor for further action.

 FINAL EVALUATION: Using the criteria listed on the evaluation sheet, your instructor will grade your performance.

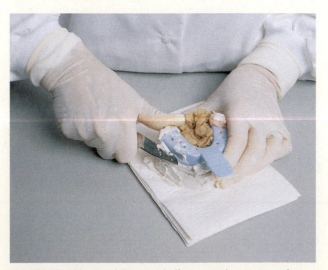

FIGURE 19–55I Use a laboratory knife or spatula to remove dry plaster from the impression tray before lifting the tray off the model.

Pouring a Stone Model

Equipment and Supplies

Alginate or polysulfide impression; mixing bowl; hard spatula; stone powder; metric graduate and scale; vibrator; glass slab or tile; water; personal protective equipment (gloves, gown, face mask, and eye protection)

Procedure

1. Assemble equipment.

2. Wash hands. Put on personal protective equipment (PPE).

   Precaution

   CAUTION: Observe standard precautions while working with an impression.

3. Prepare an alginate impression or use a polysulfide impression a doctor has prepared. Blot excess disinfecting solution from the impression.

4. Measure the water. Use 30 milliliters (mL) (following manufacturer's instructions). The water should be room temperature (70°F or 21°C) or slightly cooler.

5. Pour the water into the bowl.

6. Weigh the stone. Use 100 grams or follow the manufacturer's instructions (**Figure 19–56**).

7. Sift the powder into the bowl. Allow the powder to absorb the water.

   NOTE: Place the bowl on the vibrator platform for 5–10 seconds to aid mixing.

8. Use a wiping and scraping motion to mix the stone powder and water until a uniform, creamy mixture is obtained.

   Safety

   CAUTION: Avoid using a whipping motion, because this causes air bubbles.

9. Place the bowl on the vibrator platform. Hold the bowl firmly in place to remove air bubbles from the mix.

10. To pour the model, follow steps 11–20 of Procedure 19:10C, Pouring a Plaster Model.

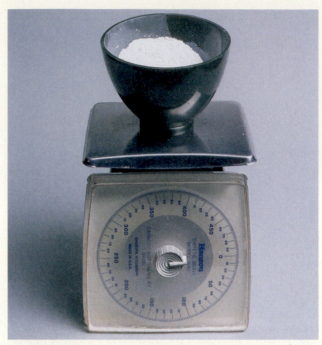

FIGURE 19–56 A small scale is used to weigh the correct amount of stone material, usually 100 grams.

11. Clean and replace all equipment. Place excess stone in a trash container. Do *not* wash stone material down the sink drain because it will clog the plumbing. Scrub the bowl, spatula, and countertop thoroughly. Disinfect or sterilize the bowl and spatula. If they are disposable, place them in an infectious-waste container.

12. Remove PPE. Wash hands.

PRACTICE: Go to the workbook and use the evaluation sheet for 19:10D, Pouring a Stone Model, to practice this procedure. When you believe you have mastered this skill, sign the sheet and give it to your instructor for further action.

Check

FINAL EVALUATION: Using the criteria listed on the evaluation sheet, your instructor will grade your performance.

Trimming a Model

Equipment and Supplies

Prepared model, model trimmer, bowl of water, safety glasses, personal protective equipment (PPE)

Procedure

1. **Math** Assemble equipment. Study the diagram in **Figure 19–57** to become familiar with the correct measurements for trimming a model.

2. Wash hands. Put on personal protective equipment (PPE).

   CAUTION: Observe standard precautions at all times while working with impressions and models.
   Precaution

3. Soak the model in a bowl of water for 5 minutes.

   NOTE: A wet model is easier to trim and less likely to break.

4. Put on safety glasses.

5. Turn on the water supply to the model trimmer. Turn on the model trimmer. Check to ascertain water is flowing freely over the grinding wheel.

6. Use light, even pressure to hold the model and trim the base so it is smooth and even (**Figure 19–58A**). The base should be parallel to the biting surfaces. It should be at least ½ inch thick and ⅓ the entire height of the model.

   CAUTION: Keep fingers away from the wheel at all times. Use steady pressure to hold the model.
   Safety

7. Trim the back, or heel, of the model. Approximately ¼ inch should remain behind the third molars. The heel should be perpendicular to the base (**Figure 19–58B**).

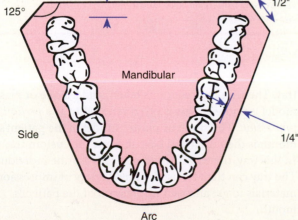

FIGURE 19–57 Measurements for trimming a model.

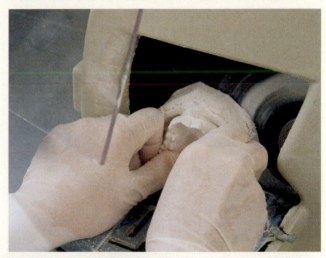

FIGURE 19–58A Use light, even pressure to hold the model and trim the base so it is smooth and even.

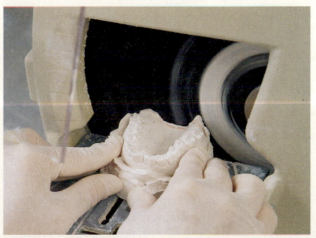

FIGURE 19–58B Trim the back, or heel, of the model so it is perpendicular to the base.

(continues)

NOTE: If working on a set of models, first trim the mandibular model. Then, hold the two models together so they are in occlusion and fit together. Trim the maxillary model parallel to the base of the mandibular model (**Figure 19–58C**).

8. Trim the sides of the model. On the maxillary model, form a 63-degree angle with the heel. Cut to within ¼ to ⅜ inch of the bicuspids (refer to Figure 19–57). On the mandibular model, form a 55-degree angle with the heel. Cut to within ¼ to ⅜ inch of the bicuspids.

9. Trim the heel points to approximately ½ inch in length to form a 125-degree angle with the heel.

10. On the maxillary model, draw a line from the center of the central incisors to the cuspid (**Figure 19–58D**). Make two cuts, one on each side, to form a point between the two central incisors. On the mandibular model, mark the cuspids and make an arc cut.

11. Label the model(s) with the patient's name and the date. Recheck both the maxillary and mandibular model to make sure they are trimmed correctly (refer to Figure 19–50).

12. Clean the trimmer thoroughly. Use a brush to clean the wheel. Remove the platform to wash and dry the inside of the trimmer.

13. Use large amounts of water to rinse the sink drain.

14. Replace all equipment.

15. Remove PPE. Wash hands.

PRACTICE: Go to the workbook and use the evaluation sheet for 19:10E, Trimming a Model, to practice this procedure. When you believe you have mastered this skill, sign the sheet and give it to your instructor for further action.

 FINAL EVALUATION: Using the criteria listed on the evaluation sheet, your instructor will grade your performance.

Check

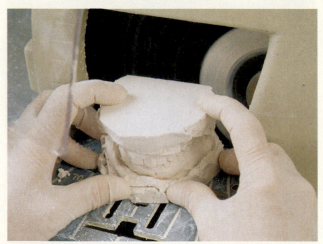

FIGURE 19–58C Hold the two models together in occlusion to align the heel cuts.

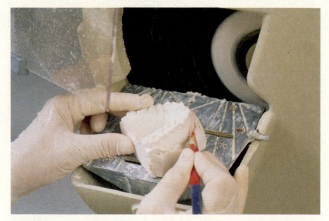

FIGURE 19–58D Draw a line from the center of the central incisors to the cuspid to mark the anterior cut.

19:11 MAKING CUSTOM TRAYS

Making custom trays for impressions may be one of the responsibilities of the dental assistant. **Custom trays** are impression trays made to fit a particular patient's mouth. To obtain exact impressions, a tray must be exactly fitted to the patient's mouth. Thus, a custom tray is produced.

To make a custom tray, the first step is to make a model or cast of the patient's mouth from a standard impression tray. Then, an impression is taken, and a stone or plaster model is poured. This is often referred to as a *preliminary impression*. The stone or plaster model of the patient's mouth is then used as a base to form the custom tray. In this way, the tray is fitted perfectly for the individual. The tray can then be used with a variety of impression materials to get an exact impression of the patient's mouth.

 Various materials are used to make custom trays. Acrylic resins are the most popular because they produce a stronger tray that can be used with all types of impression

Science

materials. The acrylic resins are supplied as a liquid catalyst and a powder that are mixed together. A process known as curing (polymerization) causes the material to become pliable so it can be fitted to the contour of the preliminary model. As curing continues, an exothermic reaction occurs in which the material gives off heat and becomes rigid or hard. Acrylic resins can be self-curing or light-curing. The light-cured resins do not set or become hard until they are exposed to a light in a special curing oven.

Because acrylic resins are difficult to remove from mixing jars or containers, a plastic- or wax-lined disposable paper cup and tongue blades are used to mix the material. Coating the fingers lightly with petroleum jelly helps prevent the material from sticking to the hands.

Acrylic resins are also supplied as sheets that can be vacuum formed. A vacuum-form unit with a heating element is used to make this type of custom tray. The preliminary model is placed on the platform of the unit. Acrylic resin sheets are positioned in a frame located under the heater at the top of the unit. As the unit heats the acrylic sheets, they begin to droop down from the frame (**Figure 19–59A**). When the sheets are 1 inch below the holding frame, the frame is dropped into position over the model (**Figure 19–59B**). Vacuum pressure is used to shape the resin sheets to the model to form the custom tray. After the material has cooled, the tray can be separated from the model and trimmed with scissors (**Figure 19–59C**).

 Custom trays must be labeled with the patient's name and used exclusively for that patient. Most manufacturers of acrylic resins suggest allowing the material to set for 24 hours before use to be sure it is completely stable. Any of the impression materials can be used in the tray to get an exact impression of the patient's mouth.

Comm

checkpoint

1. How long should most resin trays set before they are used for an impression?

PRACTICE: Go to the workbook and complete the assignment sheet for 19:11, Making Custom Trays. Then return and continue with the procedure.

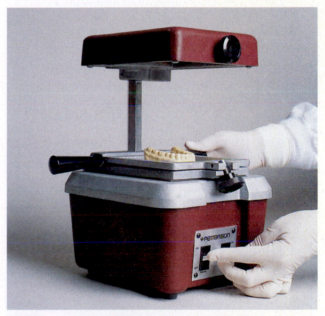

FIGURE 19–59B When the acrylic sheet sags 1 inch below the frame, the frame is positioned over the model. Vacuum pressure is then used to mold the custom tray.

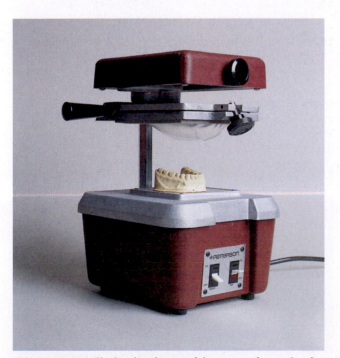

FIGURE 19–59A The heating element of the vacuum-form unit softens the acrylic sheet so it sags or droops down from the tray.

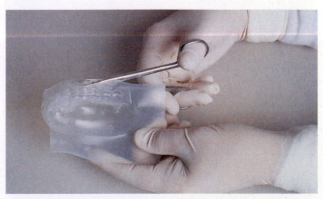

FIGURE 19–59C After it has cooled, the vacuum-formed custom tray can be trimmed with scissors.

Making Custom Trays

Equipment and Supplies

Powder and liquid catalyst tray materials, measuring devices, paper cups and tongue blades, petroleum jelly, glass slab, base-plate wax, wax knife, acrylic bur or stone, plaster or stone model, safety glasses, gloves

Procedure

1. Assemble equipment.

2. Wash hands. Put on gloves.

3. Use a single layer of baseplate wax to cover the teeth and other specified areas of the model (**Figure 19–60A**). This serves as a spacer for the tray. Cover the wax spacer with aluminum foil or coat it with a separating liquid.

   NOTE: Use very warm water to warm the wax to make it more pliable.

   NOTE: Special rolls of liner material are also available to cover the teeth. The liner material is cut to size, moistened, and then placed over the teeth.

4. Pour the required amount of liquid (follow manufacturer's instructions) into a paper cup. A wax- or plastic-lined paper cup is preferred.

Measure the correct amount of powder and add it to the liquid in the cup.

 CAUTION: Never use a rubber bowl for mixing. Paper cups provide for easier cleanup because they can be discarded.

5. Use a tongue blade for mixing. Mix thoroughly for approximately 1 minute until the mix is uniform.

6. Allow the mixture to stand until it is not sticky to the touch and is stringy when pulled, approximately 2–3 minutes.

7. Coat the model, glass slab, and your hands with petroleum jelly to prevent the material from sticking.

8. Remove the mixture from the cup and knead it gently (**Figure 19–60B**).

9. Place the material on the glass slab. Roll or form it into a wafer with a uniform thickness of approximately ¹⁄₁₆ to ⅛ inch.

10. Remove the wafer from the tray. Slowly adapt it to the model. Start at the palate area and extend to the sides (**Figure 19–60C**).

11. For a mandibular tray, trim off the excess material to form the arch. Form a handle on the tray (**Figure 19–60D**). Extra material can be applied by using a small amount of the resin liquid at the point of attachment.

12. Use a knife to remove excess material from the sides.

13. Allow the tray to cure for 7–10 minutes. Then, gently remove the tray from the model.

14. Remove the aluminum foil and wax spacer, unless the doctor wants it left in place. Label the tray with the patient's name.

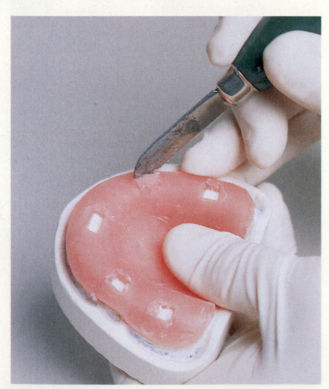

FIGURE 19–60A Use baseplate wax to cover the teeth of the model and form a spacer.

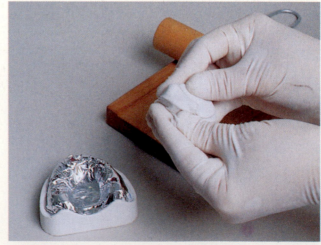

FIGURE 19–60B When the mixture is not sticky to the touch, remove the material from the cup and knead it gently.

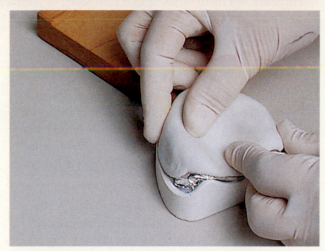

FIGURE 19–60C Start at the palate area to adapt the wafer of custom tray material to the model.

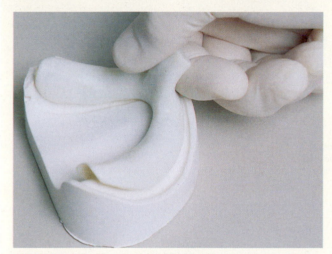

FIGURE 19–60D After the tray is trimmed for a mandibular arch, a handle is attached to the front of the tray.

15. Use special acrylic burs or an arbor band on a lathe to trim and smooth the tray (**Figure 19–60E**).

 CAUTION: Wear safety glasses while trimming the tray.

16. Clean and replace all equipment. The liquid catalyst can be used to remove mix from surfaces, but it should be used sparingly.

17. Remove gloves. Wash hands.

PRACTICE: Go to the workbook and use the evaluation sheet for 19:11, Making Custom Trays, to practice this procedure. When you believe you have mastered this skill, sign the sheet and give it to your instructor for further action.

 FINAL EVALUATION: Using the criteria listed on the evaluation sheet, your instructor will grade your performance.

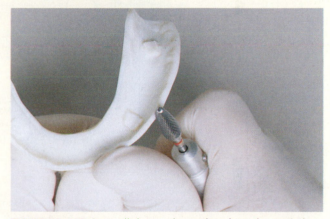

FIGURE 19–60E An acrylic bur can be used to trim and smooth the edges of a custom tray.

19:12 MAINTAINING AND LOADING AN ANESTHETIC ASPIRATING SYRINGE

 Anesthesia is used in many dental procedures to decrease pain or discomfort. Some responsibilities of the dental assistant with regard to anesthesia are discussed in this section. It is important to note, however, that the degree of responsibility may vary from state to state. It is your responsibility to learn exactly what you are legally permitted to do.

Pain control is an important part of any dental procedure. **Anesthesia**, which means "absence of feeling," is the term used to describe the condition that exists when the sensation of feeling pain has been decreased or eliminated. The type of anesthesia used depends on the needs of the patient. Different types of anesthesia include:

- **General anesthesia:** This type renders the patient unconscious. It is usually used in a hospital and administered by an anesthesiologist. It is seldom used in dental offices.

- **Analgesia or sedation:** This type causes loss of ability to feel pain but not loss of consciousness. In dental offices, analgesia is usually given by having the patient inhale a mixture of nitrous oxide and oxygen gases. This causes the patient to feel pleasantly relaxed but remain awake and able to cooperate. The effects wear off very quickly after the administration is stopped. Other forms of sedation are also used. These include oral doses or injections of mild sedatives, or tranquilizers.

- **Local anesthesia**: This is the form of anesthesia used most frequently in dental offices. An anesthetic is injected into the area where loss of sensation is desired. This decreases or eliminates the sensation of pain in the specific area but has no effect on the patient's level of consciousness.

- **Topical anesthesia**: Topical anesthetics are frequently used to reduce the pain or discomfort caused by the injection for local anesthesia. These anesthetics are applied to the mucous membrane to desensitize the area where another anesthetic is to be injected. Topical anesthetics are available as liquids,

sprays, gels, and ointments. In some states, the dental assistant is allowed to apply the topical anesthetic.

There are two main kinds of injections used to produce local anesthesia in the oral cavity (**Figure 19–61**):

- **Block**: The anesthetic is injected near a main nerve trunk. This kind of injection is used primarily for mandibular teeth. Several teeth are anesthetized.

- **Infiltration, or field**: The anesthetic is injected around the terminal nerve branches of the teeth. This kind of injection is used mainly for maxillary teeth, but it can be used for anterior mandibular teeth. Each tooth usually requires a separate injection.

 Science A variety of medications are used to produce local anesthesia. The main local/anesthetic medication is lidocaine (Xylocaine). It decreases

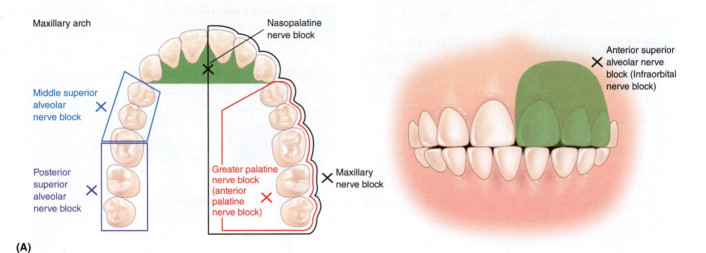

(A)

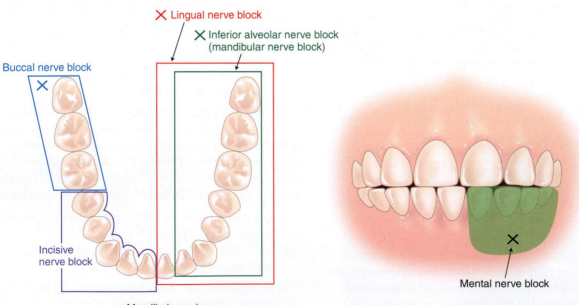

(B)

FIGURE 19–61 Types of injections for dental anesthesia: (A) maxillary infiltration and (B) mandibular block.

nerve sensation. Other anesthetics that may be used include mepivacaine (Carbocaine) and prilocaine (Citanest). Procaine (Novocain) is used infrequently. Vasoconstrictors are often added to anesthetics. Vasoconstrictors decrease the size of the blood vessels in the area and, thus, keep the blood from rapidly carrying away the anesthetic. In this way, the anesthesia effect is prolonged. Vasoconstrictors also help reduce bleeding at the site. Epinephrine is a common vasoconstrictor.

CAUTION: *Vasoconstrictors can be dangerous for patients with heart disease, hyperthyroidism, and hypertension (high blood pressure). It is important to review the patient's health history and follow the doctor's directions before epinephrine is used.*

Safety

Anesthetic carpules (cartridges) are glass cylinders that contain premeasured amounts of anesthetic solutions (**Figure 19–62**). The carpule fits into the barrel of a syringe. This is the most common delivery system for local-anesthetic injection. The following points must be observed when using carpules:

- **Check the glass:** Do not use if cracks or chips are present.
- **Check the expiration date on the cartridge or container:** Do not use the cartridge if the medication expiration date has passed.
- **Check the solution:** It should be clear in color. If it is yellow or straw colored, this may mean that the epinephrine has broken down. Do *not* use a carpule containing discolored solution.
- **Check the rubber plunger:** It should be level with or just slightly below the top of the cartridge.
  (1) An extruded (pushed-out) plunger with a large air bubble usually means that the cartridge was frozen. Do *not* use.
  (2) An extruded plunger with no air bubble usually means that the cartridge was left in a disinfecting solution too long. The disinfecting solution passed through the rubber diaphragm and entered the carpule. Do *not* use.

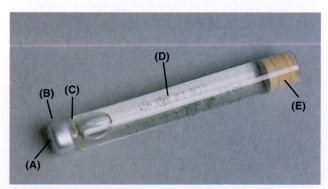

FIGURE 19–62 Parts of an anesthetic carpule (cartridge): (A) rubber diaphragm, (B) aluminum cap, (C) neck, (D) glass cylinder, and (E) rubber plunger or stopper.

- **Check the bubbles:** Small bubbles (1–2 mm) are normal. Large bubbles are usually caused by freezing. Return a carpule containing large bubbles to the supplier for replacement.
- **Check the aluminum cap:** A thin diaphragm is in the center of the cap to allow for the insertion of the needle. Rust from the container can contaminate the caps. It is best not to use a carpule having rust on the cap.
- **Care of carpules:** Do *not* autoclave carpules. They are sterile on the inside. It is best *not* to soak any carpule for a long time because the disinfecting solution can pass into the rubber diaphragm and contaminate the solution inside. Prior to using any carpule, use a sterile pad moistened with 70-percent ethyl alcohol or 91-percent isopropyl alcohol to rub the aluminum cap end and rubber-plunger end. Cartridge dispensers are available for conveniently storing carpules.

Aspirating syringes are commonly used to inject local anesthetic. *Aspiration* means "drawing back by suction." After penetrating the mucous membrane with the syringe, the doctor draws back on the syringe to be sure the needle has not penetrated a blood vessel and to be sure it is properly inserted in the tissues before injecting the medication.

Parts of the anesthetic aspirating syringe are shown in **Figure 19–63** and include:

- **Needle adaptor:** threaded area at the end of the syringe where a disposable needle is attached to the syringe
- **Barrel:** cylinder with one open side to allow for the insertion of the anesthetic carpule (cartridge)
- **Guide bearing:** stabilizes the movement of the piston and harpoon
- **Spring:** allows for the advancement and retraction of the piston and harpoon
- **Piston with harpoon:** a metal shaft with a barbed tip to allow the harpoon to be inserted in the rubber plunger of the carpule
- **Finger grip:** supports the index and middle fingers as the anesthetic solution is being injected into the tissues
- **Thumb ring:** area of insertion for the thumb to allow for aspiration and injection

After each use, the syringe must be washed thoroughly and rinsed. It must then be autoclaved. After each five uses, the syringe should be dismantled, or taken apart. All parts should be checked carefully. Worn or defective parts should be replaced. Threaded areas should be lubricated.

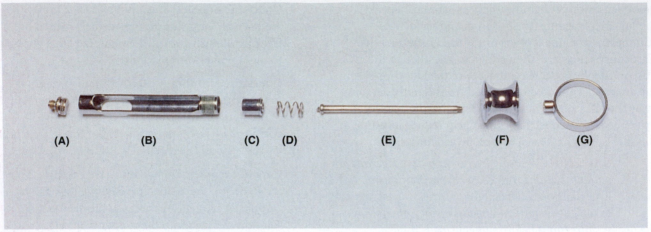

FIGURE 19–63 Parts of the aspirating syringe: (A) needle adaptor, (B) barrel, (C) guide bearing, (D) spring, (E) piston with harpoon, (F) finger grip, and (G) thumb ring.

Technology

A newer method of administering dental anesthesia is a computer-controlled local anesthetic delivery system, commonly called "the wand." This system uses a disposable tip on a handpiece that is connected to a computerized processor. The computerized processor compensates for different tissue densities and determines the exact amount of anesthesia needed. As the needle of the wand enters the tissues, the computer delivers a flow of anesthetic directly ahead of the needle. This numbs the site of insertion and eliminates most of the discomfort experienced with a standard injection of dental anesthetic. In addition, the computerized wand can direct the anesthesia to the exact area where it is needed and decrease the collateral numbness of the tongue, lips, and facial muscles. This technology is more expensive, but provides the patient with a more comfortable anesthetic injection.

Precaution

Standard precautions must be followed while handling the disposable needle after an injection has been given. Handle the needle carefully to avoid needlesticks. The needle must be removed from the syringe and placed in a leak-proof, puncture-resistant sharps box. It must not be bent, broken, or recapped. If the needle must be recapped during the procedure, a one-handed scoop technique must be used. The needle guard or cover must be placed on a tray or in a special recap device designed to hold the guard in position. The used needle should then be inserted into the guard or cap. Fingers must be kept off of the guard until the end of the needle is covered. Once the needle end is covered by the guard or cap, it is safe to pick up the guard and slip it firmly into position over the needle.

Correct care of carpules and syringes, and correct loading of syringes are part of the responsibilities of a dental assistant. Procedures 19:12A and 19:12B provide additional information.

checkpoint

1. What are the two (2) main kinds of injections used to produce local anesthesia in the oral cavity?

PRACTICE: Go to the workbook and complete the assignment sheet for 19:12, Maintaining and Loading an Anesthetic Aspirating Syringe. Then return and continue with the procedures.

Procedure 19:12A

Maintaining an Anesthetic Aspirating Syringe

Equipment and Supplies

Soap, water, aspirating syringe, pliers, lubrication, personal protective equipment (PPE)

Procedure

1. Assemble equipment.

2. Wash hands. Put on personal protective equipment (PPE).

Precaution

CAUTION: Observe standard precautions while working with a contaminated aspirating syringe.

3. Use pliers and gentle pressure to unscrew the parts of the syringe.

4. Use the manufacturer's instructions to identify all of the following parts:

   - thumb ring
   - finger grip
   - spring
   - guide bearing
   - piston with harpoon
   - barrel
   - needle adaptor

   NOTE: Parts may vary slightly depending on the manufacturer.

5. Use soap and water to clean all parts thoroughly. Rinse all parts.

6. Inspect the piston and harpoon. Make sure the harpoon is sharp and *not* damaged.

7. Check the needle adaptor. Make sure the hole is open and *not* plugged.

8. Check all other parts. Make sure they are *not* damaged or defective.

   NOTE: Parts can be replaced. This is more economical than replacing the entire syringe.

9. Lubricate all of the threaded joints: thumb ring, piston top, barrel, and adaptor.

10. Put the syringe back together. First, put the needle adaptor on the barrel. Then, place the guide bearing narrow end down on the piston. Next, place the spring on top. Screw on the finger grip and thumb ring. Finally, place on the barrel and secure.

11. Check the syringe to make sure it is secure and correctly assembled.

12. After each use, wash the syringe thoroughly. Rinse and dry the syringe. Sterilize it in the autoclave.

13. After each five uses, repeat steps 1–11 of this procedure to check the anesthetic aspirating syringe and keep it in good condition. Replace any defective parts. Then, sterilize by autoclaving prior to use.

14. Replace all equipment.

15. Remove PPE. Wash hands thoroughly.

PRACTICE: Go to the workbook and use the evaluation sheet for 19:12A, Maintaining an Anesthetic Aspirating Syringe, to practice this procedure. When you believe you have mastered this skill, sign the sheet and give it to your instructor for further action.

 FINAL EVALUATION: Using the criteria listed on the evaluation sheet, your instructor will grade your performance.

Loading an Anesthetic Aspirating Syringe

Equipment and Supplies

Aspirating syringe, needles, carpules, cartridge dispenser, gauze with disinfectant solution, sharps container, personal protective equipment (PPE)

Procedure

1. Assemble equipment (**Figure 19–64A**). Check with the doctor to determine the type of cartridge and needle length and gauge to use.

    CAUTION: The doctor will determine the type of medication after checking the patient's medical history. If the patient has allergies, hyperthyroidism, heart disease, or hypertension, epinephrine (a vasoconstrictor) is usually *not* used.

2. Wash hands. Put on personal protective equipment (PPE).

    CAUTION: Observe standard precautions while working with an aspirating syringe.

3. Check the carpule. Note color of solution, medication expiration date, location of plunger, condition of aluminum cap, presence of bubbles, and condition of glass. Use gauze containing 70-percent ethyl alcohol or 91-percent isopropyl alcohol to wipe the rubber diaphragm on the aluminum cap end and the plunger end of the carpule.

    CAUTION: Never use a defective or expired carpule. Discard or return it to the supplier.

4. Check the syringe. Note condition of the harpoon and other parts.

(continues)

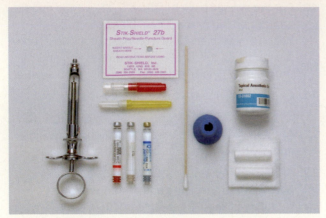

FIGURE 19–64A Equipment and supplies for loading an anesthetic aspirating syringe.

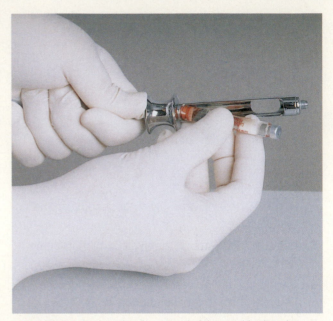

FIGURE 19–64B Place the plunger end of the cartridge into the barrel first, and the aluminum cap end will then fall into place.

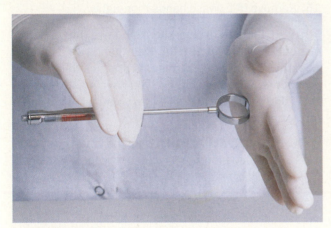

FIGURE 19–64C Use moderate pressure on the thumb ring to engage the harpoon into the rubber plunger.

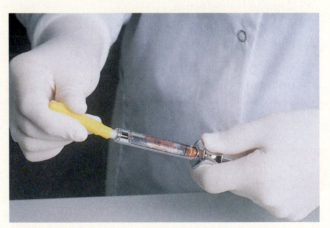

FIGURE 19–64D Attach the needle to the needle adaptor by screwing it in place.

5. Place fingers and thumb on the thumb ring and finger grip. Retract the piston all the way back.

6. Place the carpule in the syringe, with the plunger end going into the harpoon end first (**Figure 19–64B**). The aluminum cap end will then fall into place.

    CAUTION: Never force the carpule into place; it will break.

   Safety

7. Engage the harpoon into the rubber plunger. Use moderate pressure on the thumb ring to push the piston forward until the harpoon is firmly engaged in the plunger (**Figure 19–64C**). Make sure not to push too far.

8. Attach the needle to the needle adaptor by screwing it in place (**Figure 19–64D**). Make sure the needle is engaged in the center of the rubber diaphragm on the cap of the carpule.

   NOTE: Size (gauge and length) of the needle used will be determined by the doctor.

   NOTE: The needle can be attached before the harpoon is engaged in the rubber plunger.

CAUTION: Always leave the cover on the needle end to prevent contamination and accidental needlestick injuries.

Safety

9. Prior to administration of the injection, use a recap device to remove the protective cap from the needle. Expel a few drops of the solution to make sure the eye of the needle is open.

10. Expel all air bubbles from the carpule. Using extreme caution, use a recap device to replace the protective cap on the needle loosely so it can be easily removed.

11. When the doctor is ready for the anesthesic, first pass a gauze sponge to dry the injection area. Then, pass topical anesthetic as needed (**Figure 19–65A**). Position the needle with the beveled side toward the patient's teeth. A guard can be placed over the needle cap to prevent a needlestick when the cap is removed (**Figure 19–65B**). Direct the entire syringe toward the path of insertion. Use a palm-grasp position (hold syringe in palm of hand with fingers grasping syringe) to place the syringe in the doctor's hand. As the doctor grasps the syringe, carefully remove the protective cap from the needle. Some doctors prefer to remove the cap with a recap device.

    NOTE: Keep the syringe out of the patient's sight by passing it at the patient's chin level or below.

12. To unload the syringe, carefully unscrew the needle and place it in a sharps container. Then, use one hand to hold the carpule in position and use the other hand to disengage the harpoon.

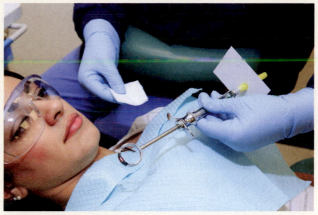
FIGURE 19–65B The syringe is passed to the doctor with the guard in position.

Invert the syringe so that the carpule falls out. Keep the piston retracted.

CAUTION: Never recap the needle by hand after use. If it must be recapped to protect the doctor or the dental assistant, use a one-handed scoop technique. Put the needle cap, cover, or guard on a tray or in a special recap device that holds the cover securely. Insert the needle into the cap without touching the cap. When the needle end is covered by the cap, push the cap firmly in place over the needle. At the end of the procedure, remove the needle with the cap in place from the syringe and discard the needle and cap in a sharps container.

Safety

13. Record the type and amount of local anesthetic used on the patient's chart.

    Comm

14. Care for the syringe as instructed in Procedure 19:12A. Place the empty carpule in a sharps container.

15. Replace all equipment.

16. Remove PPE. Wash hands thoroughly.

PRACTICE: Go to the workbook and use the evaluation sheet for 19:12B, Loading an Anesthetic Aspirating Syringe, to practice this procedure. When you believe you have mastered this skill, sign the sheet and give it to your instructor for further action.

FINAL EVALUATION: Using the criteria listed on the evaluation sheet, your instructor will grade your performance.

Check

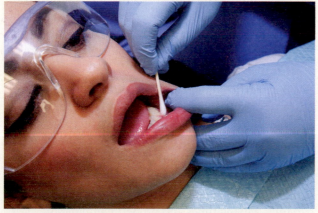
FIGURE 19–65A A topical anesthetic is frequently applied before injecting the anesthetic.

MIXING DENTAL CEMENTS AND BASES

Cements and bases are used in a variety of dental procedures. They are used to line or prepare a tooth for a restoration and/or as *luting* agents to cause materials to stick together. Important terminology includes the following:

- **Liner**: Material used to cover, line, or seal exposed tooth tissue, such as dentin. It is usually in the form of a varnish.

- **Base**: Protective material that is placed over the pulpal area of a tooth to reduce irritation and thermal (heat) shock. Used under large restorations.

- **Cement**: Material used to permanently seal inlays, orthodontic appliances, crowns, and bridges in place. It is sometimes used as a temporary filling or as a base for restorations when sedation is necessary.

- **Temporary**: Material used as a restorative material for a short time and only until permanent restoration can be done.

A large variety of products are available. Some products have several uses and can act as a base, cement, or temporary, depending on the need. Always read manufacturer's directions for mixing and use. Some of the types available are as follows:

- **Varnish** acts as a liner to protect exposed surfaces of dentin from thermal shock and irritation. It is placed under a restoration. If the varnish contains an organic solvent such as ether, acetone, or chloroform, it cannot be used under composite restorations because it interferes with the setting of the restoration. Many brands of varnish are available, including Copal, Copalite, Varnal, and Handi-Liner.

- **Zinc oxide eugenol (ZOE)** has a sedative effect when placed under a restoration.

  Science When it is reinforced with other substances, ZOE is also used as a base under metallic restorations or as a temporary cement or restoration. It is not recommended as a base material for resins or composites (anterior restorations) because it interferes with the setting reaction of these materials. ZOE is available as a powder/liquid mix, two-pastes mix, or prepared capsules (**Figure 19–66**). Some brand names for ZOE are I.R.M. and Cavitec.

- **Calcium hydroxide** is used as a base in larger restorations and for pulp capping. It stimulates the formation of secondary dentin to protect the pulp. Because it is water soluble, calcium hydroxide is not

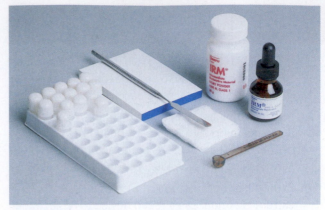

FIGURE 19–66 Zinc oxide eugenol is available as a powder/liquid mix or prepared capsules.

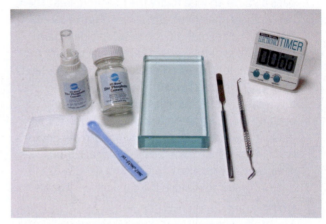

FIGURE 19–67 Zinc phosphate is a thermally protective base and a cement for crowns, inlays, bridges, and orthodontic bands and brackets.

used for temporary restorations. Some brand names include Dycal, Hypocal, and Dropsin.

- **Zinc phosphate** is used as a thermally protective base under metallic fillings and as a cement to retain gold restorations such as inlays, crowns, and bridges (**Figure 19–67**). Tenacin and Fleck's are two examples of brand names.

- **Polycarboxylate** is also called *zinc polyacrylate* or *carboxylate*. It is used as a cement for orthodontic bands and brackets, crowns, and bridges, and as a base under some restorations. Some brand names include Durelon, Hybond, and Tylock-Plus.

Correct mixing techniques must be followed when using bases or cements. Amounts must be measured carefully. Mixing times and proper manipulation techniques must be followed. Improper mixing techniques can lead to a poor base or cement and shorten the life of the restoration that is placed on top. Read the instructions carefully for each type.

Cements and bases are available in many different forms. Sometimes, a liquid and paste are used. Other times, liquids and powders or two pastes are used. In most cases, care must be taken to avoid mixing the substances in their containers because a small amount of liquid added to a powder in a container can ruin or destroy the entire contents of the container. Therefore, it is important to follow precautions that prevent mixing the containers of material together and to use clean measuring devices.

Some brands of cements and bases require light curing. A visible light source is held close to the preparation for a brief time, usually about 20 seconds for each 1-millimeter layer. This causes the material to "cure" or set and become hard. Light shields must be used by the dentist, the patient, and assistant to prevent eye irritation from the visible light source.

Procedures for mixing some types of cements and bases are described on the following pages. These procedures provide a basic introduction.

checkpoint

1. In light curing, about how long is the light source held close to the preparation?

PRACTICE: Go to the workbook and complete the assignment sheet for 19:13, Mixing Dental Cements and Bases. Then return and continue with the procedures.

Procedure 19:13A

Preparing Varnish

Equipment and Supplies

Cavity varnish, varnish solvent or thinner, cotton pliers, cotton pellets, special applicators (with some products), air syringe, personal protective equipment (PPE)

NOTE: Copal, Copalite, Varnal, and Handi-Liner are brand names of varnish.

Procedure

1. Assemble equipment. Read and follow the manufacturer's instructions for the specific varnish being used.

2. Wash hands. Put on personal protective equipment (PPE).

    CAUTION: Observe standard precautions while assisting with any dental procedure.

3. Check the bottle of varnish. If the contents are too thick, add thinner if directed to do so by the manufacturer (**Figure 19–68A**). Loosen caps slightly, but leave in place until ready for use.

   NOTE: Evaporation occurs if caps are left off bottles.

4. When the doctor has completed the cavity preparation, pass the air-water, or tri-flow, syringe to the doctor. The cavity preparation must be dry before varnish is applied.

5. Put two cotton pellets in the cotton pliers. Dip the pellets into the varnish to saturate them (**Figure 19–68B**). Remove the excess varnish by placing both pellets on a 2 × 2 gauze pad. Pick up one saturated cotton pellet with the cotton pliers and pass it to the doctor.

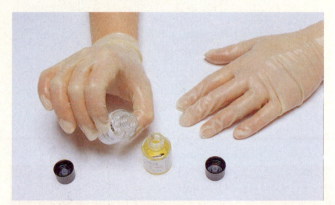

FIGURE 19–68A Some types of varnish must be thinned with a thinner solution when they become thick.

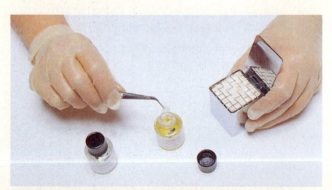

FIGURE 19–68B Cotton pliers can be used to hold the cotton pellet while saturating the pellet with varnish.

NOTE: Two pellets are saturated at the same time to avoid contamination of the varnish with the cotton pliers. To prepare the pellets one at a time, two pairs of cotton pliers must be used.

(continues)

NOTE: Special applicators are sometimes used. Cotton fibers are placed on the end of the applicator, and the applicator is then dipped in the varnish. A second applicator must be used for the second pellet.

6. The doctor paints the dentin surface with the varnish. The dental assistant should be ready to receive the pliers.

7. Pass the air syringe to the doctor. The area is dried with warm air for approximately 15–30 seconds.

8. Discard the used cotton pellet. Pick up the second saturated cotton pellet with the cotton pliers. Pass the pliers to the doctor.

9. The doctor will apply a second coat of varnish. Very porous teeth sometimes require three applications. If a third coat is necessary, use clean, uncontaminated cotton pliers to saturate a new cotton pellet with varnish.

Science

NOTE: Varnish acts as a liner and sealer. It protects against thermal shock and protects the dentin from acids in the restoration materials.

10. When you receive the pliers, discard the pellet. Close the lid on the varnish bottle immediately to avoid evaporation.

NOTE: The thinner can be used to clean the screw threads on the top of the varnish bottle. This helps prevent the lid from sticking on the varnish bottle.

11. Thinner can be used as a solvent to clean varnish from instruments. It can also be used to clean varnish from the enamel of the tooth being prepared.

12. Clean and replace all equipment. Scrub and sterilize all instruments.

13. Remove PPE. Wash hands thoroughly.

PRACTICE: Go to the workbook and use the evaluation sheet for 19:13A, Preparing Varnish, to practice this procedure. When you believe you have mastered this skill, sign the sheet and give it to your instructor for further action.

Check

FINAL EVALUATION: Using the criteria listed on the evaluation sheet, your instructor will grade your performance.

Procedure 19:13B

Preparing Calcium Hydroxide

Equipment and Supplies

Base, catalyst, ball-pointed mixing instrument, mixing pad, personal protective equipment (PPE)

NOTE: Brand names for calcium hydroxide include Dycal, Hypocal, and Dropsin.

Procedure

1. Assemble equipment. Read and follow the manufacturer's instructions for the brand being used.

2. Wash hands. Put on personal protective equipment (PPE).

Precaution

CAUTION: Observe standard precautions while assisting with any dental procedure.

3. Place equal small dots of the base and the catalyst on the mixing pad side by side. Close the caps on the tubes immediately after dispensing the material.

Safety

CAUTION: Take care that neither substance contaminates the tube of the other substance. If the catalyst mix enters the base tube, it can destroy the base material.

4. When the doctor is ready for the base, use the ball-pointed mixing instrument to mix the two pastes together (**Figure 19–69**). The mix should be uniform in color. Mixing should be completed in 10 seconds.

5. Immediately place a small amount of the mix on the end of the mixing instrument. Pass the mixing instrument to the doctor.

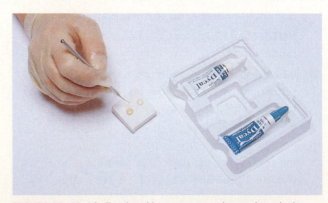

FIGURE 19–69 A ball-pointed instrument can be used to mix the base and catalyst together.

NOTE: Calcium hydroxide is used as a base under restorations. It serves as a protective barrier between the dentin and pulp and between cements and restorative materials. Because it is water soluble, it cannot be used as a temporary filling material.

6. Reapply the mix to the mixing instrument until the doctor has used the required amount of base. The mixing pad of material can also be held near the patient's chin so that the doctor can obtain mix as needed.

   NOTE: Calcium hydroxide sets in approximately 2½ to 3 minutes. In the mouth, it sets faster because of moisture and mouth temperature. Therefore, it is important to work quickly and efficiently.

   NOTE: Some brands of calcium hydroxide are light-cured. A visible light source is used to cure or set these materials.

7. Hand instruments to the doctor to remove excess material.

8. Clean and replace all equipment. A 10-percent sodium hydroxide solution or orange solvent can be used to remove the calcium hydroxide from instruments. Instruments must then be scrubbed and sterilized. Check to be sure the caps are secure on both tubes. Clean the outsides of the tubes, if necessary. Tear the used sheet off of the mixing pad and discard the sheet in a waste container.

9. Remove PPE. Wash hands thoroughly.

PRACTICE: Go to the workbook and use the evaluation sheet for 19:13B, Preparing Calcium Hydroxide, to practice this procedure. When you believe you have mastered this skill, sign the sheet and give it to your instructor for further action.

 FINAL EVALUATION: Using the criteria listed on the evaluation sheet, your instructor will grade your performance.

Preparing Polycarboxylate

Equipment and Supplies

Powder, scoop, liquid, mixing pad or glass slab, flexible stainless steel or plastic spatula, personal protective equipment (PPE)

NOTE: Durelon, Hybond, and Tylock-Plus are brands of polycarboxylate. They are used as a cement and as a base under restorations. This procedure is written for Durelon.

Procedure

1. Assemble equipment. Read and follow the manufacturer's instructions for the brand being used.

2. Wash hands. Put on personal protective equipment (PPE).

    CAUTION: Observe standard precautions while assisting with any dental procedure.

3. With the lid in place, fluff the powder by gently inverting the container several times. Open the lid carefully to avoid inhaling the powder.

4. Press the measuring scoop down into the powder. Use firm pressure to fill the scoop. Withdraw the scoop. Use the spatula to remove excess powder from the outside of the scoop. Use the spatula to level the powder.

5. Invert the scoop over the mixing pad (or glass slab). Tap the side with the spatula to release all of the powder.

   NOTE: If a glass slab is used, first cool it by placing it under cold, running water. Dry it thoroughly.

6. Hold the bottle of liquid in a vertical position. Squeeze the required number of drops of liquid onto the pad and beside the powder. Follow the manufacturer's recommendations for amount. Sample measurements are as follows:

   a. Cement: Use three drops of liquid for one scoop of powder.

   b. Base: Use two drops of liquid for one scoop of powder.

   NOTE: Some manufacturers provide calibrated, syringe-type liquid dispensers (**Figure 19–70A**). Follow instructions to use this type of dispenser. Usually, the plunger is moved from one full calibration to the next calibration to obtain each

(continues)

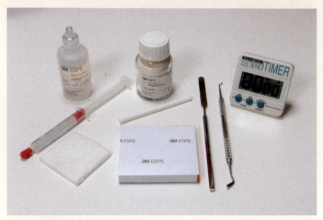

FIGURE 19–70A Some polycarboxylates use calibrated syringe dispensers for the liquid while others use a bottle of liquid.

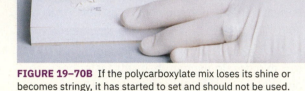

FIGURE 19–70B If the polycarboxylate mix loses its shine or becomes stringy, it has started to set and should not be used.

drop of liquid required. If two drops of liquid are needed, the plunger would be moved through two calibrations on the syringe.

7. Use the spatula to add all of the powder to the liquid at one time. Mix vigorously. The mix should be completed in 30 seconds. The final mix should appear glossy.

 CAUTION: Do not start mixing until the doctor is ready. Dispense the liquid only when you are ready to use it.

Safety

8. The final mix should be used while it is glossy. If the mix loses its shine or becomes stringy, it has started to set and should not be used (**Figure 19–70B**). The doctor has approximately 2–3 minutes of manipulation time, so it is important to work quickly and efficiently.

9. Close the lid on the bottles of liquid and powder immediately after use. The opening of the dropper bottle must be kept clean.

10. Use water to wipe the mixing spatula and instruments clean immediately after use. If the material has set, a 10-percent sodium hydroxide solution or orange solvent can be used to clean the instruments.

11. Clean and replace all equipment. Wash all instruments thoroughly and then sterilize them correctly. Tear the used sheet off of the mixing pad and discard the sheet in a waste container.

12. Remove PPE. Wash hands thoroughly.

PRACTICE: Go to the workbook and use the evaluation sheet for 19:13C, Preparing Polycarboxylate, to practice this procedure. When you believe you have mastered this skill, sign the sheet and give it to your instructor for further action.

 FINAL EVALUATION: Using the criteria listed on the evaluation sheet, your instructor will grade your performance.

Check

Procedure 19:13D

Preparing Zinc Oxide Eugenol (ZOE)

Equipment and Supplies

Containers of powder and liquid, mixing pad, small spatula, measuring devices, personal protective equipment (PPE)

 NOTE: I.R.M. is a brand of a reinforced zinc oxide eugenol (ZOE). Another brand is Cavitec. This procedure is written for I.R.M. It is used as a

Science

base under amalgam restorations and as a temporary cement or restoration. It cannot be used under resin or composite restorations because it interferes with the setting reaction of these materials.

Procedure

1. Assemble equipment. Read and follow the manufacturer's instructions for the brand being used.

2. Wash hands. Put on personal protective equipment (PPE).

 CAUTION: Observe standard precautions while assisting with any dental procedure.

Precaution

3. Fluff the powder by gently shaking the container. This ensures uniform bulk density of the contents. Open the lid carefully to avoid inhaling the powder.

4. Fill the powder scoop to excess without packing. Use the spatula to level the scoop (**Figure 19–71A**). Place the powder on the mixing pad.

5. Dispense one drop of liquid for each scoop of powder used or follow manufacturer's instructions. Dispense the drop of liquid on the pad next to the powder (**Figure 19–71B**).

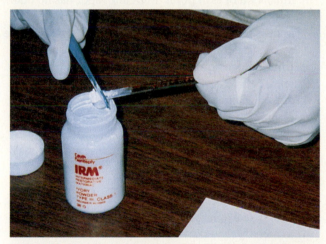

FIGURE 19–71A Use a spatula to level the powder in the scoop.

 CAUTION: Do not drop the liquid *into* the powder.

Safety

6. Return the empty dropper into the holder on the outside of the bottle. Close the cap of the bottle containing the liquid immediately.

NOTE: Prolonged contact between the dropper and the liquid eugenol will cause deterioration of the dropper, so the dropper is not stored in the liquid. If the cap is left off the bottle, evaporation of the liquid will occur.

7. Use the spatula to mix half of the powder and all of the liquid (**Figure 19–71C**). Use a stropping action with the spatula to thoroughly combine this powder with the liquid.

8. Add the rest of the powder to the mix in two or three increments. Spatulate thoroughly to mix.

NOTE: Some manufacturers recommend mixing all of the powder with the liquid at one time. Others recommend dividing the powder into four equal amounts. For this reason, it is essential to follow manufacturer's directions.

9. When all of the powder has been added, whip the mix vigorously for 5–10 seconds. The final mix should be smooth and adaptable.

NOTE: Total mixing should be complete in 1 to 1½ minutes.

10. Pass the mix and the preferred instrument to the doctor. The initial set occurs approximately 3–5 minutes from the start of mixing, so work quickly and efficiently.

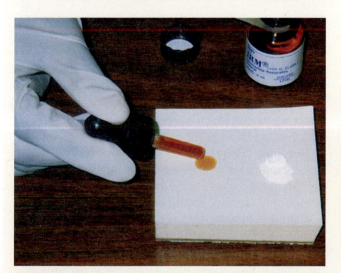

FIGURE 19–71B Dispense the liquid onto the pad next to the powder.

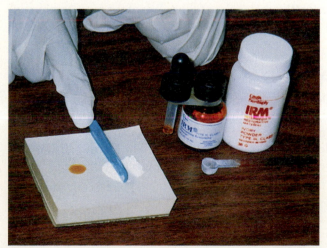

FIGURE 19–71C To begin mixing the powder and liquid, use the spatula to add half the powder to the liquid and mix thoroughly.

(continues)

11. Clean and replace all equipment. Check to be sure the lids on the bottles of powder and liquid are secure. Tear the sheet off of the mixing pad and discard the sheet in a waste container. Use orange solvent or alcohol to clean the spatula and other instruments. Scrub and sterilize all instruments.

12. Remove PPE. Wash hands thoroughly.

PRACTICE: Go to the workbook and use the evaluation sheet for 19:13D, Preparing Zinc Oxide Eugenol (ZOE), to practice this procedure. When you believe you have mastered this skill, sign the sheet and give it to your instructor for further action.

✅ **FINAL EVALUATION:** Using the criteria listed on the evaluation sheet, your instructor will grade your performance.

Check

19.14 PREPARING RESTORATIVE MATERIALS— AMALGAM AND COMPOSITE

A main method of treating dental caries is restoration by the placement of filling materials. **Restoration** is defined as the process of replacing a diseased portion of a tooth or a lost tooth by artificial means. This may include filling material, a crown, bridge, denture, partial denture, or implant.

Dental caries, or decay, is a disease process that attacks the hard tissues of the teeth, demineralizing and eventually destroying these tissues. When the enamel, dentin, and/or cementum are destroyed, a hollow space called a **cavity** is created in the tooth. To repair the damage caused by a carious lesion, the doctor removes the decayed and damaged tissue and fills the cavity preparation with a restorative material, or filling. Two of the most commonly used restorative materials are amalgam and composite.

AMALGAM

Dental **amalgam** is a restorative material used primarily on posterior teeth. Most dental offices do not use amalgam because it is mixed with mercury, but the dental assistant must still be familiar with amalgam because it is still used in some procedures.

- Dental amalgam is a mixture of metals (an alloy) combined with the metal mercury.

- Science Amalgam alloy contains four main metals: silver, tin, copper, and zinc. Each metal has certain properties that help form a durable restoration. To ensure a uniform product, the American Dental Association has established percentages by weight for each of these metals.

- **Mercury** is a metal that is a liquid at room temperature. It is added to other metals to form amalgam. It must be handled with care because it is highly toxic. It can vaporize (evaporate and float freely in the air) and be absorbed into the body through inhalation or skin pores. Mercury vapor has no odor, color, or taste, and is extremely difficult to detect. Many sources can produce a vapor. Examples include a leaking capsule, a mercury spill, air exposure while preparing and dispensing amalgam, particle release while polishing a restoration or removing old amalgam restorations, and/or improper storage of amalgam scraps. Even carpeting in a treatment room can retain amalgam particles; vacuuming can cause the mercury to vaporize into the air. Personal protective equipment (PPE), including disposable gloves, a gown, a face mask, and eye protection (glasses or a face shield) must be worn while working with dental amalgam. If skin is accidentally exposed to mercury, the skin should be scrubbed with soap and water and rinsed thoroughly. Mercury must be stored in well-sealed, unbreakable containers.

- Mercury spills should be cleaned up immediately by an *authorized* individual. The correct cleaning procedure is discussed in detail in Section 14:2 under *Environmental* Safety. Spill kits, containing gloves, a mercury-vapor respirator (to prevent inhalation of the mercury), a sulfur solution (to coat the droplets), a syringe with a large needle (to draw in the mercury), and polyethylene bags are used to clean up spills (**Figure 19–72**). In addition, proper cleanup is essential after working with dental amalgam. Mercury-contaminated items, such as gloves, masks, or used capsules should be discarded in a labeled and sealed polyethylene bag. Scrap amalgam should be submerged in a tightly sealed, unbreakable jar containing sulfur water, glycerin, or mineral oil. Most dental offices have a program of mercury hygiene to control mercury hazards. The dental assistant must become familiar with this program and follow established regulations.

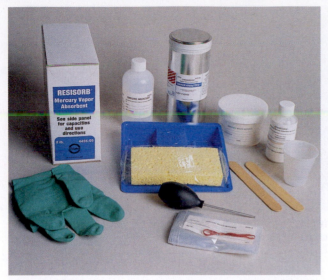

FIGURE 19–72 A mercury spill kit should be used to clean up mercury to prevent mercuric poisoning.

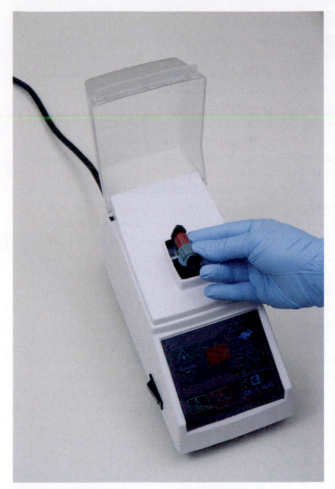

FIGURE 19–73 Place the capsule in the amalgamator. Read the manufacturer's instructions for correct trituration time.

- **Amalgamation** is the process that occurs when amalgam alloy is mixed with mercury. A new alloy is formed, which becomes the restorative (filling) material, called *dental amalgam*.

- **Trituration** is the mixing process used to combine mercury with the amalgam alloy. It is done with a mechanical amalgamator (a mixing machine) (**Figure 19–73**). It is important to follow the manufacturer's instructions regarding mixing (trituration) time.

- Dental amalgam alloy is purchased in disposable capsules containing premeasured amounts of amalgam alloy powder and mercury (**Figure 19–74**). The American Dental Association (ADA) encourages the use of these premeasured capsules because they eliminate mercury dispensers and decrease the possibility of a mercury spill, accidental inhalation of mercury vapor, or skin contact with the mercury. A membrane inside the capsule separates the amalgam alloy powder and mercury until the capsule is used. Usually, the capsule must be twisted or pressed to break the membrane and combine the alloy powder and mercury before the capsule is placed in the amalgamator for trituration.

- After amalgam has been triturated, it must be used immediately to produce a good restoration. The doctor uses an amalgam carrier to place the amalgam in the prepared cavity. The amalgam is then condensed, or packed, into the cavity preparation, after which the restoration is carved to correct occlusion (alignment between maxillary and mandibular teeth) and tooth contour.

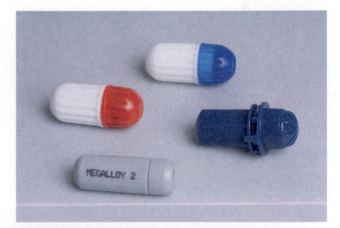

FIGURE 19–74 Dental amalgam alloy is purchased in disposable capsules containing premeasured amounts of amalgam alloy and mercury.

- Amalgam bonding agents are used for many restorations. These agents help the amalgam adhere to the tooth surfaces and increase the retention of the restoration. It is important to follow the manufacturer's recommendations while using any bonding agents.

COMPOSITE

Composite is the restorative material used most frequently in the repair of anterior teeth, but it also is used to restore posterior teeth. In comparison to other, older resins, composite offers improved appearance, increased strength, and the ability to withstand chemical actions caused by mouth fluids. It has an organic polymer matrix, such as dimethacrylate, and inorganic filler particles such as quartz, silica, and/or lithium aluminum silicate.

Self-curing, or *chemical-curing*, or *dual polymerization*, *composite* is supplied as two pastes or two cartridges that are mixed together to cause a chemical reaction. One paste or cartridge is a *base*, and the other is an *accelerator* (catalyst). When the composite base and accelerator are mixed together, substances present in the base and accelerator cause the reaction called *polymerization*, which results in a hardening of the material.

Light-cured composite is the most widely used type of composite. It is sensitive to light, and polymerization does not occur until the composite is exposed to a curing light (**Figure 19–75**). Light-cured composite is available in a premixed, syringe form. It is available in various shades to blend with the teeth. The amount needed is dispensed from the syringe and then placed in the tooth cavity. When the restoration is in place, a curing light is used on the composite, and the material sets (polymerizes). Both the doctor and the dental assistant must wear light-filtering glasses or use light-screening paddles while using the curing light to prevent eye damage. The patient should also be given light-filtering glasses or asked to close their eyes when the curing light is used.

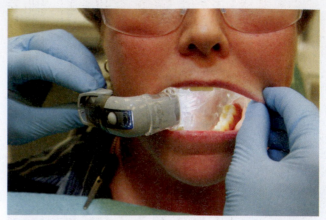

FIGURE 19–75 A curing light is used on light-cured composite to cause polymerization or hardening.

Before the composite is placed in the prepared cavity, the cavity is etched, and a bonding agent, or resin, is applied. The etching solution roughens the surface so that the composite will adhere (stick) and bond more securely to the tooth tissue. The bonding agent is then applied to help the composite material adhere to the tooth. Before using any composite, etching, or bonding materials, read and follow the manufacturer's instructions.

checkpoint

| **1.** What are dental caries?

PRACTICE: Go to the workbook and complete the assignment sheet for 19:14, Preparing Restorative Materials—Amalgam and Composite. Then return and continue with the procedures.

Procedure 19:14

Preparing Composite

Equipment and Supplies

Etching liquid, resin (universal and catalyst), composite (universal and catalyst) or light-cured composite syringe, cotton pellets, cotton pliers, mixing pads, mixing stick, plastic composite instruments, personal protective equipment (PPE)

Procedure

1. Assemble equipment (**Figure 19–76A**).
2. Wash hands. Put on personal protective equipment (PPE).

   CAUTION: Observe standard precautions while assisting with any dental procedure.

3. Assist doctor as required for the cavity preparation. A color match is usually performed to determine the shade of composite that should be used to restore the tooth and match the color of the tooth (**Figure 19–76B**).

4. When cavity preparation is complete, open the bottle of etching liquid. Dispense one to two drops on a mixing pad. Moisten a cotton pellet in the liquid. Pass cotton pliers and the moistened pellet to the doctor.

   NOTE: Etching liquid can also be dispensed into a disposable, plastic well and placed on a disposable brush for placement in the cavity. Wells and brushes are supplied with certain brands of etching liquid.

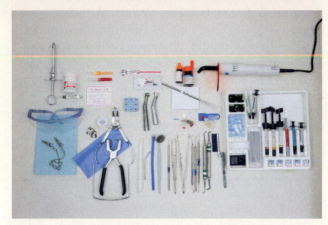

FIGURE 19–76A Equipment for a composite restoration.

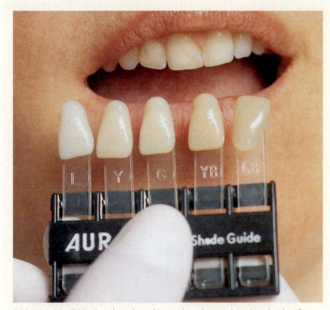

FIGURE 19–76B A color chart is used to determine the shade of composite required to restore the tooth.

NOTE: The doctor etches the surface for approximately 1 minute. This roughens the tooth surface to increase bond strength.

NOTE: If dentin is exposed, a calcium hydroxide base may be placed on the area prior to etching.

5. Pass the tri-flow syringe. The restorative area must be washed thoroughly with oil-free water and then dried after etching.

6. Prepare the bonding agent (resin). Place equal amounts (one to two drops) of universal and catalyst on a mixing pad or in a disposable, plastic well. Mix thoroughly for 5–10 seconds with a fine brush or plastic placement instrument. The doctor will apply this to the tooth surface.

NOTE: The bonding agent (resin) helps the composite material adhere to the tooth.

 CAUTION: Take care to avoid contaminating the contents of the universal container with those of the catalyst container. Such contamination may cause a reaction that destroys the contents of both containers.

7. Prepare the composite:

   a. If self-curing composite is being used, place an amount of universal paste equal to approximately half the size of the cavity on the mixing pad. Then place an equal amount of catalyst on the mixing pad. Mix the two pastes together for approximately 20 seconds and until the mix is smooth and well blended.

    CAUTION: Again, take care to avoid contaminating the contents of the universal container with those of the catalyst container. Such contamination may cause a reaction that destroys the contents of both containers.

   b. If a premixed, light-cured composite is used, dispense the amount required from the syringe. This type of composite material does not have to be mixed.

8. Use plastic composite instruments to pass the prepared composite paste to the doctor.

   NOTE: Plastic instruments will not discolor the mix. They also reduce the tendency of the composite to stick to the instruments.

9. Refill the instruments with composite mix as needed. Work quickly but efficiently.

   NOTE: Setting usually occurs 4 minutes after mixing. This allows approximately 1–2 minutes for placement.

   NOTE: If light-sensitive composite resin is used, the curing light is given to the doctor when the restoration is in place. The material will not harden, or set, until it is exposed to this light.

    CAUTION: The doctor and the dental assistant must wear light-filtering glasses or use light-screening paddles while using the curing light. The patient must also be given light-filtering glasses or asked to close their eyes.

(continues)

10. Have composite finishing and polishing strips ready for use.

11. Clean materials from instruments immediately. The mixing sticks are usually disposable. Discard these immediately to avoid contaminating the containers. Scrub and sterilize all instruments.

12. Replace all equipment. Check to make sure the lids on all containers are securely in place.

13. Remove PPE. Wash hands.

PRACTICE: Go to the workbook and use the evaluation sheet for 19:14, Preparing Composite, to practice this procedure. When you believe you have mastered this skill, sign the sheet and give it to your instructor for further action.

 Check   **FINAL EVALUATION:** Using the criteria listed on the evaluation sheet, your instructor will grade your performance.

19:15 DENTAL RADIOGRAPHS (X-RAYS)

Dental radiographs are important in diagnosing dental conditions. They are used to locate carious lesions, or dental decay; reveal tooth abscesses, cysts, or tumors; find cracks or damage in existing restorations; reveal bone loss from periodontal (gum) disease; determine if sufficient bone is present for dental implants; plan orthodontic treatments required to straighten teeth; check the condition of crowns and root canal treatments; and calculate placement of bridges or dentures.

 Technology   Digital dental radiography is a technique that is being used in most dental offices. Digital radiography eliminates the need for X-ray film and developing processes. An electronic pad or sensor is positioned in the mouth and beams of radiation are directed toward the sensor. A computer picks up the electronic image from the sensor and displays it on the screen for immediate viewing. A color contrast can also be used for the image. The radiographic image can be printed or stored electronically in the patient's electronic health record (EHR), also known as an electronic dental record (EDR). Another advantage of digital radiography is that the computer can compare the current image with previous images. Everything that is the same is eliminated and a clear image of anything new or different appears on the screen. This is called subtraction radiography and it allows the doctor to immediately note any changes in the structure of the teeth or oral cavity. Digital radiography also decreases an individual's exposure to radiation by as much as 80–90 percent. However, the amount of radiation from dental radiographs is minimal, usually about 800 times less radiation than a chest X-ray, so the benefit is slight.

In some dental offices, standard dental X-rays are still taken and developed. In most cases, an automatic film processor is used for the developing process. It is essential to read and follow the manufacturer's instructions for using the automatic processor and for performing proper maintenance on it.

Dental **radiographs** are negatives taken of the teeth, similar to the negatives received when photographs are taken. X-ray beams are passed through the teeth and tissues. A series of shadows are then produced on film. Images on the developed film are described as radiolucent or radiopaque:

- **Radiolucent**: These areas appear dark on radiographs. This means that the X-rays penetrate through the structures. Examples of these areas are the pulp and caries.

- **Radiopaque**: These areas appear light or white on radiographs. This means that the structures stop the X-rays, or that the X-rays are unable to penetrate the structures. Most tooth structures, including enamel and dentin, are radiopaque. Metallic restorations also appear very white, or radiopaque, on X-rays.

A full-mouth series of radiographs (**Figure 19–77**) shows all of the teeth and all of the surrounding bone, helping to diagnose cavities, cysts or tumors, abscesses, impacted teeth, and gum disease. A full mouth usually

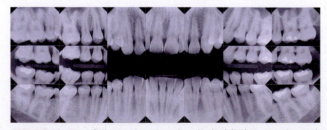

FIGURE 19–77 A full-mouth series of periapical (PA) X-rays shows the crowns and roots of all the teeth. © iStock.com/Martin Alfaro

consists of 14–20 individual radiographs and is generally recommended during the first visit with a new dentist to aid in proper diagnosis and treatment planning.

There are several different types of dental radiographs:

- **Bite-wings** (BWXR): These show only the crowns of the maxillary and mandibular teeth (**Figure 19–78**). They are called cavity-detecting radiographs because they are primarily used to detect inter-proximal (between the teeth) decay and recurring decay under restorations. They do not show root-end infection or abscess. Usually, two to four bite-wings are taken of the posterior teeth. Sometimes two to four bite-wings are taken of anterior teeth in adults. Two common sizes of bite-wing film include: size *1* used for anterior teeth, and size *3* used for posterior teeth.

- **Periapical films** (PA): These show the tooth and the surrounding area, and can show root-end infection. They are also used to determine the number and shape of roots, the condition of supporting structures of the teeth, and the relationship of a tooth to other teeth. Usually, 14 periapical radiographs are taken for a full-mouth series. This shows the complete dentition (refer to Figure 19–77). Size 2 film is usually used for periapical films, but a size *1* film can be used for adults with small mouths or children over 6 years of age.

- **Pedodontic (child) films**: These are smaller films, usually size 0, used on children to show disease or other conditions of the teeth. Both bite-wings (BWs) and periapicals (PAs) are taken.

- **Occlusal films**: These films, size *4*, are approximately twice the size of a number *2* film. They are used to view the occlusal (chewing) planes of the maxilla or mandible.

- **Panoramic**: This is a special type of radiograph that shows the entire dental arch, or all of the teeth, on one film. The film is placed in a film cassette in a panoramic X-ray unit that rotates around the

patient's head (**Figure 19–79A**). One developed film shows complete dentition, bone structure, and surrounding tissues (**Figure 19–79B**).

Radiographs are placed in special mounts for viewing or positioned in a specific way on the computer screen. The most common positioning for a full-mouth series of X-rays is shown in **Figure 19–80**. If nondigital X-rays are placed in a special mount or on a viewing box, they must be positioned correctly. Basic principles are as follows:

- Each film contains a dimple. This dimple points toward the X-ray machine. One side of the film shows a concave (pointing inward) dimple. The other side shows a convex (pointing outward) dimple.

- In one mount, all dimples must be facing the same direction.

- When all the dimples are convex (pointing outward), you are viewing the facial surface (buccal or labial). When the films are placed in the mount in this manner, the films on your left are the patient's right teeth, and the films on your right are the patient's left teeth. This is the most widely used method for mounting X-rays because most dental charts use this facial view of the teeth.

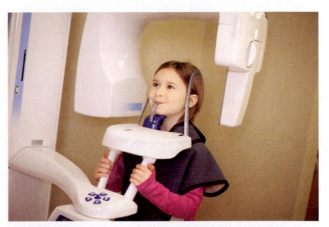

FIGURE 19–79A After a patient is positioned in a panoramic X-ray machine, the unit rotates around the patient's head. © iStock.com/Martin Alfaro

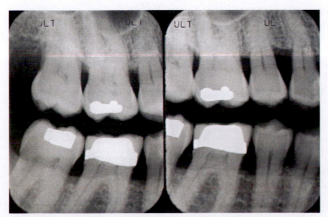

FIGURE 19–78 Bite-wing (BW) X-rays show only the crowns of the maxillary and mandibular teeth. © iStock.com/lawcain

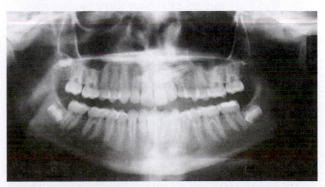

FIGURE 19–79B A panoramic X-ray shows complete dentition, bone structure, and surrounding tissue. Photo courtesy of Dr. Steve Gregg

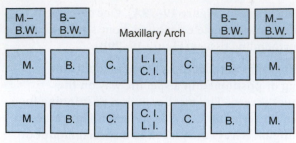

Maxillary Arch

| M.–B.W. | B.–B.W. | | | B.–B.W. | M.–B.W. |

| M. | B. | C. | L.I. C.I. | C. | B. | M. |

| M. | B. | C. | C.I. L.I. | C. | B. | M. |

Mandibular Arch

Abbreviations:
B.W.   Bite-wings
C.I.   Central incisors
L.I.   Lateral incisors
C.   Cuspids
B.   Bicuspids
M.   Molars

FIGURE 19–80 Correct placement for a full-mouth series of X-rays.

- When all the dimples are concave (pointing inward), you are viewing the lingual (tongue) surface. Thus, the films on your right are the patient's right teeth, and the films on your left are the patient's left teeth.

- The doctor determines the manner in which films should be mounted.

- Review the following facts about dentition. They are essential for mounting or positioning films:

  a. Bite-wing X-rays show only the crowns of maxillary and mandibular teeth.

  b. Periapical films show the crowns and roots of teeth.

  c. Maxillary films often have a hazy or swirly area, which is the maxillary sinus.

  d. Maxillary central incisors are larger than mandibular central incisors.

  e. Maxillary lateral incisors are larger than mandibular lateral incisors.

  f. Mandibular lateral incisors are wider than mandibular central incisors.

  g. Maxillary cuspids are the longest teeth in the mouth.

  h. Maxillary molars each have three blurred roots.

  i. Mandibular molars each have two distinct roots.

- Locate the four (or two) bite-wings (BW). Position these in the correct areas (refer to Figure 19–80). The bicuspid views should be placed closer to the center of the mount.

- Locate the two central incisor (CI) and lateral incisor (LI) films. Look at the size of the teeth to determine which are maxillary films and which are mandibular

films. Position the maxillary films with the roots pointing upward. Position the mandibular films with the roots pointing downward.

- Locate the four cuspid (C) films. The larger or longer cuspids are maxillary. Note the incisors and bicuspids on either side of the cuspids. Position the cuspid films in the correct areas.

- Locate the four bicuspid (B) films. The maxillary 1st bicuspid is the only bicuspid that is bifurcated (having two roots). Note the two maxillary films. Place them in the mount by noting cuspids and molars on either side. Do the same for the mandibular bicuspids.

- Locate the four molar (M) films. Note the blurred, trifurcated (three) roots of the maxillary molars. Look for hazy or swirly areas that indicate the maxillary sinuses. Note the arch curvature in the back of the mouth. Place these films in the correct positions. Note the bifurcated (two) roots of the mandibular molars. Use the arch and bicuspid locations to place these films in the correct mount positions.

- Check whether there are radiopaque restorations on the films, for purposes of comparison and verification of placement accuracy. Restorations can also serve as clues to placement when the quality of one film is poor or the film has been taken incorrectly.

- When all of the X-rays have been positioned correctly, they are ready for the doctor to review.

Safety **CAUTION:** *Even though radiation levels are minimal while taking dental radiographs, radiation is still being generated and safety practices should always be observed. Leaded aprons can minimize exposure to the abdomen and a thyroid collar covering can protect the thyroid from radiation. Both can be used to protect the patient. Dental assistants and staff must stay behind the barrier wall while the image is being taken. Safety factors are always paramount in any health care practice.*

checkpoint

1. How many types of dental radiographs are there? What does each type show?

PRACTICE: Go to the workbook and complete the assignment sheet for 19:15, Dental Radiographs (X-Rays).

Tissue Engineering of Pulp to Replace Endodontics?

Pulp is the soft tissue made up of blood vessels and nerves in the innermost area of the tooth. Cells within the pulp help produce dentin, which makes up the main bulk of the tooth. When the pulp is damaged by dental disease or injury to the tooth, the usual therapy is an endodontic root canal. This therapy involves removing the entire pulp area and replacing it with a gutta-percha filling. Even though this therapy prevents the loss of the tooth, the tooth is much weaker because there is a significant loss of dentin. In addition, without pulp, there is no additional production of dentin. An ideal therapy would be to remove the diseased or damaged pulp and replace it with regenerated pulp tissue that will maintain the tooth as a functioning tissue.

Researchers in many different countries are attempting to use tissue engineering to replace damaged pulp. Tissue engineering applies the principles of engineering and life sciences to develop biological substitutes that can restore, maintain, or improve tissue function. Three major factors are required: stem cells, scaffolds, and growth factors.

Researchers have been able to isolate dental pulp stem cells (DPSCs) readily from extracted third molars. These molars are commonly called wisdom teeth and are frequently extracted because they form incorrectly or put pressure on other teeth in the mouth. In order for the DPSCs to grow, they must be attached to a scaffold or structure specifically created to support the stem cells. The scaffold must be biocompatible (not toxic to a living tissue), biodegradable (capable of being broken down), and have adequate physical strength. Using polymers such as collagen or gelatin, or synthetic materials, researchers have designed different three-dimensional scaffolds that appear to allow the attachment of the DSCPs. After the DSCPs are attached to the scaffold, researchers must provide an environment that transports nutrients and oxygen to the cells and removes waste material from the cells so they can develop into pulp tissue. Early research in mice showed that the stem cells developed into odontoblasts, or cells that form dentin. In initial trials, however, the regenerated pulp tissue had limited function when transplanted into a tooth. Researchers are now working with a collagen scaffold for the DSCPs and implanting it in the root canal of teeth in mice. Initial studies have shown that within a 6-week period, the teeth had developed pulp-like tissues with blood vessels to sustain the pulp.

Even though many more years of research will be necessary before this concept becomes a reality, researchers already know that engineering a complex tissue such as dental pulp is no longer an unachievable goal. There is a strong possibility that in the near future dentists will be able to repair damaged teeth so that they function for the entire life of an individual.

Case Study Investigation Conclusion

LaTonya was hired by Dr. Green because she possessed the personal characteristics and dental assisting skills that fit in with her practice. What skills and characteristics were on your list? How were those skills documented or observed (lab check off, job experience, or some other way)? Which skills/characteristics are the most important?

CHAPTER 19 SUMMARY

- Many different skills are performed by the dental assistant. Some of the more common skills were discussed in this chapter.

- A knowledge of the structure, names, and surfaces of the teeth is essential. The dental assistant must also be familiar with the Universal/National Numbering System and the Federation Dentaire International System for identifying teeth.

- Taking impressions and pouring models of the teeth are tasks frequently performed when dental restorative or orthodontic treatment is necessary.

In addition, custom trays are made to obtain more exact models of patients' mouths.

- A knowledge of basic dental instruments allows the dental assistant to assist the doctor when basic dental restorative procedures are performed. The dental assistant helps by preparing dental anesthetic materials, mixing bases and cements, and preparing restorative materials. After procedures are complete, the dental assistant is often responsible for the maintenance and care of the equipment and instruments used.

REVIEW QUESTIONS

1. Draw a diagram of a tooth. Label the four sections or divisions of the tooth, the four tissues of the tooth, and the structures of the periodontium.

2. Name the five (5) surfaces, eight (8) line angles, and four (4) point angles for both anterior and posterior teeth.

3. Identify both the Universal/National Numbering System and the Federation Dentaire International System code for each of the following permanent teeth:
   a. maxillary right central incisor
   b. maxillary left 2nd molar
   c. mandibular left cuspid
   d. mandibular right 1st bicuspid

4. Explain the maintenance and disinfection requirements for each of the following types of dental equipment:
   a. dental chair
   b. dental light
   c. tri-flow or air-water syringe
   d. low-speed handpiece

5. List the main dental instruments that would be placed on the tray for each of the following procedures:
   a. prophylactic and oral examination
   b. amalgam restoration
   c. composite restoration
   d. surgical extraction

6. Differentiate between general anesthesia, analgesia or sedation, local anesthesia, and topical anesthesia.

7. State the main function of a dental varnish, base, cement, and temporary.

8. Draw a diagram of the 14 periapical films for a full-mouth series of radiographs. Identify the teeth that are shown in each film.

■ CRITICAL THINKING

1. If teeth are brushed correctly, why must they be flossed?

2. Why is mercury dangerous?

   2a. List four safety precautions that must be observed while working with mercury and dental amalgam.

■ ACTIVITIES

1. You are assigned to teach brushing and flossing to second graders at your local elementary school. Create a dental model that you can use to demonstrate the Bass method of brushing. Using clear language, video a lesson on brushing and flossing that the elementary nurse can broadcast.

2. With a partner, create a shoebox example of the perfect dental practice. Keep in mind safety, efficiency, and customer/patient comfort.

   For additional information on dental careers, contact the following associations:

- American Dental Assistants Association
  www.adaausa.org

- American Dental Association
  www.ada.org

- American Dental Education Association
  www.adea.org

- American Dental Hygienists' Association
  www.adha.org

- Dental Assisting National Board, Inc.
  www.danb.org

- National Association of Advisors for the Health Professions, Inc.
  www.naahp.org

- National Association of Dental Laboratories
  www.nadl.org

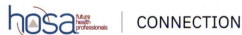 | CONNECTION

Competitive Event: Dental Science

Event Summary: Dental Science provides members with the opportunity to gain knowledge and skills required for dental careers. This competitive event consists of 2 rounds. Round One is a written, multiple choice test and the top scoring competitors will advance to Round Two for the skills assessment. This event aims to inspire members to learn more about careers in the dental field.

Details on this competitive event may be found at:

www.hosa.org/guidelines

Case Study Investigation

Madison, Jane, and Lee were friends that got jobs at the grocery store. They needed to have a drug screening test done before they could be put on the store schedule. This was each friend's first job, and they were nervous because they didn't know what to expect.

When the friends got to the clinic, they were met by Aika. She explained what would happen. At the end of this chapter, you will be asked how Aika would describe the test and how she could put Madison, Jane, and Lee at ease.

■ LEARNING OBJECTIVES

After completing this chapter, you should be able to:

- Operate the microscope and identify its parts.
- Obtain a culture specimen without contaminating it.
- Streak an agar plate or slide.
- Stain a bacterial slide using the Gram's stain technique.
- Puncture the skin to obtain blood, observing all safety factors.
- Perform a microhematocrit.
- Perform a hemoglobin test.
- Prepare and stain a blood smear using Wright's stain.
- Test blood for type and Rh factors using antiserums.
- Perform an erythrocyte sedimentation rate (ESR).
- Measure blood-sugar (glucose) level.
- Test urine using a reagent strip.
- Measure specific gravity of urine.
- Prepare urine for microscopic examination.
- Define, pronounce, and spell all key terms.

KEY TERMS

agar plate
antibody screen
anticoagulant *(an"-tie-coh-ag'-you-lant)*
antigen *(an'-tih-jen")*
anuria *(ah-nur'-ree"-ah)*
blood smear
culture specimen
differential count
direct smear
erythrocyte sedimentation rate (ESR)
erythrocytes *(eh-rith'-row-sites")*
fasting blood sugar (FBS)
glucose

glucose tolerance test (GTT)
glycohemoglobin test
glycosuria *(gly'-coh-shur'-ee-ah)*
Gram's stain
hematocrit (Hct) *(hih'-mat'-on-krit)*
hematuria *(hee"-mah-tyour'-ee-ah)*
hemoglobin (Hgb) *(hee'-mow-glow"-bin)*
hemolysis *(hih"-mall'-ah-sis)*
hyperglycemia *(high"-purr-gly-see"-me-ah)*
hypoglycemia *(high"-poh-gly-see'-me-ah)*
leukocytes

microscope
oliguria *(oh"-lih-goo'-ree-ah)*
polyuria
reagent strips
refractometer *(ree-frack-tum'-ee-ter)*
resistant
sensitive
skin puncture
specific gravity
typing and crossmatch
urinalysis *(your'-in-al"-ee-sis)*
urinary sediment
urinometer
venipuncture

Career Highlights

Career

Medical, or clinical, laboratory personnel work under the supervision of doctors, usually pathologists. They are important members of the health care team. They perform laboratory tests on body tissues, fluids, and cells to aid in the detection, diagnosis, and treatment of disease. Levels of personnel are the technologist, technician, laboratory assistant, and phlebotomist. Clinical laboratory scientists (CLS) or medical technologists (MT) perform more complex tests and have a bachelor's or master's degree. Clinical laboratory technicians (CLT) or medical laboratory technicians (MLT) perform less complex tests and usually have an associate's degree. Medical laboratory assistants perform basic laboratory tests and usually have specialized health science education (HSE) training. Phlebotomists, or venipuncture technicians, collect blood and prepare it for testing. They usually have 1–2 years of on-the-job experience or specialized health science education (HSE) training. Some states require laboratory personnel to be licensed or registered. Certification can be obtained from the National Credentialing Agency for Laboratory Personnel (NCA), the American Society for Clinical Pathology (ASCP), or the American Medical Technologists Association (AMT), each of which has specific requirements.

Legal

Any medical laboratory or physician office laboratory (POL) that performs tests on human specimens is regulated by a federal amendment, the Clinical Laboratory Improvement Amendment (CLIA) of 1988. CLIA established standards, regulations, and performance requirements based on the complexity of a test and the risk factors associated with incorrect results. The purpose is to ensure quality laboratory testing. Levels of complexity include waived tests, moderately complex tests including provider performed microscopic procedures (PPMP), and highly complex tests. Each of these levels has different requirements for personnel and quality control. Laboratories are certified by the U.S. Department of Health and Human Services (USDHHS) based on these levels. In addition, only Food and Drug Administration (FDA) approved equipment or self-contained kits may be used to perform waived tests. The FDA maintains an up-to-date listing of approved equipment and self-contained kits for waived tests at *www.fda.gov* in the search for *waived analytes* (substances whose chemical components are being identified and measured). Therefore, *medical laboratory assistants/medical assistants must follow all legal requirements before performing any laboratory test*. Some examples of waived tests, or tests that can be performed by assistants if the agency where they are working has a CLIA waiver certificate and if the equipment or self-contained test kits are FDA approved, include:

- Most urinary reagent strip (dipstick) or reagent tablet tests

- Hematocrit and spun microhematocrit

- Erythrocyte sedimentation rate (nonautomated)

- Blood cell counts, such as white blood cells and platelets

- Ovulation and pregnancy tests by visual color comparison

- Hemoglobin: automated by single analyte instruments with self-contained components to perform specimen/reagent interaction and provide direct measurement and readout

- Blood glucose

- Fecal occult blood

- Cholesterol monitoring

- Rapid tests for specific substances, such as streptococcus, adenovirus, respiratory viruses, hepatitis antibodies, and HIV antibodies

- Gastric occult blood

- Specific drug screening, such as nicotine, methadone, oxycodone, and methamphetamines

- Specified automated blood chemistry analysis

- Triglyceride test

- Provider-performed microscopy procedures (PPMP), such as pin-worm, nasal smear, and fecal leukocyte examinations if lab is certified for PPMP

Many of the waived tests are discussed in this chapter. In addition to the knowledge and skills presented in this chapter, medical laboratory assistants must also learn and master skills such as:

- Presenting a professional appearance and attitude

- Obtaining knowledge regarding health care delivery systems, organizational structure, and teamwork

- Meeting all legal responsibilities

- Communicating effectively

- Being sensitive to and respecting cultural diversity

- Comprehending human anatomy, physiology, and pathophysiology with an emphasis on cells, tissues, and body fluids, especially blood and urine

(continues)

- Learning medical terminology
- Observing all safety precautions
- Practicing all principles of infection control
- Performing business and accounting duties,

such as answering the telephone, scheduling appointments, preparing correspondence, completing insurance forms, and maintaining accounts and patient records

- Using computer and technology skills
- Cleaning and maintaining laboratory equipment
- Ordering and maintaining supplies and materials

LEGAL ALERT

Legal Before performing any procedures in this chapter, know and follow the standards and regulations established by the scope of practice; federal laws and agencies; state laws; state or national licensing, registration, or certification boards; professional organizations; professional standards; and agency policies.

It is your responsibility to learn exactly what you are legally permitted to do and to perform only procedures for which you have been trained.

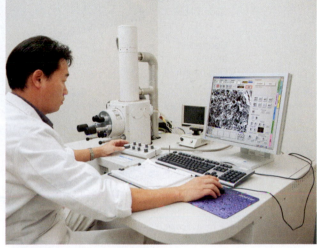

FIGURE 20–1A An electron microscope uses electron beams instead of a light source to view objects. Wake Forest Institute for Regenerative Medicine

20:1 OPERATING THE MICROSCOPE

Science The **microscope** is an instrument used to magnify and visualize objects too small to be seen with the naked eye. It is a valuable tool used in many health professions. To obtain the desired results when working with the microscope, it is important to first become familiar with its parts and how to use them correctly.

Many different models of microscopes are available. A *monocular microscope* has one eyepiece, and a *binocular microscope* has two eyepieces. The quality of microscopes also varies, according to the type of lenses, attachments, and magnification ability. The *compound*, bright-field microscope, described in this chapter, is one of the most commonly used microscopes. An *epifluorescence microscope* is used to detect antibodies and specific organisms by using a fluorescent dye stain. An *electron microscope*, which is extremely expensive and requires special expertise to operate, uses electron beams instead of a light source to view objects (**Figure 20–1A**). The beam is passed

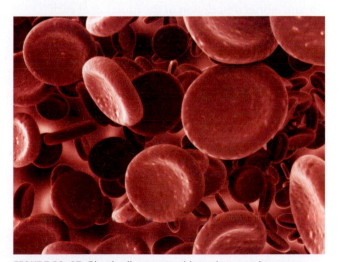

FIGURE 20–1B Blood cells as seen with an electron microscope.
© Jezper/Shutterstock.com

through the specimen and the image is projected onto a screen where it may be enlarged and/or photographed. Electron microscopes are used to view extremely small objects, such as cell organelles, viruses, and blood cells (**Figure 20–1B**).

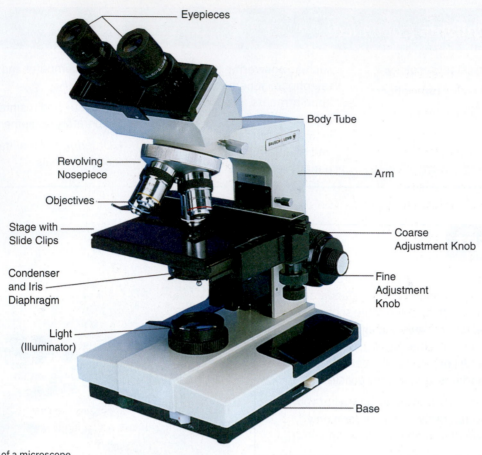

Eyepieces

Body Tube

Revolving
Nosepiece

Arm

Objectives

Stage with
Slide Clips

Coarse
Adjustment Knob

Condenser
and Iris
Diaphragm

Fine
Adjustment
Knob

Light
(Illuminator)

Base

FIGURE 20–2 Parts of a microscope.

Most microscopes contain the same basic parts. A list and a brief description of the function of each part follows. The parts of a microscope are shown in **Figure 20–2**.

- **Base**: This is the solid stand on which the microscope rests.

- **Arm**: This is the long, back stem of the microscope. In most cases, the arm is used to carry the microscope.

- **Eyepiece(s)**: This is the part(s) of the microscope through which the eye views the object or slide. The eyepiece usually has a magnification power of 10× (10 times). This means that it makes the object on the slide appear 10 times larger than normal. Some microscopes have zoom lenses. On these, the magnification can range from 10× to 20×, depending on how the eyepiece is positioned. Special lens paper should be used to clean the eyepiece to avoid scratching the lenses. The eyepiece is also called the *ocular viewpiece*.

- **Objectives**: Objectives are the parts of the microscope that magnify the object being viewed. They work with the eyepiece. A microscope may have three or four objectives, and they can vary. Some of the more common objectives are:

(1) The low-power objective is the shortest in length. It magnifies the object being viewed four times (4×).

(2) Another low-power objective magnifies the object 10 times (10×).

(3) The high-power objectives magnify the object 40 or 45 times (40× or 45×).

(4) The oil-immersion (OI) objective usually has a magnification power of 95× to 100×. Oil must be used with this objective because the image is usually too dark to be seen otherwise. The oil concentrates the light. A drop of immersion oil is placed on the slide. The oil-immersion objective is carefully rotated into the drop of oil. Care must be taken to prevent the oil from coming in contact with any of the other objectives on the microscope.

NOTE: *Smaller specimens require greater magnification. However, the high-power objectives have small openings. Therefore, to view small specimens, use a high-power objective and more light.*

For large specimens, use low-power objectives and less light. Special lens paper should be used to clean the objectives.

- **Revolving nosepiece**: This is the section to which the objectives are attached. It is turned to change the objective being used.

- **Stage**: The stage is the flat platform for the slide. Slide clips are located on the stage to hold the slide in place.

- **Coarse adjustment**: This is the larger knob on the arm. It moves the objectives up and down and also brings the slide into rough focus. The coarse adjustment should be used only on the low-power (10×) objective. It is important to watch the stage while moving the objectives to avoid breaking the slide and/or objectives.

- **Fine adjustment**: This is the smaller knob on the arm. It moves the objectives slowly for a precise and clear image. The fine adjustment is used on the low-power (10×), high-power (40–45×), and oil-immersion (95–100×) objectives.

- **Condenser and iris diaphragm**: This structure is directly underneath the stage. The condenser controls the intensity of light that passes through to the specimen on the stage. It contains an iris diaphragm that regulates the amount of light. The diaphragm is turned to a larger or smaller hole to increase or decrease the amount of light.

- **Illuminating light**: Located under the stage, the illuminating light provides the necessary light for viewing; the amount of light is controlled by the iris diaphragm.

- **Body tube**: This section connects the eyepiece and the objectives.

Math
To determine total magnification of an object (how many times you are magnifying or enlarging the object), multiply the power of the eyepiece times the power of the objective in use.

- **Example 1**: If the eyepiece is 10× and the objective is 4×, multiply the 10 and the 4.

$$10 \times 4 = 40$$

The object is magnified or enlarged 40 times its original size.

- **Example 2**: Eyepiece is 20× and objective is 40×.

$$20 \times 40 = 800$$

The object is magnified or enlarged 800 times its original size.

Proper care and cleaning of any microscope is important because dirt and dust can interfere with proper viewing and damage the delicate glass on the eyepiece

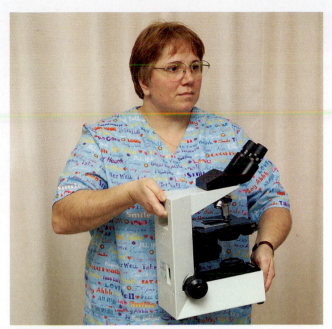

FIGURE 20–3 To carry a microscope, place one hand firmly on the arm and the other hand under the base.

and objectives. The glass in the eyepiece and objectives should be cleaned with special lens paper. Paper towels, tissues, and cloths can scratch the delicate glass. The rest of the microscope should be wiped clean with a damp, soft cloth after use. If a biological specimen such as urine or blood is examined, standard precautions must be observed (see Section 15:4). In addition, a disinfectant should be used to wipe the stage of the microscope. When oil is used with an oil-immersion objective, the oil should be wiped off immediately after use because it can seep into the lens case. Before storing the microscope, the low-power objective should be in place, and the nosepiece should be moved to its lowest position. When the microscope is not in use, it should be covered with a dust cover or stored in a dust-free cabinet. It is also important to avoid jarring or bumping the microscope because it is a delicate instrument. To carry or move a microscope, one hand should be placed firmly on the arm and the other hand under the base (**Figure 20–3**). The microscope must be put down gently when it is placed on a desk or counter. It is important to read and follow the specific operating instructions provided by the manufacturer before using any microscope.

check**point**

1. Instead of a light source, what does an electron microscope use to view objects?

PRACTICE: Go to the workbook and complete the assignment sheet for 20:1, Operating the Microscope. Then return and continue with the procedure.

Operating the Microscope

Equipment and Supplies

Microscope; lens paper; slide and coverslip; hair, paper, or other small object; drop of water; immersion oil; gloves for a biological specimen

Procedure

1. Assemble equipment.

2. Wash hands. Put on gloves if needed.

    CAUTION: Wear gloves and observe standard precautions while handling any specimen contaminated by blood or body fluids, or while examining pathogenic organisms. If splashing of the specimen is possible, wear a gown, mask or face shield, and eye protection.

3. Use a prepared slide or get a clean slide. Place a human hair, shred of paper, or other small object on the slide. Add a drop of water or normal saline. Cover with a clean coverslip by holding the coverslip at an angle and allowing it to drop on the specimen.

   NOTE: Make sure there are no air bubbles between the slide and coverslip. If air bubbles are present, remove the coverslip and position it again.

4. Use lens paper to clean the eyepiece (ocular viewpiece) and the objectives (**Figure 20–4A**).

    CAUTION: Do not use any other material to clean these surfaces. Towels, rags, and tissues can scratch these surfaces.

5. Turn on the illuminating light. Open the iris diaphragm so that the largest hole is located directly under the hole in the stage platform.

6. Turn the revolving nosepiece until the low-power objective clicks into place.

7. Place the slide on the stage. Fasten it with the slide clips (**Figure 20–4B**).

   NOTE: Avoid getting fingerprints or smudges on the slide.

8. Watch the stage and slide. Turn the coarse adjustment so that the objective moves down close to the slide.

    CAUTION: Do not look into the eyepiece while moving the objective down. The objective could crack the slide and/or be damaged.

9. Now, look through the eyepiece. Slowly turn the body tube upward until the object comes into focus.

10. Change to the fine adjustment. Turn the knob slowly until the object comes into its sharpest focus (**Figure 20–4C**).

11. Do the following while still using low power:

    a. Move the slide to the right while looking through the eyepiece. In which direction does the image move?

    b. Move the slide to the left. In which direction does the image move?

    c. Open and close the iris diaphragm. How does this affect the image?

12. Without moving the body tube, turn the revolving nosepiece until the high-power objective is in place. Focus with the fine adjustment only.

    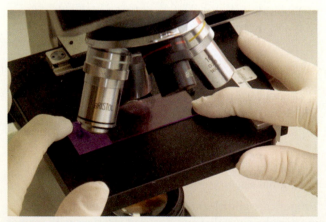 **CAUTION:** Watch the slide while turning the objectives to avoid breaking the slide or objectives.

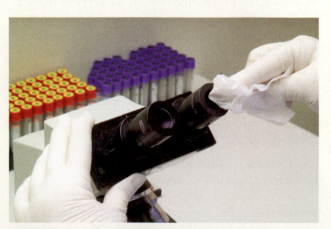

FIGURE 20–4A Use lens paper to clean the eyepiece and objectives.

FIGURE 20–4B Place the slide on the stage and fasten it in place with the slide clips.

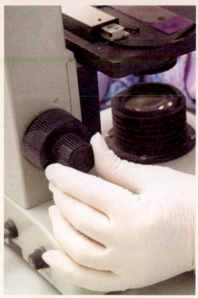

FIGURE 20–4C Turn the fine adjustment slowly until the object is in its sharpest focus.

13. Under high power, make the following observations:

   a. How does the amount of light compare with that needed under low power? (You may need to adjust the diaphragm for better viewing.)

   b. Do you see a larger or a smaller area of the object than was seen under low power?

14. If the microscope has an oil-immersion objective, do the following:

   a. Turn the revolving nosepiece until the oil-immersion objective is in position. Focus with fine adjustment only.

    CAUTION: Watch the slide while turning the objectives to avoid breaking the slide or objectives.

   b. Move the oil-immersion objective slightly to either side so that no objective is in position.

   c. Place a small drop of immersion oil on the part of the slide that will be directly under the objective (**Figure 20–4D**).

    CAUTION: Use the oil sparingly.

   d. Move the oil-immersion objective back into position, taking care that no other objective comes in contact with the oil. Make sure that the oil-immersion objective is touching the drop of oil.

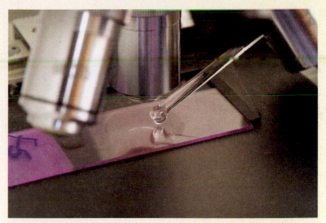

FIGURE 20–4D After moving the oil-immersion objective slightly to the side, place a drop of oil on the slide.

   e. Look through the eyepiece and use the fine adjustment to bring the slide into focus.

   f. Move the diaphragm as necessary to adjust the amount of light for viewing the slide.

   g. When you are done viewing the slide, turn the revolving nosepiece until the low-power objective is in position.

    CAUTION: Make sure no other objective comes in contact with the oil on the slide.

   h. Use lens paper to carefully remove all the oil from the oil-immersion objective (**Figure 20–4E**).

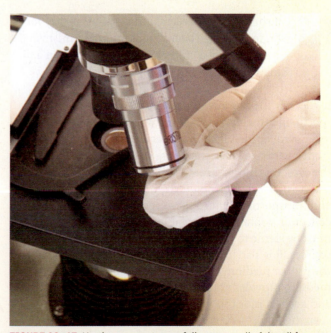

FIGURE 20–4E Use lens paper to carefully remove all of the oil from the objective.

(continues)

15. When you are done viewing the slide, remove the slide and the coverslip. Wash and dry both items.

CAUTION: Handle both with care. They break easily.

16. Use the special lens paper to clean the eyepiece and the objectives.

CAUTION: Do not use any other material to clean these parts. Towels, rags, and tissues can scratch these surfaces.

17. Use a damp, soft cloth to wipe the other parts of the microscope. If a biological specimen or pathogenic organisms were on the slide, wipe the microscope stage with a disinfectant.

18. Using the coarse adjustment, move the low-power objective so that it is in its lowest position, down close to the stage.

19. Turn off the illuminating light.

20. Place the cover back on the microscope. This protects it from dust in the room. The microscope can also be stored in a dust-free cabinet.

CAUTION: Remember to place one hand on the arm and the other hand under the base while moving the microscope.

21. Make sure that the microscope is kept away from the counter's edge. This prevents the microscope from being knocked to the floor.

22. Clean and replace all equipment.

23. Remove gloves if worn. Wash hands.

PRACTICE: Go to the workbook and use the evaluation sheet for 20:1, Operating the Microscope, to practice this procedure. When you believe you have mastered this skill, sign the sheet and give it to your instructor for further action.

✅ **FINAL EVALUATION:** Using the criteria listed on the evaluation sheet, your instructor will grade your performance.

20:2 OBTAINING AND HANDLING CULTURES

🧪 *Science*

In some health careers, it may be necessary for you to obtain a specimen of microorganisms, grow them on a culture medium, and stain a small sample.

A **culture specimen** is obtained when a doctor wants to identify the causative agent of a disease. The sample specimen is then either examined promptly or grown and examined for identification. Specimens may be obtained from a variety of sites, including lesions on the skin or from the eyes, ears, nose, throat, or other body openings. A wide variety of collection containers are available for obtaining and transporting culture specimens (**Figure 20–5**). The collection container and swab used to collect the culture must be sterile to prevent contamination from other sources. It is also important to select a container that has the proper medium for the type of culture obtained. The medium provides nourishment for the cultured organism and keeps it moist so that it can be examined. The specimen must not be allowed to be in contact with any other substances or objects once it has been obtained.

Sometimes, the specimen is placed immediately on a slide. This is called a **direct smear**, or bacteriological smear. The swab containing the culture specimen is

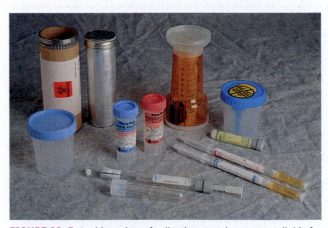

FIGURE 20–5 A wide variety of collection containers are available for obtaining and transporting culture specimens.

rolled across the surface of the slide to place a thin film of culture material on the slide. The smear is air dried and heat fixed, or passed through a flame, so the organisms will adhere, or stick, to the slide. After the direct smear is stained so that organisms are visible, it is examined by a qualified individual, and the organism causing the disease is tentatively identified.

Other times, the specimen is placed or streaked on an **agar plate**, also called a *culture plate* or *petri dish*, or in a culture media tube (**Figure 20–6**). Agar is a special solid medium that provides both nourishment and moisture for the organism. The agar plate is placed in an incubator at

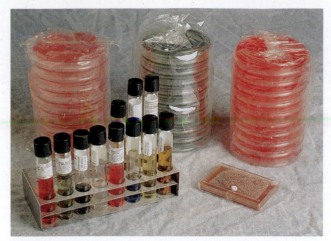

FIGURE 20–6 There are many different types of agar plates and media tubes.

35°C–37°C (95°F–99°F) for 24–36 hours, and the organism is grown. This is called *culturing an organism*. A small sample of the cultured organism (called a *colony*) is placed on a slide, stained, and then examined for identification. Exact identification sometimes requires growing a sample of the cultured organism (the colony) on another special medium, which helps differentiate the microorganisms. In this manner, the organism can be isolated.

In some instances, a *culture and sensitivity* (C&S) study is done. One method of performing a C&S is done using small, sterile disks containing different antibiotics that are placed on the agar plate after the organism has been applied (**Figure 20–7**). If the organisms grow up to the edge of a particular disk, this means the organism is **resistant** to that antibiotic. The antibiotic would *not* work against the organism and would not help cure the disease.

If the organisms do not grow close to the disk, this means the organisms are **sensitive** to the antibiotic on the disk. This antibiotic would work against the organism and aid in the curing of the disease. In this manner, a doctor is better able to determine which antibiotic or medication to give a patient for the disease or infection.

After an organism has been grown in an agar medium, a small sample can be transferred to a slide so that it can be examined and identified. The slide must be stained with some type of dye so that the organism can be seen with a microscope. However, before the slide can be stained, the slide must be fixed. To fix a slide, it must be held over a source of heat, such as an electric incinerator or Bunsen burner, for a very brief period of time. The heat causes the organisms to stick to the slide (**Figure 20–8**). As a result, the organisms will not wash off of the slide when various solutions or stains are applied to the slide.

A common technique for staining cultures is **Gram's stain**. This staining technique not only colors the organisms so that they are visible but also provides another method of identifying organisms. The Gram's stain technique involves the following four steps:

1. Gentian violet or crystal violet stain is applied to the slide for approximately 1 minute. This is called the *primary dye*. It is purple. Any organism that keeps the purple color at the end of the procedure is a gram-positive organism.

2. Iodine is applied to the slide for approximately 30–60 seconds. This solution sets the gentian violet or crystal violet stain, or makes the primary dye adhere to the organisms on the slide.

3. A 95-percent solution of ethyl alcohol or an acetone-alcohol decolorizer is applied to the slide until the solution running off the slide is no longer purple. This alcohol solution removes the purple color of the gentian violet or crystal violet stain from gram-negative organisms. Only gram-positive organisms retain the purple color after this step.

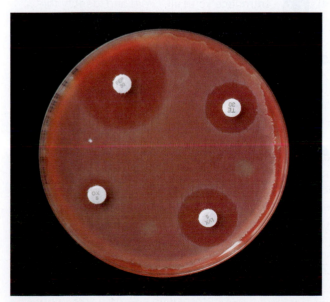

FIGURE 20–7 An agar plate prepared for a sensitivity study with small antibiotic disks positioned on the plate. © iStock.com/ksass

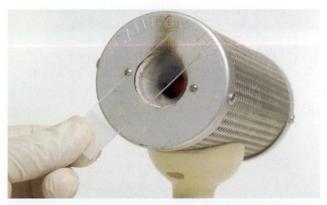

FIGURE 20–8 The slide is fixed with heat from an electric incinerator so organisms will adhere (stick) to the slide.

4. Safranin solution is applied to the slide for approximately 30–60 seconds. This solution is a counter-stain. It stains the gram-negative organisms red so that they can be seen under a microscope.

NOTE: *Times may vary depending on the type of stain used. Read and follow the manufacturer's instructions.*

After the slide is stained, organisms on the slide are identified as *gram-positive* if they retain the purple color of the gentian violet or crystal violet stain and *gram-negative* if they retain the red color of the safranin solution. A qualified lab technologist or physician examines the slide. By noting the shape of the organism and whether it is gram positive or negative, a preliminary identification of the type of organism can be made. Common gram-positive bacteria are *streptococcus* and *staphylococcus*. Common gram-negative bacteria are *Escherichia coli (E. coli)* and *Acinetobacter*.

Growing and isolating organisms on culture plates does take time, usually 3–5 days. With certain types of infections, such as a streptococcus throat infection, this delay can allow the organisms to damage the heart valves and/or kidneys. For this reason, *rapid identification test kits* have been developed for many common bacterial infections. If streptococcus is identified by a rapid identification test, antibiotics that are effective against streptococcus can be started immediately. Other rapid tests include influenza, MRSA, *E. coli*, drug screening tests, and pregnancy tests. During the COVID-19 pandemic, enormous effort was put into developing a rapid test to detect infection quickly. The rapid test systems are easy to use and have a high level of accuracy, but the manufacturer's instructions must be followed to eliminate false positives. Most rapid tests also require that a positive and negative control test be conducted at the same time as the patient's test to ensure accuracy.

Because any culture may contain pathogenic (disease-producing) organisms or be contaminated with blood and body fluids, standard precautions (see Section 15:4) must be observed at all times while handling cultures. Hands must be washed frequently and thoroughly, and gloves must be worn. Protective clothing, such as lab coats or lab aprons, must be worn. If splashing of specimens is possible, a mask or face shield and protective eyewear must be worn. All culture specimens and disposable equipment contaminated with the culture are placed in an infectious-waste bag for disposal according to legal requirements for infectious waste. Any lab counter or contaminated area must be wiped immediately with a disinfectant solution.

check**point**

1. How many days does it usually take to grow and isolate an organism on a culture plate?

PRACTICE: Go to the workbook and complete the assignment sheet for 20:2, Obtaining and Handling Cultures. Then return and continue with the procedures.

Procedure 20:2A

Obtaining a Culture Specimen

Equipment and Supplies

Sterile cotton applicator swabs, culture medium (some prepacked with sterile swabs), sterile test tube with medium (if no prepacked medium), label, pen or pencil for marking, disposable gloves, mask or face shield, protective eyewear, gown, infectious-waste bag

Procedure

1. Check physician's written order or obtain an order from your immediate supervisor.

2. Assemble equipment.

3. Wash hands. Put on gloves.

    CAUTION: Observe standard precautions while obtaining and handling the culture specimen. If splashing of specimens is possible, a gown, mask or face shield, and eye protection must be worn.

4. Introduce yourself. Greet and identify the patient. Explain the procedure to the patient. Obtain the patient's consent.

5. Check the body area where the specimen is to be obtained. The order should state the site for taking the specimen.

   NOTE: Specimens can be taken from the nose, throat, or other body areas, or from open wounds.

6. Remove the sterile applicator from its package. Pick it up by the non-applicator end only. Make sure you do not touch the sterile cotton tip to any surface or contaminate it in any way (**Figure 20–9A**).

   CAUTION: If the tip does not remain sterile, the test will be inaccurate.

7. Place the sterile tip on the area to be cultured. Use a gentle yet firm rotating motion to cover the tip of the applicator with a sample specimen (**Figure 20–9B**).

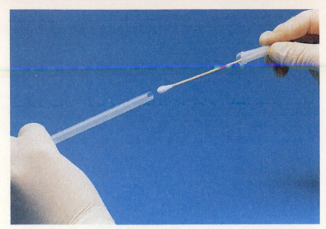

FIGURE 20–9A Take care not to contaminate the sterile tip as you remove the sterile applicator from its package.

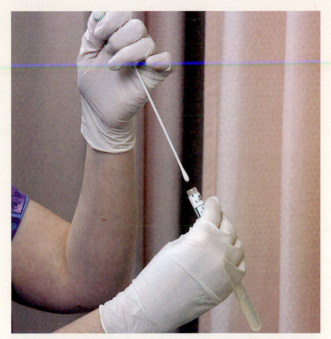

FIGURE 20–9C Take care not to touch the sides of the culture container as you place the applicator into the container.

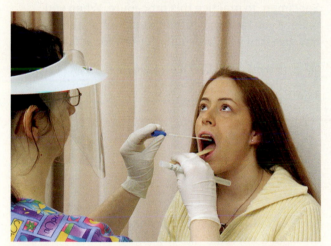

FIGURE 20–9B Rotate the applicator tip to obtain a specimen from the site.

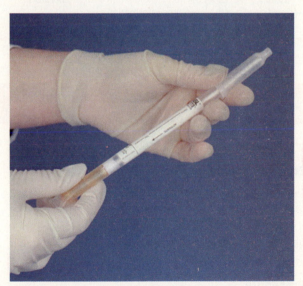

FIGURE 20–9D If the culture container has a separator, squeeze the container gently to crush the glass and release the culture medium.

8. Remove the applicator from the culture site. Be careful not to contaminate the tip.

9. Place the applicator into the sterile tube or culture-medium container (**Figure 20–9C**).

    CAUTION: Take care not to touch the sides of the container because the specimen will smear against the sides of the container instead of being placed in the medium.

   NOTE: Brace your arms against your body to keep your hands steady while inserting the applicator swab.

10. Check to be sure the tip is in the medium.

    NOTE: This keeps the specimen sterile and moist for examination.

NOTE: Some culture-medium tubes contain a liquid culture medium separated from a gauze layer by a thin layer of glass or other material. To saturate the gauze layer with the liquid medium, it is necessary to squeeze the container gently to break the glass or other material (**Figure 20–9D**). Read and follow the manufacturer's instructions when using any culture-medium container.

(continues)

11. Label the specimen with the patient's name, address, identification number, doctor's name, the date, the type of test ordered, and the site from which the specimen was obtained (**Figure 20–9E**). If a laboratory requisition form is required, complete this form. In many laboratories or offices, information is entered into a computer program to record it in the patient's electronic

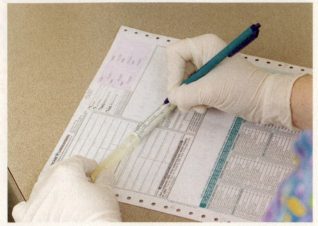

FIGURE 20–9E Label the culture specimen and/or laboratory requisition slip with all required information.

health record (EHR). Computer-generated specimen labels and/or laboratory requisitions are then printed and used to label and identify the specimen.

12. Take or send the specimen to the laboratory. If you will be transferring the specimen to a slide or an agar plate, place the specimen in a safe location until you are ready to use it. Keep it away from direct sunlight and sources of heat.

13. Clean and replace all equipment. Place all contaminated disposable materials in the infectious-waste bag. Use a disinfectant to wipe the counter and any contaminated areas.

14. Remove gloves. Wash hands thoroughly.

PRACTICE: Go to the workbook and use the evaluation sheet for 20:2A, Obtaining a Culture Specimen, to practice this procedure. When you believe you have mastered this skill, sign the sheet and give it to your instructor for further action.

 FINAL EVALUATION: Using the criteria listed on the evaluation sheet, your instructor will grade your performance.

Procedure 20:2B

Preparing a Direct Smear

Equipment and Supplies

Culture specimen for direct smear, clean glass slide, electric incinerator or Bunsen burner, staining rack, rubber-tipped hemostats or slide clamps, disposable gloves, mask or face shield, protective eyewear, gown, infectious-waste bag

Procedure

1. Assemble equipment.

2. Wash hands. Put on gloves.

 CAUTION: Observe standard precautions while handling any culture specimen. If splashing of specimens is possible, a gown, mask or face shield, and eye protection must be worn.

3. Clean the slide thoroughly. Avoid touching the top of the slide once it has been cleaned.

4. Carefully remove the specimen from the medium tube. Handle the applicator by the non-applicator end only.

 CAUTION: Avoid contaminating the applicator tip.

5. Use the thumb and forefinger of one hand to pick up the clean slide. Hold it securely. The slide can also be placed on a table or counter and held securely.

6. Place the tip of the applicator swab containing the culture on the slide approximately ½ inch away from the thumb holding the slide.

7. Hold the applicator tip firmly on the slide and roll it toward the opposite end of the slide. Use firm, even pressure to allow for the transfer of the organisms to the slide (**Figure 20–10**). Stop ½ inch from the end of the slide.

8. Allow the slide to dry at room temperature.

CAUTION: If the slide does not dry prior to being fixed, the heat from fixing the slide will drive the moisture out of the organisms and distort their shape.

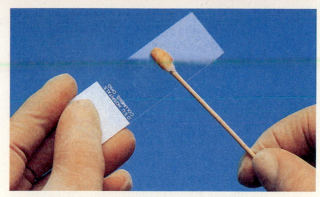

FIGURE 20–10 Roll the applicator tip across the slide to transfer the organisms to the slide.

9. Dispose of the contaminated applicator swab by placing it in an infectious-waste bag.

    CAUTION: Handle the swab carefully to avoid infecting yourself or contaminating other surfaces.

10. When the slide is dry, place it in a set of rubber-tipped hemostats or slide clamps. Make sure the smear side is facing upward.

11. Turn on the electric incinerator or Bunsen burner.

     CAUTION: If a match is used to turn on the flame, extinguish the match and then hold it under water before putting it in a trash container.

12. Hold the clamped slide 1–2 inches above the flame for 1–2 seconds. Do this three to four times. Do *not* get the slide too hot. Check the temperature by touching the bottom of the slide lightly on your hand. It should feel warm but not too hot.

    NOTE: This is called *fixing*. The heat causes the organisms to stick to the slide.

     CAUTION: Excess heat will shrink the organisms, and they will no longer be identifiable.

13. Place the slide on the staining rack; the slide must be stained prior to being viewed.

14. Label the slide with the patient's name, doctor's name, address, identification number, and any other necessary information, or attach a computer-generated label.

15. Clean and replace all equipment. Place all contaminated disposable materials in the infectious-waste bag. Use a disinfectant to wipe the counter and any contaminated areas.

16. Make sure the electric incinerator is turned off or the Bunsen burner is extinguished.

17. Remove gloves. Wash hands thoroughly.

PRACTICE: Go to the workbook and use the evaluation sheet for 20:2B, Preparing a Direct Smear, to practice this procedure. When you believe you have mastered this skill, sign the sheet and give it to your instructor for further action.

✅ **FINAL EVALUATION:** Using the criteria listed on the evaluation sheet, your instructor will grade your performance.

Procedure 20:2C

Streaking an Agar Plate

Equipment and Supplies

Agar plate with correct medium, specimen for direct smear, label, pen or marker and/or computer, incubator, disposable gloves, mask or face shield, protective eyewear, gown, infectious-waste bag

Procedure

1. Assemble equipment.

2. Wash hands. Put on gloves.

    CAUTION: Observe standard precautions while handling any culture specimen. If splashing of specimens is possible, a gown, mask or face shield, and eye protection must be worn.

3. Remove the applicator containing the culture specimen from its container. Hold it by the non-applicator end. Take care to avoid contaminating the applicator tip. Look at the tip to be sure it is still moist.

   NOTE: If the specimen is dry, the organisms have probably died, and the results will not be accurate.

4. The agar plate is made up of two parts: the lower disk, which contains the agar, and the upper lid. Open the agar plate. Take care not to touch the inside of the plate. Invert the lid; that is, place the lid with the top against the counter. In this way, the inside of the lid faces up and stays clean.

(continues)

NOTE: The agar plate can also be placed upside down, with the agar on top. The agar plate should then be lifted. The lid will remain on the table, with the inside facing up.

5. Hold the plate firmly in one hand (**Figure 20–11A**) or place it on a flat surface.

6. Starting at the top of the agar, gently place the applicator tip in one corner. Using a rotary motion, turning the top of the tip so that all sides of the tip touch the agar, go from side to side approximately one-quarter of the way down the plate. To cover the second quadrant of the plate, turn the plate one-quarter turn and repeat the side-to-side motion of the applicator tip, crossing the first quadrant two to three times. Turn the plate one-quarter turn and use the same motion to cover the third quadrant. To cover the fourth quadrant, turn the plate one-quarter turn, and cross into the third quadrant one or two times. Note the sample streaking pattern in **Figure 20–11B**. This streaking method helps isolate the colonies of organisms in the fourth quadrant (**Figure 20–11C**).

NOTE: This is only one type of streaking pattern. Use the streaking pattern preferred by your employer.

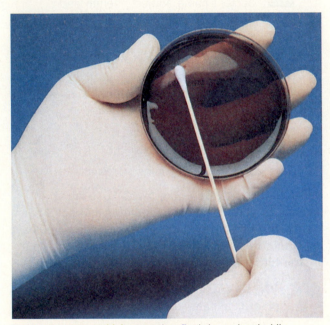

FIGURE 20–11A Hold the agar plate firmly in one hand while streaking it with the specimen.

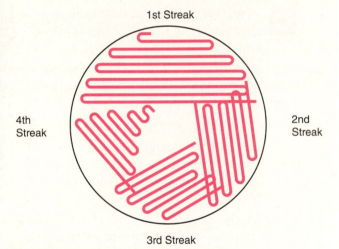

1st Streak

4th Streak

2nd Streak

3rd Streak

FIGURE 20–11B A sample streaking pattern.

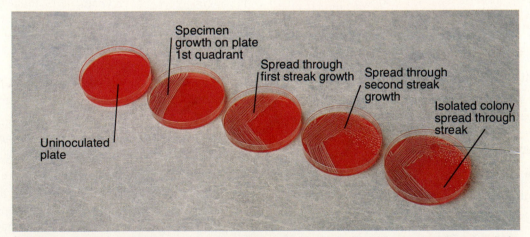

Specimen growth on plate 1st quadrant

Spread through first streak growth

Spread through second streak growth

Isolated colony spread through streak

Uninoculated plate

FIGURE 20–11C Note the isolated colonies of organisms in the fourth quadrant after the culture has grown in the incubator.

CAUTION: Be gentle. Do not break into the agar.

NOTE: An inoculating loop can also be used to streak the agar. After each quadrant is streaked, the loop is placed in a flame and cooled. Use the method the laboratory or physician prefers.

NOTE: Cover the agar only one time in each area. Do *not* go back over areas already covered.

7. Check to be sure all areas of the agar have been streaked. Different streaking methods can be used. Use the one the laboratory or physician prefers.

8. Discard the applicator swab in the infectious-waste bag or a biohazard container. Some laboratories require the swab to be placed in a container of disinfectant prior to disposal in an infectious-waste bag.

9. If a sensitivity study is to be done, place antibiotic disks on the agar. You can use an automatic dispenser of medicated disks to do so. If an automatic dispenser is not available, use sterile thumb forceps. Place the disks around the agar. Leave spaces between the disks. Make sure that the disks are not too close to the edge of the agar plate (refer to Figure 20–7).

   NOTE: The agar plate must be streaked heavily and completely for a sensitivity study.

10. Pick up the agar plate lid by the side edges. Take care not to touch the inside. Place the lid on top of the agar plate.

    NOTE: The agar plate can be placed into the lid instead, but be careful not to contaminate the insides.

11. Label the bottom of the agar plate with the patient's name, doctor's name, address, identification number, date, time, site of specimen, and other required information. In many laboratories or offices, information is entered into a computer to record it in the patient's electronic health record (EHR) and a label is printed for the agar plate.

12. Invert the agar plate and place it in the incubator at 35°C–37°C (95°F–99°F) for 24–36 hours

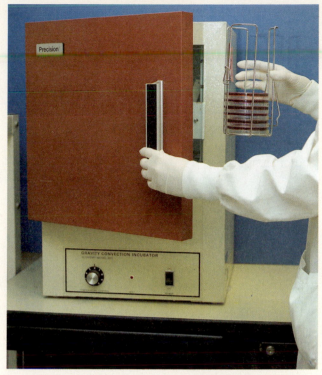

FIGURE 20–11D Invert the agar plate and place it in the incubator for 24–36 hours at 35°C–37°C.

(**Figure 20–11D**). Check the temperature of the incubator. Be sure the plate is upside down with the agar on top. This prevents moisture from settling on the agar.

NOTE: The incubator provides darkness and warmth for growth of the organism. The agar provides food and moisture to stimulate growth.

13. Clean and replace all equipment. Place all contaminated disposable equipment in the infectious-waste bag. Use a disinfectant to wipe the counter and any contaminated areas.

14. Remove gloves. Wash hands thoroughly to prevent infection and spread of the disease.

PRACTICE: Go to the workbook and use the evaluation sheet for 20:2C, Streaking an Agar Plate, to practice this procedure. When you believe you have mastered this skill, sign the sheet and give it to your instructor for further action.

FINAL EVALUATION: Using the criteria listed on the evaluation sheet, your instructor will grade your performance.

Transferring Culture from Agar Plate to Slide

Equipment and Supplies

Agar plate or slant tube with growth, inoculating loop, electric incinerator or Bunsen burner, rubber-tipped hemostat or slide clamps, slide, normal saline solution, staining rack, disposable gloves, mask or face shield, protective eyewear, gown, infectious-waste bag, pen and/or computer

Procedure

1. Assemble equipment.

2. Wash hands. Put on gloves.

    CAUTION: Observe standard precautions while handling any culture specimen. If splashing of specimens is possible, a gown, mask or face shield, and eye protection must be worn.

3. Prepare the electric incinerator or light the Bunsen burner.

    CAUTION: If a match is used, wet the match before discarding it in a trash can.

4. Open the agar plate or slant tube. Handle only the outside of the plate or tube. To prevent contamination, place the lid with the top against the counter (that is, with the inside facing up).

   NOTE: The agar plate can also be placed upside down, with the agar on top. The agar plate should then be lifted. The lid will remain on the table, with the inside facing up.

5. Place the inoculating loop in the electric incinerator or flame until the loop end gets red hot (**Figure 20–12A**).

   NOTE: This kills organisms that might be present on the loop.

6. Cool the loop by dipping it into an area of agar that has no organisms present.

   NOTE: A hot loop will destroy the shape of the organisms, making them unidentifiable.

7. Dip the loop into a small portion of the colony growth (**Figures 20–12B** and **12C**). Skim the top of the growth to get some organisms on the loop.

   NOTE: Only a small sample is needed. If too large a mass is obtained, the slide will be too concentrated.

8. Immediately place the lid on the agar plate or slant tube to prevent contamination to yourself or the environment from the organism.

9. Place a small drop of normal saline on a clean glass slide.

   NOTE: Normal saline provides a liquid medium for the organisms.

10. Mix the specimen (on the loop) and the saline on the slide (**Figure 20–12D**). This loosens the organisms and suspends them in liquid.

     CAUTION: Do not rub the mixture against the slide because doing so could damage the shape of the organisms.

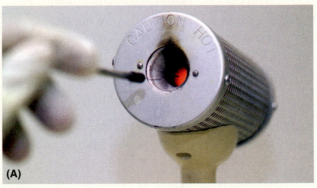

(A)

FIGURE 20–12A Sterilize the inoculating loop by putting it into an electric incinerator until the loop gets red hot.

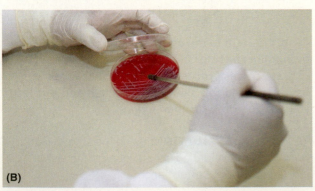

(B)

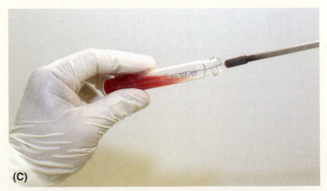

(C)

FIGURES 20–12B AND C Dip the loop into a small portion of an isolated growth of the cultured organism from (B) an agar plate or (C) an agar slant tube.

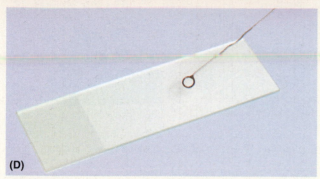

(D)

FIGURE 20–12D Mix the specimen with the saline by gently moving the loop through the saline solution.

11. Starting at one end of the slide, spread the solution thinly over the slide. Cover the entire width of the slide with the culture.

12. Place the slide on the staining rack to air-dry. Fix as previously taught.

13. Place the loop in the flame until red hot. This destroys all organisms.

14. Label the slide with the patient's name, doctor's name, address, identification number, and other required information. In many laboratories or offices, information is entered into the patient's electronic health record (EHR) and a computer-generated label is attached to the slide.

15. Clean and replace all equipment. Place all contaminated disposable equipment in the infectious-waste bag. Use a disinfectant to wipe the counter and any contaminated areas.

16. Remove gloves. Wash hands thoroughly.

PRACTICE: Go to the workbook and use the evaluation sheet for 20:2D, Transferring Culture from Agar Plate to Slide, to practice this procedure. When you believe you have mastered this skill, sign the sheet and give it to your instructor for further action.

 FINAL EVALUATION: Using the criteria listed on the evaluation sheet, your instructor will grade your performance.

Procedure 20:2E

Staining with Gram's Stain

Equipment and Supplies

Slide with fixed smear, staining rack, gentian violet or crystal violet stain, Gram's iodine, 95-percent ethyl alcohol or acetone-alcohol decolorizer, safranin solution, distilled water, asepto syringe or plastic squeeze bottle, disposable gloves, mask or face shield, protective eyewear, gown, infectious-waste bag

 NOTE: Timing may vary with types of solutions used. Read the instructions provided with the solutions or follow agency policy.

Procedure

1. Assemble equipment.

2. Wash hands. Put on gloves.

 CAUTION: Observe standard precautions while handling any culture specimen. If splashing of specimens is possible, a gown, mask or face shield, and eye protection must be worn.

3. Use your thumb and forefinger to pick up the fixed slide. Place the slide on the staining rack. Check to be sure the smear side is facing up.

 CAUTION: Avoid touching the top of the slide with your fingers.

4. Cover the slide with gentian violet or crystal violet stain (**Figure 20–13**). Leave the stain in place for the recommended time, usually 1 minute. Stain only the smeared side of the slide. This is the primary dye.

NOTE: To avoid staining the sink, it is best to let water run during the entire procedure.

 NOTE: The primary stain is purple and will dye all gram-positive organisms. Thus, any organisms that remain purple at the end of this procedure are gram-positive organisms.

5. Rinse the slide thoroughly with distilled water. Use an asepto syringe or plastic squeeze bottle to rinse gently.

6. Use Gram's iodine solution to cover the slide. Tilt the slide to allow the iodine and remaining water to run off. Then, cover the slide again with iodine. Leave in place for the recommended time, usually 30–60 seconds. This sets the primary dye.

(continues)

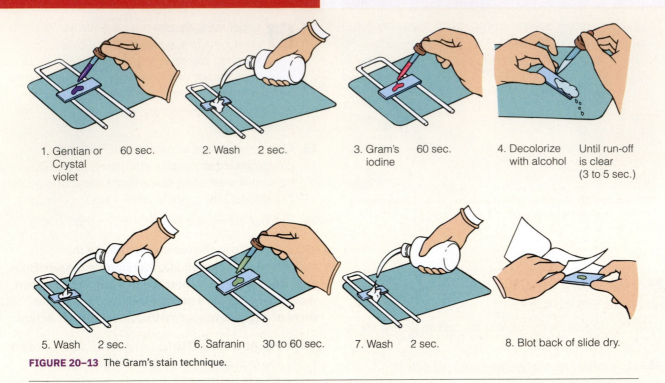

1. Gentian or Crystal violet   60 sec.

2. Wash   2 sec.

3. Gram's iodine   60 sec.

4. Decolorize with alcohol   Until run-off is clear (3 to 5 sec.)

5. Wash   2 sec.

6. Safranin   30 to 60 sec.

7. Wash   2 sec.

8. Blot back of slide dry.

FIGURE 20–13 The Gram's stain technique.

NOTE: The first application of iodine is allowed to run off the slide so that the second application will result in a full-strength iodine covering.

NOTE: Any gram-positive organisms will now have the purple primary dye set into them. After this step, gram-negative organisms will also be dyed purple. This dye must be removed.

7. Use an asepto syringe or plastic squeeze bottle to rinse the slide thoroughly with distilled water.

8. Use 95-percent ethyl alcohol or acetone-alcohol to decolorize the slide. Apply the alcohol to the slide. Immediately tilt the slide to allow the decolorizer to run off. Reapply the alcohol and again tilt the slide to allow the alcohol to run off. After each application, check the color of the alcohol as it runs off the slide. Stop immediately when the decolorizer is no longer purple. This usually occurs in 3–5 seconds.

NOTE: This step removes the primary dye from the gram-negative organisms. Only the gram-positive organisms remain purple.

CAUTION: This is a crucial step. Too many applications of alcohol can also decolorize gram-positive organisms. Stop as soon as the alcohol is no longer purple.

9. Rinse the slide well with distilled water to remove any remaining decolorizer.

10. Use safranin solution to counterstain the slide. Apply the safranin, tilt the slide to allow the safranin and remaining water to run off, and then reapply the safranin. This stain should remain on the slide for the recommended time, usually 30–60 seconds.

NOTE: Safranin stains gram-negative organisms red so that they can be seen and identified under a microscope.

11. Use distilled water to rinse the slide.

12. Use a paper towel to dry the *back* of the slide. Do *not* dry the front, or smear, side because rubbing it can remove the smear from the slide. Allow the front of the slide to air-dry.

13. Once dry, the slide is fairly permanent and is ready for microscopic examination. A laboratory technologist or doctor can examine the slide and identify the type of organism present by noting the shape and color. If purple, the organism is gram-positive; if red, it is gram-negative.

14. Clean the area thoroughly. Replace all equipment.

NOTE: The dyes can permanently stain the counter if not removed immediately.

15. Remove gloves. Wash hands.

20:3 PUNCTURING THE SKIN TO OBTAIN CAPILLARY BLOOD

Science

Blood tests are often done to assist a physician in making a diagnosis. Depending on your chosen health career, you may be responsible for performing some basic blood tests. Blood must be obtained to do these tests. This section provides basic facts on performing a skin puncture to obtain blood. *No procedures should be attempted without classroom instruction and supervision.*

Blood for testing can be obtained in various ways. For many routine tests, a simple **skin puncture** provides a sufficient amount of blood. Skin punctures are used only for tests requiring small quantities of blood. This blood is obtained from the capillaries and is often called *peripheral blood.* For other tests requiring larger quantities of blood, a **venipuncture** is performed. In a venipuncture, the blood is taken from a vein. The most common site used is the antecubital space (anterior part of the elbow on the inside of the arm). In the antecubital area, three veins are commonly accessed. The median cubital vein is first choice. It is usually large and visible, and it doesn't bruise easily. The cephalic vein is the second choice for blood collection; it is just a little more difficult to find. Finally, the basilic vein is the third choice and should only be considered after ruling out the other two. It has closer proximity to nerves and bruises more easily. Factors that impact the choice of site include the arm on the side of a mastectomy, the presence of edema or trauma, an IV cannula, or a scarred area.

For still other tests, blood is taken from an artery. *Arterial blood* is used for specific tests such as those that measure the amount of blood gases (oxygen and carbon dioxide) or determine acid-base balance.

Legal

Responsibility for obtaining blood for various blood tests varies. Liability should be checked for individual states. *In some states, health science career students are not permitted to perform any procedure involving obtaining blood. It is vital that you determine what you are legally permitted to do.*

The procedure that follows discusses only the skin puncture. If you are required to do a venipuncture or to draw arterial blood, you need specific training in these procedures. Only legally qualified individuals should perform venipunctures and arterial punctures (**Figure 20–14**).

Careful aseptic technique must be followed while performing a skin puncture. The skin must be cleaned thoroughly with 70-percent isopropyl alcohol or a similar antiseptic. The lancet used to puncture the skin must be sterile. Finally, the puncture site should be covered with sterile gauze after the skin puncture is complete.

Common puncture sites used to obtain capillary blood include the fingers, heels, and ear lobes (**Figure 20–15A**). The heel is frequently used for infants until they learn to walk. A finger is usually used for children and adults. When a finger puncture is performed, care must be taken in the selection of the finger. The thumb, index finger, or pinkie finger should not be used because they have arteries close to the surface. In addition, they are used most frequently, and the chance for infection is greater. The finger to be used must be examined closely. Avoid fingers with edema (swelling), calluses, scars, rashes, or sores. Make sure the skin is warm and pink. If the finger is cyanotic (blue), do not use it. Cyanosis indicates poor circulation.

The skin puncture should be 2–4 millimeters deep to reach the capillary beds under the skin. The puncture should be made across the grain of lines in the finger,

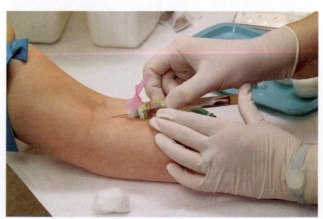
FIGURE 20–14 Only legally qualified individuals should perform a venipuncture to obtain blood.

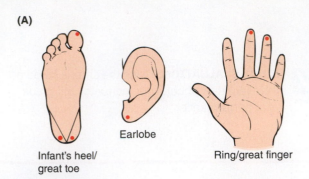

(A)

Infant's heel/
great toe

Earlobe

Ring/great finger

(B)

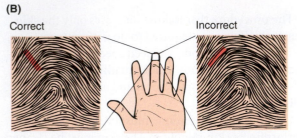

Correct

Incorrect

FIGURES 20–15A AND B (A) Common skin puncture sites for obtaining capillary blood. (B) Skin punctures should be made across the grain of lines in the finger.

or at right angles to the fingerprint striations (**Figure 20–15B**). This type of puncture heals more rapidly in most cases.

The first drop of blood obtained is always removed. It is contaminated with alcohol, perspiration, excess tissue fluid, and other substances on the skin that can dilute the blood and cause inaccurate test results. The second or succeeding drops of blood can be used for the various blood tests.

After performing a skin puncture, the health care provider must remain with the patient until the blood stops flowing. When sufficient blood has been obtained, sterile gauze should be held firmly against the puncture

for at least 1–3 minutes. If the patient is taking an anticoagulant, a medication such as aspirin or warfarin sodium (COUMADIN®) that prevents clotting of the blood, pressure should be held against the puncture site for at least 3–5 minutes to help stop the bleeding.

Precaution

Standard precautions (Section 15:4) must be observed at all times while obtaining and handling blood. Many diseases, including hepatitis B (HBV), hepatitis C (HCV), and acquired immune deficiency syndrome (AIDS), can be transmitted by blood. Hands must be washed thoroughly and gloves must be worn at all times. If splashing of the blood is possible, masks or face shields, protective eyewear, and gowns must also be worn. Any blood spills must be wiped up immediately with a disinfectant solution. All contaminated disposable materials or supplies and any remaining blood samples are placed in an infectious-waste bag prior to being disposed of as infectious waste according to legal requirements. Any sharps, such as lancets or needles, must be placed in a leakproof puncture-resistant sharps box. They should *not* be bent, broken, or recapped. It is important for the health care provider to observe all precautions established by their agency for team members who handle blood samples. All blood must be regarded as hazardous because many illnesses can be transmitted through improper handling of blood samples.

checkpoint

1. How deep should a skin puncture be to reach the capillary beds under the skin?

PRACTICE: Go to the workbook and complete the assignment sheet for 20:3, Puncturing the Skin to Obtain Capillary Blood. Then return and continue with the procedure.

Procedure 20:3

Puncturing the Skin to Obtain Capillary Blood

Equipment and Supplies

Sterile lancet, 70-percent isopropyl alcohol, sterile gauze pads, disposable gloves, mask or face shield, protective eyewear, gown, sharps box, infectious waste bag

Procedure

1. Assemble equipment.

2. Wash hands. Put on gloves. If splashing of blood is possible, put on a gown, mask or face shield, and protective eyewear.

Precaution

CAUTION: Observe all standard precautions while obtaining and testing blood.

3. Comm

Introduce yourself. Identify the patient. Explain the procedure. Obtain the patient's consent.

NOTE: It is usually best to seat the patient in a comfortable position.

4. Select a finger. Make sure it is free from edema, cyanosis, scars, sores, and calluses. Do *not* use the thumb, index finger, or pinkie finger. If the hand and fingers are cold to the touch, wrap them in a warm cloth or hold them under warm water for a few minutes to stimulate circulation.

NOTE: Check the circulation in the finger. The finger should be warm and pink for good blood supply. Check the color of the nail bed.

NOTE: Although this procedure describes a finger puncture, the same principles should be observed when using any skin site to obtain capillary blood.

5. Cleanse the finger thoroughly with a sterile alcohol swab or a sterile gauze pad saturated with 70-percent isopropyl alcohol. Allow the area to air-dry.

NOTE: Do *not* allow the finger to touch anything.

6. Grasp the finger firmly with your thumb and forefinger. Hold the sterile lancet in the other hand. Use a quick, clean, stabbing stroke to puncture the finger with the sterile lancet (**Figure 20–16**). Make the cut at right angles to the fingerprint striations, near the top of the finger but not too close to the fingernail.

NOTE: The puncture should be 2–4 millimeters deep.

NOTE: Most agencies use automatic lancet devices. The lancet is positioned over the skin site and activated to allow the lancet to puncture the skin (**Figure 20–17A**). Most manufacturers produce color-coded lancets that puncture the skin to different depths (**Figure 20–17B**). Read and follow the manufacturer's instructions when using an automatic device.

 CAUTION: Do not squeeze or milk the finger because doing so will cause tissue fluid to mix with the blood. If necessary, use gentle pressure at a distance from the puncture site to start the blood flow.

 CHECKPOINT: Your instructor will check the puncture to be sure it is at a correct angle and is free flowing.

7. Immediately place the lancet in a puncture-resistant sharps container. Do *not* bend or break the lancet before discarding it.

8. Use sterile gauze to remove the first drop of blood. This blood is contaminated with alcohol, perspiration, and other substances from the skin that can dilute the blood and cause inaccurate test results. Discard the gauze in the infectious-waste bag.

9. Use the second and succeeding drops of blood to perform the blood tests ordered (for example, hemoglobin). Work quickly to avoid cessation of bleeding.

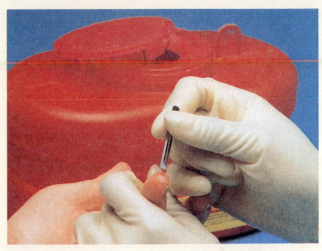

FIGURE 20–16 A sterile lancet is used to puncture the skin 2–4 millimeters deep.

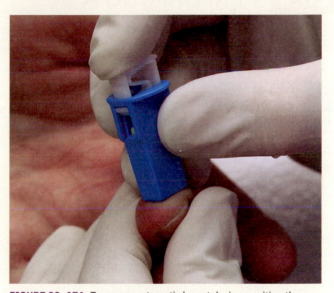

FIGURE 20–17A To use an automatic lancet device, position the lancet over the skin and depress the plunger to make the puncture.

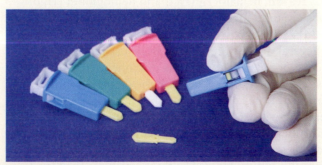

FIGURE 20–17B Lancets are color coded for different depths of skin punctures.

(continues)

10. When sufficient blood has been obtained, instruct the patient to hold sterile gauze firmly against the puncture for at least 1–2 minutes.

    CAUTION: If the patient is taking an anticoagulant, pressure should be held against the puncture site for at least 3–5 minutes.

   Safety

    CAUTION: Remain with the patient until the bleeding stops. You must be certain that bleeding has stopped before you leave the area.

   Safety

11. Clean and replace all equipment. Put all contaminated disposable supplies in the infectious-waste bag. Use a disinfectant to wipe the counter and any contaminated equipment.

12. Remove gloves and discard in an infectious-waste bag. Wash hands thoroughly.

PRACTICE: Go to the workbook and use the evaluation sheet for 20:3, Puncturing the Skin to Obtain Capillary Blood, to practice this procedure. When you believe you have mastered this skill, sign the sheet and give it to your instructor for further action.

 FINAL EVALUATION: Using the criteria listed on the evaluation sheet, your instructor will grade your performance.

Check

20:4 PERFORMING A MICROHEMATOCRIT

Science

One of the basic blood tests you may be required to perform is the microhematocrit. A **hematocrit (Hct)** or "crit," is a blood test that measures the volume of packed red blood cells (RBCs), or erythrocytes, in the blood. It is often described as a measurement of the percentage of RBCs per volume of blood. **Erythrocytes** are the blood cells that carry oxygen from the lungs to the body cells. They also carry carbon dioxide from the body cells to the lungs, where it is eliminated from the body. An average normal count for erythrocytes (red blood cells) is 4.5–6.0 million per cubic millimeter of blood for males, and 4.0–5.5 million per cubic millimeter of blood for females. Most erythrocyte counts are performed on computerized cell counters. Manual counts can be performed, but they are difficult to do accurately. For this reason, hematocrit (Hct) and hemoglobin (Hgb) tests are used much more frequently to determine the status of the erythrocytes in the blood.

Several different methods can be used to perform an Hct. A popular method is the microhematocrit. This test requires less blood and can be done in a shorter period of time compared to other methods. A special centrifuge is used for the microhematocrit. This machine spins the blood tubes at approximately 10,000 revolutions per minute with a centrifugal (driving away from the center) force. The force separates the blood into three main layers: RBCs, a buffy coat, and plasma (**Figure 20–18**). The buffy coat is a very thin, whitish layer consisting of white blood cells (WBCs) and platelets.

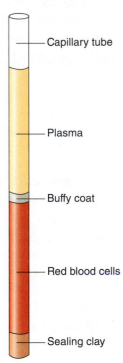

FIGURE 20–18 The microhematocrit centrifuge separates the blood into three main layers: erythrocytes (red blood cells), a buffy coat, and plasma.

Labels on figure: Capillary tube, Plasma, Buffy coat, Red blood cells, Sealing clay

Math

Leukocytes (white blood cells or WBCs) are important for fighting infections in the body. The average normal count for leukocytes is 4,500–11,000 per cubic millimeter of blood. Leukocyte counts can be performed manually or by a computerized cell counter. However, the buffy coat can provide an estimate of the number of leukocytes because each 0.1 millimeter (mm) thickness of the buffy coat equals approximately 1,000 WBCs. For example, a thickness of 0.6 mm would equal approximately 6,000 WBCs:

$$0.6 \div 0.1 = 6$$

$$6 \times 1,000 = 6,000$$

A thickness of 1 mm would equal approximately 10,000 WBCs:

$$1 \div 0.1 = 10$$
$$10 \times 1,000 = 10,000$$

A graphic reading device on the microhematocrit centrifuge is used to measure the depth of the buffy coat and the percentage of RBCs (**Figure 20–19A**). If the centrifuge does not have a graphic reading device, the manufacturer will provide a reader card to obtain the correct measurements. Follow the manufacturer's instructions to use the reader card. Some centrifuges have digital tube readers that measure and display the hematocrit level (**Figure 20–19B**).

Special capillary tubes are used in the microhematocrit centrifuge. The tubes are usually lined with an anticoagulant, such as heparin. An **anticoagulant** is a substance that prevents the blood from clotting. The tubes are filled to the indicated level with blood from a free-flowing skin puncture. The empty (that is, without blood) ends of the tubes are sealed with special plastic sealing clay (**Figure 20–20**). This clay keeps the blood from running out of the tube during centrifuging. Extreme care must be taken to avoid contaminating the clay block with the blood. Self-sealing tubes are available for use. These tubes contain a plug with a small air channel to allow air to escape when blood is drawn into the tube. When the blood touches the plug, the air channel seals automatically.

Math In some agencies, two tubes are filled for the test and the readings of the two tubes are averaged to determine the specific hematocrit (Hct) of a patient. For example, if one tube registers at 41 percent and the second tube registers at 44 percent, the two numbers are added together:

$$41 + 44 = 85$$

The total is divided by 2 to obtain the average:

$$\begin{array}{r} 42.5 \\ 2\overline{)85.0} \\ \underline{-8} \\ 05 \\ \underline{-4} \\ 10 \\ \underline{-10} \\ 0 \end{array}$$

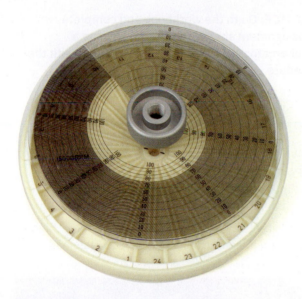

FIGURE 20–19A By using the graphic reading device on the microhematocrit centrifuge, the percentage of erythrocytes (red blood cells) can be measured. Courtesy, Unico®

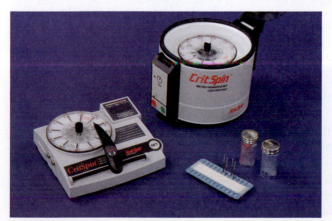

FIGURE 20–19B Some microhematocrit centrifuges have digital tube readers as shown in the lower left corner. Courtesy, Iris Sample Processing

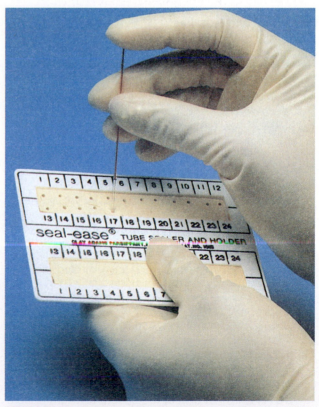

FIGURE 20–20 The empty end of the capillary tube is sealed with clay to prevent the blood from running out of the tube during centrifuging.

The Hct reading for the two tubes would be recorded as 42.5 percent. In other agencies, one tube is used to obtain the Hct reading for a patient. The reading obtained from the single tube is recorded as the Hct percentage.

Normal values for the test vary slightly depending on the types of microhematocrit centrifuge and capillary tube used. An average value for adults is 36–46 percent for women and 40–55 percent for men. In other words, 36–46 percent of the total blood volume is RBCs in female individuals, and 40–55 percent of the total blood volume in male individuals is RBCs. Newborns have an average value of 51–61 percent, children 1 year old average 32–38 percent, and children 6 years old average 34–42 percent.

A low hematocrit often indicates *anemia*. A high hematocrit reading can indicate *polycythemia*. Anemia is a low number of RBCs, and polycythemia is a high number of RBCs. Because there are several different types of each of these conditions, the physician usually conducts other, more extensive blood tests to evaluate the condition. Patients with burns or dehydration can also have a high hematocrit level, but their red blood cell counts will be normal. Patients with severe bleeding may have a low hematocrit level.

Accuracy is essential while performing this test because the test is used to diagnose disease. False results can lead to improper diagnosis and care.

CAUTION: *If any results are questionable, do not hesitate to repeat the test.*

Safety

Careful recording of the test is also essential. Hematocrit is often abbreviated *Hct*. The recording of a test might look like this: *Hct 38%*. Double-check all readings to make sure they are accurate.

Comm

It is the physician's or other authorized individual's responsibility to interpret the results of this test to the patient.

Legal

checkpoint

1. What are two (2) ways used to seal the empty end of the capillary tube?

PRACTICE: Go to the workbook and complete the assignment sheet for 20:4, Performing a Microhematocrit. Then return and continue with the procedure.

Procedure 20:4

Performing a Microhematocrit

Equipment and Supplies

Sterile lancet, alcohol swabs, microhematocrit capillary tubes, microhematocrit centrifuge, capillary tube, sealing clay (if the tube is not self-sealing), sterile gauze, disposable gloves, mask or face shield, protective eyewear, gown, sharps container, infectious-waste bag, paper, pen and/or computer

NOTE: The following procedure is for the Readacrit centrifuge. Follow specific manufacturer's instructions when using other equipment.

Procedure

1. Assemble equipment (**Figure 20–21A**).

2. Wash hands. Put on gloves. If splashing of blood is possible, put on a gown, face mask or face shield, and protective eyewear.

   CAUTION: Observe standard precautions while obtaining and testing blood.

   Precaution

3. Introduce yourself. Identify the patient. Explain the procedure. Obtain the patient's consent.

   Comm

   NOTE: It is best to seat the patient in a comfortable position.

4. Perform the procedure for a skin puncture (**Figure 20–21B**). Put the used lancet in the sharps container immediately (**Figure 20–21C**).

5. Use sterile gauze to remove the first drop of blood. Discard the gauze in the infectious-waste bag.

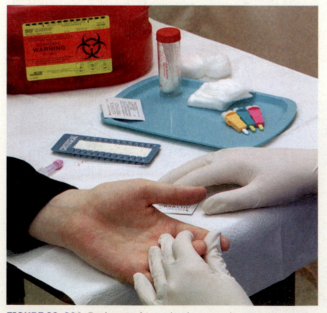

FIGURE 20–21A Equipment for a microhematocrit.

6. Allow a second well-rounded drop of blood to form at the puncture site (**Figure 20–21D**). Hold the capillary tube at a slight angle to the skin. Place the end without the indicator mark into the drop of blood (**Figure 20–21E**). Do *not* touch the skin. Allow the blood to flow into the tube until it reaches the indicator mark. Check to make sure there are no air bubbles in the tube.

   NOTE: If the tube does not have an indicator mark, fill it to within 2 millimeters of the end, or approximately three-quarters full.

 CAUTION: Do *not* use blood that has started to clot.

7. Hold a gloved finger over the end of the tube to prevent the blood from flowing out. Seal the opposite end (the one without blood) by tapping the tube into a tray of sealing clay (refer to Figure 20–20). Check the seal to be sure there are no openings. If a self-sealing tube is used, check to make sure that the plug has expanded to close the air channel and seal the tube.

 CAUTION: Avoid applying pressure while sealing the tube because the tube may break.

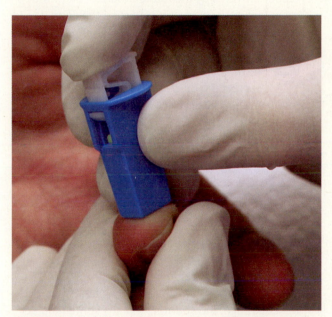

FIGURE 20–21B Perform a skin puncture to obtain capillary blood.

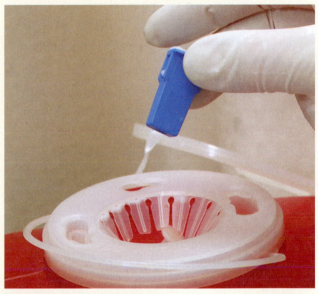

FIGURE 20–21C Immediately put the used lancet into the sharps container.

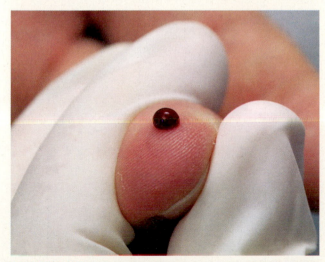

FIGURE 20–21D Allow a second well-rounded drop of blood to form at the puncture site.

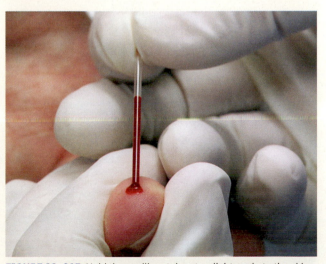

FIGURE 20–21E Hold the capillary tube at a slight angle to the skin to fill the tube with blood to the indicator mark.

(continues)

8. If your agency requires two capillary tubes for the test, fill and seal the second tube.

9. When sufficient blood has been obtained, instruct the patient to hold sterile gauze firmly against the puncture for at least 1–2 minutes.

 CAUTION: If the patient is taking an anticoagulant, pressure should be held against the puncture site for at least 3–5 minutes.
Safety

 CAUTION: Remain with the patient until the bleeding stops.
Safety

10. Place the tube into the microhematocrit centrifuge. Make sure the tube end with the clay seal is against the rubber buffer (**Figure 20–21F**). The open end of the tube should face the center of the centrifuge. If slots are designated for male or female, place the tube in the correct slot. If one tube is used, many manufacturers recommend placing an empty tube in the opposite slot to balance the centrifuge. If two tubes are used, they can be placed on opposite sides.

NOTE: Read specific manufacturer's instructions regarding loading the centrifuge.

 CAUTION: Handle tubes carefully to avoid breakage.
Safety

NOTE: Check to be sure the tube is in the correct slot.

11. Lock the centrifuge cover by turning it to the marked angle. Be sure the outside lid is also securely closed. Set the timer to the recommended time (usually 3–5 minutes) and turn the machine on.

 CAUTION: Recheck the lids. If they are not secure, the tube could fly out.
Safety

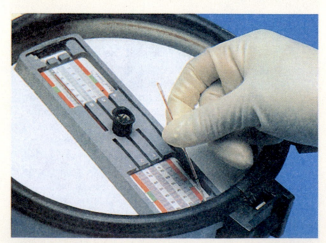

FIGURE 20–21F Place the sealed end of the capillary tube against the rubber buffer on the outer edge of the microhematocrit centrifuge.

12. When spinning stops completely, open the lid. Push the tube upward so the top of the clay line is at zero. Read the number at the top of the RBC layer (**Figure 20–21G**).

NOTE: Remember that three layers are present in the tube. The lower layer is RBCs; the middle layer is a thin, buffy coat of WBCs and platelets; and the top, clear layer is plasma (refer to Figure 20–18).

NOTE: If you are using a centrifuge without a built-in scale, carefully remove the tubes from the centrifuge. Position the tubes on the microhematocrit reader card or in the digital reader provided by the manufacturer. Follow the manufacturer's instructions to read the correct value for the hematocrit.

13. ± Double-check the accuracy of your reading. If two tubes are used, obtain a reading for
Math each of the tubes. Add the two readings together. Divide the sum by 2. This number is the hematocrit reading.

NOTE: The final reading for two tubes is an average reading of both tubes.

14. Record your reading.

15. Check the patient to be sure bleeding from the puncture has stopped.

16. Clean and replace all equipment. Put the capillary tube(s) in the sharps container. Place any contaminated disposable supplies in the infectious-waste bag. Use a disinfectant to wipe the centrifuge, the counter, and any contaminated areas.

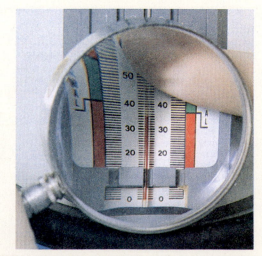

FIGURE 20–21G After positioning the tube so the top of the clay line is at zero, read the percentage number at the top of the red blood cell layer.

17. Remove gloves and discard in an infectious-waste bag. Wash hands thoroughly.

18.
   Comm

   Record required information on the patient's chart or enter it into the computer. For example: date, time, Hct: 45%, and your signature and title. Report any abnormal readings immediately.

   EHR

   NOTE: In laboratories or offices using electronic health records (EHRs), the information is entered into the patient's record on a computer.

PRACTICE: Go to the workbook and use the evaluation sheet for 20:4, Performing a Microhematocrit, to practice this procedure. When you believe you have mastered this skill, sign the sheet and give it to your instructor for further action.

✅ **FINAL EVALUATION:** Using the criteria listed on the evaluation sheet, your instructor will grade your performance.
Check

20:5 MEASURING HEMOGLOBIN

Science

The **hemoglobin (Hgb)** test is used to determine the oxygen-carrying capacity of the blood. Hemoglobin is a substance found in erythrocytes or red blood cells (RBCs). It is composed of two parts: heme, an iron-containing portion, and globin, a protein. The hemoglobin combines with oxygen and transports it to the body cells. Hemoglobin also assists in carrying carbon dioxide from the body cells to the lungs.

Before hemoglobin concentration can be determined, the blood must be hemolyzed. **Hemolysis** is the destruction of RBCs. When RBCs are destroyed, the hemoglobin is released into the solution that surrounds the cells. Whole blood is normally red and cloudy in appearance. When the cells rupture during hemolysis and hemoglobin is released, however, the blood becomes clear, or transparent. Hemolysis solutions contain special chemicals that cause this reaction outside the body.

A *hemoglobinometer* is a special instrument used to measure the hemoglobin concentration in blood. Many different CLIA-approved handheld hemoglobinometers can be used to check the level of hemoglobin (**Figure 20–22A**). A disposable cuvette (also called a *microcuvette*), test slide, or test strip/card, filled with a hemolyzing solution, is used to obtain a blood sample (**Figure 20–22B**). The hemolyzing solution in the cuvette, slide, or strip/card hemolyzes the blood and releases the hemoglobin. The cuvette, slide, or strip/card with the hemolyzed blood sample is then placed in the hemoglobinometer, which automatically measures the hemoglobin level and displays it on the screen (**Figure 20–22C**). For accurate readings, it is

important to read and follow the instructions provided by the manufacturer of the hemoglobinometer.

Normal values for hemoglobin vary with the type of test. An average range is 12–18 grams of hemoglobin per 100 milliliters of blood. Males average 13–18 grams,

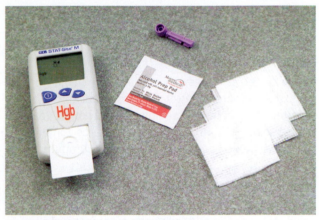

FIGURE 20–22A Handheld hemoglobinometers can be used to check the level of hemoglobin in the blood.

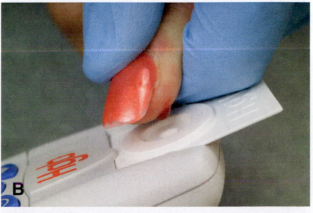

FIGURE 20–22B A drop of blood is placed into the slide reservoir of a card placed on the hemoglobinometer.

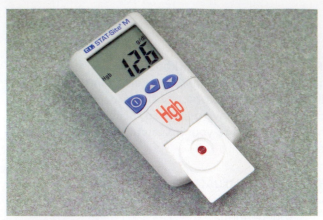

FIGURE 20–22C In less than one minute, the hemoglobin level is displayed on the screen.

females average 12–16 grams, newborns average 16–23 grams, and children from 1–10 years of age average 10–14 grams of hemoglobin per 100 milliliters of blood.

A low hemoglobin level can indicate anemia. A high level can indicate polycythemia, which is characterized by a high hemoglobin concentration and number of RBCs.

Accuracy is essential while performing this test. Care must be taken to follow the procedure exactly. The reading should be double-checked. If any results are questionable, the test should be repeated.

 It is the physician's or other authorized individual's responsibility to interpret the results of this test to the patient.

Legal

checkpoint

1. What information about the blood is provided by a hemoglobin test?

PRACTICE: Go to the workbook and complete the assignment sheet for 20:5, Measuring Hemoglobin. Then return and continue with the procedure.

Procedure 20:5

Measuring Hemoglobin with a Hemoglobinometer

Equipment and Supplies

Sterile lancet, alcohol swab, sterile gauze pads, hemoglobinometer, control cuvette, disposable cuvette, tissue or lens paper, disposable gloves, mask or face shield, eye protection, gown, sharps container, infectious-waste bag, paper, pen and/or computer

 NOTE: This procedure describes the use of the HemoCue® Hemoglobinometer. Other types of hemoglobinometers may use test slides or test strips. Always read and follow the manufacturer's instructions.

Comm

Procedure

1. Assemble equipment. Read the manufacturer's instructions provided with the hemoglobinometer.

2. Wash hands. Put on gloves. If splashing of blood is possible, put on a gown, mask or face shield, and protective eyewear.

    CAUTION: Observe all standard precautions while obtaining and testing blood.

   Precaution

3. Check the hemoglobinometer to make sure it is calibrated correctly:

   a. Press the power button to turn the hemoglobinometer on.

   b. Pull out the cuvette holder to the load position. The display will show the letters *Hb*.

   c. When the indicator displays *Ready*, insert the red control cuvette into the cuvette holder. Gently push the holder into the unit. When the holder is inserted correctly, the hemoglobinometer will display *Measuring* followed by three dashes.

   d. In 10–15 seconds, the hemoglobinometer will display a value for the control cuvette. Compare this value with the assigned value on the control cuvette card provided with the unit. The value displayed should not be more than ±0.3 g/dL (grams per deciliter) from the value on the control cuvette card. If the value is within this range, the hemoglobinometer is calibrated correctly.

    CAUTION: If the hemoglobinometer is *not* calibrated correctly, notify your instructor or refer to the troubleshooting guide in the manual provided with the hemoglobinometer. *Do not use the hemoglobinometer if the calibration is not correct.* Inaccurate test results would be obtained.

   Safety

4. Introduce yourself. Identify the patient. Explain the procedure to the patient. Obtain the patient's consent.

   Comm

5. Perform a skin puncture. Put the used lancet in the sharps container immediately.

6. Wipe off the first and/or second drop of blood. Use the second or third drop. Use your gloved

index finger and thumb to hold the cuvette at the square end (**Figure 20–23A**). Place the angled tip end into the middle of the drop of blood (**Figure 20–23B**). Hold the cuvette steady to allow capillary action to completely fill the cavity at the tip end with blood. Check the filled cuvette to make sure no air bubbles are present in the optical eye. If air bubbles are present, discard the cuvette in the sharps container. Obtain a new cuvette and repeat the filling process with another drop of blood.

 CAUTION: Never touch or handle the angled filling tip end of the cuvette. Finger marks or smudges will cause an inaccurate reading.

Safety

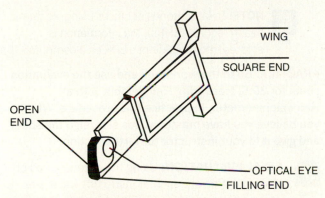

FIGURE 20–23A Always hold the disposable cuvette at the square end to prevent fingerprints or smudges from contaminating the optical eye at the filling end. Image courtesy of HemoCue®, Inc.

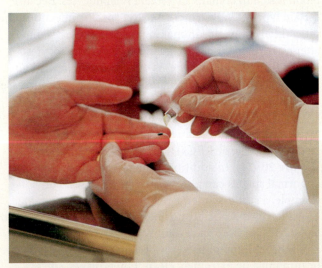

FIGURE 20–23B Place the tip end of the cuvette in the middle of the drop of blood. Image courtesy of HemoCue®, Inc.

 NOTE: The reagent inside the cavity of the cuvette will hemolyze the erythrocytes and release the hemoglobin.

Science

7. When sufficient blood has been obtained, instruct the patient to hold sterile gauze firmly against the puncture site for at least 1–2 minutes.

 CAUTION: If the patient is taking an anticoagulant, pressure should be held against the puncture site for at least 3–5 minutes.

Safety

8. Use clean, lint-free tissue or lens paper to wipe off the excess blood on the outside of the cuvette. Make sure you do *not* draw blood out of the cuvette tip while you are cleaning the outside surface.

9. Check to make sure the hemoglobinometer is displaying *Ready*. Immediately place the filled cuvette into the cuvette holder (**Figure 20–23C**). Gently push the holder into the unit. If the holder is inserted correctly, *Measuring* followed by three dashes will appear on the display.

NOTE: Obtain the hemoglobin measurement as quickly as possible after filling the cuvette. *Never* wait more than 10 minutes or test results will be inaccurate.

10. Within 60 seconds, the unit will display the hemoglobin reading in grams per deciliter (g/dL) of blood (**Figure 20–23D**). Record the reading on the display.

NOTE: Normal values for hemoglobin are 12–18 g/dL of blood.

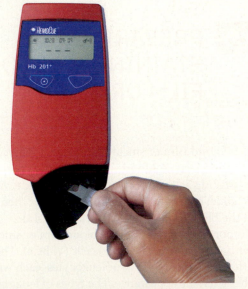

FIGURE 20–23C Place the filled cuvette into the cuvette holder and gently push the holder into the hemoglobinometer. Image courtesy of HemoCue®, Inc.

(continues)

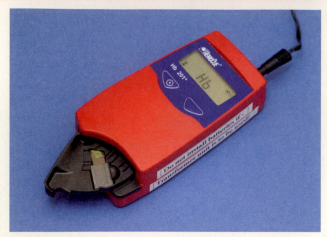

FIGURE 20–23D The hemoglobinometer displays the hemoglobin reading in grams per deciliter (g/dL) of blood. Image courtesy of HemoCue®, Inc.

11. Record your reading as in the following example: *Hgb 12.8 g.*

12. Recheck the reading to be sure it is accurate. Pull the cuvette holder out to the load position, wait until flashing dashes and *Ready* appear on the display, and then gently push the cuvette holder back into the unit. Within 60 seconds, the reading will appear.

13. Remove the cuvette from the hemoglobinometer. Immediately place the used cuvette in the sharps container. Turn the hemoglobinometer off.

14. Check the patient to be sure the skin puncture has stopped bleeding.

15. Clean and replace all equipment. Use a disinfecting solution to wipe off the outside of the hemoglobinometer or follow manufacturer's recommendations for cleaning. Place all contaminated disposable materials in the infectious-waste bag. Use a disinfectant to wipe the counter and any contaminated areas.

16. Remove gloves and discard in an infectious-waste bag. Wash hands thoroughly.

17. Comm Record the required information on the patient's chart or enter it into the computer. For example: date, time, Hgb: 12.8 g, and your signature and title. Report any abnormal readings immediately.

NOTE: In laboratories or offices using electronic health records (EHRs), the information is entered into the patient's EHR on a computer.

PRACTICE: Go to the workbook and use the evaluation sheet for 20:5, Measuring Hemoglobin with a Hemoglobinometer, to practice this procedure. When you believe you have mastered this skill, sign the sheet and give it to your instructor for further action.

 FINAL EVALUATION: Using the criteria listed on the evaluation sheet, your instructor will grade your performance.

20:6 PREPARING AND STAINING A BLOOD FILM OR SMEAR

Science A blood film or smear is used for a variety of blood tests. A **blood smear** or film is prepared by placing a small drop of blood on a slide. Another slide, coverslip, or special spreader is then used to spread the blood in a thin layer across the slide.

An important test that uses the blood film or smear is the **differential count** of white blood cells (WBCs). There are five different types of WBCs, or leukocytes, each with its own characteristic appearance. The types of leukocytes are discussed in detail in Section 7:8. In a differential count, 100 WBCs are counted. As the count is performed, a total is kept of each type of leukocyte seen by using a differential counter or calculator. The percentage of each type is then calculated. For example, if 33 lymphocytes are counted, the blood is said to contain 33 percent lymphocytes. Because certain types of WBCs increase after specific infections, the differential count aids in making diagnoses. For example, after certain viral illnesses, an increase in lymphocytes (a specific type of leukocyte) is often noted. Likewise, an infection involving certain parasites can lead to an increase in the number of eosinophils, another type of leukocyte.

The blood film or smear is also used to examine the form, structure, and relative number of erythrocytes (red blood cells, or RBCs), leukocytes, and platelets (**Figure 20–24**). In addition to abnormal blood counts, abnormal shapes can also be signs of diseases. For example, a sickle-shaped RBC can indicate the presence of sickle-cell anemia. Abnormal shapes and an increase in leukocytes are seen in certain types of leukemia.

All the equipment used for preparing the blood smear or film must be extremely clean. Fingerprints, smears, stains, and other similar contaminants will interfere with, and in some cases even distort, the appearance of the cells. Wiping the slide and spreader with alcohol is one way to remove contaminants.

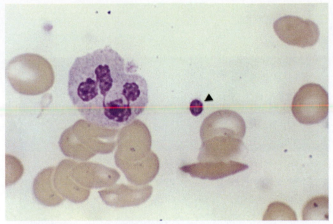
FIGURE 20–24 A photomicrograph of a stained slide showing a round cluster or aggregate of platelets (arrow), a polymorphonuclear leukocyte, and erythrocytes. Courtesy CDC/Dr F Gilbert

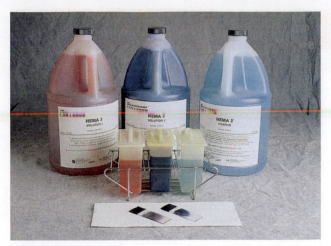
FIGURE 20–25 A quick stain, or three-step method, is another way of staining blood smear slides.

Before the slide can be viewed under a microscope, the cells must be stained so that they are visible. A common stain is Wright's stain. The stain fixes the smear, or makes the cells in the blood adhere to the slide. When a buffer is then added, the stain colors or dyes the blood cells so that they become visible under the microscope.

Another common stain is a quick stain, or three-step method. The blood smear slide is dipped into a fixative solution for about 1 second. It is then dipped into two separate staining solutions for approximately 1 second each (**Figure 20–25**). This three-step procedure is repeated four to five times following the manufacturer's instructions. Then, the slide is gently rinsed with water and allowed to air-dry before it is examined.

This method is faster and requires less than 1 minute to complete. It is important to read and follow the manufacturer's instructions to obtain a properly stained blood smear.

checkpoint

1. Describe the quick stain process and what else it is called.

PRACTICE: Go to the workbook and complete the assignment sheet for 20:6, Preparing and Staining a Blood Film or Smear. Then return and continue with the procedures.

Procedure 20:6A

Preparing a Blood Film or Smear

Equipment and Supplies

Lancet, alcohol swab, sterile gauze, alcohol, slide, coverslip or spreader slide, disposable gloves, mask or face shield, protective eyewear, gown, sharps container, infectious-waste bag, pen or pencil

Procedure

1. Assemble equipment.

2. Wash hands. Put on gloves. If splashing of blood is possible, put on a gown, mask or face shield, and protective eyewear.

    CAUTION: Observe standard precautions while obtaining and testing blood.
   Precaution

3. Use an alcohol swab to clean the slide and coverslip (spreader slide). Check both for defects or chips. Any defects could interfere with the smear pattern.

4. Introduce yourself. Identify the patient. Explain the procedure. Obtain the patient's consent.
   Comm

5. Perform a skin puncture. Wipe off the first drop of blood. Put the used lancet in the sharps container immediately.

6. Place a small drop of blood on the slide by touching the slide to the blood (**Figure 20–26A**). The drop of blood should be placed approximately ¾ inch from the end of the slide and centered on the slide.

    CAUTION: Do *not* touch the slide to the skin because doing so will cause the blood to smear.
   Safety

   NOTE: The blood drop should be approximately 2 millimeters in diameter, or the size of a match head.

(continues)

7. When sufficient blood has been obtained, instruct the patient to hold sterile gauze firmly against the puncture site for at least 1–2 minutes.

 CAUTION: If the patient is taking an anticoagulant, pressure should be held against the puncture site for at least 3–5 minutes.

Safety

 CAUTION: Remain with the patient until the bleeding stops.

Safety

8. Place the edge of the coverslip or spreader slide in front of the blood on the slide.

9. Hold the spreader slide at a 30–35-degree angle. Pull the spreader back until it touches the blood. Hold it steady while the blood spreads evenly to the edges of the spreader slide (**Figure 20–26B**).

10. Using a firm, steady movement, push the spreader to the opposite end of the slide (**Figure 20–26C**). Use a smooth, continuous motion. Keep the spreader in contact with the slide at all times. Finish by raising the spreader in a smooth, low arc. If the coverslip or spreader slide is disposable, put it in the sharps container. If it is not disposable, wash it thoroughly and clean or soak it in a disinfecting solution.

11. Allow the slide to air-dry. It is now ready for staining.

NOTE: The smear should be approximately 1½ inches long, smooth, thin, and have an even margin on all sides (**Figure 20–26D**).

NOTE: If the slide cannot be stained immediately, immerse the dried smear in methanol for 30–60 seconds to fix the slide and preserve the smear. Remove the slide from the methanol solution and allow it to air-dry.

12. Check the patient to be sure that the skin puncture has stopped bleeding.

13. Label the slide with the patient's name, doctor's name, address, identification number, and any other necessary information, or attach a computer-generated label.

Comm

14. Clean and replace all equipment. Put all contaminated disposable supplies in the infectious-waste bag. Use a disinfectant to wipe the counter and any contaminated areas.

15. Remove gloves and discard in an infectious-waste bag. Wash hands.

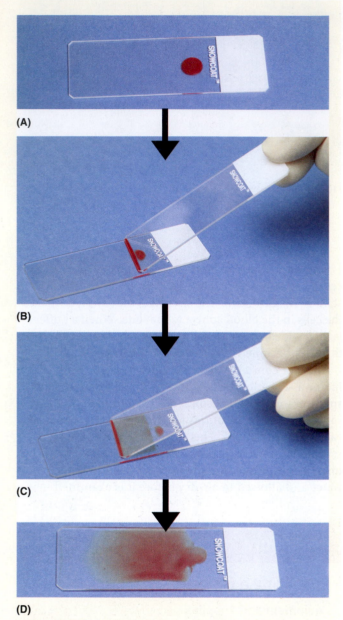

(A)

(B)

(C)

(D)

FIGURE 20–26 To prepare a blood smear: (A) place a drop of blood on the slide; (B) place the edge of the spreader slide in front of the drop of blood at a 30–35-degree angle and pull it back until it touches the drop of blood; and (C) use a firm, steady movement to push the spreader slide to the opposite end of the slide to create (D) an even smear of blood.

PRACTICE: Go to the workbook and use the evaluation sheet for 20:6A, Preparing a Blood Film or Smear, to practice this procedure. When you believe you have mastered this skill, sign the sheet and give it to your instructor for further action.

✓ **FINAL EVALUATION:** Using the criteria listed on the evaluation sheet, your instructor will grade your performance.

Check

Staining a Blood Film or Smear

Equipment and Supplies

Blood smear film slide, staining rack, Wright's stain with distilled water/buffer solution or quick stain kit, timer, disposable gloves, mask or face shield, protective eyewear, gown, infectious-waste bag

Procedure

1. Assemble equipment.

2. Wash hands. Put on gloves. If splashing of blood is possible, put on a gown, mask or face shield, and protective eyewear.

    CAUTION: Observe standard precautions while obtaining and testing blood.

3. Prepare a blood smear film (described in Procedure 20:6A) if you have not already done so.

   NOTE: The slide should be smooth and have an even margin on all sides. There should be no streaks, hesitation marks, or holes.

4. Place the slide with the smear side up on a staining rack. Make sure the rack is level.

5. To stain the slide with Wright's stain:

   a. Use Wright's stain to completely cover the dry smear (**Figure 20–27A**). Count the number of drops of the stain as you apply it. Leave the stain in place for 1–3 minutes.

   NOTE: The time and number of drops may vary with different stains; read and follow manufacturer's instructions.

   b. Add an equal amount of distilled water or buffer (**Figure 20–27B**). Place it on the slide one drop at a time. Between drops, blow gently along the length of the slide to mix the stain and water. Allow it to stand 2–4 minutes.

   NOTE: The solutions are well mixed when an oily, greenish sheen appears.

    NOTE: Some buffer solutions require doubling the amount of buffer solution compared to the amount of Wright's stain. Read the manufacturer's instructions for the solutions to determine correct amounts.

    CAUTION: Make sure none of the mixture runs off of the slide.

   c. Wash the slide by flooding it gently with distilled water. Allow the stain mixture to flow off of the slide.

6. To stain the slide with a quick stain kit:

   a. Read the manufacturer's instructions.

   b. Dip the slide into the fix solution for about 1 second.

   c. Quickly dip the slide into each of the two staining solutions for about 1 second each.

   NOTE: Touch the end of the slide on a paper towel between solutions to remove excess solution. Do *not* allow the slide to dry between solutions.

   d. Repeat the three-step dip process approximately four to five times, following manufacturer's instructions.

   e. Rinse the slide gently with water (if required by the manufacturer).

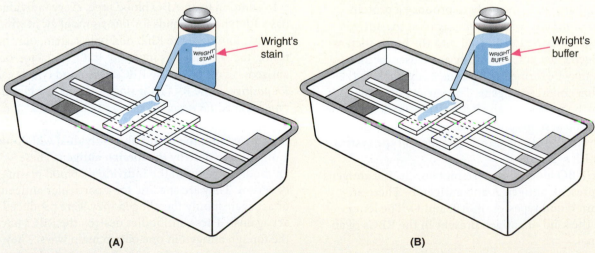

FIGURE 20–27 (A) Use Wright's stain to cover the dry smear. (B) After waiting 1–3 minutes, add an equal amount of distilled water or buffer solution.

(continues)

7. Wipe the dye from the back of the slide. Observe which part of the slide has the heaviest concentration of blood smear. Stand the slide on its end (vertically) to dry. Place the part with the heaviest concentration downward and allow the dye to flow down from the less concentrated (thinner) area. In an emergency, the front of the slide can be blotted dry, but this is not recommended. It is best to allow the slide to air-dry at room temperature.

8. The finished smear should have a lavender-pink color. If it appears too purple, hold the slide under gently running cold water until the desired color is obtained. Let the water strike the slide above the thick portion of the smear and flow downward.

   NOTE: The slide is now ready to be examined. A differential count of leukocytes is usually done with this type of stain. Examinations of erythrocytes and platelets can also be done.

9. Clean and replace all equipment. Put all contaminated disposable supplies in the infectious-waste bag. Use a disinfectant to wipe the counter and any contaminated areas.

10. Remove gloves and discard in an infectious-waste bag. Wash hands.

PRACTICE: Go to the workbook and use the evaluation sheet for 20:6B, Staining a Blood Film or Smear, to practice this procedure. When you believe you have mastered this skill, sign the sheet and give it to your instructor for further action.

 FINAL EVALUATION: Using the criteria listed on the evaluation sheet, your instructor will grade your performance.

Check

20:7 TESTING FOR BLOOD TYPES

Science

Human beings inherit a certain blood type from their parents. The type of blood is determined by the presence of certain factors, called *antigens*, on red blood cells (RBCs), or erythrocytes. An **antigen** is a substance, usually a protein, that causes the body to produce a protein, called an *antibody*, which reacts against the antigen. An antigen may be introduced into the body, such as the antigens that enter the body as viruses, or an antigen may be formed within the body, such as the RBCs that contain antigens. The variety of antigens that may be present on the RBCs serve as the basis for blood group systems and blood types. Two of the major systems are called the ABO blood type system and the Rh system.

In the ABO blood type system, two specific antigens can be present: antigen A and antigen B. There are four main blood types: A, B, AB, and O. The letters refer to the kind of antigen present in the RBCs of an individual.

- **Type A** contains antigen A on the RBCs.
- **Type B** contains antigen B on the RBCs.

- **Type AB** contains both antigen A and antigen B on the RBCs.
- **Type O** contains neither antigen A nor antigen B on the RBCs.

Red blood cells are not the only body cells with the A and B antigens. Most other cells also have them. Thus, in forensic (legal) medicine, a piece of skin or other tissue found at a crime scene can be typed. In this way, the blood type of the victim and/or criminal can be determined.

In addition to an ABO blood type, every individual has a Rh type. Rh stands for *Rhesus* monkey, in which it was first found. In the Rh blood type system, only one factor, the D antigen, is involved. If the Rh factor, or D antigen, is present on the RBCs, the blood type is called *Rh positive*. If the Rh factor is *not* present, the blood type is called *Rh negative*.

If an antigen not present in a person's RBCs is introduced into the blood, the individual will produce antibodies to destroy the foreign antigen. These antibodies remain in the individual's blood plasma or serum. They are specific for a particular antigen, or act against only the antigen they were produced to act against. These antibodies destroy the RBCs having the foreign antigen in one of two main ways. They cause the RBCs to either *hemolyze* (dissolve and go into solution, releasing hemoglobin) or to *agglutinate* (clump together). Because RBCs carry oxygen and carbon dioxide to maintain vital body functions, their destruction can lead to death.

Before anyone can receive a transfusion (transfer of blood from one individual to another), a **typing and crossmatch** must be performed on the blood. The blood typing reveals the ABO, Rh factors, and other, rarer blood type systems. Crossmatching consists of a series of tests performed on the blood of the donor (the person giving blood) and on the blood of the recipient (the person receiving blood). The purpose is to detect any possible incompatibility or difference that would make the blood unsuitable for transfusion between the recipient's serum and the cells of the donor. Most blood banks also do an **antibody screen** of blood prior to a transfusion being performed. This screening is performed to check for unexpected antibodies that may be present in the blood and that could lead to an incompatibility reaction. Only when the two types of blood are compatible, or identical in antigens and antibodies present, can the blood from one individual be given to another individual.

Blood typing is also performed on pregnant women. A Rh incompatibility between a pregnant woman and the fetus (developing infant) can cause *hemolytic disease of the newborn* (HDN). The problem occurs when the woman is Rh negative and the fetus is Rh positive. The Rh antigen, or D antigen, enters the mother's bloodstream through the placenta. The mother's bloodstream then produces anti-D antibodies against the D antigen. When these antibodies enter the developing infant's bloodstream through the placenta, the antibodies can hemolyze or destroy the infant's red blood cells. Fortunately, a medicine called RhoGAM can be given to the pregnant woman to prevent the formation of the anti-D antibodies. The RhoGAM injection is usually given to the woman once or twice during the pregnancy and within 72 hours after delivery if the infant is Rh positive.

The procedure that follows demonstrates blood typing using an anti-A serum and an anti-B serum; the Rh factor is checked using an anti-Rh, or anti-D, serum. The three serums are designed to cause an agglutination reaction if the antigens are present in the blood. Thus, if the blood reacts to the anti-A serum by agglutinating, but does not react to the anti-B serum, only antigen A is present, and the blood type is type A (**Figure 20–28**). Conversely, if the blood reacts to the anti-B serum but does not react to the anti-A serum, only antigen B is present, and the blood type is B. If the blood reacts to both the anti-A serum and the anti-B serum, both antigen A and antigen B are present, and the blood

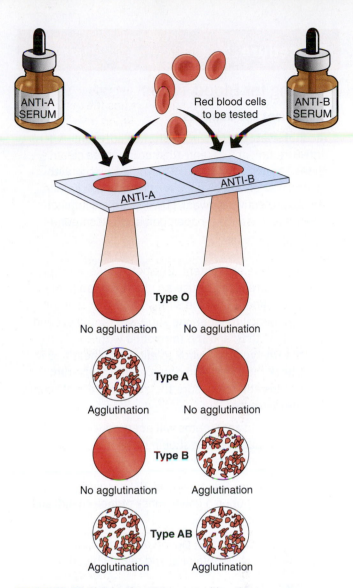

FIGURE 20–28 Blood typing ABO groups with antiserums.

type is AB. If the blood reacts to neither the anti-A serum nor the anti-B serum, neither antigen is present, and the blood type is O. If the blood reacts to the anti-Rh serum, the Rh factor is present, and the blood is Rh positive. If the blood does not react to the anti-RH serum, the Rh factor is not present, and the blood type is Rh negative. This test is used only for screening purposes. Additional and more extensive laboratory tests are performed on blood before a transfusion is given.

checkpoint

| **1.** How many blood types are there?

PRACTICE: Go to the workbook and complete the assignment sheet for 20:7, Testing for Blood Types. Then return and continue with the procedure.

Testing for Blood Types

Equipment and Supplies

Alcohol swab, sterile lancet, sterile gauze, anti-A serum, anti-B serum, anti-D (anti-Rh) serum, three clean slides, three mixing sticks, Rh-typing viewbox with heater, wax pencil, disposable gloves, mask or face shield, protective eyewear, gown, sharps container, infectious-waste bag, paper, pen and/or computer

Procedure

1. Assemble equipment. Check to make sure the slides are clean or use an alcohol swab to clean each slide. Allow the slides to air-dry. Use the wax pencil to label one slide with A, the second slide with B, and the third slide with Rh. Turn on the Rh-typing viewbox to allow it to heat to 37°C. Check the expiration dates on the antiserum bottles and make sure the solutions are at room temperature.

   NOTE: Old antiserums will not produce accurate test results. Serums should be discarded on their expiration dates.

2. Wash hands. Put on gloves. If splashing of blood is possible, put on a gown, mask or face shield, and protective eyewear.

    CAUTION: Observe standard precautions while obtaining and testing blood.

3. Introduce yourself. Identify the patient. Explain the procedure. Obtain the patient's consent.

4. Perform a skin puncture as previously instructed. Wipe off the first drop of blood. Put the used lancet in the sharps container immediately.

5. Place one drop of blood on the slide labeled A, a second drop on the slide labeled B, and a third drop on the slide labeled Rh.

    CAUTION: Take care *not* to touch the skin to the slide.

6. When sufficient blood has been obtained, instruct the patient to hold sterile gauze firmly against the puncture site for at least 1–2 minutes.

    CAUTION: If the patient is taking an anticoagulant, pressure should be held against the puncture site for at least 3–5 minutes.

 CAUTION: Remain with the patient until the bleeding stops.

7. Place one drop of anti-A serum next to the first drop of blood on the slide labeled A (**Figure 20–29A**). Immediately mix the blood and serum with a mixing stick. Discard the stick in the sharps container.

    CAUTION: Work quickly, before the blood clots.

8. Place one drop of anti-B serum next to the second drop of blood on the slide labeled B. Mix immediately with a second mixing stick. Discard the stick in the sharps container.

9. Place one drop of anti-Rh or D serum next to the third drop of blood on the third slide labeled Rh. Mix immediately with a third mixing stick. Discard the stick in the sharps container. Place this slide on the Rh-typing viewbox. The viewbox will heat the slide to body temperature and gently rock the slide back and forth for 2 minutes to mix the solutions.

   NOTE: The blood must be at body temperature to obtain an accurate reaction to the anti-D or Rh serum.

10. Gently rock the slides containing the anti-A and anti-B serums back and forth for at least 1–2 minutes. Keep the slides separate to make sure the drops of blood do not mix together. The rocking motion allows the antigens in the blood to react with the serums. Using a strong light, check for an agglutination, or clumping, reaction in the two drops of blood. Agglutination indicates

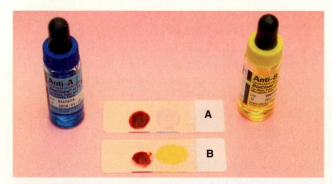

FIGURE 20–29A Place a drop of blood on each slide and mix with antiserums. The top slide contains anti-A serum and the bottom slide contains anti-B serum.

a positive reaction. If the reaction is positive, the cells will clump together. If the reaction is negative, the blood will remain unchanged (**Figure 20–29B**).

11. At the end of 2 minutes, check the Rh slide on the viewbox. Use a strong light and observe for agglutination (**Figure 20–29C**). If the cells have agglutinated, the reaction is positive, and the Rh factor is present in the blood. If the blood remains unchanged, the reaction is negative, and the Rh factor is not present in the blood.

12. Use the following chart to determine blood type based on serum agglutination reactions.

Type of Blood	Anti-A	Anti-B	Anti-Rh or Anti-D
O	Negative	Negative	
A	Positive	Negative	
B	Negative	Positive	
AB	Positive	Positive	
Rh positive			Positive
Rh negative			Negative

13. Recheck any questionable results. Correctly record the information.

    NOTE: Blood type is noted as A positive (A+), AB negative (AB−), and so forth for the various blood types.

14. Check the patient to make sure the skin puncture has stopped bleeding.

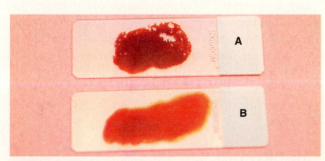

FIGURE 20–29B The top slide containing anti-A serum has agglutinated. which means the blood contains antigen A. The bottom slide containing anti-B serum did not agglutinate, which means antigen B is not present.

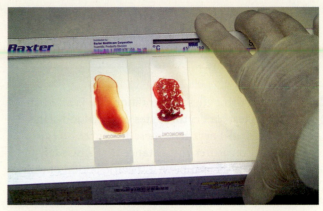

FIGURE 20–29C The slide on the left did not react with anti-Rh or D serum, so the blood is Rh negative. The slide on the right agglutinated, so the blood is Rh positive.

15. Clean and replace all equipment. If the slides are disposable, put them in the sharps container. If the slides are not disposable, wash them thoroughly and then clean or soak them in a disinfecting solution. Put all contaminated disposable supplies in the infectious-waste bag. Use a disinfectant to wipe the counter, viewbox, and other contaminated areas.

16. Remove gloves and discard in an infectious-waste bag. Wash hands.

17. Record all required information on the patient's chart or enter it into the computer. For example: date, time, Blood Type AB+, and your signature and title. Report any abnormal readings immediately.

    NOTE: In laboratories or offices using electronic health records (EHRs), the information is entered into the patient's EHR on a computer.

PRACTICE: Go to the workbook and use the evaluation sheet for 20:7, Testing for Blood Types, to practice this procedure. When you believe you have mastered this skill, sign the sheet and give it to your instructor for further action.

 FINAL EVALUATION: Using the criteria listed on the evaluation sheet, your instructor will grade your performance.

20:8 PERFORMING AN ERYTHROCYTE SEDIMENTATION RATE

Science

An erythrocyte sedimentation rate is another blood test for erythrocytes or red blood cells (RBCs). An **erythrocyte sedimentation rate (ESR)** measures the distance that RBCs fall and settle in a special glass tube in a specific period of time. The test is also called a *sedimentation rate*, or *sed rate*. Venous blood is used for this test. An anticoagulant, such as oxalate or sequestrene, is added to the blood to prevent clotting. The blood is then placed in a special tube. The RBCs fall and settle in the tube. The distance is measured in millimeters by using graduated marks on the tube or rack. The measurement is taken at the point where the clear plasma line is noted above the settled RBCs (**Figure 20–30**).

In order for the RBCs to fall and settle correctly, the tube containing the blood must be placed in a special rack. The rack is designed to hold the tube in an exact vertical position. Many sedimentation racks contain a level indicator. This indicator must be adjusted so that the rack is 100 percent level with it. The sedimentation rack must also be placed on a counter that is free of vibrations and not exposed to a heating/cooling vent or direct sunlight. The test must be conducted at room temperature to obtain accurate results.

Measurements of ESR are usually taken at specific time periods. Some laboratories check the distance at 20-minute intervals. A measurement is always taken at the 1-hour period. The various readings and times are then placed on a graphic chart. By reading the chart, the physician can determine both the rate and distance of fall for the RBCs.

Two main methods are used to perform an ESR: the Wintrobe and the Westergren. Both methods provide the same results, but the National Committee for Clinical Laboratory Standards recommends the Westergren system. This system is a completely closed system and eliminates the manual transfer of blood that can result in leakage, overfilling, and spraying from the transfer pipette. The method used will depend on the preference of the health care facility. No matter which method is used, it is essential to read and follow the manufacturer's instructions to obtain accurate results.

Normal values for ESR can vary slightly. The normal range depends to some extent on the test kit or method used. Most normal values for the Wintrobe method are 0–20 millimeters per hour (mm/hr) for adult women and 0–9 mm/hr for adult men. Most normal values for the Westergren method are 0–20 mm/hr for adult women younger than 50 years, 0–30 mm/hr for women 50 years or older, 0–15 mm/hr for adult men younger than 50 years, and 0–20 mm/hr for men 50 years or older.

A faster-than-normal sedimentation rate signifies that inflammation and/or cell destruction has taken place. This may occur in conjunction with many medical conditions, including infections, cancers (such as certain carcinomas and leukemia), inflammatory processes (such as rheumatic fever and rheumatoid arthritis), and acute viral hepatitis. Pregnant or menstruating female individuals may also have an increased sedimentation rate. A slower-than-normal sedimentation rate can occur in conjunction with polycythemia (a high number of RBCs), sickle-cell anemia, certain types of heart disease (such as congestive heart failure), and severe liver disease.

checkpoint

1. What are the two (2) main methods used to perform an ESR?

PRACTICE: Go to the workbook and complete the assignment sheet for 20:8, Performing an Erythrocyte Sedimentation Rate. Then return and continue with the procedure.

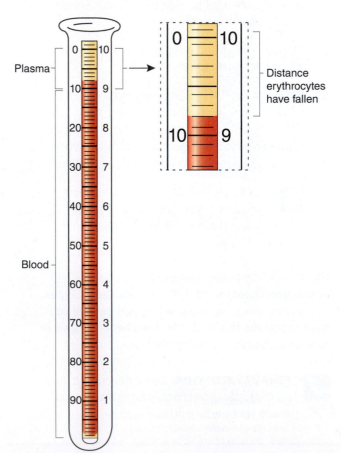

FIGURE 20–30 Read the level at the marked line between the cells and the plasma of the blood. The example shown is 8 millimeters (mm).

Procedure 20:8

Performing an Erythrocyte Sedimentation Rate

Equipment and Supplies

Venous blood with oxalate or sequestrene (anticoagulant), sedimentation rack, sedimentation-rate tubes, transfer pipette, timer, disposable gloves, mask or face shield, protective eyewear, gown, infectious-waste bag, paper, pen and/or computer

Procedure

1. Assemble equipment. Read the manufacturer's instructions carefully.

2. Wash hands. Put on gloves. If splashing of blood is possible, put on a gown, mask or face shield, and protective eyewear.

    CAUTION: Observe standard precautions while obtaining and testing blood.

3. Check the sedimentation rack. Make sure the rack is level. Check the bubble or level indicator for the level mark if one is present. Make sure the rack is on a counter that is free of vibrations and not exposed to direct sunlight or a heating/cooling vent.

   NOTE: If the rack has a level indicator, turn the platform knobs located near the feet to center the bubble in the indicator and level the rack (**Figure 20–31**).

4. Obtain venipuncture blood that has been mixed with an anticoagulant. Blood should be at room temperature. Make sure the stopper is secure on the test tube containing the blood. Invert the tube and shake it gently for 3–5 minutes to thoroughly mix the blood.

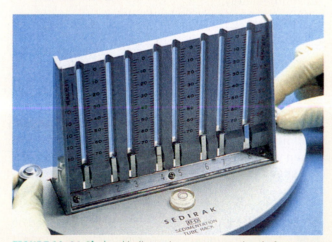

FIGURE 20–31 If a level indicator is present, turn the platform knobs to center the bubble in the indicator and to level the sedimentation rack.

 NOTE: Health science career students are *not* permitted to obtain blood by venipuncture unless they receive special training.

5. To perform an ESR by the Wintrobe method:

   a. Place the sedimentation tube in the rack. Make sure the black line on the tube is at the zero on the rack.

      NOTE: The tube must be clean and dry for an accurate measurement.

      NOTE: The tube can also be filled with the proper amount of blood first and then placed in the rack.

   b. With a transfer pipette, withdraw blood from the blood tube into the pipette and place the filled pipette in the bottom of the sedimentation-rate tube (**Figure 20–32**). Gradually withdraw the pipette while expelling the blood to prevent air bubble formation. Fill the tube to the zero mark.

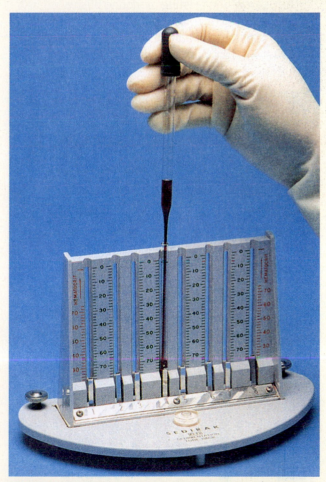

FIGURE 20–32 For the Wintrobe method, transfer the blood from the pipette to the sedimentation-rate tube, taking care to keep the pipette below the level of the blood at all times to prevent air bubble formation.

(continues)

NOTE: Self-filling tubes are available for the Wintrobe method. Follow the manufacturer's instructions to use these tubes.

NOTE: Check the filled tube. If air bubbles are present, start over.

6. To perform an ESR using the Sediplast Westergren method:

   a. Remove the stopper on the diluting vial. Fill the vial with the venipuncture blood to the line indicated on the vial.

   NOTE: The diluting vials contain a 3.8-percent sodium citrate solution that dilutes the blood sample.

   b. Replace the stopper and gently invert the vial three to six times to mix the blood and dilutent.

   c. Place the vial in the Sediplast rack.

   d. Use a gentle twisting motion to push a disposable pipette through the pierceable stopper on the vial. Push down until the pipette touches the bottom of the vial (**Figure 20–33**).

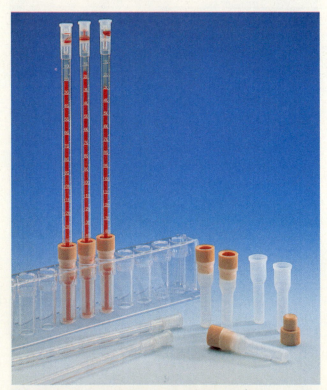

FIGURE 20–33 For the Sediplast Westergren method, gently push the disposable pipette down into the diluting vial. The pipette will fill automatically. Note the empty diluting vials with stoppers on the right. Image courtesy of Polymedco, Inc. Sediplast is a trademark of Polymedco, Inc.

The pipette will fill automatically to the zero mark. Excess diluted blood will flow into the sealed reservoir compartment.

7. Recheck the level of the rack.

8. The RBCs will fall and settle. At the time(s) specified, read the level to which the RBCs have fallen. Most tests are done at 20-, 40-, and 60-minute intervals. Many laboratories record only a 60-minute reading.

   NOTE: Read at eye level. Take the reading at the marked line between the cells and plasma of the blood (refer to **Figure 20–30**).

9. Record the readings in millimeters (mm). Note the time of each reading. Make sure all readings are recorded.

   NOTE: Normal readings vary. Check the manufacturer's instructions to determine normal values for the test kit used.

10. Clean and replace all equipment. Most tubes are disposable. Place disposable tubes in a sharps container. Put other contaminated disposable supplies in the infectious-waste bag. Use a disinfectant to wipe the rack, counter, and any other contaminated areas.

11. Remove gloves and discard in an infectious-waste bag. Wash hands thoroughly.

12. Record required information on the patient's chart or enter it into the computer. For example: date, time, ESR Westergren: 12 mm/hr, and your signature and title. Report any abnormal readings immediately.

     NOTE: In laboratories or offices using electronic health records (EHRs), the information is entered into the patient's EHR on a computer.

PRACTICE: Go to the workbook and use the evaluation sheet for 20:8, Performing an Erythrocyte Sedimentation Rate, to practice this procedure. When you believe you have mastered this skill, sign the sheet and give it to your instructor for further action.

FINAL EVALUATION: Using the criteria listed on the evaluation sheet, your instructor will grade your performance.

20:9 MEASURING BLOOD-SUGAR (GLUCOSE) LEVEL

Science

Glucose is a form of sugar found in the bloodstream. Insulin, which is produced by the islets of Langerhans in the pancreas, normally allows glucose to cross cell membranes so that it can be metabolized. In a disease known as *diabetes mellitus*, however, there is an insufficient amount of insulin. Individuals with diabetes, therefore, cannot metabolize glucose, or convert it into energy. Glucose builds up in the bloodstream. Excess amounts are filtered out by the kidneys and eliminated from the body in the urine. **Hyperglycemia**, or high blood sugar, and **glycosuria**, or sugar in the urine, are two main signs of diabetes.

Individuals with diabetes control their disease by following calculated diets that meet nutritional needs while controlling blood-sugar levels. In some cases, diet control can regulate blood-sugar level. However, many individuals with diabetes must also take insulin injections to control blood-sugar levels. Correct insulin dosage and proper diet can maintain normal blood-sugar level. However, the dosage of insulin required can vary depending on body metabolism, food intake, amount of exercise, other illness, and stress. For this reason, many diabetics are taught to check blood-sugar levels and regulate insulin dosages based on glucose levels. Because too much insulin can lead to severe **hypoglycemia**, or low blood sugar, and a condition called *insulin shock*, proper insulin dosage is essential.

A variety of blood tests can be used to check the level of glucose. One method of checking blood-sugar level is a **fasting blood sugar (FBS)**. This test is usually performed in medical laboratories. The patient does not eat or drink anything (fasts) for 8–12 hours before the test. A venipuncture is done to obtain a sample of blood, and the amount of glucose is checked. Normal fasting blood sugar varies according to the testing method used, but an average is 70–100 milligrams per deciliter (mg/dL) of blood.

Another test called the **glucose tolerance test (GTT)** evaluates how well a person metabolizes a calculated amount of glucose. The GTT is frequently used to diagnose diabetes. The patient fasts for 8–12 hours before the GTT. Blood and urine specimens are obtained and tested for fasting levels. The patient then drinks a calibrated amount of glucose. Blood and urine specimens are usually obtained and tested at 30 minutes, 1 hour, 2 hours, and 3 hours, but test times vary. Normally, the glucose ingested would be metabolized by the end of the GTT, and blood and urine levels of glucose would be in normal ranges. In a person with diabetes mellitus, the levels would remain elevated.

Another blood test that is performed on individuals with diabetes is the **glycohemoglobin test** (HbA1C or HbA1, commonly called A1C). This test measures the amount of glucose that attaches to the hemoglobin on red blood cells (RBCs). Because RBCs live approximately 120 days, or 4 months, this test provides information on the average blood-sugar levels for the previous 2–3 months. Although normal values depend on the test used, a common normal range is 4.0–5.6 percent. A range of 5.7–6.4 percent indicates an increased risk for diabetes, or prediabetes. A reading above 6.5 indicates diabetes. A person with well-controlled diabetes averages 6–7 percent. A person with untreated or uncontrolled diabetes might have levels of 10–12 percent or even higher. If the glycohemoglobin level rises, it indicates that the patient's diabetic management plan must be improved. This can be accomplished by more frequent evaluations of daily glucose levels, changes in the type or dosage of insulin, and/or stricter dietary control. The American Diabetes Association recommends that individuals with diabetes with good glucose control be tested for glycohemoglobin levels once or twice a year. Diabetics with poor control should have the test four times a year.

In past years, most individuals with diabetes checked the level of glucose in the urine. A high level of glucose in the urine can indicate a high blood-sugar level because excess glucose is filtered out of the blood by the kidneys. However, urine tests do *not always* accurately indicate a current blood-sugar level because the urine may show glucose that was excreted several hours earlier. Therefore, individuals with diabetes are now encouraged to check blood-glucose levels rather than urine-glucose levels. Advantages of checking blood glucose include increased accuracy compared to urine tests, unlimited flexibility with regard to timing of the test, ability to detect both low and high glucose levels, better regulation of insulin dosage, and improved control of diabetes.

Technology

Reagent strips are an easy way to test daily blood-sugar levels. These are plastic strips with a chemical-reagent pad or pads. A drop of blood from a skin puncture is placed on the pad. When glucose in the blood reacts with the chemicals on the pad, color changes occur. The amount of glucose present can be determined by comparing the color on the chemical-reagent pad to a color chart usually located on the bottle of reagent strips. This method is not as accurate because it relies on the operator performing a color match. Usually, the strips are placed in a special instrument called a glucose meter, glucose analyzer, or glucometer that measures the refractions of light created by the presence of glucose. The glucose meter provides a more accurate reading of the reagent strip and shows the amount of glucose in milligrams by way of numbers that light up on the screen.

The following steps should be taken to obtain the most accurate results:

- Store all reagent strips properly. Reagent strips are very sensitive to heat, light, and moisture. They should be stored in a dark, dry, cool area, but should not be refrigerated. The bottle containing the strips is usually made of dark or light-resistant glass. To prevent contamination from moisture in the air, close the bottle immediately after use.

- Handle the reagent strips carefully. Never touch the chemical-reagent pad(s). Chemicals and moisture on the skin can cause inaccurate results. In addition, the chemicals on the strips can burn or injure the skin.

  Safety

- Read all instructions carefully. Times and procedure methods vary with different strips. A few require rinsing before a reading is taken. Others must be blotted at a set time interval. If a glucose meter is used, it is important to use the strip designed for that particular brand of meter.

  Comm

- Read all instructions provided with the glucose meter. To ensure accuracy, meters have to be calibrated before use. Test strips or solutions are used to calibrate the meter. Different time intervals and procedures are used for different meters.

  Comm

- Some new glucose meters do not require the use of reagent strips. An example is the HemoCue glucose meter (**Figure 20–34**). A disposable cuvette is filled with a drop of blood and the cuvette is inserted into the holder on the side of the unit. When the cuvette holder is pushed into the unit, the photometer measures the glucose level in 15–240 seconds and displays the reading on the monitor. The cuvette is then discarded in a sharps container. It is important to measure the sample of blood within 40 seconds to obtain the most accurate results.

- Glucose meters must be cleaned carefully after each use. Accumulation of dirt, dust, or other residue can lead to inaccurate readings. Most manufacturers recommend specific cleaning procedures. Lens paper is frequently recommended to prevent scratching the screen. Water is usually the only solution used for cleaning because alcohol can damage many meters. If possible, disinfect the meter.

   The FDA has recently approved several models of *continuous glucose monitoring devices.* These devices do not require drops of blood and eliminate the need for frequent finger punctures. A small sensor is attached to the skin, usually on the upper arm. A special reader device is

  Technology

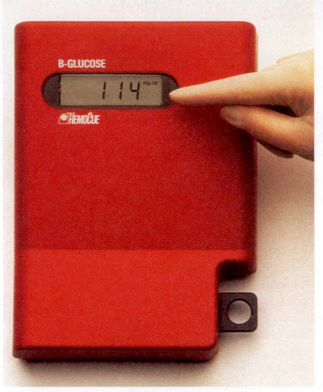

FIGURE 20–34 A disposable cuvette is filled with blood and inserted into the HemoCue glucose meter. The glucose level is displayed on the screen in 15–240 seconds. Reagent strips are not used with this type of glucose meter. Photo courtesy of HemoCue®, Inc.

then held over the sensor and the blood glucose level is displayed on the screen. This allows an individual to check blood glucose levels frequently with minimal effort and can alert a patient to high or low glucose levels quickly. The devices are more expensive than standard glucose meters, but some insurance policies will cover the cost.

 Most patients check their own blood-glucose levels. Even children can be taught to monitor their own blood-sugar levels. Patients must be given complete instructions on the correct procedure to use. Correct skin puncture techniques must be taught. Asepsis must be stressed. Proper use and storage of reagent strips and operation and cleaning of the glucose meter must be demonstrated. Patients frequently are taught to determine insulin dosages based on glucose levels, so their determinations of glucose levels must be as accurate as possible.

Comm

check point

| 1. What information is provided by an A1C test?

PRACTICE: Go to the workbook and complete the assignment sheet for 20:9, Measuring Blood-Sugar (Glucose) Level. Then return and continue with the procedure.

Measuring Blood-Sugar (Glucose) Level

Equipment and Supplies

Sterile lancet, alcohol swabs, sterile gauze, glucose reagent strips or disposable cuvette (depending on which glucose meter is used), glucose meter, lens paper, tissues or blotter paper, watch or timer with second hand, disposable gloves, mask or face shield, protective eyewear, gown, sharps container, infectious-waste bag, paper, pen and/or computer

NOTE: The method used varies slightly depending on the type of reagent strip and/or glucose meter used. Follow the specific manufacturer's instructions.

Procedure

1. Assemble equipment. Carefully read instructions provided with the glucose reagent strips and the glucose meter. Make sure the reagent strips are compatible with the meter. Note times that must be observed during each step of the procedure.

    Comm

2. Wash hands. Put on gloves. If splashing of blood is possible, put on a gown, mask or face shield, and protective eyewear.

     CAUTION: Observe standard precautions while obtaining and testing blood.

    Precaution

3. Calibrate the glucose meter for accuracy (**Figure 20–35A**). Follow the manufacturer's instructions. Most meters have test reagent strips or solutions that are placed on a reagent strip to check calibration.

4. Introduce yourself. Identify the patient. Explain the procedure. Obtain the patient's consent.

    Comm

NOTE: It is best to seat the patient in a comfortable position.

5. Perform the procedure for a skin puncture. Place the used lancet in the sharps container immediately.

6. Use sterile gauze to remove the first drop of blood.

7. Remove one reagent strip from the bottle, being careful not to touch the chemical-reagent pad on the strip. Immediately close the lid of the bottle.

    ⚠ **CAUTION:** If the chemical reagent pad touches the skin, injury or burns can occur, as can inaccurate readings.
    Safety

8. Press the start button on the glucose meter. A beep or light usually indicates the correct time for placing a large drop of blood on the reagent strip (**Figure 20–35B**). Make sure the drop of blood completely covers the chemical-reagent pad. Hold the strip level to avoid spilling the blood. Do not allow the chemical-reagent pad to touch the skin while applying the drop of blood.

NOTE: If the glucose meter uses a disposable cuvette instead of a reagent strip, place the tip end of the cuvette into the middle of the drop of blood. Hold the cuvette steady to allow the chamber to fill completely through capillary action. Use a lint-free tissue or lens paper to wipe off excess blood on the outside of the cuvette. Immediately place the cuvette into the holder on the side of the glucose meter (refer to Figure 20–34). Gently push the cuvette holder into the glucose meter. Within 15–240 seconds, the glucose reading will be displayed on the screen. Steps 10 and 11 of this procedure are not used with this type of glucose meter.

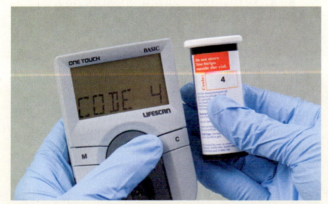

FIGURE 20–35A Calibrate the glucose meter for accuracy following the manufacturer's instructions. This meter uses a test strip.

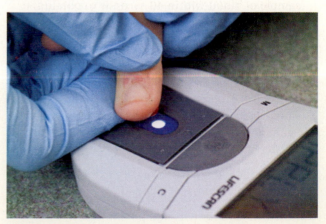

FIGURE 20–35B Place the drop of blood on the strip.

(continues)

NOTE: In some glucose meters, the reagent strip is inserted into the meter first. Then, the end of the strip is placed in the drop of blood. The strip uses capillary action to draw the blood into the meter where the glucose is measured and the value displayed.

9. When sufficient blood has been obtained, instruct the patient to hold sterile gauze firmly against the skin puncture for at least 1–2 minutes.

 CAUTION: If the patient is taking an anticoagulant, pressure should be held against the puncture site for at least 3–5 minutes.

 CAUTION: Remain with the patient until the bleeding stops.

10. The glucose meter signals with a beep or light when the blood has been on the strip for the required period of time. If necessary, blot the strip gently by placing it between a fold of tissue or blotter paper. Some glucose meters do not require blotting of the reagent strip, so it is important to follow the manufacturer's instructions.

NOTE: Blood usually remains on the strip for 10–60 seconds. It is important to follow the time period established by the manufacturer because this is a crucial step.

 CAUTION: Never wipe the strip while blotting it. Wiping removes too much of the blood and causes inaccurate results.

11. Immediately insert the strip into the correct position in the meter. Most manufacturers require that the reagent pad face the window on the meter. Check to be sure the strip is in the correct position. Follow the manufacturer's instructions to obtain an accurate reading. Most glucose meters display the glucose level automatically (**Figure 20–35C**).

12. Record the reading in milligrams (mg), for example, *102 mg*. Be sure to include the date, time, glucose test, your name or initials, and other required information. Double-check the reading for accuracy.

13. Check the patient to make sure that bleeding from the skin puncture has stopped.

14. Clean and replace all equipment. Place the reagent strip and any contaminated disposable

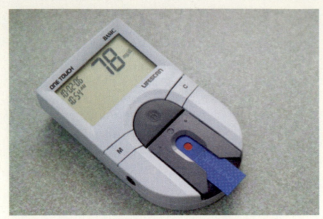

FIGURE 20–35C Most glucose meters display the glucose level automatically.

equipment in the infectious-waste bag. If a disposable cuvette was used, place the cuvette in the sharps container. Use a disinfectant to wipe the counter and any contaminated areas. Follow the manufacturer's instructions for proper cleaning of the glucose meter.

NOTE: Most manufacturers recommend using lens paper and water to clean the window, strip slot, and other areas on the meter. A disinfectant solution should then be put on these areas unless prohibited by the manufacturer.

15. Remove gloves and discard in an infectious-waste bag. Wash hands thoroughly.

16. Record all required information on the patient's chart or enter it into the computer. For example: date, time, Blood Glucose: 102 mg, and your signature and title. Report any abnormal readings immediately.

NOTE: In laboratories or offices using electronic health records (EHRs), the information is entered into the patient's EHR on a computer.

PRACTICE: Go to the workbook and use the evaluation sheet for 20:9, Measuring Blood-Sugar (Glucose) Level, to practice this procedure. When you believe you have mastered this skill, sign the sheet and give it to your instructor for further action.

 FINAL EVALUATION: Using the criteria listed on the evaluation sheet, your instructor will grade your performance.

20:10 TESTING URINE

Science

Urine tests are often done to determine the physical condition of a patient. Abnormal urine tests are often the first indications of a disease process. **Table 20–1** provides the main facts regarding urine, specifically normal and abnormal characteristics of urine. Refer to this table as you perform the basic urine tests.

A **urinalysis** is an examination of urine and consists of three main areas of testing: physical, chemical, and microscopic.

- **Physical testing** of urine is usually done first and consists of observing and recording color, odor, transparency, and specific gravity. The urine specimen should be fresh and mixed gently prior to being checked for physical characteristics.

- **Chemical testing** of urine is performed to check pH, protein, glucose, ketone, bilirubin, urobilinogen, and blood. Reagent strips, described in detail in Section 20:11, are usually used for chemical testing.

- **Microscopic testing** of the urine is done to examine formed elements in the urine, such as cells, casts, crystals, and amorphous deposits. To do a microscopic examination, the urine is centrifuged

TABLE 20–1 Characteristics of Urine

Characteristic	Normal	Abnormal
Volume or amount	1,000–2,000 mL daily	Polyuria—increased amount, more than 2,000 mL in 24 hours Oliguria—decreased amount, less than 500 mL in 24 hours Anuria—no formation
Color	Some shade of yellow; straw-yellow to amber	Pale or colorless—dilute Dark yellow, orange, or brown—concentrated Yellow or beer-brown—bilirubin or bile pigment, can precede jaundice and indicate hepatitis Cloudy-red—caused by presence of red blood cells (RBCs) (*hematuria*) Clear-red—hemoglobin, due to increased RBC destruction
Transparency	Clear	Cloudy because of pus, mucus, white blood cells (WBCs), and/or old specimen Milky because of fats or lipids
Odor	Faintly aromatic	Ammonia—old specimen Foul/putrid—bacteria or infection Fruity or sweet—acetone or ketones, diabetes mellitus
pH reaction	Range 5.0–8.0, average 6 (mildly acidic)	Alkaline—infection, chronic renal failure, or old specimen High acidity—diarrhea, starvation, and ketones (diabetes mellitus)
Specific gravity	1.005–1.030	Increased—diabetes mellitus, concentrated urine, low fluid intake, dehydration Decreased—renal disease, diluted urine, high fluid intake, diuretic medications (water pills)
Glucose	None	Presence, *glycosuria*, may mean diabetes mellitus
Albumin, protein	None to trace	Presence, *proteinuria* or *albuminuria*, can indicate kidney disease
Acetones-ketones	None	Presence, *ketonuria*, can indicate starvation, diabetes mellitus, or a high-fat diet
Blood	None	Presence, *hematuria*, indicates kidney, ureter, or bladder disease or infection
Pus	None	Presence, *pyuria*, indicates infection in urinary system
Bacteria	None in catheter specimen Small amount in routine specimen is normal	Large amount may indicate infection
Red blood cells (Erythrocytes)	None to less than 2–3/hpf (high-power field)	Presence may indicate disease of kidneys, bleeding in the urinary tract
White blood cells (Leukocytes)	Few normal; less than 4–5/hpf	Large number indicates infection
Bilirubin	None	Presence, *bilirubinuria*, can indicate liver disease, hepatitis, or bile duct obstruction
Urobilinogen	0.1–1.0 mg/dL (milligrams per deciliter)	Presence can indicate liver disease, destruction of red blood cells (RBCs) (hemolytic diseases)

to spin out the solid particles and form urinary sediment. This procedure is described in detail in Section 20:13. The sediment is then examined under a microscope and checked for the presence of blood cells, bacteria, casts (formed in the kidney tubules and expelled during kidney damage), and other elements.

A variety of specimen containers are available for collecting urine. Most containers are clear, calibrated in milliliters (mL), and disposable. The container should have a secure lid to prevent spillage (**Figure 20–36**). Most routine urine specimens can be collected in a nonsterile container. Sterile containers are required if the urine is being cultured or tested for the presence of organisms such as bacteria. All specimen containers must be labeled with the patient's name, date, time of collection, and test ordered. Some facilities also require a patient identification number and the doctor's name on the label. Different methods of collecting urine are discussed in detail in Section 22:10.

For the most accurate results, a urinalysis should be performed on fresh, warm urine. If possible, a urine specimen should be examined within 1 hour after it is collected. If this is not possible, the specimen can be refrigerated. After refrigeration, it should be returned to room temperature before being examined.

Precaution

Urine is a body fluid, so standard precautions (Section 15:4) must be observed while collecting and handling urine. Hands must be washed frequently, and gloves must be worn at all times. If splashing of the urine is possible, a mask or face shield, protective eyewear, and protective clothing must be worn. Urine should be discarded in a toilet but is sometimes poured down a sink. If this is done, the sink must be flushed with water and wiped with a disinfectant. Any areas contaminated by the urine must be wiped with a disinfectant. The specimen containers and other contaminated disposable supplies must be discarded in the infectious-waste bag prior to being discarded as infectious waste according to legal requirements.

checkpoint

1. Identify six (6) characteristics of urine that a urinalysis can detect?

2. What color is normal urine?

PRACTICE: Go to the workbook and complete the assignment sheet for 20:10, Testing Urine.

20:11 USING REAGENT STRIPS TO TEST URINE

Science

A urine reagent strip (dipstick) test is frequently used as a screening test for urine. Many different types of reagent strips are available, and all work according to the same basic principles. Read the label of the reagent strip container for directions.

Excess amounts of many substances in the blood are eliminated from the body by the kidneys as part of urine. By testing the urine for the presence of these substances, certain diseases in the body can be detected. The most common method of testing for the presence or absence of these substances is the use of the urine reagent strip, or dipstick.

Urine **reagent strips** are firm, plastic strips. Small pads containing chemical reactants are attached to the strip. Each pad reacts to a specific substance. If the substance is present in the urine, it reacts with the chemical reactant on the strip and produces a color change. In addition to showing the presence of the substance, most of the chemical reactants will also measure the amount of the substance present by producing different color changes according to the amount of substance present.

Safety

Most urine reagent strips are sensitive to light, heat, and moisture. They must be stored in a dry, cool, dark area. The bottle containing the strips is usually made of dark or light-resistant glass. A moisture-absorbent pad or pack is usually present in the bottle. The bottle must be closed immediately after use. Care must be taken not to touch or handle any of the chemical-reactant pads on the strip.

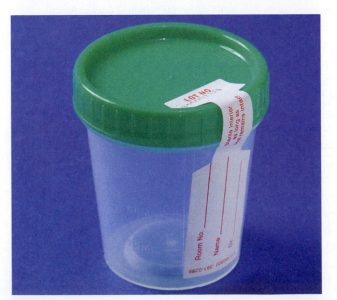

FIGURE 20–36 Urine specimen containers should have a secure lid to prevent spillage.

Chemicals and moisture on the skin can lead to an inaccurate test. In addition, many of the chemicals on the strip are poisonous and can burn or injure the skin. Many patients use reagent strips in their homes for specific urine tests, so it is important to make sure that the patient understands the importance of correct storage and handling of reagent strips. The patient should be cautioned against storing the strips in a bathroom, on windowsills, or close to sources of heat. The strips must also be stored out of the reach of children.

Chemical reactants on the pads of the strips are effective only for a certain period of time. An expiration date is printed on every bottle of strips. Reagent strips should never be used after the expiration date because inaccurate test results will occur. In an agency where many bottles of strips are kept in stock, it is important to rotate the strips so that the bottle with the closest expiration date is used first.

Reagent strips can be used to test for a variety of substances present in the urine. Some of the more common ones include the following:

- **pH** is a measure of the acidity or alkalinity of urine. pH is measured on a scale of 1–14. A neutral pH is 7. A pH below 7 indicates acidic urine, and a pH above 7 indicates alkaline urine. Urine is usually slightly acidic, with a pH range of 5.0–8.0. Diet, medications, kidney disease, starvation, and diabetes can each change pH.

- **Protein** should be retained in the blood, and it is not normally found in the urine. Its presence, *proteinuria*, usually in the form of albumin, *albuminuria*, may indicate kidney disease.

- **Glucose** is usually metabolized to produce energy and is not normally found in the urine. If the level of glucose in the blood is high, glucose will be eliminated in the urine, a condition called *glycosuria*. The presence of glucose can indicate diabetes mellitus.

- **Ketones** and **acetones** are the end products of the metabolism of fat in the body. They are not normally found in the urine. Their presence, *ketonuria*, can indicate diabetes mellitus, starvation, fasting, dieting, a high-fat diet, and metabolic disorders.

- **Blood** is not normally found in the urine. A test sometimes shows positive for blood when the patient is menstruating. If blood is detected in the urine, a microscopic examination of the urine should be performed. Blood in the urine is called **hematuria**. Its presence can indicate injury, infection, or disease in the kidneys and/or urinary tract.

- **Bilirubin** is not usually present in the urine. It is a breakdown product of the hemoglobin on red blood cells (RBCs) and is usually eliminated through the intestines. Its presence, *bilirubinuria*, in the urine can indicate liver disease, such as hepatitis or bile duct obstruction.

- **Urobilinogen** is bilirubin that has been converted by intestinal bacteria. It is usually excreted by the intestines. Small amounts of 0.1–1.0 milligrams per deciliter (mg/dL) of urine are normal. The presence of larger amounts usually indicates heart, spleen, liver, or hemolytic (destruction of blood cells) disease.

- **Phenylalanine** is an amino acid (protein) that is excreted in the urine when it is not metabolized by the body. Its presence indicates *phenylketonuria* (PKU), a congenital disease that causes intellectual disabilities if not detected early. For this reason, most states require a PKU blood and/or urine test for all newborns.

Many different types of reagent strips are available. Some of the more common types and the substances they test for include:

- Albustix: protein
- Bili-Labstix: pH, protein, glucose, ketone, bilirubin, and blood
- Clinistix: glucose
- Combistix: pH, glucose, and protein
- Diastix: glucose
- Hemastix: blood
- Keto-Diastix: glucose and ketone
- Ketostix: ketone
- Labstix: pH, specific gravity, glucose, protein, ketone, and blood
- Multistix: pH, specific gravity, glucose, protein, ketone, blood, bilirubin, urobilinogen, nitrite, and leukocytes
- Phenistix: phenylalanine or phenylketonuria (PKU)
- Uristix: protein, glucose, nitrites, and leukocytes

Comm

It is important to read the instructions carefully when using any type of reagent strip. A color comparison chart is usually located on the bottle of reagent strips or on a paper enclosed in the box. This chart lists the substances to be tested and the correct time interval for reading each reaction. The exact time for reading each chemical reaction must be followed for the most accurate results. Adequate lighting is essential to correctly match colors.

Most laboratories and offices perform quality-control checks on reagent strips to make sure the strips produce accurate results. A urine control solution, with predetermined results, is tested with a reagent strip. If the results do not meet the predetermined range, the strips must not be used. Quality-control checks should be run at least once a day, whenever a new container of strips is opened, and any time test results seem questionable.

Automated strip readers or analyzers are available (**Figure 20–37**). The strip readers, or spectrophotometers, analyze the color change and intensity for each reagent on the strip. The results are displayed on a lighted screen and/or printed. The automated strip readers are more accurate than the human eye, but they are more expensive.

Fresh urine specimens should be used to obtain the greatest degree of accuracy with a reagent strip. Urine should be tested within 1 hour of collection. If this is not possible, the urine specimen should be refrigerated. However, refrigerated specimens should be allowed to return to room temperature prior to being tested. Results are most accurate if testing can be done immediately after collecting the specimen, while the specimen is still warm.

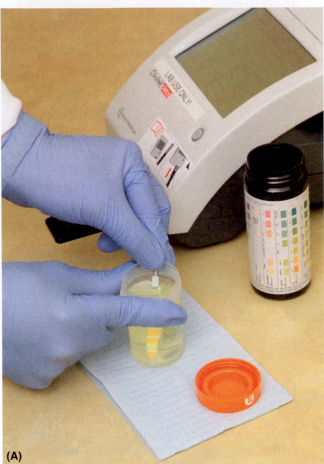
(A)

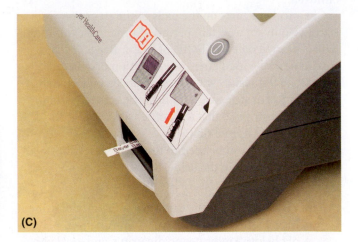
(C)

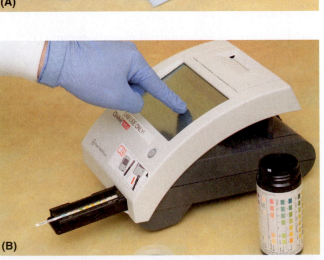
(B)

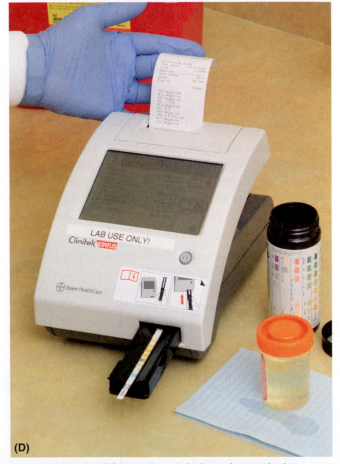
(D)

FIGURE 20–37 Steps for using an automated urine analyzer: (A) dip the reagent strip in the urine; (B) insert the strip in the analyzer and select desired urine tests; (C) allow the machine to pull in the strip and analyze it; and (D) obtain the printed results of the urine analysis.

Comm
When results of the test are recorded, the type of test used must be specified, for example, Labstix or Multistix. All substances tested must be listed along with the results for each. The date and time of the test should also be noted. Put your name or initials near the recording. A sample charting is as follows:

1/30/—9:00 a.m. Miss Smith
Labstix Test: pH: 6
                     Specific gravity: 1.022
                     Protein: neg.
                     Glucose: 1%
                     Ketone: mod.
                     Blood: neg.

checkpoint

1. What are urine reagent strips?

PRACTICE: Go to the workbook and complete the assignment sheet for 20:11, Using Reagent Strips to Test Urine. Then return and continue with the procedure.

Procedure 20:11

Using Reagent Strips to Test Urine

Equipment and Supplies

Fresh, early-morning urine specimen, if possible; urine-specimen container; reagent strips and color comparison chart; disposable gloves; mask or face shield; protective eyewear; gown; infectious-waste bag; paper; pen and/or computer, watch with second hand or timer

Procedure

1. Assemble equipment. Read instructions for the reagent strip.

2. Wash hands. Put on gloves.

    Precaution **CAUTION:** Observe standard precautions while obtaining and testing urine. If splashing of urine is possible, put on a gown, mask or face shield, and protective eyewear.

3. Introduce yourself. Identify the patient. Explain the procedure. Obtain the patient's consent.

4. Obtain a fresh urine specimen in a urine-specimen container.

   NOTE: An early-morning, first-voided specimen is the most concentrated and, therefore, is preferred.

5. Gently rotate the container between your hands to mix the urine specimen.

6. Hold a reagent strip by the clear end (**Figure 20–38A**). Immerse the strip in the urine specimen, making sure all reagent areas are submersed.

7. Remove the strip immediately. Tap the edge of the strip lightly on a paper towel or against the side of the specimen container to remove excess urine (**Figure 20–38B**).

   NOTE: This will prevent urine from dropping on the color comparison chart during color matching.

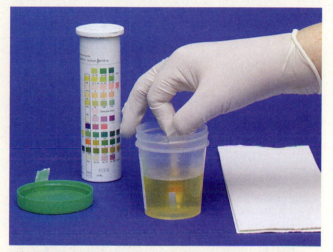

FIGURE 20–38A Hold the reagent strip by the clear end to immerse the strip in the urine specimen.

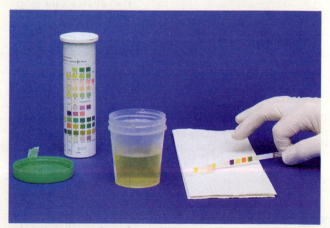

FIGURE 20–38B Tap the edge of the strip lightly on a paper towel or against the side of the specimen container to remove excess urine.

8. Turn the strip so that the reagent areas are facing you. Hold the strip horizontally near the color comparison charts on the bottle (**Figure 20–38C**).

(continues)

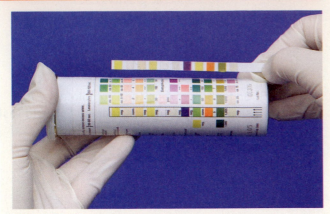

FIGURE 20–38C Under good lighting, compare the strip to the color charts to determine correct readings.

9. Note the time. A watch or clock with a second hand is essential because many readings are done in a period of seconds.

10. Start at the center of the strip. Read any reagent areas that require immediate readings. Record these readings.

11. Watch the time and read additional reagent areas at the correct time intervals. Some are read at 10 seconds, 15 seconds, 30 seconds, or 60 seconds. Record all readings.

    NOTE: The time lapses between readings are usually sufficient to allow you to read readily down the strip.

12. Recheck all readings. Using a second reagent strip to check the accuracy of results is sometimes required.

13. Discard the strip and any contaminated disposable supplies in the infectious-waste bag. Pour the urine into a toilet or down a sink. If a sink is used, flush the sink with water and wipe with a disinfectant. Use a disinfectant to wipe the counter and any contaminated areas. Clean and replace all equipment.

14. Remove gloves and discard in an infectious-waste bag. Wash hands.

15. Record all required information on the patient's chart or enter it into the computer. For example: date, time, Labstix: pH: 6, Specific gravity: 1.022, Protein: neg., Glucose: 1%, Ketones: Tr., Blood: Neg, and your signature and title. Report any abnormal readings to your supervisor immediately.

    NOTE: In health care agencies using electronic health records (EHRs), the information is entered directly into the patient's EHR on a computer.

PRACTICE: Go to the workbook and use the evaluation sheet for 20:11, Using Reagent Strips to Test Urine, to practice this procedure. When you believe you have mastered this skill, sign the sheet and give it to your instructor for further action.

 FINAL EVALUATION: Using the criteria listed on the evaluation sheet, your instructor will grade your performance.

20:12 MEASURING SPECIFIC GRAVITY

 Specific gravity is defined as the weight of a substance compared to the weight of distilled water, in equal volumes. Specific gravity of urine, then, is the weight of urine compared to the weight of an equal amount of distilled water. The weight of distilled water is 1.000. Its specific gravity is expressed as: *SpGr 1.000.* Specific gravity of urine, therefore, is a measurement of the concentration of urine.

The normal range for specific gravity of urine is 1.005–1.030 with most specimens ranging between 1.010 and 1.025. Variations occur as follows:

- **Low specific gravity**, below 1.005, is usually caused by diluted urine possibly resulting from excessive fluid intake, kidney disease in which the kidneys cannot concentrate urine, diuretic medications, or diabetes insipidus.

- **High specific gravity**, above 1.030, is usually caused by concentrated urine possibly resulting from low fluid intake, dehydration, excessive fluid loss through other body parts, kidney disease in which too many substances are excreted, and/or diabetes mellitus in which sugar is present in the urine.

One way to determine specific gravity is to measure it with a **urinometer**. Urine is poured into a urinometer jar or cylinder. The urinometer, which is a float with a calibrated stem, is placed in the urine with a spinning motion. The urine collects at a line at a curved angle on the urinometer float. This line is known as the *meniscus*. The reading for specific gravity is taken at the lower part of the meniscus. It must be read at eye level to be accurate. Each calibration on the urinometer float is in thousandths. The top line represents 1.000, the specific gravity of distilled water, and each small line below it represents 0.001. The calibrations read 1.000, 1.001, 1.002, 1.003, 1.004, and so forth. It is important that the urinometer be free floating and away from the sides and bottom of the jar or cylinder when the reading for specific gravity is taken.

Another way to determine specific gravity is with a **refractometer** (**Figure 20–39A**). One drop of well-mixed urine is placed on the refractometer. Specific gravity is read by looking through an ocular, or eyepiece. The degree of concentration of the urine forms a line on the refractometer scale (**Figure 20–39B**). It is important to follow the manufacturer's instructions and to calibrate the refractometer with distilled water when it is used.

Digital refractometers are also available. An eye dropper is used to place drops of urine on the prism at the center of the stainless-steel stage (**Figure 20–40**). The refractometer then reads the specific gravity and displays the value on the screen. This eliminates the chance of human error in reading the scale.

All refractometers must be tested for accuracy before use. Most manufacturers provide test strips or test solutions

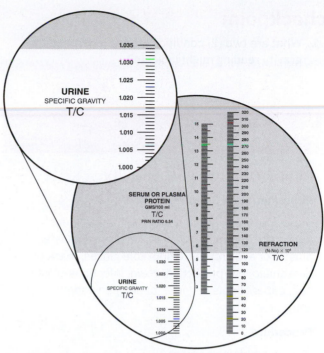

FIGURE 20–39B The urine forms a line on the refractometer scale. This specimen shows a specific gravity of 1.034.

that show a preset reading. Distilled water can also be used to check the refractometer because it should show a specific gravity of 1.000. The manufacturer's instructions will also provide information on how to calibrate the refractometer if the test reading is not accurate.

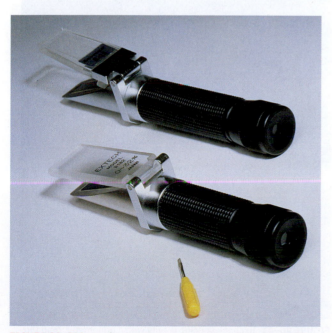

FIGURE 20–39A A refractometer can be used to calculate specific gravity of urine.

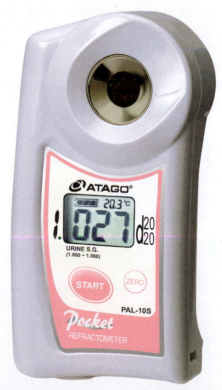

FIGURE 20–40 A digital refractometer automatically reads specific gravity when drops of urine are placed on the prism. Courtesy, Atago USA, Inc.

checkpoint

1. What are two (2) conditions that a low specific gravity reading might indicate?

PRACTICE: Go to the workbook and complete the assignment sheet for 20:12, Measuring Specific Gravity. Then return and continue with the procedure.

Procedure 20:12

Measuring Specific Gravity

Equipment and Supplies

Urine specimen in a container, urinometer float, urinometer jar or cylinder, refractometer, transfer pipette or eye dropper, disposable gloves, mask or face shield, eye protection, gown, infectious-waste bag, paper towels or gauze, paper, pen and/or computer

Procedure

1. Assemble equipment.

2. Prepare the equipment:

    a. Urinometer: Clean the urinometer float and cylinder or jar thoroughly and make sure they are dry.

    b. Refractometer: Place one drop of distilled water on the glass plate and close the lid gently. Look through the eyepiece and read the specific gravity to make sure it is 1.000. If it is not, the refractometer must be calibrated according to the manufacturer's instructions. Use lens paper to dry and clean the glass plate.

    NOTE: Dirty equipment will interfere with the reading.

3. Wash hands. Put on gloves.

    Precaution

    CAUTION: Observe standard precautions while obtaining and testing urine. If splashing of urine is possible, put on a gown, mask or face shield, and protective eyewear.

4. **Comm**

    Introduce yourself. Identify the patient. Explain the procedure. Obtain the patient's consent.

5. Obtain a fresh urine specimen. Do *not* refrigerate the specimen because this can alter the test results. It is best to perform the test as soon as possible after obtaining the urine. The most accurate results are obtained when the urine is at room temperature.

    NOTE: An early-morning, first-voided specimen is the most concentrated and is, therefore, preferred.

6. To check specific gravity using a urinometer, proceed as follows:

    a. Fill the urinometer jar or cylinder with urine to within 1 inch from the top.

    NOTE: Make sure the urine is mixed well.

    b. Using paper or a piece of gauze, remove any bubbles from the top of the urine.

    c. Grasp the urinometer stem at the top and slowly insert it into the jar or cylinder containing the urine. Avoid wetting the top of the stem. As you insert the urinometer float, twirl it slightly so that it does not stick to the sides.

    NOTE: A spinning float will not stick to the sides of the urinometer jar or cylinder.

    d. Make sure the float is away from the sides of the jar and that it is *not* touching the bottom of the jar or cylinder. The urinometer must be free floating.

    e. When the urinometer float stops spinning, take the reading at eye level at the lower line of the meniscus (**Figure 20–41**).

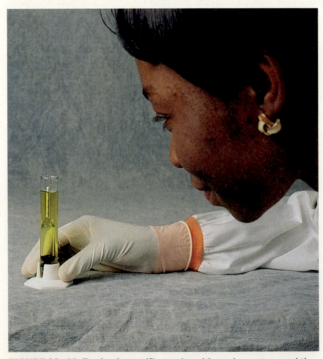

FIGURE 20–41 To check specific gravity with a urinometer, read the specific gravity of urine at eye level at the lower line of the meniscus.

NOTE: Do *not* read above the meniscus. This is inaccurate.

NOTE: Normal specific gravity is 1.005–1.030.

CHECKPOINT: Your instructor will check the accuracy of your reading.

7. To check specific gravity using a refractometer, proceed as follows:

   a. Use a transfer pipette or eye dropper to place one drop of well-mixed urine on the glass plate of the refractometer (**Figure 20–42A**).

   b. Close the lid gently.

   c. Look through the eyepiece and read the specific gravity on the scale (**Figure 20–42B**).

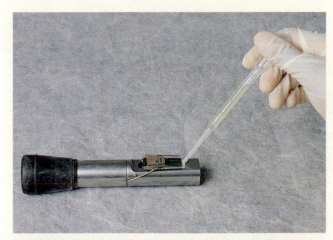

FIGURE 20–42A Place one drop of well-mixed urine on the glass plate of the refractometer.

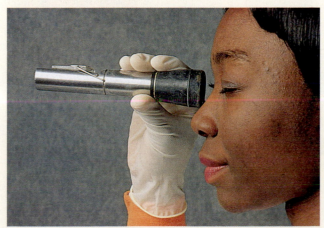

FIGURE 20–42B Look through the eyepiece to read the specific gravity on the refractometer scale.

CHECKPOINT: Your instructor will check the accuracy of your reading.

8. Record the reading.

9. Recheck the reading, if necessary.

10. Clean and replace all equipment:

    a. Urinometer: Pour the urine into a toilet or sink. If a sink is used, flush the sink with water and wipe with a disinfectant. Wash the urinometer and jar or cylinder thoroughly, rinse or soak with a disinfectant, and dry both pieces completely.

    b. Refractometer: Follow manufacturer's instructions. Most manufacturers recommend using lens paper on the glass to prevent scratches. A disinfectant can be put on the lens paper to clean the glass, and another sheet of lens paper can be used to dry the glass.

    c. Put all contaminated disposable supplies in the infectious-waste bag.

    d. Use a disinfectant to wipe the counter and any contaminated areas.

11. Remove gloves and discard in an infectious-waste bag. Wash hands thoroughly.

12. Record all required information on the patient's chart or enter it into the computer. For example: date, time, SpGr: 1.011, and your signature and title. Report any abnormal readings to your supervisor immediately.

NOTE: In laboratories or offices using electronic health records (EHRs), the information is entered into the patient's EHR on a computer.

PRACTICE: Go to the workbook and use the evaluation sheet for 20:12, Measuring Specific Gravity, to practice this procedure. When you believe you have mastered this skill, sign the sheet and give it to your instructor for further action.

FINAL EVALUATION: Using the criteria listed on the evaluation sheet, your instructor will grade your performance.

20:13 PREPARING URINE FOR MICROSCOPIC EXAMINATION

Science

Microscopic testing of urine is done to examine all the solid materials suspended in the urine. These materials are called **urinary sediment**. Presence of certain substances, such as blood cells, casts, and bacteria, can indicate disease conditions of the kidneys, urinary tract, and/or blood.

A fresh, early-morning, first-voided specimen is preferred. This type of specimen is usually the most concentrated; thus, it is more likely to contain abnormal substances. The specimen should be examined immediately, if at all possible. Certain elements, such as red cells and casts, disintegrate rapidly in warm specimens. If the urine cannot be examined immediately, it should be kept cold to preserve these substances.

Only a portion of the urine specimen is actually examined under a microscope. The entire specimen is first mixed well. A small amount, usually 10–15 milliliters (mL), is then placed in a centrifuge tube. This tube is then put into a centrifuge. The centrifuge spins the urine, causing any solid materials to settle to the bottom of the tube. These solid materials are called *sediment*. The clear urine on the top of the tube is poured off, leaving approximately 1 milliliter (mL) of sediment in the bottom of the tube. This procedure results in concentrated urine, which is then examined under a microscope.

Some health care facilities add a dye stain to the urine to color various elements and make it easier to identify them. Usually one to two drops of a urine stain are added to the sediment before placing the sample on the slide.

The size of the drop of concentrated urine examined is important. The drop of sediment placed on a slide for viewing will be covered with a coverslip. The drop should be large enough so that there is no empty space under the coverslip but not so large as to cause the coverslip to float.

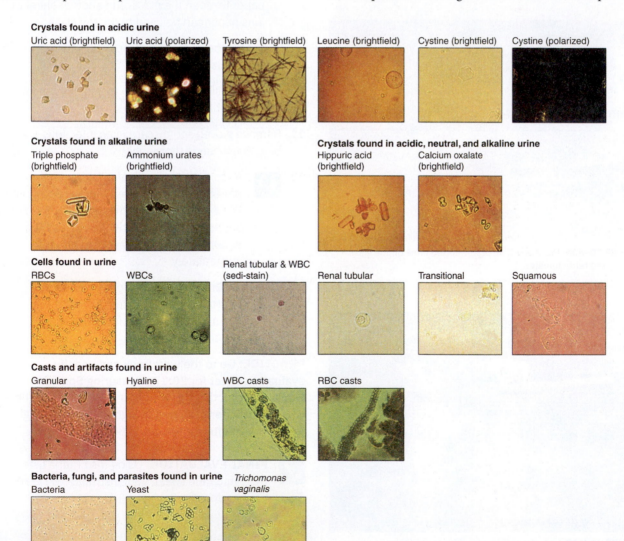

FIGURE 20–43 Some elements that may be found in urinary sediment.

The urinary sediment should be examined immediately after it is placed on the slide. Drying of the specimen occurs quickly, and this can result in distortions in the shapes and sizes of any substances present.

Learning to identify various substances detected during a microscopic examination of the urine requires training and experience. Some of the substances that may be seen in urinary sediment are shown in **Figure 20–43**. Elements, such as epithelial cells and certain casts, can be seen with the low-power objective. Other elements, such as blood cells, bacteria, and crystals, can be seen only with the high-power objective. When recording the elements seen, it is important to note the objective used. This is usually recorded as *per low-power field* (lpf) or *per high-power field* (hpf). For example, a recording might state, *epithelial cells: mod/lpf*.

Legal Microscopic examination of urinary sediment is not a CLIA-waived test. It is classified as a moderately complex test. Only legally qualified individuals can perform the actual examination of the sediment. However, centrifuging the specimen and preparing the slide is within the realm of duties for laboratory or medical assistants in most states. *It is the responsibility of the health care provider to know and follow state regulations.* In many settings, the laboratory assistant prepares the urine for microscopic examination and a specially trained individual examines the sediment and identifies the elements present. Follow your agency's policy regarding this procedure.

checkpoint

1. What time of day is the preferred time to obtain a urine specimen?

PRACTICE: Go to the workbook and complete the assignment sheet for 20:13, Preparing Urine for Microscopic Examination. Then return and continue with the procedure.

Procedure 20:13

Preparing Urine for Microscopic Examination

Equipment and Supplies

Urine specimen in a container, centrifuge, small measuring cup, centrifuge tube, microscopic slide, coverslip, transfer pipette, urinary-sediment chart, disposable gloves, mask or face shield, protective eyewear, gown, infectious-waste bag, paper, pen and/or computer

Procedure

1. Assemble equipment.

2. Wash hands. Put on gloves.

   Precaution **CAUTION:** Observe standard precautions while obtaining and testing urine. If splashing of urine is possible, put on a gown, mask or face shield, and protective eyewear.

3. Introduce yourself. Identify the patient. Explain the procedure. Obtain the patient's consent.
   Comm

4. Obtain a fresh, early-morning, first-voided specimen. This type of specimen is preferred because it is the most concentrated and yields the most accurate results.

5. Mix the urine well to suspend any sediment that has settled to the bottom.

6. Pour 10–15 milliliters (mL) of urine into a small measuring cup.

7. Pour the measured urine into a clean centrifuge tube.

   NOTE: Residue or dirt in the tube can cause inaccurate results.

8. Place the centrifuge tube in the centrifuge (**Figure 20–44A**). Make sure there is another tube containing an equal amount of urine or water opposite this centrifuge tube; the second tube acts to counterbalance the weight of the first.

9. Centrifuge the urine for 4–5 minutes at approximately 1,500 revolutions per minute.

10. Carefully pour off 9–14 mL of the clear urine. Leave 1 mL of urine and the sediment in the bottom of the tube (**Figure 20–44B**).

11. Gently shake the tube to resuspend the sediment in the bottom of the remaining 1 mL of urine.

    NOTE: If a urine stain is used to color the elements, add one to two drops of the stain to the sediment. Gently shake the tube to mix the sediment and stain.

12. Using care, transfer one drop of the well-mixed sediment to a clean glass slide (**Figure 20–44C**).

    NOTE: The size of the drop is important. If it is too large, it will cause the coverslip to float. If it is too small, it will not fill the area under the coverslip.

13. Hold the coverslip at an angle to the drop of urine. Carefully drop the slip into place (**Figure 20–44D**). Make sure that *no* air bubbles are present.

    NOTE: Air bubbles will interfere with the examination. If any air bubbles are present, discard the drop on the slide and use another drop of the urine.

(continues)

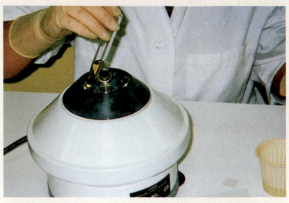

FIGURE 20–44A After pouring 10–15 milliliters (mL) of urine into the centrifuge tube, place the tube in the centrifuge.

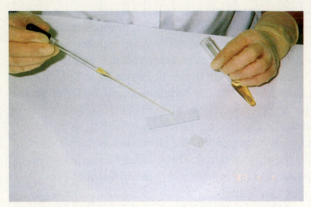

FIGURE 20–44C Transfer one drop of well-mixed sediment to a clean glass slide.

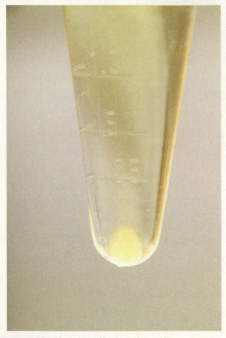

FIGURE 20–44B After centrifuging, the sediment accumulates at the bottom of the centrifuge tube.

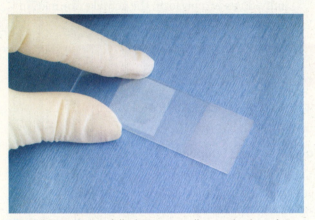

FIGURE 20–44D Carefully drop a cover slip over the drop of urinary sediment on the slide.

14. Place the slide on the microscope stage. Hold it in place with slide clips.

 CAUTION: Hold the slide level at all times to prevent the urine from running off the slide.

15. Inform the physician or laboratory technologist that the slide is ready to be examined. Examination of the sediment is *not* a CLIA-waived test. The following steps for examining the sediment are included only for practice examination.

    a. Use the low-power (10×) objective and the coarse adjustment to bring the slide into focus.

 CAUTION: Watch the stage while using the coarse adjustment to move the objective down toward the slide.

    b. Adjust the lighting to allow the best viewing of the slide. A dimmer light usually provides a clearer view under low power.

    c. Use a chart on urinary sediment or refer to Figure 20–43 to identify some of the substances present in the urinary sediment.

    NOTE: The examination should be completed within 3 minutes. Drying occurs after this time and can lead to inaccurate identification.

    d. Switch to the high-power objective and examine the specimen again. Note which substances are best viewed under high power according to the chart.

16. When the slide has been examined by a legally qualified individual, clean and replace all equipment. Pour the urine into a toilet or down a sink. If a sink is used, flush the sink with water and

wipe with a disinfectant. Place all contaminated disposable supplies in the infectious-waste bag. Use a disinfectant to wipe the counter and any contaminated areas. Cover the microscope.

17. Remove gloves and discard in an infectious-waste bag. Wash hands thoroughly.

18. Check that all required information has been recorded on the patient's chart or enter it into the computer. For example: date, time, Microscopic Exam: epithelial: few/lpf, WBCs: 4–6/hpf, RBCs: few/hpf, casts: neg, crystals: few/hpf, and your signature and title.

 NOTE: In laboratories or offices using electronic health records (EHRs), the information is entered into the patient's EHR on a computer.

PRACTICE: Go to the workbook and use the evaluation sheet for 20:13, Preparing Urine for Microscopic Examination, to practice this procedure. When you believe you have mastered this skill, sign the sheet and give it to your instructor for further action.

✅ **FINAL EVALUATION:** Using the criteria listed on the evaluation sheet, your instructor will grade your performance.

Today's Research   Tomorrow's Health Care

No More Blood and Urine Tests? Just Use Tears, Sweat, and Saliva!

Tests on blood and urine are used to diagnose many different diseases and to check the health status of the body. However, obtaining blood can be painful, and collecting urine can be messy. In addition, when urine is required for drug testing, the close supervision required to ensure that the sample is from the patient can invade the patient's privacy. Now, thanks to biotechnology, it may be possible to use tears, sweat, and saliva to perform diagnostic tests.

An estimated 402 million diabetics worldwide need to monitor blood-sugar levels several times a day by puncturing their fingers with a lancet to obtain blood. In initial research, engineers used a small biochip containing thousands of light-measuring devices to measure the amount of glucose in water. Researchers found this is similar to levels found in saliva. Other researchers found they could measure glucose levels in the tears of rats with a similar biosensor. If diabetics could use tears or saliva to measure glucose, it would allow them to avoid the discomfort associated with repeated finger punctures. However, one problem found by researchers was the fact that they could not always correlate blood glucose levels with glucose levels in saliva and tears.

Latest research has developed biosensors that can be applied to the skin. These sensors measure glucose levels in interstitial fluid (fluid surrounding cells). A small transmitter attaches to the sensor. When a recorder is held over the sensor, the glucose reading is displayed on a screen. FDA has currently approved some of these devices, and more are being evaluated in trial studies. By using these devices, diabetics can avoid frequent finger punctures to obtain blood. In addition, they can check glucose levels easily and frequently. Another device currently being evaluated that is also applied to the skin contains minuscule holes at its base to collect sweat. The sweat is transferred to tiny reservoirs in the device, and each reservoir contains a sensor that reacts with a specific chemical in the sweat, such as glucose for diabetics, lactate for people with cystic fibrosis, and even oxygen levels for people with respiratory diseases. Similar research is being performed on the sweat on fingers. Fingerprints have been used to determine a person's identity for years. Now, researchers have developed a portable device called a Drug Screening Cartridge that can determine the presence of drugs, such as cocaine, opiates, and amphetamines, in a person's body by analyzing the sweat in fingerprints. Initial studies show more than 90 percent accuracy when compared with blood and urine samples. Results can be obtained in 10 minutes or less. This would eliminate the privacy concerns associated with urine tests and, at the same time, make it almost impossible to dispute the identity of the individual taking the drug test. In the future, the device could be used for drug screening, criminal forensic work, and measuring other health markers, such as the level of therapeutic medications.

Bioengineers are now building sensors that specifically measure a wide range of substances, from biological substances such as anthrax to different chemical compounds. It will be many years before many of the sensors are available for commercial use, but if they prove successful, the sensors will provide an easier way to perform many medical tests.

Madison, Jane, and Lee were very much reassured by Aiko's explanation of the drug screening procedure. What do you think she said to the girls?

What kind of body language and communication skills should she use?

CHAPTER 20 SUMMARY

- Laboratory assistant skills are utilized not only in medical laboratories but also in medical offices and nursing care facilities. The microscope is used in many laboratory tests, so the health care provider should be familiar with how to operate it.

- Obtaining culture specimens and preparing them for examination helps the health care professional determine the cause of a disease and, often, the proper way to treat the disease. Many of the specimens contain communicable pathogens (germs capable of spreading disease), so care must be taken while performing these procedures.

- Blood tests are performed for a variety of reasons. Some of the more common tests include blood typing, hemoglobin, hematocrit, erythrocyte sedimentation rate, blood smear or film, and blood glucose. Following proper techniques and striving for accuracy are essential because these tests are used to determine the presence or absence of disease. Urine tests are performed to check the function of various body organs. The presence of abnormal substances in the urine is frequently the first indication of disease.

- Standard precautions must be followed at all times while performing laboratory tests. Many diseases are transmitted by blood and body fluids, so extreme care must be taken while handling these substances.

REVIEW QUESTIONS

1. Differentiate between *sensitive* and *resistant* organisms.

2. List six (6) points that must be checked prior to performing a skin puncture to obtain blood.

3. Differentiate among an erythrocyte count, hematocrit, and hemoglobin.

4. State the normal values or ranges for each of the following tests:
   a. microhematocrit
   b. hemoglobin
   c. erythrocyte count
   d. leukocyte count
   e. erythrocyte sedimentation rate
   f. specific gravity of urine

5. List five (5) precautions that must be observed while storing and/or using urinary reagent strips.

6. Briefly list the components or tests performed during a physical, chemical, and microscopic examination of the urine.

7. List all of the standard precautions that must be observed while performing culture studies, blood tests, or urine tests.

For additional information about laboratory careers, contact the following associations:

- American Medical Technologists' Association
  www.americanmedtech.org

- American Society for Clinical Laboratory Science
  www.ascls.org

- Clinical Laboratory Management Association
  www.clma.org

- National Accrediting Agency for Clinical Laboratory Sciences
  www.naacls.org

- State Society for Medical Technology

- State Society for Medical Technologists

CRITICAL THINKING

1. Why is it important to evaluate the Rh status of a pregnant woman?

2. What is the purpose of a culture and sensitivity test?

ACTIVITIES

1. Create a dialogue between a laboratory assistant obtaining a capillary blood puncture in order to check blood glucose and a patient.

2. Using your pen and plate template, draw the pattern of streaking an agar plate.

   2a. Using a marker and an empty agar plate, draw the streaking pattern while manipulating the actual plate.

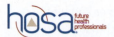 | CONNECTION

Competitive Event: Biomedical Laboratory Science

Event Summary: Biomedical Laboratory Science provides members with the opportunity to gain knowledge and skills required for a medical laboratory setting. This competitive event consists of 2 rounds. Round One is a written, multiple choice test and the top scoring competitors will advance to Round Two for the skills assessment. This event aims to inspire members to learn more about biotechnology careers.

Details on this competitive event may be found at

www.hosa.org/guidelines

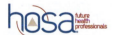 | CONNECTION

Biochemistry

Summary: The goal of the Academic Testing Center is to provide as many International Leadership Conference HOSA delegates as space permits with the opportunity to demonstrate their basic knowledge in preparation to become future health professionals.

The series of events in the Academic Testing Center are written tests based on items from the identified text specific to each event. Competitors will recognize, identify, define, interpret, and apply knowledge in a 50-item multiple choice test with a tie-breaker question. The written test will measure knowledge and understanding at the recall, application, and analysis levels. Higher-order thinking skills will be incorporated.

Details on this event may be found at

www.hosa.org/guidelines

Case Study Investigation

Max and Molly are medical assistants at the hectic Hill Country Medical Clinic. The six doctors conduct many examinations, immunizations, procedures, and medication refills. Both Molly and Max like to be busy and assist with a variety of patient needs. Molly has been at the clinic for 15 years and Max just graduated from medical assisting training last year. Molly is glad to work as a team with Max to deliver excellent care for Hill Country patients. At the end of the chapter, you will be asked what kind of skills Max and Molly will need to know in order to assist the doctors in providing competent and caring support for Hill Country Medical Clinic patients.

■ LEARNING OBJECTIVES

After completing this chapter, you should be able to:

- Measure and record height and weight.
- Position and properly drape a patient in horizontal recumbent, prone, Sims', knee–chest, Fowler's, lithotomy, dorsal recumbent, Trendelenburg, and jackknife positions.
- Use a Snellen chart to screen for vision problems.
- Prepare for and assist with an eye, ear, nose, and throat examination.
- Prepare for and assist with a gynecological examination.
- Prepare for and assist with a general physical examination.
- Set up a minor surgery tray without contaminating equipment or supplies.
- Set up a suture removal tray without contaminating equipment or supplies.
- Record and mount an electrocardiogram.
- Use the *Physicians' Desk Reference* (PDR) website to find basic information about various drugs.
- Identify methods of administering medications and safety rules that must be observed.
- Define, pronounce, and spell all key terms.

■ KEY TERMS

auscultation *(oss"-kull-tay'-shun)*

Ayer blade *(a'-ur)(A as in "say")*

bandage scissors

cervical spatula

dorsal recumbent

electrocardiogram (ECG) *(ee-leck"-trow-car'-dee-oh-gram)*

Fowler's

hemostats *(hee'-mow"-stats)*

horizontal recumbent (supine)

hyperopia *(high"-puh-row'-pee-ah)*

jackknife (protologic)

knee–chest

laryngeal mirror *(lar"-ren-gee'-ul)*

leads

left lateral

lithotomy *(lith"-ought'-eh-me)*

medication

myopia *(my"-oh'-pee-ah)*

needle holder

observation

ophthalmoscope *(op-thayl'-mow-skope")*

otoscope *(oh'-toe-skope")*

palpation

Papanicolaou *(pah"-pan-ee'-cow-low)*

percussion

percussion (reflex) hammer

Physicians' Desk Reference (PDR)

Prone

Retractors

scalpels *(skal'-pelz)*

sigmoidoscope *(sig-moy'-doh-skope")*

Sims'

Snellen charts

speculum *(speck'-you-lum)*

sphygmomanometer *(sfig"-moh-ma-nam'-eh-ter)*

splinter forceps

stethoscope

supine *(sue-pine')*

surgical scissors

suture removal sets

sutures

tissue forceps

tongue blade/depressor

towel clamps

Trendelenburg *(Tren'-dell-en"-burg)*

tuning fork

visual acuity

Career

Medical assistants work under the supervision of physicians, and they are important members of the health care team. Educational requirements vary from state to state but can include on-the-job training (less frequent), 1- or 2-year health science education (HSE) programs, and/or an associate's degree. Certification (CMA) can be obtained from the American Association of Medical Assistants (AAMA), and registered credentials (RMA) can be obtained from the American Medical Technologists (AMT) Association, each of which has specific requirements. The duties of medical assistants vary depending on the size and type of practice, and on the legal requirements of the state in which they work. Duties are often classified as administrative or clinical. Administrative, or "front office," duties may include

tasks such as answering telephones, greeting patients, scheduling appointments, maintaining records, handling correspondence, and bookkeeping. These duties are usually performed by medical administrative assistants who can obtain certification. Clinical, or "back office," duties may include taking medical histories, recording vital signs, preparing patients for and assisting with examinations and treatments, and performing basic laboratory tests. Some medical assistants perform both administrative and clinical duties; others specialize in either administrative or clinical work. The procedures discussed in this chapter represent clinical duties. Administrative duties are discussed in Chapter 24 of this textbook. In addition to the knowledge and skills presented in this chapter, medical assistants must also learn and master skills such as:

- Presenting a professional appearance and attitude
- Obtaining knowledge regarding health care delivery systems, organizational structure, and teamwork
- Meeting all legal responsibilities
- Communicating effectively
- Being sensitive to and respecting cultural diversity
- Comprehending human anatomy, physiology, and pathophysiology

- Learning medical terminology
- Observing all safety precautions
- Practicing all principles of infection control
- Taking and recording vital signs
- Performing CLIA-waived laboratory tests
- Administering first aid and cardio-pulmonary resuscitation
- Promoting good nutrition and a healthy lifestyle to maintain health

- Using computer and technology skills
- Performing administrative duties such as answering the telephone, scheduling appointments, preparing correspondence, completing insurance forms, maintaining accounts, recording medical histories, and maintaining patient records
- Ordering and maintaining supplies and materials

21:1 MEASURING/ RECORDING HEIGHT AND WEIGHT

OBRA

Height and weight measurements are taken in many health care fields. Height and weight measurements are used to determine whether a patient is overweight or underweight. Either of these conditions can indicate disease. Height–weight charts can be used to determine averages, but in most cases body mass index (BMI) is calculated to determine if a patient is underweight or overweight. BMI is discussed in detail in Section 11:5. Height–weight measurements must be accurate. Always recheck your calculations.

Height–weight measurements are a part of the general physical examination in a physician's office. They are also usually done routinely when a patient is admitted to a hospital, long-term care facility, or other health care agency. In addition, the measurements provide necessary

information in performing and evaluating certain laboratory tests and in calculating dosages of certain medications.

The height, weight, head circumference, and, at times, chest circumference measurements of infants and toddlers is monitored frequently because growth is rapid. Usually infants are checked every two months to detect any changes that may indicate problems with growth and development. The measurements are usually recorded on a National Center for Health Statistics (NCHS) growth graph (**Figure 21–1**). The graphed information allows the physician to check the child's growth and compare it to the average percentiles of other children the same age. Abnormal growth patterns may indicate nutritional deficiencies or genetic diseases.

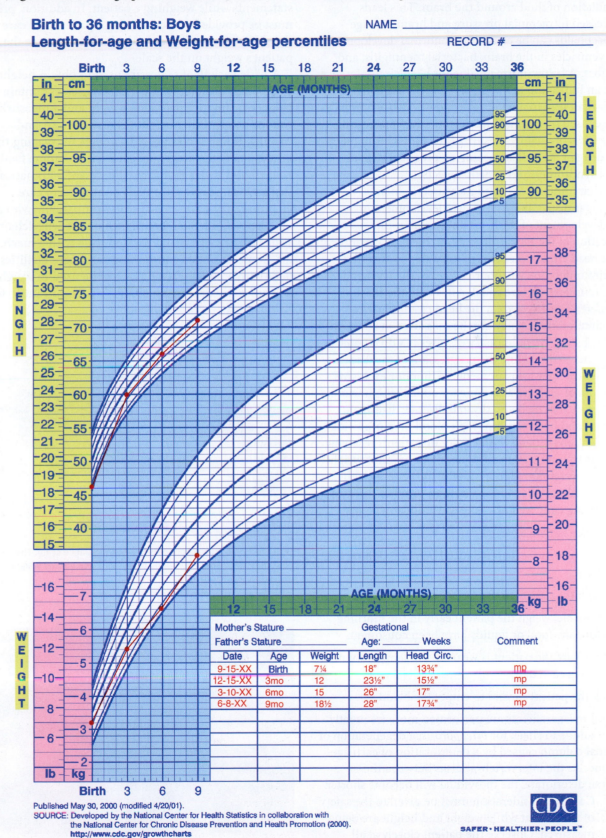

Birth to 36 months: Boys
Length-for-age and Weight-for-age percentiles

NAME _____

RECORD # _____

Date	Age	Weight	Length	Head Circ.	Comment
9-15-XX	Birth	7¼	18"	13¾"	mp
12-15-XX	3mo	12	23½"	15½"	mp
3-10-XX	6mo	15	26"	17"	mp
6-8-XX	9mo	18½	28"	17¾"	mp

Mother's Stature _____   Gestational
Father's Stature _____   Age: _____ Weeks

Published May 30, 2000 (modified 4/20/01).
SOURCE: Developed by the National Center for Health Statistics in collaboration with the National Center for Chronic Disease Prevention and Health Promotion (2000).
http://www.cdc.gov/growthcharts

CDC
SAFER · HEALTHIER · PEOPLE™

FIGURE 21-1 The National Center for Health Statistics (NCHS) growth graph is used to monitor the growth and development of infants and toddlers.

Source: Kuczmarski RJ, Ogden CL, Guo SS, et al. 2000 CDC growth charts for the United States: Methods and development. National Center for Health Statistics. Vital Health Stat 11(246), 2002.

The head circumference in infants can be an early indication of abnormal development of the brain. Any head circumference that measures above the 95th percentile usually indicates *hydrocephalus*, an accumulation of fluid around the brain. This leads to increased intracranial pressure and brain damage. Hydrocephalus can be caused by abnormal development of the ventricles in the brain, bacterial meningitis, and/or tumors. A below-normal value for head circumference can be an indication of *microencephaly*, or a small brain. This too can lead to mental retardation. Microencephaly can be caused by a congenital defect, infections during pregnancy, a premature closure of the fontanels in the brain, drug or alcohol abuse during pregnancy (fetal alcohol syndrome), and genetic defects.

Chest circumference is also measured in infants, especially if suspicion exists of overdevelopment or underdevelopment of the heart and/or lungs or a calcification of the rib cartilage. From birth to 1 year of age the head circumference is usually greater than the chest circumference. At about 1–2 years, the head and chest circumferences are equal. After that, the chest circumference is larger than the head circumference. Chest circumferences may also be measured in adults with chronic obstructive pulmonary diseases (COPDs) such as emphysema to determine the progression of the disease.

Frequent weight measurements to monitor excessive weight loss or gain are also done for adults with hormone disorders such as diabetes, thyroid disease, digestive disorders, and hypertension (high blood pressure) with fluid retention. Patients with cancer or patients receiving chemotherapy are weighed frequently to monitor weight loss. Daily weights are often ordered for patients with edema (swelling) due to heart, kidney, or other diseases. When taking daily weights, note the following points:

- Use the same scale each day.
- Make sure the scale is balanced before weighing the patient.
- Weigh the patient at the same time each day.
- If possible, weigh the patient early in the morning before any food or liquids have been consumed.
- Make sure the patient is wearing the same amount of clothing each day.
- Ask the patient to void to empty the bladder.

Height measurements are performed more frequently in older adults to check for *osteoporosis*, a degeneration of the spinal column caused by a deterioration of cartilage and bone. As the intervertebral disks between the vertebrae deteriorate, the individual will become shorter.

 Careful consideration must be given to the safety of the patient while weight and height are being measured. Observe the patient closely at all times. Prevent falls from the scale and possible injury from the protruding height lever.

 Most patients are very weight conscious. Parents may also worry about the weight of their children. Therefore, it is very important for the health care provider to make only positive statements while weighing a patient. In addition, privacy must be provided while weighing a patient and care should be taken so other individuals cannot see the patient's weight on the scale.

A wide variety of scales are used to obtain height and weight measurements. Most clinical scales contain a balance beam for measuring weight and a measuring rod for determining height (**Figures 21–2A** and **21–2B**). Infant scales provide an area for placing the infant in a lying-down, or flat, position. Some facilities have digital scales that show the weight automatically. Institutions, such as hospitals or long-term care facilities, may have special scales for patients who are unable to stand. Such scales include the wheelchair scale (**Figure 21–3**) and the bed scale with a mechanical lift. Some hospitals and/or long-term care facilities have beds with a built-in scale that can be used to weigh comatose or paralyzed patients. It is important to follow

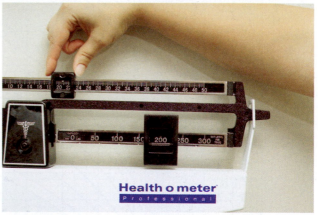

FIGURE 21-2A The weight bars of a beam-balance scale. The bottom weights are in 50-pound increments and the top weights are in 1/4-pound increments.

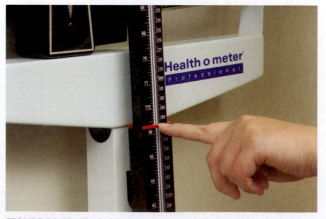

FIGURE 21-2B The height bar of a beam-balance scale. The height is read at the break point on the movable bar.

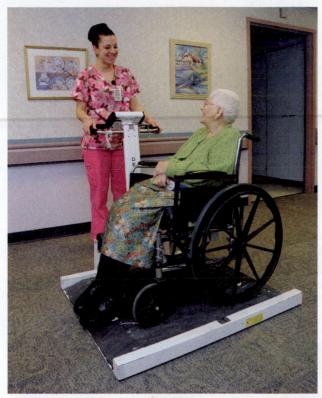

FIGURE 21-3 A wheelchair scale is a convenient scale for weighing a patient who may have difficulty standing on a beam-balance scale.

the manufacturer's instructions while using any special scale to obtain accurate weight measurements.

Math

Weight is recorded as pounds and ounces or as kilograms (1.0 kilogram = 2.2 pounds). Most scales measure pounds in ¼-pound increments. Metric scales measure in kilograms and have 0.1-kilogram increments. At times, it may be necessary to convert kilograms (kg) to pounds (lb) or pounds to kilograms.

To convert kilograms to pounds, use the following formula:

$$\text{Kilograms(kg)} \times 2.2 = \text{pounds (lb)}$$

Example: Convert 60 kilograms to pounds.

$$60 \text{ kg} \times 2.2 = 132 \text{ lb}$$

To convert pounds to kilograms, use the following formula:

$$\text{Pounds (lb)} \div 2.2 = \text{kilograms(kg)}$$

Example: Convert 110 pounds to kilograms.

$$110 \text{ lb} \div 2.2 = 50 \text{ kg}$$

Math

Height is recorded as feet and inches or as centimeters. The measuring bar measures inches and fractions of ¼-inch increments. A metric measuring bar has 1-centimeter increments. One inch equals 2.5 centimeters. At times, it may be necessary to convert centimeters (cm) to inches (in) or inches to centimeters.

To convert centimeters to inches, use the following formula:

$$\text{Centimeters (cm)} \div 2.5 = \text{inches (in)}$$

Example: Convert 95 centimeters to inches.

$$95 \text{ cm} \div 2.5 = 38 \text{ in}$$

To convert inches to centimeters, use the following formula:

$$\text{Inches (in)} \times 2.5 = \text{centimeters (cm)}$$

Example: Convert 24 inches to centimeters.

$$24 \text{ in} \times 2.5 = 60 \text{ cm}$$

checkpoint

1. What brain condition does a head circumference above the 95th percentile usually indicate?

PRACTICE: Go to the workbook and complete the assignment sheet for 21:1, Measuring/Recording Height and Weight. Then return and continue with the procedures.

Procedure 21:1A

Measuring/Recording Height and Weight

Equipment and Supplies

Balance scale, paper towel, paper, pen and/or computer

Procedure

1. Assemble equipment.

2. Wash hands.

3. Prepare the scale. Place a paper towel on the foot stand of the scale (**Figure 21–4A**). Move both weights to the *zero* position. If the end of the balance bar swings freely, the scale is balanced. If the scale is *not* balanced, follow the manufacturer's instructions to balance the scale.

   NOTE: Most scales have a small screw by the end of the balance bar. By adjusting the screw, the scale can be balanced.

   NOTE: The paper towel prevents spread of disease.

(continues)

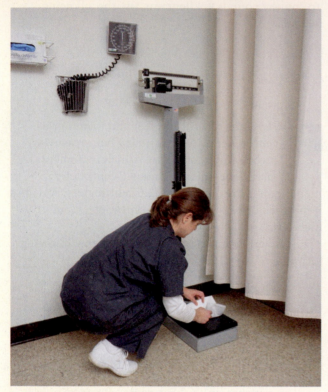

FIGURE 21-4A Place a paper towel on the foot stand of the scale.

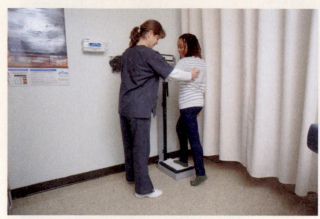

FIGURE 21-4B Assist the patient onto the scale with her feet centered on the platform.

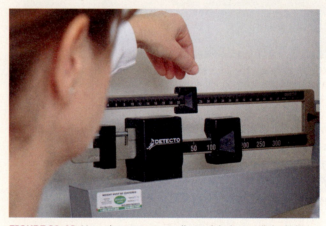

FIGURE 21-4C Move the upper or smaller weight bar until the balance bar swings freely halfway between the upper and lower guides.

4. Introduce yourself. Identify the patient. Explain the procedure. Remember to make only positive statements.
   Comm

5. Ask the patient to remove shoes, jackets, heavy outer clothing, purses, and heavy objects that may be in the pockets of clothing.

   NOTE: In a hospital or long-term care facility, the patient is usually weighed in a gown or in pajamas.

6. Assist the patient onto the scale (**Figure 21–4B**). The patient should stand unassisted, with their feet centered on the platform and slightly apart.

   ⚠ **CAUTION:** Watch closely at all times to prevent falls.
   Safety

7. Move the large 50-pound weight to the right until the balance bar drops down on the lower guide. Then move this weight back one notch.
   Math Move the smaller ¼-pound weight until the balance bar swings freely halfway between the upper and lower guides (**Figure 21–4C**). Add the two weights together to determine the patient's correct weight. Recheck your reading. Record the weight correctly.

   ✅ **CHECKPOINT:** Your instructor will check your reading for accuracy.
   Check

NOTE: If the scale has a digital display, wait until the display is stationary and record the number shown.

8. Help the patient get off the scale. Raise the height bar higher than the height of the patient (**Figure 21–5A**). Help the patient get back on the scale with their back to the scale.

   ⚠ **CAUTION:** Watch closely at all times to prevent falls.
   Safety

9. Instruct the patient to stand as erect as possible. Ask the patient to look straight ahead to keep the head level.

10. Move the bar of the measuring scale down until it just touches the top of the patient's head (**Figure 21–5B**).

    ⚠ **CAUTION:** Move slowly. Do *not* hit the patient with the bar.
    Safety

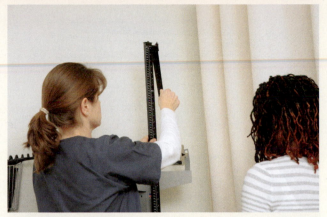

FIGURE 21-5A Raise the height bar of the scale higher than the height of the patient.

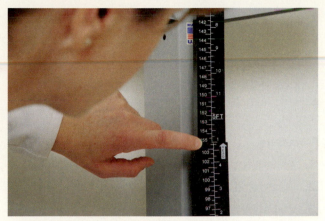

FIGURE 21-5C Read the height at the point of the break by reading in a downward direction on the upper bar.

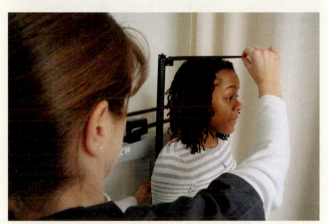

FIGURE 21-5B Move the bar of the measuring scale down until it just touches the top of the patient's head.

11. Read the measurement in inches or centimeters. Recheck your reading. Record the height correctly.

   NOTE: If the height is difficult to read, assist the patient off the scale without moving the height bar. Then read the correct height measurement.

   NOTE: If the reading is in inches, it can be converted to feet and inches after the patient is off the scale.

   NOTE: If the height bar is extended above the break point of the movable bar, remember to read the height at the point of the break by reading in a downward direction on the upper bar (**Figure 21–5C**).

    CHECKPOINT: Your instructor will check your reading for accuracy.

12. Elevate the height bar.

13. Help the patient get off the scale.

    CAUTION: Watch the patient closely to prevent falls.

14. Replace all equipment. Throw the paper towel in a waste can.

15. Return both weight beams to the zero positions. Lower the measurement bar.

16. Convert the inches to feet and inches by dividing by 12. For example, 64½ inches divided by 12 equals 5 feet, 4½ inches.

17. Wash hands.

18. Record all required information on the patient's chart or enter it into the computer. For example: date, time, Wt: 132½ lb, Ht: 5 ft, 4¼ in, and your signature and title.

   NOTE: In offices with electronic health records (EHRs), information is entered directly into the patient's record on a computer.

PRACTICE: Go to the workbook and use the evaluation sheet for 21:1A, Measuring/Recording Height and Weight, to practice this procedure. When you believe you have mastered this skill, sign the sheet and give it to your instructor for further action.

 FINAL EVALUATION: Using the criteria listed on the evaluation sheet, your instructor will grade your performance.

Measuring/Recording Height and Weight of an Infant

Equipment and Supplies

Infant scale, towel or scale paper, tape measure, growth graph, patient's chart or paper, pen and/or computer

Procedure

1. Assemble equipment.

2. Wash hands.

3. Prepare the scale. Place a towel or scale paper on the scale to protect the infant from the shock of the cold metal and pathogens (germs). Then balance the scale. Move both weights to the *zero* position. If the end of the balance bar swings freely, the scale is balanced. If the scale is *not* balanced, follow the manufacturer's instructions to balance the scale.

   NOTE: Most scales have a small screw by the end of the balance bar. By adjusting the screw, the scale can be balanced.

   NOTE: Many health care facilities use digital scales for infants. The infant is placed on the scale and the digital display shows the weight. This type of scale is safer for infants.

4. Introduce yourself. Explain the procedure to the parent. Identify the infant by asking the parent for the infant's name. Ask the parent to undress the infant.

   NOTE: An undershirt or pajama is sometimes left on the infant.

5. Pick up the infant. Use one arm to support the neck and shoulders and the other arm to support the back and hips.

6. Place the infant on the scale.

   ⚠️ **Safety** **CAUTION:** Watch closely at all times. To prevent falls, keep one hand over the infant while adjusting the scales (**Figure 21–6**).

7. ➕ **Math** Move the large weight to the right until the balance bar drops down on the lower guide. Then move this weight back one notch. Move the smaller weight until the balance bar swings freely halfway between the upper and lower guides. Add the two weights together to determine the infant's correct weight.

   NOTE: If the infant scale contains only one bar and one weight, move the weight to the right until the balance bar swings freely halfway between the upper and lower guide. Read the weight on the bar.

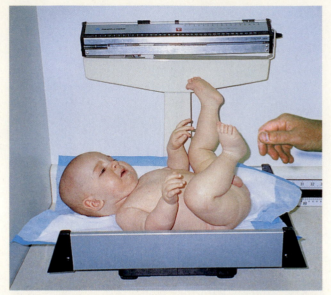

FIGURE 21-6 Always keep one hand close to the infant to prevent the infant from falling off the scale.

NOTE: Many offices have scales with digital readouts. The weight is measured automatically when the infant is placed on the scale. However, it is important to make sure that you are not touching the infant when you read and record the weight.

8. Record the weight in pounds and ounces or in kilograms. Recheck your reading.

   ✅ **Check** **CHECKPOINT:** Your instructor will check your reading for accuracy.

9. Pick up and place the infant on a flat surface.

   ⚠️ **Safety** **CAUTION:** Watch closely at all times. Do not leave the infant unattended. If it is necessary to reach for anything nearby, use one hand to hold the infant and the other hand to reach.

10. Place the zero mark of the measuring tape or rod at the infant's head. If the measuring bar is a part of the examination table, position the infant so that the infant's head is at the zero mark (**Figure 21–7A**). Ask the parent or an assistant to hold the head at this mark. Gently straighten the infant's legs. If a measuring tape is used, measure to the infant's heel (**Figure 21–7B**). If a bar is used, position the heel on the bar while holding the leg straight.

    NOTE: If the infant is lying on examining table paper, mark the paper at the infant's head and heel. Then measure the marked area.

11. Record the height correctly in inches or centimeters. Recheck your reading.

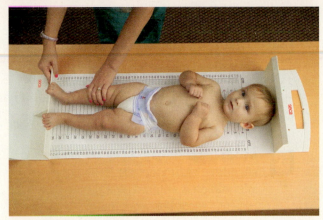

FIGURE 21-7A Position the infant's head against the zero mark bar and gently straighten the legs to measure the infant's height.

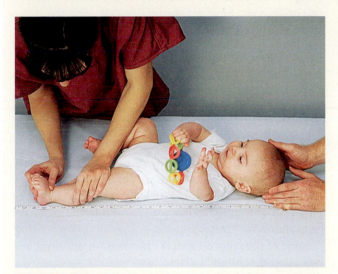

FIGURE 21-7B Hold the tape measure in a straight line to measure an infant's height.

 CHECKPOINT: Your instructor will check your reading for accuracy.

12. The head circumference is frequently measured on an infant. To measure head circumference:

   a. Position the infant on the examination table or ask the parent to hold the infant.

   b. Use a thumb or finger to hold the zero mark of the tape measure against the infant's forehead just above the eyebrows.

   c. Use your other hand to bring the tape around the infant's head, just above the ears, over the occipital bone at the back of the head, and back to the forehead to meet the zero mark on the tape (**Figure 21–8**).

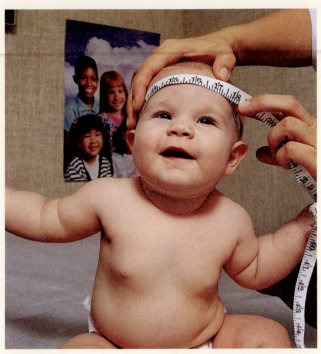

FIGURE 21-8 To measure head circumference, bring the tape around the infant's head, just above the ears, and back to the forehead.

   d. Pull the tape snug to compress the hair, but not too tight.

   e. Read the tape measure to the nearest ½ inch or 0.1 centimeter.

   f. Record the reading.

 CHECKPOINT: Your instructor will check your reading for accuracy.

13. To measure chest circumference of the infant:

   a. Lay the infant flat on their back.

   b. Use the thumb of one hand to hold the zero mark of the tape at the middle of the sternum.

   c. Use your other hand to wrap the tape snugly under the axillary area and around the back to meet at the midsternal area (**Figure 21–9**).

   d. Make sure the tape is at the nipple level of the chest and that it is not twisted.

   e. Read the measurement after the infant has exhaled or during the resting phase between respirations.

   f. Read the tape measure to the nearest ½ inch or 0.1 centimeter.

 CHECKPOINT: Your instructor will check your reading for accuracy.

(continues)

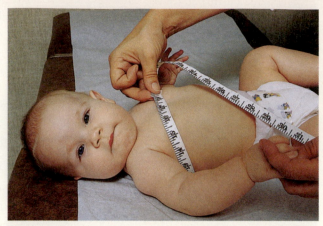

FIGURE 21-9 To measure chest circumference, wrap the tape snugly around the chest and back at the nipple line.

14. Return the infant to the parent.

15. Clean and replace all equipment. Use a disinfectant to wipe the scale. Set the weights at zero. Fold up the tape measure.

16. Wash hands.

17. Record all required information on the infant's chart or enter it into the computer. For example: date, time, Wt: 9 lb 8 oz, Ht: 23½ in, Head circumference: 16¾ in, Chest circumference: 17¼ in, and your signature and title. The measurements should also be recorded on the infant's growth graph.

 NOTE: In health care agencies using electronic health records (EHRs), the information is entered directly into the patient's record on a computer.

PRACTICE: Go to the workbook and use the evaluation sheet for 21:1B, Measuring/Recording Height and Weight of an Infant, to practice this procedure. When you believe you have mastered this skill, sign the sheet and give it to your instructor for further action.

 FINAL EVALUATION: Using the criteria listed on the evaluation sheet, your instructor will grade your performance.

21:2 POSITIONING A PATIENT

A wide variety of positions are used for different procedures and examinations. The patient may need to be positioned on a medical examination table or a surgical table. It is important to know how to operate the table before attempting to position a patient. Obtain instruction or read the manufacturer's directions carefully. After use, medical examination tables and surgical tables are usually cleaned with an antiseptic soap and/or a disinfectant solution. In addition, table paper is frequently used to cover an examination table prior to the examination and is removed and replaced after the examination.

  During any procedure or examination, reassure the patient. Make sure the patient understands what is being done and grants permission for the procedure. At all times, watch the patient closely for signs of distress. Observe all safety factors to prevent falls and injuries. Use correct body mechanics at all times to prevent injury to yourself.

It is also essential to make sure that the patient is not exposed during any examination or procedure. The door to the room should be closed, and the curtains, if present, should be drawn. Care must be taken to properly drape or cover the patient to avoid unnecessary exposure. At the same time, the drape must be applied so that the physician or technician has ready access to the area to be examined or treated.

Some of the most common examination positions are listed and described.

Horizontal Recumbent (Supine) Position

- This position is used for examination or treatment of the front, or anterior, part of the body (**Figure 21–10**).

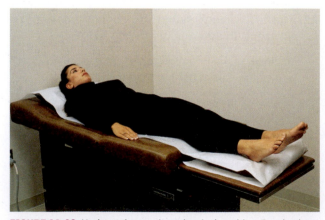

FIGURE 21-10 Horizontal recumbent (supine) position. Draping has been omitted for clarity.

- The patient lies flat on the back with the legs slightly apart
- One small pillow is allowed under the head.
- The arms are flat at the side of the body.
- The drape is placed over the patient but left loose on all sides to facilitate examination or treatment.

Prone Position

- This position is used for examination or treatment of the back or spine (**Figure 21–11**).
- The patient lies on the abdomen and turns the head to either side. A small pillow may be placed under the head.
- The arms may be flexed at the elbows and positioned on either side of the head or positioned along the side of the body.
- One sheet or drape is placed over the patient but left loose on all sides to facilitate examination or treatment.

Sims' (**Left Lateral**) Position

- This position is used for simple rectal and sigmoidoscopic examinations, enemas, rectal temperatures, and rectal treatments (**Figure 21–12**).

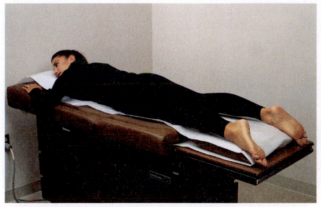

FIGURE 21-11 Prone position.

FIGURE 21-12 Sims' (left lateral) position.

- The patient lies on the left side.
- The left arm is extended behind the back.
- The head is turned to the side. A small pillow may be used.
- The right arm is in front of the patient, and the elbow is bent.
- The left leg is bent, or flexed, slightly.
- The right leg is bent sharply at the knee and brought up to the abdomen.
- Draping can be done with one large sheet or two small sheets that meet at the rectal area. A sheet with a hole at the examination site may also be used. All sheets hang free at the sides.

Knee–Chest Position

- This position is used for rectal examinations, usually a sigmoidoscopic examination (**Figure 21–13**). It is only used in rare circumstances when proctologic tables are not available.
- The patient rests the body weight on the knees and chest.
- The arms are flexed slightly at the elbows and are extended above the head.
- The knees are slightly separated, and the thighs are at right angles to the table.
- Draping can be done with one large sheet or two small sheets that meet at the rectal area. A large sheet with a hole at the rectal area can also be used. Sheets hang loose with no tucks.

⚠️ Safety **CAUTION:** *Do not place the patient in this position until the physician is ready to begin the examination.*

⚠️ Safety **CAUTION:** *Never leave a patient alone in this position. This is a difficult position for the patient to maintain and should be used only as long as absolutely necessary.*

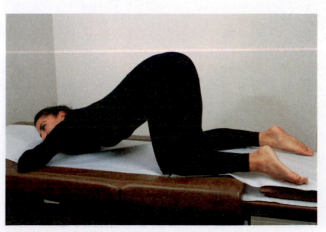

FIGURE 21-13 Knee–chest position.

Fowler's Positions

- These positions are used to facilitate breathing, relieve distress, encourage drainage, and examine the head, neck, and chest.

- The patient lies on the back.

- The head is elevated to one of three main positions:

  (1) *Low Fowler's:* the head is elevated to a 25-degree angle.

  (2) *Semi-Fowler's:* the head is elevated to a 45-degree angle (the most frequently used position) (**Figure 21–14A**).

  (3) *High Fowler's:* the head is elevated to a 90-degree angle (**Figure 21–14B**).

- The legs lie flat on the table but the knees are bent slightly and are sometimes supported on a pillow.

- One sheet is used to drape the patient. The sheet is left hanging loose.

Lithotomy Position

- This position is used for vaginal examinations, Pap tests, urinary catheterization, cystoscopic examinations, and surgery of the pelvic area (**Figure 21–15**).

- The patient is positioned on the back.

- The knees are separated and flexed, and the feet are placed in stirrups.

- The arms rest at the sides.

- The buttocks are at the lower end of the table.

- The lower end of the table is dropped down or pushed in depending on the model of the examination table.

- Draping is done with one large sheet placed over the body in a diamond shape. One corner is at the upper chest, and one corner hangs loose between legs. Each of the other two corners is wrapped around a foot.

Dorsal Recumbent Position

- This position is similar to the lithotomy position, but the patient is in bed or on a table without stirrups (**Figure 21–16**).

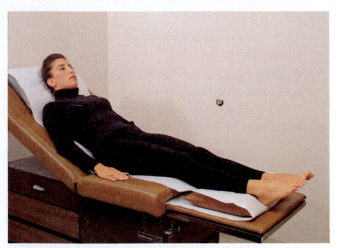

FIGURE 21-14A Semi-Fowler's (mid-Fowler's) position.

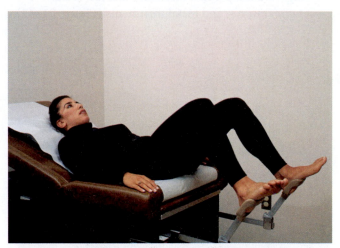

FIGURE 21-15 Lithotomy position.

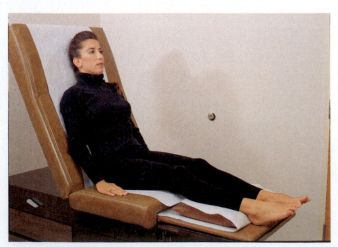

FIGURE 21-14B High Fowler's position.

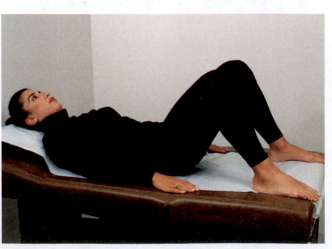

FIGURE 21-16 Dorsal recumbent position.

- The feet are separated but flat on the table/bed.
- The knees are bent.
- Draping and other points are the same as for the lithotomy position.

Trendelenburg Position

- This position increases circulation of blood to the head and brain, and can be used for circulatory shock. The entire bed or table is elevated at the feet. The patient lies in the horizontal recumbent position, with the head lower than the feet.

- The surgical Trendelenburg position (**Figure 21–17**) can be used for surgery on pelvic organs and for pelvic treatments. The patient is flat on the back. The table is lowered at a 45-degree angle to lower the head, and the feet and lower legs are inclined downward.

- Straps are frequently used to hold the patient in position.

  NOTE: *Draping for the Trendelenburg position depends on the treatment being performed; usually, one large sheet is used and left hanging loose. For surgical procedures, the patient is draped with a sheet that has a hole to expose the surgical area.*

Jackknife (Proctologic) Position

- This position is used mainly for rectal surgery or examinations and for back surgery or treatments (**Figure 21–18**).

- The patient is in the prone position.

- The table is elevated at the center so that the rectal area is at a higher elevation. A special surgical table is required for this position.

- The head and chest point downward. The feet and legs hang down at the opposite end of the table.

- The patient must be supported to prevent injury. Straps are used to hold the patient in position.

- Draping is done with a surgical sheet that has a hole to expose the surgical or treatment area. Two small sheets that meet at the surgical or treatment area can also be used.

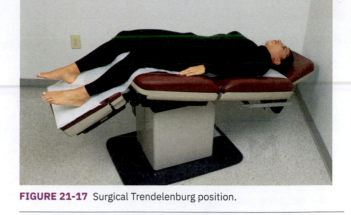

FIGURE 21-17 Surgical Trendelenburg position.

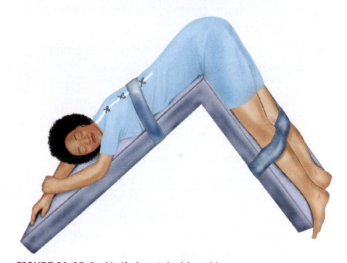

FIGURE 21-18 Jackknife (proctologic) position.

Safety

CAUTION: *It is important to use good body mechanics while positioning the patient to protect both yourself and the patient.*

checkpoint

1. What are the nine (9) most common examination positions?

PRACTICE: Go to the workbook and complete the assignment sheet for 21:2, Positioning a Patient. Then return and continue with the procedure.

Procedure 21:2

Positioning a Patient

Equipment and Supplies

Two to three sheets or disposable drapes, examination table, patient gown, two small pillows, pen and/or computer

Procedure

1. Assemble equipment. Prepare the examination table by wiping it with a disinfectant and covering it with table paper.

2. Wash hands.

(continues)

3. Introduce yourself. Identify the patient. Explain the procedure. Obtain the patient's consent.

4. Instruct the patient to remove all clothing and to put on an examining gown. Instruct the patient to leave the opening in the front or the back depending on the examination to be performed. Ask the patient to void to prevent bladder discomfort during the examination or treatment.

5. Help the patient get on table.

   NOTE: Positioning of the patient will depend on the examination, treatment, or procedure to be performed.

6. Position the patient in the horizontal recumbent (supine) position as follows:

   a. Lay the patient flat on their back.

   b. Place a small pillow under the head.

   c. Rest the arms at the sides of the body.

   d. Position the legs flat and slightly separated.

   e. Use a large sheet or disposable drape to drape the patient. Do *not* tuck the sheet in at the sides or bottom. It should hang loose.

   NOTE: Most health care agencies use disposable drapes that are discarded after use.

7. Position the patient in the prone position as follows:

   a. Ask the supine patient to turn the body in your direction until lying on the abdomen. Hold the drape up while the patient is turning.

    CAUTION: Watch the patient closely to make sure they do not roll off of the table. Do *not* leave the patient alone.

   b. Turn the head to either side to rest on a small pillow.

   c. Flex the arms at the elbows and place at the sides of the head.

   d. Use one large sheet or disposable drape to drape the patient. Do *not* tuck in at the sides or bottom.

8. Position the patient in the Sims' (left lateral) position as follows:

   a. Ask the prone patient to turn on the left side.

   b. Extend the left arm behind the back.

   c. Rest the head on a small pillow.

   d. Bend the left leg slightly.

   e. Bend the right leg sharply to the abdomen.

   f. Place the right arm bent at the elbow in a comfortable position in front of the body.

   g. Drape with one large sheet or disposable drape. Do *not* tuck in at the sides or bottom. Draping can also be done with two small sheets or disposable drapes. One sheet covers the upper part of the body and meets the second sheet, which covers the thighs and legs. A sheet with an opening at the rectal area may also be used.

9. Position the patient in the knee–chest position as follows:

   a. Ask the patient to lie on the abdomen (that is, in the prone position).

   b. Raise the buttocks and abdomen until the body weight is resting on the upper chest and knees.

    NOTE: Do *not* place the patient in this position until the physician is ready to begin the examination. It is a difficult position for the patient to maintain.

   c. Make sure the knees are slightly separated and the thighs are at right angles to the table.

   d. Rest the head on a small pillow.

   e. Flex the arms slightly and position on the sides of the head.

   f. Drape with one large, untucked sheet or disposable drape or two small sheets or disposable drapes that meet at the rectal area. A drape with a hole at the rectal area can also be used.

   CAUTION: *Never* leave the patient alone in the knee–chest position.

   g. When the examination is complete, help the patient get into the prone position. Watch closely for signs of dizziness or discomfort and report any such signs immediately after being sure that the patient is in a comfortable, safe position.

10. Position the patient in the Fowler's positions as follows:

    a. Place the patient in the horizontal recumbent position.

    b. Place a small pillow under the patient's head.

    c. Low Fowler's: elevate the head of the table/bed to a 25-degree angle.

    d. Mid-, or semi-, Fowler's: elevate the head to a 45-degree angle.

e. High Fowler's: elevate the head to a 90-degree angle.

f. Place a second small pillow under the patient's knees after flexing them slightly.

g. Use a large sheet or disposable drape to drape the patient. Do *not* tuck in the sides or end of the sheet or drape.

11. Position the patient in the lithotomy position as follows:

a. Position the patient on the back with the arms at the sides. The feet should be resting on the extension at the lower end of the table.

b. Ask the patient to slide the buttocks down on the table to where the lower end of the table folds down or pulls out.

c. Position a small pillow under the patient's head.

d. Place a sheet or disposable drape over the patient in a diamond position. One corner should be at the chest, the opposite corner at the perineal area, or between the legs. Wrap each side corner around a foot.

e. Position the stirrups and lock them in place.

NOTE: Many tables have a knob at the side that is turned to lock the stirrups in position.

f. Flex and separate the knees.

g. Place the feet in the stirrups.

h. Drop the lower end of the table, or push in the extension.

i. To get the patient out of this position, first raise the end of the table or pull out the extension so that it is level. Lift the feet out of the stirrups and place them on the table. Ask the patient to move back up on the table.

12. Position the patient in the Trendelenburg positions as follows:

 CAUTION: These positions require a special bed or table and assistance. Care should be taken to prevent the patient from sliding off the table.

a. Put the patient in the horizontal recumbent position.

b. Operate the power table or electric bed to raise the foot of the table or bed so that the patient's head is lower than the rest of the body. The lower frame of a bed is sometimes supported up on blocks.

c. For the surgical Trendelenburg position, lower the bottom end of the table so that the lower legs are inclined at a downward angle.

d. Use one large or two small sheets or disposable drapes to drape the patient, or use a drape with a hole at the surgical site.

e. Use straps to secure the patient in position.

f. Remain with the patient at all times.

13. Position the patient in the jackknife or proctologic position as follows:

 CAUTION: This position requires a special table and assistance (**Figure 21–19**). Care must be taken to prevent the patient from sliding off the table or being injured in any way.

a. Position the patient in the prone position.

b. Secure the safety straps on the table.

c. Lower the top of the table so that the head and upper body are inclined at a downward angle.

d. Lower the bottom of the table so that the feet and legs are inclined at a downward angle.

e. Use a large sheet or special drape that has an opening in it to cover the patient. Place the opening over the rectal area. You may also use two small sheets or disposable drapes that meet at the rectal area.

f. Remain with the patient at all times. Observe for any negative reactions to the position, such as dizziness, pain, or discomfort. Immediately report any such signs to your supervisor.

14. When the examination, treatment, or procedure is complete, allow the patient to sit up. Observe for signs of dizziness or weakness.

15. Help the patient get off the table. Ask the patient to get dressed or assist if necessary. Inform the patient of how and when they will be notified of test results (if tests were conducted during the examination).

 CAUTION: Watch the patient closely and prevent falls.

16. Clean and replace all equipment.

17. Wash hands.

18. Record all required information on the patient's chart or enter it into the computer. For example: date, time, positioned in semi-Fowler's for comfort, appears to be resting well, and your signature and title.

(continues)

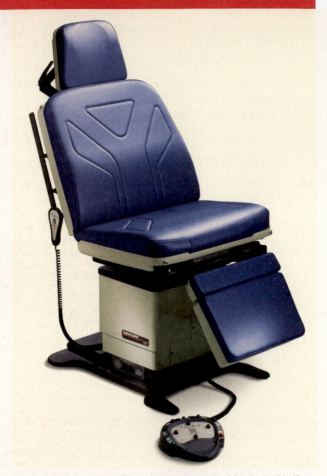

 NOTE: In health care agencies using electronic health records (EHRs), the information is entered directly into the patient's record on a computer.

PRACTICE: Go to the workbook and use the evaluation sheet for 21:2, Positioning a Patient, to practice this procedure. When you believe you have mastered this skill, sign the sheet and give it to your instructor for further action.

 FINAL EVALUATION: Using the criteria listed on the evaluation sheet, your instructor will grade your performance.

FIGURE 21-19 A special power table is required for the jackknife or proctologic position. Courtesy of Midmark Corp.

21:3 SCREENING FOR VISION PROBLEMS

Vision screening tests are given to measure an individual's **visual acuity**, or ability to perceive and comprehend the sense of sight. They are often given as part of a physical examination or to detect eye disease. Any test for visual acuity should be conducted in a well-lighted room. Natural daylight, with no direct sunlight, is preferred. During any test, it is important to watch the patient for squinting, leaning toward the eye chart, closing one eye when both eyes are being tested, excessive blinking, and/or watering of the eyes. If defects are noted on any test, the patient should be referred to an ophthalmologist for a more extensive examination.

One method of vision screening involves the use of Snellen charts. **Snellen charts** are used to test distant vision (**Figure 21–20**). They come in a variety of types. Some contain pictures for use with small

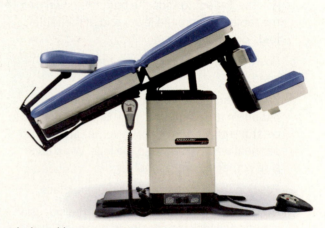

FIGURE 21-20 Snellen charts are used for vision screening.

children. Some contain the letter *E* in a variety of positions. The patient points in the direction that the *E* points. This type of chart is used for non-English-speaking people or nonreaders. Some contain letters of the alphabet. It is important to make sure the patient knows all the letters of the alphabet when using this type of chart.

Characters (that is, letters or pictures) on the Snellen chart have specific heights, ranging from small, on the bottom of the chart, to large, on the top of the chart. When standing 20 feet from the chart, a person with normal visual acuity should be able to see characters that are 20 millimeters high. Such a person is said to have 20/20 vision. When referring to 20/20 vision, the top number represents the distance the patient is from the chart. For this screening test, then, the patient is placed 20 feet from the chart. The bottom number represents the height of the characters that the patient can read at that distance.

- **Example 1**: If a patient has 20/30 vision, this means that when standing 20 feet from the chart, the patient can see characters 30 millimeters (mm) high. It can also be stated that this patient, who is standing 20 feet from the chart, can see what a patient with normal visual acuity can see standing 30 feet from the chart.

- **Example 2**: If a patient has 20/100 vision, this means that when standing 20 feet from the chart, the patient can only see characters that are 100 millimeters (mm) high. This finding represents a defect in distant vision. A person with normal visual acuity would be able to see the same figures while standing 100 feet from the chart.

It is important to note that Snellen charts test only for defects in distant vision, or for nearsightedness (myopia). Defects in close vision (problems with reading small print and seeing up close), known as farsightedness (hyperopia), are tested by the Jaeger system. This system uses a printed card with different short paragraphs. Each paragraph is printed in a different size type, ranging from 0.37 to 2.5 millimeters (mm) high. A card with different characters or pictures is available for use with small children or individuals who cannot read. The patient holds the card approximately 14–16 inches away from the eyes (**Figure 21–21**). The patient then reads printed text or identifies pictures that gradually become smaller. The smallest print or character that the patient can read or identify without error is recorded.

Defects in color vision, or color blindness, are usually tested by the Ishihara method. The Ishihara book contains a series of numbers printed in colored dots against a background of dots in contrasting color (**Figure 21–22**). Patients with normal color vision are able to readily identify the numbers. Patients with color

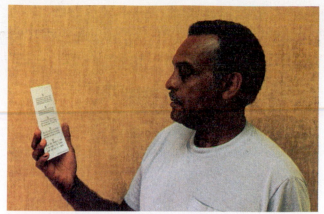

FIGURE 21-21 The patient holds the card 14–16 inches from the eyes when testing for defects in close vision.

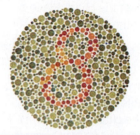 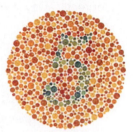

FIGURE 21-22 People with color blindness are not able to see the numbers in these Ishihara color plates.

blindness either are unable to see the numbers or identify incorrect numbers. This test is most accurate when it is conducted in a room illuminated by natural daylight but not by bright sunlight.

When screening for visual acuity, there are some special terms or abbreviations to remember:

- **OD**: abbreviation for *oculus dexter*, or right eye

- **OS**: abbreviation for *oculus sinister*, or left eye

- **OU**: abbreviation for *oculus uterque*, or each eye; both eyes

- **Myopia**: nearsightedness, defect in distant vision

- **Hyperopia**: farsightedness, defect in close vision

- **Ophthalmoscope**: instrument for checking the eye

- **Tonometer**: instrument to measure intraocular tension or pressure; increased pressure often indicates glaucoma

check**point**

1. What is the name of the chart used for vision screening?

PRACTICE: Go to the workbook and complete the assignment sheet for 21:3, Screening for Vision Problems. Then return and continue with the procedure.

Procedure 21:3

Screening for Vision Problems

Equipment and Supplies

Snellen eye chart, Jaeger card, Ishihara book with color plates, pointer, tape, eye shield or occluder, paper, pen and/or computer

Procedure

1. Assemble equipment. Check the lighting in the room to make sure there is no glare. Natural daylight is preferred.
2. Attach the Snellen chart to the wall or place it in a lighted stand. Measure a distance of 20 feet directly away from the front of the chart. Place a piece of tape on the floor at the 20-foot mark.

   NOTE: Most medical offices will have a mark on the floor to indicate the 20-foot distance.

   NOTE: Vision screening devices that are calibrated for distance are also available. The patient looks through eyepieces to see the charts and identify letters. The device allows the operator to turn off the light in an eyepiece to test vision in either the right or left eye.
3. Wash hands.
4. Comm — Introduce yourself. Identify the patient. Explain the procedure.

   NOTE: If using a chart with letters, make sure the patient knows the letters of the alphabet. If using a picture chart, make sure small children know what each picture represents.
5. Instruct the patient to stand facing the chart. Make sure the patient's toes are on the taped line; the patient's eyes will be 20 feet from the chart.
6. Point to various letters or pictures on the chart. Ask the patient to identify the letters or pictures. If the patient wears corrective lenses (glasses or contact lenses), check the vision with the corrective lenses first. Then ask the patient to remove the corrective lenses. Check the vision again. Record both readings. Observe the following points:
   a. Start with the larger letters or pictures and proceed to the smaller ones.
   b. Make sure the pointer you are using does not block the letters or pictures.
   c. Select letters or pictures at random in each row. Do *not* start at one end of the row and go straight across the line. Patients may memorize order; random sampling makes the patient focus on individual letters or pictures.

   NOTE: If you are sure the patient has not memorized the letters, you may ask the patient to read a row of letters. If the patient is able to read all letters correctly, proceed to a smaller row.

   d. Watch to be sure the patient is not leaning forward or squinting to see the letters or pictures (**Figure 21–23A**). Note whether the patient is blinking excessively or if the eyes are watering.

   NOTE: Some examiners do the left or right eye first, the opposite eye second, and both eyes last. Follow your agency's policy.
7. Ask the patient to correctly identify all the letters or pictures in the 20/20 line. If the patient is unable to do so, note the line that the patient *can* read with 100-percent accuracy.
8. Give the patient an eye shield or occluder with which to cover the left eye (**Figure 21–23B**). Warn the patient not to close the left eye while it is covered, because doing so can cause blurred vision. Repeat steps 6 and 7 to test the vision in the right eye (OD).

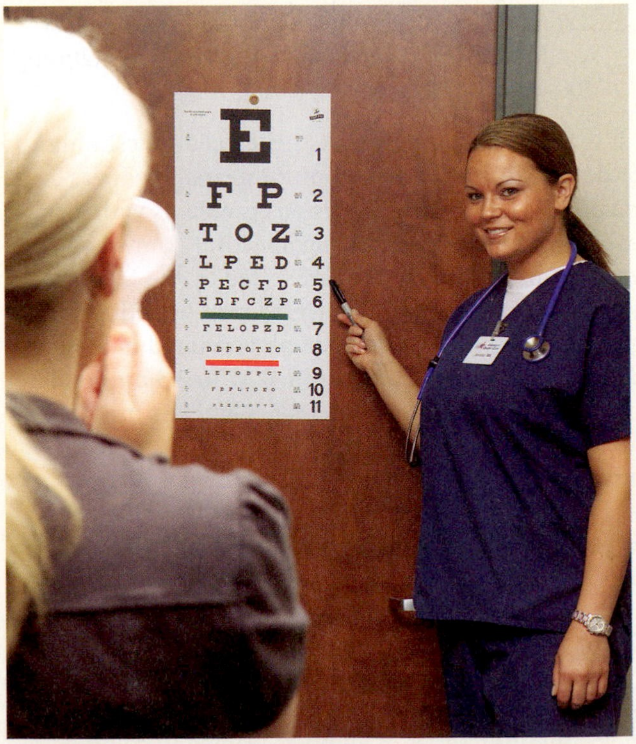

FIGURE 21-23A Watch to make sure the patient is not leaning forward or squinting to see the letters.

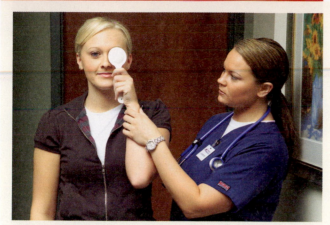

FIGURE 21-23B The patient should keep the eye open while covering it with an eye shield or occluder.

 CAUTION: Warn the patient against pressing on the covered eye to avoid injuring the eye with the occluder or shield. Do *not* use the occluder or shield on another patient until it has been disinfected. Some occluders are disposable.

9. Ask the patient to cover the right eye. Repeat steps 6 and 7 to test the vision in the left eye (OS).

   NOTE: Remind the patient to keep the right eye open while it is covered.

10. Record the test results for both eyes, the right eye, and the left eye. Use abbreviations of *OU*, *OD*, and *OS* and readings of *20/20*, *20/30*, or the correct reading.

11. To test vision by the Jaeger system:

    a. Seat the patient in a comfortable position.

    b. Ask the patient to hold the Jaeger card 14–16 inches from the eyes.

    c. Ask the patient to read the paragraphs out loud.

       NOTE: If the patient cannot read, provide a Jaeger card that contains characters or pictures.

    d. Record the smallest line of print the patient can read with both eyes.

    e. Ask the patient to cover the right eye with an occluder and then to read the paragraphs out loud. Record the smallest line of print the patient can read with the left eye.

    f. Ask the patient to cover the left eye with an occluder and then to read the paragraphs out loud. Record the smallest line of print the patient can read with the right eye.

12. To test color vision with the Ishihara plates:

    a. Seat the patient in a comfortable position.

    b. Hold the plate approximately 30 inches from the patient's eyes.

    c. Ask the patient to read the number on the plate.

       NOTE: Some plates contain color lines in place of numbers. The patient is asked to trace the color line with a finger.

    d. Show the patient all of the plates. Record the number of plates the patient identifies correctly.

    e. Ask the patient to cover the right eye with an occluder and then to identify the numbers on the plates. Record the number of plates the patient identifies correctly with the left eye.

    f. Ask the patient to cover the left eye with an occluder and then to identify the numbers on the plates. Record the number of plates the patient identifies correctly with the right eye.

    g. Report any frame that the patient misses. This allows the physician to determine which type of color blindness the patient has.

13. Thank the patient for being cooperative.

    NOTE: These are only screening tests. Unfavorable results indicate the need for additional testing or referral to an eye specialist.

14. Clean and replace all equipment. If the eye shield is not disposable, wash it thoroughly and clean it with a disinfectant solution.

15. Wash hands.

16. Record all required information on the patient's chart or enter it into the computer. For example: date, time, vision screening with Snellen chart: OU 20/30, OD 20/40, OS 20/30, Jaeger card: OU #3 (0.62 m), OD #3 (0.62 m), OS #5 (1.00 m), Ishihara plates: 10 plates correct for OU, OD, and OS, and your signature and title.

    NOTE: In health care agencies using electronic health records (EHRs), the information is entered directly into the patient's record on a computer.

PRACTICE: Go to the workbook and use the evaluation sheet for 21:3, Screening for Vision Problems, to practice this procedure. When you believe you have mastered this skill, sign the sheet and give it to your instructor for further action.

FINAL EVALUATION: Using the criteria listed on the evaluation sheet, your instructor will grade your performance.

21:4 ASSISTING WITH PHYSICAL EXAMINATIONS

A large variety of physical examinations are performed. The methods used and the equipment available vary from physician to physician. However, there are some basic principles that apply to all examinations.

Three major kinds of examinations are:

- **EENT**: This is an eye, ear, nose, and throat examination. Special equipment should be available to examine these areas of the body.

- **GYN**: This is an examination of the female reproductive organs; that is, a gynecological examination. The physician usually examines the vagina, cervix, and other pelvic organs as well as the breasts. A Pap, or **Papanicolaou**, test frequently is done to detect cancer of the cervix or reproductive organs.

- **General**, or **complete, physical**: All areas of the body are examined. Blood and urine tests frequently are done. Radiographs and an electrocardiogram (ECG) may also be part of the examination. An EENT and/or GYN examination may be performed. Necessary equipment and tests are determined by the physician performing the examination.

Four main techniques used during the examination are observation, palpation, percussion, and auscultation.

- **Observation** (inspection): The physician looks at the patient carefully to observe things such as skin color, rash, growths, swelling, scars, deformities, body movements, condition of hair and nails, and general appearance (**Figure 21–24**).

- **Palpation**: The physician uses the hands and fingers to feel various parts of the body (**Figure 21–25**). The physician can determine whether a part of the body is enlarged, hard, out of place, or painful to the touch.

- **Percussion**: The physician taps and listens for sounds coming from various body organs (**Figure 21–26**). The physician may place one or several fingers of one hand on a part of the body, then use the fingers of the other hand to tap the body part. The sounds emitted allow a trained individual to determine the size, density, and position of underlying organs.

- **Auscultation**: The physician listens to sounds coming from within the patient's body (**Figure 21–27**). A stethoscope is used in most cases. The physician listens to sounds produced by the heart, lungs, intestines, and other body organs.

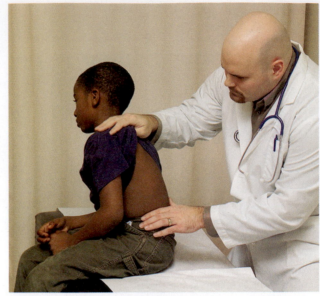

FIGURE 21-24 The physician uses observation to inspect the body for signs of disease.

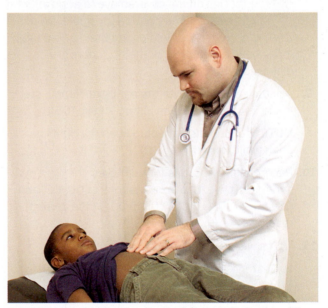

FIGURE 21-25 For palpation, the physician uses the hands and fingers to feel various parts of the body.

All necessary equipment should be assembled prior to the examination. The equipment needed will vary depending on the body areas to be examined. Try to anticipate what the physician will need, and assemble the items for convenient use. Some of the equipment and instruments used for different examinations (**Figure 21–28**) include:

- **Cervical spatula** (**Ayer blade**): a wooden or plastic blade used to scrape cells from the cervix, or lower part of the uterus; it is usually a part of a Pap kit that also contains slides, swabs, and a cytology brush; used to perform a Pap (Papanicolaou) test or smear to check for cancer of the cervix

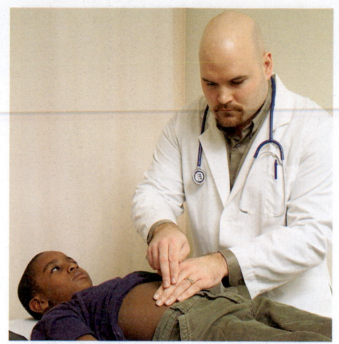

FIGURE 21-26 Percussion involves tapping on body parts and listening to sounds coming from body organs.

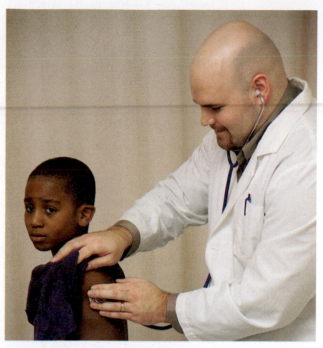

FIGURE 21-27 The physician is using a stethoscope and auscultation to listen to posterior lung and heart sounds.

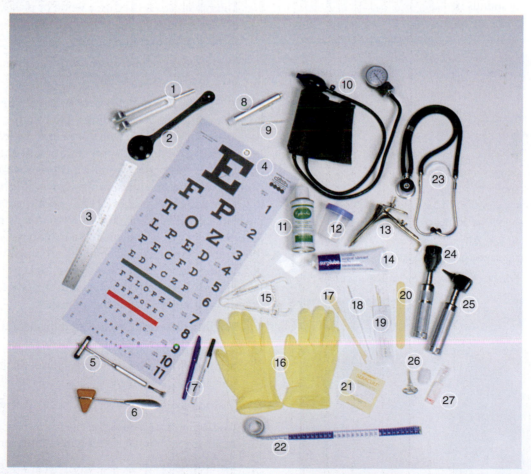

FIGURE 21-28 Instruments and equipment for physical examinations: 1. Tuning fork. 2. Visual occluder. 3. Ruler. 4. Visual acuity chart. 5. Reflex hammer with brush. 6. Percussion hammer. 7. Pen and marking pen. 8. Penlight. 9. Thermometer. 10. Sphygmomanometer. 11. Slide and fixative. 12. Specimen cup. 13. Vaginal speculum. 14. Lubricant. 15. Goniometer to measure angles. 16. Gloves. 17. Cervical spatula (Ayer blade). 18. Cervical brush (cytobrush). 19. Cotton-tip applicator. 20. Tongue depressor. 21. Guaiac material for fecal occult blood. 22. Tape measure. 23. Stethoscope. 24. Ophthalmoscope. 25. Otoscope. 26. Neurological examination key and cotton ball. 27. Sterile needle.

- **Laryngeal mirror**: an instrument with a mirror at one end; used to examine the larynx, or voice box, in the throat
- **Ophthalmoscope**: a lighted instrument used to examine the eyes (**Figure 21–29**)
- **Otoscope**: a lighted instrument used to examine the ears (**Figures 21–30A** and **21–30B**)
- **Percussion (reflex) hammer**: an instrument used to test tendon reflexes
- **Sigmoidoscope**: a lighted instrument used to examine the sigmoid colon, or inside of the lower part of the large intestine; used during sigmoidoscopic examinations
- **Speculum**: an instrument used to examine internal canals of the body; a nasal speculum is used to examine the nose; a vaginal speculum is used to examine the vagina; a rectal speculum is used to examine the rectum
- **Sphygmomanometer**: an instrument used to measure blood pressure
- **Stethoscope**: an instrument used for listening to internal body sounds

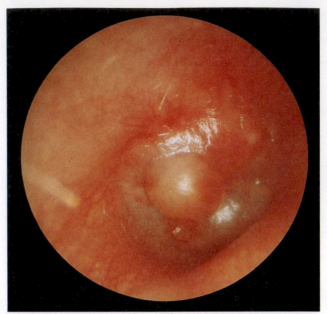

FIGURE 21-30B An otoscopic examination may reveal a bulging tympanic membrane, a sign of otitis media or middle ear infection.
Courtesy of Bruce Black, MD, Brisbane, Australia

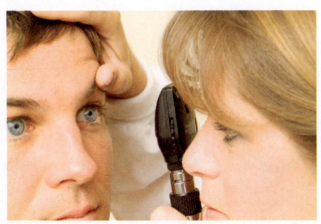

FIGURE 21-29 An ophthalmoscope is used to examine the patient's eye.

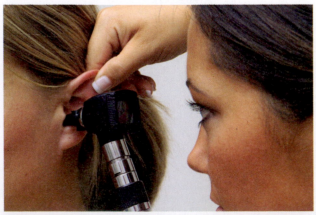

FIGURE 21-30A An otoscope is used to examine the interior of the patient's ear.

- **Tongue blade/depressor**: a wood or plastic stick used to depress, or hold down, the tongue so that the throat can be examined
- **Tuning fork**: an instrument with two prongs that is used to test hearing acuity

 Preparation of the patient must include carefully explaining all procedures. Thorough explanations can help alleviate some fear.

Comm

Patients often are apprehensive and need reassurance. The patient usually must remove all clothing and put on an examining gown. It is important to tell the patient to void before the examination so that the bladder will be empty and internal organs in the area of the bladder can be palpated. If a urinalysis is ordered, the urine specimen can be obtained at this time. Correct positioning and draping are also essential.

Some tests frequently done prior to the physical examination might include the following:

- **Height and weight**: record all information accurately
- **Vital signs**: including TPR (temperature, pulse, respiration) and BP (blood pressure); record all information accurately
- **Vision screening**: test as previously instructed
- **Audiometric screening**: a special hearing test requiring additional training to administer
- **Blood tests**: various tests may be ordered by the physician
- **Electrocardiogram**: a test to check the electrical conduction pattern in the heart; performed if ordered by the physician

During the examination, be prepared to assist as necessary. Hand equipment to the physician as needed. Position the patient correctly for each part of the examination. Pay attention so that you are ready to help with each procedure.

Precaution

Standard precautions (discussed in Section 15:4) must be followed at all times while assisting with physical examinations. Hands must be washed frequently, and gloves must be worn if contact with blood or body fluids is likely. If splashing or spraying of blood or body fluids is possible, other personal protective equipment (PPE) such as a mask or face shield, eye protection, and/or a gown must be worn. Any instruments or equipment contaminated by blood or body fluids must be correctly cleaned and disinfected or sterilized after use. The medical assistant must always be aware of and take steps to prevent the spread of infection.

checkpoint

1. What four (4) main techniques are used during an examination?

PRACTICE: Go to the workbook and complete the assignment sheet for 21:4, Assisting with Physical Examinations. Then return and continue with the procedures.

Procedure 21:4A

Eye, Ear, Nose, and Throat Examination

NOTE: This is a basic guideline. Methods and equipment will vary from physician to physician.

Equipment and Supplies

Tray covered with a towel, basin lined with a paper towel, cotton-tipped applicators, ophthalmoscope, otoscope, tuning fork, nasal speculum, tongue blades or depressors, flashlight or penlight, Snellen chart, culture tubes and slides (as needed), disposable gloves, infectious-waste bag, patient's chart, lab requisition forms, pen and/or computer

Procedure

1. Assemble equipment. Arrange the instruments on a Mayo stand or tray.

2. Wash hands. Put on gloves for any procedure that involves contact with blood or body fluids.

   Precaution

   CAUTION: Observe standard precautions at all times. If splashing of body fluids is possible, a gown, mask or face shield, and protective eyewear must be worn.

3. **Comm** Introduce yourself. Identify the patient. Explain the procedure. Remember that this procedure has multiple steps.

4. Screen for visual acuity with a Snellen chart, Jaeger card, and/ or Ishihara plates as required. Record all results accurately.

5. Place the patient in a sitting position.

   NOTE: If an eye, ear, nose, and throat examination (EENT) is the only examination being done, the patient can remain dressed.

6. Ask the patient to remove glasses and/or hearing aid(s). Tell the patient to place these items in a safe place.

   NOTE: Hearing aids are sometimes *not* removed until the actual ear examination. This is particularly true if the patient cannot hear questions without a hearing aid.

7. Notify the physician that the patient is ready. Have disposable gloves available for the physician to use. The physician may put the gloves on at the start of the examination or at the point during the examination when contact with body fluids may occur.

8. Eyes are usually examined first. The physician may use a penlight or flashlight to examine the eyes and check whether the pupils of the eyes are the same size and whether they react to light. Then, turn the ophthalmoscope light on and hand the ophthalmoscope to the physician. When the physician hands the ophthalmoscope back, turn the light off if the physician did not do so.

   NOTE: Some physicians want the room light turned off during the eye examination.

9. The nose is usually examined next. Have the nasal speculum and penlight ready for use. Also have cotton-tipped applicators ready. If a culture is taken, handle the culture stick correctly.

   NOTE: Refer to Procedure 20:2A, Obtaining a Culture Specimen, if necessary.

(continues)

10. The ears are usually examined next. Pass the otoscope with its light on to the physician. Have a cotton-tipped applicator ready for use. When the examination is done, turn off the otoscope light. Place the otoscope tip in the towel-lined basin. If the physician wants to test hearing acuity, hand the physician the tuning fork. Hold the tuning fork in the middle so the physician can grasp it at the stem end. The physician will check auditory acuity (hearing) with the tuning fork (**Figures 21–31A** to **21–31C**).

11. The mouth and throat are usually examined last. Pass the tongue blade or depressor by holding it in the center. Turn on the penlight and hand it to the physician, as needed.

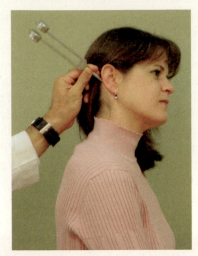

FIGURE 21-31C The physician can also check bone conduction of sound by placing the tuning fork on the mastoid bone behind the ear.

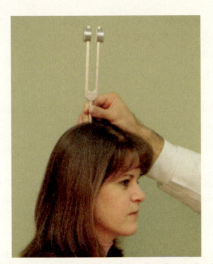

FIGURE 21-31A The physician places the vibrating tuning fork on the top of the head to ascertain whether both ears can hear the sound.

12. Have culture sticks and tubes available if a throat culture is taken. Hand these to the physician correctly.

    CAUTION: Avoid contaminating the tip of the culture stick.
   Safety

13. Take hold of the used tongue depressor in the center. Without touching either end, place it in the infectious-waste bag.

14. When the examination is complete, help the patient replace glasses, hearing aid(s), and so forth. Help the patient get off the examination table. Inform the patient of how and when they will be notified of test results.
   Comm

15. Label all specimens correctly with the patient's name, identification number, and physician's name. Print all information on the lab requisition form or use a computer-generated label. This might include date, time, patient's name, address, identification number, physician's name and identification number, type or site of specimen, and test ordered. Send all specimens to the laboratory as soon as possible.
   Comm

16. Clean and replace all equipment. Put on gloves while disinfecting and sterilizing contaminated instruments or equipment. Put all contaminated disposable supplies in the infectious-waste bag. Use a disinfectant to wipe any contaminated areas.
   Precaution

17. Remove gloves and discard in an infectious-waste bag. Wash hands.

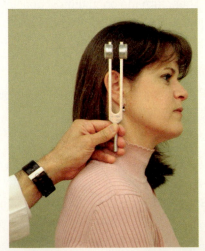

FIGURE 21-31B The physician can also test auditory acuity by placing the vibrating tuning fork about 1–2 inches away from each ear.

18.
Comm

Record all required information on the patient's chart or enter it into the computer. For example: date, time, EENT examination, throat culture sent to lab, and your signature and title. Place a copy of any lab requisitions in the patient's chart. The physician sometimes records the required information.

EHR

NOTE: In health care agencies using electronic health records (EHRs), the information is entered directly into the patient's record on a computer.

PRACTICE: Go to the workbook and use the evaluation sheet for 21:4A, Assisting with an Eye, Ear, Nose, and Throat Examination, to practice this procedure. When you believe you have mastered this skill, sign the sheet and give it to your instructor for further action.

Check

FINAL EVALUATION: Using the criteria listed on the evaluation sheet, your instructor will grade your performance.

Procedure 21:4B

Assisting with a Gynecological Examination

NOTE: The equipment and steps of this procedure can vary from physician to physician.

Equipment and Supplies

Tray covered with a towel, sheet or drape, patient gown, cotton-tipped applicators; sterile cotton-tipped applicators, gloves, lubricant, vaginal speculum, cervical spatulas (Ayer blades), cytology (cervical) brush or ThinPrep test kit, culture tubes, slides and fixative, examining light, cotton balls, basin lined with a paper towel, tissues, infectious-waste bag, patient's chart, lab requisition forms, pen and/or computer

Procedure

1. Assemble equipment and arrange on a tray or Mayo stand (**Figure 21–32**).

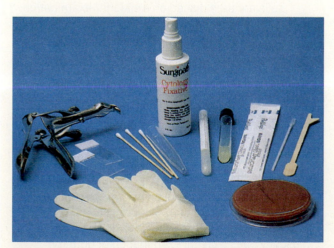

FIGURE 21-32 Basic equipment for a gynecological examination.

2. Wash hands. Put on gloves.

Precaution

CAUTION: Gloves must be worn when any contact with vaginal secretions is possible. If splashing of fluids is possible, a gown, mask or face shield, and protective eyewear must be worn.

3.
Comm

Introduce yourself. Identify the patient. Explain the procedure. Remember that this procedure has multiple steps.

4. Ask the patient to void. If a urinalysis is ordered, obtain the urine specimen at this time.

NOTE: An empty bladder makes it easier for the physician to palpate the uterus.

5. Ask the patient to remove all clothing and put on an examination gown. The gown is usually open in the front to facilitate the breast examination.

6. Make sure the extension of the examining table is pushed in or dropped down. Then assist the patient into a sitting position on the table. Use the drape to cover the patient's lap and legs.

7. Notify the physician that the patient is ready for examination.

8. The breasts are usually examined first. After the physician has examined the breasts, place the patient in the horizontal recumbent position. Drape correctly. The physician will usually complete the breast examination at this point.

Comm

NOTE: The patient should be taught how to do a breast self-examination, or BSE (refer to Figure 7–86). This can be done before or after the examination. Pamphlets describing the procedure, available from the American Cancer Society, can be given to the patient.

(continues)

9. Place the patient in the lithotomy position. Drape correctly. Position the examining light for proper lighting.

10. Warm the vaginal speculum by placing it in warm water or rubbing it with a clean towel. Hand the speculum in the closed position to the physician. Have cotton-tipped applicators ready for use.

    NOTE: Lubricant is not placed on the speculum because it can distort the shape of cervical cells for a Pap test and/or organisms if a culture is being obtained.

11. If a culture is to be taken, hand the sterile applicator to the physician. Take care to avoid contaminating the tip. Have the culture tube or slide available to receive the culture.

12. If a Pap test is to be done, hand the physician the cervical spatula (Ayer blade). Grasp the blade in the center and place the blunt end in the physician's hand. The V-shaped end is inserted in the patient by the physician.

    NOTE: A cytology (cervical) brush may be used in place of or in addition to the cervical spatula. Again, grasp the brush in the center, with the brush end directed toward the patient, to hand the brush to the physician.

    NOTE: If a ThinPrep Pap smear is being done, hand the physician the cytology (cervical) broom from the test kit (**Figure 21–33**).

    NOTE: A Pap test is done to detect cancer of the cervix.

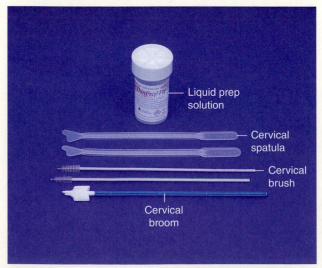

FIGURE 21-33 A cervical broom is usually used to perform a ThinPrep Pap smear, but some physicians use a cervical spatula.

13. If a conventional Pap test is being performed:

    a. Have a slide ready for use. The physician will place the smear on the slide or hand the cervical spatula or cytology brush to you. If the latter, spread the smear evenly and moderately thin on the slide.

       NOTE: If the smear is too thick, the cells cannot be seen.

    b. Put the cervical spatula or cytology brush in the infectious-waste bag.

    c. Frequently, two or three slides are prepared: a cervical smear, a vaginal smear, and/or an endocervical smear. Label each slide with the patient's name and place a *C* on the cervical slide, a *V* on the vaginal smear, and an *E* on the endocervical smear or used computer-generated labels.

    d. Apply fixative to the slide(s). The fixative is usually a spray that is applied to the entire slide. Sometimes the entire slide is placed in a specimen jar containing fixative solution.

       NOTE: Fixative makes the cells adhere (stick) to the slide until the slide is examined.

14. If a ThinPrep Pap test is being performed:

    a. Grasp the cytology broom in the middle as the physician hands it to you.

    b. Vigorously swish the cytology broom in the ThinPrep solution to wash the specimen off the brush.

       NOTE: This suspends the entire specimen in the solution. At the laboratory, the solution will be processed to eliminate blood cells, mucus, and any other substances. The remaining cervical cells are then placed on a slide for examination. By eliminating other cells and debris, the slide can be read much more accurately by either a computerized or manual method.

    c. Close the lid on the ThinPrep solution container.

    d. Discard the cytology broom in an infectious-waste bag.

15. When the physician hands you the vaginal speculum, place it in the towel-lined basin. If it is disposable, place it in the infectious-waste bag.

16. The digital (finger) examination is usually done next. Place lubricant on the physician's gloved fingers without touching the gloves. The physician usually does a digital examination of both the vagina and rectum.

17. When the examination is complete, assist the patient out of the lithotomy position. Offer tissue to the patient to remove excess lubrication. Place the tissue in the infectious-waste bag. If no signs of weakness or dizziness are noted, help the patient get off the table.

 CAUTION: Watch the patient closely to prevent falls.

18. Inform the patient how and when she will be notified of test results. Ask the patient to get dressed or assist with dressing if necessary.

19. Completely label all cultures and slides with the patient's name, identification number, and physician's name. Print all information on the lab requisition form or use a computer-generated label. This might include date, time, patient's name, address, identification number, physician's name and identification number, type or site of specimen, test ordered, date of last menstrual period, and information on any hormone therapy. Be sure you have all required information before the patient leaves the office.

20. Send all specimens to the laboratory as soon as possible.

21. Wear gloves while cleaning and sterilizing the speculum and any contaminated instruments or equipment. Put all contaminated disposable supplies in the infectious-waste bag. Use a disinfectant to wipe any contaminated areas.

22. Remove gloves and discard in an infectious-waste bag. Wash hands.

23. Record all required information on the patient's chart or enter it into the computer. For example: date, time, GYN examination, Pap smear sent to lab, and your signature and title. Place a copy of any lab requisitions in the patient's chart. The physician sometimes records the required information.

 NOTE: In health care agencies using electronic health records (EHRs), the information is entered directly into the patient's record on a computer.

PRACTICE: Go to the workbook and use the evaluation sheet for 21:4B, Assisting with a Gynecological Examination, to practice this procedure. When you believe you have mastered this skill, sign the sheet and give it to your instructor for further action.

 FINAL EVALUATION: Using the criteria listed on the evaluation sheet, your instructor will grade your performance.

Procedure 21:4C

Assisting with a General Physical Examination

NOTE: The equipment and steps of this procedure can vary from physician to physician.

Equipment and Supplies

Tray or Mayo stand and cover, patient gown, drape or sheet, basin lined with paper towels, tissues, scale, Snellen chart, thermometer, stethoscope, sphygmomanometer, ophthalmoscope, otoscope, nasal speculum, tuning fork, tongue depressors, percussion hammer, new safety pin or sensory wheel, rectal speculum or proctoscope, Pap test kit and vaginal speculum (female), culture tubes, slides, fixative solution, sterile applicators, lubricant, alcohol swabs, gloves, penlight or examining light, infectious-waste bag, patient's chart, lab requisition forms, pen, and/or computer

Procedure

1. Assemble equipment. Arrange equipment conveniently on the Mayo stand or tray (**Figure 21–34**).

2. Wash hands. Put on gloves or have gloves available for later use.

 CAUTION: Gloves must be worn anytime contact with blood or body fluids is possible. If splashing of fluids is possible, wear a gown, mask or face shield, and eye protection. Observe standard precautions at all times.

3. Introduce yourself. Identify the patient. Explain the procedure. Remember that this procedure has multiple steps.

(continues)

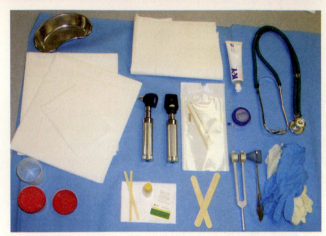

FIGURE 21-34 Equipment and supplies for a physical examination should be arranged in a convenient order.

4. Ask the patient to remove all clothing and put on an examining gown. Ask the patient to void. If a urinalysis is ordered, collect the urine specimen at this time.

5. Do any of the required following procedures:

   a. Record height and weight.

   b. Take and record TPR (temperature, pulse, respiration) and/or BP (blood pressure).

   c. Use a Snellen chart to test visual acuity; record results.

   d. Check visual acuity with a Jaeger card and/or Ishihara plates; record results.

   e. Perform an audiometric screening if ordered; record results.

   f. Run an electrocardiogram if ordered.

   g. Obtain all required blood samples for tests ordered.

6. Seat the patient on the examining table. Drape the patient correctly.

7. Notify the physician that the patient is ready.

8. Assist with eye, ear, nose, and throat examination as previously instructed.

9. Give the physician the stethoscope and/or sphygmomanometer. Remain quiet while the patient's heart and lungs are examined.

   NOTE: The physician may check the blood pressure.

   NOTE: The physician may also do an initial examination of the breasts, legs, and feet.

10. Place the patient in the horizontal recumbent or supine position. Drape correctly.

11. The physician will examine the chest and abdomen. Draw the drape down to the pubic area. Replace the drape after the abdomen has been examined.

12. The legs and feet are examined next. Have the percussion hammer ready. In addition, have an open new safety pin or sensory wheel ready in case the physician wants to use it to check sensation in the feet.

13. The back and spine are usually examined next. Turn the patient to the prone position and let the drape hang loose. Assist as needed.

    NOTE: The back and spine can also be examined with the patient in a sitting position.

14. On a female patient, a vaginal examination is usually done next. Put the patient in the lithotomy position. Drape correctly. Assist as taught for a gynecological examination. The male patient can be placed in the horizontal recumbent position for a genital organ examination.

    NOTE: Male patients should be taught how to do a testicular self-examination (refer to Section 7:14 Testicular Cancer). This can be done at this point or at the end of the examination.

15. The rectal area is examined last in most cases. A female can be examined while still in the lithotomy position or in the Sims' position. A male is usually placed in the Sims' position. Hand gloves and lubricant to the physician, as needed. Have the rectal speculum or anoscope in a closed position ready for use. If the physician wants to check fecal occult blood, put on gloves. Hand guaiac paper to the physician.

    NOTE: The physician will place a small amount of fecal material on the guaiac paper. To test the paper, add one to two drops of hemoccult developing solution to the paper. A color change indicates the presence of blood in the stool.

     CAUTION: Gloves must be worn any time contact with fecal material is possible.

    Precaution

16. When the examination is complete, assist the patient into a sitting position on the examination table. Allow the patient to rest for a few minutes. If no signs of weakness or dizziness are noted, help the patient get off the table. Inform the patient how and when they will be notified of test results. Ask the patient to get dressed or assist with dressing if necessary.

CAUTION: Watch closely to prevent falls.

Safety

17. Label all specimens and cultures with the patient's name, identification number, and physician's name. Print all information on the lab requisition form(s) or use a computer-generated form. This might include date, time, patient's name, address, identification number, physician's name and identification number, type or site of specimen, and test ordered. Send specimens to the laboratory as soon as possible.

Comm

18. Wear gloves while cleaning and sterilizing any contaminated instruments or equipment. Put all contaminated disposable supplies in the infectious-waste bag. Use a disinfectant to wipe any contaminated areas.

Precaution

19. Remove gloves and discard in an infectious-waste bag. Wash hands.

20. Record all required information on the patient's chart or enter it into the computer.

Comm

For example: date, time, physical examination, throat culture and Pap smear sent to laboratory, and your signature and title. Place a copy of any lab requisition forms in the patient's chart. The physician sometimes records the required information.

NOTE: In laboratories or offices using electronic health records (EHRs), the information is entered into the patient's EHR on a computer.

EHR

PRACTICE: Go to the workbook and use the evaluation sheet for 21:4C, Assisting with a General Physical Examination, to practice this procedure. When you believe you have mastered this skill, sign the sheet and give it to your instructor for further action.

FINAL EVALUATION: Using the criteria listed on the evaluation sheet, your instructor will grade your performance.

Check

21:5 ASSISTING WITH MINOR SURGERY AND SUTURE REMOVAL

As a health care provider, you may be required to prepare for and assist with minor surgery or suture removal in a medical, dental, or health care facility. Minor surgery includes removing warts, cysts, tumors, growths, or foreign objects; performing biopsies of skin growths or tumors; suturing wounds; incising and draining body areas; and other similar procedures.

Instruments and equipment used depend on the type of surgery or procedure being done. Some basic instruments and supplies that may be used (**Figure 21–35**) include the following:

- **Scalpels**: instruments with a handle attached to knife blades; used to incise (cut) skin and tissue; disposable scalpels with a protective retractable blade to prevent sharps injuries are also available for use (**Figure 21–36**)

- **Surgical scissors**: special scissors with blunt ends or sharp points or a combination; identified as sharp-sharp, sharp-blunt, or blunt-blunt; used to cut tissue

- **Hemostats**: special group of curved or straight instruments, usually striated at the ends; used to compress (clamp) blood vessels to stop bleeding or grasp tissue

- **Tissue forceps**: instruments with one or more fine points (or teeth) at the tip of the blades; used to grasp tissue

- **Splinter forceps**: instruments with fine-pointed ends and no teeth; used to remove splinters and other foreign objects from the skin and/or tissues

- **Towel clamps**: instruments with sharp points at the end that lock together; used to attach surgical drapes to each other; also used to clamp on to tissue that has been dissected (separated or cut into pieces)

- **Retractors**: instruments used to hold or draw back the lips, or sides, of a wound or incision; also called *skin hooks*

- **Suture materials**: special materials used for stitches (**sutures**); applied to hold a wound or incision closed; absorbable suture material such as surgical gut or vicryl is digested by tissue enzymes and absorbed by the body; nonabsorbable suture materials such as silk, nylon, Dacron, stainless steel, and metal skin clips or staples are removed after the tissue or skin has healed (**Figure 21–37**)

Surgical scissors

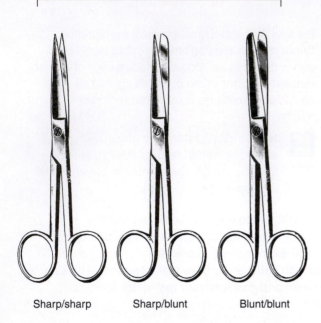

Sharp/sharp   Sharp/blunt   Blunt/blunt

Needle holder

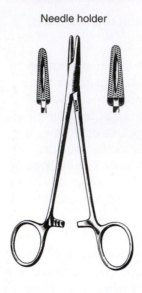

Bandage scissors

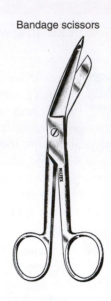

Scalpel blades and handles

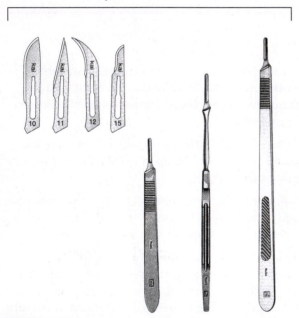

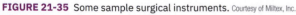

Hemostatic forceps
(curved or straight)

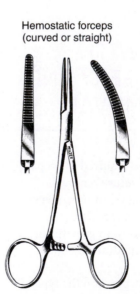

Allis tissue forceps

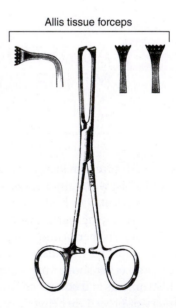

FIGURE 21-35 Some sample surgical instruments. Courtesy of Miltex, Inc.

- **Needle holder**: special instrument used to hold or support the needle while sutures are being inserted

- **Needle**: pointed, slender instrument with an eye at one end; used to hold suture material while sutures are being inserted into an incision or wound; usually curved for easier insertion into the skin; *swaged* needles have the suture material attached to the needle as one unit

- **Bandage scissors**: special scissors with blunt lower ends; used to remove dressings and bandages; the blunt ends prevent injury to the skin directly next to the dressing material

Preparation of the surgical tray requires the use of strict sterile technique to prevent infection. Instruments and supplies must be sterilized. Care must be taken to avoid contaminating the instruments and supplies when they are placed on the tray. Complete sterile setups are

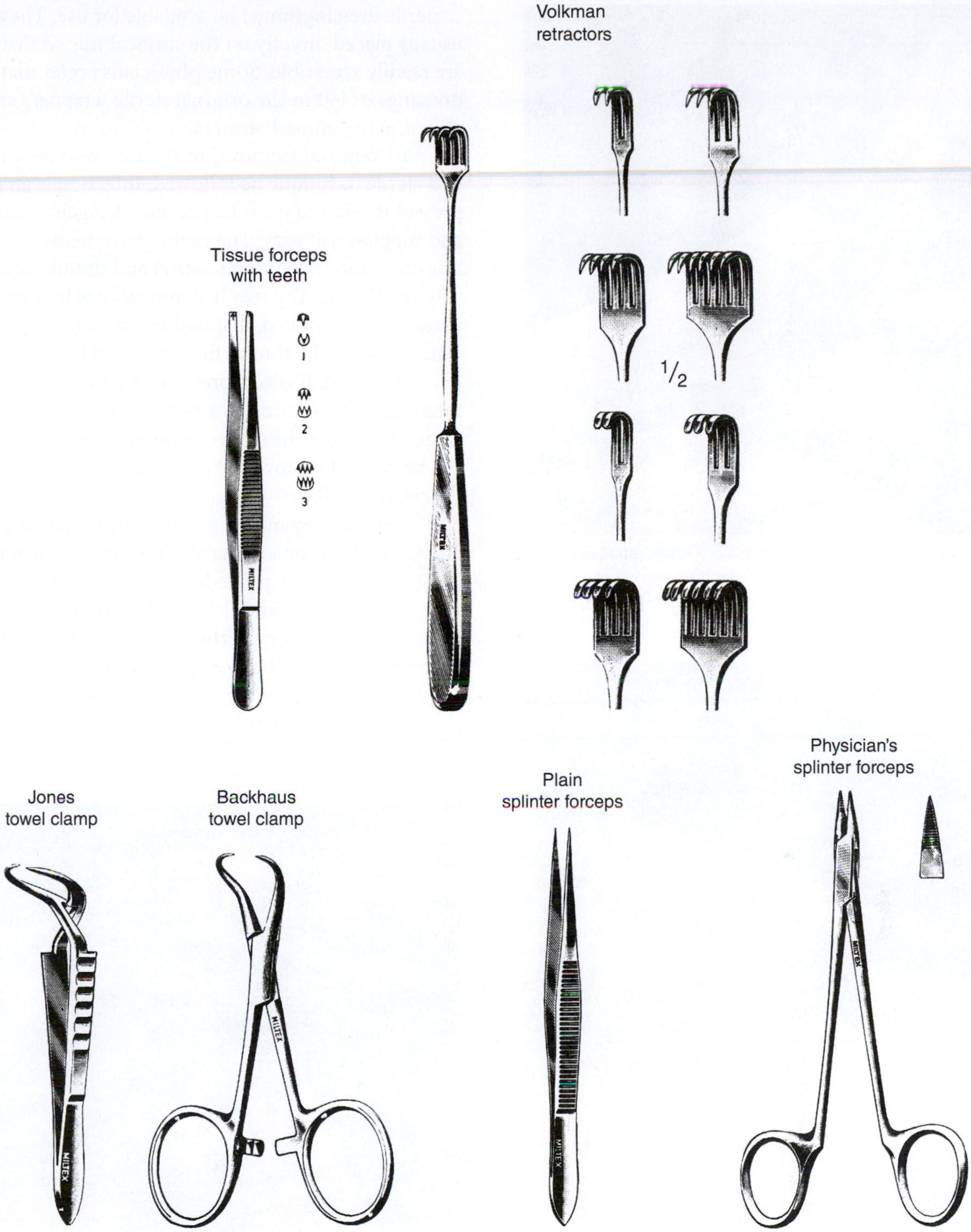

Volkman
retractors

Tissue forceps
with teeth

$\frac{1}{2}$

Jones
towel clamp

Backhaus
towel clamp

Plain
splinter forceps

Physician's
splinter forceps

FIGURE 21-35 *(continued)* Courtesy of Miltex, Inc.

also available in commercially prepared, disposable packages. Examples include setups for insertion of sutures and for removal of sutures. It is important to follow sterile technique (see Section 15:8) while opening the packages to maintain sterility of all materials in the package.

A skin prep is sometimes done before minor surgery. This means that the surgical site is cleansed thoroughly with an antiseptic soap. If the surgical area has excessive

hair, the area may be shaved. Shaving the surgical area is controversial because shaving increases the risk for abrasions leaving open areas that are prone to infection. The person doing the skin prep should wear gloves. The entire surgical area must be washed thoroughly with an antiseptic soap. If the site is shaved, the skin is held taut while a disposable razor is used to shave in the direction of hair growth. It is important to avoid nicking the patient with the razor.

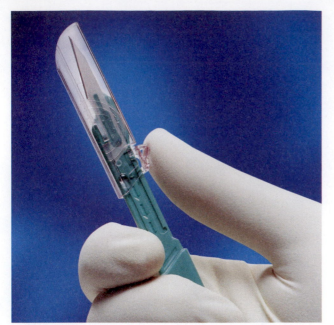

FIGURE 21-36 Disposable scalpels with a protective retractable blade help prevent sharps injuries. Photo reprinted courtesy of BD [Becton, Dickinson and Company]

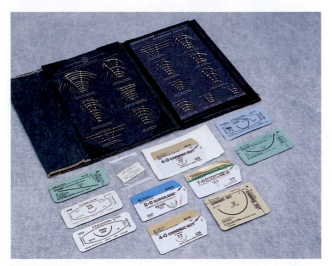

FIGURE 21-37 A wide variety of suture materials and needles are available for minor surgeries.

Before minor surgery, a local anesthetic is often administered by the physician. This numbs the surgical site and decreases pain. Before the injection of local anesthesia, the physician may apply a liquid or spray topical anesthetic to the surface of the skin to decrease the pain of the injection. Anesthetics must be available for use. They are usually placed on the side of the sterile tray. Sterile needles and syringes can be placed on the surgical tray or kept in their packages by the side of the tray.

During surgery, the medical assistant will be expected to assist as needed. The procedure will depend on the physician doing the surgery. Be alert to all points of the procedure and be ready to help as needed.

Sterile dressings must be available for use. These are usually placed directly on the surgical tray so that they are readily accessible. Some physicians prefer that sterile dressings be left in the original sterile wrappers and placed in the immediate area.

Suture removal (removal of stitches) also requires that sterile technique be followed. Infection is an ever-present threat and must be prevented. Again, instruments and supplies will vary. The main instruments used for this procedure are suture scissors and thumb forceps (**Figure 21–38**). The two instruments are frequently packaged in sterilized, disposable kits called **suture removal sets**. The thumb forcep is used to grasp and hold the suture. It is compressed with the thumb and forefinger. The suture scissors have a curved blade that is inserted under the suture material so that the stitch can be cut and removed. Basic guidelines are provided in Procedure 21:5B.

Legal

Before any minor surgery, the patient must sign a written consent form. The consent form must describe the procedure, cite alternative treatments, and list possible complications and/or risks of the surgery. If the patient is a minor or is incompetent, an authorized person must sign the form. Most offices also provide written preoperative and postoperative instructions.

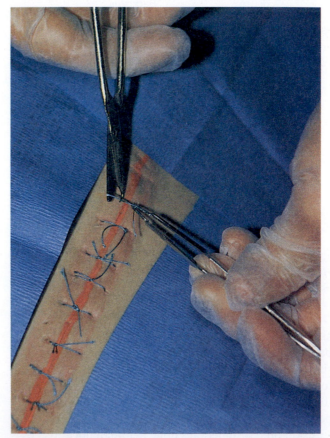

FIGURE 21-38 A suture removal set consists of suture scissors and thumb forceps.

Comm

Patients who are undergoing minor surgery or suture removal are often fearful and apprehensive. Reassure the patient to the best of your ability. Refer specific questions regarding the surgery or procedure to the physician.

Body tissues, abnormal growths, and other specimens removed during surgery are usually sent to a laboratory for examination. Each specimen must be placed in an appropriate container immediately to avoid loss. A biopsy specimen is usually placed in a formalin solution that preserves the specimen until it can be examined. Most laboratories will provide a health care facility with the required specimen containers. The containers must be labeled correctly, and the lab requisition form must be filled in completely. Many labs use computer-generated forms. The specimens should be sent to the laboratory as soon as possible.

Precaution

Because contamination from blood and body fluids is possible during minor surgical procedures, standard precautions (discussed in Section 15:4) must be observed at all times. Hands must be washed frequently, and gloves must be worn. If splashing of blood or other body fluids is possible, a gown, mask or face shield, and eye protection must be worn. Instruments and equipment must be properly cleaned and sterilized after use. Contaminated areas must be wiped with a disinfectant. Contaminated disposable supplies must be placed in an infectious-waste bag prior to being disposed of according to legal requirements. Sharp objects such as scalpel blades (or disposable scalpels) and needles must be placed in a leakproof puncture-resistant sharps container immediately after use. The medical assistant must always be aware of and take steps to prevent the spread of infection.

checkpoint

1. List four (4) basic instruments or equipment that may be used for surgery or a procedure.

PRACTICE: Go to the workbook and complete the assignment sheet for 21:5, Assisting with Minor Surgery and Suture Removal. Then return and continue with the procedures.

Procedure 21:5A

Assisting with Minor Surgery

NOTE: Instruments and procedures vary depending on the type of surgery and the physician.

Equipment and Supplies

Tray with cover or Mayo stand, infectious-waste bag, sharps container, personal protective equipment (disposable gloves, mask or face shield, eye protection, gown), tape, patient gown, patient's chart, lab requisition forms, pen and/or computer

NOTE: All the following equipment should be sterile: towels, drapes and towel clamps, two to three pairs of sterile gloves, needle and syringe, anesthetic medication, basin, antiseptic solution, gauze pads, scalpel and blades, surgical scissors, hemostat forceps (straight and curved), tissue forceps, retractors, needle holder, needle, suture material, and dressings (gauze and pads).

Procedure

1. Assemble equipment required.

2. Wash hands.

3. Check dates and sterilization indicators on all sterile supplies to make sure the supplies are still sterile. Make sure that the package has not been wet and that there are no tears or openings on the wrap.

NOTE: Many sterile supplies are good for 1 month only.

4. Place the tray or stand in an area where there is freedom of movement and limited chance of contamination.

5. Open a sterile towel and place it on the tray so that the entire tray is covered.

NOTE: Follow the correct procedure to avoid contamination (see Section 15:8).

6. Open the other sterile towels or drapes and place them on the tray.

7. Open a sterile basin. Place it on the tray. Put the sterile gauze in the basin. Obtain the correct antiseptic solution and pour a small amount of the solution in a sink or separate container to rinse the lip of the bottle. Then hold the solution bottle approximately 6 inches above the sterile basin and carefully pour the required amount of solution into the sterile basin.

NOTE: Read the label three times to be sure you have the correct solution.

Safety

CAUTION: Avoid handling the inside of the solution bottle cap. If the cap is placed on a counter, make sure the open end, or inside, is facing up. This prevents contamination of the inside of the cap.

(continues)

CAUTION: Do *not* splash the solution onto the tray.

Safety

8. Open all wrapped instruments and place them on the tray in a convenient order, usually the order of use (**Figure 21–39**).

   NOTE: Number and type of instruments will depend on the type of surgery and the physician.

9. Open the needle and syringe and place it on the tray. Unless the physician has specified a certain size, have a variety of needles of different gauges available.

10. Open the suture packages. Place them on the tray. If specific sizes and types have not been requested by the physician, a variety of materials should be made available.

11. Place the sterile dressings on the tray. The outer dressings should be placed on the bottom of the pile. This way, the dressings are in the order of use.

    NOTE: In some offices the dressings and bandages are kept in their sterile wraps and placed to the side of the tray to be opened as needed at the end of the procedure.

12. Check the tray to be sure everything is present. Use a sterile towel to cover the tray.

    CAUTION: Do *not* leave the tray unattended because contamination of the materials may occur.

    Safety

13. Place the anesthetic solution, sterile gloves, tape, and infectious-waste bag close to the tray.

    NOTE: Several pairs of gloves should be available in case one pair becomes contaminated.

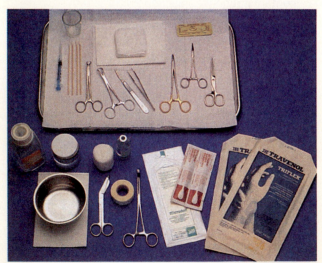

FIGURE 21-39 Instruments and supplies for minor surgery should be arranged in a convenient order. Wrapped sterile items and nonsterile items are placed by the tray.

14. Introduce yourself. Identify the patient. Confirm that the patient observed all preoperative instructions. Explain the procedure and preview postoperative orders. Ascertain that the patient has signed a written consent form.

    Comm

    NOTE: If the patient is a minor or is incompetent, an authorized person must sign the consent form.

    Legal

15. Ask the patient to empty the bladder, remove clothing as necessary for the procedure, and put on a patient gown. Provide privacy for the patient or assist if necessary.

16. Take and record the patient's vital signs.

17. Position and drape the patient according to the surgery to be performed.

18. If necessary, prep the surgical site. Wash hands and put on gloves. Wash the site thoroughly with an antiseptic soap. If a skin shave has been ordered, hold the skin taut and use a disposable razor to shave in the direction of hair growth. Discard long hairs on a gauze pad or paper towel. Rinse the area and then pat it dry with gauze.

    CAUTION: Be careful not to nick the skin.

    Safety

    NOTE: Sometimes the physician prefers to do the skin prep before the surgery. Some minor surgeries will not require a skin prep.

19. During the surgery, assist as needed:

    a. Uncover the tray when ready for use.

    b. Give the sterile gloves to the physician.

       CAUTION: If splashing of blood or body fluids is possible, a gown, mask or face shield, and eye protection must be worn. Observe all standard precautions while performing or assisting with minor surgery.

       Precaution

    c. The physician will apply sterile drapes. Have towel clamps ready for the physician to use to hold the drapes in position. The physician may cleanse the surgical site with an antiseptic.

    d. When the physician is ready to inject the anesthetic, use a gauze pad saturated with alcohol to clean the top of the anesthetic solution vial. Hold the vial in a convenient position so the physician can fill the syringe (**Figure 21–40**). The physician will then inject the anesthetic. The needle and syringe should be discarded immediately into a sharps container.

    e. If required, put on sterile gloves and assist as needed. Hold retractors, hand instruments, and assist with the procedure.

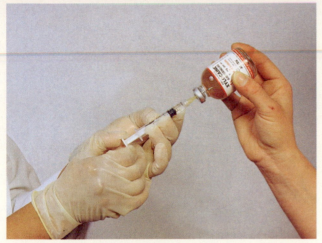

FIGURE 21-40 Hold the anesthetic solution in a convenient position so the physician can fill the syringe without contaminating the needle.

f. If tissue or a biopsy specimen is removed, open the lid of the specimen container. Hold the container close to the physician so the specimen can be placed into the container (**Figure 21–41**). Immediately close the lid on the container.

g. If the physician is going to insert sutures, have the suture material and suture needles ready for use.

h. Get additional supplies or equipment as needed.

20. After the surgery, assist as needed with placement of dressings and bandages. Observe for any signs of distress. If no signs of weakness or dizziness are noted, help the

Comm

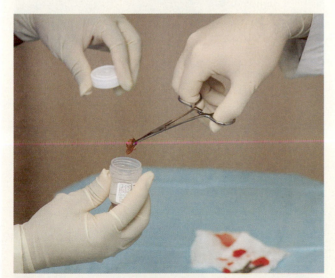

FIGURE 21-41 Tissue or biopsy specimens removed during minor surgery must be placed in the correct type of specimen container so they can be examined by a pathologist.

patient get off the table. Review postoperative orders with the patient. Provide the patient with a written copy of postoperative orders if this is office policy. Inform the patient how and when they will be notified of test results.

21. Label all specimens correctly with the patient's name, identification number, and physician's name or use a computer-generated label. Print all information on the lab requisition form. This might include date, time, patient's name, address, identification number, physician's name and identification number, type or site of specimen, and test ordered. Make sure each specimen is in the correct specimen container or bottle. Check the lids on the containers to make sure they are closed securely. Send specimens to the laboratory as soon as possible.

Comm

NOTE: Pathologists will provide special containers for most health care facilities.

22. Wear gloves to clean and sterilize all instruments and equipment. Put sharp objects such as the needle and syringe and scalpel blade (or disposable scalpel) in the sharps container immediately after use. Put contaminated disposable supplies in the infectious-waste container. Use a disinfectant to wipe any contaminated areas. Put all equipment in its correct place.

Precaution

23. Remove gloves and discard in an infectious-waste bag. Wash hands.

24. Record all required information on the patient's chart or enter it into the computer. For example: date, time, surgical removal of tumor on right forearm, specimen sent to pathology lab, verbal and written postoperative instructions given to patient, and your signature and title. Place a copy of any lab requisitions in the patient's chart. The physician sometimes records the required information.

Comm

NOTE: In health care agencies using electronic health records (EHRs), the information is entered directly into the patient's record on a computer.

EHR

PRACTICE: Go to the workbook and use the evaluation sheet for 21:5A, Assisting with Minor Surgery, to practice this procedure. When you believe you have mastered this skill, sign the sheet and give it to your instructor for further action.

FINAL EVALUATION: Using the criteria listed on the evaluation sheet, your instructor will grade your performance.

Check

Procedure 21:5B

Assisting with Suture Removal

NOTE: The procedure for suture removal varies according to the physician. The following serves as a basic guideline only.

Equipment and Supplies

Tray or Mayo stand, suture removal set, sterile towel, sterile gloves, drapes (as needed), dressings (as indicated), sterile basin, sterile gauze, antiseptic solution, tape, infectious-waste bag, sharps container, patient gown if needed, patient's chart, pen and/or computer

Procedure

1. Assemble required equipment.

2. Wash hands.

3. Check the dates and sterilization indicators on all sterile supplies to make sure the supplies are still sterile. Make sure that the package has not been wet and that there are no tears or openings on the wrap.

4. Place a sterile towel on the tray.

   NOTE: Follow the correct procedure for unwrapping and placing all supplies. Refer to Section 15:8.

5. Place a sterile basin on the tray. Put gauze and antiseptic solution in the basin.

6. Place dressings on the tray. Outer dressings should be on the bottom. This way, dressings are in order of use.

   NOTE: In some offices the dressings and bandages are kept in their sterile wraps and placed to the side of the tray to be opened as needed at the end of the procedure.

7. Place the sterile suture removal set on the tray.

8. Place a sterile towel or needed drapes on the tray.

9. Check the tray to be sure all equipment is present (**Figure 21–42**).

    CAUTION: Do *not* leave the tray unattended.
   Safety

10. Put the infectious-waste bag, tape, and sterile gloves near the tray.

11. Introduce yourself. Identify the patient. Explain the procedure. Obtain the patient's consent.
    Comm

12. If necessary, ask the patient to remove clothing and put on a patient gown. Position and drape according to location of sutures. Reassure the patient as needed.

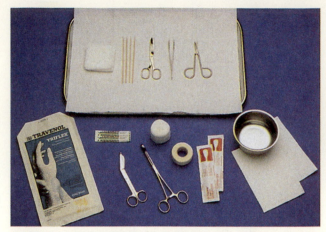

FIGURE 21-42 A sample suture removal tray setup.

13. Assist the physician as necessary during the procedure.

    🏛️ **NOTE:** Frequently, medical assistants are trained and authorized to remove sutures.
    Legal   Check the legal requirements for your state.

14. When the sutures have been removed, place a clean dressing and bandages on the wound. Use dressing forceps or wear sterile gloves to apply a sterile dressing to the site (**Figure 21–43A**). Then apply roller gauze and/or tape to anchor the dressing in place (**Figure 21–43B**).

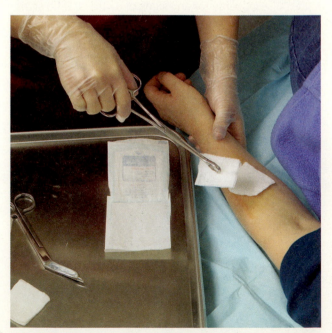

FIGURE 21-43A Use dressing forceps or wear sterile gloves to apply a sterile dressing to the site.

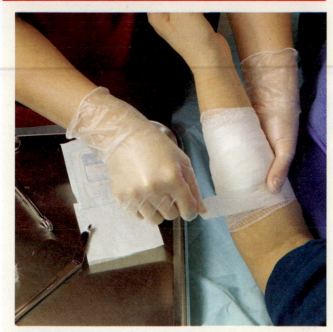

FIGURE 21-43B Anchor the dressing in place with roller gauze and/or tape.

15. Instruct the patient on wound care and provide written instructions if this is office policy. Watch closely for signs of distress. If no signs of weakness or dizziness are noted, help the patient get off the table.

Comm

16. Wear gloves to clean and sterilize all instruments. If the suture set is disposable, place it in a sharps container. Put all contaminated disposable supplies in the infectious-waste bag. Use a disinfectant to wipe any contaminated areas.

Precaution

17. Remove gloves and discard in an infectious-waste bag. Wash hands.

18. Record all required information on the patient's chart or enter it into the computer. For example: date, time, sutures removed from right forearm, sterile dressing applied, and your signature and title. The physician sometimes records the required information.

Comm

NOTE: In laboratories or offices using electronic health records (EHRs), the information is entered into the patient's EHR on a computer.

EHR

PRACTICE: Go to the workbook and use the evaluation sheet for 21:5B, Assisting with Suture Removal, to practice this procedure. When you believe you have mastered this skill, sign the sheet and give it to your instructor for further action.

FINAL EVALUATION: Using the criteria listed on the evaluation sheet, your instructor will grade your performance.

Check

21:6 RECORDING AND MOUNTING AN ELECTROCARDIOGRAM

 In order to understand an **electrocardiogram (ECG)**, it is essential to understand the electrical conduction pattern in the muscles of the heart (**Figure 21–44**). The contraction of the heart muscles is controlled by electrical impulses within the heart. The electrical impulse originates in the *sinoatrial (SA) node* of the heart, located near the top of the right atrium. The impulse moves through the atria, causing the muscles of the atria to contract. The impulse next travels to the *atrioventricular (AV) node*, through a band of fibers called the *bundle of His*, and then through the *right and left bundle branches* to the final branches,

Science

called the *Purkinje fibers.* The Purkinje fibers distribute the impulse to the muscles of the right and left ventricles, which then contract.

The movement of the electrical impulse is recorded by an electrocardiograph machine as a series of waves known as a *PQRST complex.* The P wave occurs as the impulse originates in the SA node and travels through the atria. The QRS wave represents the movement of the impulse through the AV node, bundle of His, bundle branches, and Purkinje fibers. The T wave represents the *repolarization* of the ventricles, or the period of recovery in the ventricles before another contraction occurs.

The pattern of electrical current in the heart is recorded by an electrocardiograph machine as an ECG. Each PQRST pattern represents the electrical activity that occurs during each contraction of the heart muscle; thus, each PQRST complex represents one heartbeat. Because an abnormal pattern of the electrical impulses will be evident on an ECG, the ECG can be used to diagnose disease and/or damage to the muscles of the heart.

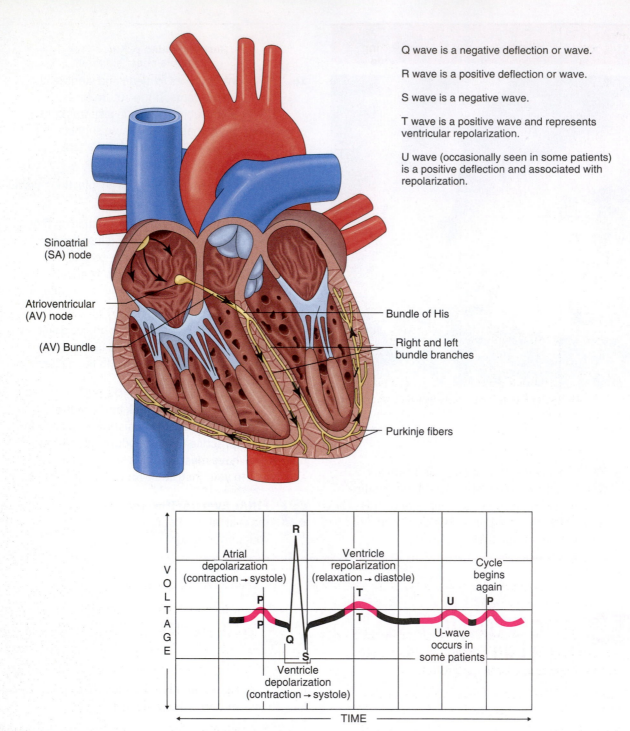

Q wave is a negative deflection or wave.

R wave is a positive deflection or wave.

S wave is a negative wave.

T wave is a positive wave and represents ventricular repolarization.

U wave (occasionally seen in some patients) is a positive deflection and associated with repolarization.

Sinoatrial (SA) node

Atrioventricular (AV) node

(AV) Bundle

Bundle of His

Right and left bundle branches

Purkinje fibers

VOLTAGE

Atrial depolarization (contraction → systole)

R

P

P

Q

S

Ventricle depolarization (contraction → systole)

Ventricle repolarization (relaxation → diastole)

T

T

Cycle begins again

U

P

U-wave occurs in some patients

TIME

FIGURE 21-44 As the electrical impulse passes through the conduction pathway in the heart, it creates a pattern recorded as an electrocardiogram.

Using special electrodes, the electrical activity is recorded from different angles, called **leads**. The different leads give the physician a more complete picture of the heart. By noting an electrical disturbance in any of the leads, the physician can determine which parts of the heart are diseased or malfunctioning.

A complete ECG normally consists of 12 leads. Electrodes are placed at specific locations on the body to pick up the voltage present. Connections between the various electrodes create the various leads. The leads are labeled as 1 (I), 2 (II), 3 (III), aVR, aVL, aVF, V_1, V_2, V_3, V4, V_5, and V_6. There are three classifications: standard, augmented, and chest leads (**Figure 21–45**).

- **Standard**, or **limb, leads**: Include leads 1 (I), 2 (II), and 3 (III) (**Figure 21–46**). Each records the voltage between two extremities.

Lead 1 (I) connects the right arm and the left arm.

Lead 2 (II) connects the right arm and the left leg.

Lead 3 (III) connects the left arm and the left leg.

Standard or bipolar limb leads	Electrodes connected	Marking code	Recommended positions for multiple chest leads (Line art illustration of chest positions)
Lead I	RA & LA	1 dot	
Lead II	RA & LL	2 dots	
Lead III	LA & LL	3 dots	
Augmented unipolar limb leads			V_1 Fourth intercostal space at right margin of sternum
aVR	RA & (LA-LL)	1 dash	V_2 Fourth intercostal space at left margin of sternum
aVL	LA & (RA-LL)	2 dashes	V_3 Midway between position 2 and position 4
aVF	LL & (RA-LA)	3 dashes	V_4 Fifth intercostal space at junction of left midclavicular line
Chest or precordial leads			V_5 At horizontal level of position 4 at left anterior axillary line
V	C & (LA-RA-LL)	(See data on right)	V_6 At horizontal level of position 4 at left midaxillary line

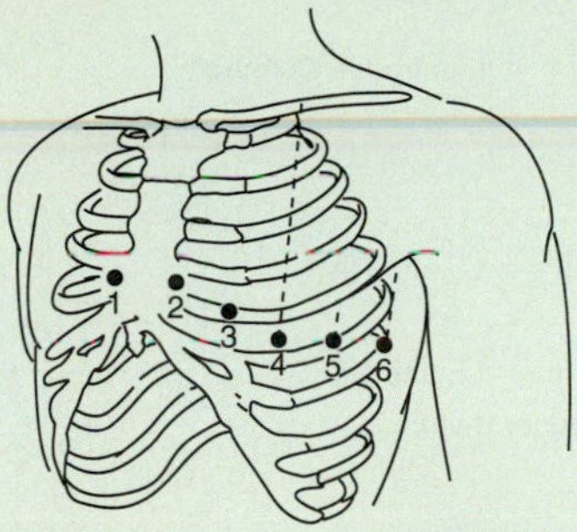

Dash—Dot

FIGURE 21-45 The lead arrangement and coding for a standard electrocardiogram. Courtesy of Quinton Cardiology, Inc.

- **Augmented voltage leads**: Include aVR, aVL, and aVF (refer to Figure 21-46). They are different angles of the standard leads 1 (I), 2 (II), and 3 (III). The aVR stands for augmented voltage right arm, aVL stands for augmented voltage left arm, and aVF stands for augmented voltage left foot.

- **Chest leads**: The six chest, or precordial, leads record angles of the electrical impulse from a central point within the heart to specific sites on the front of the chest (refer to Figure 21–46). Chest electrodes are placed at six specific locations on the chest to obtain these angles (refer to Figure 21–45).

V_1: fourth intercostal (between ribs) space on the right side of the sternum (breastbone)

V_2: fourth intercostal space on the left side of the sternum

V_3: midway between the V_2 and V_4 positions

V_4: fifth intercostal space at the junction of the midclavicular line (line drawn from the middle of the clavicle)

V_5: same level as 4 but at left anterior axillary line

V_6: same level as 4 but at left midaxillary line

Electrodes are placed on various parts of the body to record these 12 leads. The electrodes are coded so that each is put in the proper place. Codes are as follows:

- *RA* for right arm: Placed on the fleshy outer area of the upper part of the right arm

- *LA* for left arm: Placed on the fleshy outer area of the upper part of the left arm

- *RL* for right leg: Placed on the fleshy part of the lower right leg; does not record a lead but serves as a ground for electrical interference

- *LL* for left leg: Placed on the fleshy part of the lower left leg

- *C* or *V* for chest: Placed at six different locations on the chest (refer to Figure 21–45)

Electrocardiograph machines vary slightly, but most have the same basic parts. It is important to read the specific manufacturer's instructions with each machine. There are two main classes of electrocardiographs:

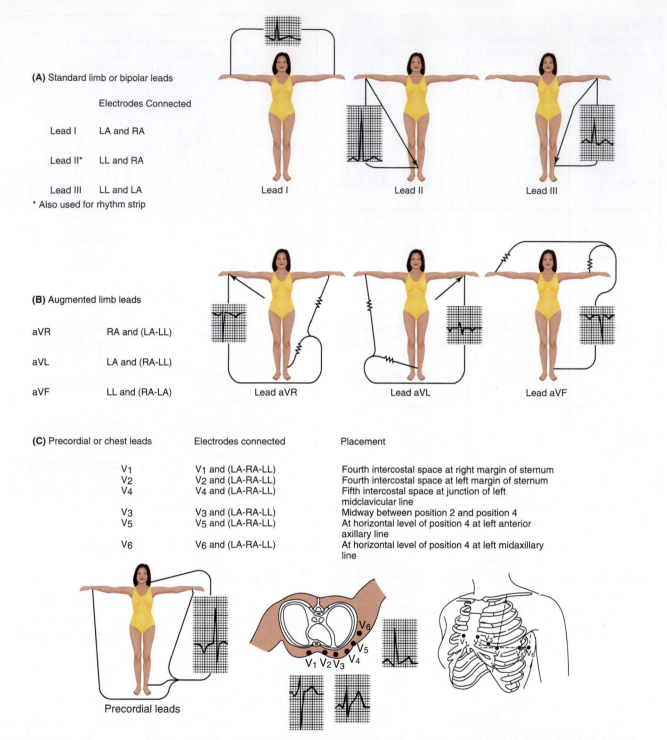

(A) Standard limb or bipolar leads

Electrodes Connected

Lead I	LA and RA
Lead II*	LL and RA
Lead III	LL and LA

* Also used for rhythm strip

Lead I   Lead II   Lead III

(B) Augmented limb leads

aVR	RA and (LA-LL)
aVL	LA and (RA-LL)
aVF	LL and (RA-LA)

Lead aVR   Lead aVL   Lead aVF

(C) Precordial or chest leads

	Electrodes connected	Placement
V1	V1 and (LA-RA-LL)	Fourth intercostal space at right margin of sternum
V2	V2 and (LA-RA-LL)	Fourth intercostal space at left margin of sternum
V4	V4 and (LA-RA-LL)	Fifth intercostal space at junction of left midclavicular line
V3	V3 and (LA-RA-LL)	Midway between position 2 and position 4
V5	V5 and (LA-RA-LL)	At horizontal level of position 4 at left anterior axillary line
V6	V6 and (LA-RA-LL)	At horizontal level of position 4 at left midaxillary line

Precordial leads

FIGURE 21-46 Lead types, connections, and placement. (A) Standard limb leads. (B) Augmented voltage (AV) leads. (C) Precordial or chest leads.

single channel and multiple channel. The single-channel electrocardiograph produces a narrow strip of paper showing one lead at a time. Most facilities use a multiple-channel electrocardiograph that produces a full sheet of paper showing all 12 leads with each lead labeled with its name (**Figure 21–47**). Multi-channel electrocardiographs can also be 3 channel machines that record 3 leads at a time until all 12 leads are recorded, or 6 channel machines.

All electrocardiographs must be calibrated correctly in order to produce an accurate electrocardiogram. A standardization check must be performed before and after every ECG for a quality-control check and to ensure that the machine is calibrated correctly to record electrical impulses. International standards require that one millivolt electrical input should cause the stylus (recording needle) to move 10 millimeters on the graph (10 small squares or 2 large

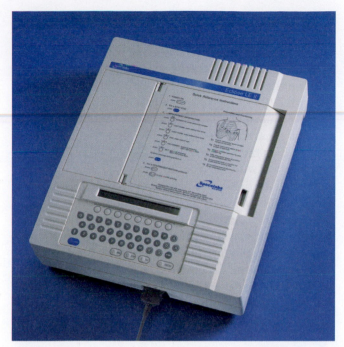

FIGURE 21-47 A multiple-channel electrocardiograph produces a full sheet of paper showing all 12 leads. Courtesy of Spacelabs Medical, Inc.

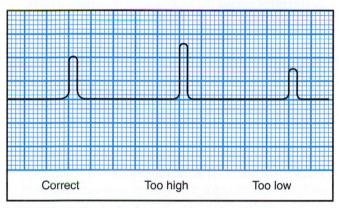

| Correct | Too high | Too low |

FIGURE 21-48 Standardization: correct, too high, too low.

25mm/SEC Chart Speed

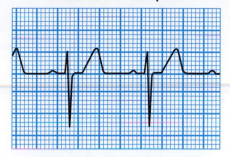

SPEED 25 engages the paper drive to run at an internationally accepted standard of 25 mm per second. This is the "normal" speed for recording.

50mm/SEC Chart Speed

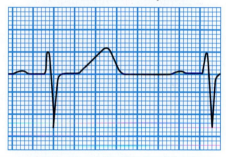

SPEED 50 doubles the speed of the paper to 50 mm per second. Useful when heart rate is rapid or when certain segments of a complex are close together, since it extends the recording to twice its normal width.

FIGURE 21-49 Speed settings for an electrocardiogram.

squares on the paper) (**Figure 21–48**). If the standard is not the correct height during the standard check, the standard control (ST'D) on the machine must be adjusted. Follow the manufacturer's instructions to adjust the standard to the proper height. Most of the newer ECG machines perform an automatic standardization when the machine is turned on and this should be checked to make sure the machine is calibrated correctly.

In addition, international standards require that the ECG paper move at a rate of 25 millimeters per second (**Figure 21–49**). However, at times complexes of the ECG are so close together that they are difficult to examine. When this occurs, the speed of the paper is increased to 50 millimeters per second, stretching the ECG out on the paper. This is often used for extremely fast tachycardias (pulse rate above 100). To make the physician aware of the increased speed, "Run 50" must be written on the paper with a pen or pencil if it is not recorded automatically by the machine.

Another problem that occurs when ECGs are recorded is the height of the PQRST complexes. A sensitivity switch is on the electrocardiograph to regulate this. Usually it is set at 1, and the standard is 10 small blocks or 2 large blocks high (**Figure 21-50**). If the complexes are very small it must be set at 2 which increases the size of the complex, making it twice as large. The standard will then be 20 small blocks or 4 large blocks high. When the complexes are so large they extend off the border of the paper, the sensitivity is set at ½. This decreases the size of the complex to one-half its normal size. The standard will then be five small blocks or one large block high. Anytime the sensitivity switch is changed, a new standard must be inserted into the recording to indicate this change.

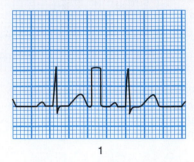
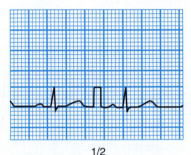
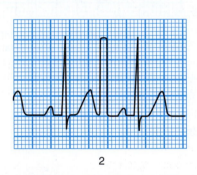
FIGURE 21-50 Sensitivity control on an electrocardiogram.

 Many patients are frightened or apprehensive about having an ECG taken. It is important to explain this procedure to the patient. Stress that it is not a painful or uncomfortable test. Position the patient comfortably with all body parts supported. Encourage the patient to relax and to avoid moving while the ECG is being taken. Muscle movement can cause electrical interference and will be displayed on the ECG recording. Nervous tension can also interfere with the recording.

After all the ECG leads have been recorded, a section of each recorded lead is mounted. Multiple-channel machines produce complete mounts. These mounts are sometimes attached to firmer backings using self-stick tape. The final mount should be neat, with each lead in the correct area on the mount. The mount should be labeled with the patient's name and address, physician's name, date, and any other pertinent information (refer to Figure 21–54).

Computerized ECG machines will retain the ECG in the computer memory so it can be viewed on the screen. Most computerized ECG machines will also provide a printed copy of an ECG. Follow the manufacturer's instructions to save the ECG correctly in the patient's electronic health record (EHR).

checkpoint

1. The electrical pulse of the heart originates from what node? Where is that node located?

PRACTICE: Go to the workbook and complete the assignment sheet for 21:6, Recording and Mounting an Electrocardiogram. Then return and continue with the procedure.

Procedure 21:6

Recording and Mounting an Electrocardiogram

 NOTE: This procedure provides basic information about recording and mounting an electrocardiogram (ECG). It is important to read the specific operating instructions provided with each electrocardiograph machine.

Equipment and Supplies

Electrocardiograph machine, electrodes, electrocardiograph cables and cords, examination gown, drape, gauze pads or disinfectant wipes, pen and/or computer

Procedure

1. Assemble required equipment.

2. Wash hands.

3. Introduce yourself. Identify the patient. Explain the procedure. Reassure the patient. Tell the patient that you will be recording the activity of the heart. Stress that the patient will not feel any discomfort from the procedure. Explain that the patient must lie perfectly still because muscle movement will interfere with the recording.

4. Ask the patient to remove clothing and put on an examination gown. The gown is usually open in the front for easy placement of the chest electrodes.

NOTE: In some offices, the patient is asked to remove clothing from the waist up and to uncover the lower legs.

5. Position the patient. Patient should be lying on a firm bed or examination table. A small pillow can be placed under the head. Use the drape to cover the patient.

6. Position the machine in a convenient location. It may be easier to work from the left side because this is where most of the chest leads are positioned.

7. Connect the power cord to the machine. Do *not* let the power cord pass under the bed or examination table. Plug it in so that it is pointing away from the patient.

CAUTION: Check the three prongs and the cord before using the power cord. Never use a defective cord for any procedure.

Safety

NOTE: Positioning the power cord away from the patient helps reduce electrical interference.

8. Obtain a package of disposable electrodes (**Figure 21–51A**). Apply the four limb electrodes. The arm electrodes are placed on the fleshy outer areas of the upper arms. The leg electrodes are placed on fleshy parts of the lower legs. Avoid bony areas. Use a gauze pad or disinfectant wipe to vigorously rub the site to stimulate circulation. If the patient's skin is oily, wipe the electrode area with alcohol and allow it to air-dry. Then, separate the electrode from the protective backing to uncover the sticky surface. Apply the electrode to the correct site using a smooth, even motion to make sure all parts of the electrode adhere to the skin. The disposable electrodes can only be used with ECG machines that have an alligator clip attached to the ends of the cable wires (**Figure 21–51B**).

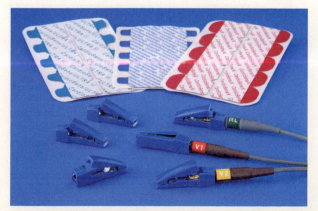

FIGURE 21-51A A disposable electrode has a sticky surface that allows the electrode to adhere to the skin. Courtesy of Spacelabs Medical, Inc.

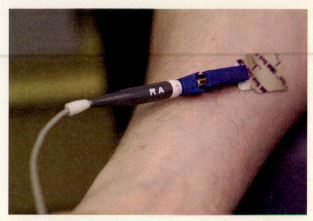

FIGURE 21-51B An alligator clip on the end of the electrocardiograph cable wire attaches to the disposable electrode.

NOTE: If the skin surface is hairy, it may be necessary to shave small areas at the application sites to allow for better attachment and conduction of the electrodes.

NOTE: Some agencies use disposable electrodes with snap connections. Use the type of electrode recommended by the manufacturer of the electrocardiograph.

9. Apply the chest electrodes. Refer to Figure 21–45 for the exact location for each electrode. Use a gauze pad or disinfectant wipe to vigorously rub the site to stimulate circulation. If the patient's skin is oily, wipe the electrode area with alcohol and allow it to air-dry. Then, separate the electrode from its protective backing to uncover the sticky surface. Apply the electrode to the site using a smooth, even motion to make sure all parts of the electrode adhere to the skin. Position all six chest electrodes in the correct locations.

NOTE: If the skin surface is very hairy, it may be necessary to shave small areas at the application sites to allow for better attachment and conduction of the electrodes.

10. Connect the cable wires to the electrodes. The lead wires should follow body contour (**Figures 21–52A** and **21–52B**). If there is excess wire, coil it in a loop and fasten with tape or a band. Pay particular attention to the labels and color codes to connect the cable ends to the correct electrodes. Make sure all connections are tight and in the same direction.

NOTE: Labels are as follows: RA for right arm; LA for left arm; RL for right leg; LL for left leg; and C or V for chest.

(continues)

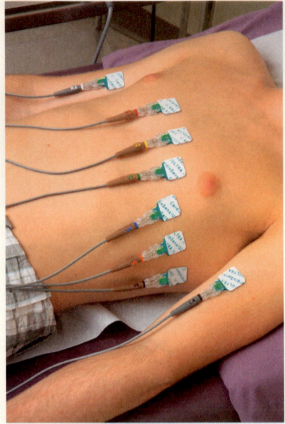

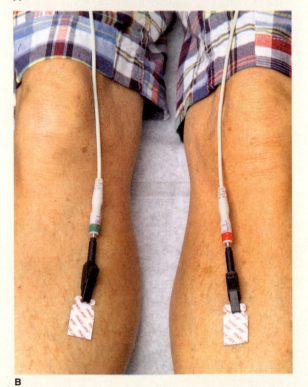

FIGURE 21-52 The lead cables should follow body contour when they are connected to the electrodes: (A) chest and arm leads and (B) leg leads.

NOTE: Color codes are as follows: white for RA, black for LA, green for RL, red for LL, and brown or multicolored for chest or V depending on the model of the ECG machine.

11. Turn on the main switch. If a computerized ECG machine is being used, enter the required patient information. The machine will print this information on the ECG.

12. Do a standardization check if the machine does not do this automatically. If the standard is not correct, adjust it to the correct height by following the manufacturer's instructions.

13. Set the control to Auto and run the 12-lead ECG. Check the ECG recording carefully as the leads are being run (**Figure 21–53**).

    NOTE: On a single-channel manual electrocardiograph, set the lead selector switch to each lead and allow the machine to record an adequate amount for each lead.

14. While running the leads, make sure the following points are noted:

    a. Make sure that the amplitude of the complexes is correct. If complexes are too small, set sensitivity to 2. If complexes are too large, set sensitivity to ½. If the sensitivity is changed, be sure to insert a standard in the lead. A standard that is five small blocks or one large block high indicates a sensitivity setting of ½. A standard that is 20 small blocks or 4 large blocks high indicates a sensitivity setting of 2.

    b. Make sure complexes are not too close together. For severe tachycardias, it is often necessary to increase the speed to Run 50. Alert the physician by marking "Run 50" on the paper

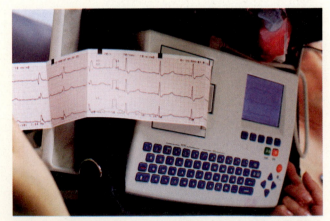

FIGURE 21-53 Check the ECG recording carefully as the leads are being run. © Kiselev Andrey Valerevich/www.Shutterstock.com

with pen or pencil unless the machine records this automatically.

c. Make sure that no electrical interference or artifact is present. Watch patient movement. Use a ground wire, as needed.

15. Run all of the leads as instructed in step 13. There is no need to turn off the machine between leads.

16. When all 12 leads have been run, turn the lead selector to the standard position. Allow all of the recording to run out of the machine. Then turn the record switch to Off.

17. Turn the power button off. Remove the electrodes from the patient and discard. Use warm water to wash the patient's skin. Dry the skin thoroughly. Help the patient get off the examination table or bed.

18. Coil all wires and replace in the proper area. Coil power cord and replace in the proper area.

NOTE: If wires are bent, they will break.

19. Write the patient's name, the date, and the physician's name on the ECG if the machine does not do this. If the ECG has been recorded with all 12 leads on one sheet of paper, it may be necessary to attach it to a self-stick mount. Follow the manufacturer's instructions. This type of ECG is sometimes simply placed in the patient's chart without mounting (**Figure 21–54**). If the ECG is one long roll from a single-channel electrocardiograph, cut it into separate leads and attach them to a mount. It is important to follow instructions provided with the mounts, and to make sure that the length for each lead is cut correctly.

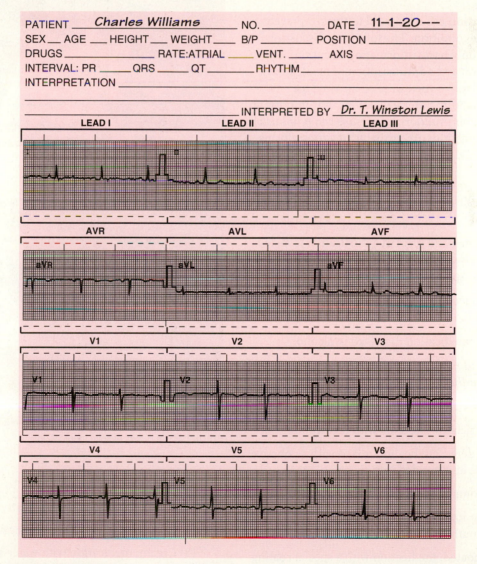

FIGURE 21-54 A mounted electrocardiogram.

(continues)

20. Wash hands.

21. Record all required information on the patient's chart or enter it into the computer. For example: date, time, ECG recorded, and your signature and title.

Comm

 NOTE: In health care agencies using electronic health records (EHRs), the information is entered directly into the patient's record on a computer.

EHR

PRACTICE: Go to the workbook and use the evaluation sheet for 21:6, Recording and Mounting an Electrocardiogram, to practice this procedure. When you believe you have mastered this skill, sign the sheet and give it to your instructor for further action.

 FINAL EVALUATION: Using the criteria listed on the evaluation sheet, your instructor will grade your performance.

Check

21:7 WORKING WITH MEDICATIONS

 A **medication** is a drug used to treat or prevent a disease or condition. The following discussion provides only basic information about the preparation and administration of medications. Even so, it should make you aware of the need for extreme care in handling all medications. It is important to remember that *only authorized persons can administer medications*. Medications are available in various forms, usually liquids, solids, or semi-solids.

Legal

- **Liquids:**

  (1) Aqueous suspension: medication is dissolved in water

  (2) Suspension: solid form of a medication is mixed with solution; usually must be shaken well before use to resuspend the medication in the solution

  (3) Syrup: concentrated solution of sugar, water, and medication

  (4) Tincture: medication dissolved in alcohol

  NOTE: *Liquid medications must be poured at eye level to ensure that the dosage is exact (**Figure 21–55**).*

- **Solids (Figure 21–56):**

  (1) Capsule: gelatin-like shell with medication inside

  (2) Pill: powdered medication mixed with a cohesive substance and molded into shape

  (3) Tablet: compressed or molded preparation

  (4) Troche or lozenge: large, flat disc that is dissolved in the mouth

  (5) Enteric coated: medication with a special coating that does not dissolve until the substance reaches the small intestine

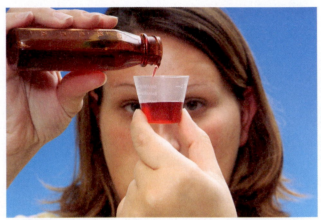

FIGURE 21-55 Liquid medications must be poured at eye level to ensure the dosage is correct.

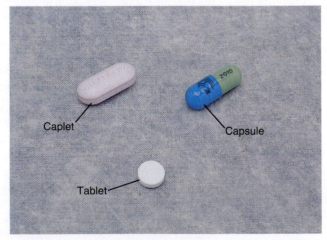

FIGURE 21-56 Types of solid medications.

- **Semi-solids:**

  (1) Ointment: medication in a fatty base

  (2) Paste: ointment with an adhesive substance

  (3) Cream: medication with water-soluble base

  (4) Suppository: a cone-shaped object that usually has a base material of cocoa butter or glycerin

mixed with the medication; usually inserted into the rectum or vagina where it melts as a result of body heat and dispenses the medication; used rectally to stimulate peristalsis and aid in expelling feces, relieve pain, decrease body temperature (aspirin suppositories), and stop vomiting (antiemetics); used vaginally to treat infection, administer hormones, or as contraceptive for birth control

Medications may be given in a variety of ways. Some of the routes of administration are:

- **Oral**: given by mouth; for liquid and solid forms
- **Rectal**: given in the rectum; liquids and suppositories
- **Injections**: given with a needle and syringe; often called *parenteral*, which means any route other than the alimentary canal (digestive tract) (**Figure 21–57**).

  (1) Subcutaneous (subQ): injected into the layer of tissue just under the skin

  (2) Intramuscular (IM): injected into a muscle

  (3) Intravenous (IV): injected into a vein

  (4) Intradermal: injected just under the top layer of skin; the skin tests for allergies and tuberculosis (TB) are examples

- **Topical or local**: applied directly to the top of the skin; ointments, sprays, liquids, and adhesive patches; transdermal adhesive patches applied to the skin can be used to provide a continuous dosage of medication for motion sickness, heart disease, hormonal imbalance, and nicotine withdrawal (for individuals who are trying to stop smoking) (**Figures 21–58A** and **21–58B**)

- **Inhalation**: inhaled, or breathed in, by way of sprays, inhalers, or special machines
- **Sublingual**: given under the tongue

Before administering any medication, it is essential to check for complete information about the medication. An excellent source of information on drugs is the ***Physician's Desk Reference* (PDR)**. It used to be published as a book annually but now is only available on the website *www.pdr.net*. Another accurate site sponsored by the National Institutes of Health is *MedlinePlus* at *www.medlineplus.gov* in the section on drugs and supplements. A site provided by the Food and Drug Administration (FDA) at *www.drugs.com/fda-consumer/* is also excellent. In addition to the websites, the packet inserts provided in medication packages also provide valuable information.

Information that must be obtained from these sources about any medication or drug before administering the drug include the following:

- **Action of drug**: tells how the drug works and what it should do
- **Uses of drug**: provides all approved reasons why the drug is used to treat specific conditions; also, frequently provides information on conditions that the drug treats that are unlabeled uses
- **Availability or how supplied**: lists all forms of the drug or routes of administration such as capsules, pills, injectables, or liquids
- **Dosage**: indicates correct dose for each form of the medication and for the specific condition for which it is being used; categorizes the dosages according to the age of the person taking the drug
- **Administration**: provides information on correct storage, special precautions such as capsules not being chewed or crushed, taking the medication with food, drinking large amount of fluid with medication, and similar factors
- **Adverse effects**: indicates all side effects that may be experienced from minor to major
- **Contraindications**: lists diseases or reasons why the medication should *not* be taken
- **Cautions for use**: emphasizes times it may be dangerous to administer this medication
- **Interactions**: provides a list of other medications that may interact with this drug and how its use would interfere with the action of other medication or decrease in effectiveness

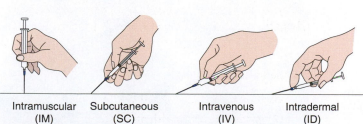

Angle of Injection for Parenteral Administration of Medications

FIGURE 21-57 Types of injections and the correct angles for administration of parenteral medications.

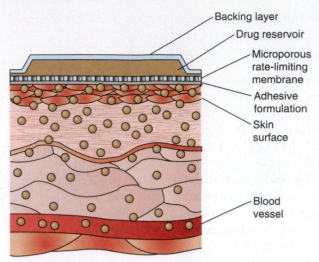

FIGURE 21-58A The layers of a transdermal patch allow the medication to be absorbed into the bloodstream over a period of time, frequently 24 hours.

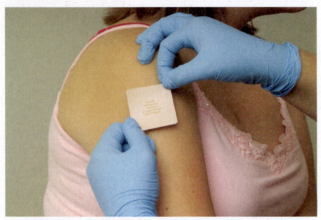

FIGURE 21-58B A transdermal patch is applied to the skin.

There are six main points to watch each and every time a medication is given. These can be called the "six rights."

- Right medication
- Right dose, or amount
- Right patient
- Right time
- Right method or mode of administration
- Right documentation

Certain safety rules must be observed when giving medication.

- Read the order carefully. Note all six *rights*.
- Check for patient allergies before administering any medication.
- Check the label three times to be sure it is the correct medication (**Figure 21–59**). The label must be read when the bottle is taken from the shelf, as the medication is poured, and when the bottle is replaced on the shelf.

- Prepare or administer medication only on the order of a physician.
- *Never* administer a medication you did not personally prepare.
- Know the action of the drug, the usual dosage, the route of administration, and the side effects.
- Store medications in a safe, cool, dry area. Make sure they are out of the reach of children.
- Check expiration dates on all medications. Medications must *never* be used beyond the expiration date and expired medications must be destroyed. Follow agency policy and federal and state laws to dispose of medications. If the policies/laws call for destruction of the medications, many states have prescription drug drop boxes at specific pharmacies or law enforcement agencies. The medications are destroyed following recommendations of the Food and Drug Administration (FDA) and the Environmental Protection Agency (EPA). Record all required information regarding the destruction of the medication according to agency policy. Expired controlled substances, such as narcotics, *must* be returned to the pharmacy as required by law. Make sure you complete all required documentation when you return expired controlled substances to the pharmacy. If a partial amount of a unit dose (single dose package) of a controlled substance is used because of the dosage ordered, witnesses must cosign when the remaining medication is destroyed.
- *Never* use medication from an unmarked bottle. Make sure the label is clear. If in doubt, throw it out.
- Do *not* return medication to a bottle. This can lead to serious errors. Discard any medication that is *not* used.

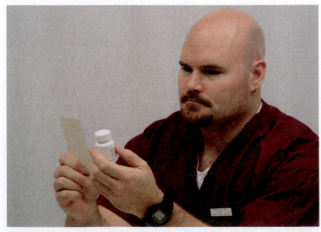

FIGURE 21-59 Check the label of any medication at least three times.

- Report all mistakes immediately.
- Concentrate while handling any medication. Avoid distractions.
- Use paper and pencil to calculate dosages. Avoid "mental" math because it can cause errors.

 Only legally authorized health care providers can administer medications. Administering medications is a major responsibility and every effort must be made to make sure the correct drug and dosage is given to the patient. Always use the *PDR* or other drug websites or the literature that comes with each medication to learn the basic information about the medication. *Question dosages or uses that do not seem correct.* It is your responsibility to determine what you are legally permitted to do.

checkpoint

1. What are the "six rights" or six (6) main points to watch every time a medication is given?

PRACTICE: Go to the workbook and complete the assignment sheet for 21:7, Working with Medications.

Today's Research   Tomorrow's Health Care

The Nose Knows Cancer?

The American Cancer Society estimates that each year in the United States over 1.8 million people will be diagnosed with some type of cancer and more than 606,520 people will die. Even though treatment for cancer has improved and many lives have been saved, some types of cancers are extremely difficult to detect at an early stage when a cure is most likely. Examples include stomach, bone, kidney, pancreatic, and ovarian cancer.

Now scientists all over the world are researching the possibility of a "smell test" for cancer. Initially, researchers in California trained five different dogs to smell breast and lung cancer on a patient's breath. The dogs were able to identify breast cancer 88 percent of the time and lung cancer 99 percent of the time. A group of researchers in Germany trained four dogs, three shepherds and a Lab, to detect lung cancer using breath samples from 100 patients with lung cancer. When the dogs were given 400 other samples from individuals without lung cancer, the dogs only had an 8 percent false positive rate. In the latest studies, Beagles detected lung cancer by smelling blood serum with an accuracy of 96.7 percent. Labrador retrievers detected colorectal cancer by smelling the watery stool from patients with the disease with an accuracy of 97 percent. Schnauzers detected cancer cells in the blood of ovarian cancer patients after treatment when they tested cancer free. In all cases, the cancer returned as a result of those residual cancer cells that only the dogs could identify. German shepherds detected prostate cancer by smelling urine with almost 100 percent accuracy.

Researchers think the dogs were able to smell the cancers by sensing minute amounts of volatile organic compounds (VOCs) that are end products of metabolism, which are excreted in breath, urine, and feces. Some researchers are isolating polyamines, molecules linked to cell growth and differentiation, because cancer raises polyamine levels and they have a distinct odor. Estimates are that a dog's sense of smell can be 10,000 to 100,000 times superior to a human's sense of smell, so the dogs can detect minute quantities of the VOCs. Does that mean that in the future every medical facility or physician's office will have a cancer-sniffing dog on staff? Of course not, but this research has created a unique way of developing tests that will detect cancer in its early stages.

Currently, many researchers are working to identify and isolate the chemical compounds associated with different types of cancers. This is very challenging because the smell of cancer is probably made up of many different chemicals. In fact, each type of cancer might have a very unique chemical combination. At the same time, researchers are trying to develop artificial noses that will be able to detect specific chemical compounds. Recently, several electronic noses (e-noses) have been produced and are being used in trial studies. Initial studies have had some success. One e-nose was able to distinguish between lung cancer patients and high-risk smoking patients without cancer 80 percent of the time. Another model was able to identify prostate cancer from the scent of urine 78 percent of the time. A third e-nose checking fecal gas identified 73–85 percent of patients with colorectal cancer. Once the compounds associated with cancer are identified, it may be possible to modify the e-nose to detect them by inserting sensors to detect the specific compounds. Eventually, it is very possible that a simple noninvasive test using scents from breathing, urine, feces, and even blood could lead to early detection of cancer. Man's best friend may have started research that will save many lives.

What skills should Max and Molly have in order to be a part of the health care team at the Hill Country Medical Clinic? If Max is unfamiliar with a procedure or skill what should he do? How can Molly help him?

CHAPTER 21 SUMMARY

- A basic knowledge of the main skills used by medical assistants is beneficial for many health care providers, because many of these skills are used in other health care areas.

- Height and weight measurements are important in evaluating basic health status of patients. Thus, knowing how to correctly measure height and weight is important for every health care provider.

- By following correct positioning techniques, the medical assistant can properly prepare patients for examinations, as well as provide patients with comfort and privacy.

- A knowledge of the basic instruments used and procedures performed during physical examinations, minor surgery, and suture removal allows the medical assistant to work with the physician to provide quality health care to the patient in an efficient manner.

- Understanding the basic principles of electrocardiography allows the medical assistant to efficiently record an electrocardiogram.

- A knowledge of how to find information on medications and of correct techniques for dispensing medications is also an important responsibility of the medical assistant.

REVIEW QUESTIONS

1. Why are height and weight measurements important?

2. Identify at least six(6) different positions that can be used for examinations and/or treatments. For each position, list at least two (2) types of treatments or examinations that are performed when a patient is in the position.

3. Differentiate between a Snellen chart, Jaeger card, and an Ishihara plate by stating the type of eye defects evaluated with each method.

4. Interpret or define each of the following:
   a. OU
   b. OS
   c. OD
   d. myopia
   e. hyperopia

5. Name the areas of the body examined and the type of tests performed during each of the following examinations:
   a. EENT
   b. gynecological
   c. general physical

6. Explain at least five (5) standard precautions that must be observed while assisting with minor surgery and/or suture removal.

7. What is the difference between a hemostat and a needle holder? What is the function of each instrument?

8. Name the twelve (12) leads for an electrocardiogram and state the location of the electrodes (for example, right arm or RA) used to record each lead.

9. List the six (6) "rights" that must be observed while administering any medication.

For additional information on medical assisting careers, contact the following associations:

- American Association of Medical Assistants
  www.aama-ntl.org

- American Medical Association
  www.ama-assn.org

- American Medical Technologists Association (AMT)
  www.americanmedtech.org

■ CRITICAL THINKING

1. Use the *Physicians' Desk Reference* (PDR) website to find the medication Celebrex. List the main action of this drug, suggested dosage, route of administration, and warnings/side effects. Create a patient information brochure about this drug.

2. Referring to Section 21:5; create a set of flashcards with a sketch of a surgical instrument on one side and on the other side write down the instrument's use. Study the flashcards to learn all of the instruments.

■ ACTIVITIES

1. In a group of four (4) create a script for the following scenario:

Mrs. Sanchez brought her baby girl, Anna, to Dr. Tran's office for her 6-week check-up. She also brought her two other children, Carlos and Robert, because they have a headache and fever. Renae is the medical assistant at Dr. Tran's clinic. She calls the Sanchez family back and processes them in. She obtains and records all measurements and their chief complaints. Dr. Tran looks in both boys and Anna's ears and orders an immunization update for everyone and antibiotics for Carlos and Robert.

1a. In the same group, role play the script. Modify the scenario by making the boys combative and not wanting to stand still for a shot.

2. Working with another student, obtain a CPR manikin to demonstrate the correct placement of a 12 lead ECG or sketch the information on a piece of paper.

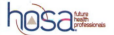 | CONNECTION

Competitive Event: Medical Assisting

Event Summary: Medical Assisting provides members with the opportunity to gain knowledge and skills required to assist in administrative and clinical tasks. This competitive event consists of 2 rounds. Round One is a written, multiple choice test and the top scoring competitors will advance to Round Two for the skills assessment. This event aims to inspire members to become allied health professionals who respond and assist efficiently in clinical settings.

Details on this competitive event may be found at

www.hosa.org/guidelines

CHAPTER 22 NURSE ASSISTANT SKILLS

Career   OBRA

Case Study Investigation

Stonybrook Hospital employs David and Imani as surgical floor nursing assistants. They work at a fast pace to keep up with the surgery schedule, procedures, and bedside care. At the end of this chapter, you will be asked about the skills David and Imani will need to work on this type of a medical/surgical unit.

◼ LEARNING OBJECTIVES

After completing this chapter, you should be able to:

- Admit, transfer, or discharge a patient, demonstrating proper care of the patient's belongings.
- Position a patient in correct alignment and with no bony prominences exposed.
- Move and turn a patient in bed, using correct body mechanics.
- Perform the following transfer techniques (using correct body mechanics): dangling, wheelchair, chair, and stretcher.
- Transfer a patient by way of a mechanical lift and observe all safety points.
- Make closed, open, and occupied beds, using correct body mechanics.
- Administer routine, denture, and special oral hygiene.
- Administer hair care and nail care.
- Administer a back rub, using the five major movements.
- Shave a patient using a safety or an electric razor, observing all safety precautions.
- Change a patient's gown or pajamas.
- Administer a partial bed bath and a complete bed bath with perineal care.
- Help a patient take a tub bath or shower, observing all safety points.
- Measure and record intake and output.
- Assist a patient with eating; feed a patient.
- Administer a bedpan or urinal.
- Provide catheter care.
- Empty a urinary-drainage unit without contaminating the catheter or unit.

LEARNING OBJECTIVES *(continued)*

- Provide ostomy care.
- Collect urine and stool specimens.
- Apply restraints, observing all safety precautions.
- Administer preoperative care as directed.
- Prepare a postoperative unit with all equipment in the correct position.
- Apply surgical (elastic) hose.
- Safely administer oxygen with an oxygen mask, nasal cannula, or tent.
- Give postmortem care.
- Define, pronounce, and spell all key terms.

KEY TERMS

alignment *(ah-line'-ment)*
anesthesia *(an-es-thee'-sha)*
bed cradle
binders
catheter
clean-catch (mid-stream) specimen
closed bed
colostomy
complete bed bath (CBB)
contracture *(kon-track'-tyour")*
dangling
defecate *(deaf'-eh-kate")*
dehydration *(dee"-high-dray'-shun)*
edema *(eh-dee'-mah)*
fanfolding

ileostomy
intake and output (I&O)
mechanical lifts
micturate *(mick'-chur-rate")*
mitered corners *(my'-terd corn"-urz)*
Montgomery straps
occult blood *(ah-kult")*
occupied bed
open bed
operative care
oral hygiene
ostomy
partial bed bath
personal hygiene
postmortem care
postoperative care

preoperative care
pressure (decubitus) ulcer *(deh-ku'-beh-tuss uhl"-sir)*
restraints
sequential compression device (SCD)
stoma
stool specimen
surgical (elastic) hose
24-hour urine specimen
ureterostomy
urinary-drainage unit
urinate
urine specimen
void
wound VAC

Career

Nurse assistants, also called nurse aides, nurse technicians, patient care technicians (PCTs), patient care assistants (PCAs), and orderlies, work under the supervision of registered nurses or licensed practical/vocational nurses. They are important members of the health care team. Educational requirements vary with states, but many assistants obtain training through health science education (HSE) programs. Assistants who work in long-term care facilities or home health must complete a minimum of 75–120 hours in a mandatory state-approved program and pass a written and/or competency examination to obtain certification or registration. Additional educational requirements include continuing education, periodic evaluation of performance, and retraining if the assistant is not employed for two or more years.

Geriatric aides or assistants provide care for patients in environments such as extended care facilities, nursing homes, retirement or assisted-living centers, and adult day care agencies.

Home health assistants or aides perform many of the duties of nurse assistants, but they provide care in the patient's home, usually for an extended period. Examples of patients who require home care include patients who have just been discharged from a hospital or long-term care facility, patients who have a disability, elderly patients who require assistance, and patients receiving hospice care. In addition to performing many of the personal care duties of the nurse assistant, home health assistants may also shop for food and prepare meals, maintain and clean the home environment, wash laundry, and accompany patients on shopping trips or to medical appointments. Throughout this chapter, special notes are provided to help a home health assistant adapt the procedure to home care.

Legal

The duties of nurse assistants vary depending on the facility in which they work and on the nursing practice laws of the state in which they work. *Every nurse assistant must know and follow the legal requirements of the state in which they are employed.* In addition to the knowledge and skills presented in this chapter, nurse assistants must also learn and master skills such as:

- Presenting a professional appearance and attitude
- Obtaining knowledge regarding health care delivery systems, organizational structure, and teamwork
- Meeting all legal responsibilities
- Communicating effectively
- Being sensitive to and respecting cultural diversity
- Comprehending anatomy, physiology, and pathophysiology
- Learning medical terminology

- Observing all safety precautions
- Practicing all principles of infection control
- Taking and recording vital signs
- Administering first aid and cardiopulmonary resuscitation
- Promoting good nutrition and a healthy lifestyle to maintain health
- Measuring and recording height and weight
- Positioning patients for and assisting with examinations and treatments

- Administering basic physical therapy including range-of-motion exercises, ambulation with assistive devices, and warm or cold applications
- Performing basic laboratory tests, such as monitoring glucose or testing urine with reagent strips
- Using computer and technology skills
- Recording information on patient records

LEGAL ALERT

Legal

Before performing any procedures in this chapter, know and follow the standards and regulations established by the scope of practice; federal laws and agencies; state laws; state or national licensing, registration, or certification boards; professional organizations; professional standards; and agency policies.

It is your responsibility to learn exactly what you are legally permitted to do and to perform only procedures for which you have been trained.

22:1 ADMITTING, TRANSFERRING, AND DISCHARGING PATIENTS

OBRA

As a health care team member in a hospital or long-term care facility, one of your responsibilities may be to admit, transfer, and discharge patients or residents. Although these procedures vary slightly in different facilities, basic principles apply in all facilities.

Comm

Admission to a health care facility can cause anxiety and fear in many patients and their families. Even a transfer from one room or unit in a facility to another room or unit can cause anxiety because the individual has to adjust to another new environment. It is essential for the health care team member to create a positive first impression. By being courteous, supportive, and kind, the health care provider can do much to alleviate fear and anxiety. Giving clear instructions about how to operate equipment and the type of routine to expect, such as mealtimes, helps the patient or resident become familiar with the environment. It is also important not to rush while admitting, transferring, or discharging a patient. Allow the individual to ask questions and express concerns. If you do not know the answers to specific questions, refer these questions to your immediate supervisor.

EHR

Most facilities have specific forms that are used during an admission, transfer, or discharge. A sample admission form is shown in **Figure 22–1**.

In most facilities, the forms are computerized, and a laptop or tablet computer is used to enter patient information. Patient records are stored electronically and are called electronic health records (EHRs). However, all of the forms list the procedures that must be performed and will vary slightly from facility to facility. It is important for the health care team member to become familiar with the information required on such forms. Much of the information on an admission form is used as a basis for the nursing care plan. Therefore, this information must be complete and accurate. If the patient is unable to answer the questions, a relative or the person responsible for the patient is usually able to provide the information. In some facilities, questions regarding medications and allergies are the responsibility of the nurse. Follow agency policy regarding these sections on the form.

When a patient is admitted to a facility, certain procedures are performed. These usually include vital signs, height and weight measurements, and collection of a routine urine specimen. Follow correct techniques while performing these procedures.

A personal inventory list is made of the patient's clothing, valuables, and personal items to protect their possessions. In a hospital, a family member frequently will take clothing home. Any clothing or personal items, such as cell phones, kept in the room should be noted on the list. The list should be checked and signed by both the health care provider and the patient (or the person responsible for the patient). At the time of transfer or discharge, the personal inventory list of clothing and personal items should be checked to make sure that the patient has all belongings.

If the family does not take valuables home, these should be put in a safe place. Most facilities require that they be kept in a safe or sent to security. A description of the valuables is usually written on a valuable's envelope, and the items are placed inside. Care should be taken when describing valuables. For example, record "a yellow-colored band with a white-colored stone," instead of "a gold band with a diamond." If money is left in the patient's wallet, it should be counted, and the exact amount recorded on the envelope. Both the health care team member and the patient (or the person responsible for the patient) should check the items and sign the valuables envelope. The valuables are then put in the safe or sent to security, and a receipt is given to the patient or put on the patient's chart. If a patient is transferred or discharged, the valuables are taken from the safe and checked by both the health care provider and the patient. Again, both individuals sign the envelope to indicate that valuables have been returned to the patient.

Comm

Patients and family members should be oriented to the facility. Instructions about how to operate the call signal, bed controls, television remote control (if present), telephone, and other similar equipment should be provided. Visiting hours, location of lounges, smoking regulations, availability of services, such as religious services and activities, mealtimes, and other rules or routines in the facility, should be explained. Many facilities give patients and family members pamphlets or papers listing such information, but it is still important to explain the main information.

Transfers are done for a variety of reasons. A transfer is sometimes related to a change in the patient's condition. For example, a person may be transferred from or to an intensive care unit. Other times, a transfer is made at the patient's request, such as a request to be moved to a private room. Agency policy must be followed during any transfer. The reason for the transfer should be explained to the patient and family. This is usually the responsibility of the physician or nurse. The new room or unit must be ready to receive the patient. Clothing, personal items, certain equipment, and medications must be transferred with the patient. The health care team member should also find out how to transport the patient. Wheelchairs, stretchers, and even the patient's bed can be used for the transfer. An organized and efficient transfer helps prevent fear and anxiety in the patient.

Legal

A written physician's order is required before a patient or resident can be discharged from a facility. If an individual plans to leave the facility without permission, report this immediately to your supervisor. Facilities have special policies that must be followed when a person leaves against medical advice (AMA). When an order for discharge has been received, the health care team member must check and pack the patient's belongings. The personal inventory list completed at the time of admission must be checked to ascertain that all of the patient's belongings have been packed. A careful check of the unit, including any drawers, closets, and storage

PATIENT PREFERS TO BE ADDRESSED AS:

_____

FROM: ❑ E.R.   ❑ E.C.F.   ❑ Home   ❑ M.D.'s Office

COMMUNICATES IN ENGLISH: ❑ Well   ❑ Minimal   ❑ Not At All   ❑ Other Language (Specify) _____

❑ INTERPRETER (Name Person)   ❑ None

_____

MODE OF TRANSPORTATION:
❑ Ambulatory   ❑ Other   Smoker: Y❑ N❑
❑ Wheelchair   _____
❑ Stretcher   _____

Home Telephone No. (   ) _____
Work Telephone No. (   ) _____

ORIENTATION TO ENVIRONMENT:

❑ Armband Checked   ❑ Call Light
❑ Bed Control   ❑ Phone
❑ TV Control   ❑ Side Rail Policy
❑ Bathroom   ❑ Visitation Policy
❑ Personal Property Policy   ❑ Smoking Policy

PERSONAL BELONGINGS: (Check and Describe)

❑ Clothing   _____
❑ Jewelry   _____
❑ Money   _____
❑ Walker   _____
❑ Wheelchair   _____
❑ Cane   _____
❑ Other   _____

DENTURES:
❑ Upper   ❑ Partial
❑ Lower   ❑ None

CONTACT LENSES:
❑ Hard   ❑ LT   ❑ RT
❑ Soft

GLASSES: ❑ Y ❑ N   **HEARING AID:** ❑ Y ❑ N
PROSTHESIS: ❑ Y ❑ N
(Describe) _____

DISPOSITION OF VALUABLES:
❑ Patient   Given To: _____
❑ Home
❑ Placed in   Relationship: _____
Safe   _____
(Claim No.)

IN CASE OF EMERGENCY NOTIFY:
Name: _____
Relationship: _____
Home Telephone No. (   ) _____
Work Telephone No. (   ) _____

VITAL SIGNS:

TEMP: _____ ❑ Oral ❑ Rectal ❑ Axillary

PULSE: _____ ❑ Radial ❑ Apical   Respiratory
Rate _____
❑ RT
B/P: _____ ❑ LT ❑ Standing ❑ Sitting ❑ Lying

HEIGHT: _____ WEIGHT: _____ ❑ Bedside
❑ Standing

ALLERGIES:

Medications: ❑ None Known   Food: ❑ None Known
❑ Tape
❑ Penicillin   ❑ Other (List)   (Shellfish, Eggs, Milk, etc.)
❑ Sulfa   _____   _____
❑ Iodine   _____   _____
❑ Aspirin   _____   _____
❑ Morphine   _____   _____
❑ Demerol   _____   _____

MEDICATIONS: (Prescription/Non-Prescription)   Dose/Frequency   Last Dose (Date/Time)
1. _____   _____   _____
2. _____   _____   _____
3. _____   _____   _____
4. _____   _____   _____
5. _____   _____   _____
6. _____   _____   _____

DISPOSITION OF MEDICATIONS:
❑ None Brought to Hospital
❑ Sent Home _____
With _____
❑ To Pharmacy: (List)
_____
_____

ADMITTING DIAGNOSIS: _____

NURSE'S SIGNATURE: _____ RN/LVN   Date _____ Time _____

FIGURE 22–1 A sample admission form.

areas, helps ensure that all items are found. Most facilities require that a staff member accompany the individual to a car. Some facilities allow patients to walk, but many prefer to transport patients by wheelchair. If a patient is to be transferred by ambulance, the ambulance attendants will bring a stretcher to the room. In this case, it is important for the health care provider to have the patient's belongings ready for the transport. Again, most agencies have forms or checklists that are used during discharge to ensure that all procedures are followed.

checkpoint

1. What should a health care team member do when a patient wants to leave against medical advice (AMA)?
2. Where should a patient's wallet be stored while in a facility?

PRACTICE: Go to the workbook and complete the assignment sheet for 22:1, Admitting, Transferring, and Discharging Patients. Then return and continue with the procedures.

Procedure 22:1A
OBRA

Admitting the Patient

Equipment and Supplies

Admission form and personal inventory list, valuables envelope, admission kit (if used), thermometer, stethoscope, sphygmomanometer, watch with second hand, scale, urine-specimen container, patient gown (if needed), paper and pen or computer

Procedure

1. Obtain orders from your immediate supervisor or check orders to obtain permission for the procedure.

2. Wash hands.

3. Assemble equipment. Prepare the room for the admission. Fanfold the top bed linen down to open the bed. If an admission kit is used, unpack the kit and place the items in the bedside stand or table. The admission kit usually includes a water pitcher, cup, soap dish, bar of soap, lotion, toothbrush, toothpaste, and mouthwash (**Figure 22–2**). Place a

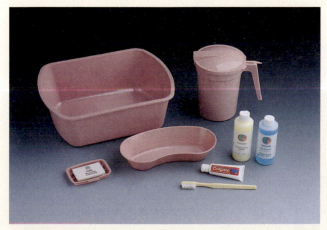

FIGURE 22–2 A sample admission kit. Courtesy of Medline Industries Inc., 1-860-MEDLINE

bedpan and/or urinal, bath basin, and emesis basin in the bedside stand. Check the room to be sure all equipment and supplies are in their proper places.

4. You may be required to go to the admissions office to get the new patient or resident, or the patient may be brought to the room by other personnel.

5. **[Comm]** Greet and identify the patient. Ask the patient if they prefer to be called by a particular name. Introduce yourself by name and title to the patient and to any family members present. If another patient is in the room, introduce the new patient. Explain the procedure and obtain consent.

   NOTE: Be friendly and courteous at all times. Do not rush or hurry the patient.

6. Ask the family or visitors to wait in the lounge or lobby while you complete the admission process, if this is facility policy.

   NOTE: If a patient is not able to answer questions, a family member or other person responsible for the patient can remain in the room to complete the admission process.

7. Close the door and pull the curtain for privacy (**Figure 22–3**). Ask the patient to change into a gown or pajamas. Assist the patient as necessary.

   NOTE: In long-term care facilities, residents usually wear street clothes during the day. In this case, gowns or pajamas are not used.

8. Position the patient comfortably in the bed or in a chair.

9. **[Comm]** Complete the admission form. Ask questions slowly and clearly. Provide time for the patient to answer the questions.

   NOTE: Observe the patient carefully during the admission process. Record all observations noted. If the patient expresses certain concerns, be sure to record and report these concerns.

(continues)

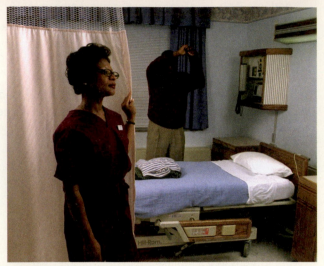

FIGURE 22–3 Close the door and pull the curtain to provide privacy while the patient undresses.

10. Measure and record vital signs. Follow the procedures outlined in Chapter 16.

11. Weigh and measure the patient. Follow Procedure 21:1A. Record the information on the admission form.

12. Complete a personal inventory list. Be sure to list all personal items that will be kept in the patient's unit, such as clothing, shoes, clocks, radios, cell phones, religious items, and books. Make sure the patient or a responsible individual checks and signs the list. Assist the patient as necessary in hanging up clothing or putting away personal items.

13. Complete a valuables list. If a family member takes the valuables home, be sure to obtain a signature on the proper form. If the valuables are to be placed in a safe or sent to security, fill out the form and obtain the patient's or a relative's signature. Follow agency policy for securing valuables.

14. Obtain a routine urine specimen if ordered. Follow Procedure 22:10A.

15. Orient the patient to the facility by demonstrating or explaining the following:

    a. Call signal or light

    b. Bed controls

    c. Television remote control and/or television rental policy

    d. Telephone

    e. Bathroom facilities and special call signal in bathroom

    f. Visiting hours

    g. Mealtimes and menu selections

    h. Activities or services available

    i. Health care facility regulations

    NOTE: Many health care facilities provide pamphlets or printed forms with the required information. However, it is still important to explain the main information to the patient and family.

16. Fill the water pitcher, if the patient is allowed to have liquids.

17. Observe all checkpoints before leaving the patient. Make sure the patient is comfortable and in good body alignment; the siderails are up, if indicated; the bed is at its lowest level; the call signal and supplies are in easy reach; and the area is neat and clean.

18. Clean and replace all equipment.

19. Wash hands.

20. When the admission process is complete, allow family members to return to the unit. Answer any questions they may have regarding facility policies. If you do not know the answers to their questions, obtain the correct answers from your immediate supervisor.

21. Record all required information on the patient's chart or enter it into the computer. For example, date, time, admission form complete, valuables placed in safe (or sent to security), patient tolerated procedure well, and your signature and title. Report any abnormal observations to your immediate supervisor.

     NOTE: In health care agencies using electronic health records (EHRs), the information is entered directly into the patient's record on a computer.

PRACTICE: Go to the workbook and use the evaluation sheet for 22:1A, Admitting the Patient, to practice this procedure. When you believe you have mastered this skill, sign the sheet and give it to your instructor for further action.

✅ **FINAL EVALUATION:** Using the criteria listed on the evaluation sheet, your instructor will grade your performance.

Transferring the Patient

Equipment and Supplies

Transfer checklist (if used), personal inventory list, valuables list, cart (if needed), wheelchair or stretcher, gloves, paper and pen or computer

Procedure

1. Obtain permission from your immediate supervisor or check orders to obtain permission for the procedure. Find out the new unit or room number. Check to be sure that the unit is ready or ask your immediate supervisor to check. Check the method of transport to be used and obtain a wheelchair or stretcher, or use the patient's bed.

2. Assemble equipment.

3. Knock on the door and pause before entering. Introduce yourself. Identify the patient. Explain the procedure to the patient and obtain consent.

   NOTE: Reassure the patient as necessary. Patients are often apprehensive.

4. Wash hands.

5. Collect the patient's clothing and personal items. Check all items against the admission personal inventory list to be sure all items are present. Put the items in a bag or place them on a cart for transport. If the patient wears dentures, glasses, and/or a hearing aid, make sure they have these items.

6. Put any bedside equipment to be transferred onto a cart. This may include items such as the water pitcher, cup, soap dish, soap, emesis basin, bedpan, and bath basin. Check whether special equipment or medications are to be transferred. Follow agency policy regarding transfer of equipment.

7. If valuables are to be transferred, they must be checked and signed for by both the patient and the health care provider. The valuables are usually kept in the facility safe or with security, and the room or unit number of the patient is changed on the valuables bag when the patient is transferred.

8. Assist the patient into a wheelchair or stretcher depending on their condition. Follow the appropriate procedure as outlined in Section 22:2.

9. Transport the patient and the cart of supplies to the new unit or room (**Figure 22–4**). If help is not available, the patient may be taken to the new room first and the belongings taken afterward.

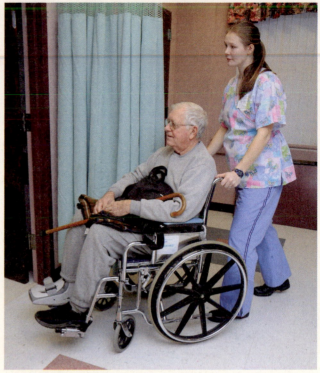

FIGURE 22–4 If the patient's condition permits, use a wheelchair to transfer the patient to the new room or unit.

⚠️ Safety **CAUTION:** Observe all safety precautions while transporting the patient.

10. Introduce the patient to the new staff members. Assist the staff members in getting the patient positioned comfortably in bed or in a chair. If another patient is in the room, introduce the patient. Orient the patient to the new room or unit by explaining or demonstrating the use of the equipment and supplies.

    NOTE: The staff members of the new unit may orient the patient.

11. Check the patient's belongings with the new staff member. Use the personal inventory and valuables checklist as needed. Be sure to obtain correct signatures according to agency policy.

12. Help put away the patient's clothing and personal items.

13. Observe all checkpoints before leaving the patient. Make sure the patient is comfortable and in good body alignment, the siderails are up (if indicated), the bed is at its lowest level, the call signal and supplies are in easy reach, and the area is neat and clean.

(continues)

14. Replace all equipment.

15. Wash hands.

16. Complete the transfer checklist. Record all required information on the patient's chart or enter it into the computer. For example, date, time, transferred to room 239-A by wheelchair, patient tolerated procedure well, transfer checklist completed, and your signature and title.

     NOTE: In health care agencies using electronic health records (EHRs), the information is entered directly into the patient's record on a computer.

17. Return to the patient's previous room. Put on gloves. Strip the bed and remove any equipment that was not transferred. Follow agency policy for cleaning the room.

     CAUTION: Wear gloves and observe standard precautions. Contact with body fluids, secretions, or excretions is possible.

NOTE: This may be the responsibility of the housekeeping department. If so, notify housekeeping that the patient has been transferred.

18. Remove gloves. Wash hands.

19. Report to your immediate supervisor that the transfer has been completed.

PRACTICE: Go to the workbook and use the evaluation sheet for 22:1B, Transferring the Patient, to practice this procedure. When you believe you have mastered this skill, sign the sheet and give it to your instructor for further action.

 FINAL EVALUATION: Using the criteria listed on the evaluation sheet, your instructor will grade your performance.

Procedure 22:1C

Discharging the Patient

Equipment and Supplies

Discharge checklist (if used), personal inventory list, valuables list, wheelchair (if needed), cart (if needed), gloves, paper and pen or computer

Procedure

1. Obtain orders from your immediate supervisor or check orders to obtain permission for the procedure. Check with the patient to determine when relatives or other individuals will be there to discharge the patient.

    NOTE: If the patient is to be discharged to another facility by ambulance, determine the time the ambulance will arrive.

2. Assemble equipment.

3. Knock on the door and pause before entering. Introduce yourself. Identify the patient. Explain the procedure and obtain consent.

4. Wash hands.

5. Close the door and pull the curtain for privacy. Help the patient dress, if assistance is needed.

6. Assemble all of the patient's personal belongings. If the patient wears dentures, glasses, and/or a hearing aid, make sure they have these items. Check drawers, closets, the bedside stand or table, and storage areas. Check all items against the personal inventory list to be sure everything is present. Obtain the patient's signature according to agency policy.

7. Assemble any equipment that is to be given to the patient. Examples include the supplies in the admission kit, such as the pitcher and cup.

8. Check to make sure that the patient has received final instructions from the nurse and/or physician. These may include discharge instructions and prescriptions.

9. Obtain the patient's valuables, if they are in a safe or with security. Check the valuables with the patient. Obtain the correct signature to indicate that the valuables were returned to the patient.

    NOTE: In some agencies, the patient or a responsible person obtains the valuables directly from the safe or security. In such a case, tell the patient how to obtain the valuables.

10. Complete a discharge checklist, if one is used, to be sure all procedures are complete.

11. Place all of the patient's belongings on a cart, if needed. Packed items sometimes are taken to the car by a relative.

12. Assist the patient into a wheelchair. Follow Procedure 22:2F.

    NOTE: Most facilities require the use of wheelchairs to transport patients. Some facilities allow patients to walk, but health care providers must accompany patients. Follow agency policy.

13. Transport the patient to the exit area. Help the patient into the car.

    NOTE: If a cart is used to transfer the patient's belongings, another staff member should take the cart to the car.

    CAUTION: Observe all safety factors while transporting the patient.

14. Help put the patient's belongings in the car.

15. Say good-bye to the patient.

16. Return to the unit. Put on gloves. Strip the bed and remove any equipment in the unit. Follow agency policy for cleaning the unit. Replace equipment.

    CAUTION: Wear gloves and observe standard precautions. Contact with body fluids, secretions, or excretions is possible.

NOTE: In some facilities, this is the responsibility of the housekeeping department. If so, notify housekeeping that the patient has been discharged.

17. Remove gloves. Wash hands.

18. Record all required information on the patient's chart or enter it into the computer. For example, date, time, patient discharged, taken to husband's car by wheelchair, tolerated procedure well, and your signature and title. Report to your immediate supervisor that the discharge has been completed.

    NOTE: In health care agencies using electronic health records (EHRs), the information is entered directly into the patient's record on a computer.

PRACTICE: Go to the workbook and use the evaluation sheet for 22:1C, Discharging the Patient, to practice this procedure. When you believe you have mastered this skill, sign the sheet and give it to your instructor for further action.

FINAL EVALUATION: Using the criteria listed on the evaluation sheet, your instructor will grade your performance.

22:2 POSITIONING, TURNING, MOVING, AND TRANSFERRING PATIENTS

As a health care provider, you may be responsible for positioning, turning, moving, and transferring many patients. If these procedures are done correctly, you will provide the patient with optimum comfort and care. In addition, you will prevent injury to yourself and the patient.

It is essential to remember that improper moving, turning, or transferring of a patient can result in serious injuries to the patient or health care provider. Some patients cannot be moved safely without special assistance or mechanical devices. Other patients who have had back, neck, or hip surgeries can only be turned certain ways. If a patient has restrictions for moving or transferring, the restrictions should be posted outside the door. If you are not sure whether a patient can be moved or transferred safely, *always* ask your supervisor before attempting any procedure. Remember, you are *legally* responsible for the safety and well-being of the patient.

Correct body mechanics are required for all procedures discussed here. Review and practice all of the rules of correct body mechanics as outlined in Section 14:1. If you are unable to move or turn a patient by yourself, always get help.

ALIGNMENT

Patient care must be directed toward maintaining normal body alignment. **Alignment** is defined as positioning body parts in relation to each other to maintain correct body posture. Benefits of proper alignment include:

- **Prevent fatigue**: Correct alignment helps the patient feel more comfortable and prevents fatigue.

- **Prevent pressure ulcers**: A pressure ulcer, also called a **decubitus ulcer**, pressure sore, or bedsore, is caused by prolonged pressure on an area of the body that interferes with circulation. Pressure ulcers are common in areas where bones are close to the skin, such as the tailbone, or coccygeal area; hips; knees; ankles; heels; and elbows. The tissue breakdown of a pressure ulcer occurs in four stages:

(1) Stage I: a red or blue-gray discoloration appears on the intact skin (**Figure 22–5A**). The discoloration does not disappear after the pressure has been relieved.

(2) Stage II: abrasions, bruises, and/or open sores develop as a result of tissue damage to the top layers of the skin (epidermis and dermis) (**Figure 22–5B**).

(3) Stage III: a deep open crater forms when all layers of the skin are destroyed and fat and muscle tissues are exposed (**Figure 22–5C**).

(4) Stage IV: damage extends into the muscle, tendon, and bone tissues (**Figure 22–5D**).

It is easier to prevent pressure ulcers than it is to treat them. In addition, if pressure ulcers are detected in early stages, immediate treatment can help prevent further damage. Effective ways to prevent pressure ulcers

include providing good skin care; using moisturizing lotions on dry skin; prompt cleaning of urine and feces from the skin; massaging in a circular motion around a reddened area; frequent turning (at least every 2 hours); positioning to avoid pressure on irritated areas; keeping linen clean, dry, and free from wrinkles; and applying protectors of sheepskin, lamb's wool, or foam to bony prominences, such as heels and elbows. Pressure relief is the most important factor in preventing pressure ulcers. Over 100 different support surfaces or pressure-reducing products are available to prevent ulcers. Alternating air pressure mattresses (**Figure 22–6**) and continuous lateral rotation beds (that constantly turn the patient side to side) are among the most advanced pressure-reducing surfaces. Careful observation of the skin during bathing or turning is essential. If a pale, reddened, or blue-gray area is noted, this should be reported and documented immediately.

- **Treatment of pressure ulcers**: Stage I and stage II pressure ulcers are often treated with special foam or hydrocolloid dressings along with

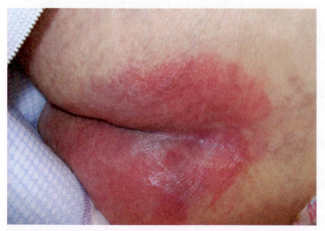

FIGURE 22–5A A stage I pressure ulcer has a red or blue-gray discoloration that does not disappear after pressure has been relieved. Used with permission of the National Pressure Ulcer Advisory Panel 2012

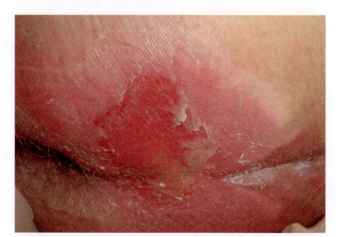

FIGURE 22–5B A stage II pressure ulcer is characterized by abrasions, bruises, and/or open sores as a result of tissue damage to the top layers of the skin. Used with permission of the National Pressure Ulcer Advisory Panel 2012

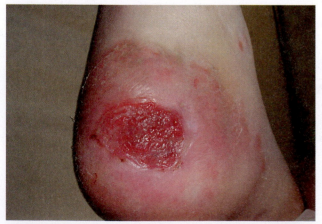

FIGURE 22–5C In a stage III pressure ulcer, a deep open crater forms when all layers of the skin are destroyed. Used with permission of the National Pressure Ulcer Advisory Panel 2012

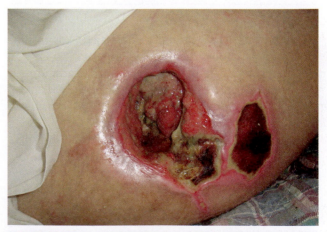

FIGURE 22–5D In a stage IV pressure ulcer, damage extends into the muscle, tendon, and bone tissues. Used with permission of the National Pressure Ulcer Advisory Panel 2012

frequent turning to keep pressure off the ulcer. Stage III and stage IV ulcers can be treated with these dressings, or they can be treated with negative-pressure wound therapy using a wound VAC (vacuum-assisted closure) (**Figure 22–7**). A foam sponge is cut to fit the size of the open wound. A transparent adhesive film is placed over the sponge, and suction tubing is placed through the film dressing. The suction tubing is attached to the suction and a disposable collection canister. This device seals the wound and applies a negative pressure to promote healing and prevent infections. It works by drawing the wound edges together and removing exudate and infectious materials. It also reduces edema (swelling) and promotes perfusion by forcing the flow of fluid in the area.

- **Prevent contractures**: A **contracture** (**Figure 22–8**) is a tightening or shortening of a muscle usually caused by lack of movement or usage of the muscle. Foot drop is a common contracture. It can be prevented in part by keeping the foot at a right angle to the leg (**Figure 22–9**). Footboards, foot supports, and high-top tennis shoes can be used to keep the foot in this position. Range-of-motion (ROM) exercises, discussed in Section 23:1, also help prevent contractures.

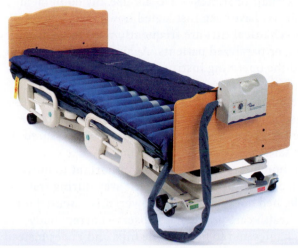

FIGURE 22–6 An alternating air pressure mattress constantly changes the pressure points against a patient's skin. Courtesy of Medline Industries Inc., 1-860-MEDLINE

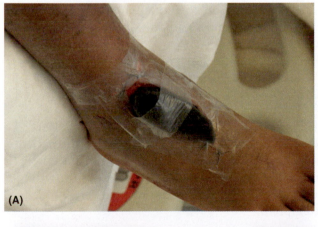

(A)

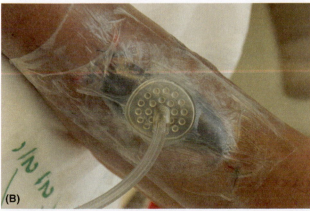

(B)

FIGURE 22–7 (A) After a pressure ulcer or wound is covered with a gauze or foam dressing, (B) the wound VAC is attached to apply negative pressure to the area to promote healing.

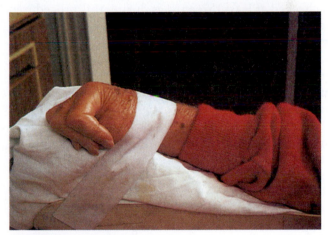

FIGURE 22–8 A contracture is a tightening of a muscle caused by lack of movement or usage of the muscle.

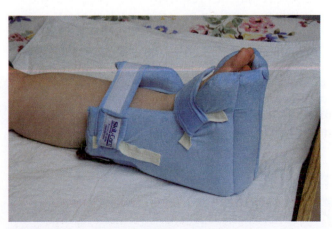

FIGURE 22–9 Foot supports can be used to hold the feet at right angles and prevent foot drop, a common contracture.

TURNING

The patient confined to bed must be turned frequently. The patient's position should be changed at least every 2 hours, if permitted by the physician. Some agencies post a turning position schedule by the patient's bed. For example: 6 am: Right side; 8 am: Back; 10 am: Left side; and 12 noon: Abdomen. Frequent turning provides exercise for the muscles. It also stimulates circulation, decreases pulmonary congestion, helps prevent pressure ulcers and contractures, and provides comfort to the patient. Correct turning procedures must be followed to prevent injury to both the patient and the health care provider.

DANGLING

If a patient has been confined to bed for a period of time, the patient is frequently placed in a dangling position before being transferred from the bed. **Dangling** means sitting with the legs hanging down over the side of the bed. This allows the patient some time to adjust to the sitting position. The pulse rate is checked at least three times during this procedure: before, during, and after the dangling period. It is taken just before the patient is moved to the dangling position; this pulse rate serves as a control, or resting, rate. The pulse rate is checked again immediately after positioning the patient in the dangling position. The third check occurs after the patient is returned to a lying-down (supine) position in the bed. By noting changes in the pulse rate, the health care provider can determine how well the patient tolerates the procedure. Blood pressure can also be checked to determine a patient's tolerance of the procedure. The blood pressure is taken while lying down, sitting, and standing. A patient might experience a drop in blood pressure with position changes, a condition called *orthostatic hypotension*. In addition to taking the pulse and blood pressure, observe the patient's respiratory rate, balance (the patient may complain of vertigo or dizziness), amount of perspiration, color, and other similar characteristics. If the pulse rate shows an abnormal increase, the blood pressure drops measurably, respirations become labored, color becomes pale, increased perspiration is noted, or the patient gets dizzy or very weak, the patient should be returned immediately to the supine, resting position.

TRANSFERS

Comm

Patients are frequently transferred to wheelchairs, chairs, or stretchers. Again, correct procedures must be followed to prevent injury to both the patient and the health care provider. Many different models of wheelchairs and stretchers are available. It is important to read the manufacturer's instructions regarding the operation of any given piece of equipment. If no instructions are available, ask your immediate supervisor to demonstrate the correct operation of a particular wheelchair or stretcher. Do *not* use any equipment until you have been instructed how to use it.

Mechanical lifts are frequently used to transfer weak or paralyzed patients. Again, it is important to read the operating instructions provided with the lift. Straps, clasps, and the sling should be checked carefully for any defects. Smooth, even movements must be used while operating the lift. Patients are often frightened of the lift and must be reassured that it is safe.

In home care situations, it is important to move unnecessary furniture out of the way during transfers. If the bed does not raise or lower, it is essential for the health care provider to observe correct body mechanics and to bend at the hips and knees instead of the waist. It is possible to rent hospital beds, wheelchairs, mechanical lifts, and other similar items for home care.

Legal

Before a patient is moved or transferred, the health care provider must obtain approval or orders from their immediate supervisor. Never move or transfer a patient without proper authorization.

Safety

During any move or transfer, it is important to watch the patient closely. Note changes in pulse rate, blood pressure, respirations, and color. Observe for signs of weakness, dizziness, increased perspiration, or discomfort. If you note any abnormal changes, return the patient to a safe and comfortable position and check with your immediate supervisor. The supervisor will determine whether the move or transfer should be attempted.

checkpoint

1. A decubitus ulcer that has abrasions, bruises, and/or open sores that develop as a result of tissue damage to the top layers of the skin is considered what stage of tissue breakdown?

2. How frequently should a patient confined to a bed be turned or repositioned?

PRACTICE: Go to the workbook and complete the assignment sheet for 22:2, Positioning, Turning, Moving, and Transferring Patients. Then return and continue with the procedures.

Procedure 22:2A

 OBRA

Aligning the Patient

Equipment and Supplies

Three pillows, two or three bath blankets, two or three large towels, two or three washcloths or small towels, protectors for bony prominences, footboard, gloves, paper and pen or computer

Procedure

1. Obtain orders from your immediate supervisor or check orders to obtain permission for the procedure.

2. Assemble equipment.

3. Comm Knock on the door and pause before entering. Introduce yourself. Identify the patient. Explain the procedure and obtain consent.

4. Provide privacy. Close the door and pull the curtain.

5. Wash hands. Put on gloves.

    Precaution **CAUTION:** Wear gloves and observe standard precautions. Contact with body fluids, secretions, or excretions is possible.

6. Lock the wheels on the bed. Elevate the bed to a comfortable height. If siderails are elevated, lower the bedrail or siderail on the side of the bed where you are working.

   ⚠ Safety **CAUTION:** If the bed does not raise to a working height, use correct body mechanics and bend from the hips and knees, not the waist, to get close to the patient.

7. Align the patient who is lying on the back in a supine position as follows (**Figure 22–10**):

   a. Position the head in a straight line with the spine.

   b. Place pillow under the head and neck to provide support.

   c. A pillow or rolled blanket may be placed under the lower legs, from the knees to 2 inches above the heels to provide support and keep the heels off the bed.

   d. Protector pads may be placed on the heels or elbows (**Figure 22–11**).

   e. Toes should point upward. You may place a footboard, pillow, or rolled blanket against the soles of the feet to achieve this. High-top tennis shoes can also be placed on the feet to keep them at this angle.

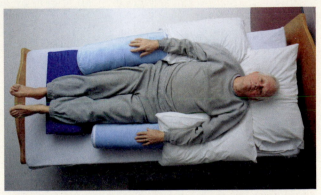

FIGURE 22–10 Correct alignment for a patient positioned on the back in the horizontal recumbent or supine position.

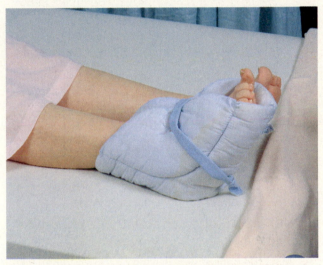

FIGURE 22–11 Foot protectors can help prevent pressure ulcers on the heels.

NOTE: Check the patient for comfort, safety, and support before leaving. Make sure no bony prominences are exposed and all body parts are supported.

8. Align the patient who is lying on the side (**Figure 22–12**) as follows:

   a. Place a small pillow under the head and neck for support.

   b. Flex the lower arm at the elbow. It can be placed in line with the face.

   c. Support the upper arm, flexed at the elbow, on a pillow or rolled blanket.

   d. Flex both knees slightly. Place a firm pillow or rolled blanket between the legs. The pillow should extend from the upper leg to the ankle.

(continues)

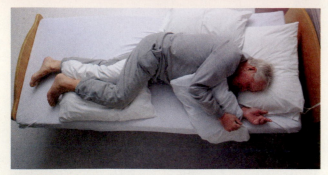

FIGURE 22–12 Correct alignment for a patient positioned on the side.

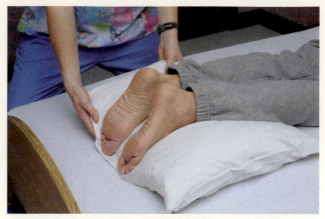

FIGURE 22–13 A large pillow can be used to support the feet when the patient is lying in the prone position.

e. Use a footboard, pillow, rolled blanket, or high-top tennis shoes to keep the feet at right angles (90 degrees) to the legs.

f. Rolled washcloths or foam rubber balls may be placed in paralyzed hands to prevent contractures.

g. Use pillows to support the back and abdomen.

h. Protector pads may be placed on the ankles, heels, and elbows.

 CAUTION: Make sure that the patient's body is not twisted and that any one body part is not applying direct pressure on any other body part.

NOTE: Check all aspects of the patient's position before leaving.

9. Align the patient who is lying on the abdomen (in the prone position) as follows:

a. Place the head in a direct line with the spine.

b. Turn the head to one side. It may be supported with a small pillow. Placing the pillow at an angle will keep it away from the patient's face.

c. A small pillow may be placed under the waist for support.

d. Place a firm pillow under the lower legs. This will slightly flex the knees.

e. The feet can be extended over the end of the mattress so that they will remain at right angles to the legs. They can also be supported in this position by pillows or rolled blankets (**Figure 22–13**).

f. Place the arms in line on either side of the head. Use pads to protect the elbows. Flex the elbows slightly for comfort.

NOTE: Check all aspects of position, comfort, and safety before leaving the patient.

10. Observe all checkpoints before leaving the patient. Make sure the siderails are elevated (if indicated), the bed is at its lowest level, the call signal and supplies are in easy reach, the patient is comfortable and in good body alignment, and the area is neat and clean.

11. Properly replace all equipment not being used.

12. Remove gloves. Wash hands.

13. Report that the procedure is complete or record all required information on the patient's chart or enter it into the computer. For example, date, time, positioned on left side in correct alignment, patient appears to be resting comfortably, and your signature and title. Note any unusual observations.

 NOTE: In health care agencies using electronic health records (EHRs), the information is entered directly into the patient's record on a computer.

PRACTICE: Go to the workbook and use the evaluation sheet for 22:2A, Aligning the Patient, to practice this procedure. When you believe you have mastered this skill, sign the sheet and give it to your instructor for further action.

 FINAL EVALUATION: Using the criteria listed on the evaluation sheet, your instructor will grade your performance.

Moving the Patient Up in Bed

Equipment and Supplies

Lift sheet, gloves, paper and pen or computer

Procedure

1. Legal   Obtain permission from your immediate supervisor or check orders to make sure that the patient can be moved. Obtain the assistance of another team member.

2. Comm   Knock on the door and pause before entering. Introduce yourself and your team member. Identify the patient. Explain the procedure and obtain consent.

3. Provide privacy. Close the door and pull the curtain.

4. Wash hands. Put on gloves.

    Precaution   **CAUTION:** Wear gloves and observe standard precautions. Contact with body fluids, secretions, or excretions is possible.

5. One person should be on each side of the bed. Lock the bed (usually by way of wheel locks) to prevent movement of the bed. Elevate the bed to a comfortable height. Lower the siderails, if elevated.

   NOTE: Locks and siderails on beds vary. If you do not know how to lock a bed or operate siderails, check with your immediate supervisor.

6. Lower the head of the bed. Remove all pillows. One pillow can be placed against the headboard of the bed to prevent injury to the patient's head while moving the patient up in bed.

   NOTE: Observe the patient for respiratory distress.

   CAUTION: If any breathing difficulty is noted, immediately raise the head of the bed. Check with your supervisor before proceeding.

   Safety

7. Position the lift sheet under the patient by turning the patient to one side (**Figure 22–14A**). The lift sheet can be fanfolded to the center of the bed. Make sure it extends under the patient's head, shoulders, hips, and thighs. Turn the patient to the opposite side and unfold the lift sheet so it covers the entire bed. Turn the patient on their back.

   NOTE: Use proper body mechanics throughout the procedure. Use the weight of your body to move the patient. Avoid back strain.

8. Two people should use the lift sheet to move the patient.

   a. One person stands on each side of the bed. Each person positions one hand on the lift sheet by the patient's shoulders and the other hand by the patient's hips.

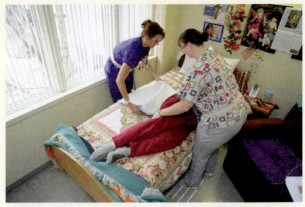

FIGURE 22–14A Turn the patient to one side to position the lift sheet under the patient.

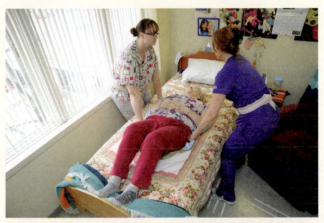

FIGURE 22–14B Both health care team members should roll the edges of the lift sheet inward close to both sides of the patient's body.

   b. Each person faces the head of the bed and gets a broad base of support by putting one foot ahead of the other. Each person should be close to the patient and the bed.

   c. If the patient's condition permits, ask the patient to flex their knees and brace both feet firmly on the bed.

   d. Each person rolls the edges of the lift sheet inward close to both sides of the patient's body (**Figure 22–14B**).

   e. At a given signal, such as *one-two-lift*, the two health care providers lift the sheet and patient, and move the patient to the head of the bed (**Figure 22–14C**).

   NOTE: Shift your weight from the rear leg to the forward leg at the same time that you slide the patient.

   f. After the patient is positioned, each team member tucks the lift sheet back into the side of the bed.

(continues)

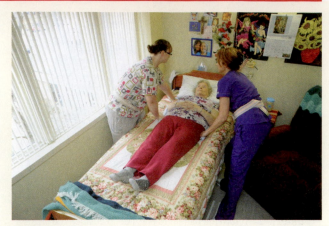

FIGURE 22–14C At a given signal, the team members lift and move the sheet and patient to the head of the bed.

9. Leave the patient in good body alignment. Make sure the patient is comfortable.

10. Elevate the siderails (if indicated). Place the call signal and any needed supplies within easy reach of the patient. Lower the bed to its lowest level.

11. Replace all equipment. Make sure the area is neat and clean.

12. Remove gloves. Wash hands.

13. **Comm** Report that the patient has been moved up in bed and/or record all required information on the patient's chart or enter it into the computer. For example, date, time, moved to head of bed, tolerated procedure well, and your signature and title. Note any unusual observations.

    EHR **NOTE:** In health care agencies using electronic health records (EHRs), the information is entered directly into the patient's record on a computer.

PRACTICE: Go to the workbook and use the evaluation sheet for 22:2B, Moving the Patient Up in Bed, to practice this procedure. When you believe you have mastered this skill, sign the sheet and give it to your instructor for further action.

 Check **FINAL EVALUATION:** Using the criteria listed on the evaluation sheet, your instructor will grade your performance.

Procedure 22:2C **OBRA**

Turning the Patient Away to Change Position

Equipment and Supplies

Paper and pen or computer, gloves

Procedure

1. Obtain permission from your immediate supervisor or check orders to make sure that the patient can be turned.

2. **Comm** Knock on the door and pause before entering. Introduce yourself. Identify the patient. Explain the procedure and obtain consent.

3. Provide privacy. Close the door and pull the curtain.

4. Wash hands. Put on gloves.

   🛑 **Precaution** **CAUTION:** Wear gloves and observe standard precautions. Contact with body fluids, secretions, or excretions is possible.

5. Lock wheels to prevent movement of the bed. Elevate the bed to a comfortable height.

6. If siderails are present and elevated, lower the siderail nearest to you. Make sure the opposite siderail is raised and locked securely.

7. The patient should be lying on the side of the bed close to you. If so, proceed to step 8. If the patient is at the center or close to the far side of the bed, move the patient as follows:

   a. Place one hand under the patient's head and neck. Place your other hand under the patient's upper back. Slide the upper part of the patient's body toward you.

   b. Place both hands under the patient's hips. Slide the hips toward you.

   c. Place both hands under the patient's upper and lower legs. Slide the legs toward you.

    Safety **CAUTION:** If you are not able to move the patient, get help.

    Safety **CAUTION:** Check the opposite siderail. Make sure it is up before proceeding.

8. Ask the patient to place their arms across the chest and move the proximal leg (the one closest to you) over the other leg.

   NOTE: This will make it easier to turn the patient and helps prevent injury.

    CAUTION: Do not cross the legs if the patient had hip replacement surgery.

9. Get close to the patient by bending your knees and keeping your back straight. Position your feet to provide a broad base of support. Place one arm under the patient's shoulders. Place your opposite hand under the patient's hips.

10. Use a smooth, even motion to roll the patient away from you and onto their side (**Figure 22–15**).

     NOTE: Explain what you are doing to the patient.

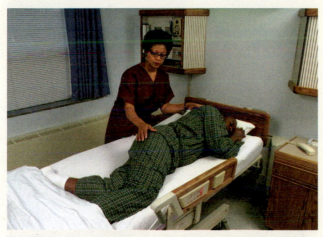

FIGURE 22–15 Put one hand under the patient's shoulder and the other hand under the patient's hip. Then use a smooth, even motion to roll the patient away from you.

11. Place your hands under the patient's head and shoulders. Draw the head and shoulders back toward the center of the bed.

12. Place your hands under the patient's hips and gently pull them back toward the center of the bed.

13. Place your hands under the patient's legs and pull them back toward the center of the bed.

14. Place a pillow behind the patient's back, between the legs to align the hips, and under the upper arm. Make sure the patient is comfortable and in good alignment.

15. Elevate the siderails (if indicated) before leaving the patient. Make sure that the call signal and other needed supplies are within easy reach of the patient. Lower the bed to its lowest level.

16. Replace all equipment. Leave the area neat and clean.

17. Remove gloves. Wash hands.

18. Report that patient has been turned and/or record all required information on the patient's chart or enter it into the computer. For example, date, time, turned on left side and positioned in correct alignment, and your signature and title. Note any unusual observations.

     NOTE: In health care agencies using electronic health records (EHRs), the information is entered directly into the patient's record on a computer.

PRACTICE: Go to the workbook and use the evaluation sheet for 22:2C, Turning the Patient Away to Change Position, to practice this procedure. When you believe you have mastered this skill, sign the sheet and give it to your instructor for further action.

 FINAL EVALUATION: Using the criteria listed on the evaluation sheet, your instructor will grade your performance.

Procedure 22:2D

Turning the Patient Inward to Change Position

Equipment and Supplies

Paper and pen or computer, gloves

Procedure

1. Obtain permission from your immediate supervisor or check orders to make sure that the patient can be turned.

2. Knock on the door and pause before entering. Introduce yourself. Identify the patient. Explain the procedure and obtain consent.

3. Provide privacy. Close the door and pull the curtain.

4. Wash hands. Put on gloves.

   CAUTION: Wear gloves and observe standard precautions. Contact with body fluids, secretions, or excretions is possible.

(continues)

5. Lock the wheels of the bed to prevent movement. Elevate the bed to a comfortable height.

6. Lower the siderail nearest to you, if present and elevated.

7. If the patient is too close to the near side of the bed, move them to the opposite side as follows:

   a. Place one hand under the patient's head and shoulders and the other hand under the patient's back. Slide the upper part of the body toward the opposite side of the bed.

   b. Place both hands under the patient's hips. Slide the hips toward the opposite side of the bed.

   c. Place both hands under the patient's legs. Slide the legs toward the opposite side of the bed.

8. Instruct the patient to cross their arms on the chest. Place the patient's leg that is farthest from you on top of the leg that is nearest to you.

   NOTE: This prevents injury to the patient's arms and legs.

    CAUTION: Do not cross the legs if the patient has had hip replacement surgery.

9. Get close to the patient by bending your knees and keeping your back straight. Position your feet to provide a broad base of support. Place your hand that is closest to the head of the bed on the patient's far shoulder. Place your other hand behind the patient's hip (**Figure 22–16A**). Use your knee to brace your body against the side of the bed. Use a gentle, smooth motion to roll the patient toward you (**Figure 22–16B**).

10. A lift sheet can also be used by one or two health care providers to turn the patient. The team members grasp the edges of the lift sheet and roll the edges inward close to the patient's body (**Figure 22–16C**). At a given signal, the team members use a smooth, even motion to turn the patient inward (**Figure 22–16D**).

     CAUTION: Observe proper body mechanics at all times.

11. Raise and secure the siderail, if indicated. Go to the opposite side of the bed and lower the siderail, if present and elevated.

12. Place your hands under the patient's head and shoulders and draw the head and shoulders back toward the center of the bed.

13. Place your hands under the patient's hips and draw them toward the center of the bed.

14. Place your hands under the patient's legs and draw them toward the center of the bed.

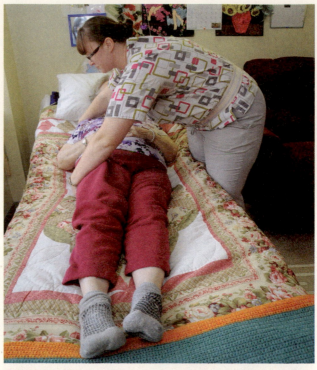

FIGURE 22–16A Position your hands on the patient's far shoulder and hip.

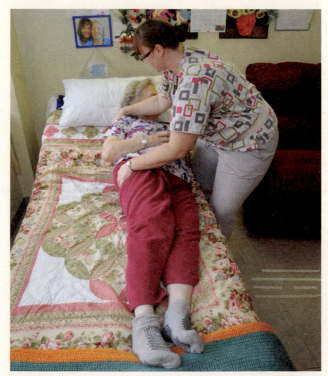

FIGURE 22–16B Use a gentle, smooth motion to roll the patient toward you.

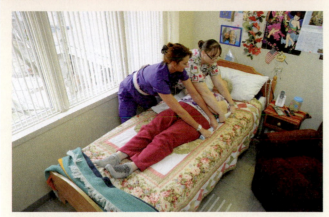

FIGURE 22–16C A lift sheet can also be used by one or two health care team members to turn the patient.

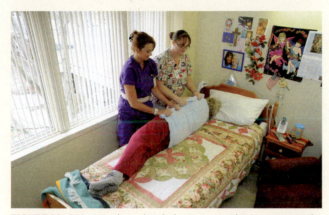

FIGURE 22–16D At a given signal, the team members use a smooth, even motion to turn the patient inward.

15. Place pillows behind the patient's back, between the legs, and under the upper arm to position the patient in good body alignment. Make sure that the patient is comfortable.

16. Elevate the siderail, if indicated. Place the call signal and other necessary supplies within easy reach of the patient. Lower the bed to its lowest level.

17. Replace all equipment. Leave the area neat and clean.

18. Remove gloves. Wash hands.

19. Report that patient has been turned and/or record all required information on the patient's chart or enter it into the computer. For example, date, time, turned on right side and positioned in correct alignment, and your signature and title. Note any unusual observations.
Comm

 NOTE: In health care agencies using electronic health records (EHRs), the information is entered directly into the patient's record on a computer.
EHR

PRACTICE: Go to the workbook and use the evaluation sheet for 22:2D, Turning the Patient Inward to Change Position, to practice this procedure. When you believe you have mastered this skill, sign the sheet and give it to your instructor for further action.

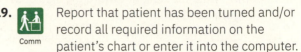 **FINAL EVALUATION:** Using the criteria listed on the evaluation sheet, your instructor will grade your performance.
Check

Procedure 22:2E
OBRA

Sitting Up to Dangle

Equipment and Supplies

Footstool (if needed), bath blanket, robe and nonskid slippers, gloves, paper and pen or computer

Procedure

1. Check orders or obtain authorization from your immediate supervisor. Orders usually state the length of time the patient should dangle.
Legal

2. Assemble equipment.

3. Knock on the door and pause before entering. Introduce yourself. Identify the patient. Explain the procedure and obtain consent.
Comm

4. Provide privacy. Close the door and pull the curtain.

5. Wash hands. Put on gloves.

 CAUTION: Wear gloves and observe standard precautions. Contact with body fluids, secretions, or excretions is possible.
Precaution

6. Lock the bed wheels to prevent movement of the bed.

7. Lower the bed to its lowest level. If siderails are present and elevated, lower the siderail on the side where the patient is to dangle.

8. Check the patient's radial pulse. This reading will serve as a guideline on how the patient tolerates the procedure.

NOTE: Blood pressure may also be checked at this time. Follow agency policy.

(continues)

9. Slowly elevate the head of the bed to a sitting position. Provide time for the patient to adjust to this position.

10. Get close to the patient by bending your knees and keeping your back straight. Position your feet to provide a broad base of support. Place your arm that is nearest to the head of the bed around the patient's shoulders. Place your other arm under the patient's knees (**Figure 22–17A**). Slowly and smoothly rotate the patient toward the side of the bed (**Figure 22–17B**).

 CAUTION: Use proper body mechanics at all times.

 CAUTION: Stand in front of the patient to prevent falls.

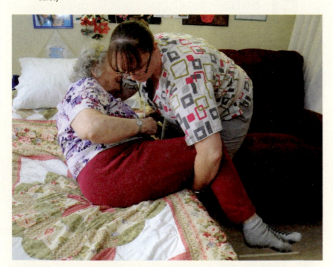

FIGURE 22–17A Place one arm around the patient's shoulders and the other arm under the patient's knees.

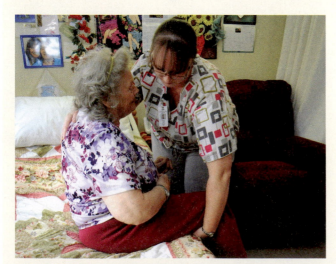

FIGURE 22–17B Slowly rotate the patient toward the side of the bed.

11. Put a robe on the patient. Prevent unnecessary exposure.

12. Use the bath blanket to cover the patient's lap and legs. Put nonskid slippers on the patient. Rest the patient's feet on a footstool (if necessary).

13. Check the patient's radial pulse. Note any signs of distress, such as pale color, increased perspiration, labored respirations, weakness, dizziness, or nausea.

    NOTE: Blood pressure may also be checked at this time. Follow agency policy.

     CAUTION: If any of these signs are noted, go immediately to step 17 and return the patient to the original position in bed.

14. Instruct the patient to flex and extend the legs and feet. This increases circulation to the area and stimulates the muscles.

15. Have the patient dangle for the time ordered or as the patient's condition permits.

16. When the time is up, remove the patient's robe, slippers, and the bath blanket.

17. Place one arm around the patient's shoulders and your other arm under the patient's knees. Gently and slowly return the patient to the bed.

     CAUTION: Use correct body mechanics.

18. Slowly lower the head of the bed.

19. Position the patient in good alignment.

20. Check the patient's radial pulse. Note any major changes. Report any changes immediately.

21. Observe all checkpoints before leaving the patient. Make sure the siderails are elevated (if indicated), the bed is at its lowest level, the call signal and other supplies are within easy reach, and the area is neat and clean.

22. Remove gloves. Wash hands.

23. Report that the patient has dangled and/or record all required information on the patient's chart or enter it into the computer. For example, date, time, sat on side of bed for 15 minutes, P 72 strong and regular at start of procedure, P 78 strong and regular at end, knees and legs flexed and extended, tolerated procedure well, and your signature and title. Note any unusual observations.

    NOTE: In health care agencies using electronic health records (EHRs), the information is entered directly into the patient's record on a computer.

PRACTICE: Go to the workbook and use the evaluation sheet for 22:2E, Sitting Up to Dangle, to practice this procedure. When you believe you have mastered this skill, sign the sheet and give it to your instructor for further action.

 FINAL EVALUATION: Using the criteria listed on the evaluation sheet, your instructor will grade your performance.

Procedure 22:2F

Transferring a Patient to a Chair or Wheelchair

 NOTE: Wheelchairs vary slightly. Read the manufacturer's instructions or ask your immediate supervisor to demonstrate correct operation of the footrests, wheel locks, and other parts.

Equipment and Supplies

Wheelchair or chair, bathrobe, transfer belt, one to two bath blankets, nonskid slippers, gloves, paper and pen or computer

Procedure

1. Obtain orders from your immediate supervisor or check physician's orders to obtain authorization.

2. Assemble equipment.

3. Knock on the door and pause before entering. Introduce yourself. Identify the patient. Explain the procedure and obtain consent.

4. Close the door and pull the curtain to provide privacy for the patient.

5. Wash hands. Put on gloves if needed.

    CAUTION: Wear gloves and observe standard precautions. Contact with body fluids, secretions, or excretions is possible.

6. Position the wheelchair or chair. It can be placed at the head of the bed facing the foot or at the foot of the bed facing the head. Positioning often depends on other equipment in the room.

   NOTE: Whenever possible, the chair should be positioned so that it is secure against a wall or solid furniture and will not slide backward.

7. Securely lock the wheels of the wheelchair. Raise the footrests so that they are out of the way (**Figure 22–18A**).

    CAUTION: Double-check the locks on the wheelchair.

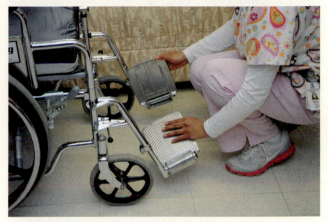

FIGURE 22–18A Lock the wheels and elevate the footrests before moving a patient to a wheelchair.

NOTE: For additional comfort and warmth, a bath blanket can be folded lengthwise and placed in the chair or wheelchair.

8. Lock the bed to prevent movement. Lower the bed to its lowest level.

9. Slowly elevate the head of the bed.

10. If siderails are present and elevated, lower the siderail on the side that the patient is to exit from the bed. Fanfold the bed linen to the foot of the bed.

    NOTE: Avoid exposing the patient during this procedure.

11. Assist the patient to a sitting position on the side of the bed with their feet flat on the floor. Observe for any signs of distress. Note color, pulse rate, breathing, and other similar signs. Put socks and shoes or slippers with nonslip soles on the patient. Put a transfer (gait) belt on the patient following Procedure 23:2A.

    NOTE: Refer to Procedure 22:2E on dangling.

     CAUTION: If the patient is weak or too heavy, get help.

(continues)

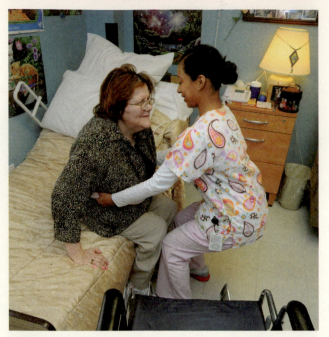

FIGURE 22–18B Lift up on the belt while the patient pushes up from the bed.

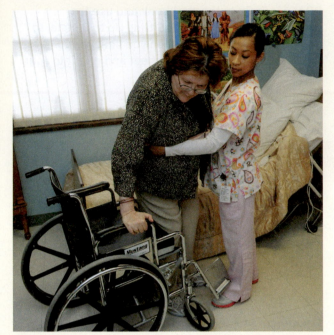

FIGURE 22–18C Help the patient turn until the backs of her legs are touching the seat of the chair.

 CAUTION: If distress is noted, return the patient to bed immediately.

Safety

 CAUTION: Use proper body mechanics.

Safety

12. If the patient needs a robe, put the robe on the patient.

13. Keep your back straight. Place one hand on each side of the belt using an underhand grasp. Face the patient and stand close to the patient. Position your feet to provide a broad base of support. If the patient has a weak leg, support the leg by positioning your knee against the patient's knee or by blocking the patient's foot with your foot.

 NOTE: If the use of a transfer belt is contraindicated, place your hands under the patient's arms and around to the back of the shoulders to provide support.

14. Arrange a signal with the patient, such as counting to three. Instruct the patient to push against the bed with their hands to rise to a standing position.

Comm

15. At the given signal, assist the patient to a standing position. Lift up on the belt while the patient pushes up from the bed (**Figure 22–18B**). Place your knees and feet firmly against the patient's knees and feet to provide support.

16. Allow the patient to adjust to the upright position. Then keeping your hands in the same position, help the patient turn by using several pivot steps until the backs of their legs are touching the seat of the chair (**Figure 22–18C**).

17. Ask the patient to place their hands on the armrests and to bend at the knees as you gradually and slowly lower the patient to a sitting position in the chair (**Figure 22–18D**).

 CAUTION: Bend at the hips and knees and keep your back straight.

Safety

18. Position the patient comfortably. Remove the transfer belt. Use a bath blanket to cover the patient's lap and legs. Lower the footrests on the wheelchair, taking care not to hit the patient's feet (**Figure 22–18E**).

 NOTE: Observe for any signs of distress.

19. Remain with the patient until you are sure there are no problems. If you leave the patient seated in a wheelchair or chair, make sure that the call signal and other supplies are within easy reach. Leave the area neat and clean. Check on the patient at frequent intervals.

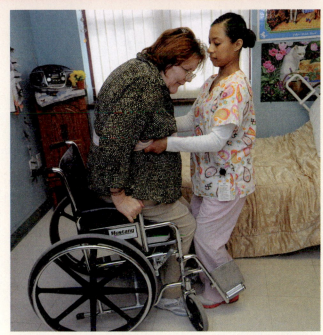

FIGURE 22–18D Gradually and slowly lower the patient to a sitting position in the chair.

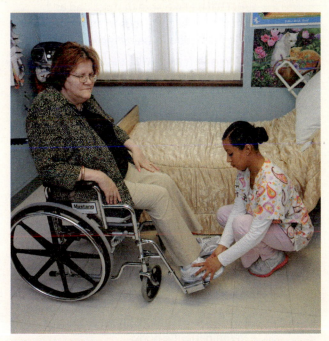

FIGURE 22–18E Lower the footrests of the wheelchair and position the patient's feet on the footrests.

20. If you are transporting the patient in the wheelchair, observe the following rules:

   a. Walk on the right side of the hall or corridor.

   b. Slow down and look for other traffic at doorways and intersections.

   c. To enter an elevator, turn the chair around and back into the elevator.

   d. To go down a steep ramp, turn the chair around and back down the ramp.

   e. Use the weight of your body to push the chair. Stand close to the chair.

   f. Watch the patient closely for signs of distress while transporting.

21. To return the patient to bed, reverse the procedure, beginning by putting a transfer belt on the patient and raising the footrests (step 18).

 CAUTION: Be sure the wheels are locked before helping the patient out of the wheelchair. Lock the bed to prevent movement.

Safety

22. Position the patient in good body alignment after returning them to bed.

23. Observe all checkpoints before leaving the patient: elevate the siderails (if indicated), lower the bed to its lowest level, and place the call signal and other supplies within easy reach of the patient.

24. Replace all equipment used. Wipe the wheelchair with a disinfectant and return it to its proper place. Leave the area neat and clean.

25. Remove gloves if worn. Wash hands.

26. Report that the patient was transferred to a wheelchair and/or record all required information on the patient's chart or enter

Comm

   it into the computer. For example, date, time, transferred to wheelchair, sat in wheelchair for 30 minutes, tolerated well, and your signature and title. Note any unusual observations.

 NOTE: In health care agencies using electronic health records (EHRs), the information is entered directly into the patient's record on a computer.

EHR

PRACTICE: Go to the workbook and use the evaluation sheet for 22:2F, Transferring a Patient to a Chair or Wheelchair, to practice this procedure. When you believe you have mastered this skill, sign the sheet and give it to your instructor for further action.

FINAL EVALUATION: Using the criteria listed on the evaluation sheet, your instructor will grade your performance.

Check

Transferring a Patient to a Stretcher

Equipment and Supplies

Stretcher with siderails and safety belt(s), bath blanket, gloves, paper and pen or computer

NOTE: Because this procedure requires more than one person, it is best to determine what tasks each of the assistants will perform before beginning the procedure.

Procedure

1. Check physician's orders or obtain authorization from your immediate supervisor for the transfer.
   Legal

2. Assemble equipment. Cover the stretcher with a clean sheet.

3. Knock on the door and pause before entering. Introduce yourself. Identify the patient. Explain the procedure and obtain consent.
   Comm

4. Provide privacy. Close the door and pull the curtain.

5. Wash hands. Put on gloves if needed.

    CAUTION: Wear gloves and observe standard precautions. Contact with body fluids, secretions, or excretions is possible.
   Precaution

6. Elevate the bed to the level of the stretcher. Lock the bed wheels to prevent movement of the bed. If siderails are present and elevated, lower the siderail on the side of the transfer.

7. Place a bath blanket over the patient. Fold bed linen to the foot of the bed.
   NOTE: Avoid exposing the patient.

8. Place the stretcher next to the bed. The bed and the stretcher should be parallel.

9. Lock the wheels of the stretcher.

    CAUTION: In addition to the locks, use the weight of your body to hold the stretcher against the bed during this procedure.
   Safety

   ⚠ **CAUTION:** Use correct body mechanics at all times.
   Safety

10. If the patient is conscious and capable of moving unassisted, proceed as follows:

    a. Reach across the stretcher and hold up the bath blanket.

    b. Ask the patient to slide from the bed to the stretcher. Hold the stretcher against the bed (**Figure 22–19**).

    c. If the patient needs assistance, help by moving first the patient's head and shoulders, then the patient's hips, and finally the patient's legs and feet.

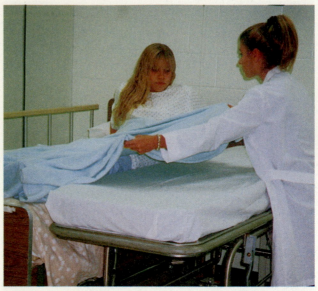

FIGURE 22–19 Hold up the bath blanket and use the weight of your body to hold the stretcher against the bed while the patient is moving to the stretcher.

 CAUTION: Make sure that the bed and stretcher wheels are locked and stabilized while the patient is being moved toward you.
Safety

 CAUTION: If the patient is too heavy or unable to assist with the move, obtain help.
Safety

11. If the patient is very weak, paralyzed, semiconscious, or unconscious, proceed as follows:

    a. Obtain the assistance of three or four other team members.

    b. Position a lifting sheet or blanket under the patient extending from the patient's head and neck to the feet.

    c. Position two or three people by the stretcher and two or three people on the open side of the bed.

    d. Roll the sides of the lifting sheet or blanket close to the patient's body.

    e. Using overhand grasps, one assistant should grasp the sheet by the patient's head and waist. The second assistant should grasp the sheet by the hip and leg. The assistants on the open side of the bed should grasp the sheet in the same areas. If a third assistant is available for one or both sides, they should be positioned so the patient's weight is equally distributed among the three.

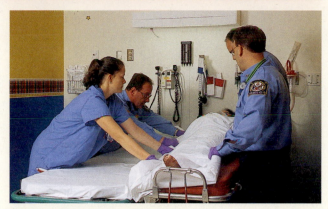

FIGURE 22–20A Team members on both sides of the stretcher should roll the sides of the lift sheet close to the patient and position themselves so all parts of the patient's body are supported.

f. At a given signal, all assistants should lift the sheet slightly to gently slide the patient from the bed to the stretcher.

   NOTE: Some facilities use slider boards instead of a lifting sheet or blanket.

12. Position the patient comfortably on the stretcher.

13. Lock the safety belt(s). Raise both siderails of the stretcher.

14. To transport the patient, two persons should direct the stretcher (one at the head and one at the foot).

    a. Unlock the wheels of the stretcher. Move slowly.

    b. The stretcher patient always travels feet first.

    c. Walk on the right side of the hall.

    d. Watch for cross traffic at doorways and intersections.

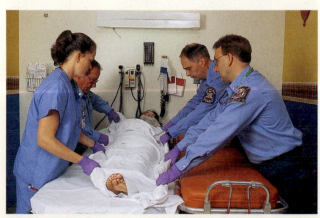

FIGURE 22–20B At a given signal, all assistants should lift the sheet slightly to gently slide the patient from the stretcher to the bed.

e. When going down an incline, the person at the foot of the stretcher should go backward and use body weight to control the stretcher.

f. To enter an elevator, push the correct button to keep the elevator door open. Back the stretcher into the elevator so that the head end enters first. To leave the elevator, push the button to keep the door open, and push the stretcher out feet end first.

15. To return the patient to bed, reverse the procedure, beginning with locking the wheels of the stretcher and bed and unlocking the safety belt(s) Then proceed as shown in **Figures 22-20A** and **22-20B**.

     CAUTION: Always check the wheel locks before transferring patients.

16. Observe all checkpoints before leaving the patient: position the patient in correct alignment, elevate the siderails (if indicated), lower the bed to its lowest level, place the call signal and other supplies within easy reach of the patient, and leave the area neat and clean.

17. Remove the sheet from the stretcher and place the sheet in a linen hamper. Use a disinfectant to wipe the stretcher. Replace all equipment used. Leave the area neat and clean.

18. Remove gloves if worn. Wash hands.

19. Report that the patient was transferred to a stretcher and/or record all required information on the patient's chart or enter it into the computer. For example, date, time, transferred to stretcher and transported to radiology department, tolerated procedure well, and your signature and title. Note any unusual observations.

     NOTE: In health care agencies using electronic health records (EHRs), the information is entered directly into the patient's record on a computer.

PRACTICE: Go to the workbook and use the evaluation sheet for 22:2G, Transferring a Patient to a Stretcher, to practice this procedure. When you believe you have mastered this skill, sign the sheet and give it to your instructor for further action.

FINAL EVALUATION: Using the criteria listed on the evaluation sheet, your instructor will grade your performance.

Procedure 22:2H
OBRA

Using a Mechanical Lift to Transfer a Patient

Comm
NOTE: Mechanical lifts vary slightly. Read the manufacturer's instructions or ask your immediate supervisor to demonstrate the correct operation of the lift.

Safety
CAUTION: The manufacturer will indicate the weight limits for the mechanical lift. Do not use the mechanical lift if the patient weighs more than the weight limit.

Equipment and Supplies

Mechanical lift with straps and sling, bath blanket, chair or wheelchair, gloves, paper and pen or computer

NOTE: If the lift is being used to transfer a patient to a bathtub or shower area, a chair or wheelchair is not required.

CAUTION: Most facilities require that two health care providers perform this procedure. One person operates the lift while the second person guides the movements of the patient. Follow agency policy for this procedure.

Procedure

1. Obtain orders from your immediate supervisor or check physician's orders to obtain authorization.

2. Assemble equipment. Read the operating instructions provided with the mechanical lift or ask your immediate supervisor to demonstrate operation of the lift. Check the straps, sling, and any clasps to make sure there are no defects. Check the hydraulic unit and look for evidence of oil leaks.

   CAUTION: Do not use the lift if straps or sling are torn or defective, if clasps are not secure, or if oil is leaking from the hydraulic unit. Serious injury may result. Label the defective mechanical lift with a warning or lock-out and notify your supervisor immediately.

3.
Comm
Obtain the assistance of another team member. Knock on the door and pause before entering. Introduce yourself and the other team member. Identify the patient. Explain the procedure and obtain consent. Reassure the patient, as needed.

   NOTE: Patients are often apprehensive about being transferred by lift. It is important that they be as relaxed as possible for the transfer. Constant reassurance and encouragement are necessary.

4. Close the door and pull the curtain for privacy during the transfer.

5. Wash hands. Put on gloves if needed.

   CAUTION: Wear gloves and observe standard precautions. Contact with body fluids, secretions, or excretions is possible.

6. Position the chair or wheelchair next to the foot of the bed, with the open seat facing the head of the bed. Lock the wheels of the wheelchair. Raise the footrests to the upright position.

7. Lock the wheels of the bed. If siderails are present and elevated, lower the siderail on the side of the transfer.

8. Turn or move the patient to position the sling under the patient. The sling should be positioned under the shoulders, buttocks, and thighs. Make sure that the sling is smooth and that the center is near the center of the patient's back (**Figure 22–21A**).

9. Position the mechanical lift over the bed (**Figure 22–21B**). Open the base of the lift to its widest position to provide a broad base of support.

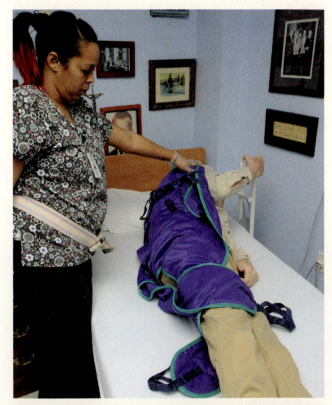

FIGURE 22–21A Position the sling under the patient's shoulders, buttocks, and thighs.

10. Attach the suspension straps to the sling. Insert the hooks from the inside of the sling to the outside to keep the open end of the hooks away from the patient's body. Make sure that the straps are not tangled or twisted. If clasps are present on the hooks, make sure they are secure.

11. Attach the straps to the frame of the lift (**Figure 22–21C**). Check to make sure that the suspension straps are locked to the frame or attached securely. Make sure that the straps are not tangled or twisted. Position the patient's arms inside the straps. Encourage the patient to keep their arms folded across the chest to keep the arms inside the straps.

12. Tell the patient that they will be lifted from the bed. Constantly reassure the patient.
     Comm

13. Turn the crank or use the hydraulic control to slowly raise the patient slightly above the bed. Check the straps, sling, and position of the patient to be sure that the patient is suspended securely by the lift.

Then continue to raise the patient as needed until you can slowly turn the lift to move the patient away from the bed and into position over the chair or wheelchair. Keep all movements as smooth and even as possible (**Figure 22–21D**).

 CAUTION: Move slowly to prevent jerking motions that may frighten the patient.
Safety

14. Slowly lower the lift to position the patient in the chair or wheelchair. Guide the patient's legs into position on the chair (**Figure 22–21E**).

15. Unhook the suspension straps from the sling (**Figure 22–21F**). Remove the sling from under the patient (**Figure 22–21G**). At times, the sling is left in position under the patient. Carefully move the lift away from the patient.

 CAUTION: Be careful not to injure the patient with the straps or lift while moving the lift away from the chair.
Safety

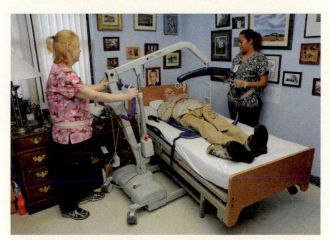

FIGURE 22–21B Position the mechanical lift over the bed.

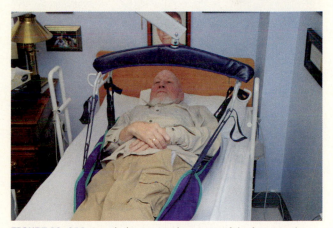

FIGURE 22–21C Attach the suspension straps of the frame to the lift, and make sure they are locked to the frame or attached securely.

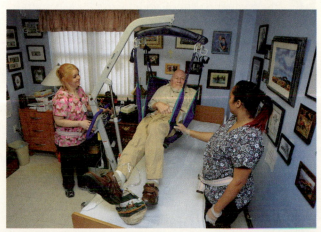

FIGURE 22–21D Use a smooth motion to lift the patient out of the bed.

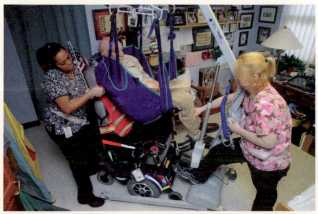

FIGURE 22–21E Lower the lift slowly to position the patient in the wheelchair.

(continues)

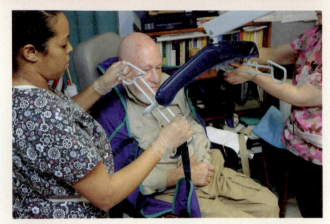

FIGURE 22–21F Unhook the suspension straps from the sling.

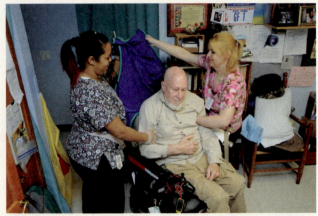

FIGURE 22–21G Remove the sling from under the patient.

16. Use the blanket to cover the patient. Lower the footrests of the wheelchair and position the patient's feet in a comfortable position. Slippers or shoes and socks can be put on the patient's feet.

17. To return the patient to bed, reverse the procedure. Begin by making sure the wheels of the chair and bed are locked. Attach the suspension straps securely to the sling.

18. Observe all checkpoints before leaving the patient: position the patient in correct alignment, elevate the siderails (if indicated), lower the bed to its lowest level, place the call signal and other supplies within easy reach of the patient, and leave the area neat and clean.

19. Use a disinfectant to wipe the mechanical lift. Properly replace all equipment used. Leave the area neat and clean.

20. Remove gloves if worn. Wash hands.

21. Report that the patient was transferred to a chair or wheelchair using a mechanical **Comm** lift and/or record all required information on the patient's chart or enter it into the computer. For example, date, time, transferred to wheelchair with mechanical lift, patient seemed slightly apprehensive at start of procedure but relaxed while in wheelchair, and your signature and title. Note any unusual observations.

 NOTE: In health care agencies using electronic health records (EHRs), the **EHR** information is entered directly into the patient's record on a computer.

PRACTICE: Go to the workbook and use the evaluation sheet for 22:2H, Using a Mechanical Lift to Transfer a Patient, to practice this procedure. When you believe you have mastered this skill, sign the sheet and give it to your instructor for further action.

 FINAL EVALUATION: Using the criteria listed on the evaluation sheet, your instructor will grade **Check** your performance.

22:3 BEDMAKING

Making beds correctly is a task that must be performed by many health care providers. A **OBRA** correctly made bed provides comfort and protection for the patient confined to bed for long periods. Therefore, care must be taken when beds are made. The bed linen must be free of all wrinkles.

Wrinkles cause discomfort and can lead to the formation of pressure ulcers.

Mitered corners are used to hold the linen firmly in place. Mitering corners is a special folding technique that secures the linen under the mattress (**Figure 22–22**). Mitered corners are also used for linen placed on stretchers and examination tables. Some agencies and homes use fitted contour sheets for bottom sheets. Mitered corners would not be used with these sheets but would be used with top sheets.

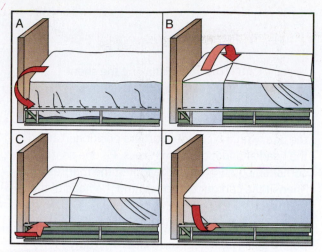

FIGURE 22–22 Steps for making a mitered corner.

Following are examples of the types of beds that you may be required to make:

- **Closed bed**: This is a bed made following the discharge of a patient and after terminal cleaning of the unit. Its purpose is to keep the bed clean until a new patient is admitted.

- **Open bed**: A closed bed is converted to an open bed by **fanfolding** (folding like accordion pleats) the top sheets. This is done to "welcome" a new patient. It is also done for patients who are ambulatory or out of bed for short periods.

- **Occupied bed**: This is a bed made while the patient is in the bed. This is usually done after the bath.

- **Bed cradle**: A cradle is placed on a bed under the top sheets to prevent bed linen from touching parts of the patient's body. A cradle frequently is used for patients with burns, skin ulcers, lesions, blood clots, circulatory disease, fractures, surgery on legs or feet, and other similar conditions.

Draw sheets, also called lift sheets or transfer sheets, are half sheets that are frequently used on beds. A draw sheet extends from the patient's shoulders to the patient's knees. The draw sheet is used to protect the mattress. If soiled, the draw sheet can be changed readily without changing the bottom sheet of the bed. In some settings, disposable bed protectors, frequently called underpads, are placed under the patient to protect the sheets instead of using draw sheets. Draw sheets are also used as lift sheets.

⚠️ **Safety** To prevent injury to yourself, you must observe correct body mechanics while making beds. It is also important to conserve time and energy. Keeping linen arranged in the order of use is one way to conserve time and energy. In addition, most beds are made completely first on one side and then on the other side. This limits unnecessary movement from one side of the bed to the opposite side.

It is also important to limit the movement of organisms and, therefore, the spread of infection while making beds. Wear gloves to handle dirty or soiled linen. Roll dirty or soiled linen while removing it from the bed. Hold dirty linen away from your body and uniform and place it in a linen hamper, cart, or bag immediately. Never place dirty linen on the floor. Some facilities do not allow linen hampers or carts in a patient's room. The hamper or cart is left in the hall. Soiled linen is placed in a pillowcase or plastic bag, carried to the hall, and placed in the hamper or cart. Remove the gloves and wash your hands after handling dirty linen and before handling clean linen. Clean linen should be stored in a closed closet or on a covered linen cart. Never allow clean linen to contact your uniform. Never bring extra linen to the patient's room because it is then considered contaminated and cannot be used for another patient. Avoid shaking clean sheets. Unfold them gently. Place the open end of the pillowcase away from the door. This looks neater and also helps prevent the entrance of organisms from the hall.

Precaution Linen may be contaminated by blood, body fluids, secretions, excretions, urine, or feces. Observe standard precautions (discussed in Section 15:4). Wash your hands frequently and wear gloves while handling linen. Gloves must be worn while removing dirty linen. Before handling clean linen, the contaminated gloves should be removed, and the hands should be washed. If there is any chance of contamination in the room, clean gloves should be applied before handling clean linen. Follow agency policy for proper disposal of linen. Many agencies have special self-dissolving plastic laundry bags that dissolve during the washing process. The contaminated linen is placed in the bag, and the bag is sealed. The bag is then placed inside another plastic bag and labeled before being sent to the laundry department. The second bag is necessary because wet linen may dissolve the water-soluble bag before it reaches the laundry department. The health care provider must be alert at all times to prevent the spread of infection by contaminated linen.

check**point**

1. Bed cradles are used for patients with what conditions?

2. What is another term for a draw sheet?

PRACTICE: Go to the workbook and complete the assignment sheet for 22:3, Bedmaking. Then return and continue with the procedure.

Making a Closed Bed

Equipment and Supplies

Two large sheets (or one large sheet and one fitted sheet); draw sheet (if used); spread (if used); pillow; pillowcase; blanket (as necessary); linen hamper, cart, or bag; gloves

Procedure

1. Assemble equipment.

2. Wash hands. Put on gloves.

    CAUTION: Wear gloves and observe standard precautions. Contact with body fluids, secretions, or excretions is possible.

3. Arrange the clean linen on a chair in the order in which the linen is to be used.

   NOTE: This simplifies the procedure and prevents excessive handling of linen.

4. Elevate the bed to a comfortable height. Lock the wheels to prevent movement.

5. Remove dirty linen from the bed. Roll it into a compact bundle. Hold the linen away from your body. Place it in the linen hamper, bag, or cart. After disposing of the dirty linen, remove the gloves and wash your hands. If there is any chance of contamination in the room, put on clean gloves.

    CAUTION: Prevent the spread of organisms and infection by wearing gloves and observing standard precautions. Linen may be contaminated with blood, body fluids, secretions, or excretions. If the mattress is soiled, wipe it with a disinfectant. After removing contaminated linen, remove the gloves and wash your hands before handling clean linen.

    CAUTION: Never place dirty linen on the floor.

   NOTE: Some facilities do not allow linen hampers or carts in a patient's room. The hamper or cart is left in the hall. Soiled linen is placed in a pillowcase or plastic bag, carried to the hall, and placed in the hamper or cart.

6. Unfold the bottom sheet right side up. Place the small hem even with the foot of the mattress (**Figure 22–23A**). The center fold should be at the center of the bed. The wide hem should be at the head of the bed.

 CAUTION: Avoid shaking the sheet because doing so spreads germs.

NOTE: If a fitted sheet is used, it is positioned on the bed, with the contour corners positioned at the head and foot of the mattress. Fit one contour corner smoothly around the foot of the mattress. Then fit the contour corner around the head of the mattress.

NOTE: Complete one side of the bed entirely before going to the opposite side. This saves time and energy.

7. Tuck 12–18 inches of the sheet under the mattress at the head of the bed (**Figure 22–23B**).

8. Make a mitered corner as follows:

   a. Pick up the sheet approximately 12 inches from the head of the bed.

   b. Form a triangle with a 45-degree angle on top of the mattress (**Figure 22–23C**).

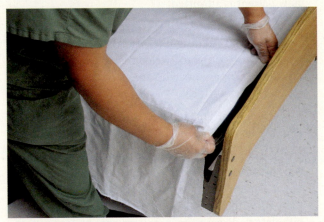

FIGURE 22–23A Position the small hem of the bottom sheet even with the foot of the mattress.

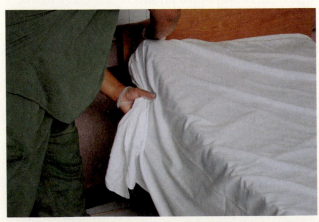

FIGURE 22–23B Tuck 12–18 inches of the sheet under the mattress at the head of the bed.

c. Tuck the lower portion under the mattress (**Figure 22–23D**).

d. Hold the fold with one hand and bring the triangle down to the side of the bed with the other (**Figure 22–23E**).

e. Tuck the folded part under the mattress (**Figure 22–23F**).

f. The mitered corner will help hold the sheet securely in place (**Figure 22–23G**).

9. Tuck in the side of the sheet by working from the head to the foot of the bed.

 CAUTION: Avoid injury. Use correct body mechanics. Work close to the bed and with a broad base of support.

10. Place a draw sheet, if used, in the center of the bed, approximately 14–16 inches from the head of the bed. Tuck the draw sheet in at the side of the bed.

NOTE: Make sure the tucks are secure and as far under the mattress as possible. This helps hold the sheets in place.

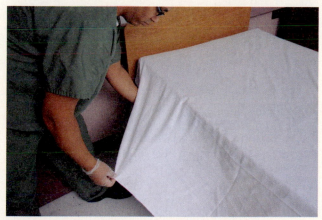

FIGURE 22–23E Bring the triangle down to the side of the bed.

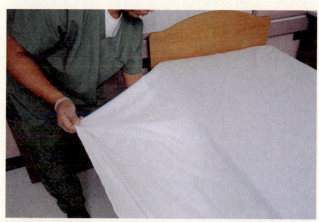

FIGURE 22–23C To make a mitered corner, pick up the sheet approximately 12 inches from the head of the bed and form a triangle with a 45-degree angle.

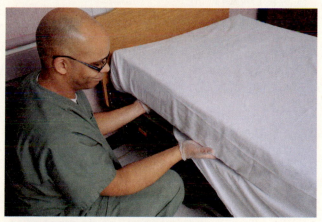

FIGURE 22–23F Tuck the sheet firmly under the mattress to finish the mitered corner.

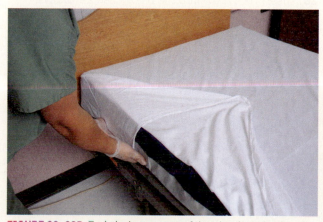

FIGURE 22–23D Tuck the bottom part of the triangle under the mattress.

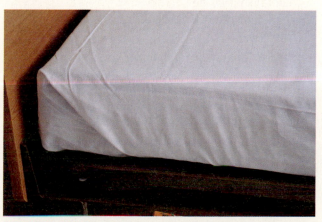

FIGURE 22–23G The finished mitered corner will help hold the sheet securely in position.

(continues)

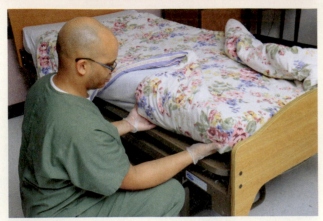

FIGURE 22–23H The top sheet, blanket, and spread can be tucked under the mattress as one unit and secured with a single mitered corner.

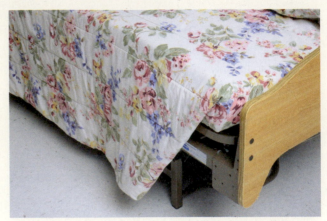

FIGURE 22–23I After making a mitered corner, allow the top sheet, blanket, and spread to hang free on the side of the mattress.

NOTE: Not all agencies use draw sheets. Underpads may be placed on the bed to prevent soiling of the linen.

11. Place the top sheet on the bed, wrong side up. Use the center fold to center the sheet. The wide hem should be even with the top edge of the mattress.

12. Tuck the top sheet over the foot of the mattress.

13. Make a mitered corner as previously instructed.

14. Tuck the side of the sheet under the mattress to the center of the bed only.

15. If a blanket is used, it can be placed on the bed in the same manner as the top sheet. The top sheet and blanket can be tucked in at the same time.

16. If a spread is used, place the spread on the bed right side up. The top edge should be even with the top edge of the mattress. Use the center fold to center the spread.

17. Tuck the spread under the mattress at the foot of the bed.

    NOTE: The top sheet, blanket, and spread can all be placed on the bed at the same time. They are then tucked in as one unit at the bottom of the bed, and a mitered corner is made with all of the linen (**Figure 22–23H**).

18. Make a mitered corner but do not tuck the final end under the side of the mattress. Let the triangle hang loose (**Figure 22–23I**).

19. Go to the opposite side of the bed. From the side, fanfold the top covers to the center of the bed so you can work with the bottom sheet.

20. Tuck the bottom sheet under the head of the mattress. Make a mitered corner.

21. Work from the head of the bed to the foot to tuck in the side of the sheet. Pull the sheet gently to remove all wrinkles before tucking in the side.

22. Grasp the draw sheet in the center. Pull gently to remove wrinkles. Tuck in firmly at the side.

23. Tuck in the top sheet (and blanket) at the foot of the bed. Make a mitered corner. Remove all wrinkles and tuck in at the side up to the center of the bed only.

24. Tuck in the spread at the foot of the bed. Make a mitered corner but do not tuck in the final fold. Let it hang free.

25. Line up all sheets so they are smooth and free of wrinkles. If a blanket is used, the top sheet can be folded back over the blanket, making a cuff. This protects the patient from the edge of the blanket.

26. Insert the pillow into the pillowcase as follows:

    a. Place hands in the clean pillowcase and loosen the corners.

    b. Use one hand to grasp the center of the end seam on the outside. Turn the case back over the hand and lower arm (**Figure 22–24A**).

    c. Using the hand that is covered by the case, grab the end of the pillow at the center of the pillow (**Figure 22–24B**).

    d. Using your free hand, unfold the case over the pillow (**Figure 22–24C**).

    e. Adjust the end corners of the pillow into the corners of the case.

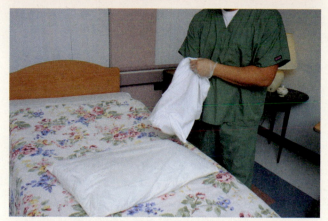

FIGURE 22–24A Grasp the center of the end seam on the pillowcase and turn the case back over the hand and lower arm.

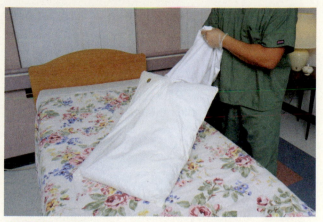

FIGURE 22–24B Using the pillowcase-covered hand, grab the end of the pillow.

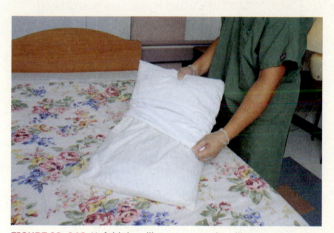

FIGURE 22–24C Unfold the pillowcase over the pillow.

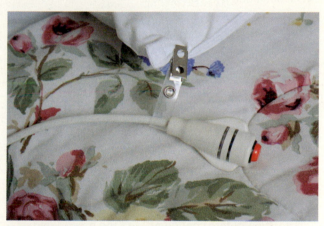

FIGURE 22–24D Make sure the call signal is firmly attached to the pillow or bed.

   f. Adjust the pillowcase on the pillow. It may be necessary to make a lengthwise pleat for a better fit.

 CAUTION: Do not hold the pillow under your chin or against your body. Rather, place it on the bed for support.

27. Place the pillow on the bed, with the open end pointed away from the door. Make sure the call signal is firmly attached to the pillow or bed (**Figure 22–24D**).

   NOTE: This position looks neater and allows fewer organisms from the hall to enter the pillow.

28. Lower the bed to its lowest position. Replace all other equipment (bedside table, call signal, chair, etc.).

29. Before leaving the area, check to make sure it is neat and clean.

30. Remove gloves if worn. Wash hands.

31. Record or report that a closed bed was made.

   Comm

PRACTICE: Go to the workbook and use the evaluation sheet for 22:3A, Making a Closed Bed, to practice this procedure. When you believe you have mastered this skill, sign the sheet and give it to your instructor for further action.

 FINAL EVALUATION: Using the criteria listed on the evaluation sheet, your instructor will grade your performance.

Check

Making an Occupied Bed

Equipment and Supplies

Laundry hamper, cart, or bag; two large sheets (or one large sheet and one fitted sheet); draw sheet (if used); spread (if used); pillow; pillowcase; blanket (if needed); bath blanket; disposable protective pads; gloves; paper and pen or computer

Procedure

1. Assemble equipment.

2. Knock on the door and pause before entering. Introduce yourself. Identify the patient. Explain the procedure and obtain consent.

3. Close the door and pull the curtain for privacy.

4. Wash hands. Put on gloves.

    CAUTION: Put on gloves and observe standard precautions. Linen on the bed may be contaminated with blood, body fluids, secretions, or excretions.

5. Arrange the clean linen on a chair in the order in which the linen will be used.

6. Lock the wheels of the bed. Elevate the bed to a comfortable working position.

7. Lower the headrest and footrest so that the bed is flat, if permissible.

   NOTE: Make sure the patient can tolerate this position before continuing with the procedure.

8. If siderails are present and elevated, lower the siderail on the side where you are working.

    CAUTION: Make sure the siderail on the opposite side is elevated.

9. Loosen the top bedclothes at the bottom of the mattress. Remove the spread and blanket. If they are to be reused, fold and place them over the chair.

10. Replace the top sheet with a bath blanket. Have the patient hold the top edge of the bath blanket, if able, while you slide the soiled top sheet out from top to bottom. Place the soiled sheet in the linen hamper, cart, or bag.

    NOTE: A bath blanket is a soft flannel or cotton blanket that is used to cover the patient and provide warmth while the other sheets are replaced.

     CAUTION: Avoid shaking the linen because doing so spreads germs. Hold the linen away from your body.

11. Remove the pillow. If this makes the patient uncomfortable, leave the pillow under the patient's head.

12. Assist the patient in turning to the opposite side of the bed.

13. Fanfold the cotton draw sheet up to the patient's body.

14. Fanfold the bottom sheet up to and under the draw sheet (**Figure 22–25A**). Make sure all of the sheets are as close to the patient as possible.

15. Place the clean bottom sheet on the bed right side up. Place the narrow hem even with the foot of the bed. Center using the center fold. Fanfold the opposite side close to patient.

     CAUTION: Avoid injury. Use correct body mechanics, including a broad base of support.

16. Tuck in the clean bottom sheet at the head of the bed. Make a mitered corner. Working from the head to the foot of the bed, tuck in the entire side (**Figure 22–25B**).

    NOTE: If a fitted sheet is used, it is positioned on the bed with the contour corners positioned at the head and foot of the mattress.

17. Place the clean draw sheet on the bed. Center using the draw sheet's center fold. Fanfold the opposite half close to the patient. Tuck the draw sheet firmly under the mattress at the side (**Figure 22–25C**).

18. Turn the patient toward you. Caution the patient that they will be turning over the top of the fanfolded linen. Elevate the siderail, if indicated.

19. Go to the opposite side of the bed. Lower the siderail, if elevated.

20. Remove the soiled bottom sheet and draw sheet (**Figure 22–25D**). Place in the linen hamper, cart, or bag.

21. Pull the clean bottom sheet into place. Tuck it under the mattress at the head of the bed. Make a mitered corner.

22. Pull gently to remove all wrinkles. Tuck the side of the sheet under the mattress, working from top to bottom.

23. Pull the clean draw sheet into place (**Figure 22–25E**). Remove all wrinkles and tuck it firmly under the side of the mattress.

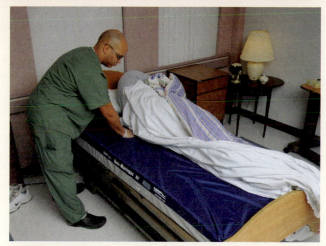

FIGURE 22-25A Fanfold the bottom sheet to the center of the bed.

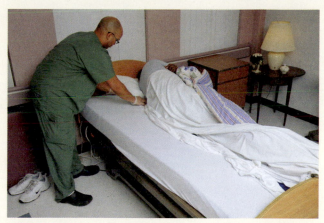

FIGURE 22-25B Position the clean bottom sheet on the bed, fanfold it at the center of the bed, make a mitered corner at the top edge, and tuck in the side of the sheet.

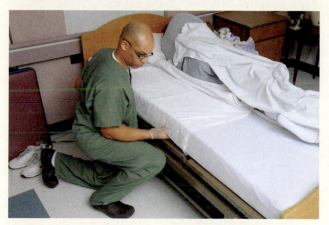

FIGURE 22-25C Fanfold the draw sheet at the center of the bed and tuck it into the side of the bed.

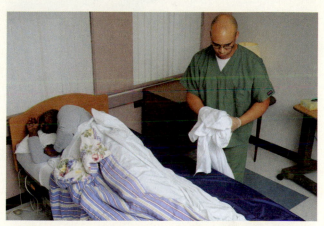

FIGURE 22-25D Go to the opposite side of the bed and remove the soiled draw sheet and bottom sheet.

24. Assist the patient to turn onto their back in the center of the bed.

25. Place the top sheet, wrong side up, over the bath blanket. Center using the sheet's center fold. Ask the patient to hold the top edge of the clean sheet. Remove the bath blanket by pulling it from the top to the bottom of the bed (**Figure 22-25F**).

 CAUTION: Avoid exposing the patient during this procedure.

26. If a blanket is to be used, place it over the top sheet.

27. If a spread is used, place the spread on top, right side up. Center it on the bed.

28. Tuck the top sheet, blanket, and spread into the bottom of the mattress. Make a mitered corner. Before tucking in the final fold, form a toe pleat by making a 3-inch fold in the top of the linen

(**Figure 22-25G**). The fold should be made toward the foot of the bed. Complete the mitered corner.

NOTE: The toe pleat provides more room for the patient's feet and toes and prevents pressure on the toes from the sheets.

29. Raise the siderail, if indicated, and go to the opposite side of the bed. Lower the siderail, if elevated, and complete the top sheets on the opposite side of the bed.

30. Fold the top edge of the spread over and under the top of the blanket. Bring the top sheet over the top of the spread and blanket, and make a 6–8 inch cuff.

31. Insert the pillow into a clean pillowcase as instructed in Procedure 22:3A.

32. Place the pillow on the bed, with the open end away from the door.

(continues)

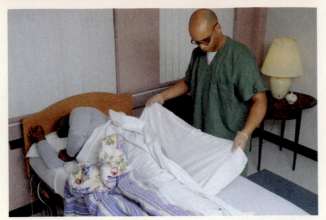

FIGURE 22-25E Pull the clean draw sheet into place and tuck it under the side of the mattress.

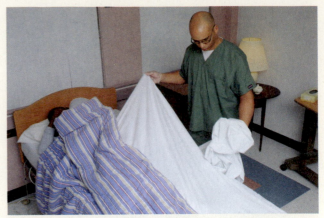

FIGURE 22-25F Position a clean top sheet on the patient and remove the bath blanket, if used, or the soiled top sheet.

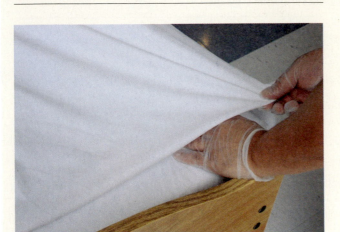

FIGURE 22-25G Make a toe pleat in the top linen to provide more room for the patient's feet and toes.

33. Position the patient comfortably in good body alignment.

34. Observe all checkpoints before leaving the patient: place the call signal and other supplies within easy reach of the patient, lower the bed to its lowest level, elevate the side-rails (if indicated), and leave the area neat and clean.

35. Dispose of dirty linen in the appropriate location. Properly replace all equipment.

36. Remove gloves. Wash hands.

37. Report that an occupied bed was made and/or record all required information on the patient's chart or enter it into the computer. For example, date, time, occupied bed made, and your signature and title. Note any unusual observations.

   NOTE: In health care agencies using electronic health records (EHRs), the information is entered directly into the patient's record on a computer.

PRACTICE: Go to the workbook and use the evaluation sheet for 22:3B, Making an Occupied Bed, to practice this procedure. When you believe you have mastered this skill, sign the sheet and give it to your instructor for further action.

 FINAL EVALUATION: Using the criteria listed on the evaluation sheet, your instructor will grade your performance.

Procedure 22:3C

Opening a Closed Bed

Equipment and Supplies

Closed bed with linen in place, paper and pen or computer

Procedure

1. Wash hands.

2. Check the closed bed to be sure it was made correctly. Lock the wheels and elevate the height of the bed to a comfortable working position.

   NOTE: For an ambulatory patient, the bed is made as a closed bed and then converted to an open bed.

3. Place the pillow on a chair or overbed table.

4. Go to the head of the bed and work from its side. Fold the top edge of the spread over and under the blanket. Fold the top sheet down over the blanket and spread to form a cuff.

5. Face the foot of the bed. Hold the upper edge of the top layers of linen (spread, blanket, and sheet) with both hands.

6. Fanfold the linen into three even layers down to the foot of the bed (**Figure 22–26**).

   NOTE: The top of the fold should be facing the head of the bed. In this manner, the patient will be able to pull the top covers up more readily after getting into the bed.

7. Place the pillow back at the head of the bed. Make sure the open end is away from the door.

8. Observe all checkpoints before leaving the area: place the call signal within easy reach of the bed, lower the bed to its lowest level, lock the bed wheels, correctly position all equipment, and leave the area neat and clean.

9. Wash hands.

10. Report that an open bed was made and/or record all required information on the patient's chart or enter it into the computer. For example, date, time, open bed made, and your signature and title.

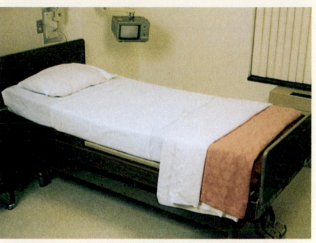

FIGURE 22–26 In an open bed, the top sheets are fanfolded to the foot of the bed.

 NOTE: In health care agencies using electronic health records (EHRs), the information is entered directly into the patient's record on a computer.

PRACTICE: Go to the workbook and use the evaluation sheet for 22:3C, Opening a Closed Bed, to practice this procedure. When you believe you have mastered this skill, sign the sheet and give it to your instructor for further action.

 FINAL EVALUATION: Using the criteria listed on the evaluation sheet, your instructor will grade your performance.

Procedure 22:3D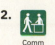

Placing a Bed Cradle

Equipment and Supplies

Laundry hamper, cart, or bag; bed cradle; two large sheets (or one large sheet and one fitted sheet); draw sheet (if used); spread (if used); pillow; pillowcase; blanket (if needed); bath blanket; gloves; paper and pen or computer

Procedure

1. Assemble equipment.

2. Knock on the door and pause before entering. Introduce yourself. Identify the patient. Explain the procedure and obtain consent.

3. Close the door and pull the curtain to provide privacy.

4. Wash hands. Put on gloves.

   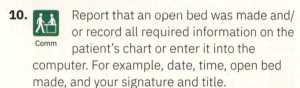 **CAUTION:** Wear gloves and observe standard precautions. Linen may be contaminated with blood, body fluids, secretions, or excretions.

5. Lock the bed wheels. Elevate the bed to a comfortable working height. If siderails are present and elevated, lower the siderail on the side of the bed where you are working.

    CAUTION: If siderails are present, check the opposite siderail to make sure it is raised and secured.

(continues)

6. Use a bath blanket to cover the patient. Remove soiled top linen and place it in the linen hamper, cart, or bag.

7. Turn the patient toward the opposite side of the bed.

8. Loosen the bottom sheet and draw sheet, and fanfold them to the center of the bed.

9. Place the clean bottom sheet and draw sheets on the bed as described in Procedure 22:3B, Making an Occupied Bed. Finish changing bottom linen on both sides of the bed.

10. Position the patient in the center of the bed and on their back.

11. Place the bed cradle into position (**Figure 22–27**).

     CAUTION: To prevent injury, make sure the cradle is not touching any part of the patient's skin.

12. Tie or anchor the cradle to the bed as necessary. Many bed cradles have metal clamps that attach to the mattress or bed frame. If no clamps are present, roller gauze or straps can be attached to the cradle and then fastened to the bedframe under the mattress.

    NOTE: A restless or confused patient may knock the cradle off of the bed. The cradle should be clamped or tied in place to prevent this.

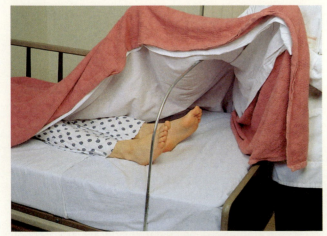

FIGURE 22–27 A bed cradle supports the top linen and prevents the linen from coming into contact with the patient's legs and feet.

13. Place the top sheet, blanket, and spread over the top of the cradle and patient. Remove the bath blanket. Tuck in the top sheets at the foot of the bed.

14. Miter the corners and tuck them into place. A larger fold can be made near the lower edge of the cradle to form a neater mitered corner.

15. Make a cuff by folding the top sheet over the blanket and spread.

16. Insert the pillow into a clean pillowcase. Position the pillow on the bed, with the open end away from the door.

17. Observe all checkpoints before leaving the patient: the patient is safe, comfortable, and in good body alignment; the call signal and other supplies are within easy reach of the patient; the siderails are elevated (if indicated); the bed is at its lowest level; and the area is neat and clean.

18. Check placement of the bed cradle at the end of the procedure and at intervals afterward. Make sure it keeps the bed linen away from the patient's legs and feet. Make sure it is securely in place.

19. Replace all equipment.

20. Wash hands.

21. Report that a bed with cradle was made and/or record all required information on the patient's chart or enter it into the computer. For example, date, time, bed with cradle made, and your signature and title. Note any unusual observations.

     NOTE: In health care agencies using electronic health records (EHRs), the information is entered directly into the patient's record on a computer.

PRACTICE: Go to the workbook and use the evaluation sheet for 22:3D, Placing a Bed Cradle, to practice this procedure. When you believe you have mastered this skill, sign the sheet and give it to your instructor for further action.

✅ **FINAL EVALUATION:** Using the criteria listed on the evaluation sheet, your instructor will grade your performance.

22:4 ADMINISTERING PERSONAL HYGIENE

OBRA Administering personal care and hygiene may be one of your responsibilities as a health care provider. Ill patients often depend on health care team members for all aspects of personal care. The health care provider must be sensitive to the patient's needs and respect the patient's right to privacy while personal care is administered.

Personal hygiene usually includes bathing, back care, perineal care, oral hygiene, hair care, nail care, and shaving, when necessary. Such care promotes good habits of personal hygiene, provides comfort, and stimulates circulation. Providing such care also gives the health care provider an excellent opportunity to develop a good and caring relationship with the patient.

TYPES OF BATHS

Different types of baths are given to patients. The type of bath depends on the patient's condition and ability to help.

- **Complete bed bath (CBB):** The health care provider bathes all parts of the patient's body and also provides oral hygiene, back care, hair care, nail care, and perineal care. A complete bath is usually given to the patient who is confined to bed and is too weak or ill to bathe.

- **Partial bed bath:** The health care provider bathes some parts of the patient's body. The term partial bath (PB) has two meanings, both related to the patient's ability to help. If the patient is too weak to help, a partial bath means that only the face, arms, hands, back, and perineal area are bathed by the health care provider. If the patient is able to wash most of their body, a partial bath means that the health care provider completes the bath, usually bathing the patient's legs and back. In both types of partial baths, the health care provider prepares the supplies needed by the patient (**Figure 22–28**).

- **Tub bath or shower:** Some patients are allowed to take tub baths or showers. The health care provider helps as needed by providing towels and supplies, preparing the tub or shower area, and assisting the patient as much as the situation demands.

- **Waterless bath:** Some facilities are using prepackaged disposable cleansing cloths instead of basins of water for baths (**Figure 22–29**). The cleansing cloths contain a rinse-free cleanser and moisturizer, and can be warmed in a microwave (follow package instructions) or in a special

warmer. The waterless bath is less tiring to the patient and helps preserve skin moisture, prevent drying, and is more gentle to the skin than most soaps. Most packages contain 8–10 cloths. Usually one cloth is used for the face, neck, and ears; one for each arm and each leg; one for the chest and abdomen; one for the perineum; and one for the back and buttocks. The solution dries quickly on the skin, but a towel can be used to gently remove excess moisture. Extreme care must be taken to avoid overheating the cloths. Read and follow manufacturer's instructions.

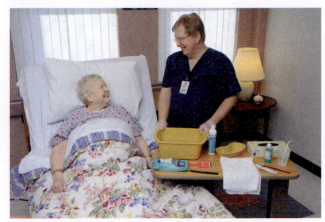

FIGURE 22–28 Position supplies conveniently when assisting a patient with a partial bath.

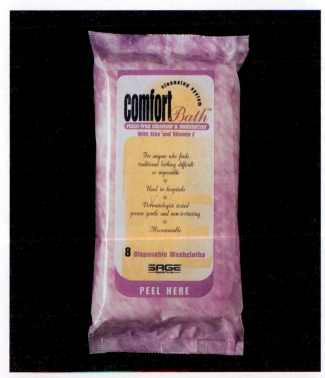

FIGURE 22–29 Packages of cleansing cloths containing a rinse-free cleaner and moisturizer can be used to give a waterless bath. Courtesy of Sage Products, Inc.

ORAL HYGIENE

Oral hygiene means care of the mouth and teeth. Oral hygiene should be administered at least three times a day. If the patient's condition requires frequent oral care, it should be administered more often, usually at least every 2 hours. Proper oral hygiene prevents disease and dental caries, stimulates the appetite, and provides comfort. In addition, it aids in the prevention of halitosis (bad breath).

- **Routine oral hygiene** refers to regular, everyday toothbrushing and flossing. Many times, patients are able to provide their own care. In such cases, the health care provider provides all of the necessary equipment and supplies. In other cases, the provider helps the patient brush and care for the teeth and mouth.

- **Denture care** is necessary when a patient has dentures or artificial teeth. In some cases, the health care provider must help clean the dentures. Patients may be sensitive about dentures. Therefore, it is important that the health care provider provide privacy and reassure the patient. Extreme care must also be taken to prevent damage to the dentures.

- **Special oral hygiene** is usually provided for the unconscious or semiconscious patient. Because many of these patients breathe through their mouths, extra care must be taken to clean all parts of the mouth. Special supplies are used for this procedure.

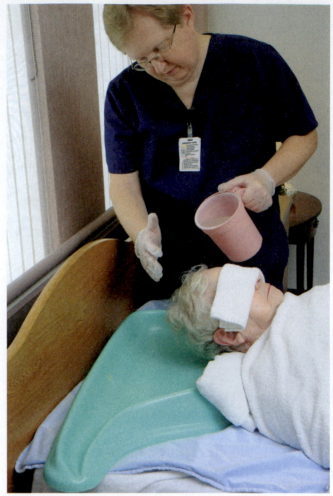

FIGURE 22–30 Special devices are available for use when shampooing the hair of a patient confined to bed.

HAIR CARE

Hair care is an important aspect of personal care that is, unfortunately, frequently neglected. Patients confined to bed often have tangles and knots in their hair. Tangles or knots can be removed by combing a small section of hair at a time and working from the ends toward the scalp. Conditioners can help prevent tangles. Braiding long hair after the tangles are removed also helps reduce the number of tangles and knots. Brushing stimulates circulation to the scalp. Brushing also removes dirt and/or lint, and helps keep the hair shiny and attractive.

It is also important to observe the condition of the hair and scalp. Signs of disease, redness, scaling, scalp irritation, or any other conditions should be reported.

Shampooing must be approved by the physician. Various types of dry or fluid shampoos are available for patients confined to bed. Read all instructions carefully before using any of these products. Special devices are also available for use while giving a shampoo to a patient confined to bed (**Figure 22–30**).

NAIL CARE

Nail care is another often-neglected area in the personal care of the patient. Nails harbor dirt, which can lead to infection and disease. In addition, rough or sharp nails can cause injury. It is important that nail care be included as a part of the daily personal care provided to the patient. However, nails should never be cut unless you receive specific orders to do so from the physician or your immediate supervisor. Cutting nails may cause injury. In some facilities, only licensed or advanced practice personnel are allowed to cut fingernails. If you are permitted to cut fingernails, use nail clippers, not scissors, and clip the nails straight across. *Never* cut below the tips of the fingers. Clip slowly and carefully to avoid accidentally damaging the skin around the nail. Then file the nails straight across to remove rough edges. *Never* cut toenails because injuries to the feet are prone to infection and slow healing. File toenails straight across. Learn and follow your agency policy on nail care.

SHAVING

Shaving is a normal daily routine for most men. It is important to provide this care when the patient is unable to shave himself. Either safety razors or electric razors may be used. The type used usually depends on the patient's personal preference. Correct technique must be used to prevent injury to the patient. Female patients usually appreciate shaving of the legs and underarms. Be sure you have specific orders from the physician or your immediate supervisor before shaving any patient. Shaving may be prohibited or special precautions may be required for patients on anticoagulants, or medications that prevent the blood from clotting.

BACK RUB

Unless contraindicated by the patient's condition, a back rub is given as part of the daily bath. It can also be given at other times during the day and should be done at least once every 8 hours for a patient confined to bed. A good back rub takes at least 4–7 minutes and stimulates circulation, prevents pressure ulcers, and leads to relaxation and comfort. It is important that the health care provider's nails be short to prevent injury.

CHANGING A GOWN OR CLOTHING

Changing a patient's gown or pajamas is also important. Most patients prefer to wear their own gowns or pajamas. However, hospital gowns are frequently used on very ill patients or on patients with limited movement. These gowns usually open down the back and are easier to position and remove. If the patient has a weak or injured arm, or if an intravenous solution is being infused in one arm, the gown or pajama top must be positioned with care. Usually, the sleeve of the soiled gown or pajama top is removed from the uninjured or untreated arm first. This allows more freedom of movement while removing the sleeve from the injured or treated arm. Likewise, the sleeve of the clean gown or pajama top is placed on the affected arm first and then is placed on the unaffected arm. It is sometimes necessary to leave one arm out of the gown and place the sleeve on the unaffected arm only. Some agencies have gowns with openings at the shoulders. Such a gown can be placed over a treated arm and then closed with snaps, ties, or Velcro strips at the shoulder area.

In home care, gowns or pajama tops can be opened at the arm seam for easy application. Velcro strips or ties can then be applied so that the gown or pajama top can be closed after being put on the patient. In long-term care facilities, most residents wear regular clothing during the day. It is important to help the resident as needed in choosing and dressing in appropriate clothing. If a resident has difficulty moving one side or is paralyzed, always put the clothing on the affected side first and remove it from the affected side last.

SUMMARY

 When administering personal hygiene, it is important that the health care team member be alert for any signs that might be unusual. When performing any personal hygiene procedure, watch for and report any unusual observations, including the following:

- **Sores, cuts, injuries**: Any injuries noted on the skin, mouth, or scalp must be reported.

- **Rashes:** Any type of rash should be reported. Many times, a rash is the first sign of an allergic reaction to a medication.

- **Color**: Any unusual color should be noted. Redness (erythema) of the skin is often the first sign of a pressure sore, or decubitus ulcer. A blue color (cyanosis) is a sign of poor circulation. A yellow color (jaundice) is a sign of liver disease, bile obstruction, or destruction of red blood cells.

- **Swelling, or edema**: This can indicate poor circulation or disease and should be reported immediately. Pay particular attention to the hands, feet, ankles, and toes.

- **Other signs of distress**: Difficult breathing (dyspnea), dizziness (vertigo), unusual weakness, excessive perspiration (diaphoresis), extreme pallor, or abnormal drowsiness or sluggishness (lethargy) should be reported immediately.

 When administering personal hygiene, standard precautions (described in Section 15:4) must be observed at all times. Hands must be washed frequently, and gloves must be worn. Contact with blood, body fluids, secretions, or excretions is possible. A gown must be worn if contamination of a uniform or clothing is likely. A mask and protective eyewear, or a face shield, must be worn if droplets of blood or body fluids are present, such as when a patient is coughing excessively. Health care team members with cuts, sores, or dermatitis on their hands must wear gloves for all patient contact. Preventing the spread of infection is a major responsibility of the health care provider.

 Always be sensitive to the patient's feelings and respect the patient's rights. Knock on the door and pause before entering a patient's or resident's room. Provide privacy during procedures by closing the door and pulling the curtain. Avoid exposing the patient when administering personal hygiene. Explain all procedures and reassure the patient as needed. Observe legal responsibilities and professional ethics at all times.

1. How frequently should oral hygiene be administered?

2. How do you get tangles or knots out of hair?

PRACTICE: Go to the workbook and complete the assignment sheet for 22:4, Administering Personal Hygiene. Then return and continue with the procedures.

Procedure 22:4A 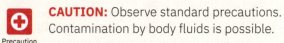 OBRA

Providing Routine Oral Hygiene

Equipment and Supplies

Toothbrush, toothpaste or powder, mouthwash solution (if used) in cup, cup of water, straw, emesis basin, bath towel, tissues, dental floss, plastic bag or plastic-lined waste can, disposable gloves, paper and pen or computer

Procedure

1. Obtain proper authorization and assemble equipment.

2. Knock on the door and pause before entering. Introduce yourself. Identify the patient. Explain the procedure and obtain consent.

Comm

3. Wash hands. Put on gloves. If spraying or splashing of oral fluids is possible, wear a gown, mask or face shield, and eye protection.

CAUTION: Observe standard precautions. Contamination by body fluids is possible.

Precaution

4. Position the patient comfortably. Close the door and pull the curtain to provide privacy. Raise the head of the bed, if permitted. Elevate the bed to a comfortable working height. If siderails are present and elevated, lower the siderail on the side where you are working. Position the overbed table containing all equipment in a convenient location (**Figure 22–31A**).

NOTE: If the patient can brush their own teeth, the overbed table is usually positioned over the patient's lap.

5. Place the bath towel on the bedclothes and over the patient's shoulders.

NOTE: A disposable bed protector can also be used to drape the patient.

6. Put water on the toothbrush. Add toothpaste. Give the brush to the patient.

NOTE: Before adding the toothpaste, ask how much the patient uses.

7. If the patient cannot brush, brush the patient's teeth (**Figure 22–31B**). Carefully insert the brush into the patient's mouth. Start at the rear of the upper teeth. Place the brush at a slight angle to the gum, rotate gently, and then use a slight vibrating motion to thoroughly clean all of the upper teeth. Repeat this process on the lower teeth.

NOTE: Refer to Procedure 19:9A, Demonstrating Brushing Technique, for guidelines on brushing the teeth.

8. Give the patient water from the cup to rinse the mouth. Provide a straw, if needed.

9. Hold the emesis basin under the patient's chin. Instruct the patient to expel the mouth secretions into the basin (**Figure 22–31C**).

10. Repeat steps 8 and 9, as necessary.

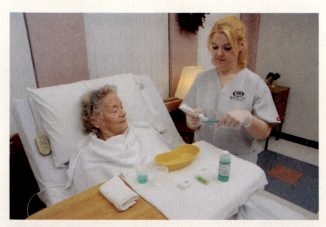

FIGURE 22–31A Position all supplies in a convenient location when assisting a patient with routine oral hygiene.

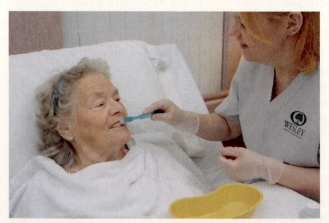

FIGURE 22–31B Assist the patient with brushing the teeth if needed.

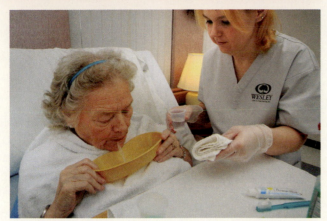

FIGURE 22–31C Instruct the patient to expectorate (spit) into the emesis basin.

11. Offer tissues to allow the patient to wipe the mouth and chin. Discard tissues in the plastic bag.

12. Provide dental floss. Allow the patient to floss the teeth. Assist as needed. If the patient is not able to floss, obtain a piece of floss about 12–18 inches long. Gently insert the floss between the teeth. Curve the floss into a C-shape. Use a gentle up-and-down motion to clean the sides of the teeth. Repeat for both sides of every tooth.

    NOTE: Refer to Procedure 19:9B, Demonstrating Flossing Technique, for guidelines on flossing the teeth.

13. Provide mouthwash, if desired by the patient. Mouthwash is sometimes diluted to a proportion of half mouthwash to half water. Use the emesis basin and tissues, as necessary, to allow the patient to expectorate the mouthwash.

14. Remove all equipment. Position the patient comfortably. Be sure the patient is in good body alignment.

15. Observe all checkpoints before leaving the patient: elevate the siderails (if indicated), place the call signal and other supplies within easy reach of the patient, lower the bed to its lowest level, and leave the area neat and clean.

16. Rinse the toothbrush thoroughly. Use cool water and towels to clean the emesis basin. Properly replace all equipment.

17. Remove gloves. Remove mask and eye protection, if worn. Wash hands.

18. Report that routine oral hygiene was given to the patient and/or record all required information on the patient's chart or enter it into the computer. For example, date, time, oral hygiene given, and your signature and title. Note any unusual observations.

    NOTE: In health care agencies using electronic health records (EHRs), the information is entered directly into the patient's record on a computer.

PRACTICE: Go to the workbook and use the evaluation sheet for 22:4A, Providing Routine Oral Hygiene, to practice this procedure. When you believe you have mastered this skill, sign the sheet and give it to your instructor for further action.

FINAL EVALUATION: Using the criteria listed on the evaluation sheet, your instructor will grade your performance.

Procedure 22:4B
OBRA

Cleaning Dentures

Equipment and Supplies

Toothbrush and toothpaste or denture brush and denture cleaner, denture cup, tissues, cup with mouthwash (if used), straw, applicators, bath towel, paper towels, emesis basin, plastic bag or plastic-lined waste can, disposable gloves, paper and pen or computer

Procedure

1. Obtain proper authorization and assemble equipment.

2. Knock on the door and pause before entering. Introduce yourself. Identify the patient. Explain the procedure and obtain consent.

    NOTE: The patient may be sensitive about dentures. Provide privacy and reassurance.

3. Close the door and pull the curtain for privacy.

4. Wash hands. Put on gloves.

     CAUTION: Observe standard precautions. If splashing of body fluids is possible, wear a gown, mask or face shield, and eye protection.

(continues)

5. Elevate the head of the bed to a comfortable working height. Raise the head of the bed, if permitted. If siderails are present and elevated, lower the siderail on the side where you are working.

6. Offer tissues to the patient. Ask the patient to remove the dentures. If the patient is unable to do so, use tissues or a gauze sponge to grasp the dentures between your thumb and index finger (**Figure 22–32A**). Gently apply downward and forward pressure to loosen and remove the top denture. Remove the lower denture by grasping it with your thumb and forefinger and turning it slightly to lift it out of the mouth.

    CAUTION: Never force dentures loose. They can break.

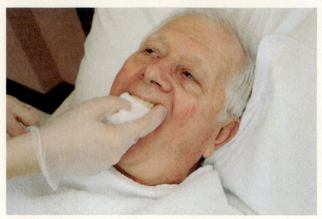

FIGURE 22–32A Use tissues or a gauze sponge to grasp the dentures and ease them down and forward to remove them from the mouth.

7. Carefully place the dentures in a denture cup. If indicated, raise the siderails for patient safety. Carry the dentures to the sink.

8. Line the sink with paper towels.

   NOTE: This provides a protective cushion for the dentures should they be dropped.

9. Put toothpaste or powder on the toothbrush. Place the dentures in the palm of one hand. Holding them under a gentle stream of cool or lukewarm water, brush all surfaces thoroughly (**Figure 22–32B**).

    CAUTION: Do *not* use hot water. This can cause breakage.

   NOTE: Clean all parts of the dentures, not just the teeth.

   NOTE: Dentures can be soaked in a solution containing a cleansing tablet prior to brushing.

10. Rinse dentures thoroughly in cool water.

     CAUTION: Do *not* use very cold water. This can also cause breakage.

11. Put clean, cool water in the denture cup. Place the cleaned dentures in the cup.

12. Return to the patient's bedside. If siderails are elevated, lower the siderail on the side where you will be working.

13. Help the patient to rinse the mouth with cool water and/or mouthwash. Use the emesis basin and tissues. Place used tissues in the plastic bag.

    NOTE: Some patients want to brush their gums with a soft toothbrush or applicator moistened with mouthwash before inserting clean dentures. Assist the patient, as necessary.

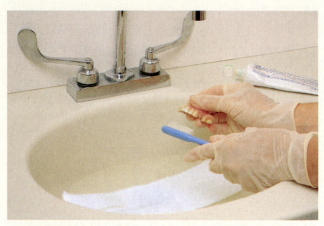

FIGURE 22–32B Hold the dentures securely while brushing all surfaces.

14. Hand the dentures to the patient. Help the patient insert the dentures, as needed. The upper denture is inserted first.

    NOTE: If the patient desires adhesive, line the palates (the sections holding the teeth) of the dentures with denture adhesive.

    NOTE: If dentures are not immediately returned to the patient, they should be stored inside the denture cup in a safe area (such as a drawer) and labeled with the patient's name and room number. At times, a denture cleansing or soaking tablet is placed in the water when dentures are stored.

15. Observe all checkpoints before leaving the patient: position the patient in correct body alignment; elevate the siderails (if indicated); lower the bed to its lowest level; place the call signal, tissues, water, and supplies within easy reach of the patient; clean and replace all equipment; and leave the area neat and clean.

16. Remove gloves. Wash hands thoroughly.

17. Report that denture care was given and/or record all required information on the patient's chart or enter it into the computer. For example, date, time, dentures cleaned, and your signature and title. Note any unusual observations.

 NOTE: In health care agencies using electronic health records (EHRs), the information is entered directly into the patient's record on a computer.

PRACTICE: Go to the workbook and use the evaluation sheet for 22:4B, Cleaning Dentures, to practice this procedure. When you believe you have mastered this skill, sign the sheet and give it to your instructor for further action.

 FINAL EVALUATION: Using the criteria listed on the evaluation sheet, your instructor will grade your performance.

Procedure 22:4C

Giving Special Mouth Care

Equipment and Supplies

Prepared mouth swabs, tissues, emesis basin, bath towel or underpad (protective pad), cotton-tipped applicator sticks, water-soluble lubricant for lips, mouth solution as ordered (optional), plastic bag or plastic-lined waste can, disposable gloves, paper and pen or computer

Procedure

1. Check physician's orders or obtain authorization from your immediate supervisor.

2. Assemble equipment.

3. Knock on the door and pause before entering. Introduce yourself. Identify the patient by checking the wristband and addressing the patient by name. Explain the procedure and obtain consent.

   NOTE: Semiconscious or unconscious patients can sometimes hear.

4. Close the door and pull the curtain for privacy.

5. Wash hands. Put on gloves.

    CAUTION: Observe standard precautions. Contamination by body fluids is possible.

6. Elevate the bed to a comfortable working height. Raise the head of the bed if permissible. If siderails are present and elevated, lower the siderail on the side where you are working.

7. Turn the patient's head to the side toward you. Place the bath towel or underpad under the patient's head and chin.

8. Open the package of prepared mouth swabs.

   NOTE: Toothette® is a common brand name of mouth swabs.

   NOTE: Prepared mouth swabs may contain lemon and glycerine, hydrogen peroxide, or sodium bicarbonate.

9. Use the prepared swab to cleanse all parts of the patient's mouth (**Figure 22–33**). Cleanse the teeth, gums, tongue, and roof of the mouth thoroughly. Work from the gums to the cutting edges of the teeth. Use a gentle motion.

10. Discard used swabs in the plastic bag. Use fresh swabs until the entire mouth is clean.

11. If the patient is able to help, have them rinse the mouth with mouthwash, if allowed. Then follow with a freshwater rinse. If the patient is unconscious, use clean applicators moistened with clear water to rinse the patient's mouth. Use a soft towel to dry the area around the mouth.

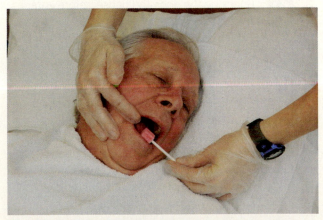

FIGURE 22–33 Use a prepared swab to cleanse all parts of the patient's mouth while providing special oral hygiene.

(continues)

CAUTION: Never give an unconscious or semiconscious patient mouthwash or any other liquids.
Safety

12. Use the cotton-tipped applicator sticks to apply water-soluble lubricant lightly to the tongue and lips.

    NOTE: This keeps the tissues soft and moist.

13. Reposition the patient in correct body alignment.

14. Replace all equipment used. A tray with supplies for special mouth care is sometimes kept at the bedside. If so, restock the supplies on the tray so it is always ready for use.

15. Observe all checkpoints before leaving the patient: elevate the siderails (if indicated), place the call signal within easy reach of the patient, lower the bed to its lowest level, and leave the area neat and clean.

16. Remove gloves. Wash hands.

17. Report that special mouth care was given and/or record all required information on the patient's chart or enter it into the computer. For example, date, time, special mouth care given, lips appear dry and chapped, and your signature and title. Immediately report any problems noted, including sores, irritated areas in the mouth, bleeding gums, or cuts.
Comm

     NOTE: In health care agencies using electronic health records (EHRs), the information is entered directly into the patient's record on a computer.
    EHR

PRACTICE: Go to the workbook and use the evaluation sheet for 22:4C, Giving Special Mouth Care, to practice this procedure. When you believe you have mastered this skill, sign the sheet and give it to your instructor for further action.

 FINAL EVALUATION: Using the criteria listed on the evaluation sheet, your instructor will grade your performance.
Check

Procedure 22:4D
OBRA

Administering Daily Hair Care

Equipment and Supplies

Comb and/or brush, towel, spray bottle of water or conditioner, baby oil, gloves, paper and pen or computer

Procedure

1. Obtain proper authorization and assemble equipment.

2. Knock on the door and pause before entering. Introduce yourself. Identify the patient. Explain the procedure and obtain consent.
   Comm

3. Close the door and pull the curtain to provide privacy.

4. Wash hands. Put on gloves if needed.

    CAUTION: Wear gloves and observe standard precautions if the scalp has open sores or infected areas. Some health care facilities require that gloves be worn while providing hair care. Follow agency policy.
   Precaution

5. Elevate the bed to a comfortable working height. Raise the head of the bed, if permissible. If siderails are present and elevated, lower the siderail on the side where you are working.

6. Cover the pillow with the towel.

7. Ask the patient to move to the side of the bed nearest to you. Assist as necessary.

    CAUTION: Use proper body mechanics, including a broad base of support. Bend from hips.
   Safety

8. Part or section the hair. Start at one side and work around to the other side.

9. Comb or brush the hair thoroughly. Keep the fingers of your hand between the scalp and comb whenever possible (**Figure 22–34**). If the hair is not tangled or knotted, begin at the scalp and work toward the ends of the hair.

   NOTE: This prevents pulling and decreases discomfort.

10. Do each section completely. To do the back of the head, turn the patient or lift the head slightly.

11. If the hair is very tangled or knotted, do the following:

    a. Spray a small amount of water on the hair.

    b. Comb or brush the hair gently starting at the ends and working toward the scalp to remove the knots and tangles.

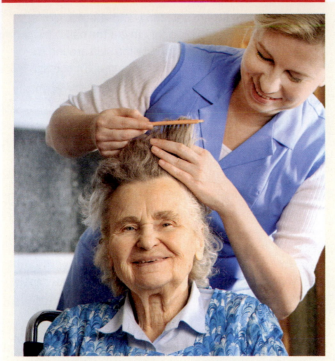

FIGURE 22–34 Keep the fingers of your hand between the patient's scalp and the comb while combing the hair. © Alexander Raths/Shutterstock.com

c. If the patient has conditioner, spraying a small amount of conditioner on the hair may also help remove the knots and tangles.

d. For very dry hair, put a very small amount of baby oil on your hands and rub it into the hair. Then comb or brush gently. Start at the ends of the hair and work toward the scalp.

12. When all areas of the hair have been brushed or combed, arrange the hair attractively according to the patient's preference. After obtaining the patient's permission, braid long hair to prevent tangling.

NOTE: Hair bands or hairpins can be used to hold the hair in place. Take care that they will not injure the scalp. Avoid the use of rubber bands whenever possible because they can break and damage the hair.

13. Throughout the entire procedure, closely observe the condition of the scalp and hair. Report any abnormal conditions immediately.

14. Observe all checkpoints before leaving the patient: position the patient in correct body alignment, elevate the siderails (if indicated), lower the bed to its lowest level, and place the call signal and supplies within easy reach of the patient.

15. Clean and replace all equipment used. It is sometimes necessary to remove hair from the brush and comb. Wash the comb and brush in a mild, soapy solution. Rinse thoroughly. Leave the area neat and clean.

16. Remove gloves if worn. Wash hands.

17. Report that hair care was given and/or record all required information on the patient's chart or enter it into the computer. For example, date, time, hair combed and braided, and your signature and title. Note any unusual observations.

 NOTE: In health care agencies using electronic health records (EHRs), the information is entered directly into the patient's record on a computer.

PRACTICE: Go to the workbook and use the evaluation sheet for 22:4D, Administering Daily Hair Care, to practice this procedure. When you believe you have mastered this skill, sign the sheet and give it to your instructor for further action.

 FINAL EVALUATION: Using the criteria listed on the evaluation sheet, your instructor will grade your performance.

Procedure 22:4E
OBRA

Providing Nail Care

Equipment and Supplies

Orange stick, emery board, nail clippers (if permitted), water and mild detergent in basin, towel, plastic bag, gloves, paper and pen or computer

CAUTION: In some facilities, only licensed or advance practice personnel are permitted to cut fingernails. In addition, cutting nails may be prohibited for some patients, such as patients who have diabetes. It is important to learn and follow agency policy regarding nail care.

Procedure

1. Check physician's orders or obtain authorization from your immediate supervisor.

2. Assemble equipment.

(continues)

3. Knock on the door and pause before entering. Introduce yourself. Identify the patient. Explain the procedure and obtain consent.

4. Close the door and pull the curtain to provide privacy.

5. Wash hands. Put on gloves.

 CAUTION: Wear gloves and observe standard precautions. Contact with nonintact skin or body fluids is possible.

6. Elevate the bed to a comfortable working height. If siderails are present and elevated, lower the siderail on the side where you are working.

7. Clean the nails by soaking them for 5–10 minutes in a solution of mild detergent and water at a temperature of 105°F–110°F (40.6°C–43.3°C). This loosens the dirt in the nail beds.

8. Use the slanted or blunt edge of the orange stick to clean dirt out of the nail beds under the nails (**Figure 22–35**). A nail brush can also be used to clean the nails. Carefully check the nails and surrounding skin while cleaning the nails.

CAUTION: Using the pointed edge of the orange stick can result in a puncture wound.

NOTE: If any redness, excessive dryness, or cracking of the skin is noted, report this to your supervisor immediately.

9. Use the emery board to file the nails and shorten them. Use short strokes. Work from the side of the nail to the top of the nail. Repeat for the opposite side.

NOTE: Do *not* use a back-and-forth motion. Such a motion can split the nails.

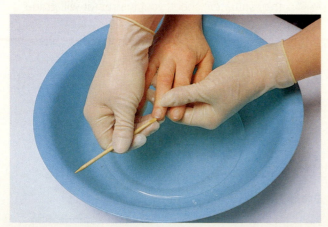

FIGURE 22–35 After soaking the nails, use the blunt edge of an orange stick to remove any dirt from under the nails.

10. If the fingernails are very long, and you are allowed to cut them, use nail clippers to cut the nails straight across. Be careful not to injure the skin around the nail. *Never* cut toenails. File them straight across.

 CAUTION: Do *not* use scissors. They can cut the patient.

 CAUTION: Make sure you are authorized to use nail clippers.

11. When the nails are the correct length, use the smooth side of the emery board to eliminate rough edges. Make sure that the nails are filed straight across.

 CAUTION: Pointed nails may cause injuries.

12. When the nails have been cleaned and filed short, apply lotion or another emollient, such as cold cream. This helps keep the nails and cuticles in good condition.

NOTE: Nail care can be carried out for fingernails and toenails.

13. Apply lotion to the hands and feet. Do *not* apply lotion between the toes because this promotes the growth of fungus.

14. Position the patient in correct body alignment.

15. Observe all checkpoints before leaving the patient: elevate the siderails (if indicated); place the call signal, water, and tissues within easy reach of the patient; lower the bed to its lowest level; and leave the area neat and clean.

16. Clean and properly replace all equipment used.

17. Remove gloves. Wash hands.

18. Report that nail care has been given and/or record all required information on the patient's chart or enter it into the computer. For example, date, time, nail care given to fingers and toes, and your signature and title. Report any observations that may signify problems.

 NOTE: In health care agencies using electronic health records (EHRs), the information is entered directly into the patient's record on a computer.

PRACTICE: Go to the workbook and use the evaluation sheet for 22:4E, Providing Nail Care, to practice this procedure. When you believe you have mastered this skill, sign the sheet and give it to your instructor for further action.

 FINAL EVALUATION: Using the criteria listed on the evaluation sheet, your instructor will grade your performance.

Giving a Back Rub

Equipment and Supplies

Lotion, bath towel, washcloth, soap and water, disposable gloves (if needed), basin, paper and pen or computer

Procedure

1. Obtain authorization from your immediate supervisor or check physician's orders.

   NOTE: Some patients *cannot* receive a back rub because of heart or lung disease or blood clots. Other patients with burns, back injuries, back surgeries, and similar conditions may not be able to tolerate a back rub.

2. Assemble equipment.

3. Knock on the door and pause before entering. Introduce yourself. Identify the patient. Explain the procedure and obtain consent.

   Comm

4. Close the door and pull the curtain to provide privacy.

5. Wash hands. Put on gloves.

   CAUTION: Wear gloves and observe standard precautions. Contact with nonintact skin or body fluids is possible.

   Precaution

6. Elevate the bed to a comfortable working height. If siderails are present and elevated, lower the siderail on the side where you are working.

7. Position the patient. The patient can lie on the abdomen (prone), or, if this is not comfortable, on their side, facing away from you.

8. Place a bath towel lengthwise next to the patient's body.

9. Fill the basin with water at a temperature of 105°F–110°F (40.6°C–43.3°C). Wash the patient's back thoroughly. Rinse and dry the back.

   NOTE: If the patient has had a bed bath, this step is not necessary because the back has already been washed.

   NOTE: Be alert for any abnormal condition of the skin. Note any red areas, rash, sores, or cuts. Pay particular attention to bony parts.

10. Rub a small amount of lotion into your hands (**Figure 22–36A**).

    NOTE: This warms the solution slightly. The container of lotion can also be placed in a basin of warm water before use.

11. Begin at the base of the spine. Rub up the center of the back to the neck, around the shoulders, and down the sides of the back. Rub down over the buttocks, around, and circle back to the starting point. Use long, soothing strokes (**Figure 22–36B**). Use firm pressure on the upward strokes and gentle pressure on the downward strokes (**Figure 22–37A**). Repeat this step four times.

     CAUTION: Long nails may scratch the patient. File your nails short before giving a back rub.

    Safety

     CAUTION: Use proper body mechanics. Get close to the patient by bending at your hips and knees, and keep your back straight. Position your feet to provide a broad base of support.

    Safety

12. Repeat the long, upward strokes, but on the downward strokes, use a circular motion (**Figure 22–37B**). Pay particular attention to bony prominences. Repeat this motion four times.

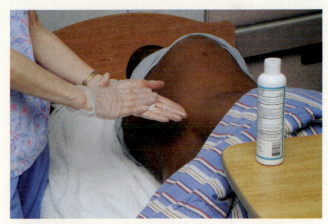

FIGURE 22–36A Rub a small amount of lotion into your hands.

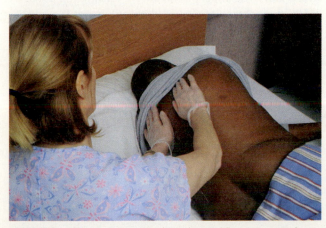

FIGURE 22–36B Use long, smooth strokes and firm pressure when giving a back rub.

(continues)

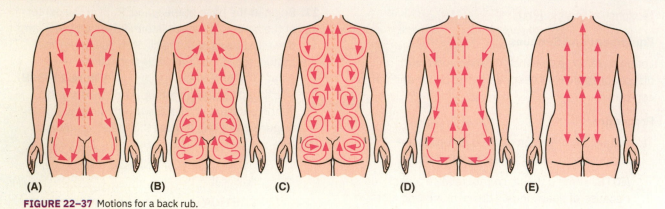

FIGURE 22–37 Motions for a back rub.

⚠ **Safety** **CAUTION:** Take care not to rub skin tags as this might cause them to bleed. Also avoid massaging directly over reddened areas. Massage around these areas. Report the presence of these areas to your supervisor immediately.

13. Repeat the long, upward strokes, but on the downward strokes, use very small circular motions (**Figure 22–37C**). Use the palm of your hand to apply firm pressure. Pay particular attention to the bony prominences. Do this motion one time.

14. Repeat the long, soothing strokes used initially (**Figure 22–37D**). Do this for 3–5 minutes.

15. End the back rub with up-and-down motions over the entire back (**Figure 22–37E**). Do this for 1–2 minutes. This provides relaxation after stimulation.

16. Dry the back thoroughly with the towel.

17. Straighten the bed linen. Change the patient's gown, if necessary.

18. Position the patient in good body alignment.

19. Observe all checkpoints before leaving the patient: elevate the siderails (if indicated); lower the bed to its lowest level; and place the call signal, water, and tissues within easy reach of patient.

20. Clean and replace all equipment. Leave the area neat and clean.

21. Remove gloves if worn. Wash hands.

22. **Comm** Report that a back rub was given and/or record all required information on the patient's chart or enter it into the computer. For example, date, time, back massage given, patient states they feel very relaxed, and your signature and title. Report any abnormal observations immediately.

 EHR **NOTE:** In health care agencies using electronic health records (EHRs), the information is entered directly into the patient's record on a computer.

PRACTICE: Go to the workbook and complete the evaluation sheet for 22:4F, Giving a Back Rub, to practice this procedure. When you believe you have mastered this skill, sign the sheet and give it to your instructor for further action.

✅ **Check** **FINAL EVALUATION:** Using the criteria listed on the evaluation sheet, your instructor will grade your performance.

Procedure 22:4G OBRA

Shaving a Patient

Equipment and Supplies

Safety razor with blade, shaving lather, gauze pad, basin with water, towel, washcloth, mirror, electric razor (for some patients), aftershave lotion (optional), disposable gloves, sharps container, paper and pen or computer

Procedure

1. Obtain proper authorization.

⚠ **Safety** **CAUTION:** If the patient is taking anticoagulants to prevent blood clots, shaving may be prohibited or restricted to the use of an electric razor. Always check with your immediate supervisor to confirm whether a patient is on anticoagulants before shaving a patient.

2. Assemble equipment. Examine the razor blade closely. Make sure there are no nicks or damaged edges. Carefully rub the razor blade over a folded gauze pad to check for damage. If it snags on the gauze, it might be damaged.

3. Knock on the door and pause before entering. Introduce yourself. Identify the patient. Explain the procedure and obtain consent.

4. Close the door and pull the curtain to provide privacy.

5. Wash hands. Put on gloves.

 CAUTION: Observe standard precautions. A razor can nick the skin and cause bleeding.

Precaution

6. Elevate the bed to a comfortable working height. Raise the head of the bed. If siderails are present and elevated, lower the siderail on the side where you are working. Put the patient in a comfortable position. Arrange all needed equipment on the overbed table.

NOTE: Allow the patient to help as much as possible.

7. Place a towel over the patient's chest and near the patient's shoulders.

8. Fill the basin with water at a temperature of 105°F–110°F (40.6°C–43.3°C). Use the washcloth to moisten the face (**Figure 22–38A**).

9. Apply lather. Put it on your fingers first and then apply it to the patient's cheek (**Figure 22–38B**).

NOTE: It is usually best to do one area of the face at a time.

10. Start in front of the ear. Hold the skin taut (stretched tightly) to prevent cuts (**Figure 22–38C**). Bring the safety razor down over the cheek and toward the chin.

 CAUTION: Always shave in the direction of hair growth.

Safety

11. Rinse the razor after each stroke. Repeat until the lather is removed and the area is shaved.

12. Repeat steps 9–11 for the opposite cheek, the chin and neck area, and under the nose. When shaving the chin and under the nose, instruct the patient to hold the skin taut. Use firm, short strokes. Rinse the razor frequently.

 CAUTION: If the skin is accidentally nicked, use a gauze pad to apply pressure directly over the area. Then apply an antiseptic or follow the policy of your agency. Be sure to report the incident to your immediate supervisor.

Safety

CAUTION: Observe standard precautions when controlling bleeding.

Precaution

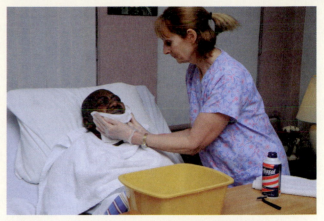

FIGURE 22–38A Use the washcloth to moisten the face.

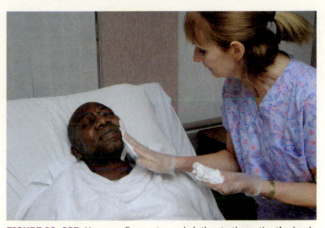

FIGURE 22–38B Use your fingers to apply lather to the patient's cheek.

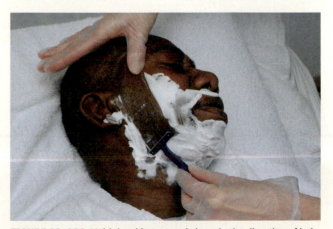

FIGURE 22–38C Hold the skin taut and shave in the direction of hair growth while shaving the patient.

13. Wash and thoroughly dry the face and neck.

14. Apply aftershave lotion, if the patient desires.

(continues)

15. To use an electric razor, read the instructions that come with the razor.

    a. Some patients prefer dry skin when using an electric razor. Others prefer to use a preshave lotion.

    b. Hold the skin taut while using the razor.

    c. Some razors require short, circular strokes. Others require short strokes in the direction of hair growth.

    d. Shave all areas of the face.

    e. Wash and dry the face thoroughly when done.

    f. Apply aftershave lotion, if desired.

    g. Clean the razor thoroughly after use. Use a small brush (which usually comes with the razor) to clean out all the hair.

16. Observe all checkpoints before leaving the patient: position the patient in correct body alignment, elevate the siderails (if indicated), lower the bed to its lowest level, and place the call signal and supplies within easy reach of the patient.

17. Clean and replace all equipment used. Wash the safety razor thoroughly. Discard the blade in a puncture-resistant sharps container. If a disposable razor was used, discard the entire razor in the sharps container (**Figure 22–38D**).

18. Remove gloves. Wash hands.

19. Report that the patient was shaved and/or record all required information on the patient's chart or enter it into the computer. For example, date, time, shaved with electric razor, and your signature and title. Report any observations that may signify problems.

     NOTE: In health care agencies using electronic health records (EHRs), the information is entered directly into the patient's record on a computer.

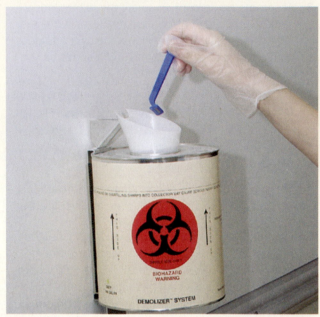

FIGURE 22–38D Discard the disposable razor in a sharps container.

NOTE: Female patients sometimes want facial, underarm, and/or leg hair shaved. Obtain proper authorization before doing any of these procedures. Follow the same steps: check the razor, moisten the area, apply lather or a soapy solution, hold the skin taut, shave in the direction of hair growth, rinse the area, do small sections at a time, and finish by thoroughly washing and drying the areas shaved.

PRACTICE: Go to the workbook and use the evaluation sheet for 22:4G, Shaving a Patient, to practice this procedure. When you believe you have mastered this skill, sign the sheet and give it to your instructor for further action.

 FINAL EVALUATION: Using the criteria listed on the evaluation sheet, your instructor will grade your performance.

Procedure 22:4H

Changing a Patient's Gown or Pajamas

Equipment and Supplies

Gown or pajamas; towel or bath blanket; linen hamper, cart, or bag; disposable gloves; paper and pen or computer

Procedure

1. Obtain proper authorization and assemble equipment.

2. Knock on the door and pause before entering. Introduce yourself. Identify the patient. Explain the procedure and obtain consent.

3. Close the door and pull the curtain to provide privacy.

4. Wash hands. Put on gloves.

   CAUTION: Wear gloves and observe standard precautions. The gown may be contaminated with blood, body fluids, secretions, or excretions, such as drainage from an incision.

5. Elevate the bed to a comfortable working height. If siderails are present and elevated, lower the siderail on the side where you are working.

   NOTE: It is easier to change the patient's clothing if you first fold the bed covers to the foot of the bed and cover the patient with a bath blanket.

6. Loosen the patient's bedclothes:

   a. If the patient is wearing a hospital gown, untie the strings by having the patient turn on their side or by reaching under the neck. Then gently pull out any part of the gown that is under the patient.

   b. If the patient is wearing a gown of their own, loosen any buttons or ties. Gently ease the gown upward from the hemline to the neck. Prevent unnecessary exposure by using the towel or bath blanket, as necessary.

   c. If the patient is wearing pajamas, first untie or unbutton the pants at the waist. Gently ease the pants down over the legs and feet. Use the towel or bath blanket to drape the patient. Avoid exposing the patient. Unbutton the pajama top.

7. Take off the soiled clothing, one sleeve at a time. Gently grasp the edge of the sleeve near the shoulder. Ease the arm out. Do the far arm first. If the patient has an affected arm (injured, paralyzed, weak, etc.) or is receiving an intravenous (IV) infusion, remove the sleeve from the unaffected arm first and from the affected arm or arm with the IV second. Place the soiled clothing on a chair or in the laundry hamper.

   NOTE: If an IV is in place, ease the sleeve off of the upper arm, taking care not to disturb the infusion site, where the needle is inserted. Then gently ease the sleeve over the tubing by keeping your hand and arm in the sleeve holding the solution bottle above the infusion site, and passing the container through the sleeve (**Figures 22–39A** and **22–39B**).

   NOTE: Many facilities use gowns that open at the shoulder when a patient has an IV. The gown is positioned over the shoulder and closed with snaps, ties, or Velcro strips.

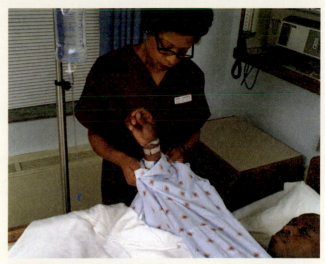

FIGURE 22–39A After removing the gown from the unaffected arm, gather the gown together on the arm with the IV infusion site.

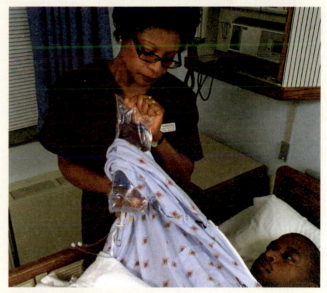

FIGURE 22–39B Keeping the IV container above the level of the infusion site, pass the IV container through the arm of the gown.

8. Unfold the clean gown or pajama top and place it over the patient.

9. Put the patient's arms into the sleeves one at a time. Gather the sleeve of the gown or pajama top into your hands. Then put your arm through the sleeve, take the patient's hand in yours, and slip the sleeve up the patient's wrist and arm and to the shoulder.

   NOTE: If one arm is affected or has an IV, do this arm first. This places less strain on the arm. For an IV, pass the solution container and tubing through the sleeve first. Keep the solution container above the level of the infusion site at all times.

(continues)

CAUTION: Sometimes, a sleeve cannot be placed because of an IV infusion machine, bulky dressing, or other similar problem. If this is the case, leave the sleeve off of the one arm, or use a gown that opens at the shoulders.

10. Pull the body of the gown down over the patient or position the pajama top correctly. Make sure that the gown or top is smooth and free from wrinkles or folds.

11. Tie the strings on the gown, or button the buttons on the pajama top. Make sure that the tied knot is not on a bony prominence.

 CAUTION: Knots or wrinkles can lead to pressure ulcers.

NOTE: Avoid exposing the patient during the procedure. Continue to use the towel or bath blanket to drape the patient.

12. If the patient is wearing pajamas, put on the pants after the pajama top. Gently ease the pants over the feet and up the legs. Adjust them into position at the waist. Use the towel or bath blanket to cover the patient during this procedure. Tie or button the pants. Make sure the pants are smooth and free from wrinkles or folds.

13. Observe all checkpoints before leaving the patient: position the patient comfortably and in good body alignment; elevate the siderails (if indicated); place the call signal, water, and supplies within easy reach of the patient; lower the bed to its lowest level; and leave the area neat and clean.

14. Place a soiled hospital gown in the laundry hamper or bag. Place a soiled personal gown or pajamas in a drawer, the closet, or other location specified by the patient.

 CAUTION: If the gown is contaminated with blood or body fluids, follow agency policy for handling contaminated linen.

NOTE: In long-term care facilities, the patient's soiled clothing is usually washed by the facility. Make sure the clothing is labeled with the patient's name and place it in the proper laundry hamper or bag.

15. Remove gloves. Wash hands thoroughly.

16. Report that the patient's gown has been changed and/or record all required information on the patient's chart or enter it into the computer. For example, date, time, pajamas changed, and your signature and title. Report any observations that may signify problems.

 NOTE: In health care agencies using electronic health records (EHRs), the information is entered directly into the patient's record on a computer.

PRACTICE: Go to the workbook and use the evaluation sheet for 22:4H, Changing a Patient's Gown or Pajamas, to practice this procedure. When you believe you have mastered this skill, sign the sheet and give it to your instructor for further action.

✅ **FINAL EVALUATION:** Using the criteria listed on the evaluation sheet, your instructor will grade your performance.

Procedure 22:4I

Giving a Complete Bed Bath

Equipment and Supplies

Bed linen (complete set); laundry hamper, bag, or cart; bath blanket; two or three washcloths; face towel; one or two bath towels; soap and soap dish; basin; bath thermometer; clean gown or pajamas; supplies for hair care; supplies for nail care; shaving supplies; oral hygiene supplies; lotion; disposable gloves; paper and pen or computer

NOTE: When packaged cleansing cloths are available, they can be used in place of the washcloths, towels, soap, and basin.

Procedure

1. Obtain authorization from your immediate supervisor or check physician's orders to obtain authorization for the procedure.

2. Assemble equipment.

3. Knock on the door and pause before entering. Introduce yourself. Identify the patient. Explain the procedure and obtain consent.

4. Close all doors, windows, and curtains. Eliminate drafts. Adjust the thermostat to a comfortable room temperature, if possible.

5. Wash hands. Put on gloves.

Precaution

CAUTION: Wear gloves and observe standard precautions. If splashing with blood, body fluids, secretions, or excretions is possible, wear a gown, mask or face shield, and eye protection.

6. Arrange all equipment conveniently. Put linen on the chair in the order of use. Position the laundry bag, hamper, or cart conveniently.

    NOTE: Proper preparation saves time and energy.

7. Elevate the bed to a comfortable working height. If siderails are present and elevated, lower the siderail on the side where you are working.

8. Replace the top linen with a bath blanket. If the same linen is to be reused, fanfold it to the bottom of the bed. If the linen is to be replaced, remove it and place it in the hamper.

9. Provide oral hygiene as previously instructed.

10. Shave the male patient, if necessary.

    NOTE: Some patients prefer to be shaved after the face is washed.

11. Fill the basin approximately two-thirds full with warm water at a temperature of 105°F–110°F (40.6°C–43.3°C). Check the temperature with a bath thermometer.

    NOTE: If cleansing cloths are used, remove them from the warmer or heat them according to instructions.

12. Help the patient move to the side of the bed nearest to you. Remove the patient's bedclothes as previously instructed.

13. Place a towel over the upper edge of the bath blanket.

14. With the washcloth, form a mitten around your hand. Tuck in the loose edges (**Figure 22–40**).

    NOTE: This prevents the loose edges of the cloth from striking the patient as you work. It also keeps water from dripping on the patient and the bed.

15. Wet the washcloth and squeeze out excess water. Wash the patient's eyes first (**Figure 22–41A**). Start at the inner area and wash to the outside of the eye. Use a different section of the cloth when you wash the second eye.

    NOTE: If using cleansing cloths, use one for the face and neck, one for the arms, one for the legs, one for the chest and abdomen, one for the back and buttocks, and one for the perineal area.

16. Rinse the washcloth. Ask whether the patient uses soap on the face and use soap if desired. Wash the face, neck, and ears. Rinse. Dry well.

17. Place a bath towel lengthwise under the patient's arm that is farthest from you. Place the basin of water on the bed on top of the towel by the patient's hand. Put the patient's hand and nails into the water. Wash, rinse, and dry the arm, from the axilla to the hand (**Figure 22–41B**). Repeat for the other arm.

    NOTE: If the patient desires deodorant, it can be applied after the axillae are clean and dry.

18. Provide nail and hand care as previously instructed.

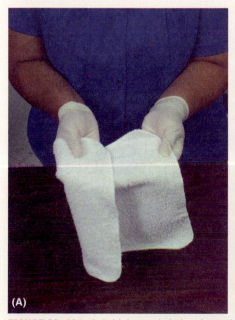
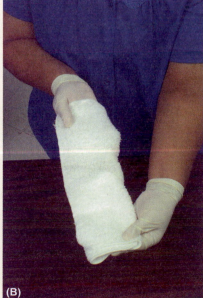
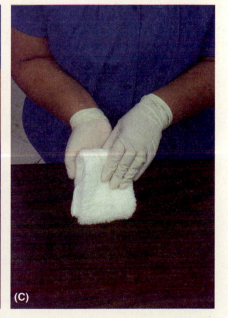

(A)   (B)   (C)

FIGURE 22–40A–C Fold the washcloth to form a bath mitten around your hand.

(continues)

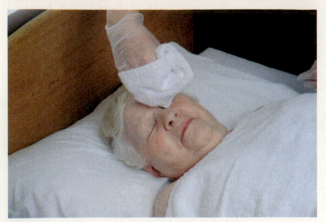

FIGURE 22–41A Wash the eyes first, starting at the inner area and moving to the outside of the eye.

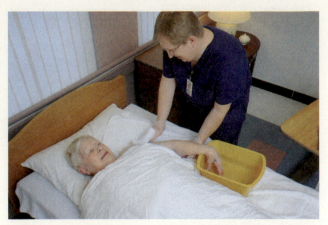

FIGURE 22–41B With the hand in the basin, wash and rinse the arm from the axilla to the hand.

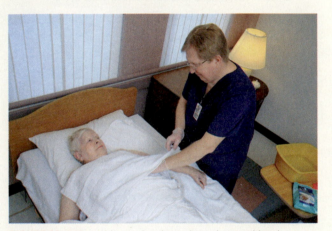

FIGURE 22–41C Avoid exposing the patient when washing the breasts.

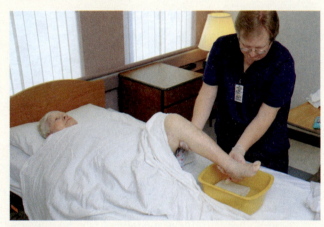

FIGURE 22–41D Support the leg and foot when placing the patient's foot in the basin.

19. Elevate the siderail, if indicated. Discard the bath water and fill the basin with clean water at a temperature of 105°F–110°F.

20. Return to the bedside and lower the siderail, if elevated. Put a bath towel over the patient's chest. Fold the bath blanket down to the patient's waist.

21. Wash, rinse, and dry the chest and breasts (**Figure 22–41C**). Pay particular attention to the areas under a female patient's breasts. Dry these areas thoroughly.

22. Turn the bath towel lengthwise to cover the patient's chest and abdomen. Fold the bath blanket down to the pubic area. Wash, rinse, and dry the abdomen. Replace the bath blanket. Remove the towel.

23. Fold the bath blanket up to expose the patient's leg that is farthest from you. Place a towel lengthwise under the leg and foot. Place the basin on the bed and on top of the towel. Place the patient's foot in the basin by flexing the leg at the knee. Wash and rinse the leg and foot, remove the basin, and dry the leg and foot. Repeat for the other leg.

NOTE: Support the patient's leg and foot with your hand and lower arm when moving the foot in and out of the basin (**Figure 22–41D**).

24. Provide nail care to the toes, as needed. *Never* cut the toenails. File them straight across. Apply lotion to the feet, if the skin is dry. *Never* put lotion between the toes because this promotes the growth of fungus.

⚠️ Safety **CAUTION:** Observe for any color changes or irritated areas that may signify problems.

25. Elevate the siderail, if indicated. Change the water in the basin.

NOTE: Water should always be changed at this point in the bath. However, it can be changed anytime it becomes too cool, dirty, or soapy.

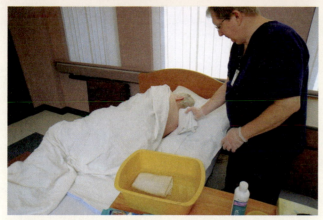

FIGURE 22–41E Turn the patient onto their side to wash, rinse, and dry the back.

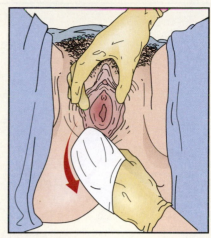

FIGURE 22–42 To provide perineal care to a female patient, separate the labia and cleanse the area with a front-to-back motion.

26. Lower the siderail, if elevated.

27. Turn the patient on their side or into the prone position. Place the towel lengthwise on the bed and along the patient's back. Wash, rinse, and dry the entire back (**Figure 22–41E**).

     CAUTION: Observe the back closely for any changes that may signify problems. Pay particular attention to bony areas and abnormal skin color. Report any abnormality to your supervisor.

28. Give a back rub as previously instructed.

29. Help the patient turn onto their back. Keep the patient draped with the bath blanket.

30. If the patient is able to wash the perineal area, place the basin with water, the soap, the washcloth, the towel, and the call signal within easy reach. Raise the siderail (if indicated) and wait outside the unit while the patient completes this procedure.

31. If the patient is not able to wash the perineal area, put on gloves. Drape and position the patient in the dorsal recumbent position. Put a towel or disposable underpad under the patient's buttocks and upper legs.

    a. For a female patient, always wash from the front to the back, or rectal, area. Separate the labia, or lips, and cleanse the area thoroughly with a front-to-back motion (**Figure 22–42**). Use a clean area of the washcloth or rinse the cloth between each wipe.

    b. For a male patient, cleanse the tip of the penis using a circular motion and starting at the urinary meatus and working outward. Cleanse the penis from top to bottom (**Figure 22–43A**).

If a male patient is not circumcised, gently draw the foreskin back to wash the area (**Figure 22–43B**). After rinsing and drying the area, gently return the foreskin to its normal position. Wash the scrotal area, taking care to clean under the scrotum. To wash the rectal area, turn a male patient on his side.

    c. Rinse and dry all areas thoroughly on both the male and female patient.

    d. When the perineal area is clean, reposition the patient on their back and remove the towel or underpad from under the buttocks. Remove gloves and wash hands.

    NOTE: In some facilities, disposable washcloths or large gauze pads are used to clean the perineal area. These are discarded in an infectious-waste bag, and a fresh washcloth or pad is used for each area. Follow agency policy.

32. Place clean bedclothes on the patient as previously instructed.

33. Provide hair care as previously taught.

34. Make the bed according to Procedure 22:3B, Making an Occupied Bed.

35. Observe all checkpoints before leaving the patient: position the patient in correct body alignment; elevate the siderails (if indicated); lower the bed to its lowest level; and place the call signal, water, tissues, and supplies within easy reach of the patient.

36. Clean and replace all equipment. Wash the emesis basin and bath basin thoroughly.

(continues)

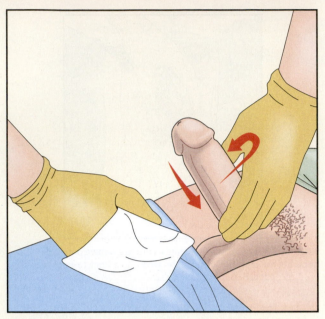

FIGURE 22–43A Use a circular motion to cleanse the penis from the top to the base.

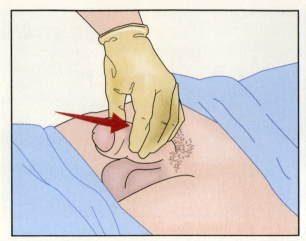

FIGURE 22–43B If a male patient is not circumcised, gently draw the foreskin back to wash the area. After rinsing and drying the area, gently return the foreskin to its normal position.

37. Put the bag or hamper of dirty linen in the proper area or send it to the laundry according to agency policy. Replace all remaining equipment.

38. Remove gloves, if worn. Wash hands.

39. Report that a complete bed bath was given and/or record all required information on the patient's chart or enter it into the computer. For example, date, time, complete bed bath given, occupied bed made, patient stated they were tired at the end of the procedure, and your signature and title. Report any observations that may signify problems.

 NOTE: In health care agencies using electronic health records (EHRs), the information is entered directly into the patient's record on a computer.

PRACTICE: Go to the workbook and use the evaluation sheet for 22:4I, Giving a Complete Bed Bath, to practice this procedure. When you believe you have mastered this skill, sign the sheet and give it to your instructor for further action.

 FINAL EVALUATION: Using the criteria listed on the evaluation sheet, your instructor will grade your performance.

Procedure 22:4J

Helping a Patient Take a Tub Bath or Shower

Equipment and Supplies

Washcloth, two or three towels, soap and soap dish, bathmat, rubber mat, bath thermometer, chair or stool (placed in bath area), bedclothes, robe, slippers, disposable gloves, paper and pen or computer

Procedure

1. Check physician's orders or obtain authorization from your immediate supervisor. A physician's order is generally required before a tub bath or shower is allowed, unless the patient is considered able to take care of this need (for example, in the case of a totally ambulatory patient).

2. Assemble equipment.

3. Knock on the door and pause before entering. Introduce yourself. Identify the patient, explain the procedure, and obtain consent. Also, check to make sure the time is appropriate for taking a shower or bath.

NOTE: If the patient has visitors or is receiving another treatment, time and energy would be wasted in preparing the tub or shower.

4. Wash hands. Put on gloves.

   CAUTION: Wear gloves and observe standard precautions. Contact with blood, body fluids, secretions, or excretions is possible.

5. Take the supplies to the bath or shower area. Make sure the tub or shower is clean. If it is dirty, put on gloves to clean the tub or shower. Wipe it with a disinfectant. When the tub or shower is clean, remove the gloves and wash your hands. If nonskid strips are not present, put a rubber mat in the tub or shower to prevent the patient from slipping. Place the bathmat on the floor. Fill the tub half full with water at a temperature of 105°F (40.6°C).

   NOTE: Many health care facilities have shower or tub chairs that are used for patients who cannot stand in a shower or climb into a tub (**Figure 22–44**). The shower chair must be cleaned and disinfected before and after every use.

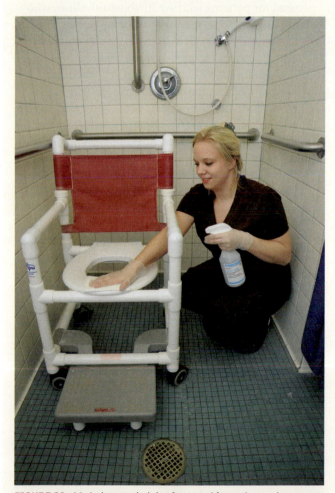

FIGURE 22–44 A shower chair is often used for patients who cannot stand in the shower or climb into a tub. It must be disinfected before and after it is used.

6. Help the patient put on a robe and slippers. Take the patient to the bath or shower area.

   CAUTION: Use a wheelchair, if necessary.

7. If necessary, help the patient undress. Help the patient into the tub or shower. If a shower chair is used, transfer the patient to the chair. Make sure the wheels on the chair are locked before transferring the patient.

   CAUTION: Before the patient enters the shower, adjust the temperature of the shower water.

8. If necessary, remain with the patient and assist with the bath or shower. If the patient can manage without assistance, explain how to use the emergency call signal, leave the room, and check on the patient at frequent intervals.

   CAUTION: If the patient shows any signs of weakness or dizziness, use the call button to get help. If the patient is in a tub, remove the plug and let the water drain. If the patient is in a shower, turn off the water and seat the patient in the chair. Keep the patient covered with a towel or bath blanket to prevent chilling.

   CAUTION: Most long-term care facilities require that you always stay with the patient.

   NOTE: In a home care situation, a small bell (such as a dinner bell) can be left with the patient.

9. When the patient is finished bathing, help as needed. Dry all areas of the patient's body thoroughly. Put clean bed clothes or clothing on the patient.

10. Assist the patient back to the bedside. Administer a back rub. Help with hair or nail care, if necessary.

11. Observe all checkpoints before leaving the patient: position the patient in correct body alignment, elevate the siderails (if indicated), lower the bed to its lowest level, place the call signal and supplies within easy reach of the patient, and leave the area neat and clean.

12. Return to the bath or shower area. Replace all supplies and equipment used. Put on gloves. Clean the tub or shower thoroughly and wipe with a disinfectant.

    NOTE: If a shower chair was used, clean and disinfect the chair.

13. Remove gloves. Wash hands.

(continues)

14.
Comm

Report that a tub bath or shower was given and/or record all required information on the patient's chart or enter it into the computer. For example, date, time, assisted with tub bath, patient tolerated procedure well, and your signature and title. Report any observations that may signify problems.

EHR

NOTE: In health care agencies using electronic health records (EHRs), the information is entered directly into the patient's record on a computer.

PRACTICE: Go to the workbook and use the evaluation sheet for 22:4J, Helping a Patient Take a Tub Bath or Shower, to practice this procedure. When you believe you have mastered this skill, sign the sheet and give it to your instructor for further action.

Check

FINAL EVALUATION: Using the criteria listed on the evaluation sheet, your instructor will grade your performance.

22:5 MEASURING AND RECORDING INTAKE AND OUTPUT

OBRA Science

A record of how much fluid is taken in and eliminated by a patient often helps a physician provide care to the patient. A large part of the body is fluid, so there must be a balance between the amount of fluid taken into the body and the amount lost from the body. In a healthy individual, the fluid balance is usually regulated by the body structures to maintain *homeostasis*, or a natural balance. However, if an individual has heart or kidney disease, or loses large amounts of fluids through vomiting, diarrhea, excessive perspiration, or bleeding, the fluid balance may be abnormal. If excessive fluid is retained by the body, swelling, or **edema**, results. If excessive fluid is lost from the body, **dehydration** occurs. Either condition can lead to death if not treated. In such cases, physicians may order that a record be kept of all fluids taken in and discharged from the body. This record is usually called an intake and output (I&O) record.

An **intake and output (I&O)** record is a means of recording all fluids a person takes in and eliminates during a certain period. Each agency has its own paper or computerized form, but most contain similar information.

INTAKE

Intake refers to all fluids taken in by the patient. The following routes and liquids must be considered:

- **Oral** is intake by way of the mouth. Liquids taken in orally include water, coffee, tea, milk, juices, and other beverages. In addition, soups, gelatin, ice cream, and other similar foods that are liquid at room temperature also qualify. The nurse assistant often measures and records or reports these amounts.

- **Tube feedings, or enteral feedings**, are recorded as oral intake or in a special column. They are used for patients who are unable to swallow, who are unconscious or comatose, or who have certain digestive diseases. The solution given contains all of the nutrients required by the body and is more nourishing than an intravenous (IV) feeding. Enteral feedings may be administered through a nasogastric tube, orogastric tube, or a gastrostomy tube. A *nasogastric (NG) tube* is a tube inserted through the nose, down the esophagus, and into the stomach (**Figure 22–45**). An *orogastric (OG) tube* takes the same route but enters through the mouth. A syringe can be used to instill food or medication into the NG or OG tube (**Figure 22–46**). A *gastrostomy tube* is surgically inserted through the abdominal skin into the stomach (**Figure 22–47**). A feeding pump is usually used to administer the

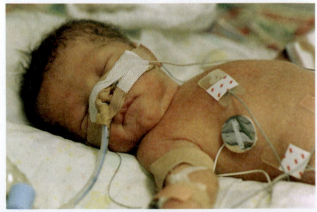

FIGURE 22–45 A nasogastric tube is inserted through the nose, down the esophagus, and into the stomach. © Steve Lovegrove/Shutterstock.com

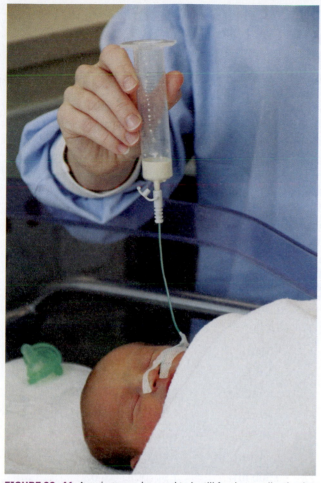

FIGURE 22–46 A syringe can be used to instill food or medication into the nasogastric (NG) tube. © andesign101/Shutterstock.com

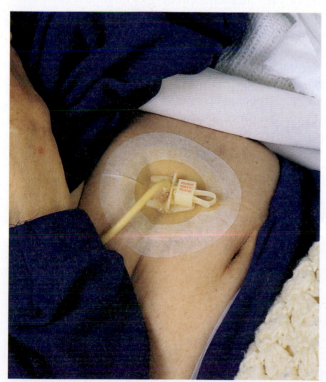

FIGURE 22–47 A gastrostomy tube is surgically inserted through the abdominal skin into the stomach.

solution (**Figure 22–48**). A nurse or another legally authorized team member will administer the enteral feeding. The nurse assistant must keep the patient's head elevated 30–45 degrees during the feeding and for approximately 30–60 minutes after the feeding; make sure there are no kinks in the tubing; use extreme caution when turning or positioning the patient to avoid dislodging the tubing; provide frequent oral hygiene; and notify the nurse immediately if the alarm sounds on the feeding pump, if the solution is not flowing through the tubing, or if the solution container is low or empty.

- **Intravenous (IV)** refers to fluids given into a vein. Blood units, IV medications, and other intravenous (IV) solutions are measured. This measurement is the responsibility of the nurse or another legally authorized team member.

-
  Math
  Tubes and drains refers to fluid placed into tubes or drains that have been inserted in the body. In some agencies, any fluid that is inserted and then removed is not considered to be intake and is not recorded. For example, if a nasogastric tube is irrigated with 80 milliliters (mL) of solution and the same exact amount is immediately drawn back out of the tube, this is not recorded as intake. However, if 60 mL is withdrawn, the intake is recorded as 20 mL (80 minus 60 equals 20). In other

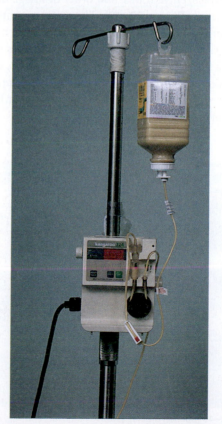

FIGURE 22–48 A feeding pump is usually used to administer tube or enteral feedings.

agencies, any fluid that is instilled is recorded under intake, and anything that comes out is output. Follow your agency policy. This measurement is also the responsibility of the nurse or another legally authorized team member.

OUTPUT

Output refers to all fluids eliminated by the patient. The following routes and liquids must be considered:

- **Bowel movement (BM)**: Liquid bowel movements are usually measured and recorded. A solid or formed BM is usually noted in the remarks column or described under feces. The nurse assistant may measure and record or report this elimination.

- **Emesis:** Anything that is vomited is measured and recorded. Color, type, and other facts are usually noted in the remarks column. The nurse assistant often measures and records or reports emesis.

- **Urine:** All urine voided or drained via a catheter is measured and recorded. This measurement may be the responsibility of the nurse assistant. A urine output of less than 30 milliliters (mL) per hour must be reported.

- **Tubes and drains**: Any irrigation or suction drainage, including drainage from nasogastric tubes, hemovacs, chest tubes, and other drainage tubes, is measured (**Figure 22–49**). The type, amount, color, and other facts about the drainage are noted in the remarks column. If an irrigating solution is injected into a tube and more solution returns, the excess amount is considered output. This measurement is the responsibility of the nurse or another legally authorized team member.

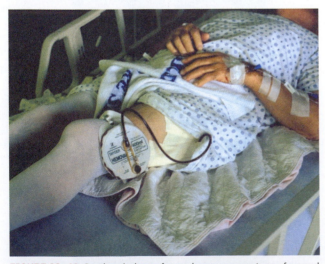

FIGURE 22–49 Suction drainage from a hemovac, one type of wound drainage system, is recorded as irrigation output on an intake and output (I&O) record.

RECORDING INTAKE AND OUTPUT (I&O)

I&O records must be accurate. All amounts must be measured in graduates. A graduate is a container that is made of plastic or stainless steel and has calibrations for milliliters/cubic centimeters and/or ounces on the side. It is similar to a measuring cup and is used to obtain accurate measurements. The graduate should be held at eye level or placed on a solid surface and viewed at eye level to accurately record amounts (**Figure 22–50**). In addition, care must be taken when adding or totaling the columns on the I&O record. Most records contain totals for 8-hour and 24-hour periods. (See **Figure 22–51** and study it carefully.) Some agencies use 12-hour periods for intake and output totals.

 For I&O records, fluids are measured in metric units called milliliters (mL). Approximate equivalents for units of the metric system are as follows:

Math

Metric		Household
1 mL	=	15 gtts (drops)
5 mL	=	1 tsp (teaspoon)
15 mL	=	1 tbsp (tablespoon)
30 mL	=	1 oz (ounce)
240 mL	=	1 cup (8 oz)
500 mL	=	1 pt (pint) (16 oz)
1,000 mL	=	1 qt (quart) (32 oz)

NOTE: A few measurement devices might use cubic centimeters (cc). However, 1 milliliter (mL) and 1 cubic centimeter (cc) are the same amount. Therefore, 30 mL equals 30 cc.

Various agencies have different policies for recording I&O. In some agencies, the I&O record is kept at the bedside. Team members note the I&O of the patient and record the measurements on the record. At times, the patient is even taught to measure and write down

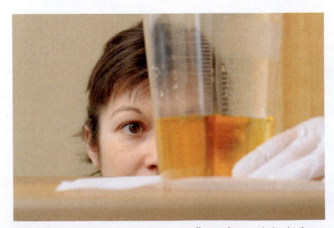

FIGURE 22–50 Place the graduate on a flat surface and obtain the reading at eye level to get an accurate measurement.

INTAKE AND OUTPUT RECORD

Family Name			First Name		Attending Physician		Room No.		Hosp. No.	
JOHNSON, ROBERT					DR. MIKE SMITH		238		54-3201	

Date 9/30	INTAKE			OUTPUT				OTHER				REMARKS
TIME	Oral	I.V.	Blood	Urine	Tube	Emesis	Feces					
7–8 AM	100											
8–9 AM	320					200						EMESIS– GREEN LIQUID
9–10 AM				420								
10–11 AM	100											
11–12 Noon			10									NG IRRIGATION NS
12–1 PM	240			310								
1–2 PM		850			200							NASOGASTRIC GOLD–BROWN
2–3 PM	60											
8 HOUR TOTAL	820	850	10	730	200	200						
3–4 PM												
4–5 PM	320	150				120						BROWN LIQUID
5–6 PM				280								
6–7 PM	180											
7–8 PM												
8–9 PM	100											
9–10 PM		500			240							NASOGASTRIC BROWNISH
10–11 PM				310								
8 HOUR TOTAL	600	650		590	240	120						
11–12 PM												
12–1 AM			10									NG IRRIGATION NS
1–2 AM	180			420								
2–3 AM												
3–4 AM						650						EMESIS– GREEN LIQUID
4–5 AM												
5–6 AM		600			180							NASOGASTRIC GOLD–BROWN
6–7 AM	100			380								
8 HOUR TOTAL	280	600	10	800	180	650						
24 HOUR TOTAL	1700	2100	20	2120	620	850	120					
	TOTAL INTAKE		3820	TOTAL OUTPUT			3170					

FIGURE 22–51 A sample intake and output (I&O) record.

the amounts. In other agencies, the I&O record is kept on the patient's chart. Measurements are noted on a slip of paper and reported. The nurse, medical secretary, health unit coordinator, or an authorized team member then records the information on the chart's I&O form. With computerized charting, totals are entered directly into the computer by the nurse or nurse assistant. Most computerized programs will automatically add all of the columns. Ascertain and follow the policy of your agency.

Comm

Patients should be given careful instructions when an I&O record is being kept. The patient must inform health care providers when they drink fluids not provided by the health care team. Sometimes, the patient records how many glasses of water or other liquids are consumed. Other times, the health care provider fills a water pitcher and then checks the quantity remaining before refilling the pitcher. The health care provider then subtracts this quantity from the total amount originally in the pitcher and records the difference as water intake. To avoid missing any amounts of oral intake, the health care team member must also think about fluid intake every time a glass, cup, or water pitcher is removed from the unit. If visitors bring milkshakes or other liquids, the amounts of these must also be recorded. Female patients should be asked to urinate in a bedpan or to use a special urine collector that can be placed under the seat of the toilet (**Figure 22–52**). Female patients must be told not to place toilet tissue or expel a bowel movement into the bedpan or urine collector. Male patients can be told to use a urinal. If patients are given correct instructions, they can cooperate and accurate records can be maintained.

Precaution

Standard precautions (discussed in Section 15:4) must be followed at all times when body fluids, such as urine, emesis, liquid bowel movements, and drainage, are measured. Gloves must be worn while the fluids are being measured and discarded. Hands must be washed frequently and must always be washed immediately after gloves are removed. If splashing or spraying of fluids is possible, a mask or face shield, eye

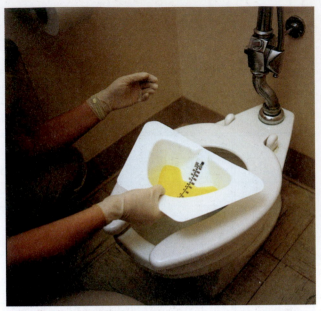

FIGURE 22–52 A specimen collector to collect urine can be placed under the seat of the toilet.

protection, and gown must be worn. The graduate or measuring device for monitoring a patient's output must be used for that patient only. It should be discarded or sterilized according to agency policy when output is no longer measured. Any areas contaminated by body fluids when measurements are being obtained must be wiped with a disinfectant. The health care provider must constantly take steps to prevent the spread of infection.

checkpoint

1. What are four (4) routes that are considered liquid output?
2. Where is a gastrostomy tube inserted?

PRACTICE: Go to the workbook and complete the assignment sheet for 22:5, Measuring Intake and Output. Then return and continue with the procedure.

Procedure 22:5
OBRA

Recording Intake and Output

NOTE: Competency will be evaluated by way of successful completion of several assignment sheets rather than by way of the usual evaluation sheet. Follow the procedure steps to complete the assignment sheets.

Equipment and Supplies

Assignment sheets for this topic (Assignment Sheets #1 to #5 for 22:5 in workbook), scrap paper and pen or computer, calculator (if permitted)

Procedure

1. Review the preceding information section, Figure 22–51, and your completed Assignment Sheet for 22:5, Measuring Intake and Output.
2. Assemble equipment.
3. Go to the workbook and carefully read Assignment Sheet #1 for 22:5, Recording Intake and Output. *It will be part of this procedure.* After reading it through once, do the assignment based on the following guidelines and instructions.

4. Use a pen to record all information or follow the software instructions on a computerized program to make entries.

   a. Find the correct time line on the intake and output (I&O) record.

   b. Find the correct column: for example, *oral intake* or *urine output*.

   c. Record the amounts stated on the assignment sheet in the correct block. Number of milliliters (mL) for a coffee cup and other containers are at the top of the I&O assignment sheet.

5. When the information on the assignment sheet has been recorded in the appropriate places on the I&O record, recheck all areas of the record.

6. Make sure you have entered observations about color, type, and other facts in the remarks columns. Make sure the observations are on the right time lines by checking the times against the assignment sheet.

7. Under intake, add each column for 8-hour totals. For example, add all of the amounts for oral intake between 7 am and 3 pm. Do the same for each of the other columns for all three 8-hour periods.

   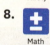 **CAUTION:** Recheck your addition. The totals must be accurate.

8. Now add the three 8-hour totals together for each column (7 am to 6 am) to get the 24-hour total at the bottom of the page. Do this for each column in intake and each column in output.

   NOTE: You should have a 24-hour total for oral intake and another total for IV intake.

9. Recheck all work.

   NOTE: If you make an error, draw one red line through the error. Place your initials in red by the error line. Then use a blue or black pen to write the correct information on the record. With computerized charting, you can modify your work and it will be marked as such. You will still be able to see what the original entry was. Follow the instructions on the computer software.

10. Give the paper to your instructor for grading. Replace all equipment used.

    NOTE: The record must be neat and legible. All figures must be recorded in metric units.

PRACTICE: Your instructor will grade Assignment Sheet #1 for 22:5, Recording Intake and Output. When it is returned to you, note all comments or corrections. Then complete Assignment Sheet #2 for 22:5, Recording Intake and Output. Give it to your instructor to grade. Again note comments or corrections. Repeat the process for Assignment Sheets #3, #4, and #5.

 FINAL EVALUATION: Using the criteria listed on the evaluation sheet, your instructor will grade your performance.

22:6 FEEDING A PATIENT

Good nutrition is an important part of a patient's treatment. It may be one of your responsibilities to make mealtimes as pleasant as possible for the patient. Mealtimes are often regarded as a time for social interaction. Most people prefer to eat with others. People who eat alone often have poor appetites and poor nutrition. In long-term care facilities, patients are encouraged to eat in the dining room. This provides an opportunity for social interaction with others. If a patient is confined to bed, it is important to talk with the patient while serving the food tray or feeding the patient.

Proper mealtime preparation is important. If the patient is ready to eat when the tray arrives, mealtime is likely to be more pleasant. Preparation before the tray is delivered includes:

- Offering the bedpan or urinal or assisting the patient to the bathroom; clearing the room of any offensive odors by using a deodorizer or opening a window

- Allowing the patient to wash their hands and face, if desired (**Figure 22–53A**)

- Providing oral hygiene, if desired; many individuals want to brush their teeth before meals, especially before breakfast

- Positioning the patient comfortably and in a sitting position, if possible

- Clearing the overbed table and positioning it for the tray

- Removing objects such as an emesis basin or bedpan from the patient's view; place such objects in the bedside stand, if they will not be needed

If a meal will be delayed because of radiographs (X-rays) or other treatments, be sure to explain this to the patient.

Check the tray carefully against the patient's name and room number and the type of diet ordered (**Figure 22–53B**). If anything seems out of place (for example, a salt shaker provided with a salt-free diet, or sugar with a diabetic diet), check with your immediate supervisor or the dietitian. Never add any food to the tray without checking the diet order first.

Allow patients to feed themselves whenever possible. If necessary, assist by cutting meat, opening beverage cartons, and buttering bread (**Figure 22–53C**). If a patient is blind or visually impaired, tell the patient what food is on the plate by comparing the plate to a clock. For example, say, "Swiss steak is at 12 o'clock, peas and carrots are at 4 o'clock, and mashed potatoes are at 9 o'clock." Make sure all food and utensils are conveniently placed.

Before feeding any patient, test the temperature of all hot foods. A small amount can be placed on your wrist to check temperature. Never blow on hot food to cool it.

Points to observe when feeding a patient include:

- Alternate the foods by giving sips of liquids between solid foods.

- Use straws for liquids unless the patient has dysphagia (difficulty in swallowing). Straws can force liquids down the throat faster and cause choking. A food thickener can be added to liquids to solidify them slightly and make them easier to swallow. A physician or dietitian must approve the use of this product.

- Offer only small bites of food at one time. Fill the spoon or fork one-third to one-half full.

- Hold the spoon or fork at right angles to the patient's mouth so you are feeding the patient from the tip of the utensil.

- Encourage the patient to eat as much as possible.

- Provide a relaxed, unhurried atmosphere.

- Give the patient sufficient time to chew the food.

 Comm Observe how much the patient eats so that a record of nutritional intake can be kept. If the patient does not like certain foods on the tray, ask your immediate supervisor or the dietitian whether a substitute can be provided. Record intake if an intake and output (I&O) record is being kept for the patient.

 Safety **CAUTION:** Always be alert to signs of choking while feeding a patient. Take every effort to prevent choking by feeding small quantities,

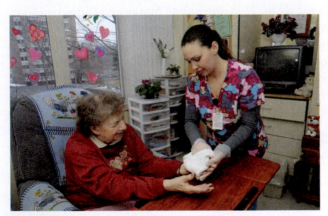

FIGURE 22–53A Allow the patient to wash her hands.

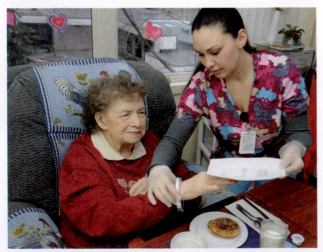

FIGURE 22–53B Check the food tray carefully against the patient's name, room number, and type of diet ordered.

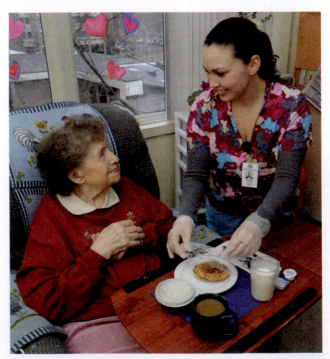

FIGURE 22–53C Assist the patient by cutting meat, opening beverage cartons, and positioning the food conveniently.

allowing sufficient time for the patient to chew and swallow, and providing liquids to keep the mouth moist and make chewing and swallowing easier. If the patient coughs or chokes frequently when swallowing, the feeding should be stopped to prevent aspiration of food. Notify your supervisor immediately. If a patient had a stroke, one side of the mouth may be affected. As you feed the patient, direct food to the unaffected side. Watch the patient's throat to check swallowing. Watch for food that may be lodged in the affected side of the mouth. If a patient chokes on food, be prepared to provide abdominal thrusts as described in Procedure 17:2E, *Performing CPR—Obstructed Airway on Conscious Adult or Child.*

checkpoint

1. What do you compare a plate to for a visually impaired or blind patient?

PRACTICE: Go to the workbook and complete the assignment sheet for 22:6, Feeding a Patient. Then return and continue with the procedure.

Procedure 22:6
OBRA

Feeding a Patient

Equipment and Supplies
Food tray with diet card, flex straws, towel, gloves, paper and pen or computer

Procedure

1. Obtain proper authorization and assemble equipment.

2. Knock on the door and pause before entering. Introduce yourself. Identify the patient. Explain that it is almost time to eat and obtain consent. Close the door and pull the curtain to provide privacy.

   Comm

3. Wash hands. Put on gloves.

    CAUTION: Wear gloves and observe standard precautions. Contact with body fluids, secretions, or excretions is possible.

   Precaution

4. Prepare the patient for mealtime. Provide oral hygiene, if desired. Help the patient use the bedpan, as needed. Position the patient in a sitting position, if permitted. Allow the patient to wash their hands and face. Position the overbed table and remove unnecessary articles.

   NOTE: Make sure the patient is not scheduled for radiographs or any other treatment requiring the tray to be withheld.

5. Check the tray. Match the name on the diet card with the patient's identification band if one is worn. Check the type of diet ordered to make sure the food on the tray is correct. Do not add anything to the tray without first checking with your supervisor.

   NOTE: If any foods seem to be incorrect for the diet ordered, check immediately with your supervisor.

   Comm

6. Place the tray on the overbed table. Place a towel or napkin under the patient's chin.

7. If the patient can feed themselves, arrange all food and silverware conveniently. Cut meat, butter bread, and open beverage cartons.

8. To feed a patient, proceed as follows:

   a. Follow the patient's preference for the order of foods eaten.

   b. Test hot liquids on your wrist before giving them to the patient. Wipe away any food placed on your wrist.

      NOTE: *Never* blow on the food to cool it. *Never* taste the patient's food. This can transmit infection.

   c. Use drinking straws for liquids unless the patient has dysphagia. Use a separate straw for each liquid offered. Give the patient a drink of water to wet the palate and make swallowing easier.

   d. Hold utensils at a right angle (90-degree angle) to the patient's mouth (**Figure 22–54**). Feed the patient from the tip of the utensil.

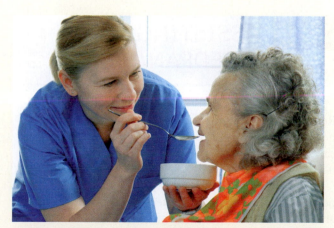

FIGURE 22–54 Hold utensils at a right angle to the mouth to feed the patient from the tip of the utensil. © Alexander Raths/Shutterstock.com

(continues)

e. Place a small amount of food on the utensil. Fill the spoon or fork about one-third to one-half full.

f. Tell the patient what they are eating.

g. If the patient had a stroke, place food in the unaffected side of the mouth. Watch the throat to make sure the patient is swallowing.

h. Allow sufficient time for the patient to chew. Do not hurry the patient.

i. Alternate foods, but don't mix foods together. Provide liquids at intervals to keep the mouth moist and make chewing and swallowing easier.

j. Allow the patient to hold bread and to help to the extent that they are able.

k. Use a towel or napkin to wipe the patient's mouth, as necessary.

 CAUTION: Be alert at all times to signs of dysphagia or choking. If the patient coughs or chokes frequently when swallowing, stop the feeding to prevent aspiration of food. Notify your supervisor immediately.

9. Encourage the patient to eat as much as possible.

NOTE: If the patient does not like a particular food, check with your immediate supervisor or the dietitian about substitute foods.

10. When the meal is complete, allow the patient to wash their hands. Provide oral hygiene. Position the patient comfortably and in correct body alignment.

11. Observe all checkpoints before leaving the patient: elevate the siderails, if indicated; lower the bed to its lowest level; place the call signal and supplies within easy reach of the patient; and leave the area neat and clean.

12. Note how much food was eaten. Record amounts on the I&O record, if one is being kept.

NOTE: In many health care facilities, the supervisor must be notified if the patient refuses food and/or liquids or eats less than 25 percent of the food.

13. Clean and replace all equipment. Place the tray in the correct area.

14. Remove gloves. Wash hands.

15. Report that the patient has been fed and/or record all required information on the patient's chart or enter it into the computer. For example, date, time, fed breakfast, ate everything except one-half slice toast, and your signature and title.

 NOTE: In health care agencies using electronic health records (EHRs), the information is entered directly into the patient's record on a computer.

PRACTICE: Go to the workbook and use the evaluation sheet for 22:6, Feeding a Patient, to practice this procedure. When you believe you have mastered this skill, sign the sheet and give it to your instructor for further action.

✅ **FINAL EVALUATION:** Using the criteria listed on the evaluation sheet, your instructor will grade your performance.

22:7 ASSISTING WITH A BEDPAN/URINAL

Regular elimination of body wastes contributes to good health. Patients confined to bed must rely on the health care provider's help in meeting this important physical need.

Elimination of body wastes is essential. Death will occur if wastes are not eliminated. The following terms are used in reference to elimination:

• **Urinate**, **micturate**, or **void**: These terms refer to emptying the bladder, which stores the liquid waste, or urine, produced by the kidney. A urinal is used by male patients when they need to urinate, micturate, or void; a bedpan is used by female patients. Two main types of bedpans are the fracture, or orthopedic, bedpan and the standard bedpan (**Figure 22–55**).

• **Defecate**: This refers to having a bowel movement, or BM; the discharge of the waste through the rectum. The material is called feces or stool.

Many patients are sensitive about using bedpans or urinals. It is important that the health care provider provide privacy by closing the door, privacy curtain, and window curtain. Make the patient as comfortable as possible during this procedure. It is also important to provide the bedpan or urinal immediately when the patient requests it. In addition, a bedpan or urinal should be offered frequently to any patient confined to bed.

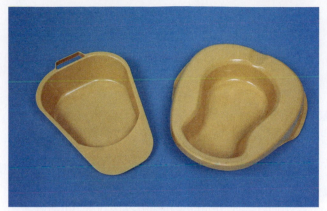

FIGURE 22–55 Two types of bedpans: the fracture, or orthopedic, bedpan (at left) and the standard bedpan (at right).

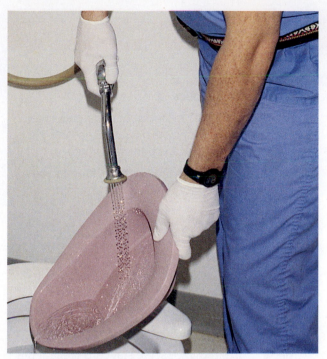

FIGURE 22–57 Some agencies have special spray units in the bathrooms to rinse and clean bedpans and urinals.

Accurate observations of the frequency, amount, and appearance of urine and stool are important. Abnormalities in any of these factors may indicate disease or complications. Any abnormality must be reported immediately, and a specimen must be saved for examination.

Before emptying a bedpan or urinal, it is the health care provider's responsibility to check whether specimens are needed. In addition, amounts must be measured and recorded if an intake and output (I&O) record is being kept for the patient. Check with your immediate supervisor or note physician's orders for this information.

Precaution Standard precautions must be observed when handling urine or feces. Hands must be washed frequently, and gloves must be worn. Eye protection and a mask or face shield must be worn if splashing or spraying is possible while emptying the bedpan. Some health care facilities require a one-glove technique to protect the environment while assisting with bedpans or urinals (**Figure 22–56**). Two gloves are worn to remove the bedpan or urinal. The bedpan or urinal is covered and placed on top of an underpad or bed protector that has been placed on a

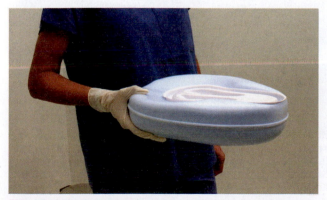

FIGURE 22–56 A one-glove technique can be used to carry a contaminated bedpan, leaving the other hand free to perform other tasks without contaminating the environment.

chair. The bedpan or urinal should never be placed on the overbed table or bedside stand. One glove is removed and held in the gloved hand. The ungloved hand is used to elevate the siderails (if indicated), open doors, and turn on faucets. A paper towel can also be used with a gloved hand to prevent contact with items in the environment. It is important to protect environmental surfaces from contamination with substances on gloved hands.

Some agencies have special spray units in the bathrooms to rinse and clean bedpans and urinals (**Figure 22–57**). After rinsing, the bedpan or urinal must be disinfected. It must be used for only one patient. After the patient is discharged, it must be sterilized according to agency policy before being used for another patient. Many bedpans are disposable and are discarded in an infectious-waste container when the patient is discharged.

Any areas contaminated with urine or feces must be wiped with a disinfectant. In addition, patients should have the opportunity to wash their hands and receive perineal care after using bedpans or urinals. Taking proper precautions can help prevent the spread of infection.

check**point**

I **1.** What three (3) words refer to emptying the bladder?

PRACTICE: Go to the workbook and complete the assignment sheet for 22:7, Assisting with a Bedpan/Urinal. Then return and continue with the procedures.

Assisting with a Bedpan

Equipment and Supplies

Bedpan with cover, bed protector or underpad, toilet tissue, basin, soap, washcloth, towel, disposable gloves, plastic waste bag, paper and pen or computer

NOTE: If cleansing cloths are available, they can be used in place of the basin, soap, and washcloth.

Procedure

1. Obtain proper authorization and assemble equipment.

2. Knock on the door and pause before entering. Introduce yourself. Identify the patient. Explain the procedure and obtain consent.
   Comm

3. Wash hands. Put on gloves.

    CAUTION: Observe standard precautions when handling urine or feces.
   Precaution

4. Close the door and pull the curtain for privacy. Put a bed protector or underpad on the chair and then place the bedpan on top. Place the tissue within easy reach of the patient. Raise the bed to a comfortable working height. Lower the head of the bed, if tolerated by the patient.

   CAUTION: Use correct body mechanics during this procedure. Bend from the hips, not the waist. Maintain a broad base of support.
   Safety

5. If the bedpan is metal, warm it by running hot water into it and then emptying it. If no water is available, rub the bedpan briskly with a cloth.

6. If siderails are present and elevated, lower the siderails on the side where you are working.

7. Fold the top bedcovers back at a right angle. Raise the patient's gown.

   NOTE: Avoid exposing the patient. If the patient is wearing pajama pants, help lower the pants.

   NOTE: The patient can also be covered with a bath blanket. The top sheets are then fanfolded to the foot of the bed.

8. Ask the patient to flex the knees and rest their weight on the heels, if able. Discuss a signal such as, "On the count of three, raise up."
   Comm

9. At the signal, assist the patient to raise their hips by putting one of your hands under the small of the patient's back.

CAUTION: If the patient is too heavy, get help.
Safety

10. With your other hand, slide the bedpan under the patient's hips. Adjust to the correct placement.

    NOTE: The patient's buttocks should rest on the rounded portion or seat of the pan.

11. The patient who is too weak to get on the pan may be rolled away from the health care provider and onto their side. The bedpan can then be placed against the patient's buttocks (**Figure 22–58**). The patient is then rolled back onto the bedpan. The bedpan must be held in place during this procedure.

    NOTE: Lower bedpans, called *fracture* (or orthopedic) *bedpans*, can also be used by patients who are unable to help (refer again to Figure 22–55).

12. Remove gloves and place them in the plastic waste bag.

13. Replace the top bedcovers. Position the patient in a comfortable position. Raise the head of the bed, as needed.

14. Place the call signal and tissue within easy reach of the patient.

    NOTE: If a urine specimen is needed or the patient is on Intake and Output, instruct the patient not to put toilet tissue in the pan. Provide a small plastic bag for discarding the soiled tissue.

15. If indicated, raise the siderail before leaving the patient.

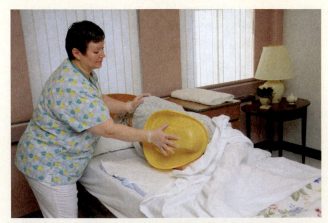

FIGURE 22–58 The patient can also turn onto their side so that the bedpan can be positioned. The patient then rolls back onto the bedpan.

16. Wash hands thoroughly.

17. Answer the patient's call signal immediately.

18. Wash hands.

19. Fill the bath basin with water at a temperature of 105°F–110°F. Place the basin on the overbed table or bedside stand. Position soap, a washcloth, and towel by the basin.

    NOTE: Cleansing cloths can be used for this step if they are available.

20. Put on gloves.

21. If elevated, lower the siderail. Ask the patient to flex the knees and put their weight on the heels. Place one hand under the small of the patient's back. Assist in raising the patient's buttocks off the pan. With your other hand, remove the bedpan carefully.

22. Cover the bedpan and place it on the underpad on top of the chair.

    NOTE: If a bedpan cover is not available, an underpad or bed protector, cloth, paper bags, or tissue paper can be used to cover the bedpan. Some bedpans have lids (refer to Figure 22–56).

23. If the patient is unable to assist in getting off the bedpan, it may be necessary to get help. Roll the patient off the bedpan and onto their side while holding the bedpan firmly in place with one hand. Cover the bedpan and place it on the underpad on top of the chair.

24. Clean the genital area, as necessary. Wipe from front to back. Drop the soiled tissue into the bedpan, unless a specimen is needed or output is being measured. In these situations, temporarily place the tissue in a plastic bag until you can discard it in the toilet or trash can in the utility room.

25. Wash the patient's perineal area, if necessary, or assist the patient as needed.

26. Remove gloves and place them in the plastic bag.

27. Replace the bedcovers. Elevate the siderails, if necessary.

28. Wash hands thoroughly.

29. Empty the bath basin and refill it with warm water or offer a clean cleansing cloth. Allow the patient to wash their hands.

30. Observe all checkpoints before leaving the patient: position the patient in correct body alignment; elevate the siderails (if indicated); lower the bed to its lowest level; and place the call signal, water, and tissues within easy reach of the patient.

31. Put on gloves. Take the bedpan to the bathroom. Note the contents. Check amount, color, and type. If an I&O record is being kept for the patient, measure and record the amount.

    NOTE: Check to see whether a specimen is needed before emptying the bedpan.

     CAUTION: Save a sample of the contents if there are any abnormalities.

32. Empty the bedpan. Use a paper towel to cover your gloved hand while turning on the faucet or flushing the toilet. Put on eye protection if spraying or splashing is possible. Rinse the bedpan with cold water and a disinfectant. Rinse and dry.

    NOTE: Follow your agency's policy for cleaning bedpans.

33. Return the covered pan to the patient's unit. Use a paper towel on the gloved hand or remove one glove. Replace all equipment used.

34. Remove gloves. Wash hands thoroughly.

35. Report and/or record all required information on the patient's chart or enter it into the computer. For example, date, time, used bedpan, voided 250 mL of straw yellow urine, and your signature and title. Always report unusual observations immediately.

     NOTE: In health care agencies using electronic health records (EHRs), the information is entered directly into the patient's record on a computer.

PRACTICE: Go to the workbook and use the evaluation sheet for 22:7A, Assisting with a Bedpan, to practice this procedure. When you believe you have mastered this skill, sign the sheet and give it to your instructor for further action.

✅ **FINAL EVALUATION:** Using the criteria listed on the evaluation sheet, your instructor will grade your performance.

Assisting with a Urinal

Equipment and Supplies

Urinal with cover, bed protector or underpad, basin, soap, washcloth, towel, toilet tissue, disposable gloves, plastic waste bag, paper and pen or computer

NOTE: If cleansing cloths are available, they can be used in place of the basin, soap, and washcloth.

Procedure

1. Obtain proper authorization and assemble equipment. Make sure the urinal has a lid or cover of some type (**Figure 22–59**).

2. **Comm** Knock on the door and pause before entering. Introduce yourself. Identify the patient. Explain the procedure and obtain consent.

3. Wash hands. Put on gloves.

   CAUTION: Observe standard precautions when handling urine or feces.

4. Close the door and pull the curtain for privacy. Elevate the bed to a comfortable working height. If siderails are present and elevated, lower the siderail on the side where you are working.

5. If the patient is weak or helpless, lift the top bedcovers and help the patient grasp the handle and position the urinal.

6. Make sure the call signal and toilet tissue are within easy reach of the patient. Leave the patient alone, if possible, to ensure privacy. Remove one glove. If necessary, elevate the siderail with the ungloved hand before leaving.

7. Remove gloves and wash hands.

8. Answer the patient's call signal immediately.

9. Wash hands.

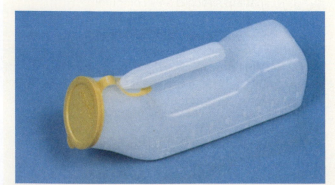

FIGURE 22–59 A urinal should have a lid or cover.

10. Fill the bath basin with water at a temperature of 105°F–110°F. Place the basin on the overbed table or bedside stand. Position soap, a washcloth, and towel by the basin.

    NOTE: If cleansing clothes are available, they can be used for this step.

11. Put on gloves.

12. Ask the patient to hand you the urinal. If the patient needs assistance, reach under the covers and take hold of the urinal handle. Close the lid or cover the top of the urinal and place it on top of the underpad on the chair.

    NOTE: Avoid exposing the patient.

13. Wash the patient's perineal area, if necessary, or assist the patient, as needed.

14. Remove gloves and place them in the plastic waste bag.

15. Replace the bedcovers. Elevate the siderails, if necessary.

16. Wash hands thoroughly.

17. Empty the basin and refill it with warm water or offer a clean cleansing cloth. Allow the patient to wash their hands or assist as needed.

18. Observe all checkpoints before leaving the patient: position the patient in correct body alignment, elevate the siderails, if indicated; lower the bed to its lowest level; and place the call signal and supplies within easy reach of the patient.

19. Put on gloves.

20. Take the urinal to the bathroom. Observe the contents. Measure and record the amount if an I&O record is being kept for the patient.

    NOTE: Check to see whether a specimen is needed before emptying the urinal.

     Safety **CAUTION:** Save a specimen if there are any abnormalities. Report unusual observations immediately to your supervisor.

21. Empty the urinal. Use a paper towel to cover your gloved hand while turning on the faucet or flushing the toilet. Put on eye protection if spraying or splashing is possible. Rinse the urinal with cold water and a disinfectant. Rinse and dry.

    NOTE: Follow agency policy for cleaning the urinal.

22. Return the urinal to the patient's unit. Use a paper towel on the gloved hand or remove one glove. Place it in the bedside stand or in the urinal holder on the bed.

23. Remove gloves. Wash hands thoroughly.

24. Report and/or record all required information on the patient's chart or enter it into the computer. For example, date, time, used urinal, voided 250 mL of straw yellow urine, and your signature and title. Always report unusual observations immediately.

 NOTE: In health care agencies using electronic health records (EHRs), the information is entered directly into the patient's record on a computer.

PRACTICE: Go to the workbook and use the evaluation sheet for 22:7B, Assisting with a Urinal, to practice this procedure. When you believe you have mastered this skill, sign the sheet and give it to your instructor for further action.

 FINAL EVALUATION: Using the criteria listed on the evaluation sheet, your instructor will grade your performance.

22:8 PROVIDING CATHETER AND URINARY-DRAINAGE UNIT CARE

 Some patients are unable to urinate, or void. In these cases, a catheter may be inserted into the bladder to drain the urine. The catheter is usually connected to a drainage unit to collect the urine.

A **catheter** is a hollow tube, usually made of soft rubber or plastic. There are different kinds of catheters. A urethral, or straight, catheter is inserted into the bladder to drain urine but is not left in the bladder (**Figure 22–60A**). It is usually used to collect a sterile urine specimen. A Foley catheter (also called an *indwelling*, or *retention*, catheter) is usually used to drain the bladder over an extended period. It has a small balloon on the end that is inserted into the bladder (**Figure 22–60B**). Once the catheter is inserted, the balloon is inflated with sterile water to keep the catheter in place. The catheter must be kept sterile at all times. Insertion of a catheter is a sterile technique performed by a nurse, physician, or other authorized person. If a

male patient requires urinary drainage, external condom catheters may be used (**Figure 22–60C**). The condom catheters eliminate the need for an internal catheter and decrease the chance of urinary infection. The condom catheter is placed on the penis and attached to the urinary-drainage tubing and collection bag. The condom must be removed at least every 24 hours, and the skin must be cleansed thoroughly and checked for any signs of irritation.

A **urinary-drainage unit** or bag is attached to the catheter to collect drained urine (**Figure 22–61A**). This is usually a closed unit to keep microorganisms from entering the catheter and, therefore, prevent infection. The unit consists of plastic or rubber tubing attached to the catheter and extending to a bag in which the urine is collected. Patients who are

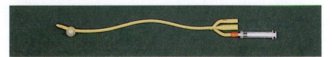

FIGURE 22–60B A Foley catheter has a small balloon on the end that is inserted into the bladder. The balloon is inflated with sterile water to hold the catheter in place.

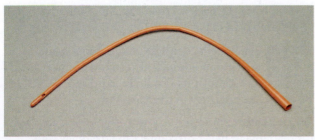

FIGURE 22–60A A straight catheter is inserted into the bladder to drain urine but is not left in the bladder.

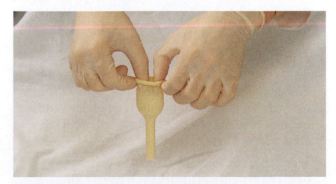

FIGURE 22–60C Condom catheters are used to provide an external urinary-drainage system for male patients.

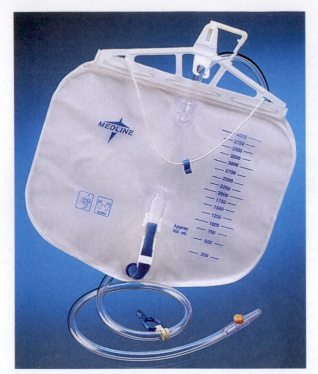

FIGURE 22–61A The urinary-drainage bag is connected to the catheter and attached to the bed frame below the level of the bladder to collect the drained urine. Courtesy of Medline Industries Inc., 1-860-MEDLINE

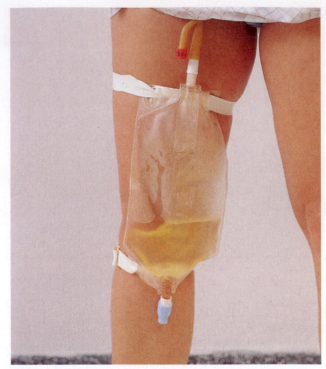

FIGURE 22–61B A leg bag may be used for ambulatory patients to collect urine drained through a catheter. It is usually attached to the leg with Velcro straps.

ambulatory may use a leg bag to collect the urine drained through the catheter (**Figure 22–61B**). The leg bag is smaller than a urinary-drainage bag and must be emptied more frequently. However, it does allow the patient more freedom of movement. Most leg bags are held in place with Velcro straps. The bag must be positioned so there is a straight drop down from the catheter. When the patient returns to bed, the leg bag is removed and the catheter is connected to a urinary-drainage bag. Most leg bags are discarded in an infectious-waste bag after one use. To prevent infection, careful aseptic technique must be used while connecting and disconnecting the catheter from either a urinary-drainage bag or a leg bag.

Careful observation of the catheter and drainage unit is required. The following should be checked frequently:

- The connection between the catheter and drainage unit is secure.

- The tubing is free from kinks or bends that stop the urine flow.

- The drainage bag is always below the level of the bladder. If it is raised above the level of the bladder, a backflow of urine into the bladder can occur. This, in turn, can lead to infection.

- The urine is flowing freely into the drainage bag. The system usually relies on gravity for drainage. Therefore, the drainage bag should be kept low enough to make use of the force of gravity.

- The catheter is secured to the patient's leg using a catheter stabilization device, or it can be taped or strapped onto the leg. This prevents pull on the catheter, which might dislodge it or cause irritation.

- The drainage unit is emptied frequently. Stagnant urine encourages the growth of microorganisms. The units are usually emptied every 8 hours, but they may be emptied more frequently, if required.

- The drainage bag and/or tubing are not lying on the floor. The drainage bag should be attached to the bed frame.

- No loops of the drainage tube are hanging below the drainage bag. Such loops interfere with the gravitational flow of urine into the bag.

- The drainage tubing leading to the drainage bag is always above the level of urine in the unit. This prevents infection and microorganisms in the urine from traveling back up the tubing and into the patient's bladder.

- Comm If a patient complains of burning, pain, irritation, or tenderness in the urethral area, the complaints should be reported immediately to the supervisor.

When a catheter and urinary-drainage unit is in place, it is preferable to never disconnect the drainage unit. However, it may sometimes be necessary to disconnect the catheter from the unit. For example, if a patient uses a leg bag during ambulation, the catheter is disconnected from the urinary-drainage unit and attached to the leg bag. If a urine-collection area is not present on the drainage unit, and a sterile or fresh urine specimen is required (because the urine in the bag is not fresh and is contaminated), the drainage unit must be disconnected. In either instance, careful sterile technique must be followed to prevent infection. Both the catheter and top connection of the drainage unit must be kept sterile. Special clamps, plugs, and other equipment are available for disconnecting the catheter (**Figure 22–62A**). Follow agency policy for disconnecting the catheter. Usually, the catheter is clamped to prevent leakage of urine. The health care provider wears gloves to disconnect the catheter from the tubing, taking care to avoid touching the ends of the catheter or tubing to any surface. A plug is inserted into the catheter, and a cap is placed on the end of the drainage tubing (**Figure 22–62B**). The drainage tubing is attached to the bed frame so it cannot touch the floor or become contaminated before it is reconnected. If a plug is not available, both the end of the catheter and the end of the drainage tubing should be covered with sterile gauze.

Most drainage units have special urine-collection areas or ports on the tubing. The catheter does not have to be disconnected when a specimen is obtained from this type of unit. Follow the specific instructions provided with the unit or follow agency policy to maintain sterility during this procedure. A clamp is usually placed on the tubing below the collection port to allow urine to collect in the tubing and/or bladder. The collection unit is wiped with a disinfectant, and a sterile syringe is inserted into the needleless port of the drainage tubing to obtain the urine specimen (**Figures 22–63A** and **22–63B**). A few health care facilities use units without needleless ports. A syringe with a sterile needle is inserted in this type of port to obtain the specimen. The urine is then placed in a sterile specimen container. Gloves must be worn during this procedure, and the contaminated syringe (and needle if one is used) must be placed in a sharps container immediately after use.

When a Foley, or indwelling, catheter is in place, the urinary meatus must be kept clean and free of secretions to help prevent bladder and kidney infections. Catheter

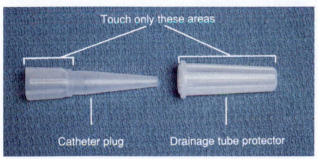

FIGURE 22–62A A sterile catheter plug and protective cap.

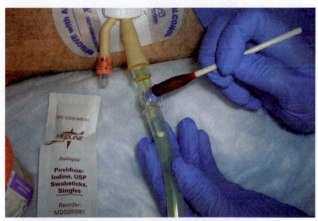

FIGURE 22–63A The urine-collection area is first wiped with a disinfectant.

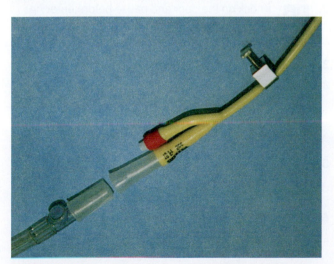

FIGURE 22–62B A catheter disconnected from the drainage tube and protected with the catheter plug. Note the protective cap on the drainage tube.

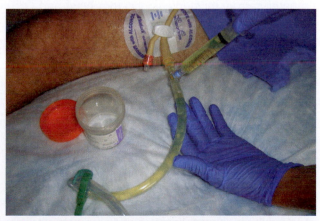

FIGURE 22–63B A sterile syringe is inserted into the port to obtain the urine specimen.

care is provided for this purpose, and it should be administered at least once every 8 hours, and more frequently if ordered. This care is usually provided during the bath and as part of perineal care. Disposable catheter-care kits containing applicators and antiseptic solution are used in many agencies. Other agencies use soap and water. Some kits also contain disposable bed protectors or underpads and gloves. Follow the instructions provided with the kit or the procedure recommended by your agency. Procedure 22:8A describes one method of catheter care.

Comm

Careful observations of the urine drained should be made. The amount, color, type, presence of other substances, and other observations should be noted. Unusual observations should be reported immediately.

Correct procedure must be followed when emptying the drainage unit to prevent contamination and infection. Procedure 22:8B describes one way of emptying a drainage unit.

If a patient has had an indwelling catheter in place for a time, a *bladder-training program* may be instituted before the catheter is removed. The purpose of a bladder-training program is to develop voluntary control of urination and prevent incontinence, or the inability to control urination. At first, the catheter is clamped for 1–2 hours at a time to allow urine to accumulate in the bladder. The clamp is then released, and urine is allowed to drain into the urinary-drainage unit bag. The time is gradually increased until the catheter is clamped for 3–4 hours at a time. After the catheter is removed, the patient is encouraged to void every 3–4 hours or whenever necessary to regain bladder control. Bladder-training programs can also be used for incontinent patients who do not have indwelling catheters in place. This type of program encourages the patient to attempt to void at regularly scheduled intervals. A record is kept of times of incontinence to establish when the patient should be encouraged to void. Staff members then assist the patient to the bathroom or offer the bedpan or urinal before the expected time of incontinence. The support, understanding, and cooperation of all team members is important when a bladder-training program is used for a patient.

Precaution

Standard precautions (discussed in Section 15:4) must be observed at all times when handling urine. Gloves must be worn when providing catheter care, obtaining urine specimens from a urine-collection unit, and emptying a urinary-drainage unit. Hands must be washed frequently and immediately after removing gloves. If splashing or spraying of body fluids is possible, eye protection, a mask or face shield, and gown must be worn. Any areas contaminated with urine must be wiped with a disinfectant. Taking proper precautions helps prevent the spread of infection.

check**point**

1. What is a catheter?

2. How is an indwelling or Foley catheter held in place?

PRACTICE: Go to the workbook and complete the assignment sheet for 22:8, Providing Catheter and Urinary-Drainage Unit Care. Then return and continue with the procedures.

Providing Catheter Care

Equipment and Supplies

Catheter-care kit (or sterile applicators, bowl, and antiseptic solution or soap and water), bath blanket, disposable underpad or bed protector, catheter stabilization device, catheter strap or tape (if needed), disposable gloves, infectious-waste bag, paper and pen or computer

NOTE: Catheter care is usually administered after the perineal area has been washed and cleaned during the bath. If administered at a different time, equipment must be obtained to wash and clean the perineal area before providing catheter care.

Procedure

1. Obtain proper authorization and assemble equipment.

2. **Comm** Knock on the door and pause before entering. Introduce yourself. Identify the patient. Explain the procedure and obtain consent.

3. Close the door and pull the curtain for privacy.

4. Wash hands. Put on gloves.

    Precaution **CAUTION:** Wear gloves and observe standard precautions when providing catheter care.

5. Elevate the bed to a comfortable working height. If siderails are present and elevated, lower the siderail on the side where you are working.

6. Cover the patient with a bath blanket. Without exposing the patient, fanfold the top bed linen to the foot of the bed.

7. Place the disposable underpad or bed protector under the patient's buttocks and upper legs.

8. Position the male patient in a supine position and the female patient in the dorsal recumbent position, if possible, with the legs separated and knees bent. Drape the patient so that only the perineal area is exposed.

9. Open the catheter-care kit and place it on the overbed table. Position the infectious-waste bag conveniently.

10. If sterile gloves are required, remove disposable gloves, wash hands, and put on sterile gloves.

   NOTE: Sterile gloves are required by some agencies. Follow agency policy.

11. Obtain a sterile applicator (usually a cotton ball or gauze pad) moistened with antiseptic solution or soap and water.

   NOTE: Some kits contain premoistened sterile applicators. Other kits contain containers of antiseptic solution that must be poured into small bowls provided with the kits. The sterile applicator is then placed in the antiseptic.

12. For a female patient:

   a. Use the thumb and forefinger of one hand to gently separate the labia, or lips, and expose the urinary meatus (opening).

   b. Wipe from front to back with the sterile applicator.

   c. Place the used applicator in the infectious-waste bag.

   d. Using a clean sterile applicator each time, continue to wipe from front to back until the area is clean.

13. For a male patient:

   a. Gently grasp the penis and draw the foreskin back.

   b. Use the sterile applicator to wipe from the meatus down the shaft.

   c. Place the used applicator in the infectious-waste bag.

   d. Using a clean sterile applicator each time, continue to wipe from the meatus down the shaft until the area is clean.

   e. After the area is clean, gently return the foreskin to its normal position.

14. Without pulling on the catheter, use a sterile applicator to clean the catheter from the meatus down approximately 4 inches. Place the used applicator in the infectious-waste bag. Repeat as necessary, using a fresh applicator for each stroke.

15. Observe the area carefully for any signs of irritation, abnormal discharge, or crusting.

16. Remove the bed protector or underpad and place it in the infectious-waste bag.

17. Remove gloves and discard in the infectious-waste bag. Wash hands.

18. Check the catheter to be sure it is secured to the leg. Tape or a strap may be used if a catheter stabilization device is not available (**Figures 22–64A**, **22–64B**, and **22–64C**).

    CAUTION: Make sure there is no strain or pull on the catheter.

19. Position the patient comfortably and in correct body alignment.

20. Replace the top bed linen and remove the bath blanket.

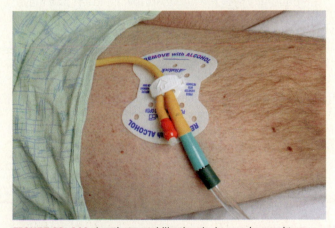

FIGURE 22–64A A catheter stabilization device can be used to secure the catheter to the leg.

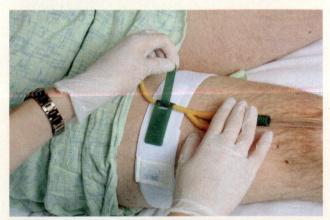

FIGURE 22–64B A strap can also be used to secure the catheter to the leg.

(continues)

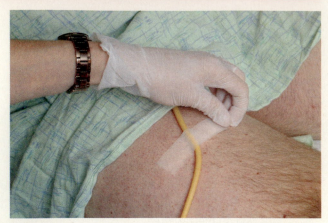

FIGURE 22–64C The catheter may also be taped to the leg. If possible, use hypoallergenic tape.

21. Observe all checkpoints before leaving the patient: elevate the siderails (if indicated); place the call signal, water, and supplies within easy reach of the patient; lower the bed to its lowest level; and leave the area neat and clean.

22. Perform a final check of the catheter and drainage unit to ensure the following:

    a. The tubing is free of kinks and bends.

    b. The tubing is positioned to allow for proper flow of urine. Do *not* allow excess tubing to hang below the drainage bag. Coil the excess tubing on the bed so the tubing hangs straight down into the drainage bag.

    c. The drainage bag is attached to the bed frame.

    d. The drainage bag is below the level of the bladder.

    e. The drainage tubing is above the level of the urine in the bag.

    f. Urine is flowing into the drainage bag.

23. Place all disposable supplies in the infectious-waste bag. Seal properly and dispose of in the correct area. Clean and properly replace any other equipment used.

24. Wash hands thoroughly.

25. Report and/or record all required information on the patient's chart or enter it into the computer. For example, date, time, catheter care given, urine flowing into drainage bag, and your signature and title. Report any unusual observations immediately.

     NOTE: In health care agencies using electronic health records (EHRs), the information is entered directly into the patient's record on a computer.

PRACTICE: Go to the workbook and use the evaluation sheet for 22:8A, Providing Catheter Care, to practice this procedure. When you believe you have mastered this skill, sign the sheet and give it to your instructor for further action.

✅ **FINAL EVALUATION:** Using the criteria listed on the evaluation sheet, your instructor will grade your performance.

Procedure 22:8B ⚖️

Emptying a Urinary-Drainage Unit

Equipment and Supplies

Paper towels, graduate or pitcher, antiseptic or disinfectant swab, disposable gloves, infectious-waste bag, paper and pen or computer

Procedure

1. Obtain proper authorization and assemble equipment.

2. Knock on the door and pause before entering. Introduce yourself. Identify the patient. Explain the procedure and obtain consent.

3. Wash hands. Put on gloves. Wear eye protection, a mask or face shield, and a gown if spraying or splashing of body fluids is possible.

 CAUTION: Observe standard precautions when measuring urine.

4. Place paper towels on the floor. Place the graduate on top of the towels.

5. Remove the drainage outlet from the drainage bag. Place the end of the outlet in the measuring pitcher or graduate.

 CAUTION: Do not allow the end of the outlet to touch the graduate.

6. Release the clamp to allow the urine to drain. Empty all the urine (**Figure 22–65A**).

    NOTE: If necessary, tilt the bag to remove all the urine.

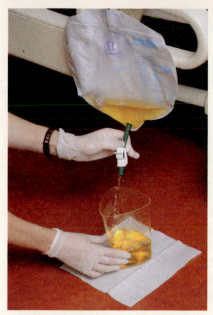

FIGURE 22–65A Drain the urine from the urinary-drainage unit.

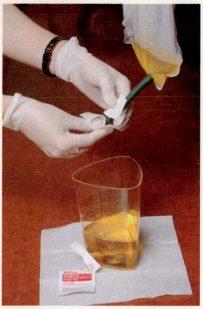

FIGURE 22–65B Wipe the drainage outlet with a disinfectant.

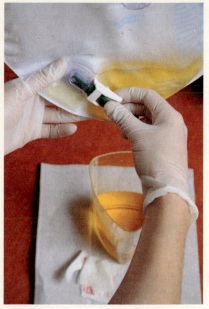

FIGURE 22–65C Replace the drainage tube in the drainage unit.

7. Clamp the drainage tube. Wipe the drainage outlet with an antiseptic or disinfectant swab (**Figure 22–65B**). Discard the antiseptic wipe in the infectious-waste bag. Replace the tube in the unit (**Figure 22–65C**).

8. Observe all checkpoints before leaving the patient: position the patient comfortably and in correct body alignment, elevate the siderails (if indicated), lower the bed to its lowest level, place the call signal and supplies within easy reach of the patient, and leave the area neat and clean.

9. Perform a final check of the catheter and unit to ensure the following:

   a. The catheter is secured to the patient's leg with a stabilization device, strap, or tape.

   b. The tubing is free of kinks and bends.

   c. The tubing does not loop down below the drainage bag. Do *not* allow excess tubing to hang below the drainage bag. Coil the excess tubing on the bed so the tubing hangs straight down into the drainage bag.

   d. The drainage bag is attached to the bed frame.

   e. The drainage bag is below the level of the bladder.

   f. The drainage tubing is above the level of the urine in the bag.

   g. Urine is flowing into the bag.

10. Pick up the graduate and paper towel. Discard the paper towel in the infectious-waste bag.

11. Take the graduate to the patient's bathroom. Place the graduate on a paper towel on a counter and read the measurement at eye level. Record the amount and color of urine in the graduate. Record any unusual observations and report such observations immediately.

    NOTE: Save a specimen if needed, or if anything unusual is noted about the urine.

12. Empty the graduate into the toilet. Rinse it with cold water. Wash with soap and warm water. Clean with a disinfectant. Rinse and dry. Return to its proper place.

    NOTE: The graduate is usually kept in the patient unit. It should be used for one patient only. Most agencies use disposable graduates. If the graduate is not disposable, it should be sterilized according to agency policy before being used for another patient.

13. Remove gloves. Wash hands.

14. Report and/or record all required information on the patient's chart or enter it into the computer. For example, date, time, emptied urinary-drainage unit, 580 mL of light yellow urine, and your signature and title. Report any unusual observations immediately.

    NOTE: In health care agencies using electronic health records (EHRs), the information is entered directly into the patient's record on a computer.

(continues)

PRACTICE: Go to the workbook and use the evaluation sheet for 22:8B, Emptying a Urinary-Drainage Unit, to practice this procedure. When you believe you have mastered this skill, sign the sheet and give it to your instructor for further action.

 FINAL EVALUATION: Using the criteria listed on the evaluation sheet, your instructor will grade your performance.

Check

22:9 PROVIDING OSTOMY CARE

An **ostomy** is a surgical procedure in which an opening, called a **stoma**, is created in the abdominal wall. This allows wastes such as urine or stool (feces) to be expelled through the opening. In most cases, an ostomy is performed because of tumors or cancer in the urinary bladder or intestine. An ostomy may also be done as a treatment for birth defects, ulcerative colitis, bowel obstruction, or injury. At times, an ostomy is permanent. At other times, an ostomy is temporary and is repaired when the injury heals or the condition necessitating the ostomy improves.

Science

There are different types of ostomies including the following:

- **Ureterostomy**: A ureterostomy is an opening into one of the two ureters that drain urine from the kidney to the bladder. The ureter is brought to the surface of the abdomen, and urine drains from the stoma, or opening.

- **Ileostomy**: An ileostomy is an opening into the ileum, a section of the small intestine. A loop of the ileum is brought to the surface of the abdomen. Because the entire large intestine is bypassed, the stools expelled are frequent and liquid, and contain digestive enzymes that irritate the skin.

- **Colostomy**: A colostomy is an opening into the large intestine, or colon. There are different kinds of colostomies, depending on the area of large intestine involved (**Figure 22–66**). Stool expelled through an ascending colostomy tends to be liquid, while stool expelled through a transverse or descending colostomy is more solid and formed. Stool expelled through a sigmoid colostomy is similar to normal stool because the digestive products have moved through most of the intestine, and water and other substances have been reabsorbed.

Most patients with ostomies wear a bag or pouch over the stoma to collect the drainage (**Figure 22–67**). The pouch is held in place with a belt or an adhesive seal. Problems that can occur include leakage, odor, and irritation of the skin surrounding the stoma. The pouch must be emptied frequently. Many pouches have areas that can be opened to allow urine or stool to drain. The drainage end of the bag is placed in a bedpan (**Figure 22–68**). If the patient is ambulatory, the patient can sit on the toilet and position the drainage end of the bag over the toilet. The clamp at the drainage end of the bag is opened to allow the stool or urine to drain. The drainage end is then cleaned to prevent odors, and the clamp is resealed. Some pouches are disposable and are removed and replaced. Used bags should be discarded in an infectious-waste bag.

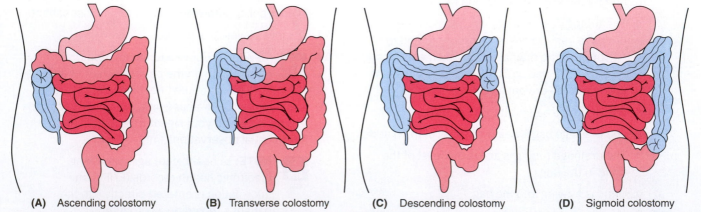

(A) Ascending colostomy   **(B)** Transverse colostomy   **(C)** Descending colostomy   **(D)** Sigmoid colostomy

FIGURE 22–66 The type of colostomy depends on which part of the intestine is removed. Areas of intestine that remain after each type of colostomy are shown in blue.

Good stoma and skin care are essential because of irritation caused by urine or stool drainage. Skin barriers such as wafers, creams, lotions, powders, and liquid films frequently are applied to the skin around the stoma to

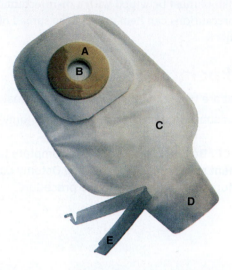

A. **Adhesive ring seals around stoma to prevent leakage**
B. **Opening placed over stoma**
C. **Collection bag**
D. **Drainage end of bag**
E. **Secures drainage end of bag to prevent leakage**

FIGURE 22–67 Most patients with ostomies wear a bag or pouch over the stoma, or opening, to collect the drainage.

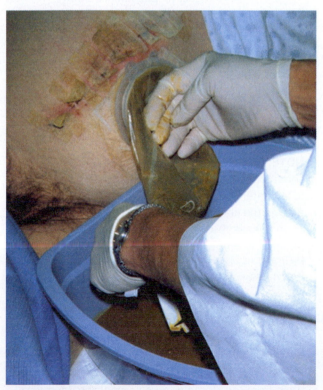

FIGURE 22–68 To empty the ostomy pouch, place the drainage end in a bedpan.

prevent irritation from the removal of the pouch. Only a thin layer of the barrier should be applied because too much lotion or cream may interfere with sealing the bag and irritate the skin.

 When an ostomy is first performed, care is provided by a registered nurse or wound care/ ostomy nurse. For "older" ostomies, other trained and qualified health care providers may provide routine stoma care. It is essential to check the policy of your facility and to know your legal responsibilities before providing ostomy care. Eventually, most patients are taught to care for their own ostomies, if they are capable.

Patients with ostomies may experience psychological reactions. They may feel loss of personal worth and dignity because they are unable to eliminate body wastes in a routine manner. Even though clothing conceals the ostomy and pouch, the patient feels different. Some individuals have difficulty maintaining normal sexual relationships. Others may feel anger, anxiety, depression, fear, or hopelessness. If the ostomy is done because of a malignant tumor (cancer), fear and anxiety can be more severe. It is essential to allow the patient to express feelings and verbalize fears. Understanding and support from all health care providers are important during the initial adjustment period. Eventually, patients realize that thousands of people with ostomies live normal lives. Through ostomy support groups, made up of people with ostomies, and help from health care providers, most individuals learn to cope and live with their ostomies.

 Careful observation is essential when providing care to the patient with an ostomy. The stoma is mucous membrane with no nerve endings. It is bright to dark red and looks wet because of the exposed mucosa (**Figure 22–69**). Rubbing or pressure can cause the stoma to bleed. Any abnormalities in appearance should be reported immediately. A blue-to-black color indicates interference with the blood supply.

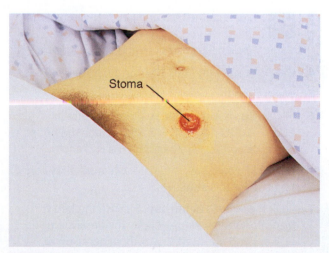

FIGURE 22–69 A stoma should be bright to dark red and look wet because of the exposed mucous membrane.

A pale or pink color can indicate a low hemoglobin level. A dry or dull appearance signifies dehydration. Profuse bleeding, ulcerations or cuts, or the formation of crystals on the stoma also indicate problems. The discharge in the ostomy bag or pouch should also be observed. It is important to note the amount, color, and type (liquid, semi-formed, formed) of discharge. Any unusual observations should be reported to your immediate supervisor and recorded on the patient's chart or the agency form.

 Standard precautions (discussed in Section 15:4) must be observed at all times when handling urine or stool. Gloves must be worn when emptying the pouch or providing stoma care. Hands must be washed frequently, and immediately after removing gloves. Eye protection, a mask or face shield,

Precaution

and a gown must be worn if splashing or spraying of body fluids is possible. The pouch must be discarded in an infectious-waste bag. If a bedpan is used, it must be cleaned and disinfected. Any areas contaminated with urine or stool must be wiped with a disinfectant. Taking proper precautions can help prevent the spread of infection.

checkpoint

1. What are two (2) characteristics of a normal stoma?
2. What substance drains from a ureterostomy?

PRACTICE: Go to the workbook and complete the assignment sheet for 22:9, Providing Ostomy Care. Then return and continue with the procedure.

Procedure 22:9

Providing Ostomy Care

Equipment and Supplies

Washcloth, towel, soap, basin, bed protector or underpad, bath blanket, ostomy pouch or bag, ostomy belt, adhesive (if needed), skin barrier or wafer (as ordered), toilet tissue, bedpan, disposable gloves, infectious-waste bag, paper and pen or computer

NOTE: If cleansing cloths are available, they can be used in place of the basin, soap, and washcloth.

Procedure

1. Check physician's orders or obtain authorization from your immediate supervisor.

   CAUTION: Know your legal responsibilities before providing ostomy care.

   Legal

2. Assemble equipment.

3. Knock on the door and pause before entering. Introduce yourself. Identify the patient. Explain the procedure and obtain consent.

   Comm

4. Close the door and pull the curtain for privacy.

5. Wash hands.

6. Fill the basin with water at a temperature of 105°F–110°F (40.6°C–43.3°C). Place the bedpan and infectious-waste bag within easy reach.

   NOTE: If cleansing cloths are available, they can be used for this step.

7. Lock the wheels of the bed. Elevate the bed to a comfortable working height. If siderails are present and elevated, lower the siderail on the side where you are working.

8. Cover the patient with a bath blanket. Without exposing the patient, fanfold the top bed linen to the foot of the bed.

9. Place a bed protector or underpad under the patient's hips on the side of the stoma.

10. Put on disposable gloves.

     CAUTION: Observe standard precautions at all times when handling urine or feces. If splashing of a body fluid is possible, wear a gown, mask or face shield, and eye protection.

    Precaution

11. Open the belt, if used, and carefully remove the ostomy bag. Be gentle when peeling the bag away from the stoma. Note the amount, color, and type of drainage in the bag. Place the bag in the bedpan or infectious-waste bag. Follow agency policy.

    NOTE: Most ostomy bags are disposable, but some are reusable. To reuse a bag, drain the fecal material (or urine from a ureterostomy) by placing the clamp end of the bag over a bedpan. Then release the clamp and allow the fecal material to empty into the bedpan. Wash the inside of the bag with soap and water and allow it to dry before reapplying the bag. Most people use a second bag while the first bag is drying.

12. Use toilet tissue to gently wipe around the stoma to remove feces or drainage. Put the tissue in the bedpan or infectious-waste bag.

    NOTE: If the patient has a ureterostomy, wipe urine from the stoma area to prevent the urine from contacting the skin.

13. Carefully examine the stoma and surrounding skin. Make sure it is bright to dark red and looks moist or wet. Check for irritated areas, bleeding, edema (or swelling), or discharge. Make sure you report any unusual observations to your immediate supervisor at the end of the procedure.

14. Wash the ostomy area gently with soap and water. Use a circular motion, working from the stoma outward.

15. Rinse the entire area well to remove any soapy residue. Dry the area gently with a towel.

    NOTE: Make sure soap is removed. It has a drying effect and may irritate the skin.

16. If ordered, apply a thin layer of barrier cream or lotion around the stoma.

     CAUTION: Avoid applying the barrier cream too thickly because it may interfere with adhesion of the wafer and/or irritate the skin.

17. Use a measuring chart to check the size of the stoma and determine the correct size barrier or wafer (**Figure 22–70A**). If the wafer is not self-adhesive, apply adhesive stoma paste to the skin around the stoma. Some pastes must dry a few minutes; follow the manufacturer's instructions. Peel the paper backing from the wafer. Position the wafer, adhesive side down, over the adhesive paste (**Figure 22–70B**).

    NOTE: The wafer serves as a barrier between the ostomy pouch or bag and the skin. It is not changed every time the pouch is changed. A new pouch can be snapped onto the existing wafer.

    NOTE: Some types of ostomy pouches and bags do not use wafers. Instead, barriers in the forms of pastes, liquids, or powders are applied to the skin to protect it. Follow the manufacturer's instructions.

18. If used, position the belt around the patient. If necessary, apply a clean belt.

19. Gently press to snap a clean ostomy bag in place over the wafer (**Figure 22–70C**). Seal the bag tightly to the wafer to prevent leakage.

20. If the pouch has a drainage area, make sure the clip or clamp sealing the drainage site is secure.

21. Remove the underpad or bed protector. If any linen on the bed is soiled, change the linen.

22. Remove gloves and discard in an infectious-waste bag.

23. Replace the top bed linen and remove the bath blanket. Make sure the patient is comfortable and positioned in correct body alignment.

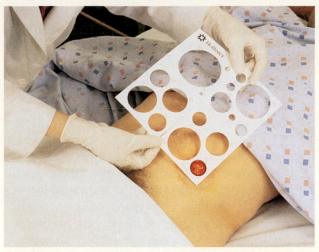

FIGURE 22–70A Check the size of the stoma to determine the correct size for the barrier or wafer.

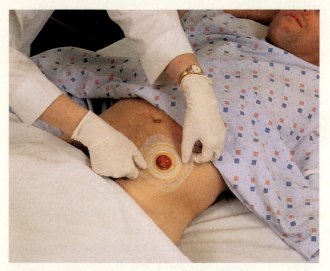

FIGURE 22–70B Position the wafer, adhesive side down, around the stoma.

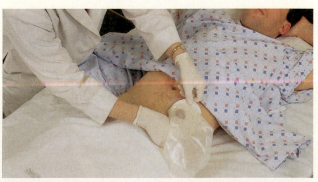

FIGURE 22–70C Gently press to snap the ostomy bag in place over the wafer.

(continues)

24. Observe all checkpoints before leaving the patient: elevate the siderails (if indicated); lower the bed to its lowest level; and place the call signal, water, tissues, and other supplies within easy reach of the patient.

25. Wash hands thoroughly and put on gloves.

26. Take the bedpan and waste bag to the bathroom. Follow agency policy for disposal of the ostomy pouch or bag. In some agencies, the bag is emptied into the bedpan. The contents of the bedpan are then flushed down the toilet. In other agencies, the bag is emptied directly into the toilet. The ostomy pouch or bag is then placed in an infectious-waste bag. In other agencies, the full bag is put in an infectious-waste bag. Rinse the bedpan with cool water and a disinfectant. Then rinse and dry it. Discard any other contaminated supplies in an infectious-waste bag.

27. Return the covered bedpan to the patient's unit. Replace all equipment used. Leave the area neat and clean.

28. Remove gloves. Wash hands thoroughly.

29. Report and/or record all required information on the patient's chart or enter it into the computer. For example, date, time, provided ostomy care, pouch three-fourths full of semi-formed light brown stool, and your signature and title. Always report unusual observations immediately.

Comm

NOTE: In health care agencies using electronic health records (EHRs), the information is entered directly into the patient's record on a computer.

EHR

PRACTICE: Go to the workbook and use the evaluation sheet for 22:9, Providing Ostomy Care, to practice this procedure. When you believe you have mastered this skill, sign the sheet and give it to your instructor for further action.

FINAL EVALUATION: Using the criteria listed on the evaluation sheet, your instructor will grade your performance.

Check

22:10 COLLECTING STOOL/ URINE SPECIMENS

As a health care provider, you may be responsible for collecting stool and urine specimens. Laboratory tests are performed on the specimens to aid in diagnosis of disease. For the tests to be accurate, the specimens must be collected correctly. Types of specimens include the routine urine specimen; clean-catch, or midstream-voided, specimen; catheterization for sterile urine specimen; 24-hour urine specimen; routine stool specimen; and stool for occult blood.

ROUTINE URINE SPECIMEN

- A routine **urine specimen** is one of the most common specimens. It is used for a variety of laboratory tests such as urinalysis (described in Section 20:10). The specimen is usually collected from the first urine voided in the morning because this urine is more concentrated and may reveal more abnormalities. In addition, a first-voided specimen usually has an acidic pH, which helps preserve any cells present. However, for some tests, such as specific gravity and checking urine with reagent strips, a fresh specimen is required. Check with

the physician, team leader, laboratory technologist, or other person in charge to find out when the specimen should be collected.

- The specimen can be collected in a bedpan, urinal, or special specimen collector positioned on a toilet under the seat. The collected urine is then poured into the specimen container (**Figure 22–71**). It may also be collected by instructing the patient to void directly into the specimen container.

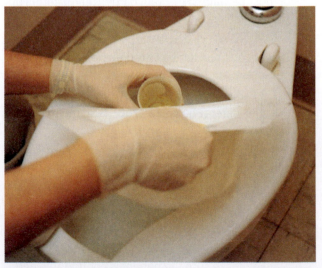

FIGURE 22–71 Carefully pour the urine from the specimen collector into a specimen container.

- Usually, 120 milliliters (mL) of urine is sufficient for this test. If the patient is unable to void this amount, obtain what is available and send this amount to the laboratory.

- The specimen should be sent to the laboratory immediately. If this is not possible, refrigerate the specimen until it can be sent to the laboratory.

- If a specimen container is not available, any clean container can be used. Wash the container thoroughly with soap and water, then rinse and dry it. Patients should be cautioned against using containers that previously held medications, however, because using such containers can alter the results of the test.

CLEAN-CATCH, OR MIDSTREAM-VOIDED, SPECIMEN

- A **clean-catch (midstream) specimen** is a urine specimen that is free from contamination. Because microorganisms are present on the genital area and on the specimen containers, special precautions are used to obtain a specimen.

- A sterile urine-specimen container, free from all micro organisms, is used to collect a midstream specimen.

- The genital area is cleansed thoroughly. This can be done by the health care team member, or the patient can be given careful instructions on how to do this procedure. Prepared wipes or clean cotton sponges or gauze squares and a mild antiseptic solution may be used.

- On a female patient, the genital area includes the perineum and the vulva. The vulva consists of two prominent folds, called the labia majora, and the structures within them: the labia minora, the urinary opening, the clitoris, and the vagina. Wipes are used to clean the external lips of the vulva. They are wiped from front to back. After each area is cleaned the wipe is discarded. The internal lips are then cleaned. Finally, the center area is cleaned from front to back. The center area contains the urinary opening (meatus).

- On a male patient, a circular motion is used. Starting at the urinary meatus (opening) at the tip of the penis, the end is cleaned thoroughly in a circular downward motion. Each wipe is discarded after each area is cleaned.

  NOTE: On uncircumcised male patients, the foreskin should be pushed back before cleaning. After the end of the penis is clean, gently push the foreskin back into its normal position.

- After the area has been cleaned, the patient is told to urinate, or void. A few drops of urine are allowed to flow into the bedpan or toilet bowl. The sterile container is then used to catch the urine that follows. The last few drops of urine should be discarded. In this way, the first and last part of the specimen are discarded, and only the middle, or midstream, urine is collected.

- The sterile lid of the container should be placed on this specimen immediately to prevent contamination. The specimen should immediately be sent to the laboratory or refrigerated.

CATHETERIZATION FOR STERILE URINE SPECIMEN

- It is sometimes necessary to obtain a sterile urine specimen from a patient. In order to do this, the patient is catheterized. A narrow, hollow, sterile tube is inserted directly into the bladder. Urine from the tube is then placed in a sterile urine-specimen container.

- Specimen collection catheters are also available for obtaining a sterile urine specimen (**Figure 22–72**). These units contain a very small catheter attached to a collection test tube. The catheter is inserted into the bladder and urine drains directly into the tube. When the tube is full, the catheter is withdrawn. The catheter is then separated from the tube and discarded in a sharps container. The tube is sealed by pressing on the spout.

- **Legal** Only a trained person should insert the catheter. However, if a catheter is already in place, you may collect a urine specimen in the sterile container (refer to Figures 22–63A and 22–63B). It is important that you work under supervision and use sterile technique to prevent contamination of the catheter when obtaining the specimen.

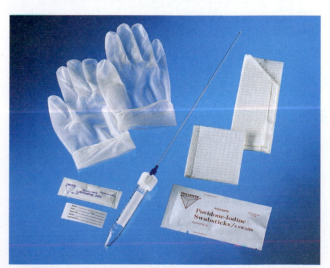

FIGURE 22–72 This Speci-Cath kit is designed to obtain a sterile urine specimen from a male patient. Courtesy of Medline Industries Inc., 1-860-MEDLINE

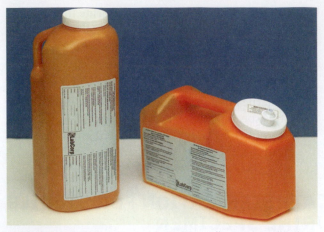

FIGURE 22–73 Different types of specimen collectors for collecting 24-hour urine specimens.

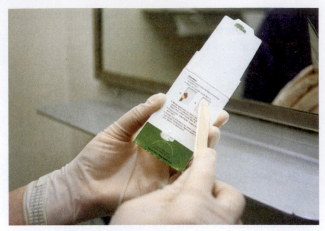

FIGURE 22–74 A small specimen of stool is placed on the Hemoccult card to test for occult blood.

24-HOUR URINE SPECIMEN

- Special tests require a **24-hour urine specimen**. This means that all of the urine produced by the patient during a 24-hour period must be saved. This urine is used to check kidney function and components such as protein, creatinine, urobilinogen, hormones, and calcium.

- The urine is preserved by chemicals or cold storage. The laboratory sends the correct container and instructions for preserving the specimen (**Figure 22–73**).

- To start, the patient voids to empty the bladder. This urine is discarded because it was produced before the start of the 24-hour period. The time of voiding is noted as the start of the 24-hour period. All urine voided in the next 24 hours is saved in the special container. At the end of the 24-hour period, the patient voids again for the final collection of urine.

- If any specimen is accidentally discarded during the 24-hour period, the test must be discontinued and restarted. In addition, toilet tissue cannot be discarded in any specimen. The tissue must be discarded in a plastic waste bag or toilet.

ROUTINE STOOL SPECIMEN

- A **stool** (feces) **specimen** is examined by the laboratory, usually to check for ova and parasites (eggs and worms). Stool can also be examined for the presence of fats, microorganisms, and other abnormal substances. A new stool test checks for a gene or a DNA mutation that is usually faulty in the earliest stages of colon cancer. One test has been approved by the FDA, and several others are in trial studies. This test can help physicians detect colon cancer at its earliest stages when it can be treated much more effectively.

- The stool is placed in a special stool-specimen container.

- The container should be kept at body temperature, and the specimen sent to the laboratory immediately. For the most accurate results, it should be examined within 30 minutes.

STOOL FOR OCCULT BLOOD

- Sometimes **occult blood** (blood from areas of the intestinal tract) can be found in the stool. Testing for occult blood requires only a small amount of stool.

- A special card is usually used for this test. The small specimen of stool is placed on a designated section(s) of the card (**Figure 22–74**).

- The card is sent to the laboratory or checked immediately by an authorized individual in some health care facilities. A few drops of a special developing solution, such as Hemoccult, is added to the area. A color change indicates a positive result.

- A positive test means that blood is present in the stool.

- The test for occult blood does not require that the stool be kept warm or that it be examined immediately. However, it should be sent to the laboratory as soon as possible so that the specimen is not misplaced.

SUMMARY

EHR

All specimens must be labeled correctly, including the kind of specimen (urine or stool), the test ordered, the patient's name, room number or identification (ID) number, the date and time, and the physician's name. It is best to label the specimen container instead of the lid because errors could occur if the lid is misplaced. All required information must also be printed on the correct lab requisition form. A lab requisition must be sent with the labeled specimen.

Health care agencies with electronic health records (EHRs) use computer-generated labels for the specimen container and lab requisition form.

Precaution

Standard precautions (discussed in Section 15:4) must be observed when obtaining and handling urine or stool specimens. Gloves must be worn. Hands must be washed frequently and are always washed immediately after removing gloves. Eye protection, a mask or face shield, and a gown must be worn if splashing or spraying of body fluids is possible. Any areas contaminated with urine or stool must be wiped with a disinfectant. To avoid contamination from spills, all urine or stool specimens are placed in special biohazard bags before being transported to the laboratory for testing. Taking proper precautions can help prevent the spread of infection.

checkpoint

1. When collecting a routine urine specimen, if a specimen cup is not available, what can be used?
2. If a urine specimen is not sent to the lab right away, how should it be stored?

PRACTICE: Go to the workbook and complete the assignment sheet for 22:10, Collecting Stool/Urine Specimens. Then return and continue with the procedures.

Procedure 22:10A

Collecting a Routine Urine Specimen

Equipment and Supplies

Bedpan with cover/urinal or specimen collector, urine-specimen container and label, toilet tissue, graduate or measuring pitcher, disposable gloves, infectious-waste bag, biohazard bag, paper and pen or computer

Procedure

1. Check physician's orders or obtain authorization from your immediate supervisor to be sure you are collecting the right type of specimen.

   NOTE: In most cases, the first-voided specimen of the day is collected.

2. Assemble equipment.

3. **Comm** Knock on the door and pause before entering. Close the door and pull the curtain for privacy. Introduce yourself. Identify the patient. Explain the procedure and obtain consent.

4. Wash hands. Put on gloves.

    Precaution **CAUTION:** Observe standard precautions when obtaining and handling urine specimens.

5. If the patient is ambulatory, assist the patient to the bathroom.

   a. Place a specimen collector on the toilet and then reposition the toilet seat.

   b. Instruct the patient to discard the toilet tissue into the toilet and not into the specimen collector. An infectious-waste bag can also be provided for the discarded tissue.

   c. Provide privacy while the patient voids. Make sure the call signal and toilet tissue are within reach.

   d. After the specimen has been collected, assist the patient back to a chair or bed.

6. If the patient is not ambulatory, offer the bedpan or urinal as previously instructed in Procedure 22:7A or 22:7B.

   a. Advise the patient not to put toilet tissue in the bedpan or urinal. Provide an infectious-waste bag for disposal of soiled toilet tissue.

   b. After the patient has voided, remove the bedpan or urinal. Place it on top of an underpad or bed protector that has been placed on the chair.

7. Remove gloves and wash hands thoroughly.

8. When the specimen has been obtained, allow the patient to wash their hands.

9. Observe all checkpoints before leaving the patient: position the patient comfortably and in correct body alignment, elevate the siderails (if indicated), place the call signal and supplies within easy reach of the patient, lower the bed to its lowest level, and leave the area neat and clean.

10. Put on clean gloves.

11. Take the bedpan or urinal to the patient's bathroom or remove the specimen collector from the toilet. Pour the urine into a measuring pitcher or graduate.

    NOTE: Record the amount if an intake and output (I&O) record is being kept for the patient (**Figure 22–75**).

12. Pour approximately 120 mL into the urine-specimen container.

13. Wash the outside of the container to remove any spilled urine. Remove gloves. Wash hands.

     Safety **CAUTION:** Do not allow water to enter the container. Water will dilute the urine specimen and affect the accuracy of the test results.

    (continues)

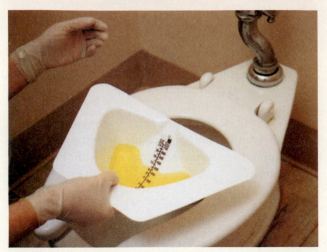

FIGURE 22–75 If an I&O record is being kept for the patient, measure the amount of urine in the specimen collector.

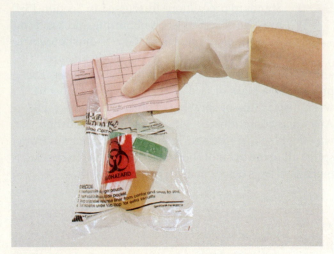

FIGURE 22–76 All specimens must be placed in protective biohazard bags before being transported to the laboratory.

14. Place the cover on the container.

15. 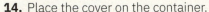 **Comm** Label the container or attach the computer-generated label. Include the date, time, patient's name, room or ID number, specimen type, test required, and physician's name. Print required information on the correct lab requisition; obtain the requisition from your immediate supervisor or use the computer-generated requisition. A lab requisition must be sent with the labeled specimen.

16. Clean and replace all equipment.

CAUTION: Remember to wear gloves and observe standard precautions when cleaning any equipment or area contaminated with urine.

Precaution

17. **Precaution** Put the specimen in a protective biohazard bag for transport (**Figure 22–76**). Take or send the specimen to the laboratory immediately. Report the arrival of the specimen to laboratory personnel. If this is not possible, refrigerate the specimen until it can be sent to the laboratory.

18. Wash hands thoroughly.

19. **Comm** Report and/or record all required information on the patient's chart or enter it into the computer. For example, date, time, routine urine specimen collected and sent to lab, and your signature and title.

NOTE: In health care agencies using electronic health records (EHRs), the information is entered directly into the patient's record on a computer.

EHR

PRACTICE: Go to the workbook and use the evaluation sheet for 22:10A, Collecting a Routine Urine Specimen, to practice this procedure. When you believe you have mastered this skill, sign the sheet and give it to your instructor for further action.

 FINAL EVALUATION: Using the criteria listed on the evaluation sheet, your instructor will grade your performance.

Check

Procedure 22:10B

Collecting a Clean-Catch (Midstream) Urine Specimen

Equipment and Supplies

Sterile urine-specimen bottle and label, prepared wipes or gauze or cotton squares with antiseptic solution, small basin, infectious-waste bag, biohazard bag, disposable gloves, underpad or bed protector (if needed), paper and pen or computer

NOTE: This procedure may vary slightly in different health care facilities or laboratories. Follow the procedure recommended by your facility.

Procedure

1. Check physician's orders or obtain authorization from your immediate supervisor to be sure you are collecting the correct type of specimen.

2. Assemble equipment.

3. Knock on the door and pause before entering. Introduce yourself. Identify the patient. Explain the procedure and obtain consent.

   Comm

4. Wash hands.

5. Close the door and pull the curtain to provide privacy for the patient. Elevate the bed to a comfortable working height. If siderails are present and elevated, lower the siderail on the side where you are working. If the patient is ambulatory, the specimen can be collected in the bathroom. If the patient is not ambulatory, provide a bedpan or urinal as instructed in Procedure 22:7A or 22:7B.

6. Provide the patient with prepared wipes. If the wipes are not available, a gauze or cotton square and antiseptic solution can be used. In many agencies, a special kit is available for collecting midstream specimens. Follow the instructions that come with the kit, if one is used.

7. Put on disposable gloves.

    CAUTION: Wear gloves and observe standard precautions when obtaining urine specimens.

   Precaution

8. Clean the genital area correctly or instruct the patient on how to do so.

   a. For a female patient, use the prepared wipes to clean the outer folds from front to back. Use a clean wipe for each area cleaned. Discard each wipe in the infectious-waste bag after one use. Clean the inner folds (lips) from front to back, using a clean wipe for each area cleaned. Discard each wipe after use. Finally, clean the innermost (middle) area from front to back. Discard soiled wipe.

   b. For a male patient, use a circular motion to clean from the urinary meatus outward and downward. Discard each wipe after one area is cleaned in the infectious-waste bag. Repeat at least two times or until the entire area is clean.

   NOTE: On uncircumcised male patients, the foreskin should be pushed back before cleaning. After cleaning, gently push the foreskin back to its normal position.

9. Instruct the patient to void. Allow the first part of the stream to escape. Catch the middle of the stream in the sterile specimen container. Allow the last part of the stream to escape.

   NOTE: If the amount must be measured because an intake and output (I&O) record is being kept for the patient, catch the first and last urine in a bedpan or urinal or in a specimen collector if the patient is on the toilet.

10. Place the sterile cap on the container immediately to prevent contamination of the specimen (**Figure 22–77**).

     CAUTION: Do not touch the inside of the specimen container or the inside of the lid because this will contaminate the specimen.

    Safety

    If the lid is placed on a counter while the specimen is being obtained, it should always have the inside of the lid facing up.

    NOTE: Some midstream-specimen containers have a funnel that aids in the collection of the specimen. This is removed and discarded in the infectious-waste bag before the sterile cap is placed on the container.

11. Allow the patient to wash their hands.

12. Observe all checkpoints before leaving the patient: position the patient in correct body alignment, elevate the siderails (if indicated), lower the bed to its lowest level, place the call signal and supplies within easy reach of the patient, and leave the area neat and clean.

    NOTE: Use a paper towel with a gloved hand or a one-glove method to avoid contaminating the environment.

13. Wash the outside of the container. Remove gloves and wash hands.

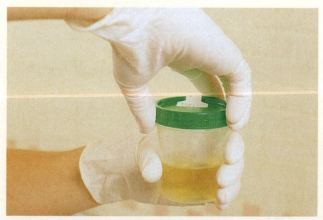

FIGURE 22–77 Place the sterile cap on the container immediately after collecting the urine specimen.

(continues)

14.
Label the container as a "Clean-Catch" or "Midstream" specimen or attach a computer-generated label. Print the name of the ordered test, the patient's name, room number or ID number, the date and time, and physician's name on the label. Print required information on the correct lab requisition. Obtain the requisition from your immediate supervisor or use a computer-generated requisition. A lab requisition must be sent with the labeled specimen.

15. Clean and replace all equipment.

CAUTION: Remember to wear gloves and observe standard precautions when cleaning any equipment or area contaminated with urine.

16. Put the specimen in a protective biohazard bag for transport. Take or send the specimen to the laboratory immediately. Report the arrival of the specimen to laboratory personnel. If this is not possible, refrigerate the specimen until it can be sent to the laboratory.

NOTE: For the most accurate results, the specimen should be examined as soon as possible.

17. Wash hands thoroughly.

18.
Report and/or record all required information on the patient's chart or enter it into the computer. For example, date, time, midstream urine specimen collected and sent to laboratory, and your signature and title.

NOTE: In health care agencies using electronic health records (EHRs), the information is entered directly into the patient's record on a computer.

PRACTICE: Go to the workbook and use the evaluation sheet for 22:10B, Collecting a Clean-Catch (Midstream) Urine Specimen, to practice this procedure. When you believe you have mastered this skill, sign the sheet and give it to your instructor for further action.

✅ **FINAL EVALUATION:** Using the criteria listed on the evaluation sheet, your instructor will grade your performance.

Procedure 22:10C

Collecting a 24-Hour Urine Specimen

Equipment and Supplies

24-hour specimen container and label, sign for patient's bed, graduate (if urine is to be measured), disposable gloves, infectious-waste bag, biohazard bag, paper and pen or computer

Procedure

1. Check physician's orders or obtain authorization from your immediate supervisor to be sure you are collecting the correct specimen.

2. Check on the type of container and preservative required.

NOTE: Some containers for certain tests contain chemical preservatives. Others must be kept on ice or refrigerated during the 24 hours. The laboratory will supply information about the correct method for preserving the specimen.

3. Assemble equipment.

4.
Label the container with the patient's name, room number or ID number, the test ordered, the specimen type, the date, and the physician's name, or attach a computer-generated label.

5.
Knock on the door and pause before entering. Close the door and pull the curtain for privacy. Introduce yourself. Identify the patient. Explain the procedure and obtain consent. Tell the patient not to discard toilet tissue in the urine specimen. Provide a plastic waste bag for disposal of toilet tissue.

NOTE: Make sure the patient understands the entire procedure. Stress the importance of saving all urine.

6. Wash hands. Put on disposable gloves.

CAUTION: Remember to wear gloves and observe standard precautions when obtaining urine and placing it in a 24-hour specimen container.

7. Allow the patient to void. Assist with the bedpan or urinal, if necessary. Measure the amount if an intake and output (I&O) record is being kept for the patient. Discard this specimen. Note the time of voiding as the start of the 24-hour period.

NOTE: Urine voided at this time has been produced before the 24-hour time period. The patient must begin the 24-hour period with an empty bladder.

NOTE: For female patients allowed to use the bathroom, a specimen collector can be placed under the seat in the toilet (refer to Figure 22–52). The patient must be told not to discard toilet tissue or defecate in the specimen collector.

8. Remove gloves. Wash hands thoroughly.

9. Place a sign on the patient's bed and/or in the bathroom to alert others that a 24-hour specimen is being collected. The sign usually states, "Save all urine—24-hour specimen."

10. During the 24-hour period, use the specimen container to collect all urine voided (**Figure 22–78**).

    NOTE: If any urine is discarded, the procedure must be stopped and started again.

    NOTE: Make sure the specimen is preserved correctly during this time. If it should be kept on ice, always check to make sure the ice is replenished as it melts and drain all water from the container holding the ice.

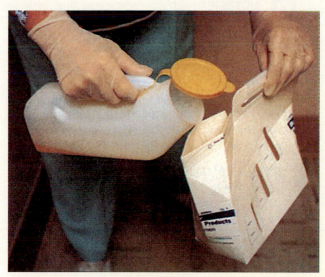

FIGURE 22–78 All urine voided during the 24-hour period must be placed in the specimen container.

11. At the end of the 24-hour period, ask the patient to void. Add this urine to the specimen container. It is the final voiding of the procedure.

12. Remove the sign from the patient's bed.

13. **Comm** Check the specimen label to make sure it is accurate and contains all the required information. Print the required information on the correct lab requisition. Obtain the requisition from your immediate supervisor or use a computer-generated requisition. A lab requisition must be sent with the labeled specimen.

14. **Precaution** Put the specimen in a protective biohazard bag for transport. Take or send the specimen to the laboratory immediately. Notify laboratory personnel of the specimen's arrival.

    NOTE: For the most accurate results, urine should go to the laboratory as soon as possible.

15. Replace all equipment used.

16. Remove gloves. Wash hands thoroughly.

17. **Comm** Report and/or record all required information on the patient's chart or enter it into the computer. For example, date, time, 24-hour urine specimen completed and sent to laboratory, and your signature and title.

    EHR **NOTE:** In health care agencies using electronic health records (EHRs), the information is entered directly into the patient's record on a computer.

PRACTICE: Go to the workbook and use the evaluation sheet for 22:10C, Collecting a 24-Hour Urine Specimen, to practice this procedure. When you believe you have mastered this skill, sign the sheet and give it to your instructor for further action.

Check **FINAL EVALUATION:** Using the criteria listed on the evaluation sheet, your instructor will grade your performance.

Collecting a Stool Specimen

Equipment and Supplies

Bedpan with cover or specimen collector, stool-specimen container, tongue blades, label, disposable gloves, infectious-waste bag, biohazard bag, paper and pen or computer

Procedure

1. Check physician's orders or obtain authorization from your immediate supervisor; verify the type of specimen needed.

2. Assemble equipment.

(continues)

3. Knock on the door and pause before entering. Close the door and pull the curtain for privacy. Introduce yourself. Identify the patient. Explain the procedure and obtain consent. Ask the patient to use the bedpan for their next bowel movement because a specimen is needed. Ask the patient not to void or place toilet tissue in the bedpan. Provide an infectious-waste bag for soiled toilet tissue.

   NOTE: In some agencies, specimen collectors that fit directly under the toilet seat are used.

4. Wash hands. Put on disposable gloves.

    CAUTION: Wear gloves and observe standard precautions when obtaining stool specimens.

5. Obtain the specimen in the bedpan or specimen collector. Allow the patient to wash their hands.

   NOTE: Assist with the bedpan, as necessary.

6. Take the bedpan to the bathroom.

7. Use two tongue blades to remove the stool from the bedpan. Place the stool in the specimen container. Discard the tongue blades in the infectious-waste bag.

8. Remove gloves and wash hands thoroughly.

   ⚠️ **CAUTION:** Avoid contaminating the outside of the container.

9. Place the lid on the container. Make sure it is tightly in place.

10. Label the container correctly, including specimen type, test ordered, patient's name, room or ID number, date and time, and physician's name, or attach a computer-generated label. Print the required information on the correct lab requisition. Obtain the requisition from your immediate supervisor or use a computer-generated requisition. A lab requisition must be sent with the labeled specimen.

11. Put on gloves to clean the bedpan. Rinse the bedpan with cool water. Clean with a disinfectant, and rinse and dry. Replace all equipment used. Leave the area neat and clean.

12. Remove gloves and wash hands.

13. Keep the specimen warm. Put the specimen in a protective biohazard bag for transport. Take or send it to the laboratory immediately. Report the arrival of the specimen to laboratory personnel.

   NOTE: The specimen should be examined within 30 minutes for most accurate results.

14. Wash hands.

15. Report and/or record all required information on the patient's chart or enter it into the computer. For example, date, time, stool specimen collected and sent to laboratory, and your signature and title.

   🔲 **NOTE:** In health care agencies using electronic health records (EHRs), the information is entered directly into the patient's record on a computer.

PRACTICE: Go to the workbook and use the evaluation sheet for 22:10D, Collecting a Stool Specimen, to practice this procedure. When you believe you have mastered this skill, sign the sheet and give it to your instructor for further action.

✅ **FINAL EVALUATION:** Using the criteria listed on the evaluation sheet, your instructor will grade your performance.

Procedure 22:10E

Preparing and Testing a Hemoccult Slide

🏛️ **NOTE:** Legal requirements regarding who can perform this procedure vary from state to state. Check your legal responsibilities before performing this procedure.

Equipment and Supplies

Bedpan with cover/specimen collector, Hemoccult slide packet, Hemoccult developer, tongue blade, paper towel, disposable gloves, infectious-waste bag, biohazard bag, paper and pen or computer

Procedure

1. Obtain proper authorization to be sure of the type of specimen needed.

2. Assemble equipment. Read the manufacturer's instructions for the use of the Hemoccult slide packet and developer.

3. Knock on the door and pause before entering. Close the door and pull the curtain for privacy. Introduce yourself. Identify the patient. Explain the procedure and obtain consent. Ask the patient to use the bedpan for their next bowel movement because a

specimen is needed. Tell the patient not to void or place toilet tissue in the specimen in the bedpan. If necessary, provide an infectious-waste bag for disposal of soiled toilet tissue.

NOTE: In some agencies, specimen collectors that fit directly under the toilet seat are used.

4. Wash hands. Put on gloves.

 CAUTION: Wear gloves and observe standard precautions when obtaining stool specimens.

5. Obtain the specimen in the bedpan or specimen collector. Assist the patient, as necessary. Allow the patient to wash their hands.

6. Take the bedpan and specimen to the bathroom.

7. Place a paper towel on the counter. Put the Hemoccult slide packet on top of the towel.

8. Open the front cover or flap of the Hemoccult packet.

9. Use the tongue blade to smear a small amount of the stool specimen on the correct areas of the slide (refer to Figure 22–74). Use different parts of the stool specimen to obtain sample smears for each of the two areas.

NOTE: Read the instructions. One or two small areas of exposed guaiac paper are present under the cover. Stool is placed on these areas.

10. Discard the tongue blade in an infectious-waste bag.

11. Remove gloves and wash hands.

12. Close the cover or flap of the Hemoccult packet.

13. 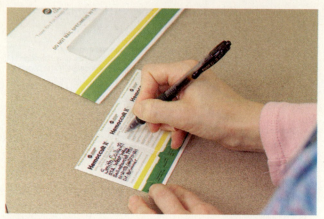 Label the outside of the Hemoccult packet with all the required information, usually the date and time, patient's name, room or ID number, and physician's name (**Figure 22–79A**), or attach a computer-generated label. Print the required information on the correct lab requisition. Obtain the requisition from your immediate supervisor or use a computer-generated requisition. A lab requisition must be sent with the labeled specimen.

14. 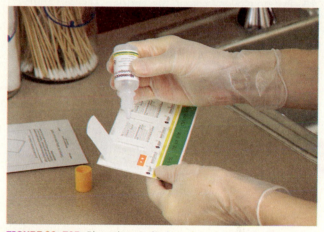 Send the Hemoccult packet to the laboratory for developing. Put the specimen in a protective biohazard bag for transport. In some agencies, you may be required to complete the test. To develop the test, proceed as follows:

a. Wash hands and put on gloves.

b. Open the back tab of the Hemoccult packet to expose the back of the guaiac paper.

FIGURE 22–79A Label the Hemoccult packet with all required information.

FIGURE 22–79B Place the required number of drops of Hemoccult developing solution on the exposed guaiac paper.

c. Place the required number of drops (usually one to two) of Hemoccult developer on the exposed guaiac paper (**Figure 22–79B**). Some packets also have test areas to which developer is applied.

NOTE: Read and follow manufacturer's instructions.

d. Wait the correct amount of time, usually 30–60 seconds.

e. Check the areas for color change. A positive test usually causes a blue or purple discoloration of the smear (**Figure 22–79C**).

NOTE: A positive test indicates the presence of blood in the stool.

f. Remove gloves and wash hands.

(continues)

READING AND INTERPRETING THE HEMOCCULT® TEST

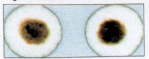

Negative Smears

Sample report: negative
No detectable blue on or at the edge of the smears indicates the test is negative for occult blood.

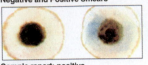

Negative and Positive Smears

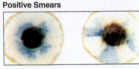

Positive Smears

Sample report: positive
Any trace of blue on or at the edge of one or more of the smears indicates the test is positive for occult blood.

FIGURE 22–79C A change in color indicates that blood is present in the stool.

15. Put on gloves to clean the bedpan. Discard any remaining stool in the toilet. Rinse the bedpan with cool water. Clean with a disinfectant, then rinse and dry. Replace all equipment used. Leave the area neat and clean.

16. Remove gloves and wash hands.

17. Report and/or record all required information on the patient's chart or enter it into the computer. For example, date, time, Hemoccult stool specimen obtained and sent to laboratory, and your signature and title.

Comm

 NOTE: In health care agencies using electronic health records (EHRs), the information is entered directly into the patient's record on a computer.

EHR

PRACTICE: Go to the workbook and use the evaluation sheet for 22:10E, Preparing and Testing a Hemoccult Slide, to practice this procedure. When you believe you have mastered this skill, sign the sheet and give it to your instructor for further action.

✅ **FINAL EVALUATION:** Using the criteria listed on the evaluation sheet, your instructor will grade your performance.

Check

22:11 APPLYING RESTRAINTS

 Although sick people are usually quiet and need encouragement to move, there are times when it is necessary to limit the movement of overactive patients. **Restraints** are used to limit movement.

OBRA

There are two kinds of restraints: chemical and physical. *Chemical restraints* are medications that affect the patient's behavior. Examples include tranquilizers, sedatives, and mood-altering medications. Licensed personnel are responsible for administering any chemical restraints.

 Physical restraints are protective devices that limit a patient's movements. They should be used only to protect patients from harming themselves or others and when all other measures to correct the situation have failed. Omnibus Budget Reconciliation Act (OBRA) legislation clearly defines the limitations of using restraints. All patient or resident behavior that may necessitate the use of restraints must be documented. Alternatives must be tried and carefully documented. If alternate solutions are not successful, a physician must write the order for the restraint, and the order must state the type of restraint, the reason for its use, the length of time it can be used, and where or when it can be used.

Legal

The least restrictive device must always be used first. A restraint applied unnecessarily can be considered false imprisonment. A health care provider should *never* apply a restraint without proper authorization.

Circumstances and conditions that may necessitate the use of restraints include:

- **Severe behavioral or cognitive issues**: Patients with a psychiatric diagnosis or in adverse mental health may demonstrate violent tendencies toward staff, self, or others. Restraints may have to be applied for their own safety and/or the safety of others.

- **Irrational or confused patients**: Patients can become irrational or confused because of anesthesia, medications, senility, sleep deprivation, and other factors. They may attempt to climb out of bed or over siderails, or they may wander about. Because they could fall and injure themselves, restraints must sometimes be applied to limit their movements.

- **Danger to self**: A patient may require restraints if they are unable to comprehend the need for treatment and are interfering with medical care or devices or attempting to pull out vital lines or tubes.

- **Skin conditions**: Patients, especially small children, with itchy skin conditions must sometimes have their hands restrained or encased in protective mittens to prevent scratching.

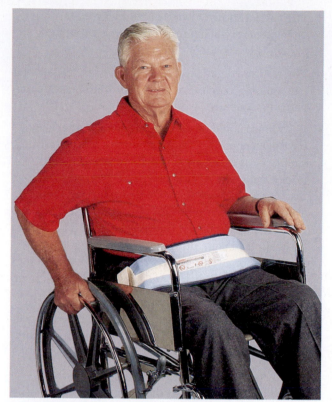

FIGURE 22–80A A belt restraint can be used to support a patient sitting in a wheelchair. Courtesy of J. T. Posey Company

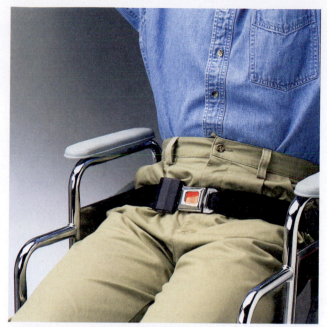

FIGURE 22–80B An alternative self-release belt sounds an alarm when the patient begins to open it. Courtesy of J. T. Posey Company

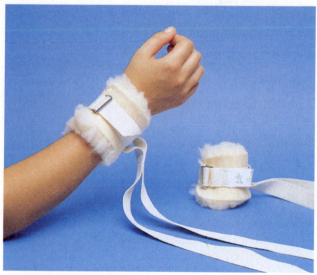

FIGURE 22–81 Place the soft edge of the limb restraint against the patient's skin. Courtesy of J. T. Posey Company

- **Paralysis or limited muscular coordination:** Patients under anesthesia or who are paralyzed by strokes are often unable to coordinate or control their muscular movements. They may require restraints.

There are different kinds of physical restraints. It is important to follow the manufacturer's recommendations when applying any kind of restraint. Some common kinds include:

- **Straps or safety belts:** Usually found on wheelchairs, some are designed to be used interchangeably on wheelchairs, beds, and stretchers (**Figure 22–80A**). A strap or safety belt is used to prevent a patient from falling out of the device. The strap or belt should not be applied too tightly because it can restrict breathing and interfere with circulation. Self-release belt restraints are also available for use. They are considered to be less restrictive because the patient can release the belt. However, when the patient does start to release the belt, an alarm sounds that alerts the staff (**Figure 22–80B**).

- **Limb restraints:** Usually, these are soft, padded restraints that are wrapped around the arm or leg to limit movement of the limb (**Figure 22–81**). The restraint straps are then attached to the movable part of the bed frame or stretcher to secure the limb into position. At least two to three fingers should be slipped between the restraint and the patient's skin to make sure the restraint is not too tight.

- **Restraint jackets:** These devices are used to prevent a patient from sitting up, rolling, getting out of bed, or falling out of a wheelchair. Jacket restraints are available in different sizes. It is important to follow manufacturer's directions and measure the patient carefully to make sure the correct size jacket restraint is used. Jacket restraints must also be applied so that they do not interfere with breathing or circulation.

- **Geriatric chair:** These are used for patients who may sit up in a chair but are at risk for falling because they are unsteady and confused. Most chairs contain a tabletop tray that locks into place to prevent patients from getting up unassisted (**Figure 22–82**).

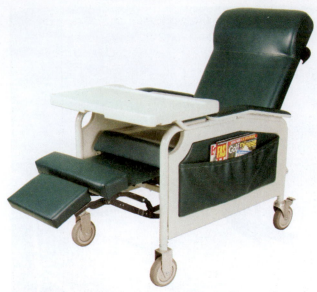

FIGURE 22–82 A geriatric chair can be used to position a patient comfortably in an upright or reclining position. When the tabletop is locked into position across the patient's lap, the patient is not able to get out of the chair. Courtesy, Winco

- **Hand mitts:** These devices are similar to mittens that are applied to the hands to prevent the patient from scratching or injuring the skin (**Figure 22–83**). They can also be used to prevent patients from pulling on lines and tubes.

There are some important points to remember when using restraints:

- Use only when all other means of obtaining the patient's cooperation have failed.

- Restraints should be as unnoticeable to the patient as possible.

- Patients should be allowed to move as much as possible without danger of self-injury.

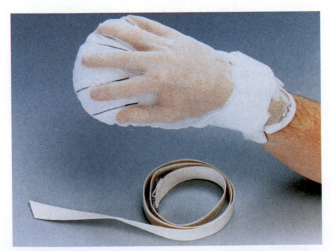

FIGURE 22–83 Hand mitts can be applied to prevent the patient from scratching or injuring the skin. Courtesy of J. T. Posey Company

- The patient should always be told why their movements are being restricted, even when the patient is irrational or confused.

- The restrained patient feels both physical and mental frustration. Therefore, it is important to reassure the patient frequently.

- Restraints should be checked frequently after they have been applied. Circulation below a limb restraint should be checked every 15–30 minutes. Signs of poor circulation include paleness; cyanosis (blue discoloration); cold skin; edema (swelling); weak or absent pulse; poor return of pink color after the nail beds are pressed lightly (or blanched); and patient complaints of pain, numbness, or tingling. If any signs of poor circulation are noted, the restraint must be removed immediately and the supervisor notified.

- All restraints *must* be removed every 2 hours for at least 10 minutes. The patient should be repositioned, and range-of-motion (ROM) exercises and skin care to the skin under the restraint should be provided.

- Remove restraints as soon as there is adequate supervision or as soon as the danger of the patient injuring themselves has passed.

Some complications that can occur when restraints are applied include:

- **Physical and mental frustration** on the part of the patient is common. The loss of freedom imposed by restraints can cause disorientation, depression, hostility, agitation, and withdrawal. Provide reassurance and supportive care to the patient.

- **Impaired circulation** can result. Check skin color and skin temperature frequently.

- **Pressure ulcers** from the pressure applied by restraint can develop.

- **Loss of muscle tone, joint stiffness, and discomfort** from immobility are common. The inability to go to the bathroom at will can lead to incontinence and constipation. Provide frequent ROM exercises and offer to take the patient to the bathroom at regular intervals.

- **Respiratory or breathing problems**, especially when jacket restraints are applied, may develop.

Legal All health care facilities have specific rules and policies regarding the use of restraints. All patients have the right to maintain their dignity and independence as much as possible. It is important for the staff to evaluate whether the risk for potential injury to the patient and/or others is greater than the risk for complications from the use of restraints. It is essential that the health care provider knows and follows all rules and policies, and is aware of legal responsibilities regarding the use of restraints.

checkpoint

1. A geriatric chair is used for what type of patient?
2. List two (2) kinds of restraints.

PRACTICE: Go to the workbook and complete the assignment sheet for 22:11, Applying Restraints. Then return and continue with the procedures.

Procedure 22:11A OBRA

Applying Limb Restraints

Equipment and Supplies

Adjustable limb restraint(s), paper and pen or computer

Procedure

1. Check physician's orders or obtain authorization from your immediate supervisor.

    CAUTION: A restraint cannot be applied without a physician's order.

   NOTE: The order must state the type of restraint and reason for its use. The least restrictive device must be used first.

2. Assemble equipment.

3. Knock on the door and pause before entering. Introduce yourself. Identify the patient. Explain the procedure even if the patient is irrational or confused, and obtain consent if possible.

4. Wash hands.

5. Close the door and pull the curtain to provide privacy. If the patient is in a bed, elevate the bed to a comfortable working height. If siderails are present and elevated, lower the siderail on the side where you are working. If the patient is in a wheelchair, lock the wheels of the chair. Position the patient in a comfortable position and in good body alignment.

6. Place the soft edge of the restraint against the patient's skin. Wrap the restraint smoothly around the limb (**Figure 22–84A**). Make sure there are no wrinkles.

7. Pull the ends of the straps through the tabs or rings on the restraint. Then pull the restraint securely, but not too tightly, against the patient's skin.

   ⚠ **CAUTION:** If applied too tightly, the restraint could stop circulation or cause a pressure sore.

8. Test for fit and comfort by inserting two to three fingers between the restraint and the patient's skin (**Figure 22–84B**).

9. Position the arm or leg in a comfortable position. Limit movement only as much as is necessary.

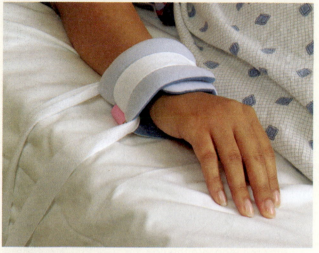

FIGURE 22–84A Wrap the restraint smoothly around the limb, making sure there are no wrinkles.

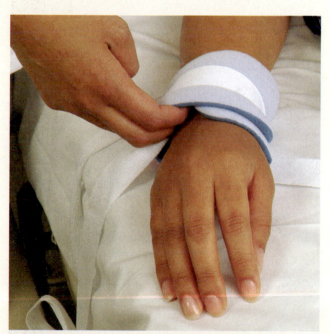

FIGURE 22–84B Insert two to three fingers between the restraint and the patient's skin to make sure the restraint is not too tight.

10. Use a quick-release tie to secure the straps to the movable part of the bed frame so the restraints move when the bed moves (**Figure 22–84C**). If the patient is in a wheelchair, tie the straps to the nonmovable arms or frame. To make the

(continues)

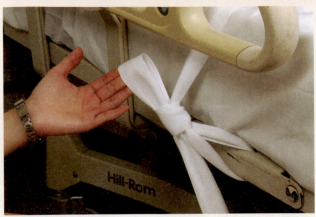

FIGURE 22–84C Restraint straps must always be tied to the movable part of the bed frame so the restraints move when the bed moves.

quick-release tie, bring the end of the strap around the frame. Then bring the loose end up behind and around the back of the strap to create a hole. Fold the loose end of the strap into a loop and tuck the loop into the hole formed. Pull up on the descending part of the strap to tighten the loop in the hole. To release the tie, simply pull on the loose, exposed end of the strap.

NOTE: Many restraints have snap closures that make them easy to attach to the bed or wheelchair.

11. Recheck the patient before leaving.

 CAUTION: Make sure the restraint is secure but not too tight.

12. Observe all checkpoints before leaving the patient: position the patient in correct body alignment, place the call signal and supplies within easy reach of the patient, elevate the siderails (if indicated), lower the bed to its lowest level, and leave the area neat and clean.

13. Check the circulation below the limb restraint every 15–30 minutes. Note color and temperature of skin; return of color after pressing lightly on nail beds; edema (or swelling); and patient complaints of pain, numbness, or tingling.

 CAUTION: If any signs of impaired circulation are noted, remove the restraint immediately and notify your supervisor.

14. Remove the restraint every 2 hours for at least 10 minutes. Reposition the patient. Provide ROM exercises to the restrained limb. Administer skin care to the skin under the restraint.

15. Remove the restraint when authorized to do so by your supervisor or the physician.

NOTE: Restraints are removed when the physician or supervisor feels that the danger of self-injury to the patient has passed. Restraints must always be removed as soon as possible.

16. Replace all equipment.

17. Wash hands.

18. Report and/or record all required information on the patient's chart or enter it into the computer. For example, date, time, limb restraints applied to both arms while patient positioned in wheelchair, P 82 strong and regular at both wrists, patient appears to be resting quietly, and your signature and title. Report any unusual observations immediately.

 NOTE: In health care agencies using electronic health records (EHRs), the information is entered directly into the patient's record on a computer.

PRACTICE: Go to the workbook and use the evaluation sheet for 22:11A, Applying Limb Restraints, to practice this procedure. When you believe you have mastered this skill, sign the sheet and give it to your instructor for further action.

✅ **FINAL EVALUATION:** Using the criteria listed on the evaluation sheet, your instructor will grade your performance.

Procedure 22:11B ⚖️

Applying a Jacket Restraint

Equipment and Supplies

Sleeveless jacket restraint, paper and pen or computer

Procedure

1. Check physician's orders or obtain authorization from your supervisor.

 CAUTION: A restraint *cannot* be applied without a physician's order.

NOTE: The order must state the type of restraint and reason for its use. The least restrictive device must be used first.

2. Assemble equipment. Obtain the correct size restraint for the patient.

CAUTION: Follow the manufacturer's instructions and carefully measure the patient to make sure the correct size jacket/vest restraint is used. If an incorrect size is used, the restraint will not provide proper support and could injure the patient.

3. Knock on the door and pause before entering. Introduce yourself. Identify the patient. Explain the procedure even if the patient is irrational or confused, and obtain consent if possible.

4. Wash hands.

5. Close the door and pull the curtain to provide privacy. If the patient is in a bed, elevate the bed to a comfortable working height. If siderails are present and elevated, lower the siderail on the side where you are working. If the patient is in a wheelchair, lock the wheels of the chair. Place the patient in a comfortable position and in good body alignment.

6. Slip the sleeves of the jacket restraint onto the patient's arms. The solid part of the jacket restraint goes on the back, and the open or V-neck part of the restraint goes on the front (**Figure 22–85A**). It is essential to follow the manufacturer's instructions.

CAUTION: A restraint applied incorrectly may cause suffocation or injury.

7. Crisscross the straps in the back. Check all of the material to make sure it is free from wrinkles.

8. Bring the loose ends of the straps through the hole in the jacket. The jacket should now completely encircle the patient.

9. Check the restraint to be sure it is not too tight against the patient.

CAUTION: Excessive tightness could interfere with breathing.

10. Place the patient in a comfortable position. Allow as much movement as possible without risk of injury.

11. On each side of a bed or stretcher, use a quick-release tie to bring the straps down and secure them to the movable part of the frame.

12. Straps should be brought down between the wheelchair and side plate. In a wheelchair, the straps can be attached to the kick bars at the rear of the wheelchair. Note that the kick bars' plastic end-caps must be in place to ensure that the ties will not slip off (**Figure 22–85B**).

CAUTION: Never attach the straps to any parts of the wheels.

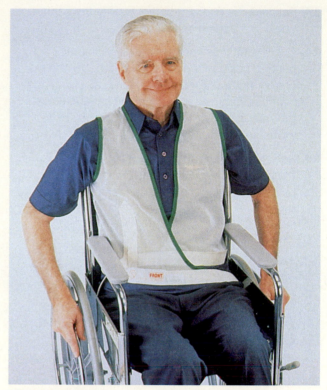

FIGURE 22–85A Follow the manufacturer's instructions to measure a patient to make sure the jacket or vest is the correct size. Position the jacket restraint with the open or V-neck part of the restraint on the front. Courtesy of J. T. Posey Company

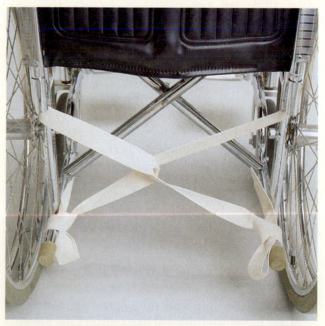

FIGURE 22–85B Use a quick-release tie to secure the straps to the back frame of a wheelchair. Courtesy of J. T. Posey Company

(continues)

13. Recheck the restraint before leaving the patient. Check the patient's respirations.

14. Observe all checkpoints before leaving the patient: position the patient comfortably and in correct body alignment, place the call signal and supplies within easy reach of the patient, elevate the siderails (if indicated), lower the bed to its lowest level, and leave the area neat and clean.

15. Return every 15–30 minutes to check the patient. Check count and character of respirations, and the color and temperature of the skin.

 CAUTION: If any signs of impaired circulation or respiration are noted, remove the restraint immediately and notify your supervisor.

16. Remove the restraint every 2 hours for at least 10 minutes. Reposition the patient. Provide ROM exercises. Administer skin care to the skin under the restraint.

17. Remove the restraint when authorized to do so by your supervisor or the physician.

NOTE: A restraint is removed when the danger of self-injury has passed. Restraints must always be removed as soon as possible.

18. Replace all equipment.

19. Wash hands.

20. Report and/or record all required information on the patient's chart or enter it into the computer. For example, date, time, jacket restraint applied, patient seated in wheelchair, and your signature and title.

 NOTE: In health care agencies using electronic health records (EHRs), the information is entered directly into the patient's record on a computer.

PRACTICE: Go to the workbook and use the evaluation sheet for 22:11B, Applying a Jacket Restraint, to practice this procedure. When you believe you have mastered this skill, sign the sheet and give it to your instructor for further action.

✅ **FINAL EVALUATION:** Using the criteria listed on the evaluation sheet, your instructor will grade your performance.

22:12 ADMINISTERING PREOPERATIVE AND POSTOPERATIVE CARE

Providing care to patients scheduled for surgery may be one of your responsibilities as a health care team member. Surgical care is divided into three phases:

- **Preoperative care** (pre-op): care provided before the surgery
- **Operative care** (peri-op): care provided during the surgery
- **Postoperative care** (post-op): care provided following surgery

NOTE: Unless you work in an operating room, your major responsibilities will likely involve the pre-op and post-op phases.

 Every patient scheduled for surgery, no matter how minor, has some fears. Fears regarding disfigurement, pain, loss of control, the unknown, length of recovery time, costs and financial problems, a poor diagnosis after surgery, and even death create concerns for many patients. It is important to provide emotional support in addition to physical care. Answer all questions you can to the best of your ability. However, specific questions about the surgery, outcome, or anesthesia should be referred to the physician or your supervisor. Be sure to report these questions and the patient's fears to your immediate supervisor.

PREOPERATIVE CARE

Preoperative care involves many aspects of care. The preparation is ordered by the physician, depending on the type of operation. Possible aspects of preparation are:

- **Operative permit:** This is a form signed by the patient to give permission for the anesthesia and surgery. If the patient is unable to sign due to a severe illness or confusion, the next of kin or an individual with a power of attorney (POA) can sign for them. Signatures must be witnessed by a legally authorized individual.

- **Laboratory tests:** These tests may include blood tests, urine tests, chest or other radiographs, electrocardiogram (ECG), and special tests ordered by the physician.

- **Enemas or vaginal irrigations**: These are ordered by the physician in preparation for certain types of surgery.
- **Baths**: Baths may be given both the night before surgery and the morning of surgery. The purpose is to remove as many microorganisms as possible in an effort to prevent infections. Some surgeries require a Hibiclens bath the night before and the morning of the surgery. Hibiclens is a cleanser that removes bacteria from the skin to prevent it from entering the surgical incision. Baths also give the patient a chance to talk and relieve some anxiety.
- **Vital signs**: These are taken and recorded. They are used as a standard to check vital signs during and after the surgery.
- **NPO**: The patient is allowed nothing by mouth for 8–12 hours before the surgery. The order usually starts at 12:00 am (midnight). A sign is usually placed on the patient's bed. Water is removed from the area at the appointed time.
- **Valuables**: All the patient's valuables, including money and jewelry, should be placed in a hospital safe or with security to prevent loss. A patient is sometimes allowed to wear a wedding ring. However, it must be taped or tied to the finger to prevent loss.
- **Remove prosthetics**: All artificial parts are removed. This includes dentures, contact lenses or glasses, artificial arms or legs, and hearing aids.
- **Remove cosmetics**: Nail polish, makeup, hair pins, and wigs are all removed before surgery. The presence of cosmetics can mask skin or nail bed color changes.
- **Clothing**: Usually, the patient must remove all clothing, including undergarments. A hospital gown is placed on the patient. Most agencies also place a surgical cap on the patient to cover the hair.
- **Name band**: Before surgery, the patient's name band or identification band should be checked for accurate information. Because the patient frequently is unconscious during surgery, the name band is the only method of identifying the patient.

  Comm
- **Voiding**: To make sure the bladder is empty during surgery, the patient should void immediately before being brought to the operating room. For some surgeries, a catheter is inserted in the bladder to constantly drain all urine. Only a legally qualified person should insert the catheter.
- **Surgical checklist**: Most agencies use surgical checklists to track most of the previously noted preparation items. As these items are completed, they are checked off the checklist. This provides a method for determining that the patient has been properly prepared for surgery. The checklist is usually attached to the patient's chart or entered into the computerized record.

Frequently, patients are not admitted to the hospital or surgical clinic until the morning of the surgery. In this case, many of the tests such as blood work, radiographs, and ECG are performed on an outpatient basis before the day of surgery.

ANESTHESIA

Anesthesia is prevention of pain by way of loss of sensation. Medication is administered by an anesthesiologist, nurse anesthetist, or physician. The type of anesthetic used and the method of administration depends on the type of surgery, the length of time needed, and the physical condition of the patient. Three main kinds are:

- **General anesthesia**: Medication is given intravenously or is inhaled through a mask. This causes unconsciousness, which continues throughout the surgery. A common postoperative problem is nausea or vomiting.
- **Local anesthesia**: Medication is injected into the area around the operative site to stop the sensation of pain. The patient is awake when local anesthesia is used.
- **Spinal anesthesia**: Medication is injected into the spinal canal and causes loss of sensation (feeling) in all areas below the injection. This is often used for abdominal surgery because it produces good muscle relaxation. Patients must be told that they will not have any feeling or movement in the legs for a period of time. Patients sometimes complain of headaches after this type of anesthesia. This symptom should be reported.

POSTOPERATIVE CARE

While the patient is in surgery, the postoperative room or bed unit is prepared in such a way that all necessary equipment will be available when the patient returns from surgery. A recovery bed is made, an intravenous (IV) pole or stand and equipment for taking vital signs is put in place, and an emesis basin and tissues are placed at the bedside. Necessary special equipment, such as a suction machine for drainage tubes or equipment for administering oxygen, is also placed in the unit. All unnecessary supplies or equipment are removed from the area. For example, the water pitcher and cup are removed until postoperative orders state that the patient can have fluids.

Postoperative care is an important aspect of surgical care. Some of the factors to be considered in immediate postoperative care are:

- **Vital signs**: These must be checked frequently and as ordered. They are sometimes taken every 15 minutes until the patient is stable. A sudden drop in blood pressure or change in pulse rate or character are often the first signs of hemorrhage or shock, so any changes or abnormal readings must be reported immediately.

- **Dressings**: These must be checked frequently (**Figure 22–86**). The color, amount, and type of drainage must be noted. Any unusual observations should be reported immediately.

- **IV**: The flow rate and injection site must be checked only by an authorized individual.

- **Level of pain**: An assessment must be made of the amount of pain a patient is experiencing. Frequently, patients are asked to describe pain on a scale of 1 to 10, with 1 being mild pain and 10 being extreme pain. *Patient-controlled analgesics (PCAs)* are often used to control pain. An analgesic pump is attached to an IV line. The patient is taught to push a button when pain is felt. The pump delivers a specific dose of pain medication directly into the bloodstream to provide immediate relief. The patient cannot overdose on the medication because the pump locks out delivery of medication for a set period. A change in position, if allowed, can also help alleviate pain. If patients do not seem to be able to get pain relief, this should be reported immediately.

- **Observations**: Restlessness, color and temperature of skin, nausea or vomiting, and similar observations should be noted and reported.

- **Position**: The patient's position must be changed when possible. Be sure you are aware of all movement restrictions. Some operations limit movement and positioning. Turn or move patients only after obtaining correct authorization.

- **Cough and deep breathe**: Most patients need to be encouraged to cough and deep breathe after general anesthesia (**Figure 22–87**). This exercise helps remove mucus from the lungs and respiratory tract and helps prevent pneumonia and other lung disorders.

- **Tubes**: Surgical patients frequently have drainage tubes in place. The tubes are connected to drainage bottles or special drainage collectors. If the tubes are not draining, if they are clamped, if the drainage solution changes or seems unusual, if a tube is not connected to a drainage source, or if any unusual observations are noted, they should be reported immediately. Care must also be taken when turning or moving the patient to make sure that the tubes are not disconnected, twisted, or pulled out.

Binders are special devices that are usually made of heavy cotton or flannelette with elastic sides or supports. They are applied to various parts of the body, but mainly to the abdomen, back, and breasts. Functions of binders include the following:

- Provide support and relief from pain following surgery
- Hold dressings in place
- Provide support for engorged breasts
- Limit motion
- Apply pressure to specific body parts

Binders must be applied smoothly to prevent pressure areas, which can lead to the formation of pressure ulcers. Binders should fit snugly for support but not be so tight as to cause discomfort. No wrinkles or creases

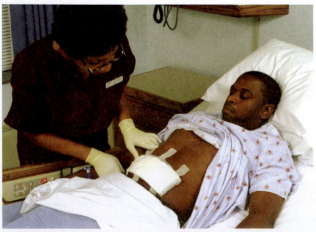

FIGURE 22–86 Dressings must be checked frequently after surgery.

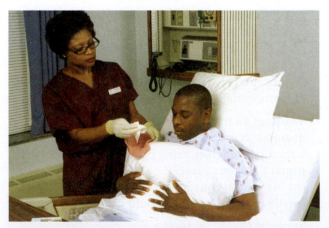

FIGURE 22–87 A pillow across the abdomen provides support when the patient is coughing and deep breathing.

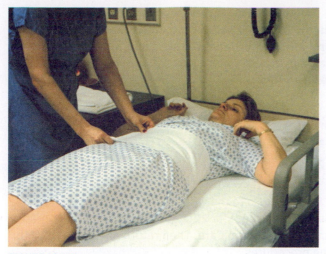

FIGURE 22-88 A straight binder provides support to the abdomen.

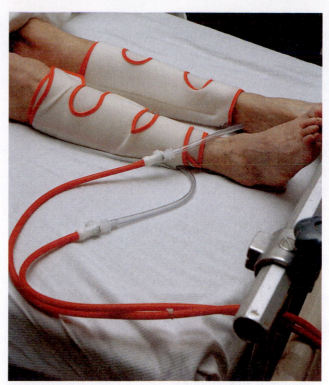

FIGURE 22-89 Compression stockings continually inflate and deflate to stimulate circulation in the legs.

should be present. The type used most frequently is a straight binder (**Figure 22-88**). It can be applied to the abdomen, back, or rib cage. Straight binders are secured using Velcro tabs. Binders are applied from bottom to top for optimal support. In this way, organs can be supported correctly. Circulation and breathing should always be checked after binders are applied. A binder that is too tight can cause severe complications. In addition, binders should be removed at intervals, and skin care should be provided to the skin under the binder.

Surgical (elastic) hose, also called support or compression hose, may be ordered to support the veins of the legs and increase circulation. These hose help prevent formation of blood clots in the legs. The hose must be applied correctly. If they are applied too tightly, they can interfere with circulation.

Compression stockings, also called **sequential compression devices (SCDs)**, are attached to a pump that continually inflates and deflates the hose. They are frequently used to stimulate circulation in the legs by mimicking the action of the leg muscles on blood vessels (**Figure 22-89**). They increase the venous blood flow and prevent the formation of blood clots, or venous thromboembolism (VTE).

Montgomery straps are special adhesive strips that are applied when dressings must be changed frequently at the surgical site (**Figure 22-90**). The skin around the surgical site is cleaned thoroughly. A skin barrier, such as a liquid or paste, is applied to the skin to protect it from being irritated by the tape. The Montgomery straps are then applied on either side of the surgical site. The centers of the straps are nonadhesive and tied together. To change dressings, the straps are untied, the dressings are changed, and the straps are then tied in place on top of the dressings. This eliminates the need to remove and reapply adhesive tape during each dressing change.

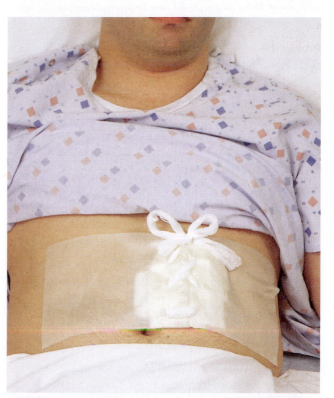

FIGURE 22-90 Montgomery straps are special adhesive strips that are applied when dressings must be changed frequently at the surgical site.

Wound VACs provide negative-pressure wound therapy that can be used for recently closed surgical incisions or ones that were left open due to excessive edema or drainage. They can also be used for incisions that were reopened for exploration or drainage (refer to Figure 22–7). This technique removes exudate and infectious material, and it reduces edema. It draws the wound edges together, promotes healing, and fights infection. It cannot be used if there are exposed vital organs or major vessels.

SUMMARY

Precaution

It is essential that the nurse assistant follow all standard precautions discussed in Section 15:4 whenever contact with blood or body fluids is possible. This helps prevent the spread of infection, including infection in the surgical patient after surgery.

It is essential for the nurse assistant to know and understand all aspects of care that have been ordered to properly care for the surgical patient. Good operative care can mean a faster recovery with fewer complications for the patient.

checkpoint

1. List the three (3) phases of surgical care.

2. How frequently are vital signs taken after surgery?

PRACTICE: Go to the workbook and complete the assignment sheet for 22:12, Administering Preoperative and Postoperative Care. Then return and continue with the procedures.

Procedure 22:12A

Administering Preoperative Care

Equipment and Supplies

Thermometer, stethoscope, sphygmomanometer, surgical gown and cap, nail polish remover, valuables envelope, tape or gauze (if needed), disposable gloves, paper and pen or computer

Procedure

1. Check physician's orders or obtain authorization from your immediate supervisor. Check the time of surgery.

   NOTE: Care should be completed 1 hour before surgery.

2. Assemble equipment.

3. Knock on the door and pause before entering. Introduce yourself. Identify the patient. Explain the procedure and obtain consent. Make sure the operative permit has been signed (**Figure 22–91A**).

   NOTE: The patient may be frightened; reassure as needed.

4. Close the door and pull the curtain for privacy.

5. Wash hands. Puts on gloves.

   Precaution
   CAUTION: Wear gloves and observe standard precautions. Contact with body fluids, secretions, or excretions is possible.

6. Elevate the bed to a comfortable working height. If siderails are present and elevated, lower the siderail on the side where you are working.

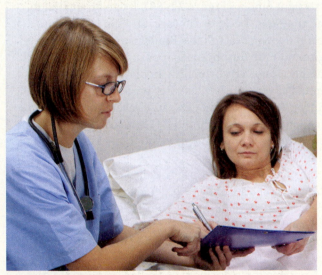

FIGURE 22–91A Explain the procedure and make sure that the operative permit is signed. Remember that only authorized individuals can witness the signature. ©iStock.com/Daniel Yordanov

7. Check the patient's identification band. Make sure it is secure. Verify name, room number, and other facts.

8. Assist with or instruct the patient to complete oral hygiene and bath.

   NOTE: Normally, the bed is not made before surgery unless a Hibiclens bath is given. Then the bed is changed when the bath is complete.

   Safety
   CAUTION: Because the patient is NPO (nothing by mouth), do not allow the patient to swallow any water when performing oral hygiene.

9. Put a surgical gown on the patient. No other clothing is permitted. Make sure the patient's underwear is removed.

10. Remove all hairpins, wigs, and other hair ornaments. Put a cap on the patient. Make sure all hair is inside the cap.

11. Remove nail polish. Check to be sure the patient is not wearing any makeup.

12. Remove all of the patient's jewelry and place it in a valuables envelope. Also place money and other valuables in the envelope. Follow hospital procedure for securing valuables.

    NOTE: Wedding rings may be tied or taped in place. Follow hospital procedure.

     CAUTION: In some agencies, only certain health care providers are permitted to handle valuables. Follow agency policy.

13. Remove full or partial dentures. Place these in a denture cup labeled with the patient's name and room number. Place the cup in a drawer or safe area to prevent breakage.

14. Have the patient remove contact lenses, glasses, hearing aids, and all other prostheses (artificial parts). Place in a safe area.

15. Offer a bedpan or assist the patient to the bathroom. Encourage the patient to void. If a catheter and urinary-drainage unit is in place, empty the urinary-drainage unit and record the measurement.

16. Take vital signs and record correctly (**Figure 22–91B**).

     CAUTION: The vital signs must be accurate and correct. If in doubt about the results, ask your supervisor to check them.

17. Elevate the siderails immediately after preoperative medication has been given by an authorized person.

    NOTE: Preoperative medication is usually given 1 hour before surgery. It helps the patient relax, and it often contains medication to dry up nose and mouth secretions. Because the patient could become drowsy and fall out of bed, the siderails must be elevated immediately.

18. Place the patient in a comfortable position. Encourage the patient to rest.

19. Observe all checkpoints before leaving the patient: make sure the water pitcher has been

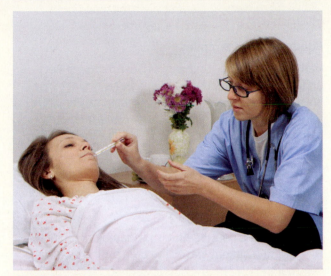

FIGURE 22–91B Vital signs must be taken and recorded as part of preoperative care. ©iStock.com/Daniel Yordanov

removed from the unit, lower the bed to its lowest level, place the call signal within easy reach of the patient, and leave the area neat and clean.

NOTE: Many hospitals use pre-op checklists, which are placed on patients' charts. If this is hospital policy, complete the checklist.

20. Clean and replace all equipment.

21. Remove gloves and wash hands.

22. Report and/or record all required information on the patient's chart or enter it into the computer. For example, date, time, pre-op care complete and noted on checklist, siderails elevated, patient resting quietly, and your signature and title. Report any unusual observations immediately.

     NOTE: In health care agencies using electronic health records (EHRs), the information is entered directly into the patient's record on a computer.

PRACTICE: Go to the workbook and use the evaluation sheet for 22:12A, Administering Preoperative Care, to practice this procedure. When you believe you have mastered this skill, sign the sheet and give it to your instructor for further action.

 FINAL EVALUATION: Using the criteria listed on the evaluation sheet, your instructor will grade your performance.

Preparing a Postoperative Unit

Equipment and Supplies

Bed linen for an unoccupied bed; extra draw sheet; underpads or protective covers; emesis basin; tissues; plastic bag and tape; gauze bandage; intravenous (IV) pole or stand; vital signs equipment (thermometer, blood pressure apparatus, watch with second hand); linen bag, hamper, or cart; gloves; paper and pen or computer

Procedure

1. Assemble equipment.

   NOTE: The post-op unit is prepared immediately after the patient leaves the area for the operating room.

2. Wash hands. Put on gloves.

   CAUTION: Wear gloves. The linen may be contaminated with blood, body fluids, secretions, or excretions. Remove the gloves and wash hands thoroughly after removing the dirty linen and before applying the clean linen.

   Precaution

3. Remove any used linen from the bed and place in the linen bag, hamper, or cart.

4. Remove gloves and wash hands.

5. Make the foundation (bottom sheet and draw sheet) of the bed as previously instructed for an unoccupied bed.

6. Place a cotton draw sheet over the head of the bed. Tuck in at the head of the bed as was done for bottom sheet. Make mitered corners and tuck in at the sides.

   NOTE: This protects the bed should the patient vomit.

   NOTE: Some agencies use underpads instead of draw sheets.

7. Place a top sheet and a spread on the bed. Let them fall loose.

8. Go to the foot of the bed and fold the top linen back. Make a cuff so that the top linen is even with the end of the mattress.

   NOTE: The top linen is not tucked in.

9. Go to the head of the bed. Make a cuff with the top linen.

10. Fanfold the top linen to the side of the bed opposite from where the patient will be brought in on the stretcher.

    NOTE: In some agencies, the sheets are folded to the foot of the bed. Follow agency policy.

11. Cover the pillow with a pillowcase. Place the pillow in an upright position at the head of the bed.

    NOTE: This protects the patient's head against injury during the transfer to the bed.

12. Estimate the height of the stretcher and elevate the bed to this height.

13. Put a cuff on the plastic bag. Tape it to the side of the bed or bedside table.

14. Place underpads on the bed near where the operated body part will be resting.

15. Remove all unnecessary articles from the bedside stand. Place the emesis basin, tissues, and equipment for taking vital signs on the stand.

    NOTE: Make sure the water pitcher and cup are not on the bedside stand. Patients may be NPO (nothing by mouth) postoperatively.

16. Position the overbed table, chair, and other furniture so it will not be in the way of the stretcher.

17. Place the IV stand or pump in the most convenient location. It should be ready for the IV when the patient is transferred to the bed.

18. Check the area before leaving. Make sure that all equipment and supplies are ready for the patient's return from surgery (**Figure 22–92**).

19. Replace all equipment used.

20. Wash hands.

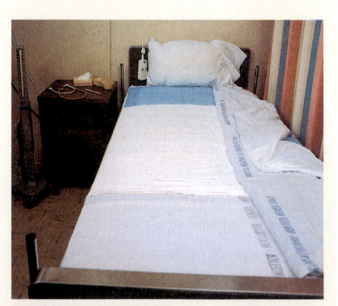

FIGURE 22–92 Before leaving the post-op unit, check to make sure that all equipment and supplies are ready for the patient's return from surgery.

21. Report and/or record all required information on the patient's chart or enter it into the computer. For example, date, time, post-op unit prepared, and your signature and title.

NOTE: In health care agencies using electronic health records (EHRs), the information is entered directly into the patient's record on a computer.

PRACTICE: Go to the workbook and use the evaluation sheet for 22:12B, Preparing a Postoperative Unit, to practice this procedure. When you believe you have mastered this skill, sign the sheet and give it to your instructor for further action.

 FINAL EVALUATION: Using the criteria listed on the evaluation sheet, your instructor will grade your performance.

Procedure 22:12C

Applying Surgical Hose and Compression Stockings

NOTE: Surgical hose and compression stockings come in various sizes and lengths. This procedure deals with the application of knee-length surgical hose and compression stockings.

Equipment and Supplies

Correct size surgical hose and compression stockings, compression pump, measuring tape, paper and pen or computer

Procedure

1. Check physician's orders or obtain authorization from your immediate supervisor.

2. Assemble equipment.

3. Knock on the door and pause before entering. Introduce yourself. Identify the patient. Explain the procedure and obtain consent.

4. Wash hands.

5. Check the hose and stockings to be sure they are clean and the correct size.

   NOTE: Hose and stockings from different companies are sized differently. Use the measuring tape and follow the instructions that came with the hose to determine the correct size for the patient.

6. Close the door and pull the curtain for privacy. Elevate the bed to a comfortable working height. If siderails are present and elevated, lower the side rail on the side where you are working. Expose the patient's legs.

7. Start with the surgical hose. Insert your hand into the top of the hose. Turn the hose so that the smooth side is on the outside.

   NOTE: This makes application easier and leaves the rough edge on the outside of the foot.

8. Grasp the heel area of the hose. Smoothly tuck the foot portion back into the hose.

9. Stretch the hose open at the heel. Support the patient's leg and slide the foot and pocket of the heel into position on the patient's foot (**Figure 22–93A**).

    CAUTION: Use correct body mechanics when applying hose. Stand with your feet apart and one leg ahead of the other, bending at the hips rather than the waist.

10. Make sure the heel of the hose is secure over the patient's heel.

11. Grasp the top of the hose. Pull it over the foot. Gather the material at the ankle. Use two hands and gentle pressure.

12. Begin gently moving the hose up the leg to the area below the knee (**Figure 22–93B**). Work slowly to prevent wrinkles. Use both hands to smooth the hose into place.

     CAUTION: Do not pull and stretch the hose. This will make it too tight and interfere with circulation.

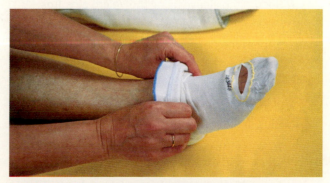

FIGURE 22–93A Slide the foot of the hose into position.

(continues)

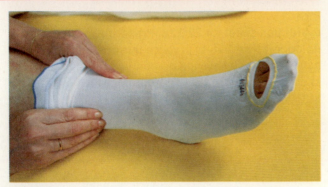

FIGURE 22–93B Draw the hose gently up the leg to the area below the knee.

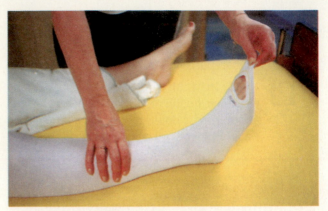

FIGURE 22–93C Pull the toe forward slightly to provide "toe room."

13. Check the position of the hose. The top should be just below the knee. Smooth any excess material with your hands.

14. Pull the toe forward slightly to provide "toe room" (**Figure 22–93C**).

15. Repeat steps 7–14 for the opposite leg.

16. Once the surgical hose are in place, put the compression stockings, also called sleeves or sequential compression devices (SCDs), on top of them.

    NOTE: Surgical hose and compression stockings/sleeves can be ordered together, or just one or the other may be ordered.

    a. Place the side of the compression sleeve with the printed instructions against the patient's leg.

    b. Position the compression sleeve so it is centered behind the calf.

    c. Wrap the sleeve securely around the calf, ensuring that two fingers can fit between the calf and the sleeve.

    d. Secure the sleeve using the Velcro closures beginning at the ankle, then calf, then thigh.

    e. Repeat the process for the other leg (refer to Figure 22–89).

    f. Attach the compression pump to the sleeves by snapping the connectors together.

    g. Plug in the pump and turn it on.

    h. Instruct the patient that they will feel the stockings inflating and deflating.

    i. Stay with the patient for several cycles to make sure they are tolerating the compression.

17. Observe all checkpoints before leaving the patient: position the patient in correct body alignment, elevate the siderails (if indicated), lower the bed to its lowest level, place the call signal and supplies within easy reach of the patient, and leave the area neat and clean.

18. Check the hose and/or compression sleeves at intervals. Look for signs of impaired circulation, including abnormal skin color or temperature, swelling, a weak pedal pulse, and other abnormalities. Report any abnormalities to your supervisor immediately. Remove the hose and/or compression sleeves at intervals, at least once every 8 hours. Administer skin care to the skin under the hose. If the surgical hose become soiled, they can be washed.

19. Wash hands.

20. Report and/or record all required information on the patient's chart or enter it **Comm** into the computer. For example, date, time, surgical hose and compression sleeves applied to both legs, and your signature and title. Report any unusual observations immediately.

    NOTE: In health care agencies using electronic health records (EHRs), the **EHR** information is entered directly into the patient's record on a computer.

PRACTICE: Go to the workbook and use the evaluation sheet for 22:12C, Applying Surgical Hose and Compression Stockings, to practice this procedure. When you believe you have mastered this skill, sign the sheet and give it to your instructor for further action.

 FINAL EVALUATION: Using the criteria listed on the evaluation sheet, your instructor will grade **Check** your performance.

ADMINISTERING OXYGEN

 CAUTION: This section provides facts about administering oxygen. *Check your legal responsibilities with regard to this procedure.* Some states prohibit administration of oxygen by a health care assistant.

Legal

 The blood must have oxygen. The blood's supply of oxygen is normally obtained from the air, which is approximately 23 percent oxygen. As a result of accident, injury, or respiratory disease, however, the body may be unable to take in enough oxygen or to use oxygen effectively. In such cases, oxygen can be given to the patient by various means.

Science

The signs of an oxygen shortage are rapid and shallow respirations, rapid pulse, restlessness, anxiety, and cyanosis. A deficiency of oxygen is called hypoxia. Lack of oxygen can cause brain damage in 4–6 minutes.

 A physician's order is usually required for the administration of oxygen. The order will include the method of administration and the concentration to be given. In cases of extreme emergency, oxygen can be started with standard concentrations, and the physician notified as soon as possible. Most rescue teams, ambulance personnel, and others involved in emergency work follow specific orders regarding oxygen administration.

Legal

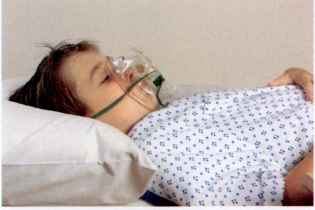

FIGURE 22–94A The oxygen mask covers the nose and mouth and provides a high concentration of oxygen. © Leah-Anne Thompson/Shutterstock.com

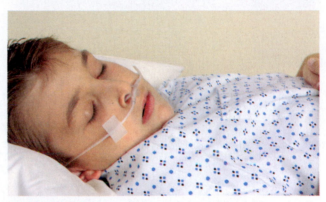

FIGURE 22–94B When a nasal cannula is used to provide oxygen, the patient must breathe through the nose. © Leah-Anne Thompson/Shutterstock.com

METHODS OF OXYGEN ADMINISTRATION

Oxygen is usually administered by one of the following methods:

- **Mask (Figure 22–94A):** The mask should cover the mouth and the nose. It should fit snugly to prevent loss of oxygen, but it should not be so tight as to cause discomfort to the patient. Oxygen by mask is the method of administration used most frequently by rescue personnel. It provides the highest concentration of oxygen. However, some patients are frightened by the mask. A careful explanation of its purpose along with constant reassurance are necessary. The rate of flow by mask is usually 6–10 liters per minute (lpm). Masks should never be used with flow rates less than 5 liters per minute because the patient will rebreathe carbon dioxide and feel smothered.

- **Nasal Cannula (Figure 22–94B):** The cannula consists of two small, curved, plastic tubes, which are placed one in each nostril. The other end of the cannula is attached to an oxygen tank or unit. The patient must be instructed to breathe through the nose. If the patient opens the mouth to breathe, the concentration of oxygen is reduced. The rate of flow by cannula is usually 2–6 liters per minute (lpm).

- **Tent:** The tent surrounds the patient with a high concentration of oxygen. It is usually used for infants and small children. Oxygen and humidity are provided. A common example is a croupette used with infants and small children. The flow rate is usually 10–12 liters per minute (lpm).

OXYGEN DELIVERY SYSTEMS

Different systems can be used to provide oxygen. Most hospitals pipe in oxygen through the wall. A flow meter for the oxygen is plugged into an adaptor in the wall (**Figure 22–95A**). When the flow meter is turned on, oxygen is delivered. Oxygen is color coded with a green label in the United States. The wall adaptor usually has a green label with the word oxygen or the symbol O_2. Portable oxygen cylinders are used while transporting patients, in emergencies, in some long-term care facilities, and in home situations (**Figure 22–95B**). Other health care facilities, such as some long-term care facilities,

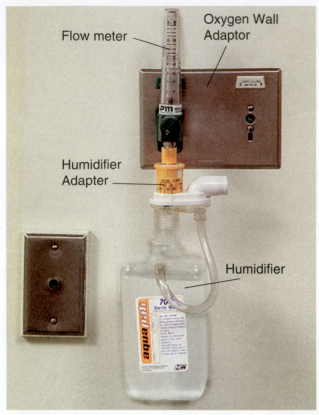

FIGURE 22–95A When oxygen is piped through a wall, the flow meter is plugged into a wall adaptor. A humidifier is used to moisturize the oxygen.

medical offices, or dental offices, may pipe in oxygen. However, in most cases, they use oxygen cylinders or oxygen concentrators. An oxygen concentrator removes impurities and other gases from room air to concentrate oxygen in the unit (**Figure 22–95C**). The oxygen concentrator cannot be used with oxygen masks because it provides only low liter flow rates, usually 2–4 liters per minute. A filter on the oxygen concentrator must be cleaned frequently by washing it with warm soapy water, rinsing it, and squeezing it dry before replacing it in the unit.

Oxygen is also available as a liquid stored in a vacuum-jacketed pressure vessel similar to a thermos bottle. An internal vaporizer turns the liquid to gas when it is released. Large amounts of oxygen can be stored in this type of reservoir (**Figure 22–95D**). In addition, patients can fill small, lightweight portable containers with liquid oxygen that can be carried like a shoulder bag. With a light, concentrated supply of oxygen that does not rely on an electrical source or batteries, a patient can have mobility for 10 or more hours.

Pure oxygen is very drying and can damage or irritate mucous membranes. The current recommendation is that any oxygen flow rate above 4 lpm should be moisturized by passing it through water before it is administered to the patient. A humidifier is used to moisturize oxygen (refer to Figure 22–95A). Most health care facilities use prefilled sterile disposable humidifiers. These units are changed and discarded when they are empty. They must be changed at least once each week or according to the

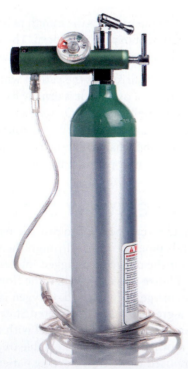

FIGURE 22–95B Portable oxygen cylinders can be used to provide oxygen in health care facilities, emergency care units, and homes. ©iStock. com/Thomas Acop

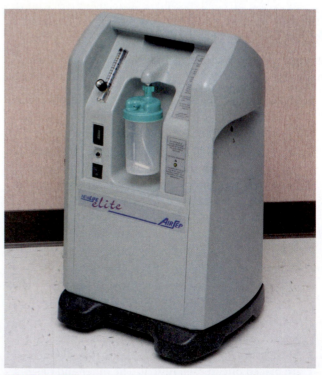

FIGURE 22–95C Oxygen concentrators remove impurities and other gases from room air to concentrate oxygen in the unit.

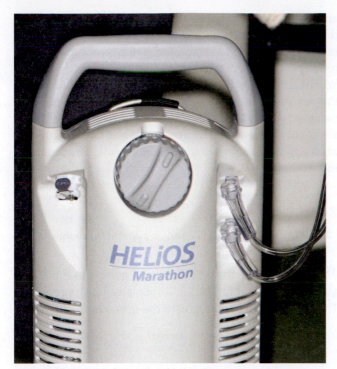

FIGURE 22–95D Liquid oxygen is available in smaller containers and delivers a high concentration of oxygen. Dr. P. Marazzi/Science Source

manufacturer's instructions. Some facilities use refillable humidifiers. These humidifiers must be filled with sterile water to the proper level, usually one-half to two-thirds of the container; most humidifiers are marked for the proper level. Sterile water is used to prevent infection from contaminants in water. Refillable humidifiers must be washed and sterilized every 24 hours to prevent infection. A label is usually placed on the humidifier to indicate the date and time it was changed. Additional water should never be added to a partially filled humidifier.

SAFETY PRECAUTIONS

Safety

Safety precautions must be observed when oxygen is in use. Although oxygen does not explode, burning is more rapid and intense in the presence of oxygen. Flammable materials (those that burn) will burn much more rapidly in the presence of oxygen. The following precautions should be taken whenever oxygen is in use:

- Smoking, lighting cigarettes or matches, burning candles, and the use of open flames are prohibited when oxygen is in use. Most health care facilities prohibit smoking in all areas. In home situations or any areas where smoking may occur, a warning sign reading, for example, "No Smoking—Oxygen" is placed on the door, in the patient's room, on the bed, or on the wall nearby. Warning labels are also sometimes placed on tanks used by emergency rescue personnel.

Comm

- The sign is not enough. The patient must be cautioned against smoking. Observers at the scene of an accident or emergency situation must also be told to avoid smoking.

- The use of electrically operated equipment, which could cause sparks, should be avoided.

- Flammable liquids, such as nail polish remover or adhesive tape remover, should never be used while oxygen is in use. Alcohol-based aftershave lotions, hairspray, perfumes, and nonapproved lip balms should not be used for patient care.

- Cotton blankets should be used in place of wool or nylon. In addition, all bed linen, bedspreads, and gowns or pajamas should be cotton instead of synthetic materials. Cotton is static-free, and its use decreases the danger of static electricity.

- Frequent inspections must be made of any area where oxygen is in use. Sources of sparks or static electricity should be removed.

PULSE OXIMETERS

Technology

Pulse oximeters may be used to monitor the patient who is receiving oxygen (**Figure 22–96**). An oximeter measures the level of oxygen in arterial blood. A photo-detector probe is clipped on the patient's finger, toe, or earlobe. The percentage of oxygen in the arterial blood is displayed on

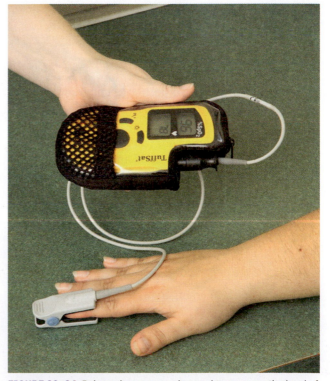

FIGURE 22–96 Pulse oximeters may be used to measure the level of oxygen in arterial blood.

the monitor screen of the oximeter. A normal range of blood oxygen saturation level is 95–100 percent. Levels below 90 are considered to be hypoxia, a deficiency of oxygen reaching the tissues. If the oxygen level falls below the minimum percentage programmed into the oximeter, an alarm will sound. Licensed personnel are responsible for programming and monitoring the oximeter. The health care assistant should make sure the probe is not disturbed and notify a supervisor if the alarm sounds.

SUMMARY

Legal

A patient who is receiving oxygen must be checked frequently. Quality of respirations should be noted. Mouth and nose care must be provided if a mask or cannula is used. The oxygen flow rate should be checked. Watch to make sure that the patient

and visitors do not change the liter flow. If a humidifier is used, the water level must be checked, and the humidifier replaced as indicated. Safety precautions must be checked frequently. In many facilities, oxygen administration is the responsibility of the respiratory therapy department. However, the health care team member, who is with the patient more frequently, should always be aware of safety precautions and check patients carefully. Any abnormal observations should be reported immediately.

checkpoint

1. List two (2) methods used to administer oxygen.

PRACTICE: Go to the workbook and complete the assignment sheet for 22:13, Administering Oxygen. Then return and continue with the procedure.

Procedure 22:13

Administering Oxygen

Equipment and Supplies

Oxygen mask, nasal cannula, or tent; tubing and gauge; oxygen tank or supply; disposable humidifier or sterile water (if refillable humidifier is used); paper and pen or computer

Legal

CAUTION: Some states prohibit the administration of oxygen by a health care assistant. Check your legal responsibilities in regard to this procedure.

Procedure

1. Read the physician's orders or obtain orders from your immediate supervisor. In emergency rescue situations, standard orders are usually provided for victims requiring oxygen. The orders should state the method of administration and liter flow per minute.

2. Assemble equipment.

3.
Comm
Knock on the door and pause before entering. Introduce yourself. Identify the patient. Explain the procedure and obtain consent. Patients are often apprehensive. Reassure as needed.

4. Wash hands. In emergency situations, this may not be possible.

5. Connect the tubing from the oxygen supply (tank or wall unit) to the tubing on the mask or cannula. If a prefilled humidifier is used, follow manufacturer's

instructions to release the seal and attach it to the flow meter. If a refillable humidifier is used, fill the container with sterile water. Replace the lid and connect it to the flow meter or oxygen outlet.

NOTE: If you are using oxygen from a wall unit, ensure that you are using the green flow meter marked oxygen. In many facilities, similar flow meters are used for air. They are yellow and marked as such.

6. Turn on the oxygen supply.

Legal

CAUTION: Do not insert the nasal cannula or apply the mask at this time. Regulate the gauge to the correct liter flow rate per minute first only if you are legally authorized to do so. If you are not authorized, notify an authorized person that the flow rate needs to be set (**Figure 22–97**).

Comm

CAUTION: Make sure to follow specific manufacturer's instructions or agency policy for connecting and turning on the oxygen supply. Do not operate any oxygen equipment until you have been specifically instructed on how to use it and are legally permitted to do so.

7. Check to be sure that oxygen is passing through the tubing. Place your hand by the outlet on the mask or cannula.

8. Put on disposable gloves.

Precaution

CAUTION: Observe all standard precautions. Contact with the patient's oral or nasal secretions is possible.

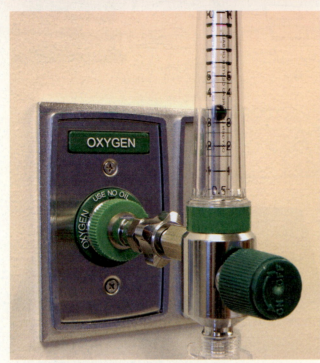

FIGURE 22–97 Regulate the gauge to provide the correct liter flow rate for oxygen. © Scott Milless/Shutterstock.com

9. With the oxygen still flowing, apply the mask or nasal cannula to the patient.

   a. If a mask is used, position it over the patient's nose and mouth. Adjust the strap so that it fits snugly but does not apply pressure to the face.

   b. If a nasal cannula is used, place the two tips in the patient's nostrils and loop the tubing around each ear. Adjust the straps at the neck so that the tips remain in position. Instruct the patient to breathe through the nose.

10. If a tent is used, it is first filled with oxygen. Then the prescribed liter flow is set. The humidifier is positioned correctly or a reusable humidifier is filled to the marked level with sterile water. Next, the tent is placed over the bed or crib, and the edges are tucked in on all sides to prevent oxygen loss. A cotton blanket, bath blanket, or sheet can be used to provide a cuff around the loose end covering the patient.

11. Check the surrounding area to make sure all safety precautions are being observed. Eliminate any sources of sparks or flames. In facilities where smoking is not already prohibited, caution any visitors and the patient against smoking while the oxygen is in use. In a home care situation, make sure a sign is posted on the door or in the immediate area.

12. Check the patient at frequent intervals. Note respirations, color, restlessness, or discomfort. Provide skin care to the face and/or nose if a mask or nasal cannula is used. Check the skin behind the ears and provide skin care if a nasal cannula is used. At times, it may be necessary to use a towel or cloth to dry the inside of the mask, because moisture will accumulate in the mask. If a nasal cannula is used, check the tips to make sure they are open and not plugged by mucus. Provide oral hygiene frequently. Check the water level, if a humidifier is used, and replace the humidifier as needed. Check the gauge and make sure the liter flow rate is correct. Report any abnormal conditions immediately.

13. When the oxygen is discontinued, make sure that the oxygen supply is turned off. Follow the specific manufacturer's instructions or agency policy. Clean and replace all equipment. Most masks and cannulas are disposable and discarded after use. If the items are not disposable, they should be cleaned and sterilized according to established agency policy.

14. Remove gloves. Wash hands.

15. Report and/or record all required information on the patient's chart or enter it into the computer. For example, date, time, oxygen per mask at 6 lpm, R 16 deep and even, and your signature and title. Report any unusual observations immediately.

NOTE: In health care agencies using electronic medical records (EMRs), the information is entered directly into the patient's record on a computer.

PRACTICE: Go to the workbook and use the evaluation sheet for 22:13, Administering Oxygen, to practice this procedure. When you believe you have mastered this skill, sign the sheet and give it to your instructor for further action.

 FINAL EVALUATION: Using the criteria listed on the evaluation sheet, your instructor will grade your performance.

GIVING
POSTMORTEM CARE

The Morgue Kit

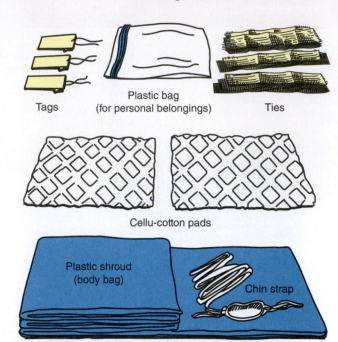

FIGURE 22–98 Supplies needed for postmortem care.

OBRA

Providing care after death is a difficult but essential part of patient care. As a health care provider, you may perform or assist with this care.

Postmortem care is care given to the body immediately after death. It begins when a physician has pronounced the patient dead.

Dealing with death and dying is a difficult part of providing care. If a health care provider has cared for a patient for a time, it is natural for the provider to feel grief and a sense of loss on the patient's death. Crying is a natural expression of grief, and you should not feel embarrassed if you cry. However, it is also important for health care providers to try to control emotions because family members and other patients will need their support.

Legal

The patient's rights continue to apply after death. The body should be treated with dignity and respect. Privacy should be provided at all times.

If family members are not present when death occurs and want to view the body before it is taken to the morgue or funeral home, the body should be prepared for viewing. The patient should be positioned naturally, with the limbs straight. Elevate the head of the bed 30 degrees to prevent discoloration of the head and neck. Follow agency policy regarding dentures and glasses. Some facilities state dentures and glasses should be placed on the patient for family viewing. After the viewing, they are removed, packed safely, and sent to the funeral home with the body. Other facilities state that the dentures and glasses must be packed immediately and not placed on the body because the items could fall off and break. The bed linen should be neat and clean, and extra equipment should be removed from the unit. Provide privacy while the family views the body unless they request that you remain with them.

After the family has viewed the body, postmortem care is completed. The procedure for this care varies in different facilities. In some facilities, morgue personnel prepare the body and remove it to the morgue. In other facilities, the body is prepared and remains in the unit until the funeral home personnel arrive. In yet other facilities, funeral home personnel remove the body and provide postmortem care. Know and follow the procedure established by your facility.

Morgue kits often are used for postmortem care (**Figure 22–98**). Each kit usually contains a shroud or body bag, a gown, chin strap, pads, gauze squares, ties, two or three tags to identify the body, and safety pins. Procedure 22:14 describes one method of using these supplies to provide postmortem care.

Care of the patient's valuables and belongings is an important part of postmortem care. Each facility has a policy that should be followed. The personal inventory and valuables lists prepared on admission are often used to make sure that all items are present. These items are checked according to facility policy. Valuables in the safe or with security usually remain there until a family member signs for them. Jewelry is usually removed from the body, listed, and placed in the safe or with security until received by a family member. A wedding ring is frequently left on the body, but it should be taped in place and noted on the chart.

Legal

Frequently, two people work together to complete postmortem care. Some aspects of care, such as removal of tubes or IVs, may be the responsibility of the nurse or another authorized person. Follow your agency's policy and know your legal responsibilities with regard to giving or assisting with postmortem care.

checkpoint

1. How high should the head of the bed be raised in postmortem care?

PRACTICE: Go to the workbook and complete the assignment sheet for 22:14, Giving Postmortem Care. Then return and continue with the procedure.

Giving Postmortem Care

Equipment and Supplies

Postmortem kit (shroud or clean sheet, gown, tags, gauze squares, cotton balls, safety pins), underpads or bed protectors, basin, towels, washcloth, personal inventory and valuables lists, disposable gloves, plastic waste bag, paper and pen or computer

NOTE: If cleansing cloths are available, they can be used in place of the basin and washcloth.

Procedure

1. Obtain proper authorization and assemble equipment.

2. Identify the patient by checking the armband.

3. Close the door and screen the unit to provide privacy.

4. Wash hands. Put on gloves.

    CAUTION: Observe all standard precautions because the body may be contaminated with blood or body fluids.

   Precaution

5. Elevate the bed to a comfortable working height. If siderails are elevated, lower the siderail on the side where you are working.

6. Position the body lying flat on the back, with the arms and legs straight. Place a pillow under the head and shoulders and elevate the bed 30 degrees.

   NOTE: The head is elevated to prevent the bluish purple discoloration of the head and neck that occurs when gravity causes blood to accumulate in the lowest areas of the body after death.

   NOTE: Handle the body gently and with respect.

7. If the eyes are open, close them by gently pulling the eyelids over the eyes and holding them shut for a few seconds (**Figure 22–99**). Put a moist cotton ball on each eye if the eyes do not remain shut.

8. Follow agency policy regarding the use of dentures and chin straps. Some agencies state that dentures should be replaced in the mouth for family viewing. Others state that they should be packed securely in a denture cup because they could fall out of the mouth and break. Some agencies use a chin strap to hold the jaw shut. Other agencies feel that the chin strap can bruise or discolor the skin and that it should not be used. Some agencies use a rolled towel or padding under the chin to keep the mouth closed.

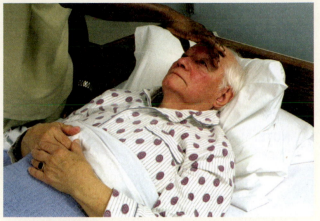

FIGURE 22–99 If the eyes are open after death, close them by gently pulling the eyelids over the eyes.

9. Remove soiled dressings and replace with clean ones, as necessary. If tubes, IVs, catheters, or drainage bags are in place, follow agency policy for removal. This is often the responsibility of the nurse. If an autopsy is to be performed, some tubes may have to be left in place.

   Legal

10. Use warm water or cleansing cloths to bathe any soiled body areas. Dry all areas thoroughly. Comb the hair, if needed.

11. Place an underpad or padding under the buttocks at the anal area.

    NOTE: The bowels and bladder may empty after death.

12. Put a clean gown on the body.

13. Remove gloves and wash hands.

14. If jewelry is present, follow agency policy. Jewelry is usually removed, listed on a valuables list, and stored in a safe or with security until signed for by a family member. A wedding ring frequently is left on the body, but it should be taped in place and noted on the chart or postmortem form.

15. If the family is to view the body, use a sheet to cover the body to the shoulders. Make sure the room is neat and clean. Provide privacy for the family unless they request that you remain with them.

16. After the family visit, remove dentures and eyeglasses (if they were placed on the patient). Pack them securely, label them with the patient's name, and send them to the funeral home.

(continues)

17. Fill out the identification card or tag. One tag is usually placed on the patient's right ankle or right big toe.

Comm

18. Place the body in the shroud or body bag. Use safety pins or tape to hold the shroud in place. If a shroud is not available, use a sheet to cover the body.

NOTE: Many facilities have plastic body bags with zippers.

⚠ **CAUTION:** Handle the body carefully. Pressure from your hands can leave marks on the body.

Safety

NOTE: Sometimes, padding is placed between the ankles and knees, and the legs are tied together lightly before the body is placed in the shroud.

19. If required, attach a second identification card or tag to the outside of the shroud or body bag.

20. Collect all belongings and make a list. This list frequently is checked against the admission personal inventory and valuables list to make sure that all items are present. Put the items in a bag or container and attach an identification card or tag. Follow agency policy for care of belongings until they are signed for by a family member.

21. Obtain assistance and transfer the body to a stretcher. Make sure doors to other patient's rooms are closed and the corridor is empty before transporting the body to the morgue.

NOTE: In some facilities, morgue personnel or orderlies transport the body to the morgue. In other facilities, the body remains in the unit until funeral home personnel arrive.

22. Return to the unit. Wash hands and put on gloves. Strip the linen from the bed. Follow agency policy for cleaning the unit and equipment. Leave the area neat and clean.

23. Remove gloves. Wash hands.

24. Report and/or record all required information on the patient's chart or enter it into the computer. For example, date, time, postmortem care given, body transported to morgue, belongings placed in locked closet by nurses' station, and your signature and title.

Comm

🖥 **NOTE:** In health care agencies using electronic health records (EHRs), the information is entered directly into the patient's record on a computer.

EHR

PRACTICE: Go to the workbook and use the evaluation sheet for 22:14, Giving Postmortem Care, to practice this procedure. When you believe you have mastered this skill, sign the sheet and give it to your instructor for further action.

 FINAL EVALUATION: Using the criteria listed on the evaluation sheet, your instructor will grade your performance.

Check

Gene Therapy That Cures Cancer?

Hepatocellular carcinoma (HCC), or liver cancer, kills many individuals. The American Cancer Society estimates that more than 42,800 new cases of liver cancer are diagnosed each year in the United States with more than 800,000 cases worldwide. About 30,160 people die of liver cancer every year in the United States, and more than 700,000 die worldwide. How can these lives be saved?

Researchers are experimenting with many different treatments for liver cancer. One treatment involves the use of gene therapy. Every human has between 50,000 and 100,000 different genes. These genes determine what a person inherits, such as hair and eye color. Genes also carry instructions that tell cells to perform certain functions, such as when to reproduce and grow. Initially, scientists researching the spread of liver cancer to the colon and rectum identified a gene called p53. This gene codes for a protein that is present in normal cells and regulates cell growth. In many types of cancer, the gene is missing or mutated (changed), allowing uncontrolled growth of the cancer cells. Another group of researchers in Japan studied hepatitis C (HVC) carriers and discovered that the presence of a gene identified as DEPDC5 SNP roughly doubles the chances that a hepatitis C carrier will develop liver cancer. Scientists also identified genes called FGF-19 and FGFR4 that become active in liver, breast, and pancreatic cancer patients, causing healthy cells to become cancerous. However, these scientists also found that when an experimental antibody inhibitor was applied, the gene's activity stopped, preventing the development of cancerous cells. Currently, several FGFR4 inhibitors are in initial trial studies. Other scientists found a gene called STAT3 that seems to protect liver cancer cells from the effects of chemotherapy (treatment with cancer drugs). Research to find a substance that blocks the action of this gene so chemotherapy is more effective has developed several potential inhibitors for STAT3. One of the most promising inhibitors is napabucasin because it seems to be efficient at blocking the action of STAT3 and allowing chemotherapy to be more effective. If scientists can find ways to replace missing genes or block the actions of genes that are causing cells to become malignant, they will be able to stop or decrease the growth of cancer so other treatments will be more effective.

One major problem of gene therapy is the way the gene has to be inserted into a person's cell. Scientists cannot simply inject genes into cells. They must be transported into the cell by using a carrier called a vector. The most common vectors used are retroviruses. Scientists inactivate the retroviruses to keep them from causing disease and then use them to carry the gene into cells. The problems that occur with this method are that the genes might alter or change other normal cells, or that the new gene might be inserted into the wrong location, causing additional damage to the body. For these reasons, scientists must identify easier and better ways to deliver genes to body cells. Scientists throughout the world are trying to solve these problems. If they are successful, many people with cancer may be cured.

Case Study Investigation Conclusion

What skills do you think David and Imani will need to have in order to deliver superior care to their patients at Stoneybrook? What skills involve asking each other for help? What communication skills will they need to use?

CHAPTER 22 SUMMARY

- Many nurse assistant skills are directed toward providing quality personal care for the patient. Examples include bathing, caring for hair and nails, gowning or dressing the patient, giving back rubs, providing oral hygiene, shaving, feeding, assisting with bedpans or urinals, and bedmaking. It is essential that the nurse assistant learn and follow correct procedures to provide for the safety, comfort, and privacy of the patient.

- Other nurse assistant skills include positioning, turning, moving, and transferring patients. During any move or transfer, the use of correct body mechanics is essential.

- Nurse assistant skills are required for other special procedures, such as measuring intake and output (I&O), collecting stool and urine specimens, assisting the surgical patient, administering oxygen, applying restraints, providing catheter care, applying surgical hose, and giving postmortem care. It is important to determine legal responsibility before performing some of these special procedures because some states or agencies do not allow all nurse assistants to perform the procedures.

- It is important to make careful observations of the patient while providing care, and to record or report these observations correctly. In this way, you will use nurse assistant skills to become an important member of the health care team.

REVIEW QUESTIONS

1. List six (6) specific tasks that must be performed while admitting a patient to a hospital or long-term care facility.

2. Name three (3) main ways to make beds and explain when each type is made.

3. Identify all the areas of care that may provide personal hygiene to a patient.

4. What is a urinary catheter? Why is it used?

5. Differentiate between a routine, clean-catch (midstream), sterile, and 24-hour urine specimen.

6. Why is stool tested for occult blood?

7. Define each of the following words:
   a. colostomy
   b. pressure ulcer
   c. edema
   d. nasogastric tube
   e. dysphagia
   f. compression sleeves

8. List four (4) specific rules that OBRA legislation has placed on the use of restraints.

9. Identify five (5) specific aspects of care for both pre-op and post-op patients.

10. Name three (3) methods for administering oxygen. Describe the use for each method.

11. Explain five (5) standard precautions that must be observed while performing any nurse assisting procedure.

For additional information about nursing careers, contact the following associations:

- All Nursing Schools
  www.allnursingschools.com

- American Health Care Association
  www.ahcancal.org

- American Nurses Association
  www.nursingworld.org

- National Association for Home Care and Hospice
  www.nahc.org

- National Association for Practical Nurse Education and Service
  www.napnes.org

- National Association of Health Care Assistants
  www.nahcacares.org

- National Federation of Licensed Practical Nurses
  www.nflpn.org

- National League for Nursing
  www.nln.org

- National Network of Career Nursing Assistants
  www.cna-network.org

- Registered Nurse, RN
  www.registerednursern.com

CRITICAL THINKING

1. Identify six (6) observations that might be indicative of a medical problem.

    1a. Why is it important to constantly observe a patient while providing personal care?

2. Describe four (4) ways to prevent pressure sores and contractures from developing.

    2a. Why is it easier to prevent a pressure ulcer or contracture than it is to treat them?

3. When transferring a patient to a stretcher or using a mechanical lift, why is it especially important to cooperate and communicate as a team?

ACTIVITIES

1. In pairs, obtain a bedpan and apply to each other. Write a paragraph describing your feelings as a care giver applying a bedpan and as a patient having this procedure done.

2. With a partner, sketch the perfect hospital room that is ready for a new admission. Create a script of a caring nurse assistant helping a new patient feel comfortable.

3. Obtain a balloon, blow it up, and draw a face on it with a permanent marker. Gather supplies for shaving. Have a partner hold up the balloon as you administer a shave (refer to Procedure 22:4G) without popping the balloon.

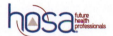 | CONNECTION

Competitive Event: Nursing Assisting

Event Summary: Nursing Assisting provides members with the opportunity to gain knowledge and skills required for patient care in medical settings. This competitive event consists of 2 rounds. Round One is a written, multiple choice test and the top scoring competitors will advance to Round Two for the skills assessment. This event aims to inspire members to be learn more about the field of nursing and how to provide quality care.

Details on this competitive event may be found at

www.hosa.org/guidelines

CHAPTER 23

PHYSICAL THERAPY SKILLS

Career   Science   OBRA

Case Study Investigation

Vincent is a physical therapy assistant at New Day Rehabilitation Center. He has been assigned a new patient, Marcus, a 17-year-old who was injured in a car wreck. Marcus was pinned in the car for a long time and suffered severe right side injuries. His right leg was broken in four places, his wrist was broken, and several ribs were cracked. His face and body are very swollen and painful with severe bruising. At the end of this chapter, you will be asked what techniques or skills Vincent may use in his care of Marcus as he progresses to independent activities of daily living (ADLs) through his physical therapy at the rehabilitation center.

After completing this chapter, you should be able to:

- Perform range-of-motion (ROM) exercises on all body joints, observing all safety precautions.

- Ambulate a patient using a transfer (gait) belt.

- Check the correct measurements of patients for canes, crutches, and walkers.

- Ambulate a patient using the following crutch gaits: four point, three point, two point, swing to, and swing through.

- Ambulate a patient using a cane.

- Ambulate a patient using a walker.

- Apply an ice bag or ice collar, observing all safety precautions.

- Apply a warm-water bag, observing all safety precautions.

- Apply an aquamatic pad, observing all safety precautions.

- Apply a moist compress, observing all safety precautions.

- Define, pronounce, and spell all key terms.

■ **KEY TERMS**

aquathermia pads *(ak"-wah-thur'-me-ah)*

cane

compresses *(cahm'-press-ez)*

contracture *(kun-track'-shure)*

crutches

cryotherapy

dry cold

dry heat

hydrocollator packs

hypothermia blanket *(high"-poh-thur'-me-ah)*

ice bags

ice collars

moist cold

moist heat

paraffin wax treatment

range of motion (ROM)

Sitz baths

thermal blankets

thermotherapy

transfer (gait) belt

vasoconstriction *(vay"-zow"-kon-strik'-shun)*

vasodilation *(vay'-zow"-di-lay'-shun)*

walker

warm-water bags

Career

Physical therapist assistants (PTAs) provide treatment to improve mobility and prevent or limit permanent disability of patients with disabling injuries or disease. They are important members of the health care team. They work under the supervision of a physical therapist who has a doctoral degree from an accredited program and is licensed (required in all states). Most physical therapist assistants have an associate's degree from an accredited program and an internship. Licensure is required in most states.

The duties of physical therapist assistants vary but usually include performing exercises; providing ultrasound or electrical stimulation treatments; administering heat, cold, or moist applications; ambulating patients with assistive devices; and informing the physical therapist of the patient's response and progress. In addition to the knowledge and skills presented in this chapter, physical therapist assistants must also learn and master skills such as:

- Presenting a professional appearance and attitude
- Obtaining knowledge regarding health care delivery systems, organizational structure, and teamwork
- Meeting all legal responsibilities
- Communicating effectively
- Being sensitive to and respecting cultural diversity
- Learning medical terminology

- Comprehending anatomy, physiology, and pathophysiology with an emphasis on the skeletal, muscular, nervous, and circulatory systems
- Observing all safety precautions
- Practicing all principles of infection control
- Administering first aid and cardio-pulmonary resuscitation
- Promoting good nutrition and a healthy lifestyle to maintain health

- Using computer and technology skills
- Cleaning and maintaining equipment
- Ordering and maintaining supplies and materials
- Performing administrative duties such as answering the telephone, scheduling appointments, completing insurance forms, and maintaining patient records

LEGAL ALERT

Legal

Before performing any procedures in this chapter, know and follow the standards and regulations established by the scope of practice; federal laws and agencies; state laws; state or national licensing, registration, or certification boards; professional organizations; professional standards; and agency policies.

It is your responsibility to learn exactly what you are legally permitted to do and to perform only procedures for which you have been trained.

23:1 PERFORMING RANGE-OF-MOTION (ROM) EXERCISES

OBRA

Activity and exercise are important for all individuals. Activity maintains the ability to perform activities of daily living (ADLs) like cooking, cleaning, dressing, shaving, and brushing hair. The muscle strength gained from exercise enables individuals to have the endurance to stand for showering and to maintain balance and mobility for taking a walk. Independent activity benefits the person's physical as well as mental and emotional outlook. When patients have limited ability to move, range-of-motion exercises help keep muscles and joints functioning.

Range-of-motion (ROM) exercises are done to maintain the health of the musculoskeletal system. Each joint and muscle in the body is moved through its full range of motion. Range-of-motion exercises are frequently ordered by physicians for patients with limited ability to move. These exercises are administered by a physical therapist, nurse, health care assistant, or other authorized person. Range-of-motion exercises can be done during the daily bath or at other times during the day.

Range-of-motion exercises are done to prevent the problems caused by lack of movement and by inactivity (**Figure 23–1**). Some of these problems include:

- **Contracture:** A contracture is a tightening and shortening of a muscle, resulting in a permanent flexing of a joint. Foot drop is a common contracture, but contractures can also affect the knees, hips, elbows, and hands (refer to Figure 22–8).

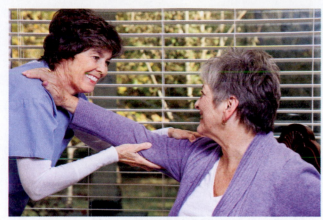

FIGURE 23–1 Range-of-motion (ROM) exercises are done to prevent problems caused by lack of movement and by inactivity. © iStock.com/Pamela Moore

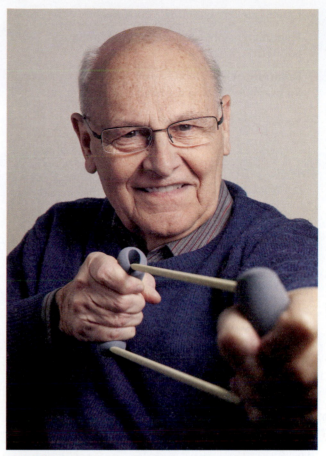

FIGURE 23–2 Patients who are able to move each joint without assistance perform active range-of-motion (ROM) exercises. © Carme Balcells/Shutterstock.com

- **Muscle and joint function**: Muscles atrophy (shrink) and become weak. Joints become stiff and difficult to move.

- **Circulatory impairment**: The circulation of blood is affected, and blood clots and pressure ulcers (pressure sores) can develop.

- **Mineral loss**: Inactivity causes mineral loss, especially of calcium from the bones. The bones become brittle, and fractures occur. As the blood calcium level increases, renal calculi (kidney stones) are more likely to form.

- **Other problems**: Lack of exercise can also cause poor appetite, constipation, urinary infections, respiratory problems, and hypostatic pneumonia.

There are four main types of ROM exercises:

- **Active ROM exercises**: These are performed by patients who are able to move each joint without assistance (**Figure 23–2**). This type of ROM exercise strengthens muscles, maintains joint function and movement, and helps prevent deformities.

- **Active assistive ROM exercises**: The patient actively moves the joints but receives assistance to complete the entire ROM. This type of ROM strengthens muscles, maintains joint function and movement, and helps prevent deformities. At times, equipment, such as a pulley, is used to complete the ROM.

- **Passive ROM exercises**: Another person moves each joint for a patient who is not able to exercise. This type of ROM maintains joint function and movement, and helps to prevent deformities. However, it does not strengthen muscles.

- **Resistive ROM exercises**: Administered by a therapist, these exercises are performed against resistance provided by the therapist. This type of ROM helps the patient develop increased strength and endurance.

 The health care provider should find out what type of ROM exercises are to be performed and determine whether any limitations to the exercises exist before administering or assisting the patient with the exercises. In some states and health care facilities, only physical therapists or registered nurses may perform ROM exercises to the head and neck, especially if stretching is involved. After hip or knee replacement surgeries, some ROM exercises may be restricted or limited. Patients with osteoporosis, a condition in which the bones become porous and are prone to fracture, may have limitations on ROMs. It is your responsibility to check legal requirements regarding ROM exercises.

 Various movements are used when performing ROM exercises. The health care provider must be aware of the terms used for movements of each joint. The main movements are shown in **Figure 23–3** and include:

- **Abduction**: moving a part away from the midline of the body

- **Adduction**: moving a part toward the midline of the body

- **Flexion**: bending a body part

- **Extension**: straightening a body part
- **Hyperextension**: excessive straightening of a body part
- **Rotation**: moving a body part around its own axis, for example, turning the head from side to side

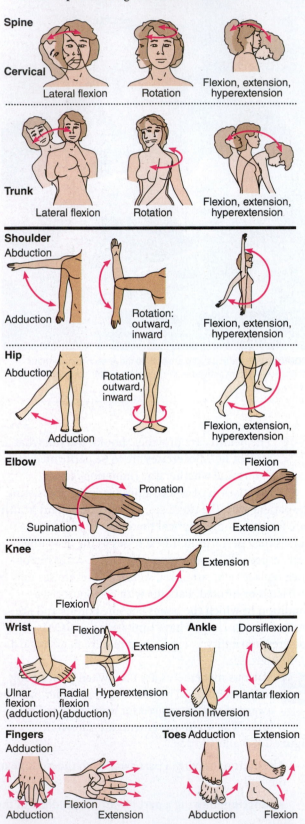

Spine

Cervical

Lateral flexion | Rotation | Flexion, extension, hyperextension

Trunk

Lateral flexion | Rotation | Flexion, extension, hyperextension

Shoulder
Abduction
Adduction
Rotation: outward, inward
Flexion, extension, hyperextension

Hip
Abduction
Rotation: outward, inward
Adduction
Flexion, extension, hyperextension

Elbow
Pronation
Supination
Flexion
Extension

Knee
Extension
Flexion

Wrist
Flexion
Extension
Ulnar flexion (adduction)
Radial flexion (abduction)
Hyperextension

Ankle
Dorsiflexion
Plantar flexion
Eversion Inversion

Fingers
Adduction
Flexion
Abduction
Extension

Toes Adduction Extension
Abduction
Flexion

FIGURE 23–3 Range-of-motion (ROM) exercises for specific joints.

- **Circumduction**: moving in a circle at a joint, or moving one end of a body part in a circle while the other end remains stationary, such as swinging the arm in a circle; involves all the movements of flexion, extension, abduction, adduction, and rotation
- **Pronation**: turning a body part downward (turning palm down)
- **Supination**: turning a body part upward (turning palm up)
- **Opposition**: touching each of the fingers with the tip of the thumb
- **Inversion**: turning a body part inward
- **Eversion**: turning a body part outward
- **Dorsiflexion**: bending backward (bending the foot toward the knee)
- **Plantar flexion**: bending forward (straightening the foot away from the knee)
- **Radial deviation**: moving toward the thumb side of the hand
- **Ulnar deviation**: moving toward the little finger side of the hand

Certain principles must be observed at all times when performing ROM exercises:

- Movements should be slow, smooth, and gentle to prevent injury.
- Support should be provided to the parts above and below the joint being exercised.
- A joint should never be forced beyond its ROM or exercised to the point of pain, resistance, or extreme fatigue.
- If a patient complains of pain, stop the exercise and report this fact to your immediate supervisor.
- If a muscle becomes rigid or muscle spasms develop, hold steady gentle pressure on the muscle until it relaxes.
- Watch the patient closely. If you notice the patient is in pain, has shortness of breath, is perspiring profusely (diaphoresis), or is pale, stop the exercise and notify your supervisor.
- Each movement should be performed three to five times or as ordered.
- The patient should be encouraged to assist as much as possible.
- Prevent unnecessary exposure of the patient. Only the body part being exercised should be exposed.
- The door should be closed and/or the curtain pulled shut to provide privacy.
- Use correct body mechanics at all times to prevent injury.

checkpoint

1. What does ROM stand for?
2. What is the most common type of contracture?

PRACTICE: Go to the workbook and complete the assignment sheet for 23:1, Performing Range-of-Motion (ROM) Exercises. Then return and continue with the procedure.

Procedure 23:1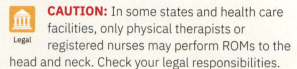

Performing Range-of-Motion (ROM) Exercises

Equipment and Supplies

Bath blanket, paper and pen and/or computer

Procedure

1. Obtain proper authorization. Determine the type of ROM exercises and any limitations to movement.

    CAUTION: Remember, it is your responsibility to check legal requirements regarding ROMs.
   Legal

2. Assemble supplies.

3. Knock on the door and pause before entering. Introduce yourself. Identify the patient. Explain the procedure and obtain consent.
   Comm

4. Close the door and pull the curtain for privacy. Lock the wheels of the bed to prevent movement.

5. Wash hands.

6. Elevate the bed to a comfortable working height. If siderails are present and elevated, lower the siderail on the side where you are working.

7. Position the patient in the supine position (on the back) and in good body alignment.

   NOTE: Some ROM exercises can be done while the patient is sitting in a chair.

8. Use the bath blanket to drape the patient. Fanfold the top bed linens to the foot of the bed.

9. Administer the exercises in an organized manner. Start at the head and move to the feet. Complete one side of the body first and then work on the opposite side of the body. Perform each movement three to five times or as ordered. Provide support for the body parts above and below the joint being exercised. *Never* force any joint beyond its ROM or cause pain while exercising a joint.

    CAUTION: Use proper body mechanics when administering ROM exercises. Get
   Safety close to the patient by bending at your hips and knees and keeping your back straight. Stand with your feet apart and one foot slightly forward to provide a good base of support.

CAUTION: If the patient complains of pain or discomfort, begins to perspire profusely, or has difficulty breathing during any exercise, stop the exercise and report the fact to your immediate supervisor.
Safety

10. Exercise the neck, if you have specific orders to do so:

    CAUTION: In some states and health care facilities, only physical therapists or registered nurses may perform ROMs to the
    Legal head and neck. Check your legal responsibilities.

    a. Support the patient's head by placing one hand under the chin and the other hand on the top-back part of the head.

       NOTE: Hands can also be placed on either side of the patient's head.

    b. Rotate the neck by turning the head gently from side to side.

    c. Flex the neck by moving the chin toward the chest.

    d. Extend the neck by returning the head to the upright position.

    e. Hyperextend the neck by tilting the head backward.

    f. Laterally flex or rotate the neck by moving the head first toward the right shoulder and then toward the left shoulder.

11. Exercise the shoulder joint nearest to you:

    a. Support the patient's arm by placing one hand above the elbow and the other at the wrist.

    b. Abduct the shoulder by bringing the arm straight out at a right angle to the body (**Figure 23–4A**).

    c. Adduct the shoulder by moving the arm straight in to the side (**Figure 23–4B**).

    d. Flex the shoulder by raising the arm in front of the body and then above the head (**Figure 23–5A**).

    e. Extend the shoulder by bringing the arm back down to the side from above the head (**Figure 23–5B**).

(continues)

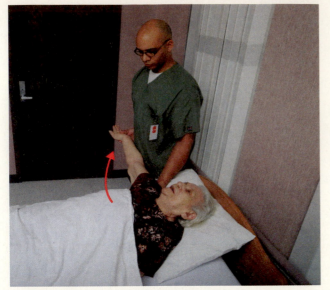

FIGURE 23–4A Abduct the shoulder by bringing the arm straight out at a right angle to the body.

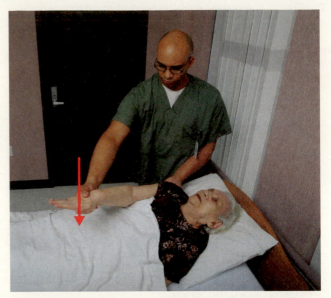

FIGURE 23–4B Adduct the shoulder by moving the arm straight in to the body.

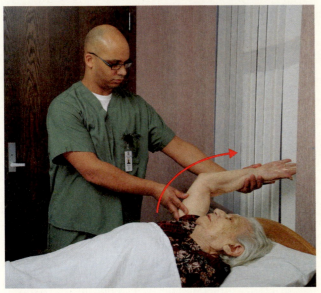

FIGURE 23–5A Flex the shoulder by raising the arm in front of the body and then above the head.

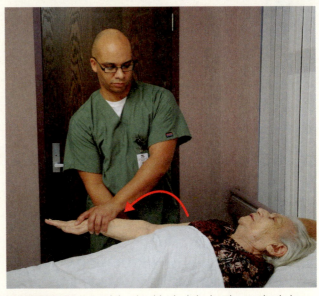

FIGURE 23–5B Extend the shoulder by bringing the arm back down to the side from above the head.

12. Exercise the elbow joint nearest to you:

   a. Support the patient's arm by placing one hand under the elbow and the other hand on the wrist.

   b. Flex the elbow by bending the forearm and hand up to the shoulder (**Figure 23–6A**).

   c. Extend the elbow by moving the forearm and hand down to the side, or straightening the arm (**Figure 23–6B**).

   d. Pronate by turning the forearm and hand so that the palm of the hand is down.

   e. Supinate by turning the forearm and hand so that the palm of the hand is up.

13. Exercise the wrist nearest to you:

   a. Support the patient's wrist by placing one hand above it and the other hand below it.

   b. Flex the wrist by bending the hand down toward the forearm (**Figure 23–7A**).

   c. Extend the wrist by straightening the hand (**Figure 23–7B**).

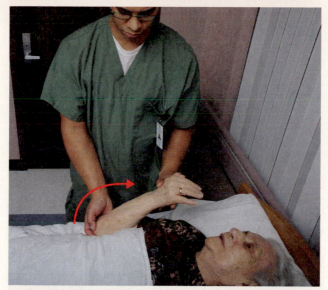

FIGURE 23–6A Flex the elbow by bending the forearm and hand up to the shoulder.

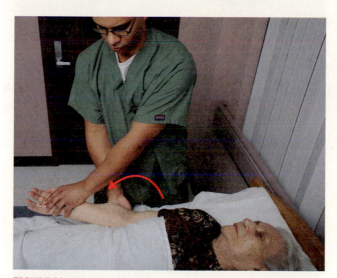

FIGURE 23–6B Extend the elbow by moving the forearm and hand down to the side.

d. Hyperextend the wrist by bending the top of the hand back toward the forearm (**Figure 23–7C**).

e. Deviate the wrist in an ulnar direction by moving the hand toward the little finger side (**Figure 23–8A**).

f. Deviate the wrist in a radial direction by moving the hand toward the thumb side (**Figure 23–8B**).

14. Exercise the fingers and thumb on the hand nearest to you:

   a. Support the patient's hand by placing one hand at the wrist.

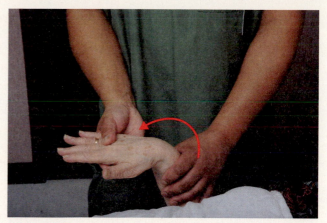

FIGURE 23–7A Flex the wrist by bending the hand down toward the forearm.

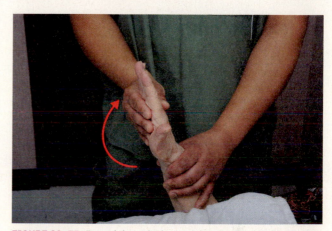

FIGURE 23–7B Extend the wrist by straightening the hand.

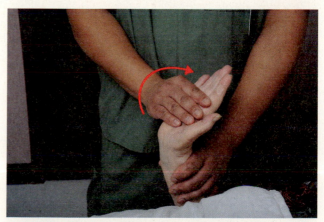

FIGURE 23–7C Hyperextend the wrist by bending the top of the hand back toward the forearm.

   b. Flex the thumb and fingers by bending them toward the palm (**Figure 23–9A**).

   c. Extend the thumb and fingers by straightening them (**Figure 23–9B**).

(continues)

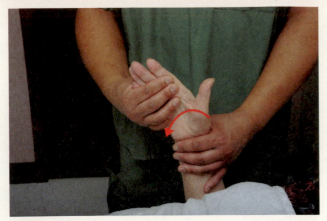

FIGURE 23–8A Deviate the wrist in an ulnar direction by moving the hand toward the little finger side.

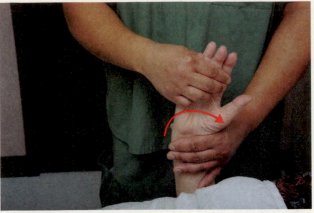

FIGURE 23–8B Deviate the wrist in a radial direction by moving the hand toward the thumb side.

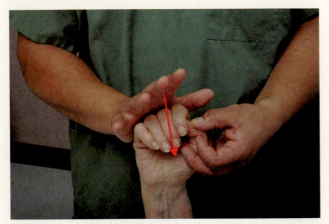

FIGURE 23–9A Flex the thumb and fingers by bending them toward the palm.

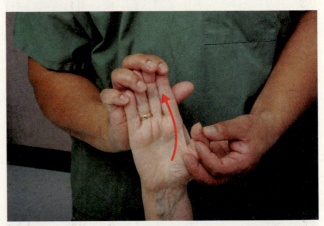

FIGURE 23–9B Extend the thumb and fingers by straightening them.

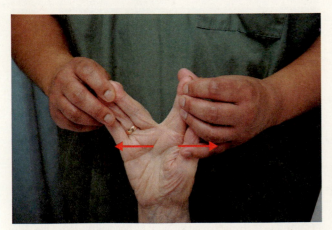

FIGURE 23–10A Abduct the thumb and fingers by spreading them apart.

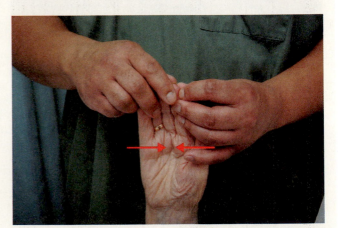

FIGURE 23–10B Adduct the thumb and fingers by moving them together.

d. Abduct the thumb and fingers by spreading them apart (**Figure 23–10A**).

e. Adduct the thumb and fingers by moving them together (**Figure 23–10B**).

f. Perform opposition by touching the thumb to the tip of each finger.

g. Circumduct the thumb by moving it in a circular motion.

15. Uncover the leg nearest to you and exercise the hip:

 Safety **CAUTION:** If the patient had hip or knee replacement surgery, check first for any limitations or restrictions to ROMs.

a. Support the patient's leg by placing one hand under the knee and the other hand under the ankle.

b. Abduct the hip by moving the entire leg out to the side (**Figure 23–11A**).

c. Adduct the hip by moving the entire leg back toward the body (**Figure 23–11B**).

d. Flex the hip by bending the knee and moving the thigh up toward the abdomen (**Figure 23–12A**).

e. Extend the hip by straightening the knee and moving the leg away from the abdomen (**Figure 23–12B**).

f. Medially rotate the hip by bending the knee and turning the leg in toward the midline.

g. Laterally rotate the hip by bending the knee and turning the leg out away from the midline.

16. Exercise the knee nearest to you:

 Safety **CAUTION:** If the patient had hip or knee replacement surgery, check first for any limitations or restrictions to ROM exercises.

a. Support the patient's leg by placing one hand under the knee and the other hand under the ankle.

b. Flex the knee by bending the lower leg back toward the thigh.

c. Extend the knee by straightening the leg.

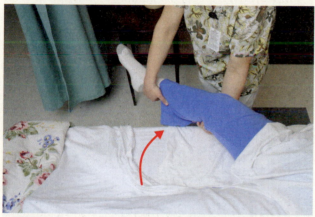

FIGURE 23–11A Abduct the hip by moving the entire leg out to the side.

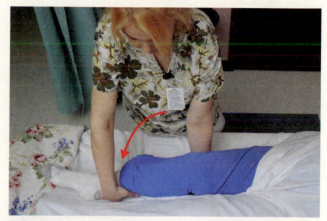

FIGURE 23–11B Adduct the hip by moving the entire leg back toward the body.

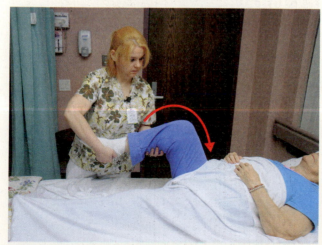

FIGURE 23–12A Flex the hip by bending the knee and moving the thigh up toward the abdomen.

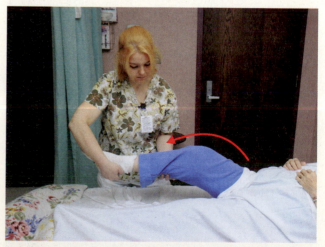

FIGURE 23–12B Extend the hip by straightening the knee and moving the leg away from the abdomen.

(continues)

17. Exercise the ankle nearest to you:

    a. Support the patient's foot by placing one hand under the foot and the other hand behind the ankle.

    b. Dorsiflex the ankle by moving the toes and foot up toward the knee (**Figure 23–13A**).

    c. Plantar flex the ankle by moving the toes and foot down away from the knee (**Figure 23–13B**).

    d. Invert the foot by gently turning it inward (**Figure 23–14A**).

    e. Evert the foot by gently turning it outward (**Figure 23–14B**).

18. Exercise the toes on the foot nearest to you:

    a. Rest the patient's leg and foot on the bed for support.

    b. Abduct the toes by separating them, or moving them away from each other.

    c. Adduct the toes by moving them together.

    d. Flex the toes by bending them down toward the bottom of the foot.

    e. Extend the toes by straightening them.

19. Use the bath blanket to cover the patient. Raise the siderail, if indicated, and move to the opposite side of the bed. Lower the siderail if it is elevated.

20. Repeat steps 11–18 on the opposite side of the body.

21. When ROM exercises are complete, comfortably position the patient in good body alignment. Replace the top bed linens and remove the bath blanket.

22. Observe all checkpoints before leaving the patient: elevate the siderails (if indicated), lower the bed to its lowest level, place the call signal and supplies within easy reach of the patient, and leave the area neat and clean.

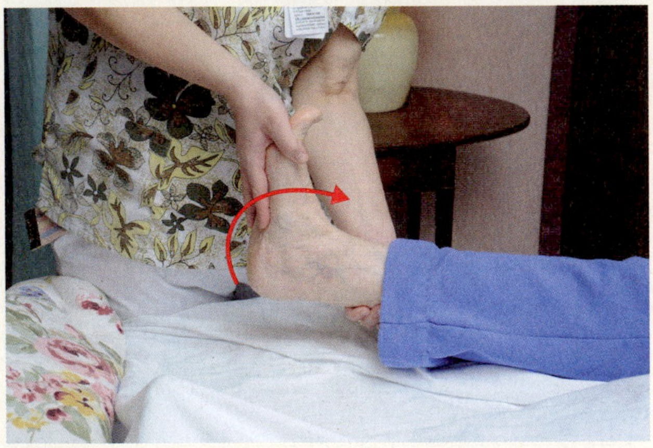

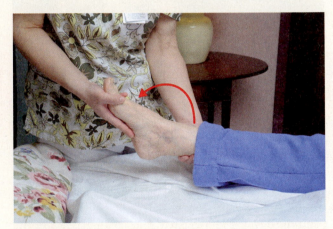

FIGURE 23–13A Dorsiflex the ankle by moving the toes and foot up toward the knee.

FIGURE 23–13B Plantar flex the ankle by moving the toes and foot down away from the knee.

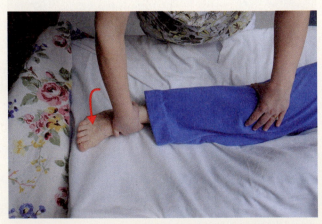

FIGURE 23–14A Invert the foot by gently turning it inward.

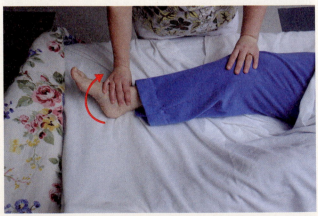

FIGURE 23–14B Evert the foot by gently turning it outward.

23. Wash hands.

24. Report and/or record all required information on the patient's chart or enter it into the computer. For example: date, time, ROM exercises performed on all joints, patient assisted with movements of arms and hands, and your signature and title. Report any unusual observations immediately.

Comm

 NOTE: In health care agencies using electronic health records (EHRs), the information is entered directly into the patient's record on a computer.

EHR

PRACTICE: Go to the workbook and use the evaluation sheet for 23:1, Performing Range-of-Motion (ROM) Exercises, to practice this procedure. When you believe you have mastered this skill, sign the sheet and give it to your instructor for further action.

✅ **FINAL EVALUATION:** Using the criteria listed on the evaluation sheet, your instructor will grade your performance.

Check

23:2 AMBULATING PATIENTS WHO USE TRANSFER (GAIT) BELTS, CRUTCHES, CANES, OR WALKERS

 Injuries and illness require many patients to use aids, or assistive devices, when ambulating. Athletes have trauma to their extremities frequently during athletic competition, requiring them to utilize aids like crutches. Although a variety of health care practitioners provide care to athletes, usually these injuries are initially assessed by athletic trainers. The trainer must arrive at a provisional diagnosis, provide initial treatment, determine if an urgent referral is needed for further evaluation, and finally, make a decision as to whether an athlete can safely return to play during the contest.

OBRA

Evaluation of on-field extremity injuries begins with a thorough history. The athletic trainer should question the athlete to learn the following information:

- identify the specific nature and location of their complaint

- determine how they were injured

- check the severity of the pain

- determine if they are able to bear weight on an injured leg or move an injured arm

- notice any instability, problems with joint motion, numbness, and/or weakness

- find out if there is any history of previous injuries to the injured and opposite extremity

The physical examination is directed to the entire injured extremity. The athletic trainer should first look for open injuries, any gross deformities, and soft tissue swelling. The surrounding joints should then be measured for active and passive range of motion and compared with the uninjured side. During this examination, any limitation of motion, point tenderness, abnormal skin temperature, discoloration, and/or a weak pulse should be noted. The injured area should be palpated carefully to identify any crepitus, swelling, or deformity. All adjacent ligaments should be examined, major tendons by the joint should be palpated, and the strength of major muscle groups in the extremity should be assessed. Those results should then be compared with the patient's uninjured side and any differences should be noted. After the athletic trainer evaluates all findings, they must then decide the type of treatment the injury requires. At times, treatment may be as simple as rest, a cold application, or supportive bandage. At other times, treatment might require a referral for x-ray imaging, medical care, and/or assistive devices such as crutches.

In addition to athletes, many other patients may require assistive devices. The type of assistive device used depends on the injury and the patient's condition. However, certain points must be observed when a patient uses crutches, canes, or a walker.

TRANSFER (GAIT) BELT

A **transfer (gait) belt** is a band of fabric or leather that is positioned around the patient's waist. During transfers or ambulation, the health care provider can grasp the transfer belt to provide additional support for the patient (**Figure 23–15**). The transfer belt helps provide the patient with a sense of security and helps to stabilize the patient's center of balance. Some important facts to remember when ambulating a patient with a transfer belt include the following:

- The transfer belt must be the proper size. It should fit securely around the waist for support but must not be too tight for comfort.

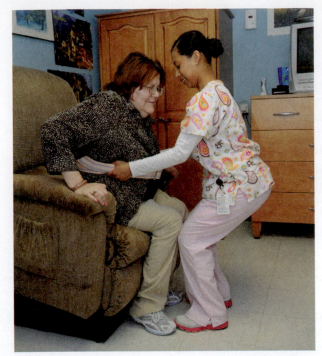

FIGURE 23–15 A transfer belt can provide support for the patient during transfers or ambulation.

- Some transfer belts contain loops that are grasped when ambulating the patient. If loops are not present, an underhand grasp should be used to hold on to the belt during ambulation. The underhand grasp is more secure than grasping the belt from the top, because the hands are less likely to slip off the belt.

- The belt should be grasped at the back during ambulation, and the health care provider should walk slightly behind the patient. When assisting a patient to stand, or during transfers such as transferring a patient to a wheelchair, grasp the belt on both sides while facing the patient.

- The transfer belt is applied over the patient's clothing. It should not be applied over bare skin because it can irritate the skin.

The use of a transfer belt is contraindicated in patients who have an ostomy, gastrostomy tube, abdominal pacemaker, severe cardiac or respiratory disease, fractured ribs, or recent surgery on the lower chest or abdominal area. It is also contraindicated for pregnant women.

CRUTCHES

Crutches are artificial supports that assist a patient who needs help walking. Crutches are usually prescribed by a physician. A physical therapist or other authorized individual fits the crutches to the patient and teaches the appropriate gait. In addition, exercises to strengthen the muscles of the shoulders, arms, and hands are frequently prescribed by the physician or therapist. Health care providers should be aware of the criteria for fitting crutches and of the gaits so that they can properly ambulate patients.

There are three main types of crutches:

- **Axillary crutches (Figure 23–16A):** These crutches are made of wood or aluminum and are used for patients who need crutches for a short period of time. The patient must be taught to bear weight on the hand bars instead of the axillary supports. If pressure is applied on the axillary bar, it can injure axillary blood vessels and nerves. They are *not* recommended for weak or elderly patients since axillary crutches require good upper body and arm strength, and a good sense of balance and coordination.

- **Forearm or Lofstrand crutches (Figure 23–16B):** These crutches attach to forearms, are used for patients with weakness or paralysis in both legs, are recommended for patients who need crutches permanently or for a long period of time, and require upper arm strength and good coordination.

- **Platform crutches (Figure 23–16C):** These crutches are used for patients who cannot grip handles of other crutches or bear weight on their wrists and hands. They do not require as much upper body strength, but do require a good sense of balance and coordination. They require that elbows be flexed at a 90-degree or right angle so the patient can bear weight on the forearm.

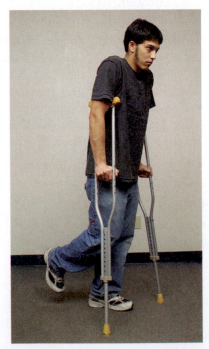

FIGURE 23–16A A patient using an axillary crutch must be taught to bear weight on the hand bars instead of on the axillary supports.

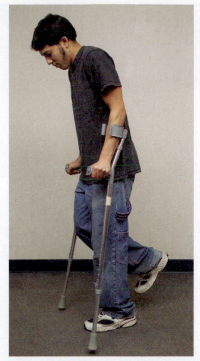

FIGURE 23–16B Forearm or Lofstrand crutches are recommended for patients who need crutches permanently or for a long period of time.

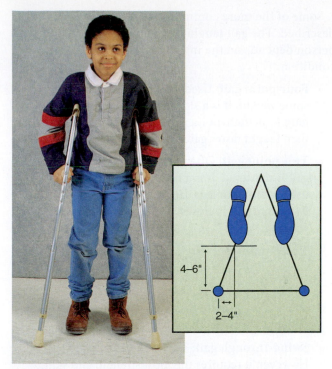

FIGURE 23–17 Crutches should be positioned 4–6 inches in front of and 2–4 inches to the side of the patient's foot.

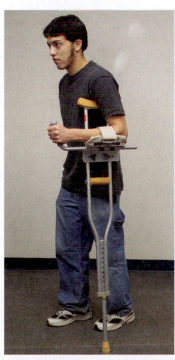

FIGURE 23–16C Platform crutches are used by patients who cannot grip the handles of other crutches or bear weight on the wrists and hands.

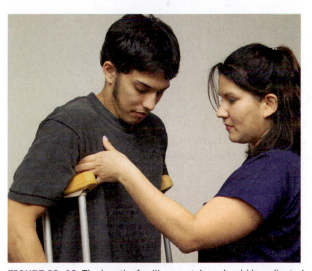

FIGURE 23–18 The length of axillary crutches should be adjusted so that there are 1 ½ to 2 inches or 2 to 3 finger widths between the axillary area and the top of the crutches.

The following points should be observed when fitting crutches to a patient.

- The patient should wear walking shoes that fit well and provide good support. The shoes should have low, broad heels approximately 1–1½ inches high and nonskid soles.

- The crutches should be positioned 4–6 inches in front of and 2–4 inches to the side of the patient's foot (**Figure 23–17**).

- The length of axillary crutches should be adjusted so that there are 1½–2 inches or 2–3 finger widths between the armpit and the axillary bar of the crutch (**Figure 23–18**).

- The handpieces of axillary or forearm crutches should be adjusted so that each elbow is flexed at a 25- to 30-degree angle.

Some of the more common crutch-walking gaits are described. The gait taught by the therapist or authorized person depends on the injury and the patient's condition.

- **Four-point gait**: Used when both legs can bear some weight. It is a slow gait. Patients often are taught the four-point gait as the first gait and are then taught faster gaits when this one is mastered.

- **Two-point gait**: Often taught after the four-point gait is mastered. It is a faster gait and is usually used when both legs can bear some weight. The two-point gait is closest to the natural rhythm of walking.

- **Three-point gait**: Used when only one leg can bear weight. It too is a gait taught initially.

- **Swing-to gait**: This is a more rapid gait. It is taught after other gaits are mastered. It requires that the patient have more shoulder and arm strength.

- **Swing-through gait**: This is the most rapid gait. However, it requires the most strength and skill. It is usually taught as a more advanced method of crutch walking.

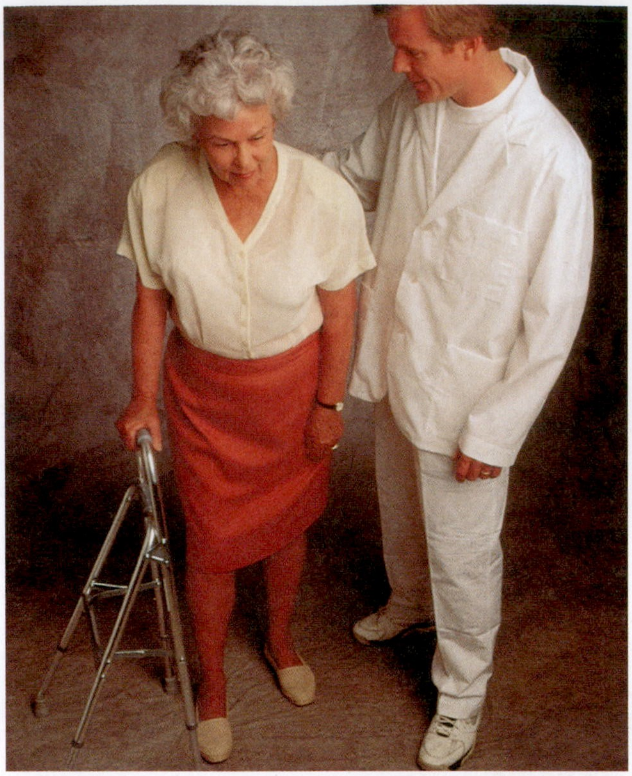

CANE

A **cane** is an assistive device that provides balance and support. There are several different types of canes (**Figure 23–19A**). *Standard* canes are single-tipped canes. They can have curved handles, T-handles, or J-handles with a handgrip. *Tripod* canes with three tips and *quad* canes with four tips provide a wider base of support and more stability for the patient. A *walkcane*, also called a *Hemiwalker*, has four legs and a handlebar

FIGURE 23–19B A walkcane has four legs and a handlebar that the patient can grip. Courtesy of Sunrise Medical

that the patient can grip (**Figure 23–19B**). It is used with patients who have *hemiplegia*, or paralysis on one side of the body. The bottom tip(s) of all canes should be fitted with a 1-inch rubber-suction tip to provide traction and prevent slipping.

Basic principles for using canes include:

- A cane is used on the unaffected (good) side (**Figure 23–19C**). In this way, a wider base of support is provided to increase stability. This prevents the patient from leaning toward the cane and falling because of the weak or injured leg. In addition, in normal walking, the leg and opposite arm move together, so the cane and leg will follow the same pattern.

- Canes must be correctly fitted. The bottom tip of the cane should be positioned approximately 6–8 inches from the side of the unaffected foot. The cane handle should be level with the top of the femur at the hip joint. The patient's elbow should be flexed at a 25- to 30-degree angle.

- Several gaits for cane walking can be taught. In a two-point gait, the patient is taught to move the cane and affected leg together, and then move the unaffected leg. In a three-point gait, the patient is taught to move the cane, then the affected or involved leg, and finally the unaffected leg. The therapist or other authorized person determines the correct gait.

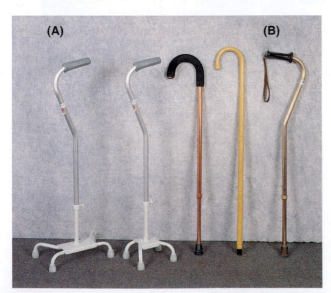

FIGURE 23–19A Different types of canes: (A) quad canes; (B) single-tipped canes.

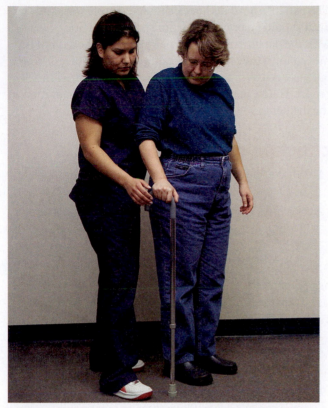

FIGURE 23–19C A cane is used on the unaffected (good) side to provide a wider base of support.

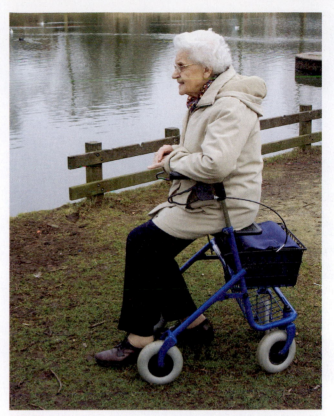

FIGURE 23–20 Some walkers have wheels and a seat, but a patient must be evaluated carefully before this type of walker is used. © iStock.com/Els van der Gun

WALKER

A **walker** is a four-legged device that provides support. Walkers are available in several styles, including standard, folding, rolling, and platform. Rolling walkers have wheels and are easily pushed by a patient who uses a walker primarily for balance. However, if a patient leans on the walker for support, the wheels can be dangerous because the walker may move away from the patient, causing the patient to fall. Some rolling walkers have brakes on the wheels that lock automatically when weight is placed downward on the walker. The patient must be evaluated carefully before a rolling walker is used (**Figure 23–20**).

Walkers often are used for weak patients who have a poor sense of balance even though no leg injuries may be present. To use a walker, patients must be strong enough to hold themselves upright while leaning on the walker. Basic principles for using a walker include:

- The walker should be fitted to the patient. The handles should be level with the top of the femurs at the hip joints. Each elbow should be flexed at a 25- to 30-degree angle.

- The patient must be taught to lift the walker and place it in front of the body. It should be positioned so that the back legs of the walker are even with the toes of the patient. The patient then walks "into" the walker.

- All legs of the walker should be fitted with rubber tips to prevent slipping.

 CAUTION: *The patient should be cautioned against sliding the walker. A sliding technique may be dangerous because it can easily tip over the walker. Most walkers are made of lightweight aluminum, so most patients are capable of lifting them.*
Safety

 CAUTION: *Patients must also be cautioned against using the walker as a transfer device. If they try to hold on to the walker while getting out of bed or up from a chair, the walker can tip forward, causing the patient to fall. Patients should be taught how to use their arms to push against the bed or arms of a chair to rise to a standing position.*
Safety

AMBULATION PRECAUTIONS

 It is essential that the health care provider remain alert at all times when ambulating a patient. Always walk on the patient's weak side and slightly behind the patient, and be alert for signs that the patient may fall. If the patient starts to fall, do *not* try to hold the patient in an upright position. Use your body to brace the patient, if at all possible. Keep your back straight, bend from the hips and knees, maintain a broad base of support, and try to grasp the patient under the axillary (armpit) areas. If the patient is wearing a transfer belt, keep a firm hold on the belt. The patient should be eased to the floor as slowly as possible (**Figure 23–21**).
Safety

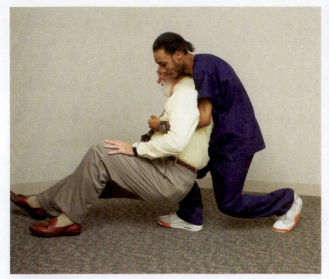

FIGURE 23–21 Ease a falling patient to the floor as slowly as possible. Try to protect the patient's head and neck.

The patient's head and neck should be protected, and the head should be prevented from striking the floor. Stay with the patient and call for help. Patients should not be moved until they have been examined for injuries. After a fall has occurred, most agencies require a written incident report. Follow agency policy for correct documentation of the incident.

checkpoint

1. What are two (2) contraindications to using a gait belt?
2. Is a cane used on the affected or unaffected side of the body?

PRACTICE: Go to the workbook and complete the assignment sheet for 23:2, Ambulating Patients Who Use Transfer (Gait) Belts, Crutches, Canes, or Walkers. Then return and continue with the procedures.

Procedure 23:2A
OBRA

Ambulating a Patient with a Transfer (Gait) Belt

Equipment and Supplies

Transfer or gait belt, paper and pen and/or computer

Procedure

1. Check orders or obtain authorization from your immediate supervisor for ambulating the patient.
2. Assemble supplies.
3. Knock on the door and pause before entering. Introduce yourself. Identify the patient, explain the procedure, and obtain consent.
   Comm
4. Close the door and pull the curtain to provide privacy.
5. Wash hands.
6. Lock the wheels on the bed to prevent movement. If siderails are present and elevated, lower the siderail on the side where you are working.
7. Assist the patient into a sitting position. If the patient is wearing bedclothes, put a robe on the patient.
8. Check to be sure the transfer belt is the correct size. Position the belt around the patient's waist and on top of the clothing (**Figure 23–22A**). Position the buckle or clasp so that it is slightly off center in the front. Make sure the belt is smooth and free of wrinkles.

    CAUTION: *Never* apply the belt over the bare skin because it will irritate the skin.
   Safety

9. Tighten the belt so that it fits snugly; secure the clasp or buckle. Place three to four fingers under the belt to make sure it is not too tight (**Figure 23–22B**). Make sure the belt is comfortable and does not interfere with breathing. On a female patient, make sure the breasts are not under the belt.

10. Put shoes or slippers on the patient. For the most security, shoes should be worn. The shoes should have low, broad heels approximately 1–1½ inches high and nonskid soles. Make sure the patient's feet are on the floor. If the patient's feet are not on the floor, move the patient closer to the side of the bed or edge of a chair.

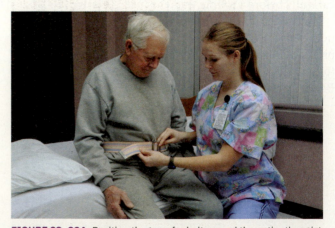

FIGURE 23–22A Position the transfer belt around the patient's waist and on top of the clothing.

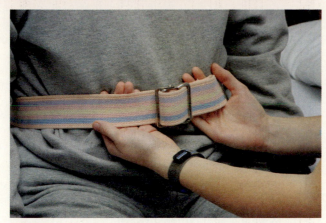

FIGURE 23–22B Check the transfer belt to make sure it is not too tight.

11.
Comm
Assist the patient to a standing position. Face the patient and get a broad base of support. Grasp the loops on the side of the belt or place your hands under the sides of the belt. Ask the patient to assist by pushing against the bed with their hands at a given signal, such as "one, two, three, stand." Bend at your knees and give the signal for the patient to stand. Keep your back straight and straighten your knees as the patient stands (**Figure 23–22C**).

⚠ Safety **CAUTION:** Use correct body mechanics at all times.

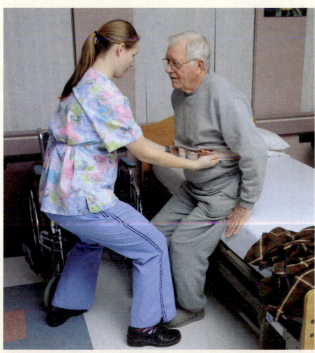

FIGURE 23–22C Place your hands under the sides of the belt and use proper body mechanics as you help the patient to a standing position.

12. To ambulate the patient, support the patient in a standing position. Keep one hand on one side of the belt while moving the other hand to the loops or the back of the belt. Then, move the second hand from the side to the loops or the back of the belt while you move behind the patient.

⚠ Safety **CAUTION:** Keep one hand firmly on the belt at all times when changing position.

13. Ambulate the patient. Encourage the patient to walk slowly and use handrails, if available. Walk slightly behind the patient at all times and keep a firm, underhand grip on the belt or keep your hands firmly in the loops.

NOTE: If the patient has a weak side, position yourself on the patient's weak side.

14. If the patient starts to fall, keep a firm grip on the belt. Use your body to brace the patient. Keep your back straight. Gently ease the patient to the floor, taking care to protect their head. Stay with the patient and call for help. Do not try to stand the patient up until help arrives and the patient has been examined for injuries.

15. When ambulation is complete, assist the patient in returning to bed. Remove the transfer belt.

16. Observe all checkpoints before leaving the patient. Make sure the patient is comfortable and in good body alignment. Elevate the siderails (if indicated), lower the bed to its lowest level, place the call signal and supplies within easy reach of the patient, and leave the area neat and clean.

17. Replace all equipment.

18. Wash hands.

19.
Comm
Report and/or record all required information on the patient's chart or enter it into the computer. For example: date, time, ambulated with a transfer belt, walked down to lounge and back, and your signature and title. Report any problems immediately.

🏢 EHR **NOTE:** In health care agencies using electronic health records (EHRs), the information is entered directly into the patient's record on a computer.

PRACTICE: Go to the workbook and use the evaluation sheet for 23:2A, Ambulating a Patient with a Transfer (Gait) Belt, to practice this procedure. When you believe you have mastered this skill, sign the sheet and give it to your instructor for further action.

✅ Check **FINAL EVALUATION:** Using the criteria listed on the evaluation sheet, your instructor will grade your performance.

Ambulating a Patient Who Uses Crutches

Equipment and Supplies

Adjustable crutches, paper and pen and/or computer

Procedure

1. Check orders or obtain authorization from your immediate supervisor. Ascertain which gait the therapist taught the patient.

2. Assemble equipment.

3. Check the crutches. Make sure there are rubber-suction tips on the bottom ends and that the tips are not worn down or torn. Check to be sure the axillary bars and hand rests are covered with padding.

   NOTE: Foam-rubber pads are usually placed on crutches.

4. Knock on the door and pause before entering. Introduce yourself. Identify the patient. Explain the procedure and obtain consent.

   Comm

5. Wash hands.

6. Help the patient put on good walking shoes. The shoes should have low, broad heels approximately 1–1½ inches high and nonskid soles.

7. Place a transfer (gait) belt on the patient. Use an underhand grasp on the belt and assist the patient to a standing position. Advise the patient to bear their weight on the unaffected leg. Position the crutches correctly.

8. Check the fit of the crutches.

   a. Position the crutches 4–6 inches in front of the patient's feet.

   b. Move the crutches 2–4 inches to the sides of the feet.

   c. Make sure there is a 1½ to 2-inch or 2 to 3 finger widths gap between the axilla (armpit) and the axillary bar or rest. If the length must be adjusted, check with your immediate supervisor.

   d. Each elbow must be flexed at a 25- to 30-degree angle. If the hand rests must be adjusted to achieve this angle, check with your immediate supervisor.

      NOTE: In some agencies, the trained health care provider is permitted to adjust the crutches as necessary. The adjustments are then checked by the therapist or other authorized person. Follow your agency policy.

      Legal

9. Assist the patient with the required gait. The gait used depends on the patient's injury and condition, and is determined by the therapist or other authorized person.

   ⚠ **CAUTION:** Remain alert at all times. Be ready to catch the patient if there are any signs of falling.
   Safety

10. Four-point gait (**Figure 23–23**):

    a. The patient can bear weight on both legs. Start the patient in a standing position, with crutches at the sides.

    b. Move the right crutch forward.

    c. Move the left foot forward.

    d. Move the left crutch forward.

    e. Move the right foot forward.

    NOTE: This is a slow gait taught initially when both legs can bear weight.

11. Three-point gait (**Figure 23–24**):

    a. The patient can bear weight on one leg only. Start the patient in a standing position, with crutches at the sides.

    b. Advance both crutches and the weak or affected foot.

    c. Transfer the patient's body weight forward to the crutches.

    d. Advance the unaffected, or good, foot forward.

    NOTE: This is a slow gait taught initially when only one leg can bear weight.

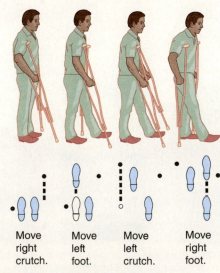

Move right crutch. | Move left foot. | Move left crutch. | Move right foot.

FIGURE 23–23 Four-point gait for crutches.

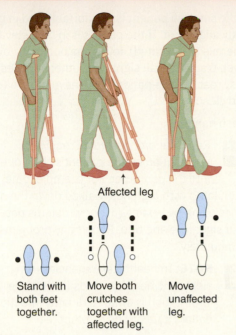

FIGURE 23–24 Three-point gait for crutches.

12. Two-point gait (**Figure 23–25**):

    a. The patient can bear weight on both legs. Start with the crutches at the sides.

    b. Move the right foot and left crutch forward at the same time.

    c. Move the left foot and right crutch forward at the same time.

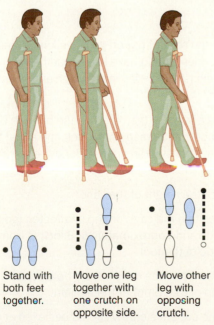

FIGURE 23–25 Two-point gait for crutches.

NOTE: This is a more advanced and a more rapid gait used when the four-point gait has been mastered.

NOTE: The two-point gait is closest to the natural rhythm of walking.

13. Swing-to gait:

    a. One or both of the patient's legs can bear weight. Start with the crutches at the sides.

    b. Balance weight on foot or feet. Move both crutches forward.

    c. Transfer weight forward.

    d. Use shoulder and arm strength to swing feet up to crutches.

NOTE: This is a more rapid gait and requires more shoulder and arm strength and a good sense of balance and coordination.

14. Swing-through gait (**Figure 23–26**):

    a. One or both of the patient's legs can bear weight. Start with the crutches at the sides. Balance weight on foot or feet.

    b. Advance both crutches forward at the same time.

    c. Transfer weight forward.

    d. Use shoulder and arm strength to swing up to and through the crutches, stopping slightly in front of the crutches.

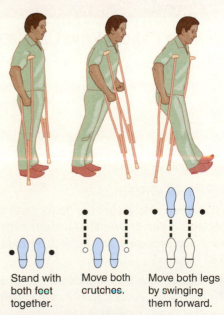

FIGURE 23–26 Swing-through gait for crutches.

(continues)

NOTE: This is the most rapid and advanced gait. It requires a great deal of shoulder and arm strength. It also requires an excellent sense of balance because at one point only the crutches are in contact with the ground.

15. When using crutches, the patient must *not* rest their body weight on the axillary rests. Shoulder and arm strength should provide movement on the crutches.

     CAUTION: Warn the patient that nerve damage can occur if weight is supported constantly on the axillary rest.

    Safety

16. Check to make sure that the patient is not moving too far forward at one time. Distances should be limited. If the patient attempts to move the crutches too far forward, they can very easily lose balance and fall forward.

17. Check the patient's progress. Report the progress to the therapist or your immediate supervisor. The therapist will determine when to teach the patient more advanced gaits.

    Comm

18. When the patient is finished using the crutches, replace all equipment.

19. Assist the patient back to bed or position the patient in a chair. Remove the transfer belt. Observe all checkpoints before leaving the patient.

Make sure the patient is comfortable and in good body alignment. If the patient is in bed, elevate the siderails (if indicated), lower the bed to its lowest level, place the call signal and other supplies within easy reach of the patient, and leave the area neat and clean.

20. Wash hands.

21. Report and/or record all required information on the patient's chart or enter it into the computer. For example: date, time, ambulated with crutches, walked down the hall two times using two-point gait, no problems noted, and your signature and title. Report any problems immediately.

    Comm

    NOTE: In health care agencies using electronic health records (EHRs), the information is entered directly into the patient's record on a computer.

    EHR

PRACTICE: Go to the workbook and use the evaluation sheet for 23:2B, Ambulating a Patient Who Uses Crutches, to practice this procedure. When you believe you have mastered this skill, sign the sheet and give it to your instructor for further action.

✅ **FINAL EVALUATION:** Using the criteria listed on the evaluation sheet, your instructor will grade your performance.

Check

Procedure 23:2C ⚖️
OBRA

Ambulating a Patient Who Uses a Cane

Equipment and Supplies

Adjustable cane, paper and pen and/or computer

Procedure

1. Check orders or obtain authorization from your immediate supervisor. Ascertain which gait the therapist taught the patient.

2. Assemble equipment.

3. Check the cane. Make sure the bottom has a rubber-suction tip. If the patient needs extra stability, use a tripod (three-legged) or quad (four-legged) cane.

4. Knock on the door and pause before entering. Introduce yourself. Identify the patient. Explain the procedure and obtain consent.

    Comm

5. Wash hands.

6. Help the patient put on good walking shoes. The shoes should have low, broad heels approximately 1–1½ inches high and nonskid soles.

7. Place a transfer (gait) belt on the patient. Use an underhand grasp on the belt and assist the patient to a standing position. Advise the patient to bear their weight on the unaffected leg.

8. Check the height of the cane:

    a. Position the cane on the unaffected (good) side and approximately 6–8 inches from the side of the foot.

    b. The top of the cane should be level with the top of the femur at the hip joint.

    c. The patient's elbow should be flexed at a 25- to 30-degree angle.

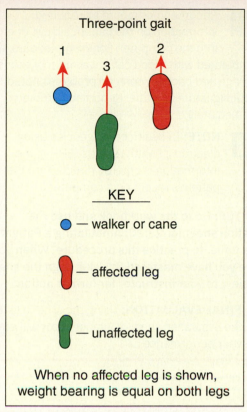

FIGURE 23–27A Three-point gait for canes.

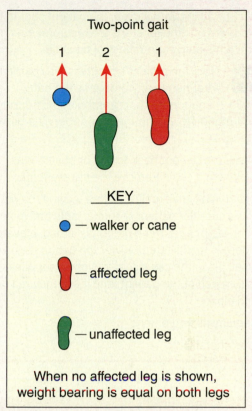

FIGURE 23–27B Two-point gait for canes.

🏛️ **Legal**

NOTE: If the height of the cane needs adjustment, follow agency policy. In some agencies, only the therapist adjusts canes. In other agencies, the trained health care provider can adjust canes.

9. Instruct the patient to use the cane on the good, or unaffected, side.

   NOTE: This prevents leaning toward the weak or affected side and provides a broader base of support.

10. Assist the patient with the gait ordered. For a three-point gait (**Figure 23–27A**):

   a. Balance the body weight on the strong or unaffected foot. Move the cane forward approximately 12–18 inches.

   b. Move the weak or affected foot forward.

   c. Transfer the weight to the affected foot and cane. Bring the unaffected foot forward.

11. For a two-point gait (**Figure 23–27B**):

   a. Balance the weight on the strong or unaffected foot.

   b. Move the cane and the weak or affected foot forward. Keep the cane fairly close to the body to prevent leaning.

   c. Transfer body weight forward to the cane.

   d. Move the good, or unaffected, foot forward.

⚠️ **Safety**

   CAUTION: Remain alert at all times. Be ready to catch the patient if there are any signs of falling.

   NOTE: Maintain an underhand grasp on the transfer belt if the patient is not steady.

12. A common sequence to follow when assisting the patient up and down stairs is as follows:

   a. Encourage the patient to hold onto the hand rail at all times and to hold the cane in the other hand.

   b. To go up steps, step up with the unaffected or strong leg first.

   c. Then bring the cane and weak or affected leg up.

   d. To go down steps, reverse this order. Move the cane and weak or affected foot down first.

   e. Then step down with the unaffected or good leg.

   NOTE: Remember this sequence by saying, "Go up with the good, down with the bad."

(continues)

13. When walking with a cane, the patient should take small steps. Smaller steps are recommended to prevent leaning and/or loss of balance.

14. Note the patient's progress. Pay particular attention to any problems the patient experiences during ambulation. Report this information to your immediate supervisor or the therapist.

15. Assist the patient back to bed or position the patient in a chair. Remove the transfer belt.

16. Observe all checkpoints before leaving the patient. Make sure the patient is comfortable and in good body alignment. If the patient is in bed, elevate the siderails (if indicated), lower the bed to its lowest level, place the call signal and other supplies within easy reach of the patient, and leave the area neat and clean.

17. Replace all equipment.

18. Wash hands.

19. Report and/or record all required information on the patient's chart or enter it into the computer. For example: date, time, ambulated with tripod cane, walked to visitor's lounge and back to room, no problems noted, and your signature and title. Report any problems immediately.

NOTE: In health care agencies using electronic health records (EHRs), the information is entered directly into the patient's record on a computer.

PRACTICE: Go to the workbook and use the evaluation sheet for 23:2C, Ambulating a Patient Who Uses a Cane, to practice this procedure. When you believe you have mastered this skill, sign the sheet and give it to your instructor for further action.

✅ **FINAL EVALUATION:** Using the criteria listed on the evaluation sheet, your instructor will grade your performance.

Procedure 23:2D

Ambulating a Patient Who Uses a Walker

Equipment and Supplies

Adjustable walker, paper and pen and/or computer

Procedure

1. Check orders or obtain authorization from your immediate supervisor for ambulating the patient.

2. Assemble equipment.

3. Check the walker. Make sure rubber-suction tips are secure on all of the legs. Check for rough or damaged edges on the hand rests.

4. Knock on the door and pause before entering. Introduce yourself. Identify the patient. Explain the procedure and obtain consent.

5. Wash hands.

6. Help the patient put on good walking shoes. The shoes should have low, broad heels approximately 1–1½ inches high and nonskid soles.

7. Place a transfer (gait) belt on the patient. Use an underhand grasp on the belt and assist the patient to a standing position. Position the walker correctly and ask the patient to grasp the hand rests securely.

8. Check the height of the walker to see whether the following requirements are met (**Figure 23–28A**):

   a. The hand rests are level with the tops of the femurs at the hip joints.

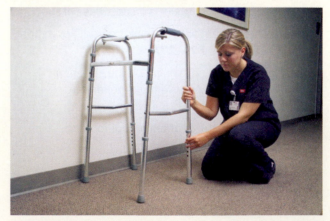

FIGURE 23–28A Check the adjustment of the walker to make sure it is the correct height for the patient.

b. The elbows are flexed at 25- to 30-degree angles.

NOTE: If the height of the walker needs adjustment, follow agency policy. In some agencies, only the therapist makes such adjustments. In other agencies, a trained health care worker may adjust walkers.

9. Start with the walker in position. The patient should be standing "inside" the walker.

10. Tell the patient to lift the walker and place it forward so that the back legs of the walker are even with the patient's toes.

CAUTION: Tell the patient to avoid sliding the walker. The walker could fall forward and cause the patient to fall.

11. Instruct the patient to transfer their weight forward slightly to the walker.

12. Instruct the patient to use the walker for support and to walk "into" the walker (**Figure 23–28B**). Do *not* allow the patient to "shuffle" their feet.

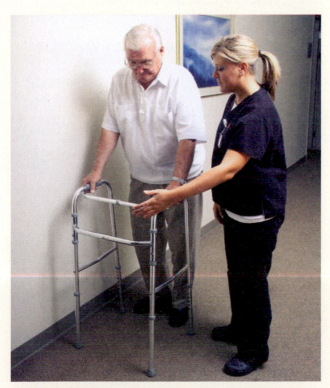

FIGURE 23–28B Instruct the patient to use the walker for support while walking "into" the walker.

13. Repeat steps 10–12. While the patient is using the walker, walk to the side and slightly behind the patient. Be alert at all times. Be ready to catch the patient if there are any signs of falling.

NOTE: If the patient has a weak side, position yourself on the patient's weak side. Keep a firm grip on the transfer belt.

14. Check constantly to make sure the patient is lifting the walker to move it forward. Also make sure the patient is placing the walker forward just to their toes and not attempting too large a step.

15. Note the patient's progress. Pay particular attention to any problems the patient experiences during ambulation. Report this information to your immediate supervisor or the therapist.

16. Assist the patient back to bed or position the patient in a chair. Remove the transfer belt.

17. Observe all checkpoints before leaving the patient. Make sure the patient is comfortable and in good body alignment. If the patient is in bed, elevate the siderails (if indicated), lower the bed to its lowest level, place the call signal and other supplies within easy reach of the patient, and leave the area neat and clean.

18. Replace all equipment.

19. Wash hands.

20. Report and/or record all required information on the patient's chart or enter it into the computer. For example: date, time, ambulated with walker, walked down the hall and back two times, needs encouragement to pick up walker and not slide it, and your signature and title. Report any problems immediately.

NOTE: In health care agencies using electronic health records (EHRs), the information is entered directly into the patient's record on a computer.

PRACTICE: Go to the workbook and use the evaluation sheet for 23:2D, Ambulating a Patient Who Uses a Walker, to practice this procedure. When you believe you have mastered this skill, sign the sheet and give it to your instructor for further action.

FINAL EVALUATION: Using the criteria listed on the evaluation sheet, your instructor will grade your performance.

ADMINISTERING
HEAT/COLD
APPLICATIONS

As a health care provider, you may be responsible for administering a variety of heat and cold applications. Some of the main principles involved are described in this section.

Cryotherapy is the use of cold for treatment. Cold applications are administered to relieve pain, reduce swelling and inflammation, reduce body temperature, and control bleeding.

- **Moist cold** applications are cold and moist or wet against the skin. Examples are cold **compresses**, packs, and soaks. These applications are more penetrating than are dry cold applications.

- **Dry cold** applications are cold and dry against the skin. Examples are ice bags, ice collars, hypothermia blankets, gel packs that are cooled in the freezer, and similar devices.

- **Ice bags** or **collars** are special containers filled with ice. Most health care facilities use disposable bags to prevent the spread of infection (**Figure 23–29**). A hit or push on the surface of the bag activates the chemical and the bag gets cold. Read and follow the instructions on the bag to activate it.

- **Hypothermia blankets**, also called *thermal blankets*, contain coils that are filled with cool fluid. They are used to reduce high body temperatures. A rectal probe is usually used to monitor the patient's temperature. When the patient's temperature reaches a preset level, the blanket decreases the circulation of the cooling fluid.

Thermotherapy is the use of heat for treatment. Heat applications are administered to relieve pain, increase drainage from an infected area, stimulate healing, increase circulation to an area, combat infection, relieve muscle spasms, and increase muscle mobility before exercise.

- **Moist heat** applications are warm and wet against the skin. These applications are more penetrating and more effective in relieving pain in deeper tissues than are dry heat applications. Examples are the Sitz bath, hot soaks, compresses, hydrocollator packs, and paraffin wax treatments.

- **Sitz baths** provide warm moist heat to the perineal and rectal area. They are used postpartum (after birth) and after rectal surgery to provide comfort and promote healing. Most agencies use portable units that are placed on the base of a toilet and filled with the correct temperature of water usually 105°F or 41°C (**Figure 23–30**).

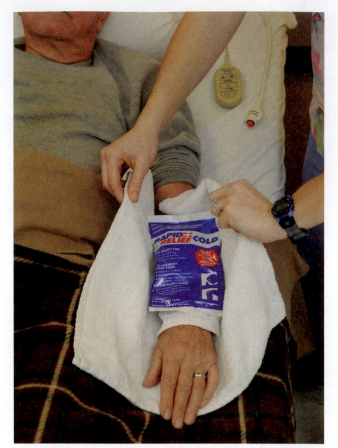

FIGURE 23–29 Most health care facilities use disposable ice bags to prevent the spread of infection. A towel or cover must be used because the bags should not be placed directly on the skin.

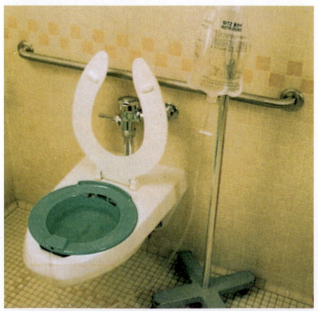

FIGURE 23–30 A portable Sitz bath unit is positioned on the base of the toilet after the seat is elevated.

- **Hydrocollator packs** are gel-filled packs that are warmed in a water bath at a temperature of 150°F–170° F, or 65.6°C–76.7° C. The gel maintains the warmth for approximately 30–40 minutes, and the pack can be contoured to fit smoothly over any area of the body (**Figure 23–31**). The pack must be covered with a thick terry cloth or flannel cover before being applied to the skin. Hydrocollator packs are frequently used prior to ROM exercises.

- **Paraffin wax treatments** are often used for chronic joint disease, such as arthritis, or prior to ROM exercises. A mixture of paraffin and a small amount of mineral oil are heated to the melting point. The physical therapist or authorized individual dips the patient's hand(s) or other body part into the warm paraffin three or four times to create a "glove" of wax (**Figure 23–32A**). The wax is left in place for 20–30 minutes before being peeled off (**Figure 23–32B**).

- **Dry heat** applications are warm and dry against the skin. Examples are warm-water bags, heating pads, thermal blankets, gel packs that are warmed in the microwave, aquamatic pads or aquathermia pads, and heat lamps.

- **Warm-water bags** are special containers filled with warm water to provide heat to body parts. Most health care agencies use disposable bags to prevent the spread of infection. A hit or push on the surface of the bag activates the chemical and the bag gets warm. Read and follow the instructions on the bag to activate it.

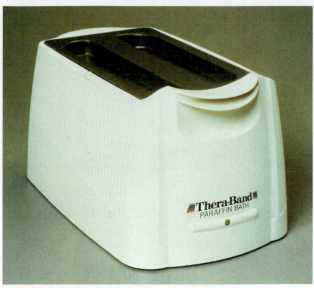

FIGURE 23–32A A body part is dipped into the paraffin bath three or four times to create a layer of warm wax on the skin. Courtesy of Briggs Corporation, Des Moines, IA

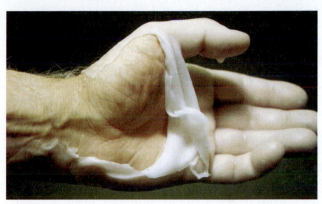

FIGURE 23–32B After the wax has been in place for 20–30 minutes, it is peeled off and discarded.

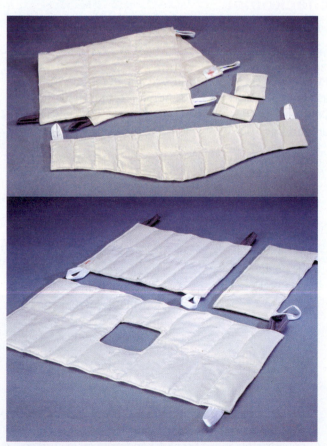

FIGURE 23–31 Hydrocollator packs are gel-filled packs that are warmed in a water bath. Courtesy of Briggs Corporation, Des Moines, IA

- **Thermal blankets** contain coils that can be filled with air or fluid to warm or cool a patient (**Figure 23–33**). Usually, a rectal probe is used to monitor the patient's temperature. The unit automatically circulates warm or cool fluid or air to maintain a preset temperature.

- **Aquathermia pads**, also called *aquamatic units* or *K-pads*, are smaller pads that contain coils that fill with warm water. A control unit maintains a constant preset temperature of the water.

 Heat and cold applications are effective because of the reactions they cause in the
Science   blood vessels.

- Heat applications cause **vasodilation**. The blood vessels in the area become larger (dilated). More blood comes to the area. Therefore, more oxygen and nutrients are available to stimulate healing. Heat applications ease pain by allowing the blood to carry away fluids that cause inflammation and pain.

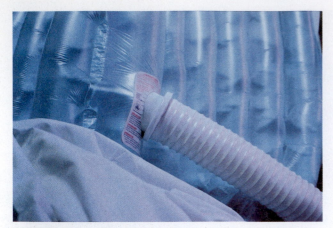

FIGURE 23–33 A thermal blanket contains coils that are filled with water or air to warm or cool the body.

- Cold applications cause **vasoconstriction**. The blood vessels become smaller (constricted). Less blood comes to the area. Swelling decreases because fewer fluids are present. The cold also has a numbing effect, which decreases local pain.

Legal A physician's order is required for a heat or cold application. The order should state the type of application, duration of treatment, temperature (if not standard), and area of application. In some states and agencies, health care assistants are not allowed to administer heat or cold applications. It is important to check your agency's policy and be aware of your legal responsibilities.

Safety **CAUTION:** *The patient must be checked frequently when an application is in place. Color and temperature of the skin, amount of pain and bleeding, effect on circulation, and other signs and symptoms must be noted. Special attention must be* given to infants, young children, and elderly patients, because the skin of these patients is less resistant and burns or injuries can occur rapidly. Metal objects, such as rings, bracelets, necklaces, watches, and zippers, readily conduct heat or cold. Patients should be asked to remove all metal objects in the treated area before a heat or cold application is administered. When administering heat or cold applications, the rubber or plastic should never come in contact with the skin. All rubber or plastic applications should be covered with a towel or special cloth cover. If any abnormal symptoms are noted, the application should be discontinued and the immediate supervisor notified. The health care provider must be alert at all times and observe all safety precautions when administering heat and cold applications.*

 Precaution Standard precautions (discussed in Section 15:4) must be observed if any contact with blood, body fluids, secretions, or excretions is possible. An example is a moist heat application placed on a draining wound. Gloves must be worn. Hands must be washed frequently and are always washed immediately after removing gloves. A gown, mask or face shield, and eye protection must be worn if splashing or spraying of body fluids is possible. A health care provider must always use proper precautions to prevent the spread of infection.

checkpoint

1. List four (4) ways to apply cryotherapy.

2. Is vasodilation caused by heat or cold applications?

PRACTICE: Go to the workbook and complete the assignment sheet for 23:3, Administering Heat/Cold Applications. Then return and continue with the procedures.

Procedure 23:3A

Applying an Ice Bag or Ice Collar

Equipment and Supplies

Ice collar or ice bag and cap, cover or towel, tape, ice in basin, scoop or paper cup, paper and pen and/or computer.

Procedure

1. Check physician's orders or obtain authorization from your immediate supervisor for the application.

2. Assemble equipment.

3. Wash hands.

4. Fill the ice bag or collar with water. Check for leaks. Empty if no leaks are present.

NOTE: Ice bags come in various sizes for different parts of the body. An ice collar is narrow and is used on the throat.

5. Use the scoop to fill the ice bag or collar half full (**Figure 23–34A**). To assist in filling, a paper cup with the bottom cut out can be placed in the neck of the bag and used as a funnel. Ice can then be scooped into the bag.

NOTE: If ice cubes are used, rinse them with water to remove sharp edges.

NOTE: In most agencies, disposable cold packs are used. To activate the chemicals in the cold pack, squeeze the pack or strike it against a solid surface. It does not need to be filled with ice. Read and follow the instructions on the bag. A cover must still be placed on the disposable cold pack because the plastic and cold can injure the skin.

CAUTION: Chemical ice packs are *not* recommended for use on the face or head because of the danger of leaking chemicals.

NOTE: Gel packs that are stored in the freezer can also be used. The gel pack must be covered because the plastic and cold can injure the skin. These packs can be reused many times for the same patient. In a health care agency, the pack should be labeled with the patient's name so it is not used on another patient.

6. Place the bag on a table or flat surface. Push gently on the bag to expel all air (**Figure 23–34B**). Tighten the cap.

   NOTE: If a rubber ring is present on the cap, make sure the ring is secure; it prevents leakage.

7. Wipe the outside of the bag dry.

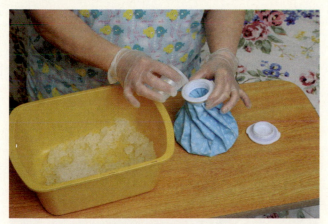
FIGURE 23–34A Fill the ice bag half full.

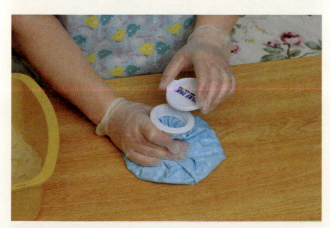
FIGURE 23–34B Push gently on the bag to expel all air before tightening the cap.

8. Place a cover on the bag. If an ice bag or ice collar cover is not available, use a towel. Tape the towel in place.

    CAUTION: The bag *must* be covered. The rubber or plastic and the extreme cold can injure the skin.
   Safety

9. Knock on the door and pause before entering. Introduce yourself. Identify the patient. Explain the procedure and obtain consent.
   Comm

10. Wash hands. Put on gloves if necessary.

     CAUTION: Wear gloves and observe standard precautions if the area to be treated has any drainage of blood, body fluids, secretions, or excretions.
    Precaution

11. Place the ice bag gently on the affected area as ordered. If the cap is metal, make sure it is not on the patient's skin.

    NOTE: Metal will intensify the cold. If the cold metal cap rests on the patient's skin, an injury can occur.

12. Make sure the patient is comfortable and the ice application is positioned correctly before leaving. Place the call signal within easy reach of the patient. Remove gloves, if worn, and wash hands before leaving the room.

13. Recheck the patient at least every 10 minutes. Make sure the bag is cold and refill it as needed. Check the condition of the skin. Check for pale or white skin, cyanosis (bluish color), or a mottled appearance. Ask the patient about numbness and pain.

     CAUTION: If the skin is mottled or very discolored, or the patient complains of pain, remove the bag immediately and inform your immediate supervisor.
    Safety

14. Leave the ice application in place for the length of time ordered. In some cases, continuous application is ordered; in others, a specific time period, such as 20 minutes, is ordered. Remove the bag when the designated time has elapsed.

15. Carefully check the condition of the patient's skin. Note any comments the patient makes about the treatment. Report these to your supervisor.
    Comm

16. Observe all checkpoints before leaving the patient: position the patient in correct body alignment, elevate the siderails (if indicated), lower the bed to its lowest level, place the call signal and supplies within easy reach of the patient, and leave the area neat and clean.

(continues)

17. If the ice bag is disposable, discard it. If it is a gel pack, wipe it with a disinfectant, label it with the patient's name, and return it to the freezer. If the ice bag is not disposable, empty it and clean it thoroughly. Wipe it with a disinfectant, rinse, and dry. Inflate it with air before storing. This prevents the sides from sticking. Replace all equipment.

18. Remove gloves, if worn. Wash hands.

19. 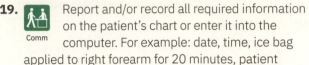 Report and/or record all required information on the patient's chart or enter it into the computer. For example: date, time, ice bag applied to right forearm for 20 minutes, patient states arm feels better, and your signature and title. Report any unusual observations immediately.

 NOTE: In health care agencies using electronic health records (EHRs), the information is entered directly into the patient's record on a computer.

PRACTICE: Go to the workbook and use the evaluation sheet for 23:3A, Applying an Ice Bag or Ice Collar, to practice this procedure. When you believe you have mastered this skill, sign the sheet and give it to your instructor for further action.

 FINAL EVALUATION: Using the criteria listed on the evaluation sheet, your instructor will grade your performance.

Procedure 23:3B

Applying a Warm-Water Bag

Equipment and Supplies

Warm-water bag, cover or towel for bag, tape, measuring graduate or pitcher, bath thermometer, paper and pen and/or computer.

Procedure

1. Check physician's orders or obtain authorization from your immediate supervisor for the application.

2. Assemble equipment.

3. Wash hands.

4. Check for leaks by filling the warm-water bag with tap water or air. Expel the water or air if no leaks are present.

5. Fill the pitcher with water at a temperature of 110°F–120°F, or 43°C–49°C. Use the bath thermometer to check the temperature (**Figure 23–35A**).

    CAUTION: The temperature should not exceed 120°F, or 49°C.

   NOTE: Temperatures may vary. Follow agency policy.

   NOTE: In most agencies, disposable heat packs are used. To activate the chemicals in the heat pack, squeeze the pack or strike it against a solid surface. It does not need to be filled with hot water. Read and follow the instructions on the bag. A cover must still be placed on the disposable heat pack because the plastic and heat can injure the skin.

 CAUTION: Chemical heat packs are *not* recommended for use on the face or head because of the danger of leaking chemicals.

NOTE: Gel packs that are heated in the microwave can also be used. Read and follow the instructions provided with the gel pack to determine microwave time. The gel pack must be covered because the plastic and heat can injure the skin. These packs can be reused many times for the same patient. In a health care agency, the pack should be labeled with the patient's name so it is not used on another patient.

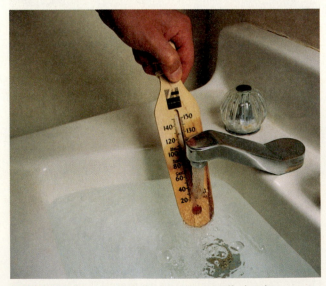

FIGURE 23–35A Use a bath thermometer to verify that the temperature of the water is 110°F–120°F.

6. Pour the measured hot water into the warm-water bag. Fill the bag one-third to one-half full (**Figure 23–35B**).

7. Expel remaining air by placing the warm-water bag on a flat surface, lifting and holding the neck portion of the bag upright, and pushing gently on the bag until the water reaches the neck (**Figure 23–35C**). Apply the screw cap or fold over the end.

   NOTE: If the bag has a fold end, note the letters *A*, *B*, and *C*. Fold *A* to *B*, *B* to *C*, and *C* to seal.

8. Wipe the outside of the bag dry. Check again for any signs of leaks.

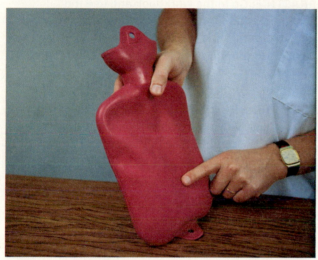

FIGURE 23–35B Fill the warm-water bag one-third to one-half full.

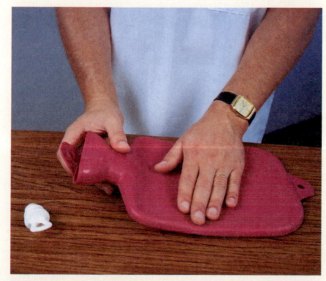

FIGURE 23–35C Expel air from the warm-water bag by placing it on a flat surface and gently pressing it until the water reaches the neck of the bag.

 CAUTION: Never use a warm-water bag or cap that leaks. The patient can be scalded.
Safety

9. Place a cover on the warm-water bag (**Figure 23–35D**). Use a standard cover, if available. If not, use a towel and tape the towel in place. The towel should be smooth and should completely cover the warm-water bag.

 CAUTION: The warm-water bag *must* be covered to prevent injury to the skin.
Safety

10. Knock on the door and pause before entering. Introduce yourself. Identify the patient. Explain the procedure and obtain consent.
Comm

11. Wash hands. Put on gloves if necessary.

 CAUTION: Wear gloves and observe standard precautions if the area to be treated has any drainage of blood, body fluids, secretions, or excretions.
Precaution

12. Apply the bag gently to the affected area as ordered. Make sure it is placed on top of the area. Never place heat under the body.

    CAUTION: Do *not* allow any part of the patient's body to lie on top of the warm-water bag. The weight of the body part could intensify the heat.
Safety

13. Before leaving, check to be sure the patient is comfortable and the bag is properly positioned. Place the call signal within easy reach of the patient. Remove gloves, if worn, and wash hands before leaving the room.

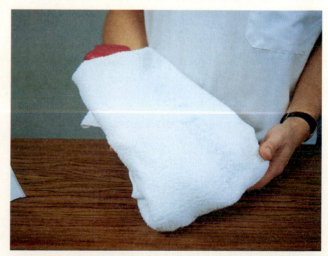

FIGURE 23–35D Cover the warm-water bag with a towel or standard cover.

(continues)

14. Recheck the patient at least every 10 minutes. Refill the bag as needed to maintain warm temperature. Note any pain, extreme redness, or other conditions.

     CAUTION: If signs of a burn are noted, remove the application immediately and report it to your immediate supervisor.

15. Remove the heat application when the time ordered has elapsed. Closely check the patient's skin.

16. Observe all checkpoints before leaving the patient: position the patient in correct body alignment, elevate the siderails (if indicated), lower the bed to its lowest level, place the call signal and supplies within easy reach of the patient, and leave the area neat and clean.

17. Discard a disposable heat pack. If a gel pack was used, wipe it with disinfectant, and label it with the patient's name before storing it. If the warm-water bag is not disposable, empty the warm-water bag and clean thoroughly. Wipe it with a disinfectant, rinse, and dry. Fill it with air before storing. This keeps the sides from sticking together. Replace all equipment.

18. Remove gloves, if worn. Wash hands.

19. Report and/or record all required information on the patient's chart or enter it into the computer. For example: date, time, warm-water bag applied to right knee for 20 minutes, patient stated pain relieved in knee, and your signature and title. Report any unusual observations immediately.

     NOTE: In health care agencies using electronic health records (EHRs), the information is entered directly into the patient's record on a computer.

PRACTICE: Go to the workbook and use the evaluation sheet for 23:3B, Applying a Warm-Water Bag, to practice this procedure. When you believe you have mastered this skill, sign the sheet and give it to your instructor for further action.

 FINAL EVALUATION: Using the criteria listed on the evaluation sheet, your instructor will grade your performance.

Procedure 23:3C

Applying an Aquathermia Pad

 NOTE: Aquathermia or aquamatic pads can vary. Read the manufacturer's instructions before using.

Equipment and Supplies

Aquathermia (K-pad) unit and pad, cover, distilled water, paper and pen and/or computer

Procedure

1. Check physician's orders or obtain authorization from your immediate supervisor for the application.

2. Assemble equipment.

3. Knock on the door and pause before entering. Introduce yourself. Identify the patient. Explain the procedure and obtain consent.

4. Wash hands. Put on gloves if necessary.

   CAUTION: Wear gloves and observe standard precautions if the area to be treated has any drainage of blood, body fluids, secretions, or excretions.

5. Place the aquathermia control unit on a solid table or stand. Check the cord. Attach the tubing to the main unit and aquathermia pad, if necessary.

   NOTE: Follow specific manufacturer's instructions. Some agencies use disposable pads. Tubing must be attached to these pads.

6. Unscrew the reservoir cap on the top of the unit. Use distilled water to fill the unit to the *fill* line.

   NOTE: Distilled water prevents formation of mineral deposits.

7. Screw the cap in place and then loosen it one-quarter turn. This allows for overflow of water and escape of steam.

8. Plug in the cord. Set the desired temperature by inserting the special key into the center of the dial or follow manufacturer's instructions. Temperature is usually set at 95°F–105°F, or 35°C–41°C. Turn the unit on.

   NOTE: Set the temperature according to physician's orders or agency policy.

    CAUTION: After setting the temperature, remove the key and store it in a safe area. Do not leave the key in position on the unit. Others could change or alter the temperature.

9. Check the pad for leaks. Also check that the unit is getting warm. Make sure the tubing is not bent or kinked. Recheck the level of water in the reservoir. A large amount of water is used when the pad is filled with water.

10. Cover the pad (**Figure 23–36**). If a custom cover is not available, a pillowcase or towel can be used. Use tape to hold the cover in place.

     CAUTION: The pad must *never* be placed directly on the patient's skin. It can cause burns.

11. Place the pad on the correct area as ordered. Coil the tubing on the bed to facilitate the flow of water through the tubing. Do not allow the tubing to hang below the level of the bed. Check that the patient is comfortable. Place the call signal within easy reach

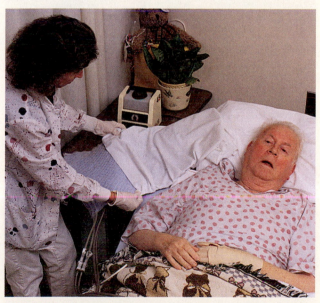

FIGURE 23–36 Cover the aquathermia pad before applying it to the patient.

of the patient. Remove gloves, if worn, and wash hands before leaving the room.

12. Recheck the patient at least every 10 minutes. Note the condition of the skin. If the skin is red or shows evidence of burns, or if the patient complains of pain, remove the pad and inform your immediate supervisor.

13. Refill the water unit with distilled water as necessary.

14. When the ordered time has elapsed, remove the pad from the patient. Note the condition of the skin. Note the patient's comments to determine whether the application was effective.

    NOTE: The physician's orders may prescribe continuous application of the pad. If so, check the patient periodically.

15. Observe all checkpoints before leaving the patient: position the patient in correct body alignment, elevate the siderails (if indicated), lower the bed to its lowest level, place the call signal and supplies within easy reach of the patient, and leave the area neat and clean.

16. Empty the pad. Empty the control unit. Clean all equipment thoroughly. Disinfect the pad and unit according to agency policy or discard the pad if it is disposable. Replace all equipment.

     CAUTION: Do *not* put the electric control unit in water.

17. Remove gloves, if worn. Wash hands.

18. Report and/or record all required information on the patient's chart or enter it into the computer. For example: date, time, aquathermia pad applied to left elbow and forearm for 20 minutes, patient stated pain relieved, and your signature and title. Report any unusual observations immediately.

     NOTE: In health care agencies using electronic health records (EHRs), the information is entered directly into the patient's record on a computer.

PRACTICE: Go to the workbook and use the evaluation sheet for 23:3C, Applying an Aquathermia Pad, to practice this procedure. When you believe you have mastered this skill, sign the sheet and give it to your instructor for further action.

 FINAL EVALUATION: Using the criteria listed on the evaluation sheet, your instructor will grade your performance.

Applying a Moist Compress

Equipment and Supplies

Basin; bath thermometer; underpads or bed protectors; wash-cloth, towel, or gauze pads (for compress); bath towel; plastic sheet; paper and pen and/or computer

Procedure

1. Check physician's orders or obtain authorization from your immediate supervisor for the application.

2. Assemble equipment.

3. Knock on the door and pause before entering. Introduce yourself. Identify the patient. Explain the procedure and obtain consent.

   Comm

4. Wash hands. Put on gloves.

   CAUTION: Observe standard precautions if any contact with blood or body fluids is likely, such as when a compress is applied to a draining wound.

   Precaution

5. Close the door and/or pull the curtain closed for privacy. Elevate the bed to a comfortable working height. Fold the sheets back to expose the area to be treated.

   NOTE: A bath blanket can be used to drape the patient during the procedure.

6. Position an underpad or bed protector near the area to be treated. This will keep the patient's bedclothes and bed linens dry.

7. Fill the basin with water at the correct temperature. Use the bath thermometer to check the temperature.

   a. If a cold compress is to be applied, fill the basin with cold water. Ice cubes are sometimes added to the water. Do not add ice cubes unless you are told to do so.

   b. If a hot compress is to be applied, fill the basin with water at a temperature of 100°F–105°F, or 37.8°C–41°C.

   NOTE: Temperatures may vary. Follow physician's orders or agency policy.

8. Put the compress (washcloth, towel, or gauze pad) in the water. Wring out the compress to remove excess liquid (**Figure 23–37A**).

9. Apply the compress to the correct area (**Figure 23–37B**). Use a plastic sheet to cover the area. Then wrap a bath towel around the treated area.

   NOTE: The plastic sheet helps keep the compress moist and hot or cold.

   NOTE: An underpad or bed protector is sometimes used instead of a plastic sheet.

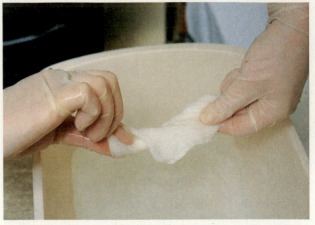

FIGURE 23–37A After putting the compress in the water, wring it out to remove excess liquid.

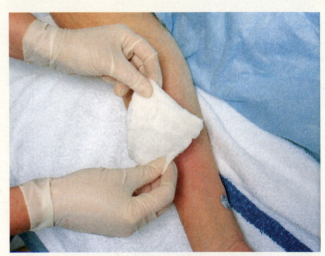

FIGURE 23–37B Apply the compress to the correct area.

10. An ice bag or aquamatic pad is sometimes placed over the compress to help maintain the temperature. Follow agency policy or physician's orders.

11. Check the compress at frequent intervals. Change the compress and remoisten it as necessary. Check the condition of the skin under the compress. If the skin is discolored or the patient complains of pain, remove the compress immediately and inform your immediate supervisor.

12. Continue the treatment for the required period of time as ordered by the physician or per agency policy. Most compresses are left in place for 15–20 minutes.

13. When the ordered time has elapsed, remove the compress from the patient. Note the condition of the skin. Note the patient's comments to determine whether the application was effective.

14. Observe all checkpoints before leaving the patient: position the patient in correct body alignment, elevate the siderails (if indicated), lower the bed to its lowest level, place the call signal and supplies within easy reach of the patient, and leave the area neat and clean.

15. Clean and replace all equipment used. Discard gauze pads used as compresses. Place linen in a hamper or the laundry area.

16. Remove gloves. Wash hands.

17. Report and/or record all required information on the patient's chart or enter it into the computer. For example: date, time, cold moist compresses applied to right knee for 20 minutes, no change in skin color noted,

patient states knee still hurts, and your signature and title. Report any unusual observations immediately.

 NOTE: In health care agencies using electronic health records (EHRs), the information is entered directly into the patient's record on a computer.

PRACTICE: Go to the workbook and use the evaluation sheet for 23:3D, Applying a Moist Compress, to practice this procedure. When you believe you have mastered this skill, sign the sheet and give it to your instructor for further action.

 FINAL EVALUATION: Using the criteria listed on the evaluation sheet, your instructor will grade your performance.

Today's Research | Tomorrow's Health Care

Rewire the Brain to Treat Tinnitus?

According to the American Tinnitus Association, tinnitus—a condition that causes people to hear a constant ringing or buzzing sound in the ear—affects nearly 45 million people in the United States. Tinnitus can range from a dull buzzing in the ear, like static on a telephone, to a loud ringing that keeps people from thinking clearly and even from sleeping. Estimates are that approximately 2 million people are severely disabled by tinnitus. The most common cause is hearing loss, especially from long exposure to loud noises. Most of the available treatments are not very effective.

Researchers know that tinnitus is a problem in the brain, not just the ear. An initial theory was that after a hearing loss, the brain remaps itself so that nerve cells that responded to a specific frequency start to respond to other frequencies. However, the nerve cells do not respond correctly to the new frequencies, so odd sounds are created. Additional research through the years showed the exact opposite. In a person with normal hearing, the sensory input controls how the nerve cells send signals to communicate with each other. When the damaged nerve cells do not receive any input, the nerve cells send signals constantly, creating the sounds associated with tinnitus. This concept is similar to "phantom limb" pain, in which an amputee feels pain or itching in the body part that is no longer there. Phantom limb syndrome is also caused by nerve cells that are sending signals even though a body part is missing. Researchers then tried to find a way to rewire

the brain so the damaged cells receive sensory input, and/or create a medication that turns off the nerve cell signals so tinnitus could be treated more effectively. Researchers examining areas of the hippocampus in the brain, a region not usually considered a part of the brain involved with hearing, found that rats exposed to loud noises for 30 minutes had nerve cells in this region that fired off signals that lasted for almost a day. They tested a substance called D-cycloserine to see if it decreased or eliminated the signals sent by these nerve cells but initial tests did not show favorable results. Researchers are still trying to find a similar substance that will work. The latest research is directed toward stimulating the vagus nerve, which passes through the outer ear to these brain regions. Initially, a small handheld neurostimulation device clipped to the outer ear was used to target the vagus nerve and modulate the brain to decrease and/or eliminate the sounds. Now they are testing an implanted lead with an external stimulator that has been effective by selectively deactivating certain regions of the brain associated with producing the tinnitus sounds. Currently, the stimulation is done at the laboratory, but researchers are determining ways an individual can do the stimulation by themselves.

Many other researchers are currently conducting studies to determine which parts of the brain are causing tinnitus, how nerve cells communicate to create the sounds, and methods that can be used to stop the abnormal electrical nerve cell signals. If the research is successful, the ringing or buzzing sounds of tinnitus may finally be turned off.

■ CHAPTER 23 SUMMARY

- Physical therapy techniques are utilized by a wide variety of health care providers. Physical therapy involves using physical means to treat the patient.

- Range-of-motion (ROM) exercises are done to maintain the health of the muscles and skeletal system. By following the correct procedures and using proper body mechanics, the health care team member can help the patient maintain as much mobility as possible.

- Proper techniques must be used when ambulating patients using transfer (gait) belts, crutches, canes, or walkers. By understanding the different gaits, proper ways of fitting the devices to patients, and safety precautions, the health care provider can provide support and guidance for patients relying on these aids.

- Heat and cold applications are administered for a wide variety of conditions. Careful observation of temperature and condition of the skin is essential to prevent injury to the patient.

- Physical therapy is an important part of the patient's treatment. By learning and understanding basic principles, the health care team member can help provide this part of the patient's care.

■ REVIEW QUESTIONS

1. What are the four (4) main types of range-of-motion (ROM) exercises? How is each type performed?

2. List eight (8) different types of joint movements and briefly describe each movement.

3. What are the basic rules that must be followed while measuring a patient for crutches?

4. You are ambulating a patient with a transfer belt. The patient starts to fall. What do you do?

5. Differentiate between a three-point and a two-point gait for canes.

6. What is the difference between moist heat and dry heat? Give two (2) examples for each type of application.

7. Define each of the following:
   a. vasodilation
   b. vasoconstriction

8. Identify five (5) safety measures or checkpoints that must be observed whenever a heat or cold application is applied to a patient.

CRITICAL THINKING

1. How do physical therapy techniques help encourage and support patients to perform their activities of daily living (ADLs) independently?

2. With a partner, practice ROM exercises. Write a paragraph about why communication between the health care team member and the patient is important.

ACTIVITIES

1. In a small group, create a video demonstrating ROM movements and exercises.

2. With a partner, interview a physical therapy rehabilitation patient about their experience in regaining the ability to perform ADLs. Write a 250–500 word essay analyzing the patient's experience.

For additional information on physical therapy careers, contact the following:

- American Physical Therapy Association
  www.apta.org

- National Athletic Trainers Association
  www.nata.org

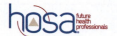 CONNECTION

Competitive Event: Physical Therapy

Event Summary: Physical Therapy provides members with the opportunity to gain knowledge and skills required for assisting patients with recovery. This competitive event consists of 2 rounds. Round One is a written, multiple choice test and top scoring competitors will advance to Round Two for the skills assessment. This event aims to inspire HOSA members to learn more about physical therapy concepts and techniques.

Details on this competitive event may be found at

www.hosa.org/guidelines

24

BUSINESS AND ACCOUNTING SKILLS ±

Case Study Investigation

Cody has been a file clerk for a doctor's practice for the last four years. The practice has ten doctors. She is quite good at her job. Cody got coronavirus and was out sick for two weeks. When she returned, files were piled everywhere! Miles is normally a scheduler but was assigned to work together with Cody to help her catch up with the filing and to show her how to schedule. At the end of the chapter, you will be asked to list the skills Miles will need to file accurately and the talents Cody will need to schedule patients.

■ LEARNING OBJECTIVES

After completing this chapter, you should be able to:

- File records using both the alphabetical and numerical systems.
- Utilize correct telephone techniques when using a business telephone.
- Schedule appointments using a standard appointment ledger or a computer program.
- Complete registration and history records.
- Compose and print letters of consultation, collection, appointment, recall, and inquiry.
- Complete basic insurance forms accurately, neatly, and thoroughly.
- Maintain a bookkeeping system.
- Write checks, deposit slips, and receipts.
- Define, pronounce, and spell all key terms.

KEY TERMS

answering service

appointments

automated routing unit (ARU)

block style

body

buffer period

cellular telephone

charge slip

check

collection

complimentary close

confidential

consultation *(con-sul-tay'-shun)*

cross-indexes/references

date line

day sheet (daily journal)

deposit slips

electronic health records (EHRs)

electronic mail

enclosure notation

endorsement *(en-dors'-ment)*

fax (facsimile) machine

filing

heading

indexed

inquiry *(in-kwy'-ree or in'-kwih-ree')*

inside address

insurance forms

ledger card

letterhead

medical history

memorandums *(meh-mow-ran'-dumbz)*

modified-block style

originator (maker)

paging system

patient portal

payee

pegboard system

recall

receipt

reference initials

salutation

screen

signature

statement–receipt

statistical data sheets

subject line

triage

voice mail

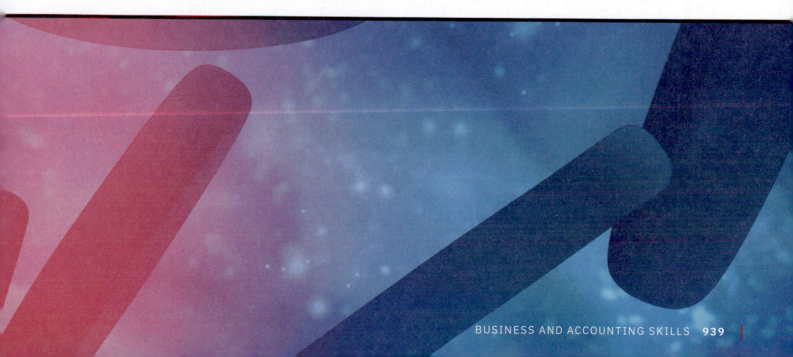

24:1 FILING RECORDS

Filing is the systematic or orderly arrangement of papers, cards, or other materials so that they are readily available for future reference. Correct filing methods for health care records and other information are necessary for two main reasons. First, it must be possible to quickly locate the material when it is needed. Second, the material must be stored safely and protected as legal records. Various filing systems are in use. It is important that you become thoroughly familiar with your agency's method and that you follow all instructions carefully.

TYPES OF FILING SYSTEMS

Four main filing systems are:

- **Alphabetical:** This is the most common method in use. Items are filed in alphabetical order according to the same rules followed in the telephone directory.

- **Numerical:** This is the second most common system. Materials to be filed, such as names, are each assigned a number. The numbers are then placed in order and filed according to numerical order. This system requires a cross-index or cross-reference list. An index card file or computer database is usually used for this purpose. The patient's name is placed on the index card or entered into the computer database along with the assigned number. The index cards or computer database are filed alphabetically according to last name. When a patient comes to the health care agency, their index card is pulled or the name is entered into the database to determine the patient's number. The patient's file is then located in the numerical file. If patients have the same name, the numerical system can eliminate errors because each patient has their own number. Previously, some health care agencies used a person's Social Security number instead of assigning another number. However, the Health Insurance Portability and Accountability Act (HIPAA) prohibits placing identifiable information, such as Social Security numbers, on the outside of a patient's chart. For this reason, random assignment of numbers is recommended. Using only numbers on the outside of a chart also helps to protect a patient from identity theft if an unauthorized person should happen to see the chart.

- **Geographic:** In this system, items are filed according to location. Cities, states, or countries are used as the key filing units. For example, in a rural agency that cares for patients from several areas, charts might be filed by area or location. Within each specific area, the charts might be filed alphabetically. A cross-reference system is usually required to prevent loss of charts. The use of geographic filing is usually reserved for large companies or corporations.

- **Subject:** In this system, material is filed by subject or topic. For example, all material concerning diabetes might be filed under the topic *Diabetes*. A cross-reference system is sometimes required. For example, if several pieces of correspondence are received on an aspect of diabetes, all the material obtained might be filed in the diabetes folder. However, another alphabetical file with the correspondent's name and a cross-reference saying "see diabetes" might be kept in case the employer wants to refer to a specific piece of correspondence.

CROSS-INDEXES OR -REFERENCES

Cross-indexes or **-references** are essential in a filing system to avoid misplacing or losing records. Some uses of cross-references were discussed in the descriptions of filing systems. Cross-references might be kept on index cards in a separate file, or colored sheets of paper might be placed in file folders. For example, if a letter contains information about three or four patients, the letter might be filed under the topic or under the name of the patient about whom the letter contains the most information. A cross-reference should be placed in each of the other patients' files. Usually on a colored sheet of paper so that it will stand out in the file, the cross-reference would state, "See… ." If a reference paper contains information about two topics, such as diabetes and glaucoma, the paper might be filed under *Diabetes*. In this case, a cross-reference that says "See diabetes" should be filed in the folder labeled *Glaucoma*. Many agencies have special cross-reference sheets that are used for this purpose.

COLOR-CODED FILING SYSTEMS

Color-coded indexing is an innovative method of filing that helps prevent errors (**Figure 24–1A**). Each folder is marked with a series of colors representing the letters in the patient's name. For example, all *A*s might be red, and all *B*s might be dark blue (**Figure 24–1B**). A series of two to eight colors is used to represent the letters in the patient's last name. The colors provide a second means of verifying placement of folders in the file. Because a chart with different color coding will stand out, a quick glance at the folders allows the person filing to immediately locate a file that is out of place.

Color-coded folder systems are frequently used in larger agencies. This system utilizes different colored file folders (**Figure 24–1C**). Some examples of color-coded folder systems include:

- **Coded by physician:** A health care agency may have several doctors. Each doctor's patients have a different color file folder. One doctor's patients have yellow file folders, a second doctor's patients have green file folders, and a third doctor's patients have red file folders.

- **Coded by type of insurance:** Each type of medical insurance has its own unique color of file folder. For example, patients on Medicare have blue file folders, patients in HMOs have yellow file folders, and patients with private insurance have green folders.

- **Coded by patient name:** Agencies use a different color folder to represent the first letter of a patient's last name. For example, last names starting with *S* are assigned a pink folder, and last names starting with *T* are assigned a green folder. This system requires 26 colors of folders, one for each letter of the alphabet.

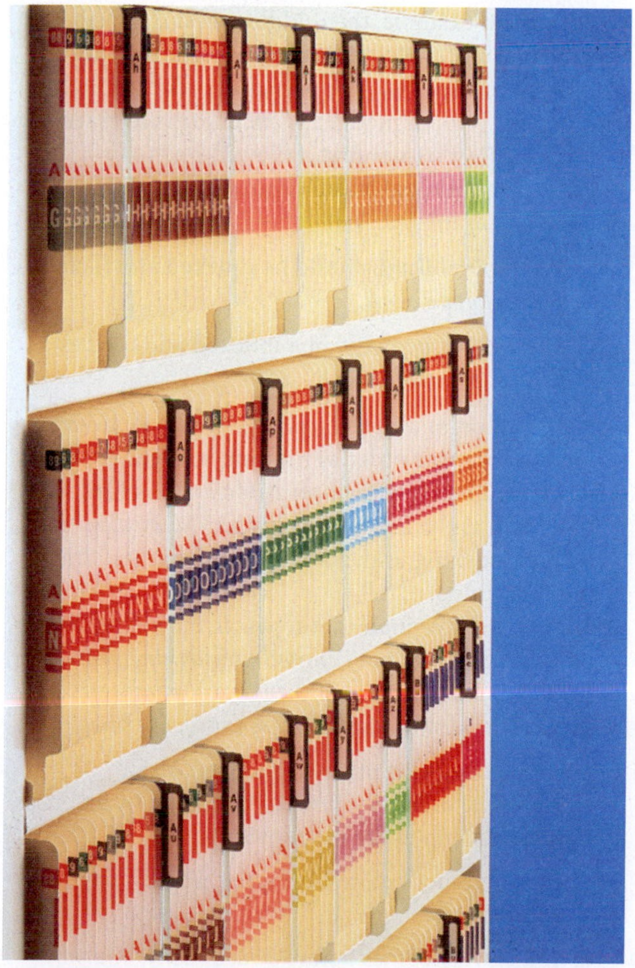

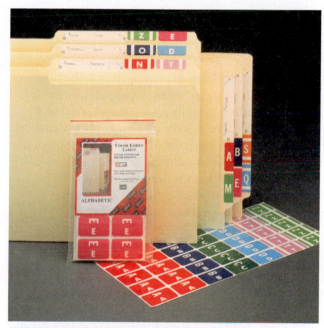

FIGURE 24–1B Color letter labels are available for both top- and side-cut files. Courtesy of Smead Manufacturing Company.

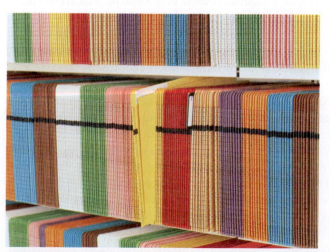

FIGURE 24–1C A color-coded folder system uses different colored file folders. Courtesy of KARDEX ® System, Inc., Marietta, OH.

FIGURE 24–1A A color-coded filing system helps prevent errors because a chart with different color-coding will stand out if placed in an incorrect position. Courtesy of Smead Manufacturing Company.

STORAGE OF FILES

In a manual filing system, records are stored in file folders and the folders are stored in filing cabinets or shelves. File folders must be durable and of good quality. Filing cabinets or shelves must be conveniently located, fireproof, and equipped with locks. Sufficient file space must be available so that records are not packed tightly in the drawers or shelves of the filing cabinets. Because thousands of records can accumulate in a busy agency, most facilities have a policy to classify records as active, inactive, or closed. An *active* record is one that is currently being used because the patient is being seen by the agency. An *inactive* record is a record for a patient who has not been seen for a number of years, usually 2–3 years. A *closed* record is usually a record for a patient who has died, transferred to another physician or facility, or a file that is no longer required.

Legel

States have different time requirements for retention of records. For this reason, most health care agencies keep all records in case they are needed for legal or research purposes. Inactive or closed records are frequently scanned and saved on an external hard drive or in a secure cloud or off-site server. The record can then be retrieved and displayed on the computer or printed in hard copy form if it is needed. It is important to note that the original record must be destroyed by shredding or burning to protect the confidentiality of the patient.

ELECTRONIC HEALTH RECORDS

EHR Technology

In an electronic filing system, agencies use computers and "paperless" files. The files are called **electronic health records (EHRs)**. A database is created with the name, address, and case number of the patient. The database will automatically file all patient names in correct alphabetical order. When the patient arrives at the agency, the patient's name is entered into the computer and the database information with the case number appears. Some computer programs will retrieve the patient's file by name; others require the case number. Once the file is retrieved, a printout can be obtained with pertinent information, or the health care provider can use a laptop computer or tablet to view and record information while providing care to the patient. When the health care provider sees the patient, current information is entered into the computerized patient file. This information can be stored on an external hard drive or in a secure cloud/off-site server so it can be retrieved when needed. Backup copies must be made frequently when an electronic system is used, because if the computer fails, or the hard drive crashes, all information would be lost. Most offices using an electronic system have automatic backups scheduled on a continuous, an

hourly, or a daily basis to prevent losing information. Maintaining the confidentiality of patients' records is also essential when an electronic system is used. Passwords, firewalls, limiting access to specific people, and using secure clouds or off-site servers are methods used to prevent access to the records by unauthorized individuals.

An efficient filing system is an important part of any health care agency. Follow all instructions carefully as you learn the system your agency uses. Ask questions when you do not understand a particular procedure.

ALPHABETICAL FILING

Alphabetical filing is one of the main methods used to file names and materials. The main rules for this system are as follows:

- Before names can be filed alphabetically, they must be put into units and indexed. Dividing a name into units simply involves separating each name. For example, the name *John Robert Davis* has three units: *John, Robert,* and *Davis*. The name *Mary K. Kasper* also has three units: *Mary, K.,* and *Kasper*. In the second example, the middle initial is considered to be one unit. After dividing the name into units, the units are **indexed**, or placed in order for filing. The most general method of indexing is to place the surname (last name) first, followed by the first name, and then the middle name or initial. Note the following examples:

  1. *John Robert Davis* would be indexed and filed as *Davis, John Robert*.

  2. *Mary K. Kasper* would be indexed and filed as *Kasper, Mary K.*

- Names of organizations and businesses are usually filed in the same order as they are written. For example, *American Medical Association* is filed with *American* as the first indexing unit, *Medical* as the second indexing unit, and *Association* as the third indexing unit.
  NOTE: *An exception is that words, such as of, at, the, on, a, and an, are not counted as indexing units. For example, The Health and Fitness Supplies would be indexed as Health (the), Fitness (and), Supplies.*

- After a name or company is indexed, strict alphabetical order is followed. Use as many letters as needed. Examples are as follows:

  1. *Brooks* comes before *Corey*, because *B* comes before *C*.

  2. *Tournovsky* comes before *Tournowsky*. *Tourno* is the same in both names. The first letter that is different is used. Because *v* comes before *w*, *Tournovsky* is filed first.

3. *Jones, Betty* comes before *Jones, Mary*. Surnames (last names) are the same, so the first letter of the first name determines the order for filing. The *B* in *Betty* comes before the *M* in *Mary*.

4. *Jones, Betty C.* comes before *Jones, Betty F.* Here, the middle initial is used to determine filing position. *C* comes before *F*.

- Nothing comes before something. For example, *Brook* comes before *Brooks* (with the additional letter *s*). Also, *Brown, W.* would come before *Brown, William*.

- Prefixes, such as *De, Del, La, Le, Mac, Mc, O, San, St., Van,* and *Von,* are treated as parts of names. They are *not* used as separate indexing units. For example, in *Van Dyke* and *O'Leary*, *Van Dyke* is one unit, not *Van* and *Dyke*; and *O'Leary* is one unit, not *O* and *Leary*. *O'Leary* would be filed before *Oliver*.

- Hyphenated names are each considered one unit, for example, *Lans-Worth*, *Miller-Jones*, and *Smith-Ville*. Therefore, *Smith-Ville* would be filed before *Smithworth*.

- Titles or degrees are usually used as the last indexing unit if names are identical. Some common titles or degrees include *MD, BS, RN, DDS, Dr.,* and *Professor*. *Dr. James A. Brown* would be indexed as *Brown, James, A., Dr.* and *James A. Brown, DDS* would be indexed as *Brown, James, A., DDS*. *Brown, James, A., DDS* would be filed before *Brown, James, A., Dr.*

- Terms of seniority, such as *Jr, Sr,* or *II,* are usually used as the last indexing unit. *Hayden Kobelak, Jr,* is indexed as *Kobelak, Hayden, Jr.* If names are identical, the seniority terms are filed in alphabetical or numerical order. For example, *Kobelak, Hayden, Jr,* is filed before *Kobelak, Hayden, Sr,* and *Kobelak, Hayden, II* is filed before *Kobelak, Hayden, III*. In addition, numerical seniority terms are filed before alphabetical terms. For example, *Kobelak, Hayden, II* is filed before *Kobelak, Hayden, Jr.*

- If names begin with numbers, the number becomes the first indexing unit and is filed in numeric order before any letters. *3rd Street Clinic* would be indexed as *3, Street, Clinic*. *40 Health Supply* would be indexed as *40, Health, Supply,* and *Sixth Avenue Radiology* would be indexed as *Sixth, Avenue, Radiology*. Correct filing order would be *3, Street, Clinic,* followed by *40, Health, Supply,* and finally *Sixth, Avenue, Radiology*.

- If two people have identical names with no titles or terms of seniority, most agencies now use birthdates to determine filing order. Follow agency policy for a situation like this.

NUMERICAL FILING

Numerical filing is also a common method of filing. Basic principles for this system are as follows:

- If a numerical system is used, cross-indexing or cross-referencing is required. Patients' names are usually indexed as for alphabetical filing. Each name is then placed on a card or in a computer database, and a number is assigned. Numbers in an agency usually run in order, and a record is kept of which numbers have been assigned. If cards are used, the card with the name and number is kept in an alphabetical file. When the patient comes to the agency, the alphabetical card is located or the patient's name is entered into the computer database to determine the patient's number. The numbered file is then located.

- In consecutive or serial filing systems, numbers always go in order from small to large. Number *23* is filed before number *230*. By simply numbering from 1 on, a large number of patients can be accommodated.

- Many offices use nonconsecutive filing or digit-numbering systems in which a series of numbers similar to Social Security numbers is used. Numbers, such as *32-444-5609,* allow for a great variety of charts. Each office establishes a preferred method that should be followed.

- If a zero falls *before* other numbers, the zero is usually disregarded when filing. For example, the number *00230* would be filed as if it were *230* and before the number *231*. Most offices use the same number of digits for each number assigned. That is why initial zeros are left in; they are used in place of other numbers.

- All of the numbers listed must be checked carefully. It is essential that numbers be written clearly if this type of system is used. Most offices prefer that numbers be typed to eliminate errors; otherwise, a written *1* can look like a *7*.

- Many systems use the same terminal, or last, digit for certain shelves or drawers. For example, a series of charts might contain 58 as the last digit. Another series might contain 62 as the last digit. Charts labeled *08-92-58, 18-99-58, 19-34-58,* and *02-41-58* are placed in one group separate from charts labeled *04-45-62, 05-98-62,* and *03-78-62*. Then, all charts with the terminal digit *58* are filed in correct numerical order. The order for the numbers listed previously is *02-41-58, 08-92-58, 18-99-58,* and *19-34-58*. These are placed on the shelf or drawer labeled *58* in the terminal system. Charts ending with *62* are then placed in numerical order. The correct order for the numbers listed previously is *03-78-62, 04-45-62,* and *05-98-62*. Therefore, in a terminal number system, first check the last digit and then put all same last digits together. Then place this series in numerical order.

checkpoint

1. List three (3) ways filing systems may use color coding.
2. When indexing a name, how is a term of seniority like Jr or Sr used?

PRACTICE: Go to the workbook and complete Assignment Sheet #1 for 24:1 Filing Records. Give the sheet to your instructor. Note any corrections or changes to the assignment sheet. Then complete Assignment Sheet #2 to be sure you understand the principles outlined in this section for filing records. Give the sheet to your instructor. Note any corrections or changes to the assignment sheet. Then complete Assignment Sheet #3. Then return and continue with the procedure.

Procedure 24:1

Filing Records

Equipment and Supplies

Labeled file folders, file drawer or index rack

Procedure

1. Assemble equipment.

2. Review the information section on filing and refer to it as necessary throughout the procedure.

   NOTE: If labeled file folders are not available for practice, make your own. Use 3-by-5-inch index cards (which are less expensive than file folders). Create three sets with 40–50 cards in each set. Make one set for alphabetical filing. Make sure you include examples of all of the rules given in the preceding information section. Make a second set of cards for numerical filing. List a variety of numbers on the cards. Be sure you include examples of the principles stated in the preceding information section. Make a third set of cards using a terminal-digit numerical filing system. Divide the cards into three or more groups. Label each group with a different terminal digit (last number). Then place a variety of numbers before the terminal digits.

3. Assemble all of the folders or cards with names in place for alphabetical filing. Check all names to be sure they are indexed correctly. Then file according to the following steps.

   a. Separate all folders or cards into letters of the alphabet. Place all *A*s together, *B*s together, and so forth through the end of the alphabet.

   b. Next, file just the *A*s. Start with the second letters of all of the *A*s and place them in alphabetical order. Proceed to the third letter, fourth letter, and additional letters as needed.

   c. When the *A*s are complete and in order, follow the same procedure for all remaining letters.

d. Recheck the files. Note common errors. Make sure that you considered prefixes, such as *Mc* or *Van*, as a part of the name and not as a separate unit. Make sure you treated any hyphenated names as one unit. Make sure that you filed any files with numbers as the first indexing unit before any letters.

 CHECKPOINT: Your instructor will check the filed folders or cards for accuracy.

4. Work with the numerical folders or cards. Note only actual numbers on each card. For example, 0023 would be regarded as a two-digit number, or 23; but 0300 would be regarded as a three-digit number, or 300. Ignore any zeros that come before the first number. Proceed as follows to file the numerical folders or cards:

   a. Divide the cards or folders into sets according to digits. Put all two-digit numbers (for example, *23, 68, 0023, 078,* and *010*) in one pile.

   NOTE: Remember to ignore any zeros *before* the number.

   b. Place all three-digit numbers in a second pile. These would include numbers, such as *893, 0938, 00567, 0800,* and *901.*

   c. Continue to separate the folders or cards in this manner. Create a four-digit stack, a five-digit stack, and so forth, as needed.

   d. Next, place all two-digit numbers in order. Start with the smallest number and proceed to the largest.

   e. Repeat step d with all remaining digit groups. Working with smaller groups of cards makes the process easier.

   f. Recheck the entire series of filed cards or folders. Make sure they are in correct order by number.

    CHECKPOINT: Your instructor will check the filed folders or cards for accuracy.

5. Work with the terminal-number system folders or cards according to the following steps:

   a. Separate the cards or folders into groups by noting the terminal digit (last number). All cards ending with the same last number will be in one group, for example, *19-52, 09-98-52, 54-19-52,* and *00-01-52.* Another group might be *05-77, 09-09-77, 00-66-77,* and *77-77.*

   b. Working with each terminal-number group, arrange each group in numerical order. Ignore any zeros that come before the first number. Order numbers from smallest to largest. For example, the series of cards ending in *52* would be filed in a group before the series of cards ending in *77.*

   c. Recheck all cards or folders filed.

    CHECKPOINT: Your instructor will check the filed folders or cards for accuracy.
   Check

6. Repeat steps 3, 4, and 5 until you master the systems. Read the preceding information section and additional references as needed. For additional practice, make up other folders or cards with names or with number systems, and file these in correct order.

7. Clean and replace all equipment used.

PRACTICE: Go to the workbook and use the evaluation sheet for 24:1, Filing Records, to practice this procedure. When you believe you have mastered this skill, sign the sheet and give it to your instructor for further action.

 FINAL EVALUATION: Using the criteria listed on the evaluation sheet, your instructor will grade your performance.
Check

24:2 USING THE TELEPHONE

BASIC TELEPHONE TECHNIQUES

Comm
The telephone is an important tool of public relations in any health agency. Because you create an impression every time you talk on the telephone, it is important that you use correct techniques.

Correct use of the telephone requires many different skills. The impression you create on the telephone will influence a patient or other caller. It is essential to be tactful, diplomatic, firm yet flexible, friendly yet professional, and courteous. You must be capable of making decisions and be willing to accept responsibility. Developing the correct tone of voice is essential. Your voice must be pleasant, low pitched, clear, and distinct. A monotone or indifferent tone should be avoided. Words must be pronounced correctly. Correct grammar should be used at all times. Courtesy and good manners must be used during the entire conversation. Don't forget to use the words *please* and *thank you.*

Always answer the telephone promptly. In addition, answer with a smile (**Figure 24–2**); doing so helps create a pleasant voice. Even though callers will not see the smile, they will be able to detect it in your voice. While talking on the phone, keep the receiver firmly against your ear. Put the mouthpiece approximately 2–3 inches away from the center of your lips. This allows the best transmission of your voice.

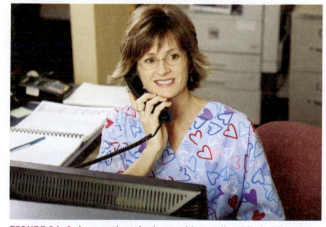
FIGURE 24–2 Answer the telephone with a smile while holding the mouthpiece 2–3 inches away from your lips. © Lisa F. Young/Shutterstock.com

Identify the office or agency—and in most cases yourself—when you answer the phone. For example, do not say "Hello," "Yes," or even just "Good morning," when answering. Use greetings, such as "Good morning, Dr. Smith's office," "Hello, Health Care Hospital, Miss Jones speaking," or "Respiratory Clinic, Miss Jones speaking, How may I help you?" In this way, callers know that they have reached the correct party.

In many agencies, it will be your responsibility to **screen** calls. This means that you must determine which calls should be referred to the doctor or other appropriate person, and which calls can be handled by you or another worker in the agency. Each agency usually has some policy regarding calls. For example, in some offices, calls from the doctor's immediate family (that is, wife or husband and children) and calls from other professionals are put through to the doctor. Other calls are screened to determine whether they are emergencies or whether the caller really must speak with the doctor. Experience in screening calls will help you make appropriate decisions.

To screen calls, you must first obtain specific information including:

- **Name of the caller**: To determine the name of the caller, you should avoid statements, such as "Who is this?" or "Who are you?" It is better to say, "May I have your name, please?" or "May I ask who is calling, please?" If the caller states, "Mrs. Jones," find out which Mrs. Jones she is. Ask for her first name. If you are unsure of the name, ask, "Would you please spell that?"

- **Birthdate**: Most offices ask for the date of birth (DOB) to help verify the identity of the person calling. In addition, this information is frequently used to find the patient's electronic health record (EHR).

- **Nature or purpose of the call**: When patients call a health care facility, they often simply ask to talk with a particular person. By asking, "May I help you?" or "May I tell Dr. Jones why you are calling?" you can usually determine the nature of the call. At times you may have to say, "Dr. Smith is with a patient at this time, may I take a message?" or "The therapist is not available at present, would you explain your problem to me so I can determine if someone else can assist you?"

Emergency calls must be evaluated. In some cases, a patient is upset and there is really no emergency. Most health care agencies establish a telephone triage procedure to deal with emergency calls. **Triage** is the process of evaluating the situation and prioritizing treatment. A list of questions is often kept by the telephone and used to assist in evaluating the situation. For example, the following questions may be used depending on the situation:

- Who is the patient?
- What happened? When did it happen?
- Is the patient breathing? conscious? bleeding?
- Is it possible the patient took or contacted a poison? If so, what, when, and how much?
- Have you called emergency medical services?

By asking pertinent questions and remaining calm, you may be able to recognize real emergencies. Most emergencies are referred to the appropriate person if they are available. If the appropriate person is not available, obtain important information so that you can help the caller obtain help from the correct source. It may be necessary to refer the patient to an emergency medical

service, emergency room, or hospital. A list of emergency numbers should be readily available so the correct number can be provided to the caller. Most agencies have procedures to follow when appropriate people are not available during emergencies.

Telephone triage can also be used to determine how quickly a patient should be scheduled for an appointment. Specific questions will help provide information on the seriousness of the patient's condition. Questions that might be asked include:

- What symptoms are you experiencing?
- How long have you had the symptoms?
- Do you have a fever or elevated temperature?
- Are you having any difficulty in breathing?
- Are you in pain? Where? How severe?

Evaluating a patient's responses will allow you to determine whether the patient should be seen immediately or the patient can be scheduled at the next convenient appointment time. Never hesitate to ask others for advice if you are not certain about the seriousness of the patient's condition.

Use discretion at all times when using the telephone. You should not say, "Doctor is having coffee down the hall," "He isn't in yet, and I don't know where he is," "The therapist is playing golf," or similar comments. Statements such as, "He is not available at present" or "I expect her to return at four o'clock; may I take a message?" are more appropriate.

Before ending any telephone conversation, repeat important information to the caller. For example, say, "Your appointment is scheduled for 10:00 am on Thursday, August 8th," or "The doctor will return your call after 4 pm today." At the end of a conversation, always close with, "Thank you for calling. Good-bye," and replace the receiver gently. If possible, allow the caller to hang up first. If you hang up first, you might miss something the patient wanted to say.

Legal

In most agencies, **memorandums**, or written messages, are made of any calls that require action. These memorandums can be handwritten or entered into a computer database or into the patient's electronic health record (EHR). In other agencies, telephone logs are kept, and every call is recorded. The log must be accurate because it can be subpoenaed as a legal record. Telephone messages should always contain the following information (**Figure 24–3A**):

- **Name of the caller**: Note the full name. Make sure it is spelled correctly.

- **Telephone number of the caller**: Be sure to note the area code and extension number, if needed. If there is a specific time when the caller can be reached, include this information.

- **Message**: Briefly summarize the reason for the call, but include all important information.

- Date and time of the call.

- **Action required**: If any action was taken, record what was done. If action must be taken, record the required action, such as "will call back," "please call back," or "please call after 3 pm."

- **Initials of the person taking the message**: If the message recipient has any questions, they will know whom to ask.

If an agency uses handwritten memorandums, it is essential to keep a pencil or pen and paper by the telephone. Most agencies use telephone message pads. If a copy of the message is needed for the patient's record or the agency's telephone log, message pads that provide a duplicate copy of each memorandum recorded can be purchased (**Figure 24–3B**). When recording any memorandum, always print clearly. Include all important facts and spell words correctly. Using a headset with the telephone frees the operator's hands and makes it easier to record telephone memorandums or key messages into a computer (**Figure 24–4**).

EHR Electronic health record systems frequently include the use of **patient portals**, or secure online websites that are established by a physician, health care facility, or other health care provider. Patients are given an access code to register for the portal

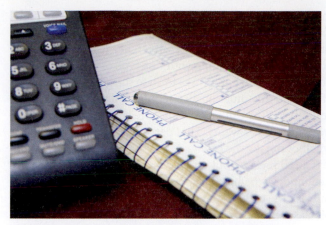

FIGURE 24–3B Message pads that provide a duplicate of each telephone memorandum can be used to create a telephone log.
© iStockphoto/Robert Simon.

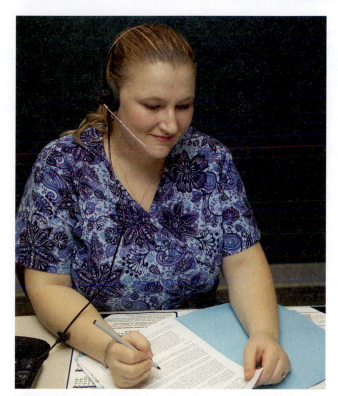

FIGURE 24–4 Using a headset with a telephone makes it easier to record memorandums.

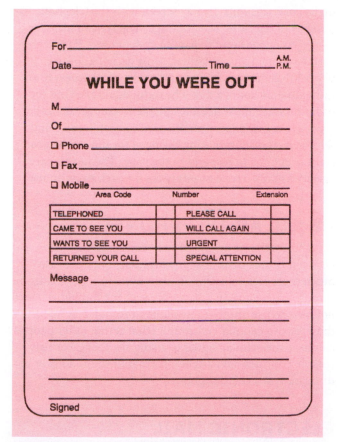

FIGURE 24–3A A sample telephone message form provides the receiver with all the information required to respond to the message.
©iStock.com/GeoPappas.

so they can log in anytime to gain electronic access to their electronic health record (EHR). This allows patients to request prescription refills, ask questions in regard to their health care, request or verify an appointment, view laboratory reports, and perform other similar tasks. When a patient request or question is sent electronically, the system sends an alert that must be answered. These requests or questions must be routed to the appropriate individual in the same manner as telephone requests or questions.

Problem calls can occur in any agency. Some individuals may refuse to give their names or state the purposes of their calls. At times, they may try to intimidate or threaten the person answering the phone. Try to remain calm and to control your temper. Do not hesitate to say, "Dr. Smith cannot be disturbed unless I can tell her who is calling." Be polite but firm in dealing with this type of caller. If a caller gives their name but refuses to state the general purpose of the call, this situation also requires tact. When in doubt, you can put the call on *hold* and check with the person whom the caller wants. That person can then determine whether to take the call.

If a call must be put on *hold* or you know there will be a slight delay before the appropriate person answers the call, ask the caller, "May I put you on hold for a moment?" Make sure the patient consents to being put on hold before placing a hold on the call. Never leave a caller on *hold* for longer than 1 minute. If there is a delay, offer to take the caller's number and have the individual return the call. Be considerate of all callers.

Correct telephone techniques require practice and experience. Think about the kind of impression you want to create; practice correct responses. At all times, think before you speak. Avoid comments that might offend a caller. Treat callers as you would want to be treated if you were the caller.

AUTOMATIC ROUTING TELEPHONE SYSTEMS

Many health care facilities have telephone systems with an **automated routing unit (ARU)**. This type of system allows many telephone calls to be answered at the same time. The ARU answers the telephone and a recorded voice provides directions to the caller. Most ARU systems provide a menu with a series of numbers. The caller presses the correct number to connect with a specific department or individual. The ARU system can be programmed so a caller with an emergency can be transferred immediately to an individual who can handle the emergency.

Voice mail is a common feature of most ARU systems. Voice mail is similar to the recording on an answering machine. If the individual is not available, the caller is instructed to leave a message and/or directed to contact another person. It is essential that individuals with voice mail check messages frequently. Most telephones will provide a signal, such as a beep, to alert the individual that messages are on the voice mail system. An individual who does not respond to voice mail messages creates poor public relations.

ANSWERING SERVICES AND MACHINES

An **answering service** is used by many health care agencies to respond to telephone calls when the agency is closed. This allows the patient to talk with an operator at the answering service who can transfer the call to

the appropriate individual, contact the individual and ask them to call the patient, or record a message. The health care agency provides the operator with procedures to follow in case of an emergency, telephone numbers of individuals who may have to be contacted, and guidelines for a variety of calls. The health care agency usually pays a monthly fee for this service.

An *answering machine* is used in some health care agencies, but it is not as efficient as an answering service. The recording on the answering machine usually identifies the agency and asks the caller to leave a message. Some health care agencies also include the hours they are open on the recording. If an answering machine is used, the message on the machine should tell patients what to do in case of an emergency. Most agencies provide an alternative number a patient can call for an emergency. The answering machine must be checked frequently for messages. A designated individual should check for messages immediately after the agency opens and at frequent intervals if the machine is used during the time the agency is open.

PAGING SYSTEMS

A **paging system** allows an individual to be contacted by using a *pager* or *beeper*. The pager can provide a voice message, a signal, such as a beep that alerts the individual to call a designated number to receive the message, or a digital message on a display screen with the telephone number of the caller or a message. The type of message received depends on the paging system used. Pagers are used to contact an individual. Most do not allow for two-way communication, but they do allow access to the individual 24 hours a day. The individual receiving the pager message must use a telephone to contact the caller. Newer two-way pagers can be used to both receive and send messages, eliminating the need for the receiver to use a telephone to respond to the page. The health care agency usually pays a monthly fee for each pager in use.

CELLULAR TELEPHONES

A **cellular telephone** allows two-way communication between people in almost any location. They provide much more flexibility for an individual to receive calls. It is more efficient than a pager because the individual does not have to use another telephone to respond. A major drawback to cellular communication is that other people can hear the cellular signal by using scanners. For this reason, confidential patient information should *never* be discussed on a cellular phone.

ELECTRONIC MAIL

Technology

Electronic mail, or e-mail, allows an individual to use an Internet connection to send, receive, and forward messages in digital form. The e-mail message can be sent to another individual in place of a telephone call or letter. Insurance companies, billing services, and health care agencies use e-mail messages to communicate with each other. In large health care agencies where computers are networked (electronically connected to each other), an e-mail message can be forwarded to many staff members at the same time and take the place of a written interoffice message. If an e-mail message is transmitted through the Internet on a modem that is not secure, it can be intercepted and read by others. For this reason, confidential patient information should *not* be sent unless a strong encryption program, firewall, and/or password protection is used. In addition, patients must sign an authorization form before any information can be sent.

FAX (FACSIMILE) MACHINES

Technology

A **fax (facsimile) machine** is used in many health care facilities to transmit data or information electronically over the telephone lines. For the system to work, the sending and receiving facilities must each have a fax machine and a telephone line designated for the fax machine. To fax information to another facility, use the telephone connected to the fax machine to dial the fax number of the other facility. Place the paper containing the information to be transmitted in the fax machine. When the fax number is answered at the other facility, the sending fax machine works similarly to a photocopy machine but transmits the information electronically. When information is being sent to a fax machine, a signal, such as a beep or light, is usually given by the receiving fax machine. The receiving fax machine then answers the fax phone and prints a copy of the information being sent.

Legal   HIPAA

Legal and confidentiality issues must be considered when faxing a patient's medical records. Many facsimile machines are password protected or allow encryption of the data. If both the sender and receiver have this type of machine, a password or encryption can be used. Material will not be transmitted until the receiver enters the password or uses the software to encrypt the data. Other ways to meet legal and confidentiality requirements include:

- Always have written authorization from the patient before records are faxed.

- Fax only to machines located in secure locations. Never fax to machines in public areas where others might gain access to the records.

- Use a cover sheet that contains a confidentiality statement, such as "This information is confidential. Be advised that you can be prosecuted under federal and state law for sharing this information with unauthorized individuals."

- Use a patient reference number instead of the patient's name when a document is sent. Inform the receiver about the number by telephone or secure e-mail. Ask others to send fax records with reference numbers instead of names.

- When in doubt, mail the records or send them by a messenger.

checkpoint

1. When taking a telephone message, what are five (5) components that messages should always contain?

PRACTICE: Go to the workbook and complete the assignment sheet for 24:2, Using the Telephone. Then return and continue with the procedure.

Procedure 24:2
Comm

Using the Telephone

Equipment and Supplies

Telephone message pad, pen or pencil, telephone setup

Procedure

1. Assemble equipment. Review the information section on telephone techniques. Prepare a list of sample triage questions to use while answering the telephone. Refer to these questions as you practice obtaining information from the caller.

2. Answer the telephone promptly and with a smile.

3. Identify yourself and the agency to the caller.

4. Determine the caller's full name, date of birth, and the purpose of the call. Be sure you have all the facts.

5. Watch your tone of voice, manners, grammar, and responses during the conversation.

6. Deal with the call or refer the call to the appropriate person if this is indicated.

7. At the end of the conversation, thank the caller and say, "Good-bye." Allow the caller to hang up the phone first. Replace the receiver gently.

8. Immediately record a memorandum of the call. Be sure to print clearly. Record all important facts.

(continues)

NOTE: In some agencies, the message is recorded during the conversation, and in other agencies the call information is entered into a computer database or into the patient's electronic health record (EHR).

9. Practice the following situations with a partner. Assume the roles of both the caller and the receptionist receiving the call.

   a. A patient calls to make an appointment.

   b. Another doctor calls to discuss his findings on a referred patient.

   c. A mother calls. Her child is ill.

   d. A salesperson calls. She has some new equipment she wants to demonstrate and discuss.

   e. A man calls. He states that his wife just fell to the floor unconscious.

   f. A mother calls and states that her 2-year-old child took an entire bottle of baby aspirin.

10. Think about other situations and role-play those situations. Use correct telephone techniques. Evaluate your partner's responses and let your partner evaluate you. Discuss different ways of dealing with the preceding and other situations.

11. Replace all equipment used.

PRACTICE: Go to the workbook and use the evaluation sheet for 24:2, Using the Telephone, to practice this procedure. When you believe you have mastered this skill, sign the sheet and give it to your instructor for further action.

 FINAL EVALUATION: Using the criteria listed on the evaluation sheet, your instructor will grade your performance.

Check

24:3 SCHEDULING APPOINTMENTS

One of the most frequent complaints that patients voice regarding doctor's offices, clinics, and other health agencies is having to spend a lot of time sitting in waiting rooms before getting to see doctors or other appropriate health personnel. To prevent this as much as possible, offices use a carefully planned appointment schedule. Correct scheduling of **appointments** is essential for good public relations.

 In most health care agencies, appointment scheduling is done by computer (**Figures 24–5A** and **Figure 24–5B**). The computer automatically locates the next available date and time, provides a record of appointments already scheduled, can be programmed to schedule a set block of time for a particular procedure, and prints out copies of the daily schedule. Although computerized scheduling can be efficient and convenient, an alternate system must exist for downtime, or times when the computer is not functioning.

Technology

If the computerized program is not working, or is not available in an office, appointment books or logs may be used. Appointment books or logs vary from office to office (**Figure 24–6**). However, most contain one or one-half page for each day. Time is usually blocked off in units of 10–15 minutes in order that all time can be used wisely. Become familiar with the type of appointment book you will use and know what block of time each line represents.

An organized approach is needed to avoid scheduling patients at times when the appropriate person is not available. Before scheduling any appointments, block out periods of time when individuals are not available. These include time periods for lunches, meetings, or afternoons off. A large *X* is usually drawn through each of these time periods so that no scheduling errors can occur.

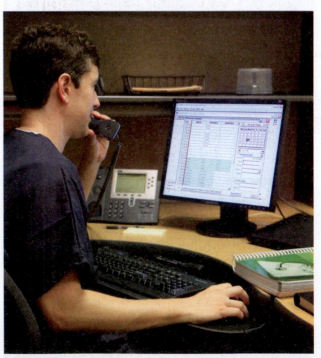

Figure 24–5A Appointment scheduling is done by computer in most health care agencies.

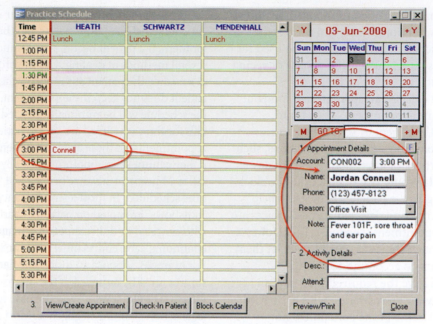

FIGURE 24–5B A sample computer screen showing an appointment that has been scheduled.

On computerized scheduling, some programs highlight the block-out times in a different color or use lines to mark off the times.

![Thursday December 7 appointment book]

![Monday February 20, Tuesday February 21, Wednesday February 22 appointment book]

FIGURE 24–6 Sample appointment books.

If an appointment book or log is used to schedule appointments, most agencies use a pencil to record the appointments. In this way, if an appointment is canceled, names can be erased, and the time can be assigned for another patient. Follow your agency's procedure.

Before scheduling any appointment, determine how long various procedures in your agency take. If an examination takes 1 hour and you schedule a 15-minute appointment, you will be 45 minutes behind for later appointments. Many agencies keep lists of standard procedures and the average time required for each near the appointment book. An example is shown in **Table 24–1**.

Appointments should be scheduled as close together as possible, but not so close that patients will feel rushed in the office or be required to wait for long periods. Long periods of unscheduled time are wasteful and cost money. Some agencies schedule a 15- to 30-minute **buffer period**

TABLE 24–1 Procedure Scheduling Times

Procedure	Time in Minutes
Amalgam Restoration	30
Composite Restoration	30
Crown Prep	45–60
Crown Placement	15–20
Denture Placement	15
Denture Prep	30–45
Examination Initial	30
Examination General	15
Extraction	30–45
Prophylactic General	30–45
Root Canal	45–60
Whitening	45–60

in the middle of each morning and afternoon. This allows time to catch up if some appointments run over. If the appointments run as scheduled, this time can be used for other business, such as returning telephone calls or seeing patients with emergencies.

When a patient calls for an appointment, find out the reason for the appointment. Then try to accommodate the patient by scheduling an appointment convenient for them. Questions, such as, "Do you prefer morning or afternoon?" "Which day is most convenient?" and "Would two o'clock or four o'clock be more convenient?" give the patient a choice and help you select the correct time and day. Sometimes, choices are limited because the appointment schedule is full. However, by giving patients as much choice as possible, you let them know that you are trying to accommodate them.

Make sure you have the required information before closing your conversation with the patient. Obtain the full name of the patient. Do not hesitate to ask the patient to spell the name if you are not sure of the correct spelling. Determine the reason for the appointment. It is also wise to get the patient's telephone number in case an emergency requires cancellation of the appointment. Writing the telephone number in the appointment ledger eliminates having to find the number in the patient's record and saves time. Repeat the date, day, and exact time of the appointment to the patient. By giving both date and day, you provide a double check and prevent errors. Make sure the patient understands all information. Before hanging up the phone, you can again repeat the information by saying, "We will expect you Friday, March 1st, at two o'clock. Thank you for calling, Mrs. Clark. Good-bye."

If a patient schedules an appointment at the health care facility, an appointment card or printed sheet should be given to the patient. The card/sheet should state the date, day, and time of the appointment. Many health care facilities also use e-mail, text messages, and/or telephone calls to send appointment reminders to their patients, so make sure you follow the policy in place at your facility.

After scheduling an appointment, make sure you mark the full amount of time in the schedule. In many agencies, arrows are used that extend down from the patient's name to fill in the entire time block the patient will require. This also prevents scheduling errors. A computerized program will usually automatically block off the time required based on the procedure entered.

If a patient calls to cancel an appointment, be polite. Ask the patient if they would like to reschedule the appointment. Delete the appointment on the computerized schedule or remove it from the printed schedule by drawing a single line through the entry. Then record all new information in the correct time block. It is not necessary to pry and ask patients why they must cancel. Many patients will offer explanations; however, if they do not, do not question them.

Chronic scheduling problems occur in every agency. Some patients schedule appointments and then do not show up for them. If a patient becomes a chronic offender, there are several methods of dealing with the problem. One method is to schedule the patient at the end of the day. This way, if the patient does not keep the appointment, other patients and the schedule will be minimally affected. In some agencies, bills for time scheduled are sent to patients who do not keep appointments. In these agencies, patients must be told that if they cannot keep appointments, they must notify the office 24 hours in advance or they will be charged for the time scheduled. In most agencies, canceled appointments or "no-shows" are noted on patients' charts. If the individual who canceled or didn't appear for an appointment needs continuing care, efforts must be made to contact the person. For example, suppose an individual had surgery and sutures must be removed; if the sutures are not removed, an infection could develop, and the individual could initiate legal action claiming negligence. Most agencies have a policy that requires calling the patient and recording the date and time of each call on the patient's chart. If there is no response from the patient after several telephone calls, a letter or e-mail is sent to the patient explaining the need for care. Documenting all efforts in the patient's chart provides legal protection if the patient files a lawsuit. The final decision on how to deal with these situations rests with the individual in charge. Be sure you know and follow their policy.

Emergencies occur in every agency. In the case of an emergency, appointments may run later than scheduled. Sometimes, it is necessary to cancel all appointments scheduled. If possible, patients should be notified by telephone before they come to the office or agency. When you call to cancel an appointment, make every effort to reschedule the patient at a time convenient to them. If a patient arrives at the office and appointments are behind schedule, offer the patient a choice between waiting or scheduling another appointment. If told that an emergency has occurred (the full nature of the emergency need not be explained) and they will have to wait, many patients will be willing to do so. However, patients should never be left waiting without an explanation.

Correctly scheduling appointments takes practice. If your present system is resulting in long waits for patients, review your system. Determine whether longer time periods are necessary for each patient. Add additional buffer times for overlap or emergency patients, if indicated. Constantly be willing to try to correct problems and create a good impression of the agency.

checkpoint

1. Why do some offices schedule a buffer period in the middle of the morning?

PRACTICE: Study the procedure for 24:3, Scheduling Appointments, before completing any assignment sheets.

Procedure 24:3

Scheduling Appointments

Equipment and Supplies

Appointment schedule ledger or worksheet, pencil, Assignment Sheets #1 and #2 for 24:3, Scheduling Appointments

Technology

NOTE: If you are using a computer program to schedule appointments, follow the instructions provided with the software. The same principles will apply, but the computer will identify available appointment times and allocate the correct amount of time based on the procedure entered.

Procedure

1. Assemble equipment. Check the appointment schedule ledger or worksheet. Note how much time each line represents. Examine the sample appointment schedule in **Figure 24–7**.

   NOTE: Appointment ledgers vary. Many contain lines that each represent a 15-minute period. In these ledgers, the line labeled *9:00* represents the time from *9:00* to *9:15*.

2. Place the day and date on the top of each of the daily columns. This provides a double check.

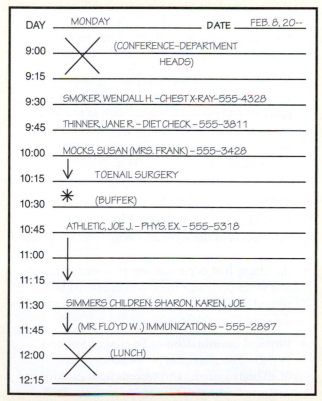

FIGURE 24–7 A sample appointment schedule.

3. Block off those periods of time when the person for whom appointments are being scheduled will not be in. Put a large *X* through each of these time periods. If the reason is known, write a brief explanation, such as *medical meeting*, to block out the time period.

4. If your agency requires a buffer time, mark this time period. It can be used for emergency patients or catch-up time.

5. Begin working with Assignment Sheet #1 for 24:3, Scheduling Appointments, in your workbook. Read each case listed. Note the time required and time preferred. Using a worksheet, schedule each of the cases. Check each case and notation to be sure of the following:

   a. Full name of the patient is listed. Spelling must be correct.

   b. The patient is in the correct time slot. Draw arrows downward from the name to indicate the time needed. Draw only to the end of the patient's appointment.

   c. The reason for the appointment is briefly listed. Abbreviations can be used.

   d. The telephone number of the patient is noted. Check to be sure the number is correct.

   e. The entry is printed and easy to read.

6. Double-check each entry. Some time periods may have to vary slightly.

7. Turn in Assignment Sheet #1 or print a copy of a computer-generated schedule to be graded. Your instructor will correct it and note changes to be made.

    CHECKPOINT: Your instructor will grade Assignment Sheet #1 according to the criteria listed on the evaluation sheet.

8. When Assignment Sheet #1 has been graded, note all changes and corrections. If you do not understand a change, be sure to ask your instructor for help before doing Assignment Sheet #2.

9. Complete Assignment Sheet #2 for 24:3, Scheduling Appointments, in your workbook. Follow steps 1–6. When you have checked all entries, turn the sheet in or print a computer-generated schedule to be graded.

10. Replace all equipment.

PRACTICE: Go to the workbook and use the evaluation sheet for 24:3, Scheduling Appointments, to practice this procedure and to complete the two assignment sheets for 24:3, Scheduling Appointments.

 FINAL EVALUATION: Using the criteria listed on the evaluation sheet, your instructor will grade your performance.

24:4 COMPLETING MEDICAL RECORDS AND FORMS

Legal   EHR   HIPAA

Medical records vary but some forms are used for certain purposes. Two common forms are statistical data sheets and medical history records. These forms can be printed and completed manually, or the information can be entered into a computer database. If records are kept electronically, they are called electronic health records (EHRs). All records are considered to be **confidential**. *No information can be released from the records without the written consent of the patient. These forms belong to the physician or agency. They should be locked up or electronically secured when not in use.*

HIPAA   EHR

Statistical data sheets are also called *patient information forms* or *patient registration forms* (**Figure 24–8**). This form is usually completed on a patient's first visit to an office or health agency. On subsequent visits, patients are asked to verify the information to be sure it is correct. The statistical data sheet contains patient demographics. The form may be a sheet of paper or the inside of the patient's folder. In most offices, the information is entered into a computer database on the patient's electronic health record (EHR). Sample computer entry screens for statistical data, insurance information, and compliance with HIPAA are shown in **Figures 24–9A**, **24–9B**, and **Figure 24–9C**. No matter what type of form is used, most contain the following information:

- Patient's name in full
- Patient's address, including city and zip code
- Patient's telephone number
- Patient's e-mail address
- Patient's marital status, sex, and birthdate
- Patient's place of employment
- Name of the person responsible for the account
- Insurance company information including name of company, address, policy and group numbers, and other pertinent information
- Name of referring physician or other person

In most agencies, this information is keyed into a computer database and a printed copy is placed in the patient's record or the information is included in the patient's electronic health record (EHR). Care must be taken to ensure that all information is accurate. Double-check numbers and spelling.

A **medical history** record is another important form used in almost all health care agencies. Information on this form helps the practitioner provide better care and, at times, even make a diagnosis. A medical history can be recorded on a form or entered into a computer database on the patient's electronic health record (EHR). These forms also vary but most forms contain the following basic parts (**Figure 24–10**):

- **General statistical data**: These data include name, address, age, and other similar information.

- **Family history**: Family history includes information on members of the patient's immediate family, including parents, grandparents, sisters, and brothers. Questions are asked regarding heart disease, cancer, mental disorders, diabetes, epilepsy, kidney disease, and allergies. If a family member has died, the cause of death and age at time of death are recorded. Only information regarding blood relatives is obtained. Information regarding relatives by marriage, such as a mother-in-law, is not obtained because the patient cannot inherit diseases from these individuals.

- **Patient's medical history**: Medical history includes past illnesses, treatments, operations, accidents, physical defects, allergies, childhood diseases, and other similar items. For each past illness, the year of the illness or the patient's age at the time of the illness is recorded. For each past operation, the date of the operation or the age of the patient at the time of the operation and the type of operation are recorded.

- **Personal/social history**: This may include questions about the patient's diet, sleep, or exercise routines and personal habits, such as smoking or alcohol use. In the case of a female patient, information regarding pregnancies, number of children, abortions, and menstrual pattern is also recorded. A list of current medications being taken by the patient is usually requested.

- **Present illness or ailment**: This is an exact description of the signs and symptoms the patient is currently experiencing. Information about when the illness first occurred, any previous treatment, and other pertinent information offered by the patient should be noted. This section is sometimes designated as *chief complaint*.

- **Physical examination or Review of Systems (ROS)**: The physician performs an examination of all body systems and records both positive and negative findings. This section may also include results from laboratory tests, although there is sometimes a separate section for laboratory tests.

PATIENT INFORMATION

DATE:

PATIENT'S NAME	MARITAL STATUS S | M | W | DIV | SEP	DATE OF BIRTH	SOCIAL SECURITY NO.

STREET ADDRESS ☐ PERMANENT ☐ TEMPORARY	CITY AND STATE	ZIP CODE	HOME PHONE NO.

CELL PHONE NUMBER	E-MAIL ADDRESS

PATIENT'S EMPLOYER	OCCUPATION (INDICATE IF STUDENT)	HOW LONG EMPLOYED?	BUSINESS PHONE NO.

EMPLOYER'S STREET ADDRESS	CITY AND STATE	ZIP CODE

IN CASE OF EMERGENCY CONTACT:	DRIVERS LIC. NO.

SPOUSE'S NAME	

CELL PHONE NUMBER	E-MAIL ADDRESS

SPOUSE'S EMPLOYER	OCCUPATION (INDICATE IF STUDENT)	HOW LONG EMPLOYED?	BUSINESS PHONE NO.

EMPLOYER'S STREET ADDRESS	CITY AND STATE	ZIP CODE

WHO REFERRED YOU TO THIS PRACTICE?

IF THE PATIENT IS A MINOR OR STUDENT

MOTHER'S NAME	STREET ADDRESS, CITY, STATE, AND ZIP CODE	HOME PHONE NO.

MOTHER'S EMPLOYER	OCCUPATION	HOW LONG EMPLOYED?	BUSINESS PHONE NO.

EMPLOYER'S STREET ADDRESS	CITY AND STATE	ZIP CODE

FATHER'S NAME	STREET ADDRESS, CITY, STATE, AND ZIP CODE	HOME PHONE NO.

FATHER'S EMPLOYER	OCCUPATION	HOW LONG EMPLOYED?	BUSINESS PHONE NO.

EMPLOYER'S STREET ADDRESS	CITY AND STATE	ZIP CODE

INSURANCE INFORMATION

PERSON RESPONSIBLE FOR PAYMENT, IF NOT ABOVE	STREET ADDRESS, CITY, STATE, AND ZIP CODE	HOME PHONE NO.

☐ COMPANY NAME & ADDRESS	NAME OF POLICYHOLDER	CERTIFICATE NO.	GROUP NO.

☐ COMPANY NAME & ADDRESS	NAME OF POLICYHOLDER	POLICY NO.

☐ COMPANY NAME & ADDRESS	NAME OF POLICYHOLDER	POLICY NO.

☐ MEDICARE	MEDICARE NO.	☐ MEDICAID	PROGRAM NO.	COUNTY NO.	ACCOUNT NO.

In order to control our cost of billing, we request that office visits be paid at the time service is rendered. We would rather control our billing costs than be forced to raise our fees.

AUTHORIZATION: I hereby authorize the physician indicated above to furnish information to insurance carriers concerning this illness/accident, and I hereby irrevocably assign to the doctor all payments for medical services rendered. I understand that I am financially responsible for all charges whether or not covered by insurance.

_____
Responsible Party Signature

FIGURE 24–8 A sample statistical data sheet or patient information form.

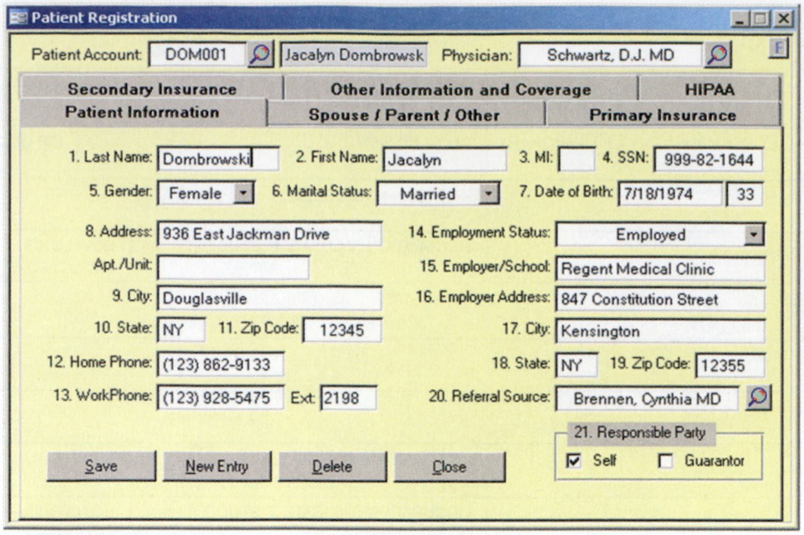

FIGURE 24–9A A sample computer database screen for statistical information.

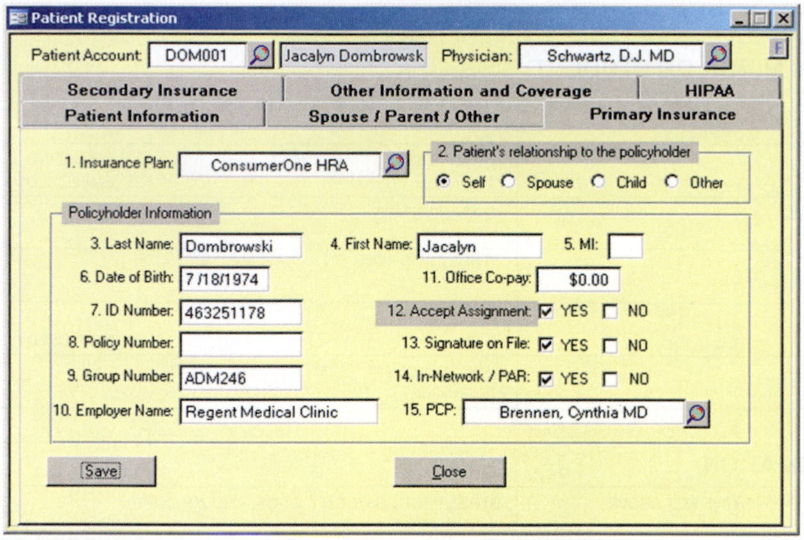

FIGURE 24–9B A sample computer database screen for insurance information.

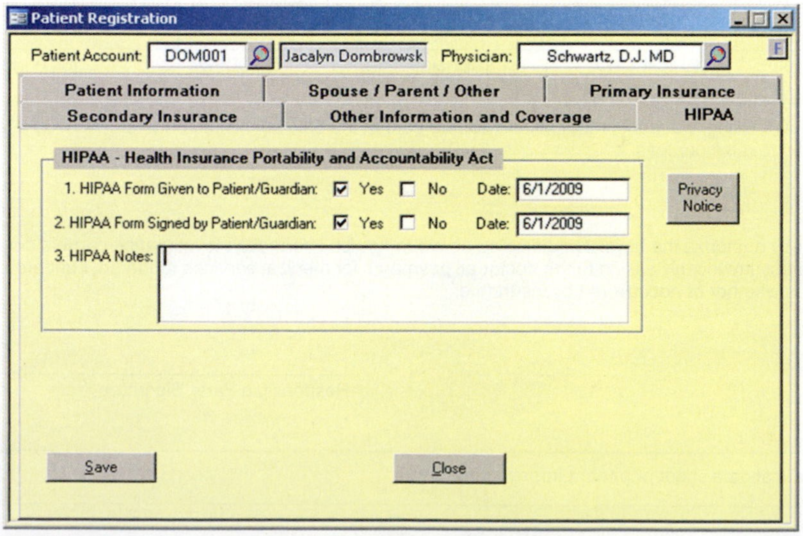

FIGURE 24–9C A sample computer database screen for HIPAA information.

MEDICAL HISTORY FORM

Date _____
Patient's name _____

Age	Date of birth	Sex	
Address	City	State	Zip code
Phone ( )	Cell phone number	E-mail address	
Insurance company	Policy number		
Place of employment	Address		
Phone ( )	Job responsibilities		
Parent/Guardian if minor			
Address	City	State	Zip code
Phone ( )	Cell phone number	E-mail address	

Family History:

List family members: (mother, father, brothers, sisters, grandparents, etc.)—ages and health status (if deceased write their age at the time of their death and the cause). List allergies and/or any conditions or diseases they may have or have had, such as asthma, arthritis, tuberculosis, diabetes, cancer, heart disease, hypertension, kidney disease, mental illness, depression, or any other health problems that you know of in your family.

_____
_____
_____

Patient's Past History: Mark the boxes to the right either "yes" or "no" for the following questions:*

Do you ever have or have you ever had any of the following: **(Yes) (No)**

SKIN
Rashes, hives, itching or other skin irritations ( ) ( )

EYES, EARS, NOSE, THROAT
Headaches, dizziness, fainting ( ) ( )
Blurred or impaired vision ( ) ( )
Hearing loss or ringing in the ears ( ) ( )
Discharge from eyes or ears ( ) ( )
Sinus trouble/colds/allergies ( ) ( )
Asthma or hay fever ( ) ( )
Sore throats/hoarseness ( ) ( )

CARDIOPULMONARY
Shortness of breath ( ) ( )
Persistent cough or coughing up blood or other secretions ( ) ( )
Chills and/or fever ( ) ( )
Night sweats ( ) ( )
Tuberculosis or exposed to TB ( ) ( )

Scarlet fever or rheumatic fever ( ) ( )
Chest pain ( ) ( )
Heart palpitations or rapid heart-beat or pulse ( ) ( )
High blood pressure ( ) ( )
Swelling of hands and/or feet ( ) ( )

GASTROINTESTINAL
Heartburn or indigestion ( ) ( )
Nausea and/or vomiting ( ) ( )
Loss of appetite ( ) ( )
Belching or gas ( ) ( )
Peptic ulcer, gallbladder or liver disease ( ) ( )
Yellow jaundice or hepatitis ( ) ( )
Diarrhea or constipation ( ) ( )
Dysentery ( ) ( )
Rectal bleeding, hemorrhoids (piles)( ) ( )
Tarry or clay-colored stools ( ) ( )

GLANDS
Weight gain or loss ( ) ( )

Diabetes ( ) ( )
Thyroid or goiter ( ) ( )
Swollen glands ( ) ( )

GENITOURINARY
Kidney disease or stones, or Bright's disease ( ) ( )
Painful, frequent or urgent urination( ) ( )
Blood or pus in urine ( ) ( )
Sexually transmitted disease (venereal disease) ( ) ( )
Been sexually active with anyone who has AIDS or HIV or hepatitis( ) ( )

NEUROMUSCULAR
Problems with becoming tired and/or upset easily ( ) ( )
Nervous breakdown/depression ( ) ( )
Poliomyelitis (infantile paralysis) ( ) ( )
Convulsions ( ) ( )
Joint and/or muscular pain ( ) ( )
Back pain or injury/osteomyelitis/rheumatism ( ) ( )

Are you currently taking any medications? Yes ( ) No ( )
If yes, please list them _____
Have you ever had or been treated for cancer or any tumors? ( ) ( )
Are you anemic or have you ever had to take iron medication? ( ) ( )
Do you use tobacco? ( ) ( )
What type? _____
Do you use IV drugs or alcohol? ( ) ( )

WOMEN ONLY
Painful menstrual periods ( ) ( )
Pregnancy/abortion/miscarriage ( ) ( )
Vaginal infection or discharge/abnormal bleeding ( ) ( )

Last menstrual period _____
Birth control _____
List dates of all operations/surgeries, injuries, and illnesses that required hospitalization:

_____

Did you ever receive benefits from a medical insurance claim due to illness or injury? Yes ( ) No ( )
Were you ever rejected from the military or for employment? ( ) ( )
Were you absent from school/work in the past 10 years because of illness or injury? ( ) ( )
Did you ever file a Workers' Compensation claim? ( ) ( )
Did you ever seek psychological or psychiatric treatment? ( ) ( )

*Please use the back of this form to explain any "yes" answers. Thank you.

FIGURE 24–10 A sample medical history form.

- **Diagnosis, prognosis, treatment rendered**: These sections can be separate or combined on the form. They are completed by the physician after all of the previous information is reviewed. The *diagnosis* is the physician's judgment regarding what disease or condition the patient has. Sometimes a tentative diagnosis is listed, or the physician may write "R/O" followed by the name of one or more diseases to indicate that tests should be done to rule out the diseases listed. The *prognosis* is the physician's opinion regarding the course and expected outcome of the disease or condition, such as "terminal in 3–6 months" or "full recovery in 1–2 weeks." Any specific treatment given is also listed.

 In most agencies, the health care assistant will complete only the statistical data information and/or family history, patient's medical history, and personal history sections. Patients may also be asked to complete a form providing this information, which can then be checked by the assistant and/or physician. The physician or another authorized person will do all other parts of the medical history.

  The patient must have privacy when being questioned. A separate room should be used, and the door to the room should be closed. Specific questions must be asked. It is essential that questions be asked in a professional rather than prying manner. It is also important to make sure the patient understands the meaning of all questions. For example, diabetes may have to be explained as "sugar." Information obtained must be accurate and complete. Facts should be rechecked as necessary. The patient should be given time to think about each question. It is important that the patient feels relaxed and at ease during the questioning. Note any additional information that the patient provides if it seems important to the overall history. If no specific areas are provided on the forms for this type of information, be sure the physician or other appropriate person is made aware of the information.

  Legal requirements must be observed while working with medical records. It is essential to remember that all information on the record is confidential and cannot be given to any other individual, agency, or insurance company without the written permission of the patient. HIPAA requires that records must be stored in a secure, locked area with limited access. Computerized records must use encryption technology, firewalls, and/or password protection. All records must be maintained for the period of time required by law. If an error is made while recording a paper medical record, the error should be crossed out in red ink, dated, and initialed. Correct information is then recorded and noted as *Corr* or *Correction*. Incorrect data on a computerized medical record must *never* be deleted or keyed over.

Follow the directions on making corrections for the particular medical office software you are using.

 An awareness of cultural diversity is essential when information is obtained. In some cultures, individuals feel it is disrespectful to speak of the dead. A patient may hesitate to discuss family history and illness if the person is deceased. A similar situation may exist in cases of adoption where biological family history is not known. An interpreter may be needed if a patient speaks a foreign language and has limited English. Patients may refuse to discuss family problems that may be causing stress and/or physical problems if they believe that this is personal information. If an individual has a cultural belief that illness is caused as a punishment for sin, the patient may not want to discuss specific symptoms or problems. In some cultures, individuals do not discuss pain. These individuals believe pain is something that must be tolerated and accepted; acknowledging pain is a sign of weakness. Many individuals may be hesitant to discuss cultural or religious remedies they have tried, such as herbal remedies, acupuncture, witchcraft, or religious rituals. The health care provider must show respect, tolerance, and acceptance of a patient's cultural and religious beliefs while obtaining information for the medical record.

The final version of the medical history record is usually keyed into a computer program and printed for the patient's permanent record or it is included in the patient's electronic health record (EHR). Make sure any handwritten copy is legible and clear. Double-check all information to make sure it has been recorded correctly.

Some common abbreviations used on medical records and forms are as follows:

- *S* for single
- *M* for married
- *W* for widowed
- *D* for divorced
- *O* for negative or none
- *l and w* for living and well
- *DOB* for date of birth
- *d* for died (year of death is usually placed after the symbol)
- *NA* or *N/A* for not applicable, or does not apply

check**point**

1. What information is contained on a statistical data sheet?

PRACTICE: Go to the workbook and complete the assignment sheet for 24:4, Completing Medical Records and Forms. Then return and continue with the procedure.

Completing Medical Records and Forms

NOTE: A blank statistical data sheet and blank medical history sheet are in the workbook. Use these sheets to practice this procedure. You may also use other varieties of the sheets and adapt the questions to the information required.

Equipment and Supplies

Statistical data sheet, medical history sheet, pen or computer

Technology

NOTE: If a computer program is used to complete medical records, follow the instructions provided with the software. Basic principles provided in this procedure are still followed when information is entered into the computer.

Procedure

1. Assemble equipment. Use a private area for questioning the patient (**Figure 24–11**).

   NOTE: A separate room with the door closed is preferred.

   Legal   HIPAA

   CAUTION: Patient information is confidential. The patient's legal right to privacy must be observed.

2.
   Comm

   Complete the statistical data sheet. Ask questions in a polite manner. Speak clearly and distinctly. Observe all of the following points:

   a. Key or print the name clearly. Check spelling.

   b. Fill in the complete address of the patient's permanent residence. Use the space provided.

   c. List the full telephone number of the patient's residence. If the patient does not have a telephone, put "none." Do not leave it blank because doing so indicates that you have omitted the question. If the phone number is not local, list the area code. If the patient has a cell phone number or e-mail address, enter them in the spaces provided.

   d. Fill in the personal information requested, including age, full birthdate (month, day, and year), and sex.

   e. Circle either *S, M, W,* or *D* to indicate the patient's marital status. The letters stand for *single, married, widowed,* or *divorced*.

   f. List the patient's full Social Security number, placing dashes (-) between sections of the number (for example, 218-00-0100).

   Safety

   CAUTION: Repeat and check numbers for accuracy.

   g. List the spouse's name (the name of the patient's husband or wife), if this is requested. If the patient is single, widowed, or divorced, put "NA" for "not applicable."

   h. List the patient's place of employment. Include address, telephone number, and other information requested. If the patient is not employed, put "none" or current work status such as "student," "homemaker," or "retired."

   i. List the full name of the person responsible for the account. If this is the patient, list "self." If it is a husband, wife, or parent, complete all requested information.

   j. List the full name of the insurance company, the address, and telephone number. Double-check the policy number to be sure it is accurate. This information is essential for billing.

   NOTE: Be sure to include dashes, letters, and other parts of the policy number.

   NOTE: Most agencies make a copy of both the front and back of the patient's insurance card to place in the patient's file or to include in their electronic health record (EHR).

   k. In the *referred by* section, place the name of the person who suggested your agency to the patient. This could be another physician, another patient, a friend, a relative, or even an Internet site.

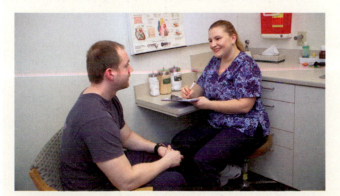

FIGURE 24–11 Make sure the patient has complete privacy while completing the medical history form.

(continues)

3. **Legal** Recheck the information on the statistical data sheet as needed. Be sure all information is printed or keyed into a computer correctly. If an error occurs on a printed paper copy, draw a single red line through any incorrect entry and put your initials and the date near the line. Then insert the correct information together with *Corr* or *Correction* to indicate it is the right information. If an incorrect entry is noted on a computer page, follow the directions for making corrections in the particular medical office software you are using.

4. **Comm** Complete the medical history form. Ask each question clearly. Obtain all pertinent information, such as dates of illnesses, treatments for illnesses, and details of complaint. Be professional. Allow the patient time to think about the answers. Be sure the patient understands all questions. Describe the various symptoms as stated. Make sure the patient has privacy when answering the questions. Note the following points:

a. Complete all parts of the form. If answers are "no" or "none," the symbol *O* is sometimes used. Some questions may not apply to the patient. An example would be menstrual history, which would not apply to a male patient. Use *NA* for "not applicable."

b. Complete the first part using information from the statistical data sheet previously completed. If no data sheet was completed, fill in as instructed.

c. Under *family history*, record information on blood relatives only. Do not include information on the patient's in-laws. Symbols can be used, such as *l and w* for "living and well"; *d. in 1960* indicates the family member died in 1960. Under *sisters and brothers*, list number of each. If any have died, list the date and cause of death. Explain the diseases listed and question the patient about any relatives who have or had the disease.

d. Under *past medical history*, record any illnesses the patient has had. List the date of the illness or the age of the patient at the time of the illness. The symbol *O* can be used if the patient has not had the disease. List types of operations and dates.

e. Under *personal history*, obtain all pertinent information. Be specific. For example, do not just put "yes" for tobacco use; instead, put "two packs per day."

f. List the *present ailment* or chief complaint in detail. For example, enter "continuous sharp pain in upper right arm" instead of "pain in arm." List any previous treatment, including treatments the patient has tried by themselves. List the date of onset (when the problem started).

 Legal **HIPAA** **NOTE:** In many agencies, the physician or other authorized person completes the medical history. Make sure that the patient and physician or other authorized person have privacy during this time. Have forms, a pen, and/or a computer readily available.

5. **Legal** Recheck the medical history record to be sure all parts are accurate because this is a legal record. Note any additional information provided by the patient. Make sure numbers, dates, spelling, and other information are correct. If an error is present on a paper copy of the medical history, draw a single red line through the incorrect entry and put your initials and the date near the line. Then insert the correct information together with *Corr* or *Correction* to indicate it is the right information. If an incorrect entry is noted on a computer page, follow the directions for making corrections in the particular medical office software you are using. A copy of a computer-generated medical history is usually printed and placed in the patient's file or the information is a part of the patient's electronic health record (EHR).

6. Prepare the patient for the physical examination, if indicated. (This procedure was explained in information Section 21:4.)

7. Replace all equipment.

PRACTICE: Go to the workbook and use the evaluation sheet for 24:4, Completing Medical Records and Forms, to practice this procedure. When you believe you have mastered this skill, sign the sheet and give it to your instructor for further action.

✅ **Check** **FINAL EVALUATION:** Using the criteria listed on the evaluation sheet, your instructor will grade your performance.

24:5 COMPOSING BUSINESS LETTERS

TYPES OF LETTERS

Comm

There are many different types of business letters. Some types of business letters you may be required to prepare include:

- **Collection** letter: Encourages a patient to pay an account that is due. Collection letters frequently are sent to patients who do not respond to bill statements.

- **Appointment** letter: Informs a patient of a scheduled appointment. All information including the day, date, and time must be included in the letter. In many agencies, appointment reminders are sent by e-mails or texts.

- **Recall** letter: Reminds a patient that it is time to return for a periodic examination. A reminder letter for a 6-month dental check-up is one example. In some agencies, recall cards, e-mails, or texts are sent to patients.

- **Consultation** letter: Sent to another professional to request an examination of a particular patient. It is sometimes used as a referral to another physician, therapist, or treatment/diagnostic agency.

- **Inquiry** letter: Seeks some information. A letter asking a patient for information about medical insurance is one example.

PARTS OF A LETTER

Every letter must include certain parts. The parts and their components are as follows:

- **Letterhead** or **heading**: In most cases, a computerized template is used to create letters and the letterhead or heading is saved in the template. The agency's name, address, and telephone number are populated in the template and will print off with the letter. Some health care agencies also include their fax number, Internet address, and/or e-mail address. In some agencies printed stationery is used, and the agency's name, address, and phone number are printed on the paper as the letterhead.

- **Date line**: The date the letter is being written is keyed under the letterhead.

- **Inside address**: This is the name, address, city, state, and zip code of the person or firm to whom the letter is being sent.

- **Salutation**: This is the name of the person to whom the letter is directed. The salutation should include the title, such as *Dear Mr., Mrs., Ms.,* or *Dr.,* followed by the last name of the person. If the letter is addressed to a title (for example, human resources manager), the salutation should read *Dear Human Resources Manager* or *To Whom It May Concern.*

- **Subject line**: Some letters may include a subject line to reference the reason for writing. This is not present in all letters.

- **Body**: This is the message of the letter. Most letters include three paragraphs. The first paragraph states why the letter is being written. The second paragraph lists the main facts. The third paragraph is the sign off or final reminder.

- **Complimentary close**: This is a courtesy, most commonly *Sincerely, Sincerely yours, Respectfully yours,* or *Yours truly*. Only the first word of the complimentary close is capitalized.

- **Signature**: The signature is the name and/or title of the person writing the letter. Leave space after the complimentary close for a handwritten signature, and then key the name and title of the person who is sending the letter.

- **Reference initials**: Reference initials are the initials of the person dictating the letter and the initials of the person preparing the letter, or the initials of just the preparer.

- **Enclosure notation**: If enclosures are included with the letter, this is noted at the end of the letter with a brief description of the material enclosed.

PROPER FORM FOR LETTERS

When keying a letter into a computer, it is important to follow specific rules and use correct spacing. Some of the main points to observe are as follows:

- All letters must be neat and professional. Spelling and punctuation must be correct. Use the spelling and grammar checks on the computer to correct errors. Use a dictionary to check medical or dental terms that might not be on the computer spell-checker.

- The style for letters varies. Follow the style desired by your agency. Two common styles are block style and modified-block style. In **block style** (**Figure 24–12**), all parts of the letter are aligned starting at the left margin of the paper. In **modified-block style** (**Figure 24–13**), certain parts of the letter are aligned at the center line of the paper and the remaining parts are aligned at the left margin of the paper.

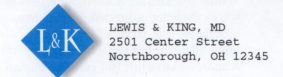

LEWIS & KING, MD
2501 Center Street
Northborough, OH 12345

Northborough
Family Medical Group

Date Line   January 12, 20____ (approximately 15th line)

Inside Address   Jeremy Brown, MD (approximately 20th line)
                          111 S Main
                          Blossom, UT 10283-1120
                              (double-space)
Salutation   Dear Dr. Brown:
                              (double-space)
Subject Line   Blossom Medical Society Meeting
                              (double-space)
Body   Thank you for inviting me to speak at the Blossom Medical Society
                          Meeting June 15, 20____. As requested, my topic will describe the
                          use of the MRI in assisting physicians to make a more accurate
                          diagnosis without resorting to invasive procedures. The exact
                          title of my speech will be sent by next Friday.
                              (double-space)
                          Please have your office manager send information regarding the
                          number of participants expected, time of meeting, location, and
                          any other details that will assist me in preparing my speech.

                          I will write or call if I have any additional questions.
                              (double-space)
**Complimentary
Closing**   Yours truly,

                          Winston Lewis, MD (4–5 line spaces)

Keyed Signature   Winston Lewis, MD
                              (double-space)
Reference Initials   WL:jg
                              (double-space)
Enclosure Notation   Enclosure: Handout on MRI

FIGURE 24–12 The form for a block-style letter. All sections are aligned at the left margin.

- If a computerized template with a populated letterhead is used, space down three to four lines below the letterhead. Begin keying at the center line for modified-block style or at the left margin for block style. Key in the month, day, and year. Do not abbreviate the month.

- If a letterhead is printed on the paper, space down approximately 15 lines from the top of the document. Begin keying at the center line for modified-block style or at the left margin for block style. Key in the month, day, and year. Do *not* abbreviate the month.

- Space down five lines and begin the inside address on the fifth line below the last line of the heading. Start at the left margin line regardless of style. The inside address should be at least three lines long. The first line is the name and title (for example, *Mr.* or *Ms.*) of the person to whom the letter is being sent. Never use a double title, such as *Dr. D. A. Jones, M.D.*; rather, use *D. A. Jones, M.D.* The second line

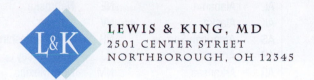

LEWIS & KING, MD
2501 CENTER STREET
NORTHBOROUGH, OH 12345

NORTHBOROUGH
FAMILY MEDICAL GROUP

January 12, 20____ (approximately 15th line)

Jeremy Brown, MD (approximately 20th line)
111 S Main
Blossom, UT 10283-1120

Dear Dr. Brown:

Blossom Medical Society Meeting

Thank you for inviting me to speak at the Blossom Medical Society
Meeting June 15, 20____. As requested, my topic will describe the use of
the MRI in assisting physicians to make a more accurate diagnosis without resorting to invasive procedures. The exact title of my speech will
be sent by next Friday.

Please have your office manager send information regarding the number of
participants expected, time of meeting, location, and any other details
that will assist me in preparing my speech.

I will write or call if I have any additional questions.

Yours truly,

Winston Lewis, MD

Winston Lewis, MD

WL:jg

Enclosure: Handout on MRI

FIGURE 24–13 The form for a modified-block style letter.

is the street number and address. The third line is the city, state, and zip code. Leave one space but no punctuation after the name of the state before keying the zip code.

- Space down two lines (double-space) and begin the salutation on the second line below the inside address. A colon (:) should follow the salutation. Start on the left margin regardless of style. Capitalize all words in the salutation, for example, *Dear Mr. Brown:, Dear Dr. Jones:,* or *Dear Director:.*

- If a subject line is included in the letter, space down two lines (double-space) below the salutation. Begin keying at the left margin to insert the subject of the letter.

- Space down two lines and begin keying the body on the second line after the salutation or subject line. Single-space within paragraphs; double-space to separate paragraphs. Start each line of the body on the left margin. In most cases, the first line of any paragraph in either modified-block style or block style is not indented. Some agencies, however, may indent the first line of each paragraph five spaces in a modified-block style letter. Follow agency policy.

- Space down two lines after the last sentence in the body and begin keying the close. Start at the center line for modified-block style or at the left margin for block style. Capitalize only the first word of the complimentary close and place a comma at the end of the close, for example, *Sincerely, Sincerely yours, Respectfully yours,* or *Yours truly.*

- Leave four to five blank lines for the written signature and begin the keyed name and title on the fifth or sixth line below the complimentary close. Start at the center line for modified-block style or at the left margin for block style. Key the name and title of the person sending the letter. Long titles may be placed on a second line under the name.

- Double-space after the keyed name and title and key the reference initials. Start at the left margin regardless of style. Key either the initials of just the preparer or the initials of the writer and the initials of the preparer. Use either capital or small letters. If two sets of initials are used, use a colon to separate capitalized initials and a slash to separate lowercased initials, for example, *LMS:WHB* or *lms/whb.* Some agencies use capital initials for the writer, lowercase initials for the preparer, and a colon to separate the two sets of initials. Follow agency policy.

- Leave neat, even margins at both sides of the paper. Margins should be wide enough to be attractive, but not too wide as to distort. An average width for margins is 1–1½ inches. Leave a bottom margin of at least 1 inch (six lines).

- At times, using the full name of a state or territory makes a letter seem unbalanced. In such cases, the name of the state or territory is abbreviated. Only the abbreviations shown in **Figure 24–14** are acceptable. They are recommended by the U.S. Postal Service. Note that both letters are capitalized and that no periods are used in the abbreviations.

AL	Alabama	NE	Nebraska
AK	Alaska	NV	Nevada
AS	American Samoa	NH	New Hampshire
AZ	Arizona	NJ	New Jersey
AR	Arkansas	NM	New Mexico
CA	California	NY	New York
CO	Colorado	NC	North Carolina
CT	Connecticut	ND	North Dakota
DE	Delaware	MP	North Mariana
DC	District of		Islands
	Columbia	OH	Ohio
FL	Florida	OK	Oklahoma
GA	Georgia	OR	Oregon
GU	Guam	PA	Pennsylvania
HI	Hawaii	PR	Puerto Rico
ID	Idaho	RI	Rhode Island
IL	Illinois	SC	South Carolina
IN	Indiana	SD	South Dakota
IA	Iowa	TN	Tennessee
KS	Kansas	TX	Texas
KY	Kentucky	TT	Trust Territory
LA	Louisiana	UT	Utah
ME	Maine	VT	Vermont
MD	Maryland	VI	Virgin Islands,
MA	Massachusetts		U.S.
MI	Michigan	VA	Virginia
MN	Minnesota	WA	Washington
MS	Mississippi	WV	West Virginia
MO	Missouri	WI	Wisconsin
MT	Montana	WY	Wyoming

FIGURE 24–14 U.S. Postal Service abbreviations for states and territories.

SUMMARY

Comm

All letters should be proofread before the sender receives them for signature. Make sure that all words are spelled correctly, and that complete sentences and correct punctuation are used. Use the spelling and grammar checks available on most word-processing programs. In most agencies, computers and word-processing software are used to prepare letters, so it is easy to correct errors on the computer screen prior to printing a hard copy of a letter.

Technology

In addition, most health care agencies have standard form letters saved in a computer database or embedded in their medical office software. When a letter is needed for a specific purpose, such as a letter of appointment, the letter of appointment form letter is retrieved. The patient's name and personal information are keyed into the form letter. If the same letter has to be sent to a large group of people, the mail merge feature (found on most word-processing programs) can be used to create a large number of personalized letters. Computer classes can help the health care assistant learn how to utilize the many features present in word-processing programs.

checkpoint

1. List four (4) types of letters that you may be required to prepare.

PRACTICE: Go to the workbook and complete the assignment sheet for 24:5, Composing Business Letters. Then return and continue with the procedure.

Procedure 24:5

Composing Business Letters

NOTE: You must have computer, word-processing software, and keyboarding skills to complete this procedure.

Equipment and Supplies

Computer with word-processing software and printer, letterhead or good quality paper, scrap paper, pen or pencil

Procedure

1. Read the preceding information section, Composing Business Letters.

2. Determine a topic for a business letter or obtain a topic from your instructor. Decide on the style of the letter (that is, modified-block or block). Your instructor may specify a style.

   NOTE: In the following steps, *MB* indicates modified-block style, and *B* indicates block style.

3. Use scrap paper to write a rough draft of the letter. Check to be sure all required information is included. Use a dictionary to ensure proper spelling.

   NOTE: Ask your instructor for assistance, as needed.

4. Open a new document. Set the margins for the document. Note the center reading.

   NOTE: Margins should be wide enough to appear attractive, but not so wide as to distort. The average width is 1–1½ inches.

5. If a computerized template is used with a populated letterhead, space down three to four lines below the letterhead and key in the month, day, and year. Begin at the center line for MB or at the left margin for B. If a letterhead is preprinted on the paper, space down to the 15th line and key in the month, day, and year. Begin at the center line for MB or at the left margin for B.

6. Space down five lines. On the fifth line, key the inside address, starting at the left margin.

7. Space down two lines (double-space). Key the salutation, starting at the left margin. Insert a colon (:) after the salutation.

8. If a subject line is included in the letter, space down two lines, begin at the left margin, and key in the subject of the letter.

9. Double-space. Start keying the body at the left margin. Single-space within paragraphs; double-space between paragraphs. Do not indent the first lines of paragraphs.

   NOTE: Most letters should contain at least three paragraphs.

10. Double-space after the body. Key the complimentary close starting at the center line for MB or at the left margin for B. If more than one word is used, capitalize only the first word. Insert a comma at the end.

11. Leave four to five blank lines for the written signature.

12. Starting at the center line for MB or at the left margin for B, key the sender's name and title. If it is long, the title can be keyed on a second line.

13. Double-space. Key the reference initials, starting at the left margin. Use either capital or lowercase letters for the initials of either just the preparer or of both the sender and the preparer. If two sets of initials are used, use a colon to separate capitalized initials and a slash to separate lowercase initials. Some agencies use capital initials for the sender, lowercase initials for the preparer, and a colon to separate the letters.

14. Read the entire letter. Perform a spelling and grammar check. Use a dictionary as necessary to check spelling of medical and dental terms not included in the computer's dictionary.

15. Print a hard copy of the letter. In most agencies, a second copy of the letter is placed in the patient's file or it is included in their electronic health record (EHR). Save the letter on the computer hard drive or on a flash drive, external hard drive, or secure cloud or off-site server.

16. Replace all equipment.

PRACTICE: Go to the workbook and use the evaluation sheet for 24:5, Composing Business Letters, to practice this procedure. When you believe you have mastered this skill, sign the sheet and give it to your instructor for further action.

 FINAL EVALUATION: Using the criteria listed on the evaluation sheet, your instructor will grade your performance.

24:6 COMPLETING INSURANCE FORMS

Because many patients rely on insurance companies to pay medical and/or dental expenses, completing **insurance forms** may be a part of your duties. To obtain prompt payment from the companies, you must complete the forms correctly.

Comm   EHR

Information regarding a patient's insurance coverage is essential. Such information is usually obtained on the patient's first visit to the agency. The information is usually recorded on the statistical data sheet, in a computer database, or in the patient's electronic health record (EHR). In addition, most agencies make a copy of both the front and back of a patient's insurance card and place the copy in the patient's file or in the patient's EHR. It is essential that all names, addresses, and contract numbers be correct. Double-check this information as it is being recorded. It is also wise to check each time the patient visits the health care agency that the patient's coverage has not changed.

HIPAA

If a patient wishes to file an insurance claim, make sure the patient has completed any parts of the form that they are required to complete. Also make sure that the patient has signed the form wherever their signature is required. If the patient is a dependent, such as a spouse or older child, it is also necessary to obtain the signature of the person to whom the insurance contract has been issued. This person is referred to as the *insured*. HIPAA requirements mandate that confidential medical information cannot be released unless a patient signs an authorization to release information to insurance companies. Because most agencies now complete insurance forms on a computer and file the claims electronically, the patient and the insured usually sign an "*Authorization to Release Information and Assign Benefits*" form. This form is kept in the patient's file and the insurance form is marked "*patient's signature on file.*" In some agencies, the form is scanned into the computer and filed electronically with the insurance form or is part of the patient's electronic health record (EHR).

A universal insurance claim form is now used in most agencies (**Figure 24–15**). This form, known as the CMS-1500, was developed by the Centers for Medicare and Medicaid Services. It must be used for any government-sponsored health care claims, such as Medicare or Medicaid. All major insurance companies will also accept this form.

CODING INSURANCE FORMS

Technology

Most insurance forms have two parts that require codes: diagnosis and procedures/services. Alphanumeric (letters and numbers) codes are used to clearly identify information in a uniform and standard manner. Most insurance companies use computers to process and pay claims, so the alphanumerical codes must be accurate. Use of an incorrect code can lead to rejection and/or delayed payment of a claim. There are two major sources of correct alphanumerical codes: the *International Classification of Diseases* and the *Current Procedural Terminology*.

The World Health Organization (WHO) has developed a coding system for diagnoses to aid in tracking the presence of the disease, maintaining morbidity (affected with disease) and mortality (causing death) statistics, and creating an international database for identifying disease. This coding system is known as the *International Classification of Diseases* (ICD). The U.S. Department of Health and Human Services (USDHHS) publishes the *International Classification of Diseases* (ICD). The USDHHS also publishes the *International Classification of Diseases Clinical Modifications* (ICD-CM), which is used for diagnosis coding. The diagnosis is the identification of the disease or condition that the patient has. If a patient is diagnosed as having more than one condition, the most important diagnosis and its corresponding ICD-CM code are listed first. Other diagnoses and their ICD-CM codes follow in order of importance.

The current codes are known as ICD-10-CM codes and can contain up to seven alphanumeric characters. This coding method is very specific for each disease or condition. The categories begin with a letter. Each level of division is a subcategory. Codes may be three, four, five, six, or seven digits. For example, the category S42 represents a fracture of the shoulder and upper arm. The code S42.2 represents a fracture of the upper end of the humerus. The code S42.20 represents an unspecified fracture of the upper end of the humerus. The sixth digit represents left or right. Therefore, S42.201 represents an unspecified fracture of the upper end of the right humerus. The seventh digit allows for more specificity. The code S42.201A represents an unspecified fracture of the upper end of the right humerus, initial encounter for a closed fracture. On the other hand, the code S42.201B indicates an unspecified fracture of the upper end of the right humerus, initial encounter for an open fracture. Note that if there are more than three digits of a code, a period separates the third digit from the fourth digit. Every diagnosis must be coded to the highest level of specificity or the claim will be rejected. Therefore, it is important to use as many digits as possible with each diagnosis.

To find a diagnosis in the code book, look up the noun or main term in the alphabetical index. For example, look up *hysterectomy* for a diagnosis of *subtotal hysterectomy*. Use the code number in the alphabetical index to find the exact ICD-10-CM number in the tabular list for a *subtotal hysterectomy*. Most computer programs will start with the noun or the three-digit category. When the noun or three-digit code is keyed into the computer, a list appears with subheadings and complete codes. By practicing using the code book or computer software, you will find

1500

HEALTH INSURANCE CLAIM FORM

APPROVED BY NATIONAL UNIFORM CLAIM COMMITTEE 08/05

☐☐ PICA PICA ☐☐

| 1. MEDICARE (Medicare #) | MEDICAID (Medicaid #) | TRICARE CHAMPUS (Sponsor's SSN) | CHAMPVA (Member ID#) | GROUP HEALTH PLAN (SSN or ID) | FECA BLK LUNG (SSN) | OTHER ☒ (ID) | 1a. INSURED'S I.D. NUMBER (For Program in Item 1): 555-55-555 |

2. PATIENT'S NAME (Last Name, First Name, Middle Initial)
MCKAY, LEO M

3. PATIENT'S BIRTH DATE MM 04 DD 01 YY 1963 **SEX** M ☒ F ☐

4. INSURED'S NAME (Last Name, First Name, Middle Initial)
MCKAY, LEO M.

5. PATIENT'S ADDRESS (No., Street)
123 W FIRST STREET
CITY ANYWHERE STATE PA

6. PATIENT RELATIONSHIP TO INSURED
Self ☒ Spouse ☐ Child ☐ Other ☐

8. PATIENT STATUS
Single ☒ Married ☐ Other ☐
Employed ☐ Full-Time Student ☐ Part-Time Student ☐

7. INSURED'S ADDRESS (No., Street)
123 W FIRST STREET
CITY ANYWHERE STATE PA

ZIP CODE 11666 TELEPHONE (Include Area Code) (824)556-6189

ZIP CODE 11666 TELEPHONE (Include Area Code) (824)556-6789

9. OTHER INSURED'S NAME (Last Name, First Name, Middle Initial)

10. IS PATIENT'S CONDITION RELATED TO:

11. INSURED'S POLICY GROUP OR FECA NUMBER
1122334

a. OTHER INSURED'S POLICY OR GROUP NUMBER

a. EMPLOYMENT? (Current or Previous) ☐ YES ☒ NO

a. INSURED'S DATE OF BIRTH MM 04 DD 01 YY 1963 **SEX** M ☒ F ☐

b. OTHER INSURED'S DATE OF BIRTH MM DD YY SEX M ☐ F ☐

b. AUTO ACCIDENT? ☐ YES ☒ NO PLACE (State)

b. EMPLOYER'S NAME OR SCHOOL NAME
ABC MANUFACTURING COMPANY

c. EMPLOYER'S NAME OR SCHOOL NAME

c. OTHER ACCIDENT? ☐ YES ☒ NO

c. INSURANCE PLAN NAME OR PROGRAM NAME
HOW MUCH INSURANCE COMPANY

d. INSURANCE PLAN NAME OR PROGRAM NAME

10d. RESERVED FOR LOCAL USE

d. IS THERE ANOTHER HEALTH BENEFIT PLAN?
☐ YES ☒ NO *If yes,* return to and complete item 9 a-d.

READ BACK OF FORM BEFORE COMPLETING & SIGNING THIS FORM.

12. PATIENT'S OR AUTHORIZED PERSON'S SIGNATURE I authorize the release of any medical or other information necessary to process this claim. I also request payment of government benefits either to myself or to the party who accepts assignment below.
SIGNED Signature on File DATE 01/14/XXXX

13. INSURED'S OR AUTHORIZED PERSON'S SIGNATURE I authorize payment of medical benefits to the undersigned physician or supplier for services described below.
SIGNED Signature on File

14. DATE OF CURRENT: MM 01 DD 10 YY XXXX ILLNESS (First symptom) OR INJURY (Accident) OR PREGNANCY(LMP)

15. IF PATIENT HAS HAD SAME OR SIMILAR ILLNESS. GIVE FIRST DATE MM DD YY

16. DATES PATIENT UNABLE TO WORK IN CURRENT OCCUPATION FROM MM DD YY TO MM DD YY

17. NAME OF REFERRING PROVIDER OR OTHER SOURCE 17a. 17b. NPI

18. HOSPITALIZATION DATES RELATED TO CURRENT SERVICES FROM MM DD YY TO MM DD YY

19. RESERVED FOR LOCAL USE

20. OUTSIDE LAB? ☐ YES ☐ NO $ CHARGES

21. DIAGNOSIS OR NATURE OF ILLNESS OR INJURY (Relate Items 1, 2, 3 or 4 to Item 24E by Line)
1. E10 .9 3. M06 .9
2. I11 .9 4.

22. MEDICAID RESUBMISSION CODE ORIGINAL REF. NO.

23. PRIOR AUTHORIZATION NUMBER

24. A. DATE(S) OF SERVICE From MM DD YY To MM DD YY	B. PLACE OF SERVICE	C. EMG	D. PROCEDURES, SERVICES, OR SUPPLIES (Explain Unusual Circumstances) CPT/HCPCS MODIFIER	E. DIAGNOSIS POINTER	F. $ CHARGES	G. DAYS OR UNITS	H. EPSDT Family Plan	I. ID. QUAL.	J. RENDERING PROVIDER ID. #
1	01 10 XXXX	3		99214	1,2,3	85 00	1		NPI	1543298760
2	01 10 XXXX	3		82270	1,2	13 00	1		NPI	1543298760
3									NPI	
4									NPI	
5									NPI	
6									NPI	

25. FEDERAL TAX I.D. NUMBER 91-1234432 SSN ☐ EIN ☒

26. PATIENT'S ACCOUNT NO. MCK111

27. ACCEPT ASSIGNMENT? (For govt. claims, see back) ☐ YES ☒ NO

28. TOTAL CHARGE $ 98 00

29. AMOUNT PAID $

30. BALANCE DUE $ 98 00

31. SIGNATURE OF PHYSICIAN OR SUPPLIER INCLUDING DEGREES OR CREDENTIALS (I certify that the statements on the reverse apply to this bill and are made a part thereof.)
Mark Wos MD 01/14/XXX
SIGNED DATE

32. SERVICE FACILITY LOCATION INFORMATION
u. NPI b.

33. BILLING PROVIDER INFO & PH # (814)555-1155
INNER CITY HEALTH CARE
222 S FIRST AVE
CANTON PA 11666
a. R09876543 b.

NUCC Instruction Manual available at: www.nucc.org APPROVED OMB-0938-0999 FORM CMS-1500 (08/05)

FIGURE 24–15 A completed medical CMS-1500 insurance claim form. Approved by National Uniform Claim Committee 8/05. NUCC Instruction Manual available at: www.nucc.org.

that it is not difficult to use. Examples of the ICD-10-CM codes for classification of diseases of the appendix are shown in **Table 24–2**.

The American Medical Association (AMA) annually publishes a professional edition of *Current Procedural Terminology* (CPT). This is the major source of numerical codes for procedures and services, called *CPT codes*. The American Dental Association (ADA) publishes a *Current Dental Terminology (CDT)* book for use in dental offices. CPT and CDT codes are also available on computer software programs for use in agencies where computers are used for billing and insurance purposes (**Figure 24–16**). It is important to use the latest edition of the book or computer software programs to be sure that the codes are accurate

| DOE, JOHN H. | | BC | BC / BS OF FLA | | BELL | BELLSOUTH | DED. | | A |

```
                              Select Diagnosis                    8,297
1    K35                                                                    K35 letter and then
2    E11.2       dia                                      ← type            bring up the
3                                                                           listing of
4            E11.0 Type 2 diabetes mellitus with hyperosmolarity            codes.
                  E11.00...... without coma
                  E11.01...... with coma
            E11.2 Type 2 diabetes mellitus with kidney complications
FROM              E11.21 Type 2 diabetes mellitus with diabetic nephropathy    INSURANC    PATIENT
11/19/08          E11.22 Type 2 diabetes mellitus with diabetic chronic kidney disease   0.00   75.00
11/26/08          E11.29 Type 2 diabetes mellitus with other diabetic kidney complication  0.00   33.00
            E11.3 Type 2 diabetes mellitus with ophthalmic complications
                  E11.31 Type 2 diabetes mellitus with unspecified diabetic retinopathy
                        E11.311...... with macular edema
                        E11.319...... without macular edema
                  E11.32 Type 2 diabetes mellitus with mild diabetic retinopathy
                        E11.321...... with macular edema
                        E11.329...... without macular edema

HOLD FOR        ENTER TO SELECT      [INS] TO ADD        [F10] TO CHANGE
                                                                               0.00        108.00
                [DEL] TO DELETE      [F6] VIEW BY NUMBER                    .00
```

| [INS] | [DEL] | [F10] | [F3] | [F4] | [F5] | [F6] | [F7] | [F8]* | [F9] |
| Next Proc. | Delete | Done | Walkout | HCFA 1500 | Payment | Transfer | Hold | Recall | Path/Lab |

FIGURE 24–16 ICD and CPT codes are available on computer software programs. Retrieved from http://www.cdc.gov/inchs/fcd/icd10cm.htm#10update.

TABLE 24–2 Sample ICD-10-CM Codes

Sample ICD-10-CM Codes Diseases of the Appendix: Classifications K35-K38 CM Codes	
K35	Acute appendicitis
K35.2	Acute appendicitis with generalized peritonitis
K35.20	• without abscess
K35.21	• with peritoneal abscess
K35.3	Acute appendicitis with localized peritonitis
K35.30	• without perforation or gangrene
K35.31	• with gangrene but no perforation
K35.32	• with perforation but no abscess
K35.33	• with perforation and abscess
K35.8	Other and Unspecified acute appendicitis
K35.80	Unspecified acute appendicitis
K35.89	Other acute appendicitis
K35.890	• without perforation or gangrene
K35.891	• without perforation, with gangrene

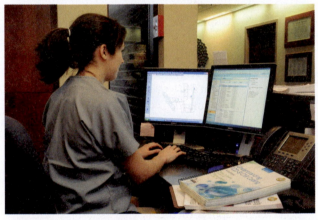

FIGURE 24–17 Use the CPT and ICD books and/or computer software programs to ensure coding is correct for both diagnoses and procedures.

and current. Each procedure or service is assigned a five-digit code without decimal points or periods. Modifiers are used to further explain or to change the meaning of a code and are separated from the code by a dash. For example, the code *44950* indicates an appendectomy, or surgical removal of the appendix. Usually, this is the only code required. However, if the appendectomy was very complex and involved much more time or care than is normally required, the modifier *-22* is added to the CPT code for a correct code of *44950-22*. The introduction in the CPT code book provides excellent instructions on the use of the book and on proper coding. By reading the introduction and practicing using the book, you can learn to correctly code procedures and services (**Figure 24–17**). In addition, most

agencies have lists containing the correct CPT codes for the common procedures and services provided. The CPT codes frequently are also printed on the communication form or superbill (discussed in information Section 24:7), which simplifies the process of completing insurance claims.

COMPLETING INSURANCE CLAIMS

Some general rules that apply to completing most insurance forms are as follows:

* Make sure you are using the correct form.

* Read the form thoroughly or review the software program on a computer to be sure you understand what is required.

```
THIS IS A PREVIOUSLY ENTERED FORM 11/19/--                                                      Pt Bal =
   Doctor [1]    Assistant [ ]    Assign? [N]                    Fee Code [A]
 MEDICARE      MEDICAID        TRICARE         GROUP          FECA        OTHER     Insured's ID Number
   [X]            [ ]              [ ]            [ ]           [ ]          [ ]     123456789A
                                                                                    Insured's Name
 Patient's Name                                Birthdate      Sex (M/F)             John H. Doe
 Doe, John H.                                  05/06/56        M                    Insured's Address
 Address
 3508 SOUTH ATLANTIC AVE                        SelfX     Spouse     Child    Other
 NEW SMRYNA BEACH FL 32771
 32771              427-0558   (904)            Single      Married        Other    Insured's Group
 Other Insured's Name                           Employed     FullTS       PartTS

 Policy Number                                 Condition Related to:               Ins. DOB                    Sex
 65913222                                      Employment  [ ] Yes   [X] No           / /
 DOB                            Sex                                          ST     Employer
   / /                                         Auto Acc.  [ ] Yes   [X] No
 Employer                                                                           Plan Name
                                               Other Acc.  [ ] Yes   [X] No         BC / BS OF FLA
 Plan Name                                                                          Date of Disability
 BELLSOUTH DED. SERV CENTR                     Local
 Date of Current                               First consulted                     Hospitalization
 Referring {F5}                                Referring ID#
                                                                                    Lab [ ] Yes [X] No
 Facility {F5}                                                                      Prior Auth
    {F10} = Next Pg       {ESC} = Back Up        {F3} = Pt Info     CTRL + ESC   Abort      11/19/--              1
```

FIGURE 24-18 A sample computer entry screen for insurance information.

- Check to be sure that the patient has completed the proper areas. Make sure their signature appears in all required spaces. If you are using a computer program to generate the form, make sure the patient and insured have signed an authorization to release information and assign benefits form. This is often kept in the patient's file or in their electronic health record. *Signature on file* is then keyed in box 12, the area designated for the patient's signature.

- Double-check for accuracy all names, addresses, and contract numbers listed on the form.

- Policy numbers or contract numbers frequently include a letter or series of letters. Make sure these numbers are accurate and appear on the form in the proper places.

- Use correct codes, if codes are required. On most forms, numerical codes are used for *place of services*. A list of the codes is available at *https://www.cms.gov/Medicare/Coding/place-of-service-codes*. For example, *11* indicates provider's office, *12* indicates home, *13* indicates Assisted Living Facility, *20* indicates urgent care center, *21* indicates inpatient hospital, *22* indicates outpatient hospital, and *32* indicates nursing home.

- Numerical codes are also used to describe *type of service*. For example, *1* indicates medical care, *2* indicates surgery, *4* indicates diagnostic X-rays, *5* indicates diagnostic laboratory, and *9* indicates other medical services. The codes required are usually listed on the form or described in the software on a computer program. Refer to these as necessary.

- Answer all questions on the form.

- Answer all questions thoroughly and list specific information. For example, instead of putting *lab tests*, list the tests that have been performed.

- Standard abbreviations are allowed on most forms. Ensure the accuracy of all abbreviations used. Do *not* use any periods with abbreviations.

- On the CMS-1500 claim forms, no punctuation, such as commas and periods, should be used. The only exception is that a hyphen may be used for a nine-digit zip code.

- Make sure the amounts charged are accurately listed. Double-check all arithmetic.

Math

- Make sure the physician or other authorized person has signed the form in the required areas. Many forms require the physician's National Provider Identifier Number (NPI) and/or the Physician's Identifying Number (PIN). Medicare requires the use of the NPI number. The NPI is a 10-digit number that is inserted in box 33 of the CMS-1500 form. Make sure this number is entered accurately.

- Note the boxed area for *assignment*. If the physician or agency will accept the amount allowed by the insurance company as payment in full, this is marked *yes*; if not, it is marked *no*.

- The form is generally copied or printed, and a copy is placed in the patient's file, or is included in their electronic health record (EHR).

- Recheck the entire form before sending electronically or mailing.

Technology In many agencies, computers programmed to complete standard insurance claim forms are used. A sample entry screen for recording information is shown in **Figure 24-18**. Information for the insurance claim is entered into the computer. The computer then prints the information in the proper areas on the insurance form. The form can be printed and mailed, but many agencies now file insurance forms electronically on a secure modem. Electronic filing results in faster processing and payment of the claim. These programs are easy to use and save a great deal of time when processing insurance forms.

checkpoint

1. What organization developed a coding system for coding diagnoses?

PRACTICE: Go to the workbook and complete the assignment sheet for 24:6, Completing Insurance Forms. Then return and continue with the procedure.

Procedure 24:6

Completing Insurance Forms

NOTE: You must have keyboarding skills to complete this procedure.

Equipment and Supplies

Computer with insurance coding software for ICD and CPT codes, sample insurance forms, *International Classification of Diseases* (ICD) book/software, *The Current Procedural Terminology* (CPT) book/software (or CDT book for dental claims)

Procedure

1. Assemble equipment. Open the insurance software program on the computer or obtain a sample insurance form from your instructor.

2. Read the insurance form or review the entry areas on the computer program. Make sure you understand all required information.

   NOTE: Ask your instructor to explain areas, as needed.

3. Make sure that the patient has completed their portions of the form and has signed an authorization to release information form. Check to be sure that correct signatures are on the form. Signatures should be written in blue or black ink. If the patient is a dependent, make sure the insured person has signed the form, if this is required.

   NOTE: If the form is computer generated or is in the patient's electronic health record (EHR), and the patient and/or insured have signed the authorization to release information forms, *Signature on file (SOF)* is keyed in the area designated for the signature.

4. Enter all patient information, usually including the full name and address of the insured (the person to whom the insurance contract is issued); the patient's name, address (including zip code), birthdate (written as numbers), sex (put an *X* in the correct box), and relationship to insured (put an *X* in the correct box); the group number or name; the contract or identifying number; and other similar data. Double-check all entries for accuracy.

   NOTE: If the contract number has letters, be sure they are included.

5. Most policies require information about other insurance the patient may have. Record this information in the correct spaces. If the patient does not have other insurance, leave this blank.

6. Most forms contain questions about whether the condition is related to employment or an accident. Workers' Compensation may cover an employment-related condition; other insurance may cover a condition caused by an accident. Therefore, it is important to answer these questions correctly. Mark *yes* or *no*, or insert an *X* in the correct box.

7. Enter information regarding dates of care. Correct information is usually obtained from the patient's chart, electronic health record, or the physician or supervisor. Be sure the sources are accurate.

8. Many forms require dates of total or partial disability. This is determined by the physician or other authorized person (for example, a therapist). The time a patient is disabled and unable to work usually begins with the date of the onset of the condition. Insert this date in the correct area. An authorized person then determines an approximate date when the patient's disability will end and the patient will be able to return to work. Insert this date as the final date. If no disability is determined, leave the blocks blank.

9. If the patient was referred by another physician or agency, insert the full name of the referring source. The NPI number of the referring physician is placed in the *ID Number* space. If there was no referring source, leave the block blank.

10. If services were provided to the patient in a hospital, record the dates of hospitalization in the correct blanks. If a laboratory outside the hospital or health care facility performed tests, note this information along with the charges for the tests.

11. Leave line 19 blank unless a public or private payer is requesting additional claim codes from the National Uniform Claim Committee (NUCC).

12. In the *diagnosis* section of the form, list the ICD code for the main or primary diagnosis first followed by other diagnoses in order of importance. Use the *International Classification of Diseases* to find the correct ICD code for each diagnosis. Make sure each diagnosis is coded to the highest level of specificity. Double-check all entries for accuracy.

NOTE: Payment on a claim can be delayed or rejected if an incorrect or nonspecific ICD code is used.

13. The CPT codes for any services or procedures provided should be listed in the *services* or *treatment* section of the form. Each service or procedure should be listed separately with the most important service listed first. Dates should be obtained from the patient's chart, electronic health record, or from an authorized person. Numerical codes are frequently used to indicate place of service. Common codes include *11* for office, *21* for inpatient hospital, *22* for outpatient hospital, *12* for patient's home, *31* for skilled-nursing facility, and *32* for nursing home. Numerical codes are also used to describe types of service. Common codes include *1* for medical care, *2* for surgery, *3* for consultation, *4* for diagnostic X-rays, *5* for diagnostic laboratory, and *9* for other medical services. Codes for both type and place of service are listed on the form or defined in the computer software. Use the *Current Procedural Terminology* to find the correct CPT code for each procedure or service. Double-check the code before inserting it in the correct area. The *diagnosis code* column refers to the diagnoses listed in the *diagnosis* section. The corresponding number of the diagnosis for which the service was given should be inserted in this column.

14. List the charges for services rendered. Make sure the numbers for dollars are lined up in the correct spaces. Place the amounts for cents or *00* in the correct columns. Total all charges. Recheck all math, especially addition. If the patient has paid an amount, note this in the correct place.

15. Insert the physician's Social Security or tax identification number in the space provided. Mark the appropriate box.

16. Insert the patient's account number in the appropriate space.

17. A boxed area is usually provided for information regarding assignment, or whether the physician or agency will accept the amount allowed and paid by the insurance company. Check either *yes* or *no*, as determined by the physician or agency.

18. Insert all required information regarding the physician or supplier, including full name and title, address, telephone number (if requested), NIP, PIN, Social Security and/or ID or license number, and other required information. Be sure the physician or authorized person signs in the correct area.

 CAUTION: Double-check all numbers for accuracy.

19. Recheck all information on the form. Make sure that all required information is recorded and all answers are provided.

20. Before filing the form electronically or mailing the form to the insurance company, place a copy in the patient's file for reference or include it in the patient's electronic health record, in accordance with the policy of your agency.

21. Replace all equipment.

PRACTICE: Go to the workbook and use the evaluation sheet for 24:6, Completing Insurance Forms, to practice this procedure. When you believe you have mastered this skill, sign the sheet and give it to your instructor for further action.

FINAL EVALUATION: Using the criteria listed on the evaluation sheet, your instructor will grade your performance.

24:7 MAINTAINING A BOOKKEEPING SYSTEM

PEGBOARD SYSTEM

 Most facilities and offices are moving to electronic bookkeeping, but some still use the pegboard system. Both systems use the same concepts to track cash flow. The **pegboard system** is also called a *"write-it-once"* system. Various records are noted simultaneously. The pegboard system usually encompasses the following series of records:

- **Day sheet** or **daily journal**: This is a daily record of all **patients** seen, all charges incurred, and all payments received (**Figure 24–19**). Each day sheet also provides a total column, which can be used for bank deposit slips; a business analysis summary;

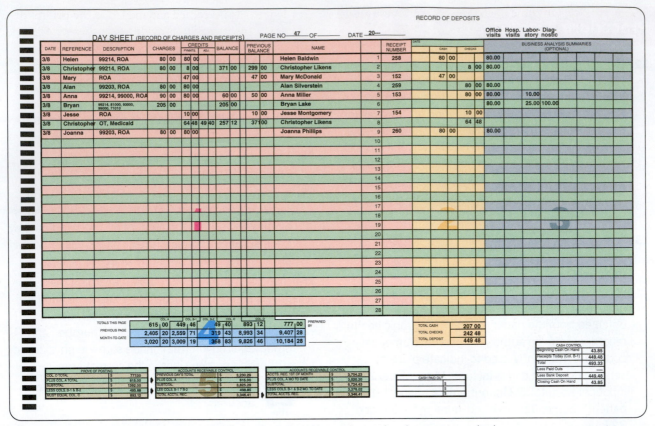

FIGURE 24–19 The day sheet provides a daily record of patients seen, charges incurred, and payments received.

a section for daily and monthly account totals; a proof of posting section for verifying that account totals are accurate; and a section to record accounts receivable, or total amounts owed by patients. When a month's supply of day sheets is compiled in one folder, a monthly record of all business is available.

- **Statement–receipt** record: This contains information on past balance due, charges for treatment, payment received, and current balance (**Figure 24–20**). Many slips also have a space to note the patient's next appointment. When complete, the statement–receipt can be given to the patient to provide a record of payment or of balance due. In some agencies, another version of this record is being used. This version is usually a three-layer form that notes all the previous information as well as specific services and corresponding insurance code numbers. Called a *communication form*, or a *superbill* (**Figure 24–21**), this version serves as a statement for the insurance company. One copy can be retained by the agency; the second copy can be sent to the insurance company (or attached to an insurance form) to serve as a claim form; and the third copy can be given to the patient to serve as a payment receipt, a record of treatment or services, a bill for the balance due on the account, and an appointment card, if another appointment is scheduled.

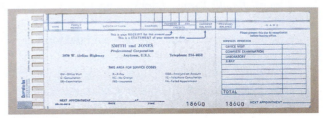

FIGURE 24–20 A statement–receipt provides information on past balance due, charges, payment received, and current balance. Courtesy of Control-O-Fax Office Systems, Waterloo, IA.

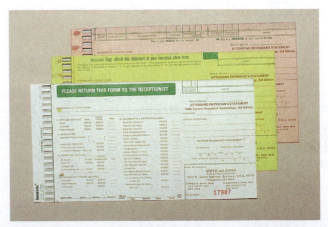

FIGURE 24–21 A three-layer version of the statement–receipt form, the communication form, or superbill also lists treatments and insurance codes. It can be used as the form for insurance claims or attached to insurance forms. Courtesy of Control-O-Fax Office Systems, Waterloo, IA.

- **Charge slip**: On some pegboard systems, these are a part of the statement–receipt record. When the patient arrives at the agency, their name is entered at the top. This section of the record is torn off the statement–receipt and attached to the patient's chart. The physician or other authorized individual then notes the treatments and charges on this slip while treating the patient. The slip is given back to the receptionist, who can then use it to post charges.

- **Ledger card**: This is a total record of care provided to a patient. It is also a financial record of the patient's account. A brief description of services, charges, payments made, and current balance due is noted on the card. In some agencies, copies of the ledger cards are used in place of separate bills. The

ledger card is copied and mailed to the patient or sent as an e-mail to provide a monthly statement (**Figure 24–22**).

The procedure for recording patient visits, treatments, charges, and payments on the pegboard system is described in Procedure 24:7. In addition to recording patients' visits and charges, the pegboard system is also used to record payments received. One example is an insurance company check for payment for services. The same steps are followed, but in place of a treatment, *ROA*, for "received on account," is usually noted under *description*. Balances are then determined, and all information is simultaneously noted on the day sheet and ledger card. A receipt may be mailed or sent electronically to the patient.

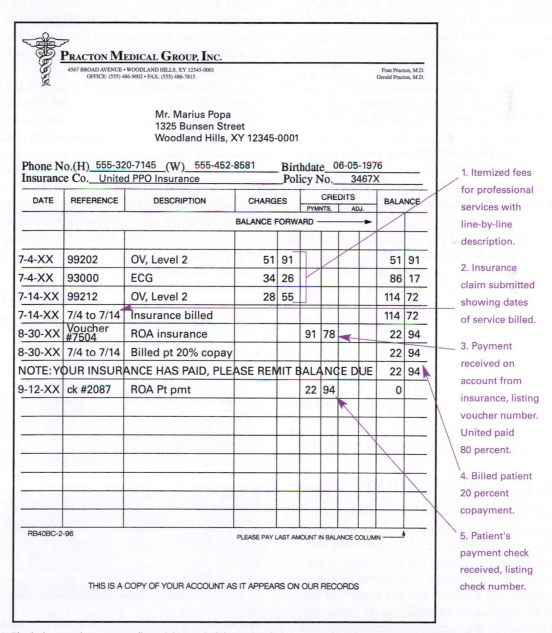

FIGURE 24–22 The ledger card serves as a financial record of the patient's account and can be copied and mailed to the patient as a monthly statement.

Many insurance companies have contracts with health care providers that specify amounts that will be paid for services. When the insurance company sends payment, it usually sends an *Explanation of Benefits* (EOB) form. This form lists the amount charged by the health care provider, the negotiated or allowed amount according to the contract, the amount the insurance company pays, and the amount of money owed by the patient. If the negotiated or allowed amount is less than the charged amount, an adjustment must be made to the patient's account. For example, a patient is charged $150 for a physical examination. The EOB form shows that the negotiated or allowed amount for this procedure is $100. The insurance company pays $80 and the patient must pay $20. An adjustment of $50 ($150 charge minus $100 allowed equals $50 adjustment) must be credited to the patient's account. This is usually done at the same time the insurance payment is recorded by putting $50 in the adjustment column on the day sheet and subtracting it from total charges.

At the end of a business day, the day sheet provides a total record of all charges and payments and a method of checking accounts. Daily totals are obtained by adding the amounts of each column on the day sheet. The accuracy of the records can be checked immediately. Small total boxes in the *Proof of Posting* section at the bottom of the sheet provide the correct formulas for determining that all entries are correct. A bank deposit slip is also provided if payments received are to be deposited.

Legal

Because a series of records is recorded at one time, it is important for the recorder to use a ballpoint pen and print neatly while pressing hard enough for all copies to record. If an error is made, it must be lined out neatly. Neither erasers nor correction fluid should be used because these are financial records that may be audited for tax or legal purposes. If a major error is made, it may be best to void the statement–receipt record and start a new record. Neatness and accuracy are essential when using the pegboard system. These are bookkeeping records; therefore, they must be stored for reference. Special folders can be purchased for this purpose.

COMPUTERIZED BOOKKEEPING SYSTEMS

Technology

Most health care facilities use computerized bookkeeping systems. There are many types of software available, but most provide the same basic functions. Most systems begin with the creation of a patient's account history or a computerized ledger card. Information including the name and address of the patient, the person responsible for the account, family members in the account, and insurance information is entered for each patient. These patient demographics form the database for the system. ICD and CPT codes used in the agency are also programmed into the computer along with a description of the codes and the fees charged for each. Most software is programmed to indicate a source of payment, such as cash, check, or insurance. When a patient receives a service, the patient's account history is retrieved. Information about the service is entered on a daily transaction screen (**Figure 24–23**). When the correct CPT codes are entered, the software automatically calculates the current balance by using the past balance in the account history and adding it to the new charges. If payment is made, the software deducts the payment and calculates the new balance. The account history or computerized ledger card is updated automatically as entries are made. Printed copies of the account can be given to the patient or electronic copies can be sent to the patient to show all charges, payments made, and the current balance due. In addition, the account history can be used for billing patients at regular intervals.

In addition to handling patient accounts, bookkeeping software will also create a daily journal (**Figure 24–24**). This provides a financial record showing patients seen, services provided, charges, payments made, and outstanding balances. Most software will generate a deposit slip created from the totals entered as payment is made.

Most computerized billing systems are easy to use. The computer guides the user through each step of entering financial information by providing directions or asking the user questions. However, the health care team member must still understand the basic principles of financial management used in the manual bookkeeping method to use the computerized program. In addition, safeguards must be in place when this type of system is used. Most agencies use password protection so

FIGURE 24–23 A daily transactions entry screen allows the health care provider to enter information about a patient's treatments and maintain the patient's account.

			DAILY CHARGES AND RECEIPTS REPORT - March 8, 20--											

Page 1

DATE	ACCNT #	ACCOUNT NAME	PAT NAME PMT. SOURCE	DOCTOR	PROC	DIAG	VOUCHER	CHARGES	RECEIPTS	TODAYS BALANCE	BILLED P	I	INS
03/08/--	2	Brown	Rachael	1	82996	V22.2	2	$18.00	$0.00	$134.00	N	N	Y
03/08/--	4	Gonzales	Joseph	1	93000	785.1	1	$36.00	$0.00	$36.00	N	N	Y
03/08/--	6	O'Brien	Janet	1	85022	285.9	3	$23.00	$23.00	$75.00	N	N	N
03/08/--	9	Williams	Ryan	1	90071	780.7	7	$44.00	$0.00	$144.00	N	N	Y
03/08/--	1	Takamoto	Credit Adj.	1	MO2		5	–$18.00	$0.00	$78.00	N	N	Y
03/08/--	10	Young	David	2	73090	848.9	6	$54.00	$54.00	$0.00	N	N	N
03/08/--	15	Anderson	Nancy	1	86300	075	4	$18.00	$0.00	$62.00	N	N	Y
03/08/--	12	Lightfoot	James	2	92551	389.9	8	$36.00	$0.00	$36.00	N	N	Y
03/08/--	11	Roberts	Debit Adj.	1	MO1		9	$0.00	–$25.00	$75.00	N	N	N
03/08/--	13	Paulson	Jon	2	95000	477.9	10	$44.00	$0.00	$144.00	N	N	Y
03/08/--	14	Bond	PAYMENT	1	M91		11	$0.00	$75.00	$200.00	N	N	Y

TOTALS $255.00 $127.00

Total interest included in Charges $0.00
Total Debit Adjustments - $25.00
Total Credit Adjustments - $18.00
Mode of operation - Daily data only

FIGURE 24–24 Computerized bookkeeping systems will provide a daily transactions report similar to the day sheet.

only authorized individuals are allowed access to the financial information. In addition, all systems should be programmed to record deleted transactions to prevent someone from deleting a transaction and stealing the money. A final important point is to make sure frequent backups are made of all information in case of computer failure.

Procedure 24:7
Math

Maintaining a Bookkeeping System

Equipment and Supplies

Pegboard base, day sheet, ledger cards, statement–receipt forms or communication forms, ballpoint pen, Assignment Sheet #1 for 24:7, Maintaining a Bookkeeping System

NOTE: This procedure describes a manual pegboard system of bookkeeping. Computerized bookkeeping systems require the same type of entries. If you are using a computerized program, follow the instructions provided with the software to enter the information and balance the accounts.

Procedure

1. Assemble equipment. Review the various forms and note the areas on each.

2. Place the day sheet on the pegboard. Use the pegs to secure it in position.

checkpoint

| **1.** What is a superbill?

PRACTICE: Go to the workbook and complete the assignment sheet for 24:7, Maintaining a Bookkeeping System. Then return and continue with the procedure.

3. Place a supply of statement–receipt forms or a communication form on top of the day sheet. Position these so that the top line of each form lines up with the first recording line on the day sheet.

4. Prepare the patient ledger cards. In most agencies, this is done according to the name of the person responsible for paying the account. If this is the case, record the last name and then first name of this individual on each card. Complete the full address. Be sure to include the zip code because it is frequently used for billing purposes. If the agency requires a separate ledger card for each patient, fill out the ledger card for each individual patient.

5. If the patient is new, enter two zeros *(00)* under *Current Balance*. If this is a second card for a patient whose first card is full, place the current balance from the old card in this space.

(continues)

6. Follow the instructions on Assignment Sheet #1 for patients seen and charges incurred. As each patient "enters" the office, do the following:

   a. Pull the correct ledger card for the patient.

   b. Insert the ledger card in position. Make sure the last line of information is above the statement–receipt form.

   c. Fill in the date and the patient's name.

   d. Put the current balance (the amount the patient owes for previously rendered services) noted on the ledger card in the space labeled *Previous Balance* on the charge slip.

   e. Put the receipt number on the statement–receipt form on the day sheet.

   f. Tear off the charge slip or remove the communication form. Attach this to the patient's chart. The person rendering treatment will complete the slip or form when they see the patient.

7. As each patient "leaves" the office, do the following:

   a. Record the treatments and total charges listed on the charge slip or communication form.

   b. Insert the patient's ledger card in the correct position between the day sheet and statement–receipt form (**Figure 24–25**). Be sure to use the correct statement–receipt form.

   c. Under *Description*, list the services or treatments noted on the charge slip. Services or treatments are already noted on communication forms. Abbreviations are usually used. These often are listed on the statement–receipt form.

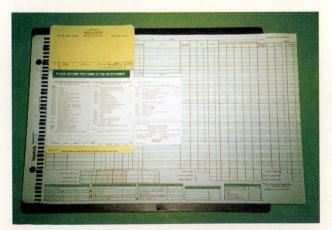

FIGURE 24–25 The ledger card is inserted between the statement–receipt record and the day sheet on the pegboard. Courtesy of Control-O-Fax Office Systems, Waterloo, IA.

d. Put the charges or amount due in the *Charges* space. Put dollars to the left of the line and cents to the right.

e. If the patient pays an amount, note this in the *Payment* area.

f. If an adjustment must be made to the charges, put the amount in the *Adj* column. Adjustments may be made for discounts or credits, but they are usually made because of contracts between health care providers and insurance companies. The amount of the adjustment is shown on the *Explanation of Benefits* (EOB) form provided by the insurance company. It is the difference between the health care provider's charge and the amount negotiated or allowed by the insurance company. Adjustments are subtracted from charges.

g. Record the payment on the day sheet. If a bank deposit slip is to be used, make sure it is folded back under the *Receipts* area of the day sheet or positioned correctly for posting. If the payment is by check, record the amount in the column labeled *Checks*. If the payment is by cash, record the amount in the column labeled *Cash*. Double-check all figures.

   NOTE: Print numbers clearly so there is no chance of error.

h. If no payment is made, draw lines through these areas.

i. **⊕ Math** Add the previous balance and charges together. Double-check your addition.

j. Subtract any payment made from the total amount due (the amount obtained in step 7i). Record your final figure in *Current Balance*.

k. Remove the ledger card and check to be sure all entries are clear and correct.

l. Tear off the statement–receipt record or remove the communication form and give it to the patient. If the patient needs an appointment, the next appointment can be recorded on this receipt.

   NOTE: If a communication form is used, one copy is given to the patient. The insurance copy of the communication form can be either given to the patient to use for filing a claim or sent to the insurance company by the agency. The third copy is retained by the agency.

m. Check to make sure all information has been recorded on the day sheet.

8. If money is received on an account, follow the same steps as before. However, record *ROA* (for "received on account") under *Description*. Note the amount as a payment.

9. At the end of the day, total all account columns on the day sheet. Enter the figures in the *Proof of Posting* box and follow the instructions given to catch any possible errors. Total the deposit slips and check these for accuracy.

10. Replace all equipment.

PRACTICE: Use the evaluation sheet for 24:7, Maintaining a Bookkeeping System, to practice this procedure. Complete Assignment Sheet #1 in the workbook and give it to your instructor. Note any corrections made to this sheet before completing Assignment Sheet #2. Make up additional practice sessions, as needed. When you believe you have mastered this skill, sign the evaluation sheet and give it to your instructor for further action.

 FINAL EVALUATION: Using the criteria listed on the evaluation sheet, your instructor will grade your performance.

24:8 WRITING CHECKS, DEPOSIT SLIPS, AND RECEIPTS

Math

Maintaining accurate financial records may be part of your responsibilities as a health care provider. Checks and receipts are important documents, and they must be filled in accurately. Checks and receipts help provide a record of financial transactions.

A **check** is a written order for payment of money through a bank. A check is used in place of cash for payment. Terms associated with checks include the following:

- **Payee**: the person receiving payment
- **Originator** or **maker**: the person writing the check, or issuing payment
- **Endorsement**: the signature of the payee; this is usually posted to the back of the check and is required before payment will be made by the bank

Basic rules for completing checks include the following:

- Checks must be written in ink or printed on a computer printer. Using pencil allows alterations by a dishonest person.
- Writing must be legible. All names and numbers must be clear.
- Spaces should be avoided in name or amount lines. Begin writing to the far left of the line. This prevents another person from adding another name or increasing the amount of money.

- Check stubs or registers should be recorded before the check is written. A check stub or register is a record of information about a check. It states the number of the check, the date, the person to whom the check was written, and the amount of the check.

- Use fractions in place of decimals to indicate number of cents. For example, instead of writing $100.00 (easily changed to $1,000.00), write $100 00/100.

-
Legal
The check must include the correct signature of the maker, or originator. This signature is recorded at the bank when a checking account is opened. In an agency, the signature is usually that of the person in authority (for example, the physician, dentist, therapist, or agency head). Only this individual is allowed to sign their name. If any other person signs the name, this is forgery.

- Before issuing a completed check, all information should be checked again for accuracy and completeness.

When a check is received from a patient, it should be checked closely. Make sure the amount is correct and noted the same way on both parts of the check showing amount. Make sure the patient has listed the correct individual or agency name as the payee. Check the date for accuracy. Make sure the check has been signed by the patient. Patients sometimes want to write checks for more than the amounts due to obtain extra cash. It is usually not wise to accept these types of checks. If the person has insufficient funds in their checking account, the agency will lose not only the amount due, but also the additional cash given to the patient. Sometimes a patient will write *Payment in Full* on a check. Do not accept such a check unless it does pay the entire balance due, including previous charges and current charges. In addition, most agencies will not accept third-party checks (a check written to the patient from another person). An exception may be if the check is from an insurance company. In this case, if the check is made out to the patient, the patient must write *Pay to the Order of. . .* on the back of the check and endorse or sign the check.

Legal Checks received by an agency are usually stamped *For Deposit Only to the Account of. . . .* This prevents anyone from cashing a check if it is stolen. It also serves as a means of endorsing the check. If the payee wishes to cash the check, it must be endorsed with their written signature. If an endorsed check is lost before it can be taken to the bank, however, anyone who finds the check will be able to cash it. If a written signature is used as an endorsement, the check should not be endorsed until the person takes it to the bank. Federal regulations now require that all endorsements be within 1 inch of the "trailing edge" (on the back and directly behind the left side of the front of the check) of all checks. If an endorsement extends below this area, the financial institution may refuse payment on the check.

A **receipt** is a record of money or goods received. If a patient makes a payment, a receipt can be given to the patient as proof of payment. The receipt stub or a register entry provides the agency with proof that payment has been received. All information must be completed accurately and legibly. Again, ink must be used to prevent any alteration of the receipt. In some agencies, a separate receipt book is used. In other agencies, receipts are part of the daily log record or pegboard system. In agencies with computerized bookkeeping systems, receipts are printed by the computer.

NOTE: *Specific instructions for writing checks and receipts are included in Procedures 24:8A and 24:8C. Each step is important. All work should be checked for accuracy.*

Deposit slips are also important in maintaining accurate financial records (**Figure 24–26**). Any cash monies or checks received should be deposited in the bank as soon as possible. Most agencies deposit monies on a daily basis. This prevents loss or theft. In addition, most agencies keep a copy of each deposit slip with the financial records. This can be used to verify deposits and/or ascertain that a specific check has been deposited. Deposit slips must be accurate. All addition must be double-checked. Terms used on these slips include the following:

- **Currency:** Currency is any money in bill form, such as $1 bills, $10 bills, and other bills. All currency to be deposited is added together and entered as one entry in this section.

- **Coins:** All coins to be deposited are added together and entered as one entry in this section.

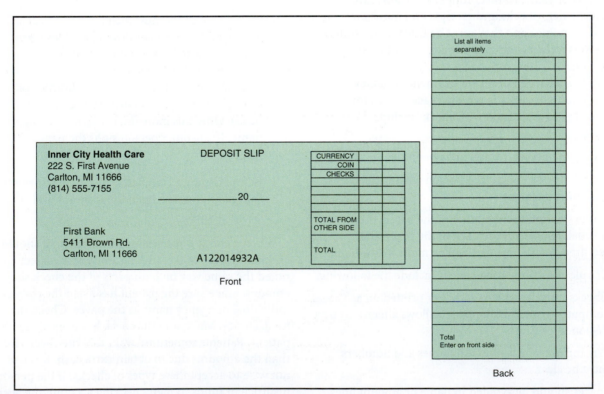

FIGURE 24–26 Deposit slips usually have an area on the back for recording a large number of checks.

- **Checks:** Checks are usually listed separately and then added together for the total. Most deposit slips have a series of lines on the back for a large number of checks. Here, the checks are again listed separately and are added together for a subtotal, which is then transferred to the front of the deposit slip in the space indicated.

Technology

NOTE: Some agencies use online banking to deposit checks to their account using money transfer apps. By using a check scanner or making an image of the front and back of endorsed checks, the check can be deposited electronically without making a trip to the bank.

NOTE: *Specific rules for completing deposit slips are noted in Procedure 24:8B.*

checkpoint

1. Define endorsement.
2. Who is responsible for signing checks?

PRACTICE: Go to the workbook and complete Assignment Sheet #1 for 24:8, Writing Checks, Deposit Slips, and Receipts. Then return and continue with the procedures.

Procedure 24:8A Math

Writing Checks

NOTE: This procedure is to be completed using the problems found in Assignment Sheets #2 and #3 in the workbook.

Equipment and Supplies

Sample blank checks (copies provided in workbook); Assignment Sheets #2 and #3 for 24:8, Writing Checks, Deposit Slips, and Receipts; pen

Technology

NOTE: This procedure describes the manual writing of checks. Computerized check writing systems require the same types of entries. If you are using a computerized program, follow the instructions provided with the software.

Procedure

1. Assemble equipment. Review preceding information about writing checks. Use only ink or a computer printer to write checks.

2. Follow the directions on Assignment Sheet #2 for 24:8, Writing Checks, Deposit Slips, and Receipts.

3. First complete the check stub or register entry (**Figure 24–27**) so that you do not accidentally issue a check without making a written record.

   a. Make sure that the current balance of the checking account is noted in the *Balance Brought Forward* section.

No.	444	$	23 ³⁹/100
Date	MARCH 8 20__		
To	ACE SUPPLY CO.		
For	ECG PAPER		
Balance Brought Forward		442	06
Deposits		–	–
Balance		442	06
Amount this check		23	39
Balance Carried Forward		418	67

Happy Doctor, M.D.
1 Healthy Lane
Fitness, OH 11133

No. 444

Date MARCH 8   20 --

Pay to the Order of   ACE SUPPLY COMPANY $ 23 ³⁹/100

TWENTY-THREE AND   ³⁹/100   dollars

First Money Bank
1 Rich Lane
Wealthy, OH 11133
0098-5567

Memo EKG PAPER   By *Happy Doctor, M.D.*

⑆0119⑈00044⑆ 268 8495⑈ 0101

FIGURE 24–27 A sample check with the check stub or register at the left.

(continues)

b. Fill in the number of the check. Most preprinted checks have the number printed on both the check and the check stub.

c. In the dollar ($) space, print in the amount of the check. Write the dollar amount close to the dollar sign. Write cents as a fraction, for example, *.50* as *50/100*, *no cents* as *no/100* or *00/100*.

d. Fill in the month, day, and year.

e. In the *To* space, write the name of the person or company to whom the check is being written. This is the payee.

f. In the *For* space, write a brief reason for the payment, for example, *computer supplies* or *rent*.

g. In the *Deposits* space, note the amount of any deposit you make to the account. Add this amount to the balance brought forward to obtain the new total balance. If no deposit has been made since the last check was written, put dashes in this space. Write the new total balance in the *Balance* space.

h. Fill in the amount of the check you are writing.

i. Subtract the amount of the check you are writing from the new total balance. Record the difference in the *Balance Carried Forward space*.

NOTE: Double-check all addition and subtraction.

j. Immediately place the final balance amount in the *Balance Brought Forward* space of the next check stub so that the balance will be there when you write the next check.

4. Once the stub has been completed, write the check. Print or write legibly. Use only ink or a computer printer.

a. If the number is not preprinted on the check, write the number of the check in the *No.* space.

b. Put the month, day, and year in the *Date* space.

c. Write the payee's name in the *Pay to the Order of* space. Write the person's name or company name completely. Begin writing to the far left of the line.

d. In the *$* space, print the amount of the check in numbers. Place the dollar amount numbers close to the dollar sign. Print cents amount as a fraction. Do *not* leave blank spaces where other numbers could be inserted.

e. In the *dollars* space, write out in words the amount of the check. Start at the far left of the line. Write the number of dollars; express cents as a fraction. Draw a line from the end of your notation to the printed word *dollars* to avoid leaving space for any alterations, for example, *Two hundred thirty-six and 30/100——dollars*.

f. If there is a *For* or *Memo* space on the check, fill in a brief explanation of why the check is being written, for example, *office supplies*, *rent*, or *insurance payment*.

g. The check must be signed on the signature line by the person to whom the checking account belongs. Only the authorized person is permitted to sign the check. After you have completed all parts of the check, double-check all entries. If they are accurate, obtain the appropriate signature. The check will *not* be valid without this signature.

 CAUTION: Never sign a check unless you are specifically authorized to do so and your signature is on the account at the bank. Otherwise, signing the check is considered forgery.

Legal

h. Recheck all parts of the check and stub for accuracy.

5. If you make an error on any part of the check, do not erase. Write *void* on both the check and the stub. Then start over with a new check and stub.

6. Follow steps 3–5 to complete all parts of assignment sheet number 2. Then turn it in to your instructor for grading.

7. Replace all equipment.

PRACTICE: Use the evaluation sheet for 24:8A, Writing Checks, to practice this procedure. Note any changes or corrections to the graded Assignment Sheet #2. Then follow the steps in the procedure to complete Assignment Sheet #3 for 24:8, Writing Checks, Deposit Slips, and Receipts. When you believe you have mastered this skill, sign the evaluation sheet and give it to your instructor for further action.

 FINAL EVALUATION: Using the criteria listed on the evaluation sheet, your instructor will grade your performance.

Check

Writing Deposit Slips

Equipment and Supplies

Assignment Sheets #2 and #3 for 24:8, Writing Checks, Deposit Slips, and Receipts; sample deposit slips (copies provided in workbook); pen

Procedure

1. Assemble equipment. Record all information in ink.

2. Read Assignment Sheet #2 for 24:8, Writing Checks, Deposit Slips, and Receipts, to note the amount of the deposit to be made to the checking account.

3. On the deposit slip (**Figure 24–28**) fill in the correct date. Put the month, day, and year.

4. Write the total amount in bills in the *Currency* space. Because no cents are involved, place two zeros in the far right hand column.

5. Count the total amount in coins. Write this amount in the *Coin* column.

    NOTE: Write dollar amounts to the left of the line and cent amounts to the right of the line.

6. List each check separately on the *Checks* lines. If additional space is needed, most deposit slips have areas on the back to note checks. The subtotal from the back is then noted on the front of the slip.

7. Add the amounts for currency, coins, and checks together, and write the sum in the *Total* space. If none of the total is to be kept as cash (that is, all of the money is to be deposited), enter this total amount two lines down in the *Total Deposit* space.

NOTE: If some of the total is kept as cash, place this amount in the *Less Cash* space. Subtract this amount from the total to obtain the amount of the total deposit.

NOTE: If cash is retained, a signature is usually required on the deposit slip. The person to whom the account belongs must sign in the space indicated.
Legal

8. Recheck all amounts for accuracy. Recheck all addition and subtraction. Make a copy of the deposit slip to keep with financial records. Take the original deposit slip, cash, and checks to the bank for deposit. Make sure to obtain a deposit receipt from the bank.

9. Note the amount deposited on the check stub of the next check to be written. Add the balance and amount deposited together to get the total current balance. The checkbook and stubs will then be up to date and ready to use.

10. Replace all equipment.

PRACTICE: Use the evaluation sheet for 24:8B, Writing Deposit Slips, to practice this procedure. Review any changes or corrections to the graded Assignment Sheet #2. Then follow the steps in the procedure to complete Assignment Sheet #3 for 24:8, Writing Checks, Deposit Slips, and Receipts. When you believe you have mastered this skill, sign the evaluation sheet and give it to your instructor for further action.

FINAL EVALUATION: Using the criteria listed on the evaluation sheet, your instructor will grade your performance.
Check

Happy Doctor, M.D.
1 Healthy Lane
Fitness, OH 11133

Date _____ March 8 _____ 20 --

Signature _____
(If cash received)

First Money Bank
1 Rich Lane
Wealthy, OH 11133
0098-5567

Currency	21	00
Coin	2	38
Checks	24	50
	182	06
TOTAL	229	94
Less Cash	—	—
TOTAL DEPOSIT	229	94

FIGURE 24–28 A sample deposit slip.

Writing Receipts

Equipment and Supplies

Assignment Sheets #2 and #3 for 24:8, Writing Checks, Deposit Slips, and Receipts; sample receipts; pen

Procedure

1. Assemble equipment. Review preceding information on writing receipts. Use ink to record all transactions.

2. Obtain information to be recorded on the receipts from Assignment Sheet #2, for 24:8, Writing Checks, Deposit Slips, and Receipts.

3. First complete the stub or register (**Figure 24–29**). In this way, you will not forget to record this information and will have a record of the receipt issued.

   a. In the *No.* space, write the number of the receipt. On preprinted receipts, this is often already done, and all receipts are numbered consecutively.

   b. In the *Date* space, print the month, day, and year.

   c. In the *To* space, print the name of the person or company to whom the receipt is being issued.

   d. In the *For* space, write a brief explanation of why the receipt is being issued, for example, *POA* (for "payment on account"), *office supplies*, or *ROA* (for "received on account").

   e. In the *Amount* space, print the dollar amount for which the receipt is being issued. Most offices also note whether the payment was made by check or cash.

4. Complete the receipt as follows:

   a. Place the correct number of the receipt in the *No.* space. This number may be preprinted.

   b. Fill in the full date, including month, day, and year.

   c. Write the full name of the person or company from whom payment was received in the *Received From* space. Write legibly. Start at the far left of the line.

   d. On the *Dollars* line, write out in words the amount received. Start at the far left of the line. Note any cents as a fraction. Draw a line from the end of your notation to the printed word *dollars*.

   e. In the *For* space, write a brief reason for the payment.

   f. In the *$* space, fill in the amount in numbers. Write close to the dollar sign. Record cents as a fraction. Note whether payment was made by check or cash.

   g. Sign your name to show that you received the money or items.

5. Recheck all parts of the receipt and stub before issuing the receipt. Make sure the amounts are accurate in both places. Be sure all writing is clear, legible, and accurate.

6. Replace all equipment.

PRACTICE: Use the evaluation sheet for 24:8C, Writing Receipts, to practice this procedure. Note any changes or corrections to the graded Assignment Sheet #2. Then follow the steps in the procedure to complete Assignment Sheet #3 for 24:8, Writing Checks, Deposit Slips, and Receipts. When you believe you have mastered this skill, sign the evaluation sheet and give it to your instructor for further action.

Check

FINAL EVALUATION: Using the criteria listed on the evaluation sheet, your instructor will grade your performance.

No. _____481_____	No. ___481___	MARCH 8	20 _ _
Date _____3/8/—_____	Received From JOHN W. SMITH		
To ___JOHN W . SMITH___	ONE HUNDRED TWENTY AND 10/100 —————— Dollars		
For ___POA___	For PAYMENT ON ACCOUNT		
Amount ___120 10/100 (ck)___	$ ___120 10/100 (ck)___ *Louise M. Simmers*		

FIGURE 24–29 A sample receipt with the receipt stub or register at the left.

Bionic Peepers?

In the United States, approximately 1 in 4,000 people or more than 100,000 people have retinitis pigmentosa (RP). RP is the name given to a group of inherited eye diseases that cause a gradual loss of vision leading to blindness. These diseases affect the retina, the nerve sensitive layer of the eye that contains the photoreceptor cells called *cones* and *rods*. Cones are sensitive to color and are used mainly to provide vision when it is light. Rod cells are used for vision in dark or dimly lit environments and to capture images to provide peripheral or side vision. RP causes a gradual deterioration of these cells, eventually leading to blindness. This disease is usually diagnosed in adolescents and young adults, and most people with the condition are legally blind by age 40.

Researchers have helped individuals with RP see some images by creating an artificial retina. The first artificial retina contained 16 electrodes and was implanted in six patients. The patients were able to distinguish some light patterns and locate some objects. This success led to the development of an Argus II implant, which contains 60 electrodes. The system uses glasses with a video camera to capture the scene, processes the information on a computer the size a wallet that is worn around the patient's neck or on a belt, and sends a signal to the electrodes implanted in the retina. The electrodes then stimulate the photoreceptors to transmit the signal to the brain through the optic nerve to create the images of sight. It was implanted in 30 patients for the first clinical trials that ran for almost 4 years. The device did not restore normal vision, but the patients were able to see colors, recognize large letters, and locate objects. Two patients were even able to read short sentences. This has been approved for use by the FDA and research continues to increase the number of electrodes in the implant to allow patients to interpret more images.

Now major research is being directed toward creating a retinal implant using a conductive polymer material that is covered with a semiconducting polymer, which bends and flexes like normal tissues when it is implanted in the eye. The semiconducting polymer absorbs photons when light enters the eye and directs electrical signals to surviving retinal neurons, which then send the impulses to the brain for interpretation as vision. This implant does not need an external camera or computer because it acts like healthy retinal tissue. Initial trials are being conducted to determine how effective the implant is in restoring vision.

The artificial retina or retinal implants will not help patients with optic nerve damage, but they may help restore vision to patients with RP and the more than 6 million people in the United States who suffer from age-related macular degeneration, another disease that destroys the photoreceptors of the eye.

Case Study Investigation Conclusion

When Cody and Miles are scheduled to cross-train in scheduling and filing, what skills will they need? What are some of the filing tips Cody would tell Miles as she is training him? What points will Cody need to be aware of when she schedules patients and takes messages?

CHAPTER 24 SUMMARY

- Business and accounting skills are used in many health care careers. In addition, many of the skills can be used in the personal life of the health care team member.

- Proper use of the telephone, composing professional business letters, completing insurance forms, and writing checks, receipts, and deposit slips are skills that can be utilized by any individual. They are also essential skills for those who work in medical or dental offices, private health care facilities, or business offices of major health care providers.

- Proper filing techniques result in excellent organization and allow for easy access to records.

- Proper scheduling of appointments helps a health care facility function efficiently.

- Maintaining patient records, such as statistical data sheets and medical histories, is an important aspect of patient care. Accuracy is essential because medical records are considered legal documents.

- Bookkeeping systems are used to maintain financial records for health care facilities, including records of services rendered, payments made, and balances due on accounts.

- By learning business and accounting skills, the health care team member can choose from a variety of health care careers.

REVIEW QUESTIONS

1. List five (5) rules that must be observed while filing records alphabetically. Create one (1) example to describe each of the rules.

2. File the following numbers in correct numerical order: 08532, 008553, 03251, 0325, 0008564, 00038, 081000, and 0566.

3. Identify security measures that must be followed when using electronic mail, cellular phones, and fax machines.

4. List five (5) sections on a medical history form. Briefly describe the type of information in each section.

5. Differentiate between a modified-block and a block style letter.

6. What is an ICD code? a CPT code? an NPI number?

7. Kaleigh Nartker visits the office with a complaint of abdominal pain. Her previous account balance is $234.55. Charges for the office visit are: consultation $85.00, complete blood count $64.00, urinalysis $38.00, and ECG $120.50. She pays $125.00 by check. What is her new account balance?

For additional information on health careers in medical records, contact the following organizations:

- American Academy of Professional Coders
  www.aapc.com

- American Health Information Management Association
  www.ahima.org

- Association for Healthcare Documentation Integrity
  www.ahdionline.org

- Professional Association of Healthcare Coding Specialists
  www.pahcs.org

CRITICAL THINKING

1. Research and obtain patient medical history forms from a hospital, a medical office, and a dental office. Interview another student in class and fill out each form based on the information they tell you.

   1a. Write a paragraph detailing the differences in the forms. Why did each type of facility choose the type of form they used?

2. You work in a medical office for four (4) different doctors. Create a list of triage questions that you can use to determine whether a patient needs an immediate appointment.

3. Research specific insurance companies, health maintenance organizations, and preferred provider organizations to determine their requirements for processing claims.

ACTIVITIES

1. Complete the statistical data sheet and medical history form in Figures 24–8 and 24–10 based on the following case:

   Mr. Martin Epstein and Mrs. Carla Epstein came into Dr. Chang's practice for the first time today. They are late for their appointment because they live at 630 Live Oak and Uber went to 630 Oak instead. The Uber driver had to go across the whole city of Cincinnati. They are both retired and have Medicare, but only Mrs. Epstein had her card and could tell them her number which was wa456372. They share an e-mail of Epsteinx2@gmail.com. Their phone number is 708-812-2345. Carla Epstein has a history of headaches, blurry vision, coughing, and asthma, and just got over a urinary tract infection. She does not take any medication except for Tylenol when she gets a headache. Martin Epstein has a history of shortness of breath, chest pain, and heartburn. He takes Tums and Valstartan 350 mg for high blood pressure. He is a two-pack-a-day smoker. Neither of the Epsteins have ever had cancer or sought psychiatric treatment.

2. Create a sample business letter for each of these purposes:
   a. recall letter
   b. consultation letter
   c. collection letter

3. Obtain a blank check. Fill in the check made out to your instructor for $7,349.22. In the memo line write why they deserve so much money from you.

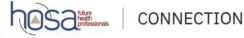 | CONNECTION

Competitive Event: Health Informatics

Event Summary: Health Informatics provides members with the opportunity to gain knowledge and skills regarding the management of health information and the assimilation of technology in health care. This competitive event consists of a written test and aims to inspire members to learn about concepts related to the study of informatics.

Details on this competitive event may be found at www.hosa.org/guidleines

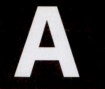

Career and technical student organizations (CTSOs) provide both secondary (high school) and postsecondary (after high school) career/technical students with the opportunity to associate with other students enrolled in the same programs or career areas. Some purposes of these organizations are to:

- Develop leadership abilities, citizenship skills, social competencies, and a wholesome attitude about life and work
- Strengthen creativity, thinking skills, decision-making abilities, and self-confidence
- Enhance the quality and relevance of education by developing the knowledge, skills, and attitudes that lead to successful employment and continuing education
- Promote quality of work and pride in occupational excellence through competitive activities
- Obtain scholarships for postsecondary education from corporations that recognize the importance of these organizations

The U.S. Department of Education recognizes and supports the following career and technical student organizations:

- Business Professionals of America (BPA)
- DECA (Distributive Education Clubs of America)
- Future Business Leaders of America (FBLA)
- Future Educators Association
- National FFA Organization (Agriculture Science Education)
- Family, Career, and Community Leaders of America (FCCLA)
- HOSA: Future Health Professionals
- Technology Student Association (TSA)
- SkillsUSA

Two organizations that supplement health science education are discussed: HOSA and SkillsUSA.

HOSA: Future Health Professionals

HOSA (pronounced *Ho'sa*) is the national organization for secondary and postsecondary/collegiate students enrolled in health science education (HSE) programs. HOSA is endorsed by the U.S. Department of Education and the Health Science Education Division of the Association for Career and Technical Education (ACTE). Membership begins at the local level, where students, who are enrolled in an HSE program or students who are interested in health professions, join together under the supervision of their classroom instructor, who serves as the HOSA local chapter advisor. Local chapters associate with the HOSA state association and the HOSA national organization.

Members of HOSA are involved in community-oriented, career-related, team-building, and leadership-development activities. All HOSA activities relate to the classroom instructional program and the health care delivery system. Furthermore, HOSA is an integral part of the HSE program, meaning that HOSA activities motivate students and enhance what the students learn in the classroom and on the job.

The mission of HOSA is "to enhance the delivery of compassionate, quality health care by providing opportunities for knowledge, skill, and leadership development of all health science education students, therefore, helping the student meet the needs of the health care community." The HOSA motto is: "The hands of HOSA mold the health of tomorrow." The HOSA slogan is: "Health Science and HOSA: A Healthy Partnership." Goals that HOSA believes are vital for each member are:

- To promote physical, mental, and social well being
- To develop effective leadership qualities and skills
- To develop the ability to communicate more effectively with people
- To develop character
- To develop responsible citizenship traits
- To understand the importance of pleasing oneself as well as being of service to others
- To build self-confidence and pride in one's work
- To make realistic career choices and seek successful employment in the health care field
- To develop an understanding of the importance of interacting and cooperating with other students and organizations
- To encourage individual and group achievement

- To develop an understanding of current health care issues, environmental concerns, and survival needs of the community, the nation, and the world

- To encourage involvement in local, state, and national health care and education projects

- To support health science education instructional objectives

- To promote career opportunities in health care

In addition to providing activities that allow members to develop occupational skills, leadership qualities, and fellowship through social and recreational activities, HOSA also encourages skill development and a healthy competitive spirit through participation in the National Competitive Events Program. Competition is held at the local, district/regional, state, and national levels. Examples of the different competitive events in specific categories include:

- *Health Science Events*: dental terminology, medical spelling, medical terminology, medical math, medical reading, and knowledge tests

- *Health Professions Events*: biomedical laboratory science, clinical nursing, clinical specialty, dental science, home health aide, medical assisting, health history form, medical office registration form, nursing assisting, personal care, physical therapy, sports medicine, and veterinary science

- *Emergency Preparedness Events*: CERT skills, CPR/first aid, emergency medical technician, epidemiology, life support skills, MRC partnership, and public health

- *Leadership Events*: extemporaneous health poster, extemporaneous writing, healthy lifestyle, interviewing skills, job seeking skills, medical photographer, prepared speaking, researched persuasive speaking, and speaking skills

- *Teamwork Events*: biomedical debate, community awareness, creative problem solving, forensic medicine, health career display, health education, HOSA bowl, medical innovation, parliamentary procedure, and public service announcement

The HOSA handbook provides detailed information about the structure, purposes, competitive events, and activities of HOSA. Students interested in further details

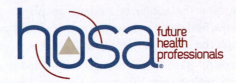

FIGURE A–1 **The HOSA emblem.** Reprinted with permission of HOSA

should refer to this handbook or obtain additional information from the Internet by contacting HOSA at *www.hosa.org*.

SkillsUSA

Students in HSE programs can also participate in SkillsUSA. SkillsUSA is a partnership of students, teachers, and industry working together to ensure America has a skilled workforce. It is a national organization for secondary and postsecondary/collegiate students enrolled in training programs in technical, skilled, and service occupations, including health careers. Examples of these programs include auto services, cosmetology, carpentry, collision repair, computer-aided drafting, electronics, masonry, precision machining, welding, and health science careers. Membership begins with local chapters that affiliate with a state association and then the national organization.

All SkillsUSA programs are in some way related to these seven major goals: professional development, community service, employment, ways and means, championships, public relations, and social activities.

The SkillsUSA motto is: "Preparing for leadership in the world of work." Some of the purposes include:

- To unite in a common bond all students enrolled in trade, industrial, technical, and health science education

- To develop leadership abilities through participation in educational, technical, civic, recreational, and social activities

- To foster a deep respect for the dignity of work

- To assist students in establishing realistic goals

- To help students attain purposeful lives

- To create enthusiasm for learning

- To promote high standards in trade ethics, workmanship, scholarship, and safety

- To develop the ability of students to plan together, organize, and carry out worthy activities and projects through the use of the democratic process
- To develop patriotism through a knowledge of our nation's heritage and the practice of democracy

To achieve these purposes, SkillsUSA offers a *Professional Development Program (PDP)* and SkillsUSA Championships. The *PDP* is a self-paced curriculum for students to obtain skills in areas such as effective communication, management, teamwork, networking, workplace ethics, and job interviewing. The *PDP* is designed to help students develop the skills they need to make a smooth transition to the workforce or higher education.

SkillsUSA Championships offer skill competition in both leadership and occupational areas. Competition is held at the local, district/regional, state, and national levels. Examples of leadership contests include prepared and extemporaneous speech, SkillsUSA opening and closing ceremonies, chapter business procedure, action skills, career pathway showcase, job interview, employment application process, American spirit, chapter display, community action project, community service, and occupational health and safety. Examples of career contests for HSE students include basic health care skills, medical assisting, dental assisting, nurse assisting, practical nursing, basic health care skills, first aid and CPR, job skill demonstration, medical math, medical terminology, health, occupations professional portfolio, and a health knowledge bowl.

The ceremonial emblem of SkillsUSA is shown in Figure A–2. The shield represents patriotism, or a belief in democracy; liberty; and the American way of life. The torch represents knowledge. The orbital circles represent modern technology and the training needed to master new technical frontiers along with the need for continuous education. The gear represents the industrial society and the cooperation of the individual working with labor and management for the betterment of humankind. The hands represent the individual and portray a search for knowledge along with the desire to acquire a skill.

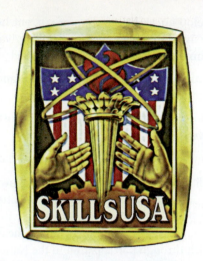

FIGURE A–2 The SkillsUSA emblem. Reprinted with permission of SkillsUSA

The colors of the SkillsUSA organization are red, white, blue, and gold. Red and white represent the individual states and chapters. Blue represents the common union of the states and chapters. Gold represents the individual, the most important element of the organization.

The SkillsUSA Leadership Handbook and other SkillsUSA publications provide more information on the various activities and programs. Students interested in further details should refer to these sources of information or obtain additional information from the Internet by contacting SkillsUSA at *www.skillsusa.org*.

Other Sources of Information

- HOSA: Future Health Professionals
  548 Silicon Drive, Suite 101
  Southlake, TX 76092
  800-321-HOSA
  www.hosa.org
- SkillsUSA
  14001 SkillsUSA Way
  Leesburg, Virginia 20176
  703-777-8810
  www.skillsusa.org

CORRELATION TO NATIONAL HEALTH CARE FOUNDATION STANDARDS

TABLE B–1 Correlation to National Health Care Foundation Standards

Health Science Chapter	Health Care Core Standards	Therapeutic Services	Diagnostic Services	Health Informatics	Support Services	Biotechnology Research and Development
History and Trends of Health Care	X	X	X	X	X	X
Health Care Systems	X	X	X	X	X	X
Careers in Health Care	X	X	X	X	X	X
Personal and Professional Qualities of a Health Care Worker	X	X	X	X	X	X
Legal and Ethical Responsibilities	X	X	X	X	X	X
Medical Terminology	X	X	X	X	X	X
Anatomy and Physiology	X	X	X	X	X	X
Human Growth and Development	X	X	X	X	X	X
Geriatric Care	X	X	X	X	X	X
Cultural Diversity	X	X	X	X	X	X
Nutrition and Diets	X	X	X	X	X	X
Computers and Technology in Health Care	X	X	X	X	X	X
Medical Math	X	X	X	X	X	X
Promotion of Safety	X	X	X	X	X	X
Infection Control	X	X	X	X	X	X
Vital Signs	X	X	X	X	X	X
First Aid	X	X	X	X	X	X
Preparing for the World of Work	X	X	X	X	X	X
Dental Assistant Skills		X	X			
Laboratory Assistant Skills		X	X	X		X
Medical Assistant Skills		X	X			
Nurse Assistant Skills		X	X			
Physical Therapy Skills		X	X			
Business and Accounting Skills	X	X	X	X	X	X

METRIC CONVERSION CHARTS

The metric system, frequently called the International System of Units, or simply SI, is used in many health care fields. The following information and charts will assist you in converting measurements between the metric system and the U.S. customary system, commonly called the English or household system of measurement.

1. *Temperature measurements:*

   - To convert Fahrenheit (F) temperatures to Celsius (centigrade) (C) temperatures, subtract 32 from the Fahrenheit temperature and then multiply the result by ⅚, or 0.5556. Use one of the following formulas:

     $$C = (F - 32) \times \tfrac{5}{9} \text{ or } C = (F - 32) \times 0.5556$$

   - To convert Celsius (C) temperatures to Fahrenheit (F) temperatures, multiply the Celsius temperature by 9/5, or 1.8, and then add 32 to the total. Use one of the following formulas:

     $$F = (\tfrac{5}{9} \times C) + 32 \text{ or } F = (1.8 \times C) + 32$$

   - The chart on the following page provides some major temperature equivalents.

2. *Linear measurements:*

   - To convert inches to centimeters, multiply the number of inches by 2.54 (1 inch = 2.54 centimeters).

   - To convert feet to centimeters, multiply the number of feet by 30.48 centimeters (1 foot = 30.48 centimeters).

   - To convert centimeters to inches, divide the number of centimeters by 2.54.

   - To convert centimeters to feet, divide the number of centimeters by 30.48.

   - The chart on the following page provides additional linear metric equivalents.

3. *Weight measurements:*

   - To convert pounds to kilograms, divide the number of pounds by 2.2 (1 kilogram = 2.2 pounds).

   - To convert kilograms to pounds, multiply the number of kilograms by 2.2.

4. *Liquid measurements:*

   - Note that 1 cubic centimeter (cc) is equal to 1 milliliter (mL).

   - To convert household measurements (for example, cups, ounces, quarts, or pints) to metric measurements, multiply the household measurement by the equivalent number of milliliters (mL). For example, 1 teaspoon equals 5 mL. Therefore, 3 teaspoons converted to metric would be 3 × 5, or 15 mL.

   - To convert metric measurements to household measurements, divide the metric measurement by the number of metric units in one of the household units. For example, there are 30 mL in 1 ounce. Therefore, 180 mL converted to ounces would be 180 ÷ 30, or 6 ounces.

5. The chart on the following page provides additional liquid metric equivalents.

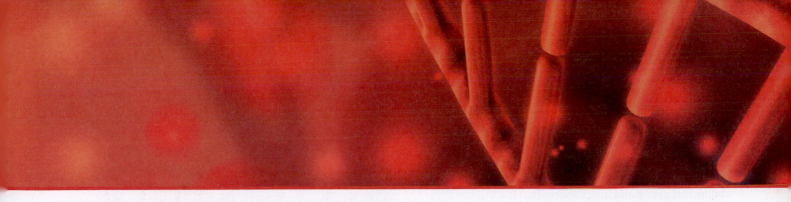

Fahrenheit–Celsius (Centigrade) Equivalents

F°	C°	F°	C°	F°	C°
32	0	102	38.9	116	46.7
70	21.1	103	39.4	117	47.2
75	23.9	104	40	118	47.8
80	26.7	105	40.6	119	48.3
85	29.4	106	41.1	120	48.9
90	32.2	107	41.7	125	51.7
95	35	108	42.2	130	54.4
96	35.6	109	42.8	135	57.2
97	36.1	110	43.3	140	60
98	36.7	111	43.9	150	65.6
98.6	37	112	44.4	212	100
99	37.2	113	45		
100	37.8	114	45.6		
101	38.3	115	46.1		

Linear English–Metric Equivalents

1 inch (in) = 0.0254 meters (m) = 2.54 centimeters (cm)

12 inches = 1 foot (ft) = 0.3048 meters (m) = 30.48 centimeters (cm)

3 feet = 1 yard (yd) = 0.914 meters (m) = 91.4 centimeters (cm)

5,280 feet = 1 mile = 1,609.344 meters (m)

39.372 inches = 3.281 feet = 1 meter (m)

1.094 yards = 1 meter (m)

0.621 miles = 1 kilometer (km)

Liquid English–Metric Equivalents

1 drop (gtt) = 0.0667 milliliter (mL)

15 drops (gtts) = 1.0 milliliter (mL)

1 teaspoon (tsp) = 5.0 milliliters (mL)

3 teaspoons = 1 tablespoon (tbsp) = 15.0 milliliters (mL)

1 ounce (oz) = 30.0 milliliters (mL)

8 ounces (oz) = 1 cup (cp) = 240.0 milliliters (mL)

2 cups (cp) = 1 pint (pt) = 500.0 milliliters (mL)

2 pints (pt) = 1 quart (qt) = 1,000.0 milliliters (mL)

GLOSSARY

A

abbreviations—Shortened forms of words, usually just letters.

abdominal cavity—a body cavity consisting of the upper abdominal cavity and lower abdominal (pelvic) cavity. The upper abdominal cavity contains the stomach, small intestine, most of the large intestine, appendix, liver, gallbladder, pancreas, and spleen. The lower abdominal cavity contains the urinary bladder, the reproductive organs, and the last part of the large intestine.

abdominal regions—Division of the abdominal cavity into nine sections. The center regions are the epigastric, umbilical, and hypogastric, or pelvic. On either side of the center the regions are the hypochondriac, lumbar, and iliac, or inguinal.

abduction—Movement away from the midline.

abrasion—Injury caused by rubbing or scraping the skin.

absorption—Act or process of sucking up or in; taking in of nutrients.

abuse—Any care that results in physical harm or pain, or mental anguish.

acceptance—The process of receiving or taking; approval; belief.

acceptance of criticism—A personal/professional characteristic required in health care careers; tolerance of feedback that is constructive and enables improvement.

acculturation—Process of learning the beliefs and behaviors of a dominant culture and assuming some of the characteristics.

acquired immune deficiency syndrome (AIDS)—A disease caused by the human immunodeficiency virus (HIV) which attacks the immune system destroying the body's ability to fight infections.

adduction—Movement toward the midline.

adenosine stress test—A cardiac test used by a physician to determine how heart responds to stress; used for patients who cannot exercise; a medication that simulates the effect of exercise is given to increase the blood flow and heart rate; *see also* **dobutamine stress test**.

admitting officers/clerks—Individuals who work in the admissions department of a health care facility and responsible for obtaining all necessary information when a patient is admitted to the facility, assigning rooms, maintaining records, and processing information when the patient is discharged.

adolescence—Period of development from 12 to 18 years of age; teenage years.

adrenal glands—One of two endocrine glands located one above each kidney.

advance directives—Legal document designed to indicate a person's wishes regarding care in case of a terminal illness or during the dying process.

aerobic—Requiring oxygen to live and grow.

affection—A warm or tender feeling toward another; fondness.

agar plate—Special laboratory dish containing agar, a gelatinous colloidal extract of a red alga, which is used to provide nourishment for growth of organisms.

Agency for Healthcare Research and Quality (AHRQ)—A federal agency established to improve the quality, safety, efficiency, and effectiveness of health care for Americans.

agent—Someone who has the power or authority to act as the representative of another.

agnostic—Person who believes that the existence of God cannot be proved or disproved.

air compressor—Machine that provides air under pressure; used in dental areas to provide air pressure to operate handpieces and air syringe.

airborne precautions—Methods of infection control that must be used for patients known or suspected to be infected with pathogens transmitted by airborne droplet nuclei.

albino—Absence of all color pigments.

alginate—Irreversible, hydrocolloid, dental impression material.

alignment—Positioning and supporting the body so that all body parts are in correct anatomical position.

alimentary canal—The digestive tract from the esophagus to the rectum.

alopecia—Baldness.

alternative therapies—Methods of treatment used in place of biomedical therapies.

alveolar process—Bone tissue of the maxilla and mandible that contains alveoli (sockets) for the roots of the teeth.

alveoli—Microscopic air sacs in the lungs.

Alzheimer's disease—Progressive, irreversible disease involving memory loss, disorientation, deterioration of intellectual function, and speech and gait disturbances.

amalgam—Alloy (mixture) of various metals and mercury; restorative or filling material used primarily on posterior teeth.

amputation—The cutting off or separation of a body part from the body.

anaerobic—Not requiring oxygen to live and grow; able to thrive in the absence of oxygen.

anatomy—The study of the structure of an organism.

anesthesia—The state of inability to feel sensation, especially the sensation of pain.

anesthetic carpules (cartridges)—Glass cylinders containing premeasured amounts of anesthetic solutions.

anger—Feeling of displeasure or hostility; mad.

angles—Measurements in degrees of the distance between a reference plane and a line drawn from a point on the plane.

anorexia nervosa—Psychological disorder involving loss of appetite and excessive weight loss not caused by a physical disease.

answering service—Service that responds to telephone calls when the agency is closed; the patient talks with an operator who can transfer the call to the appropriate individual, contact the individual and ask them to call the patient, or record a message.

anterior—Before or in front of.

antibody screen—Test that checks for antibodies in the blood prior to a transfusion.

anticoagulant—Substance that prevents clotting of the blood.

antigen—Substance that causes the body to produce antibodies; may be introduced into the body or formed within the body.

antioxidants—Enzymes or organic molecules; help protect the body from harmful chemicals called *free radicals*.

antisepsis—Aseptic control that inhibits, retards growth of, or kills pathogenic organisms; not effective against spores and viruses.

anuria—Without urine; producing no urine.

anus—External opening of the anal canal, or rectum.

aortic valve—Flap or cusp located between the left ventricle of the heart and the aorta.

apex—The pointed extremity of a conelike structure; the rounded, lower end of the heart, below the ventricles; the bottom tip of a tooth.

apical foramen—The opening in the apex of a tooth; allows nerves and blood vessels to enter tooth.

apical pulse—Pulse taken with a stethoscope and near the apex of the heart.

apnea—Absence of respirations; temporary cessation of respirations.

apoplexy—A stroke; *see* **cerebrovascular accident**.

apothecary system—A system used for weighing drugs and solutions, brought to the United States from England during the colonial period.

appendicular skeleton—The bones that form the limbs or extremities of the body.

application forms—Forms or records completed when applying for a job.

appointment—A schedule to do something on a particular day and time.

aquathermia pads—Temperature-controlled units that circulates warm liquid through a pad to provide dry heat.

aqueous humor—Watery liquid that circulates in the anterior chamber of the eye.

arrhythmia—Irregular or abnormal rhythm, usually referring to the heart rhythm.

arteriosclerosis—Hardening and/or narrowing of the walls of arteries.

artery—Blood vessel that carries blood away from the heart.

arthritis—Inflammation of a joint.

asepsis—Being free from infection.

aspirating syringes—Special dental anesthetic syringes designed to hold carpules or cartridges of medication.

assault and battery—Assault includes a threat or attempt to injure, and battery includes the unlawful touching of another person without consent.

assistant's carts—Carts that contain drawers or sliding tops with storage areas; usually contain a tri-flow syringe, a saliva ejector, and a high-velocity oral evacuator.

assisted living facilities—Long-term care facilities that allow individuals who can care for themselves to rent or purchase an apartment in the facility; provide services such as meals, housekeeping, laundry, transportation, social events, and basic medical care (such as assisting with medications); also known as *independent living facilities*.

associate's degree—Degree awarded by a vocational-technical school or community college after successful completion of a two-year course of study or its equivalent.

atheist—Person who does not believe in any deity.

atherosclerosis—Form of arteriosclerosis characterized by accumulation of fats or mineral deposits on the inner walls of the arteries.

athletic trainers certified (ATCs)—Prevent and treat athletic injuries and provide rehabilitative services to athletes; frequently works with a physician who specializes in sports medicine; teach proper nutrition, assess the physical condition of athletes, give advice regarding physical conditioning programs to increase strength and flexibility or correct weaknesses, put tape or padding on players to protect body parts, treat minor injuries, administer first aid for serious injuries, and help carry out any rehabilitation treatment prescribed by sports medicine physicians or other therapists.

audiologist—Individual specializing in diagnosis and treatment of hearing disorders.

auditory canal—A tube in the ear; contains special glands that produce cerumen, which protects the ear; sound waves travel through this canal to the eardrum; also called the *external auditory meatus*.

aural temperature—Measurement of body temperature at the tympanic membrane in the ear.

auricle—Also called the *pinna*; external part of the ear.

auscultation—Process of listening for sounds in the body.

autoclave—Piece of equipment used to sterilize articles by way of steam under pressure and/or dry heat.

autocratic leader—An individual who maintains total rule, makes all of the decisions, and has difficulty delegating or sharing duties; often called a "dictator."

automated routing unit (ARU)—System that answers the telephone and a recorded voice provides directions to the caller.

autonomic nervous system—That division of the nervous system concerned with reflex, or involuntary, activities of the body.

autonomy—Self-governance or the ability to decide for oneself by making choices and pursuing a course of action.

avulsion—A wound that occurs when tissue is separated from the body.

axial skeleton—The bones of the skull, rib cage, and spinal column; the bones that form the trunk of the body.

axillary temperature—Temperature taken in the armpit, under the upper arm.

Ayer blade—Wooden or plastic blade used to scrape cells from the cervix of the uterus; used for Pap tests.

B

bachelor's degree—Degree awarded by a college or university after a person has completed a four-year course of study or its equivalent.

bacteria—One-celled microorganisms, some of which are beneficial and some of which cause disease.

bandages—Materials used to hold dressings in place, secure splints, and support and protect body parts.

bandage scissors—Special scissors with a blunt lower end used to remove dressings and bandages.

bargaining—Process of negotiating an agreement, sale, or exchange.

Bartholin's glands—Two small mucous glands near the vaginal opening.

basal metabolic rate (BMR)—The rate at which the body uses energy to maintain life when the subject is at complete rest.

base—Protective (dental) material placed over the pulpal area of a tooth to reduce irritation and thermal shock.

base of support—Standing with feet 8–10 inches apart to provide better balance.

bed cradle—A device placed on a bed to keep the top bed linens from contacting the legs and feet.

bias—A preference that inhibits impartial judgment.

bicuspids—Also called *premolars;* the teeth that pulverize or grind food and are located between cuspids and molars.

bilateral—Affecting both sides of the body.

binders—Devices applied to hold dressings in place, provide support, apply pressure, or limit motion.

biological (medical) scientists—Individuals who study living organisms and assist in the development of vaccines, medicines, and treatments for diseases; evaluate the relationship between organisms and the environment; and administer the programs for testing food and drugs.

biomedical (clinical) engineers—Individuals who combine the knowledge of engineering with the knowledge of biology and biomechanical principles to assist in the operation of health care facilities.

biomedical equipment technicians (BETs)—Individuals who work with the many different machines used to diagnose, treat, and monitor patients.

biotechnology—The use of the genetic and biochemical processes of living systems and organisms to develop or modify useful products.

bioterrorism—The use of biological agents, such as pathogens, for terrorist purposes.

bite-wings—Also called a *cavity-detecting X-rays;* a dental radiographs that shows only the crowns of the teeth.

bladder—Membranous sac or storage area for a secretion (gallbladder); also, the vesicle that acts as the reservoir for urine.

bland diet—Diet containing only mild-flavored foods with soft textures.

block style—Letter format in which all parts of the letter start at the left margin.

blood—Fluid that circulates through the vessels in the body to carry substances to all body parts.

blood pressure—Measurement of the force exerted by the heart against the arterial walls when the heart contracts (beats) and relaxes.

blood smear—A drop of blood spread thinly on a slide for microscopic examination.

bloodborne—An infectious disease or pathogenic organism that is transmitted through blood.

Bloodborne Pathogen Standard—Standard that has mandates to protect health care providers from diseases caused by exposure to body fluids.

body—Main content, or message part, of a letter.

body cavities—Spaces within the body that contain vital organs.

body mass index (BMI)—A calculation that measures weight in relation to height and correlates this with body fat; used to determine if an individual is underweight, has ideal weight, or is overweight.

body mechanics—The way in which the body moves and maintains balance; proper body mechanics involves the most efficient use of all body parts.

body planes—Imaginary lines drawn through the body at various parts to separate the body into sections.

Bowman's capsule—Part of the renal corpuscle in the kidney; picks up substances filtered from the blood by the glomerulus.

bradycardia—Slow heart rate, usually below 60 beats per minute.

bradypnea—Slow respiratory rate, usually below 10 respirations per minute.

brain—Soft mass of nerve tissue inside the cranium.

breast—Mammary, or milk, gland located on the upper part of the front surface of the body.

bronchi—Two main branches of the trachea; air tubes to and from the lungs.

bronchioles—Small branches of the bronchi; carry air in the lungs.

bronchitis—Acute or chronic inflammation of the bronchial tubes, or air tubes in the lungs.

buccal—Outside surface of the posterior teeth; surface facing the cheek; facial surface of bicuspids and molars.

buccal cavity—Mouth.

budget—An itemized list of income and expected expenditures for a period of time.

buffer period—Period of time kept open on an appointment schedule to allow for emergencies, telephone calls, and other unplanned situations.

bulimarexia—Psychological condition in which a person eats excessively and then uses laxatives or vomits to get rid of the food.

bulimia—Psychological condition in which a person alternately eats excessively and then fasts or refuses to eat.

burn—Injury to body tissue caused by heat, caustics, radiation, and/or electricity.

burs—Small, rotating instruments of various types; used in dental handpieces to prepare cavities for filling with restorative materials.

C

calcaneus—Large tarsal bone that forms the heel.

calculus—Also called *tartar;* hard, calcium-like deposit that forms on the teeth; a stone that forms in various parts of the body from a variety of different substances.

calorie—Unit of measurement of the fuel value of food.

calorie-controlled diets—Types of diets that include both low-calorie and high-calorie diets. Low-calorie diets are frequently used for patients who are overweight. High-calorie diets are used for patients who are underweight or have anorexia nervosa, hyperthyroidism (overactivity of thyroid gland), or cancer.

cancer—A group of diseases caused by abnormal cell division and/or growth.

cane—A rod used as an aid in walking.

capillary—Tiny blood vessel that connects arterioles and venules and allows for exchange of nutrients and gases between the blood and the body cells.

carbohydrates—Group of chemical substances including sugars, cellulose, and starches; nutrients that provide the greatest amount of energy in the average diet.

cardiac muscle—Type of muscle that forms the walls of the heart and contracts to circulate blood.

cardiopulmonary resuscitation—Procedure of providing oxygen and chest compressions to a victim whose heart has stopped beating.

cardiovascular technologist—An individual who assists with cardiac catheterization and angioplasty procedures, monitors patients during open-heart surgery, and performs tests to check circulation in blood vessels.

carious lesions—Occurrences of tooth decay.

carpal—Bone of the wrist.

cataract—Condition of the eye where the lens becomes cloudy or opaque, leading to blindness.

catheter—A rubber, metal, or other type of tube that is passed into a body cavity and used for injecting or removing fluids.

caudal—Pertaining to any tail or tail-like structure.

cavitation—The cleaning process employed in an ultrasonic unit; bubbles explode to drive cleaning solution onto article being cleaned.

cavity—A hollow space, such as a body cavity (which contains organs) or a hole in a tooth.

cell—Mass of protoplasm; the basic unit of structure of all animals and plants.

cell membrane—Outer, protective, semipermeable covering of a cell.

cellular respiration—Cells use of oxygen and nutrients to produce energy, water, and carbon dioxide.

cellular telephone—Telephone that allows two-way communication between people in almost any location.

cellulose—Fibrous form of carbohydrate.

Celsius—A scale of temperature on which water freezes at 0 degrees and boils at 100 degrees under standard conditions.

cement—Dental material used to seal inlays, crowns, bridges, and orthodontic appliances in place.

cementum—Hard, bonelike tissue that covers the outside of the root of a tooth.

Centers for Disease Control and Prevention (CDC)—A division of the USDHHS; concerned with the causes, spread, and control of diseases in populations.

centigrade—A scale of temperature on which water freezes at 0 degrees and boils at 100 degrees under standard conditions.

central nervous system (CNS)—The division of the nervous system consisting of the brain and spinal cord.

centrosome—That area of cell cytoplasm that contains two centrioles; important in reproduction of the cell.

cerebellum—The section of the brain that is dorsal to the pons and medulla oblongata; maintains balance and equilibrium.

cerebrospinal fluid—Watery, clear fluid that surrounds the brain and spinal cord.

cerebrovascular accident—Also called a *stroke* or *apoplexy*; an interrupted supply of blood to the brain, caused by formation of a clot, blockage of an artery, or rupture of a blood vessel.

cerebrum—Largest section of brain; involved in sensory interpretation and voluntary muscle activity.

certification—The issuing of a statement or certificate by a professional organization to a person who has met the requirements of education and/or experience and who meets the standards set by the organization.

cervical spatula—A wooden or plastic blade used to scrape cells from the cervix; usually part of a Pap kit.

cervix—Anatomical part of a tooth where the crown joins with the root; entrance to or lower part of the uterus.

chain of infection—Factors that lead to the transmission or spread of disease.

character—The quality of respirations (for example, deep, shallow, or labored).

charge slip—A record on which charges or costs for services are listed.

check—A written order for payment of money through a bank.

chemical abuse—Use of chemical substances without regard for accepted practice; dependence on alcohol or drugs.

chemical disinfection—Chemicals used for aseptic control.

Cheyne-Stokes—Periods of difficult breathing (dyspnea) followed by periods of no respirations (apnea).

cholesterol—Fatlike substance synthesized in the liver and found in body cells and animal fats.

choroid coat—The middle of the eye, which is interlaced with many blood vessels that nourish the eyes.

chromatin—A part of a cell located in the nucleus and made of deoxyribonucleic acid and protein; during cell reproduction, condenses to form chromosomes.

cilia—Hairlike projections.

circulatory system—The "transportation" system of the body; consists of the heart, blood vessels, and blood; transports nutrients and wastes, oxygen and carbon dioxide, hormones, and antibodies contained in the blood; also known as the cardiovascular system.

circumduction—Moving in a circle at a joint, or moving one end of a body part in a circle while the other end remains stationary.

cisterna chyli—Part of the lymphatic system; serves as a storage area for purified lymph before this lymph returns to the bloodstream.

civil law—Laws that focus on the legal relationships between people and the protection of a person's rights.

clavicle—Collarbone.

clean—Free from organisms causing disease.

clean-catch (mid-stream) specimen—A urine specimen that is free from contamination.

clinic—Institution that provides care for outpatients; a group of specialists working in cooperation.

clinical account managers—Individuals who promote, sell, and educate clients, sales associates, and the public about health care products and services.

clinical account technicians (CATs)—Individuals who assist patients that have questions about their bill or need help to make payment arrangements.

clinical laboratory scientists (CLSs)—Individuals who study the tissues, fluids, and cells of the human body to help determine the presence and/or cause of disease; perform complicated chemical, microscopic, and automated analyzer/computer tests; work under the supervision of pathologists; see also **medical laboratory technologists (MTs)**.

clinical laboratory technicians (CLTs)—Individuals who perform many of the routine tests that do not require the advanced knowledge held by a medical technologist; see also **medical laboratory technicians (MLTs)**.

clinical thermometers—Thermometers consisting of a slender glass tube containing mercury or a heat-reactive mercury-free liquid such as alcohol, which expands when exposed to heat.

closed bed—Bed that is made following the discharge of a patient.

cochlea—Snail-shaped section of the inner ear; contains the organ of Corti for hearing.

cognitive—Relating to intellectual activity such as solving problems, making judgments, and dealing with situations.

collection—To receive; a letter requesting payment on an account.

colon—The large intestine.

colostomy—An artificial opening into the colon; allows for the evacuation of feces.

communicable disease—Disease that is transmitted from one individual to another.

communication—Process of transmission; exchange of thoughts or information.

compensation—Something given or received as an equivalent for a loss, service, or debt; defense mechanism involving substitution of one goal for another goal to achieve success.

competence— A personal/professional characteristic required in health care careers; qualified and capable of performing a task.

complementary therapies—Methods of treatment used in conjunction with biomedical therapies.

complete bed bath (CBB)—A bath in which all parts of a patient's body are bathed while the patient is confined to bed.

complimentary close—Courtesy closing of a letter (for example, *Sincerely*).

composite—The dental restorative or filling material used most frequently on anterior teeth.

compress—A folded wet or dry cloth applied firmly to a body part.

computer literacy—A basic understanding of how a computer works that allows an individual to feel comfortable using a computer.

computer-aided design (CAD)—Software that is used to create precision drawings, technical illustrations, or two- or three-dimensional models.

computer-assisted instruction (CAI)—Teaching method in which a computer and computer programs are used to control the learning process and deliver the instructional material to the learner.

computerized tomography (CT)—A scanning and detection system that uses a minicomputer and display screen to visualize an internal portion of the human body; formerly known as *CAT (computerized axial tomography)*.

concierge medicine—A type of personalized health care where an enhanced level of care is provided by a primary care physician for a monthly or annual fee.

confidential—Not to be shared or told; to be held in confidence, or kept to oneself.

confidentiality—Information about the patient must remain private and can be shared only with other members of the patient's health care team.

congenital—Acquired during development of the infant in the uterus and present at birth.

conjunctiva—Mucous membrane that lines the eyelids and covers the anterior part of the sclera of the eye.

connective tissue—Body tissue that connects, supports, or binds body organs.

constrict—To contract or narrow; to make smaller.

consultation—Process of seeking information or advice from another person.

Consumer Bill of Rights and Responsibilities—A list of patient's rights, implemented by the Department of Health and Human Services, that must be recognized and honored by health care providers.

contact precautions—Methods of infection control that must be used for patients known or suspected to be infected with epidemiological microorganisms that can be transmitted by either direct or indirect contact.

contaminated—Containing infection or infectious organisms or germs.

continuing education units (CEUs)—Additional hours of training required to renew licenses or maintain certification or registration in many states.

contra angle—Attachment used on dental handpieces to cut and polish.

contract—To shorten, decrease in size, or draw together; an agreement between two or more persons.

contractibility—Property of muscles; becoming short and thick when muscle fibers are stimulated by nerves, or become short and thick; causes movement.

contracture—Tightening or shortening of a muscle.

convulsion—Also called a *seizure*; a violent, involuntary contraction of muscles.

cornea—The transparent section of the sclera; allows light rays to enter the eye.

cortex—The outer layer of an organ or structure.

cost containment—Procedures used to control costs or expenses.

cover letter—Letter written with the purpose of obtaining an interview; *see also* **letter of introduction**.

Cowper's (bulbourethral) glands—The pair of small mucous glands near the male urethra.

cranial—Pertaining to the skull or cranium.

cranial cavity—Section of the dorsal cavity that contains the brain.

cranium—Part of the skull; the eight bones of the head that enclose the brain.

criminal law—Law that focuses on behavior known as crime; deals with the wrongs against a person, property, or society.

cross-index/reference—A paper or card used in filing systems to prevent misplacement or loss of records.

crown—The anatomical portion of a tooth that is exposed in the oral cavity, above the gingiva, or gums.

crust—A scab; outer covering or coat.

crutches—Artificial supports that assist a patient in walking.

cryotherapy—Use of cold applications for treatment.

cultural assimilation—Absorption of a culturally distinct group into a dominant or prevailing culture.

cultural diversity—Differences among individuals based on cultural, ethnic, and racial factors.

culture—Values, beliefs, ideas, customs, and characteristics passed from one generation to the next.

culture specimen—A sample of microorganisms or tissue cells taken from an area of the body for examination.

cuspids—Also called a *caniness* or *eyeteeth*; the type of teeth located at angle of lips and used to tear food.

custom trays—Dental impression trays specially made to fit a particular patient's mouth.

cyanosis—Bluish color of the skin, nail beds, and/or lips due to an insufficient amount of oxygen in the blood.

cyst—A closed sac with a distinct membrane that develops abnormally in a body structure; usually filled with a semi-solid liquid.

cytoplasm—The fluid inside a cell; contains water, proteins, lipids, carbohydrates, minerals, and salts.

D

dangling—Positioning the patient in a sitting position with his or her feet and legs over the side of the bed prior to ambulation.

database—An organized collection of information stored in a computer.

date line—The date the letter is being written is keyed under the letterhead.

day sheet (daily journal)—A daily record of all patients seen, all charges incurred, and all payments received.

daydreaming—Defense mechanism of escape; dream-like musing while awake.

decimals—One way of expressing parts of numbers or anything else that has been divided into parts, with the parts being expressed in units of 10.

deductions—Things subtracted or taken out (for example, monies taken out of a paycheck for various purposes).

deep—Internal; term that relates to structures within the body.

defamation—Slander or libel; a false statement that causes ridicule or damage to a reputation.

defecate—To evacuate fecal material from the bowel; to have a bowel movement.

defense mechanisms—Physical or psychological reactions of an organism used in self-defense or to protect self-image.

degenerative—Disease type, caused by a deterioration of the function or structure of body tissues and organs either by normal body aging or lifestyle choices such as diet and exercise.

degrees—A unit of measurement.

dehydration—Insufficient amounts of fluid in the tissues.

delirium—Acute, reversible mental confusion caused by illness, medical problems, and/or medications.

dementia—Loss of mental ability characterized by decrease in intellectual ability, loss of memory, impaired judgment, and disorientation.

democratic leader—An individual who encourages the participation of all individuals in decisions that have to be made or problems that have to be solved.

denial—Declaring untrue; refusing to believe.

dental assistants (DAs)—Individuals who work under the supervision of dentists to prepare a patient for dental procedures and assist with the procedures.

dental chair—Special chair designed to position a patient comfortably while providing easy access to the patient's oral cavity.

dental hygienist (DH)—A licensed individual who works with a dentist to provide care and treatment for the teeth and gums.

dental laboratory technicians (DLTs)—Individuals who make and repair a variety of dental prostheses such as dentures, crowns, bridges, and orthodontic appliances.

dental lights—Lights used in dental units to illuminate the oral cavity.

dental offices—Provide dental services, which can include general care provided to all age groups or specialized care offered to certain age groups or for certain dental conditions like orthodontics (straighten teeth). Dental offices vary in size from offices that are privately owned by one or more dentists to dental clinics that employ a group of dentists. In some areas, major retail or department stores operate dental clinics.

dentin—Tissue that makes up the main bulk of a tooth.

dentists (DMDs or DDSs)—Doctors who specialize in diagnosis, prevention, and treatment of diseases of the teeth and gums.

dentition—The number, type, and arrangement of teeth in the mouth.

dependability—Accepting the responsibility required by one's position; being prompt in reporting to work and maintaining a good attendance record; performing assigned tasks on time and accurately.

deposit slips—Bank records listing all cash and checks that are to be placed in an account, either checking or savings.

depression—Psychological condition of sadness, melancholy, gloom, or despair.

dermis—The skin.

development—Changes in the intellectual, mental, emotional, social, and functional skills that occur over time.

diabetes mellitus—Metabolic disease caused by an insufficient secretion or utilization of insulin and leading to an increased amount of glucose (sugar) in the blood and urine.

diabetic coma—An unconscious condition caused by an increased level of glucose (sugar) and ketones in the bloodstream of a person with diabetes mellitus.

diabetic diet—Type of diet used for patients with diabetes mellitus; a carbohydrate-controlled diet in which approximately 40–60 percent of calories are from carbohydrates.

diagnosis—Determination of the nature of a person's disease.

diagnostic related groups (DRGs)—Method of classifying diagnoses into specific payment or reimbursement categories.

dialysis technicians—Individuals who operate the kidney hemodialysis machines used to treat patients with limited or no kidney function.

diaphoresis—Profuse or excessive perspiration, or sweating.

diaphysis—The shaft, or middle section, of a long bone.

diastole—Period of relaxation of the heart.

diastolic—Measurement of blood pressure taken when the heart is at rest; measurement of the constant pressure in arteries.

diencephalon—The section of the brain between the cerebrum and midbrain; contains the thalamus and hypothalamus.

dietetic assistants/dietetic technicians (DTs)—Individuals who work under the supervision of dietitians and assist with food preparation and service, help patients select menus, clean work areas, and assist other dietary workers; also called *food service workers*.

dietitians (RD)—Individuals who specializes in the science of diet and nutrition.

differential count—Blood test that determines the percentage of each kind of leukocyte (white blood cell).

digestion—Physical and chemical breakdown of food by the body in preparation for absorption.

digestive system—The body system that is responsible for the breakdown of food so that it can be taken into the bloodstream and used by body cells and tissues; also called the *gastrointestinal system*.

dilate—Enlarge or expand; to make bigger.

direct smear—A culture specimen placed on a slide for microscopic examination.

disability—A physical or mental handicap that interferes with normal function; incapacitated, incapable.

discretion—Ability to use good judgment and self-restraint in speech or behavior.

disease—Any condition that interferes with the normal function of the body.

disinfection—Aseptic-control method that destroys pathogens but does not usually kill spores and viruses.

dislocation—Displacement of a bone at a joint.

displacement—Defense mechanism in which feelings about one person are transferred to someone else.

distal—Most distant or farthest from the trunk, center, or midline.

dobutamine stress test—A cardiac test used by a physician to determine how heart responds to stress; used for patients who cannot exercise; a medication that simulates the effect of exercise is given to increase the blood flow and heart rate; *see also* **adenosine stress test**.

Doctor of Chiropractic (DC)—Classification of physician who focuses on ensuring proper alignment of the spine and optimal operation of the nervous and muscular systems to maintain health.

Doctor of Medicine (MD)—Classification of physician who diagnoses, treats, and prevents diseases or disorders.

Doctor of Osteopathic Medicine (DO)—Classification of physician who treats diseases/disorders, placing special emphasis on the nervous, muscular, and skeletal systems, and the relationship between the body, mind, and emotions.

Doctor of Podiatric Medicine (DPM)—Classification of physician who examines, diagnoses, and treats diseases/disorders of the feet or of the leg below the knee.

doctorate/doctoral degree—Degree awarded by a college or university after completion of a prescribed course of study beyond a bachelor's or master's degree.

doctor's carts—Carts that usually contain air-water syringes and a variety of handpieces and rheostats.

dorsal—Pertaining to the back; in back of.

dorsal cavity—One long, continuous cavity located on the back of the body; divided into the cranial cavity and spinal cavity.

dorsal recumbent—The patient lies on the back with the knees flexed and separated; used for vaginal and pelvic examinations.

dorsiflexion—Bending backward or bending the foot toward the knee.

dressing—Covering placed over a wound or injured part.

droplet precautions—Methods of infection control that must be used for patients known or suspected to be infected with pathogens transmitted by large particle droplets expelled during coughing, sneezing, talking, or laughing.

dry cold—Application that provides cold temperature but is dry against the skin.

dry heat—Application that provides warm temperature but is dry against the skin.

duodenum—First part of the small intestine; connects the pylorus of the stomach and the jejunum.

Durable Power of Attorney (POA)—A legal document that permits an individual (principal) to appoint another person to make any decisions regarding health care if the principal becomes unable to make decisions.

dysphagia—Difficulty in swallowing.

dyspnea—Difficult or labored breathing.

E

early adulthood—Period of development from 19 to 40 years of age.

early childhood—Period of development from 1 to 6 years of age.

Ebola—A filovirus that causes hemorrhagic fever disease.

echocardiogram—A cardiac test that uses technology to direct ultra-high-frequency sound waves through the chest wall and into the heart; a computer then converts the reflection of the waves into an image of the heart; usually a reading is taken while the patient is at rest and then another reading is taken after exercise when the heart rate rises to a target level; used to evaluate cardiac function, reveal valve irregularities, show defects in the heart walls, and visualize the presence of fluid between the layers of the pericardium or bleeding.

edema—Swelling; excess amount of fluid in the tissues.

ejaculatory duct—In the male, duct or tube from the seminal vesicle to the urethra.

elasticity— Property of muscles; allows the muscle to return to its original shape after it has contracted or stretched.

electrocardiogram (ECG)—Graphic tracing of the electrical activity of the heart.

electrocardiograph (ECG) technicians—Individuals who operate electrocardiograph machines, which record electrical impulses that originate in the heart.

electroencephalographic (EEG) technologist—Individual who records the electrical activity of the brain as an electroencephalogram, which is used by neurologists and other physicians to diagnose and evaluate diseases and disorders of the brain.

electroneurodiagnostic technologist (END) —An individual who performs nerve conduction tests, measures responses to stimuli, measures brain responses, and operates monitoring devices to assist with diagnosing disorders and diseases of the brain and nervous system.

electronic health records (EHRs)—Also called an *electronic medical record (EMR)*; a computerized version of all of a patient's medical information.

electronic mail—Also called *e-mail*; a form of communication that is sent, received, and forwarded online from one computer to another by means of an Internet connection.

electronic thermometers—Types of thermometers that use a heat sensor to record temperature and display the temperature on a viewer in a few seconds; can be used to take oral, rectal, axillary, and/or groin temperatures.

embalmers—Individuals who prepare the body of a deceased person for interment or burial.

emergency care services—Provide special care for victims of accidents or sudden (acute) illness.

emergency medical responder (EMR)—The first person to arrive at the scene of an illness or injury; interviews and examines the victim to identify the illness or cause of injury, calls for emergency medical assistance as needed, maintains safety and infection control at the scene, and provides basic emergency medical care.

emergency medical technician (EMT)—An individual who provides emergency prehospital care to victims of accidents, injuries, or sudden illness.

emotional—Pertaining to feelings or psychological states.

empathy—Identifying with another's feelings but being unable to change or solve the situation.

emphysema—A chronic respiratory condition that occurs when the walls of the alveoli deteriorate and lose their elasticity resulting in poor exchanges of gases in the lungs.

enamel—Hardest tissue in the body; covers the outside of the crown of a tooth.

enclosure notation—If enclosures are included with a letter, this is noted at the end of the letter with a brief description of the material enclosed.

endocardium—Serous membrane lining of the heart.

endocrine gland—Ductless gland that produces an internal secretion discharged into the blood or lymph.

endocrine system—Body system that consists of a group of these ductless endocrine glands that secrete hormones directly into the bloodstream.

endodontics—Branch of dentistry involving treatment of the pulp chamber and root canals of the teeth; root canal treatment.

endogenous—Infection or disease originating within the body.

endometrium—Mucous membrane lining of the inner surface of the uterus.

endoplasmic reticulum—Fine network of tubular structures in the cytoplasm of a cell; allows for the transport of materials in and out of the nucleus and aids in the synthesis and storage of protein.

endorsement—A written signature on the back of a check; required in order to receive payment.

endosteum—Membrane lining the medullary canal of a bone.

energy conservation—Monitoring the use of energy to control costs and conserve resources.

enthusiasm—Intense interest or excitement.

entrepreneur—Individual who organizes, manages, and assumes the risk of a business.

environmental services facilities managers—Individuals who oversee buildings, grounds, equipment, and supplies.

epidemic—An infectious disease that affects a large number of people within a population, community, or region at the same time.

epidemiologists—Individuals who identify and tract diseases as they occur in a group of people.

epidermis—The outer layer of the skin.

epididymis—Tightly coiled tube in the scrotal sac; connects the testes with the vas or ductus deferens.

epiglottis—Leaf-shaped structure that closes over the larynx during swallowing.

epiphysis—The end or head at the extremity of a long bone.

epithelial tissue—Tissue that forms the skin and parts of the secreting glands, and that lines the body cavities.

eponyms—Terms used in medicine that are named after people, places, or things.

ergonomics—An applied science used to promote the safety and well-being of a person by adapting the environment and using techniques to prevent injuries.

erythema—Redness of the skin.

erythrocyte—Red blood cell (RBC).

erythrocyte sedimentation rate (ESR)—Blood test that determines the rate at which red blood cells settle out of the blood.

esophagus—Tube that extends from the pharynx to the stomach.

essential nutrients—Those elements in food required by the body for proper function.

esteem—Place a high value on; respect.

estimating—Calculating the approximate answer.

ethicists—Individuals who study and review the history, philosophy, theology, medical research, and sociology of health care to make judgments about treatment options and the effectiveness of these options as they relate to ethical standards regarding patient rights, quality of life, privacy, death, and how health care funds and resources should be allocated.

ethics—Principles of right or good conduct.

ethnicity—Classification of people based on national origin and/or culture.

ethnocentric—Belief in the superiority of one's own ethnic group.

etiology—The study of the cause of a disease.

eustachian tube—Tube that connects the middle ear and the pharynx, or throat.

excitability—Property of muscles; irritability, the ability to respond to a stimulus such as a nerve impulse.

excretory system—Body system responsible for removing certain wastes and excess water from the body and for maintaining the body's acid–base or pH balance; *see also* **urinary system**.

exercise stress test—A cardiac test involving an ECG run while the patient is exercising; usually involves walking a treadmill or riding an exercise bike until a target heart rate is reached; allows the physician to evaluate the function of the patient's heart during activity.

exocrine glands—Gland with a duct that produces a secretion.

exogenous—Infection or disease originating outside of or external to the body.

expiration—The expulsion of air from the lungs; breathing out air.

expressed consents—Consents stated in distinct and clear language, either orally or in writing.

extended family—A family group that includes the nuclear family plus grandparents, aunts, uncles, and cousins.

extensibility—Property of muscles; the ability to be stretched.

extension—Increasing the angle between two parts; straightening a limb.

external respiration—The exchange of oxygen and carbon dioxide between the lungs and bloodstream.

externships—Learning opportunities offered by educational institutions to give students short, practical experiences in their field of study.

F

fainting—Partial or complete loss of consciousness caused by a temporary reduction in the supply of blood to the brain.

Fahrenheit—A scale of temperature on which water freezes at 328 and boils at 2128 under standard conditions.

Fallopian tubes—Oviducts; in the female, passageway for the ova (egg) from the ovary to uterus.

false imprisonment—Restraining an individual or restricting an individual's freedom.

fanfolding—Folding in accordion pleats; done with bed linens.

fascia—Fibrous membrane covering, supporting, and separating muscles.

fasting blood sugar (FBS)—Blood test that measures blood serum levels of glucose (sugar) after a person has had nothing by mouth for a period of time.

fat-restricted diets—Diets with limited amounts of fats, or lipids.

fats—Also called *lipids*; nutrients that provide the most concentrated form of energy; highest-calorie energy nutrients.

fax (facsimile) machine—Machine used in many to transmit data or information electronically over the telephone lines.

Federation Dentaire International (FDI) System—Abbreviated means of identifying the teeth that uses a two-digit code to identify the quadrant and tooth.

feedback—A method used to determine if communication was successful which occurs when the receiver of a message responds to the message.

fee-for-service compensation—A health payment plan in which doctors or providers are paid for each service they render.

femur—Thigh bone of the leg; the longest and strongest bone in the body.

fertilization—Conception; impregnation of the ovum by the sperm.

fever—Elevated body temperature, usually above 101°F, or 38.3 °C, rectally.

fiber diets—Types of diets usually classified as high fiber or low fiber. A high-fiber diet usually provides at least 30 grams of fiber without seeds or nuts and is used to stimulate activity in the digestive tract. A low-fiber diet containing less than 10–15 grams of fiber per day eliminates or limits foods that are high in bulk and fiber and is used for patients who have digestive and rectal diseases, such as colitis or diarrhea.

fibula—Outer and smaller bone of the lower leg.

fields—Specific data categories within a computer database, for example, the entry of an address in a patient information database.

file—A group of related records that have been combined together.

filing—Arranging in order.

fire extinguishers—Devices that can be used to put out fires.

firewalls—Software programs or hardware devices designed to prevent unauthorized access to a computer system.

first aid—Immediate care given to a victim of an injury or illness to minimize the effects of the injury or illness.

fixed expenses—Those items in a budget that are set and usually do not change (for example, rent and car payments).

flexion—Decreasing the angle between two parts; bending a limb.

fomites—Substances or objects that adheres to and transmits infectious material.

fontanel—Area between the cranial bones where the bones have not fused together; "soft spots" in the skull of an infant.

Food and Drug Administration (FDA)—A federal agency responsible for regulating food and drug products sold to the public.

foramina—A passage or opening; a hole in a bone through which blood vessels or nerves pass.

forensic science technicians—Individuals who investigate crimes by collecting and analyzing physical evidence.

Fowler's—The patient lies on the back with the head elevated at one of several different angles.

fractions—A way of expressing numbers that represent parts of a whole.

fracture—A break (usually, a break in a bone or tooth).

frontal (coronal) plane—Imaginary line that separates the body into a front section and a back section.

frostbite—Actual freezing of tissue fluid resulting in damage to the skin and underlying tissue.

funeral directors—Individuals who manage and operate a funeral home; also called *morticians or undertakers*.

fungi—Group of simple, plantlike animals that live on dead organic matter (for example, yeast and molds).

G

gallbladder—Small sac near the liver; concentrates and stores bile.

genes—The structures on chromosomes that carry inherited characteristics.

genetic counseling centers—Centers that work with couples or individuals who are pregnant or considering a pregnancy; perform prenatal screening tests, check for genetic abnormalities and birth defects, explain the results of the tests, identify medical options when a birth

defect is present, and help the individuals cope with the psychological issues caused by a genetic disorder.

genetic counselors—Individuals who provide information to patients and/or their families on genetic diseases or inherited conditions.

geneticists—Individuals who study genes and how they are inherited, mutated, and activated, or inactivated.

genome—The total mass of genetic instruction humans inherit from their parents.

geriatric aides/assistants—Individuals who acquire additional education to provide care for older patients in environments such as extended care facilities, nursing homes, retirement centers, adult day care facilities, and other similar agencies.

geriatric care—Care provided to older individuals.

geriatrics, gerontology—The study of the aged or old age and treatment of related diseases and conditions.

gingiva—The gums (tissues surrounding the teeth).

glaucoma—Eye disease characterized by increased intraocular pressure.

glomerulus—Microscopic cluster of capillaries in Bowman's capsule of the nephron in the kidney.

glucose—The most common type of sugar in the body.

glucose tolerance test (GTT)—A diagnostic test that evaluates how well a person metabolizes a calculated amount of glucose.

glycohemoglobin test—A blood test that measures the amount of glucose that attaches to hemoglobin on red blood cells to determine the average blood-sugar levels for the previous 2 to 3 months; commonly called HbA1C or AIC test.

glycosuria—Presence of sugar in the urine.

goal—Desired result or purpose toward which one is working.

Golgi apparatus—That structure in the cytoplasm of a cell that produces, stores, and packages secretions for discharge from the cell.

Gram's stain—Technique of staining organisms to identify specific types of bacteria present.

gross income—Amount of pay earned before deductions are taken out.

growth—Measurable physical changes that occur throughout a person's life.

H

halitosis—Bad breath.

hard palate—Bony structure that forms the roof of the mouth.

heading—That section of a letter containing the address of the person sending the letter and the date of writing.

health care administrators—Individuals who plan, direct, coordinate, and supervise the delivery of health care in a health care facility.

health care–associated infection (HAI)—An infection acquired by an individual in a health care facility such as a hospital or long-term care facility.

health care records—Records that contain information about the care provided to the patient; considered privileged communications.

health care risk managers—Individuals who assess risks in order to reduce potential safety, financial, and patient problems.

health departments—Provide health services as directed by the U.S. Department of Health and Human Services (USDHHS); the public health system in the United States is a complex network of people and organizations in both public and private sectors that collaborate in various ways at national, state and local levels to promote and protect public health; may offer clinics for pediatric health care, treatment of sexually transmitted diseases, treatment of respiratory disease, immunizations, and other special services.

health information exchange (HIE)—A federally established system that allows all health care agencies to readily transfer patient electronic health records (EHRs) between agencies in a national network.

health educators—Individuals who teach people the behaviors that promote wellness by evaluating, designing, presenting, recommending, and disseminating culturally appropriate health education information and materials.

health information (medical records) administrators (HIAs)—Individuals who develop and manage the systems for storing and obtaining information from records, prepare information for legal actions and insurance claims, compile statistics for organizations and government agencies, manage medical records departments, ensure the confidentiality of patient information, and supervise and train other personnel.

health information (medical records) technicians (HITs)—Individuals who organize and code medical records, gather statistical information, and monitor records to ensure confidentiality.

health insurance plans—Plans that enable many people to pay for the costs of health care; when the insured individual incurs health care expenses covered by the insurance plan, the insurance company pays for the services. The amount of premium payment and the type of services covered vary from plan to plan.

Health Insurance Portability and Accountability Act (HIPAA)—Set of federal regulations adopted to protect the confidentiality of patient information and the ability to retain health insurance coverage.

health maintenance organizations (HMOs)—A type of health insurance that provides a health care delivery system which administers health care directed toward preventive care.

health science education (HSE)—Secondary education programs that prepare a student for immediate employment in many health care careers or for additional education after graduation.

heart attack—*See* **myocardial infarction**.

heat cramp—Muscle pain and spasm resulting from exposure to heat and inadequate fluid and salt intake.

heat exhaustion—Condition resulting from exposure to heat and excessive loss of fluid through sweating.

heat stroke—Medical emergency caused by prolonged exposure to heat, resulting in high body temperature and failure of sweat glands.

helminths—A parasitic worm (for example, a tapeworm or leech).

hematocrit (Hct)—Blood test that measures the percentage of red blood cells per a given unit of blood.

hematuria—Blood in the urine.

hemoglobin—The iron-containing protein of the red blood cells; serves to carry oxygen from the lungs to the tissues.

hemolysis—Disintegration of red blood cells, causing cells to dissolve or go into solution.

hemorrhage—Excessive loss of blood; bleeding.

hemostats—Instruments used to compress (clamp) blood vessels to stop bleeding.

hepatitis B—A virus caused by the HBV virus and is transmitted by blood, serum, and other body secretions; affects the liver and can lead to the destruction and scarring of liver cells; also called serum hepatitis.

hepatitis C—A virus caused by the hepatitis C virus, or HCV; transmitted by blood and blood-containing body fluids; any individuals who contract the disease are asymptomatic; others have mild symptoms that are often diagnosed as influenza or flu; can cause serious liver damage that may result in death.

high-speed handpiece—A piece of dental equipment that is held in the hand and used to do most of the cutting and preparation of the tooth during dental procedures.

high-velocity oral evacuator (HVE)—Dental handpiece used to remove particles and large amounts of liquid from the oral cavity.

hilum—A notched or indented area through which the ureter, nerves, blood vessels, and lymph vessels enter and leave the kidney.

holistic care—Care that provides for the well-being of the whole person and meets not only physical needs, but also social, emotional, and mental needs.

holistic health care—Care that promotes physical, emotional, social, intellectual, and spiritual well-being.

home health care—Any type of health care provided in a patient's home environment.

home health care assistants—Individuals who are trained to work in the patient's home and may perform additional duties such as meal preparation or cleaning.

homeostasis—A constant state of natural balance within the body.

honesty—Truthfulness; integrity.

horizontal recumbent (supine)—*See* **supine position**.

hormone—Chemical substance secreted by an organ or gland.

hospice—Program designed to provide care for the terminally ill while allowing them to die with dignity.

hospitals—Institutions that provides medical or surgical care and treatment for the sick or injured.

household system—A system of units developed so patients could measure out dosages at home using ordinary containers found in the kitchen.

housekeeping workers/sanitary managers—Individuals who help maintain the cleanliness of the health care facility to provide a pleasant, sanitary environment; also called *environmental service workers*.

humerus—Long bone of the upper arm.

hydrocollator packs—Gel-filled packs that are warmed in a water bath to provide a moist heat application.

hyperglycemia—Presence of sugar in the blood; high blood sugar.

hyperopia—Farsightedness; defect in near vision.

hypertension—High blood pressure.

hyperthermia—Condition that occurs when body temperature exceeds 104°F, or 40°C, rectally.

hypodermis—The innermost layer of the skin, made of elastic and fibrous connective tissue and adipose (fatty) tissue and connects the skin to underlying muscles; *see also* **subcutaneous fascia**.

hypoglycemia—Low blood sugar.

hypotension—Low blood pressure.

hypothalamus—That structure in the diencephalon of the brain that regulates and controls many body functions.

hypothermia—Condition in which body temperature is below normal, usually below 95°F (35°C) and often in the range of 78°F – 95°F (26°C – 35° C).

hypothermia blanket—Special blanket containing coils filled with a cooling solution; used to reduce high body temperature.

I

ice bags/collars—Plastic or rubber devices filled with ice to provide dry-cold application.

ileostomy—A surgical opening connecting the ileum (small intestine) and the abdominal wall.

ileum—Final section of small intestine; connects the jejunum and large intestine.

image-guided surgery (IGS)—A surgical procedure in which a surgeon uses preoperative and intraoperative images to guide or direct the surgery.

immunity—Condition of being protected against a particular disease.

impaction—A large, hard mass of fecal material lodged in the intestine or rectum; a tooth that does not erupt into the mouth.

implied consents—Obligations that are understood without verbally expressed terms.

implied contracts—A contract or agreement that creates obligations without verbally expressed terms.

impression—Negative reproduction of a tooth or dental arch.

improper fractions—Fractions that have numerators that are larger than the denominators.

incisal—The cutting or biting surface of anterior teeth.

incision—Cut or wound of body tissue caused by a sharp object; a surgical cut.

incisors—Teeth located in the front and center of the mouth; used to cut food.

income—Total amount of money received in a given period (usually a year); salary is usually the main source.

incontinence—The inability to control urination.

independent living facilities—*See* **assisted living facilities**.

index—To put names in proper order for filing purposes.

industrial health care centers—Clinics found in large companies or industries; provide health care for employees of the industry or business by performing basic examinations, teaching accident prevention and safety, and providing emergency care. Also called *occupational health clinics*.

industrial hygienists—Individuals who identify and analyze workplace hazards.

infancy—Period of development from birth to 1 year of age.

infection—Invasion by organisms; contamination by disease-producing organisms, or pathogens.

infectious—Disease type, caused by a pathogenic organism such as a bacteria or virus.

infectious agent—A pathogen, such as a bacterium or virus that can cause a disease.

informed consent—Permission granted voluntarily by a person who is of sound mind and aware of all factors involved.

inherited—A disease transmitted from parents to child genetically.

initiative—Ability to begin or follow through with a plan or task; determination.

inquiry—Search for information.

insertion—End or area of a muscle that moves when the muscle contracts.

inside address—That section of a letter that contains the name and address of the person or firm to whom the letter is being sent.

inspiration—Breathing in; taking air into the lungs.

insulin shock—Condition that occurs in individuals with diabetes when there is an excess amount of insulin and a low level of glucose (sugar) in the blood.

insurance forms—Forms used to apply for payment by an insurance company.

intake and output (I&O)—A record that notes all fluids taken in or eliminated by a person in a given period of time.

integrative (integrated) health care—A form of health care that uses both mainstream medical treatments and complementary and alternative therapies to treat a patient.

integumentary system—Pertaining to the skin or a covering.

internal respiration—The exchange of carbon dioxide and oxygen between the tissue cells and the bloodstream.

Internet—Worldwide computer network.

internships—On-the-job training that provides students with an opportunity to gain experience in their field of study.

invasion of privacy—Revealing personal information about an individual without his or her consent.

involuntary—Independent action not controlled by choice or desire.

iris—Colored portion of the eye; composed of muscular, or contractile, tissue that regulates the size of the pupil.

J

jackknife (proctologic)—The patient lies on the abdomen with both the head and legs inclined downward and the rectal area elevated.

jaundice—Yellow discoloration of the skin and eyes, frequently caused by liver or gallbladder disease.

jejunum—The middle section of the small intestine; connects the duodenum and ileum.

job interview—A face-to-face meeting or conversation between an employer and an applicant for a job.

joint—An articulation, or area where two bones meet or join.

K

kidney—Bean-shaped organ that excretes urine; located high and in back of the abdominal cavity.

knee–chest—The patient rests his or her body weight on the knees and chest; used for sigmoidoscopic and rectal examinations.

L

labia majora—Two large folds of adipose tissue lying on each side of the vulva in the female; hairy outer lips.

labia minora—Two folds of membrane lying inside the labia majora; hairless inner lips.

labial—Crown surface of the anterior teeth that lies next to the lips; facial surface of the anterior teeth.

laboratories—Rooms or buildings where scientific tests, research, experiments, or learning takes place.

laceration—Wound or injury with jagged, irregular edges.

lacrimal—Pertaining to tears; glands that secrete and expel tears.

lacrimal glands—Glands in the eye that produce tears.

lacteal—Specialized lymphatic capillary that picks up digested fats or lipids in the small intestine and transports them to the thoracic duct.

laissez-faire leader—An individual who believes in noninterference in the affairs of others, strives for only minimal rules or regulations, and allows the individuals in a group to function in an independent manner with little or no direction.

large intestine—The final section of the alimentary canal; its functions include absorption of water and any remaining nutrients; storage of indigestible materials before they are eliminated from the body; synthesis (formation) and absorption of some B-complex vitamins and vitamin K by bacteria present in the intestine; and transportation of waste products out of the alimentary canal.

laryngeal mirror—An instrument with a mirror at one end; used to examine the larynx, or voice box, in the throat.

larynx—Voice box, located between the pharynx and trachea.

lasers—Light beams that can be focused precisely.

late adulthood—Period of development beginning at 65 years of age and ending at death.

late childhood—Period of development from 6 to 12 years of age.

lateral—Pertaining to the side.

leads—Angles or views of the heart that is recorded in an electrocardiogram.

leader—An individual who leads or guides others, or who is in charge or in command of others.

leadership—Ability to lead, guide, and direct others.

ledger card—A card or record that shows a financial account of money charged, received, or paid out.

left atrium—One of the four chambers of the heart; receives oxygenated blood from the lungs.

left lateral—*See* **Sims' position**.

left ventricle—One of the four chambers of the heart; receives blood from the left atrium and pumps the blood into the aorta for transport to the body cells.

legal—Authorized or based on law.

legal disability—A condition in which a person does not have legal capacity and is therefore unable to enter into a legal agreement (for example, as is the case with a minor).

lens—Crystalline structure suspended behind the pupil of the eye; refracts or bends light rays onto the retina; also, the magnifying glass in a microscope.

letter of introduction—Letter written with the purpose of obtaining an interview; *see also* **cover letter**.

letterhead—Preprinted heading at the top of paper used for written correspondence.

leukocytes—White blood cells (WBC).

libel—False written statement that causes a person ridicule or contempt or causes damage to the person's reputation.

licensed practical/vocational nurses (LPNs/LVNs)—Individuals who work under the supervision of physicians or registered nurses and provide patient care requiring basic technical knowledge.

licensure—Process by which a government agency authorizes individuals to work in a given occupation.

life stages—Stages of growth and development experienced by an individual from birth to death.

ligament—Fibrous tissue that connects bone to bone.

line angles—Areas on crown surfaces of a tooth formed by a line drawn between two surfaces.

liner—Dental material that covers or lines exposed tooth tissue, usually in the form of a varnish.

lingual—The crown surface of teeth that is next to the tongue.

lipids—Organic compounds commonly called fats and oils; provide the most concentrated form of energy for the body.

liquid diets—Types of diets that include both clear liquids and full liquids; both are nutritionally inadequate and should be used only for short periods of time; all foods served must be liquid at body temperature.

listen—To pay attention, make an effort to hear.

lithotomy—The patient lies on the back with the feet in stirrups and knees flexed and separated.

liver—Largest gland in the body; located in the upper right quadrant of the abdomen; two of its main functions are excreting bile and storing glycogen.

living wills—Legal documents stating a person's desires on what measures should or should not be taken to prolong life when his or her condition is terminal.

long-term care facilities (LTCs or LTCFs)—Mainly provide assistance and care for elderly patients, usually called residents but also provide care for individuals with disabilities or handicaps and individuals with chronic or long-term illnesses.

low-cholesterol diet—Diet that restricts foods high in saturated fat.

low-speed handpiece—Slower handpiece in dental units; used to remove caries and for fine finishing work.

lung—Organ of respiration located in the thoracic cavity.

lymph—Fluid formed in body tissues and circulated in the lymphatic vessels.

lymph node—A round body of lymph tissue that filters lymph.

lymphatic capillaries—Part of the lymphatic system; small, open-ended lymph vessels that act like drainpipes.

lymphatic system—Body system that consists of lymph, lymph vessels, lymph nodes, and lymphatic tissue.

lymphatic vessels—Thin-walled vessels that carry lymph from tissues.

lysosomes—Those structures in the cytoplasm of a cell that contain digestive enzymes to digest and destroy old cells, bacteria, and foreign matter.

M

macule—A discolored but neither raised nor depressed spot or area on the skin.

magnetic resonance imaging (MRI)—Process that uses a computer and magnetic forces, instead of X-rays, to visualize internal organs.

mainframe computer—Largest type of computer; many users can access this computer at the same time.

malnutrition—Poor nutrition; without adequate food and nutrients.

malpractice—Providing improper or unprofessional treatment or care that results in injury to another person.

mandibular—Lower (relating to teeth).

massage therapists—Individuals who use massage, bodywork, and therapeutic touch to provide pain relief, improve circulation, and relieve stress and tension.

master's degree—Degree awarded by a college or university after completion of one or more years of prescribed study beyond a bachelor's degree.

matriarchal—Social organization in which the mother or oldest woman is the authority figure.

maxillary—Upper (relating to teeth).

mechanical lifts—Special devices used to move or transfer a patient.

medial—Pertaining to the middle or midline.

Medicaid—Government program that provides medical care for people whose incomes are below a certain level.

medical administrative assistants—Individuals who perform general administrative duties as well as tasks that are specific to the health care industry.

medical assistants (MAs)—Individuals who work under the supervision of physicians and perform tasks to assist physicians with patient care.

medical (clinical) laboratory assistants—Individuals who—working under the supervision of medical technologists, technicians, or pathologists— perform basic laboratory tests, prepare specimens for examination or testing, and perform other laboratory duties such as cleaning and helping to maintain equipment.

medical coders—Individuals who identify diagnoses, procedures, and services shown in a patient's health care record and assign specific codes to each; also called *coding specialists.*

medical history—A record that shows all diseases, illness, and surgeries that a patient has had.

medical illustrators—Individuals who use their artistic and creative talents to produce illustrations, charts, graphs, and diagrams for health textbooks, journals, magazines, and exhibits.

medical interpreters/translators—Individuals who assist cross-cultural communication processes by converting one language to another. Interpreters convert the spoken word while translators convert written material.

medical laboratory technicians (MLTs)— Individuals who perform many of the routine tests that do not require the advanced knowledge held by a medical technologist; *see also* **clinical laboratory technicians (CLTs).**

medical laboratory technologists (MTs)—Individuals who study the tissues, fluids, and cells of the human body to help determine the presence and/or cause of disease; perform complicated chemical, microscopic, and automated analyzer/computer tests; work under the supervision of pathologists; *see also* **clinical laboratory scientists (MTs).**

medical librarians—Individuals who organize books, journals, and other print materials to provide health information to other health care professionals; also called *health sciences librarians.*

medical offices—Provide medical services such as diagnosis, treatment, examination, basic laboratory testing, minor surgery, and other similar care.

medical secretaries/health unit coordinators—Individuals who are employed in hospitals, extended care facilities, clinics, and other health facilities to record information in records, schedule procedures or tests, answer telephones, order supplies, and work with computers to record or obtain information.

medical transcriptionists—Individuals who use a computer and word-processing software to enter data that has been dictated on a recorder by physicians or other health care professionals.

Medicare—Government program that provides medical care for elderly and/or disabled individuals.

medication—Drug used to treat a disease or condition.

medication aides/assistants—Individuals who receive special training such as a 40-hour or more state-approved medication aide course to administer medications to patients or residents in long-term care facilities or patients receiving home health care.

Medigap policy—An insurance plan that serves as supplemental insurance to Medicare; usually pays deductible for Medicare and co-payments of care.

medulla—Inner, or central, portion of an organ.

medulla oblongata—The lower part of the brainstem; controls vital processes such as respiration and heartbeat.

medullary canal—Inner, or central, portion of a long bone.

meiosis—The process of cell division that occurs in gametes, or sex cells (ovum and spermatozoa).

melanin—Brownish black pigment found in the skin, hair, and eyes.

memorandums—Short, written statements or messages.

meninges—Membranes that cover the brain and spinal cord.

mental—Pertaining to the mind.

mental health facilities—Treat patients who have mental disorders and diseases; examples include guidance and counseling centers, psychiatric clinics and hospitals, chemical abuse treatment centers, and physical abuse treatment centers.

mesial—The side surface of teeth that is toward the midline of the mouth.

metabolism—The use of food nutrients by the body to produce energy.

metacarpal—Bone of the hand between the wrist and each finger.

metatarsal—Bone of the foot between the instep and each toe.

metric system—A decimal measuring system based on the meter, liter, and gram as units of length, capacity, and weight or mass.

microcomputer—Desktop or personal computer found in the home or office.

microorganism—Small, living plant or animal not visible to the naked eye; a microbe.

microscope—Instrument used to magnify or enlarge objects for viewing.

micturate—Another word for *urinate*; to expel urine.

midbrain—That portion of the brain that connects the pons and cerebellum; relay center for impulses.

middle adulthood—Period of development from 40–65 years of age.

midsagittal (median) plane—A sagittal plane that runs down the midline of the body and divides the body into equal halves.

military time—A convention of time keeping in which the day runs from midnight to midnight and is divided into 24 hours.

minerals—Inorganic substances essential to life.

mitered corners—Special folding technique used to secure linen on a bed.

mitochondria—Those structures in a cell that provide energy and are involved in the metabolism of the cell.

mitosis—Process of asexual reproduction by which cells divide into two identical cells.

mitral valve—Flap or cusp between the left atrium and left ventricle in the heart.

mode of transmission—A way that the infectious agent can be transmitted to another reservoir or host where it can live.

model—Also called a *cast*; a positive reproduction of the dental arches or teeth in plaster or similar materials.

modified-block style—Formatting style of a letter in which certain parts of the letter are aligned at the center line of the paper and the remaining parts are aligned at the left margin of the paper.

moist cold—An application that provides cold temperature and is wet against the skin.

moist heat—An application that provides warm temperature and is wet against the skin.

molars—Teeth in the back of the mouth; largest and strongest teeth; used to grind food.

monotheists—Individuals who believe in the existence of one God.

Montgomery straps—Special adhesive strips that are applied when dressings must be changed frequently at a surgical site.

mortuary assistants—Individuals who, working under the supervision of the funeral director and/or embalmer, assist with preparation of the body, drive the hearse to pick up the body after death or take it to the burial site, arrange flowers for the viewing, assist with preparations for the funeral service, help with filing and maintaining records, clean the funeral home, and other similar duties.

motivated—Stimulated into action; incentive to act.

mouth—Oral cavity; opening to the digestive tract, or alimentary canal.

multicompetent/multiskilled worker—An individual who can perform a variety of health care tasks.

muscle tissue—Body tissue composed of fibers that produce movement.

muscle tone—State of partial muscle contraction providing a state of readiness to act.

muscular system—More than 600 muscles, bundles of muscle fibers held together by connective tissue.

myocardium—Muscle layer of the heart.

myopia—Nearsightedness; defect in distant vision.

myths—False beliefs; an established beliefs with no basis.

N

nasal cavity—Space between the cranium and the roof of the mouth.

nasal septum—Bony and cartilaginous partition that separates the nasal cavity into two sections.

National Institutes of Health (NIH)—A federal agency that is involved in research on disease.

need—Lack of something required or desired; urgent want or desire.

needle holder—Instrument used to hold or support a needle while sutures (stitches) are being inserted.

negligence—Failure to give care that is normally expected, resulting in injury to another person.

nephron—Structural and functional unit of the kidney.

nerve—Group of nerve tissues that conducts impulses.

nerve tissue—Body tissue that conducts or transmits impulses throughout the body.

nervous system—A complex, highly organized system that coordinates all the activities of the body.

net income—Amount of pay received for hours worked after all deductions have been taken out; take-home pay.

networks—Connections of two or more computers to share data and hardware.

neuron—Nerve cell.

nocturia—Excessive urination at night.

nomenclature—A method of naming.

noncontact infrared thermometer—Type of thermometer that uses light wavelength technology to measure the thermal energy radiating from the skin without requiring any physical contact with the person.

nonpathogens—Microorganisms that are not capable of causing disease.

nonprofit agencies—Agencies supported by donations, membership fees, fundraisers, and federal or state grants; provide health services at the national, state, and local levels; see also **voluntary agencies**.

nonverbal communication—The use of facial expressions, body language, gestures, eye contact, and touch to convey messages or ideas; communication that is not spoken.

nose—The projection in the center of the face; the organ for smelling and breathing.

nuclear family—A family group that usually consists of a mother, father, and children, but can consist of a single parent and children.

nuclear stress test—A cardiac test in which a small amount of a radioactive substance such as thallium is given intravenously; a special camera is used to identify the rays emitted from the substance while the patient is at rest and then during exercise; allows the physician to evaluate which parts of the heart are healthy and function normally and which parts are not.

nucleolus—The spherical body in the nucleus of a cell that is important in reproduction of the cell.

nucleus—The structure in a cell that controls cell activities such as growth, metabolism, and reproduction.

nurse assistants—Individuals who work under the supervision of registered or licensed practical nurses to provide basic patient care.

nutrition—All body processes related to food; the body's use of food for growth, development, and health.

nutritional status—The state of one's nutrition.

O

obesity—Excessive body weight 20 percent or more above the recommended weight, or a BMI equal to or greater than 30.

observation—To look at, watch, perceive, or notice.

occlusal—The chewing or biting surface of posterior teeth.

occlusal films—Films used to view the occlusal (chewing) planes of the maxilla or mandible.

occult blood—Blood that is hidden; also, a test done on stool to check for the presence of blood.

Occupational Exposure to Hazardous Chemicals Standard—Standard that requires that employers inform employees of all chemicals and hazards in the workplace.

Occupational Safety and Health Administration (OSHA)—A federal agency that establishes and enforces standards that protect workers from job-related injuries and illnesses.

occupational therapists (OTs)—Individuals who help people who have physical, developmental, mental, or emotional disabilities overcome, correct, or adjust to their particular problems.

occupational therapy assistants (OTAs)—Individuals who, working under the guidance of occupational therapists, help patients carry out programs of prescribed treatment—including arts and crafts projects, recreation, and social events; rehabilitation activities and exercises; games that develop balance and coordination; and mastering the activities of daily living.

occupied bed—A bed that is made while the patient is in bed.

odontology—Study of the anatomy, growth, and diseases of the teeth.

Office of the National Coordinator for Health Information Technology (ONC)—Leads national efforts to build a private and secure nationwide health information exchange; its goal is to improve health care by allowing health information to be exchanged quickly among providers.

olfactory—Pertaining to the sense of smell.

oliguria—Decreased or less-than-normal amounts of urine secretion.

ombudsman—Specially trained individual who acts as an advocate for others to improve care or conditions.

Omnibus Budget Reconciliation Act (OBRA) of 1987—Federal law that regulates the education and testing of nursing assistants.

open bed—A bed with the top sheets fanfolded to the bottom.

operative care—Care that is provided before, during, and after a surgical procedure.

ophthalmic assistants (OAs)—Individuals who work under the supervision of ophthalmologists, optometrists, and/or ophthalmic medical technologists or technicians to prepare patients for examinations, measure visual acuity, perform receptionist duties, help patients with frame selections and fittings, order lenses, perform minor adjustments and repairs of glasses, and teach proper care and use of contact lenses.

ophthalmic laboratory technicians—Individuals who cut, grind, finish, polish, and mount the lenses used in eyeglasses, contact lenses, and other optical instruments such as telescopes and binoculars.

ophthalmic medical technologists (OMTs)—Individuals who, working under the supervision of ophthalmologists, obtain patient histories, perform routine eye tests and measurements, fit patients for contacts, administer prescribed treatments, assist with eye surgery, perform advanced diagnostic tests such as ocular motility and biocular function tests, administer prescribed medications, and perform advanced microbiological procedures.

ophthalmic technicians (OTs)—Individuals who, working under the supervision of ophthalmologists and optometrists, prepare patients for examinations, obtain medical histories, take ocular measurements, administer basic vision tests, maintain ophthalmic and surgical instruments, adjust glasses, teach eye exercises, measure for contacts, instruct patients on the care and use of contacts, and perform receptionist duties.

ophthalmologists (MD)—Medical doctors specializing in diseases, disorders, and injuries of the eyes.

ophthalmoscope—An instrument used to examine the eye.

opioids—Substances that work in the nervous system of the body or in specific receptors in the brain to reduce the intensity of pain.

opportunistic—Characterizes infections that occur when the body's defenses are weak.

optical centers—Provide vision examinations, prescribe eyeglasses or contact lenses, and check for the presence of eye diseases; can be individually owned by an ophthalmologist or optometrist, or they can be part of a large chain of stores.

optician—An individual who makes or sells lenses, eyeglasses, and other optical supplies.

optometrist (OD)—A licensed, nonmedical practitioner who specializes in the diagnosis and treatment of vision defects.

oral hygiene—Care of the mouth and teeth.

oral surgery—Surgery on the teeth, mouth, and/or jaw and facial bones; also called *maxillofacial surgery*.

oral temperature—Temperature taken in the mouth.

oral-evacuation system—Special machine that uses water to form a suction or vacuum system to remove liquids and particles from the oral cavity.

orbital cavity—Body cavity that contains the eyes.

organ—Body part made of tissues that have joined together to perform a special function.

organ of Corti—Structure in the cochlea of the ear; organ of hearing.

organelles—Structures in the cytoplasm of a cell, including the nucleus, mitochondria, ribosomes, lysosomes, and Golgi apparatus.

organizational structure—A line of authority or chain of command that indicates areas of responsibility and leads to the efficient operation of a facility.

origin—End or area of a muscle that remains stationary when the muscle contracts.

originator (maker)—The person who writes a check to issue payment.

orthodontics—The branch of dentistry dealing with prevention and correction of irregularities of the alignment of teeth.

orthopnea—Severe dyspnea in which breathing is very difficult in any position other than sitting erect or standing.

os coxae—The hip bone; formed by the union of the ilium, ischium, and pubis.

ossicles—Small bones, especially the three bones of the middle ear that amplify and transmit sound waves.

osteoporosis—Condition in which bones become porous and brittle because of lack or loss of calcium, phosphorus, and other minerals.

ostomy—A surgically created opening into a body part.

outpatient services–Services provided to patients who have not been admitted to hospitals or other care facilities.

otoscope—An instrument used to examine the ear.

ovary—Endocrine gland or gonad that produces hormones and the female sex cell, or ovum.

overweight—A body weight that is 10–20 percent greater than the average recommended weight for a person's height, or a BMI from 25 to 29.9.

P

paging system—System that allows an individual to be contacted by using a pager or beeper; a pager can provide a voice message, a signal such as a beep that alerts the individual to call a designated number to receive the message, or a digital message on a display screen with the telephone number of the caller or a message.

pain—An unpleasant sensation that is perceived in the nervous system when illness or injury occurs.

palpation—The act of using the hands to feel body parts during an examination.

pancreas—Gland that is dorsal to the stomach; secretes insulin and digestive juices.

pandemic—An infectious disease that affects many people over a wide geographic area; a worldwide epidemic.

panoramic—Dental radiograph that shows the entire dental arch, or all of the teeth and related structures, on one film.

Papanicolaou—Also called a *Pap test*; a test to classify abnormal cells obtained from the vagina or cervix.

papule—Solid, elevated spot or area on the skin.

paraffin wax treatment—Heated mixture of paraffin and mineral oil; used to provide a moist heat application.

paramedic (EMT-P)—An individual who can perform all of the basic emergency medical technician duties in addition to in-depth patient assessment and care; the highest level of an emergency medical technician.

parasite—Organism that lives on or within another living organism.

parasympathetic—A division of the autonomic nervous system.

parathyroid glands—One of four small glands located on the thyroid gland; regulates calcium and phosphorus metabolism.

parliamentary procedure—A set of rules or guidelines that determine the conduct and order that is followed during a meeting.

partial bed bath—Bath in which only certain body parts are bathed or in which the health care provider bathes those parts of the body that the patient is unable to bathe.

patella—The kneecap.

pathogens—Disease-producing organisms.

pathophysiology—Study of how disease occurs and the responses of living organisms to disease processes.

patience—Ability to wait, persevere; capacity for calm endurance.

patient care technicians (PCTs)—Individuals who, working under the supervision of RNs or LPNs/LVNs, provide patient care such as baths, bed making, and feeding; assist in transfer and ambulation; and administer basic treatments.

patient portals—Secure online websites are established by a physician, health care facility, or other health care provider.

Patient Protection and Affordable Care Act (PPACA)—A federal statute signed into law and designed to expand access to affordable health coverage in the United States.

Patient Self-Determination Act (PSDA)—A federal law that mandates that every individual has the right to make decisions regarding medical care, including the right to refuse treatment and the right-to-die.

patients' rights—Factors of care that all patients can expect to receive.

patriarchal—Social organization in which the father or oldest male is the authority figure.

payee—Person receiving payment.

pedodontic (child) films—Smaller films used on children to show disease or other conditions of the teeth.

pedodontics—The branch of dentistry dealing with treatment of teeth and oral conditions of children.

pegboard system—Method of maintaining financial accounts and records in an office.

pelvic cavity—The lower abdominal cavity; contains the urinary bladder, the reproductive organs, and the last part of the large intestine.

penis—External sex organ of the male.

percentages—Numbers used to express either a whole or part of a whole.

percussion—Process of tapping various body parts during an examination.

percussion (reflex) hammer—Instrument used to check reflexes.

perfusionists—Individuals who are members of the open-heart surgical team and operate the heart-lung machines used in coronary bypass surgery.

periapical films—Around the apex of a root of a tooth; dental X-ray that shows the entire tooth and surrounding area.

pericardium—Membrane sac that covers the outside of the heart.

peripheral nervous system (PNS)—A main division of the nervous system; consists of the nerves and has two divisions: the somatic nervous system and the autonomic nervous system.

perineum—Region between the vagina and anus in the female and between the scrotum and anus in the male.

periodontal ligament—Dense fibers of connective tissue that attach to the cementum of a tooth and the alveolus to support or suspend the tooth in its socket.

periodontics—The branch of dentistry dealing with the treatment of the gingiva (gum) and periodontium (supporting tissues) surrounding the teeth.

periodontium—Structures that surround and support the teeth.

periosteum—Fibrous membrane that covers the bones except at joint areas.

peristalsis—Rhythmic, wavelike motion of involuntary muscles.

permanent (succedaneous) teeth—The 32 teeth that make up the second, or permanent, set of teeth.

personal computer—A type of computer that can sit on a desktop.

personal hygiene—Care of the body including bathing, hair and nail care, shaving, and oral hygiene.

personal protective equipment (PPE)—Protective barriers such as a mask, gown, gloves, and protective eyewear that help protect a person from contact with infectious material.

personal space—The distance people require to feel comfortable while interacting with others; also called *territorial* space.

phalanges—Bones of the fingers and toes.

pharmaceutical services—Link health science with chemical science, as pharmacist prepares and dispenses medications, provides expertise on drug therapy, and ensures patient safety through education.

pharmaceutical/clinical project managers—Individuals who plan and manage all aspects of scientific research studies. Pharmaceutical project managers direct drug clinical trials while clinical project managers direct trials to obtain information to help prevent, screen, diagnose, and/or treat disease or medical conditions.

pharmacists (PharmDs)—Individuals who dispense medications per written orders from physicians, dentists, and other health care professionals authorized to prescribe medications.

pharmacologists—Medical researchers that work with patients and doctors to test and evaluate effectiveness as well as safety of new drugs.

pharmacy technicians—Individuals who work under the supervision of pharmacists to help prepare medication for dispensing and perform other duties as directed by pharmacists.

pharynx—The throat.

phlebotomist—Also called a *venipuncture technician*; individual who collects blood and prepares it for tests.

physical—Of or pertaining to the body.

physical therapist assistants (PTAs)—Individuals who, working under the supervision of physical therapists, help carry out prescribed plans of treatment. They perform exercises and massages; administer applications of heat, cold, and/or water; assist patients to ambulate with canes, crutches, or braces; provide ultrasound or electrical stimulation treatments; inform therapists of patients' responses and progress; and perform other duties, as directed by therapists.

physical therapists (PTs)—Individuals who provide treatment to improve mobility and prevent or limit permanent disability of patients who have disabling joint, bone, muscle, and/or nerve injuries or diseases; often work under the direction of a physiatrist.

physicians—Doctors who examine patients, obtain medical histories, order tests, make diagnoses, perform surgery, treat diseases/disorders, and teach preventive health.

physician assistants (PAs)—Individuals who work under the supervision of physicians and take medical histories, perform routine physical examinations and basic diagnostic tests, make preliminary diagnoses, treat minor injuries, and prescribe and administer treatments.

Physicians' Desk Reference (PDR)—Reference book that contains essential information on medications.

physiological needs—Basic physical or biological needs required by every human being to sustain life.

physiology—The study of the processes or functions of living organisms.

pineal body—An endocrine gland; a small structure attached to the roof of the third ventricle in the brain.

pinna—Also called the *auricle*; external portion of the ear.

pinocytic vesicles—Pocketlike folds in the cell membrane that allow large molecules such as proteins and fats to enter the cell.

pituitary gland—Small, rounded endocrine gland at the base of the brain; regulates function of other endocrine glands and body processes.

placenta—Temporary endocrine gland created during pregnancy to provide nourishment for the fetus; the afterbirth.

plantar flexion—Bending forward or bending the foot away from the knee.

plaque—Thin, tenacious, filmlike deposit that adheres (sticks) to the teeth and can lead to decay; made of protein and microorganisms.

plasma—Liquid portion of the blood.

plaster—A gypsum material used to form dental models.

pleura—A serous membrane that covers the lungs and lines the thoracic cavity.

point angles—Areas on the crown surface of a tooth that is formed when three surfaces meet.

poisoning—Condition that occurs when contact is made with any chemical substance that causes injury, illness, or death.

polysulfide—Also called rubber-base, is an elastomeric impression material that is elastic and rubbery in nature and used in taking dental impressions.

polytheists—Individuals who worship and believe in many Gods.

polyuria—Increased production and discharge of urine; excessive urination.

pons—That portion of the brainstem that connects the medulla oblongata and cerebellum to the upper portions of the brain.

portal of entry—A way for the infectious agent to enter a new reservoir or host.

portal of exit—A way for the infectious agent to escape from the reservoir in which it has been growing.

positron emission tomography (PET)—Computerized body scanning technique in which the computer detects a radioactive substance injected into a patient.

posterior—Toward the back; behind.

postmortem care—Care given to the body immediately after death.

postoperative care—After surgery.

preferred provider organization (PPO)—A type of managed care health insurance plan usually provided by large industries or companies to their employees.

prefix—An affix attached to the beginning of a word.

prejudice—Strong feeling or belief about a person or subject that is formed without reviewing facts or information.

preoperative care—Before surgery.

pressure (decubitus) ulcer—A pressure sore; a bedsore.

primary (deciduous) teeth—Also called *deciduous teeth*; the first set of 20 teeth.

privileged communications—All personal information given to health personnel by a patient; must be kept confidential.

process technicians—Individuals who operate and monitor the machinery that is used to produce biotechnology products.

professionalism—A blending of many different personal qualities such as good judgment, proper behavior, courtesy, good communication skills, honesty, politeness, responsibility, integrity, competence, and a proper appearance to meet the standards expected in a health care career.

prognosis—Prediction regarding the probable outcome of a disease.

projection—Defense mechanism in which an individual places the blame for his or her actions on someone else or circumstances.

pronation—Turning a body part downward; turning "palm down."

prone—The patient lies on the abdomen, with the legs together and the face turned to the side.

prophylaxis angle—Dental handpiece attachment that holds polishing cups, disks, and brushes used to clean the teeth or polish restorations.

proportion—A statement of equality between two ratios, or the relationship of one part to another part.

prostate gland—In the male, gland near the urethra; contracts during ejaculation to prevent urine from leaving the bladder.

prosthodontics—The branch of dentistry dealing with the construction of artificial appliances for the mouth.

protective isolation—*See* **reverse isolation**.

protein diets—Types of diets that include both low-protein and high-protein diets; low-protein diets are ordered for patients who have certain kidney or renal diseases and certain allergic conditions; high-protein diets may be ordered for children and adolescents, if growth is delayed; for pregnant or lactating women; before and/or after surgery; and for patients suffering from burns, fevers, or infections.

proteins—Basic components of all body cells; one of six essential nutrients needed for growth and repair of tissues.

protoplasm—Thick, viscous substance that is the physical basis of all living things.

protozoa—Microscopic, one-celled animals often found in decayed materials and contaminated water.

proximal—Closest to the point of attachment or area of reference.

psychiatric/mental health technicians—Individuals who, working under the supervision of psychiatrists or psychologists, help patients and their families follow treatment and rehabilitation plans.

psychiatrists—Physicians who specialize in diagnosing and treating mental illness.

psychiatry—The branch of medicine dealing with the diagnosis, treatment, and prevention of mental illness.

psychologists—Individuals who study human behavior and use this knowledge to help patients deal with the problems of everyday living.

puberty—Period of growth and development during which secondary sexual characteristics begin to develop.

pulmonary valve—Flap or cusp between the right ventricle of the heart and the pulmonary artery.

pulp—Soft tissue in the innermost area of a tooth and made of nerves and blood vessels held in place by connective tissue.

pulse—Pressure of the blood felt against the wall of an artery as the heart contracts or beats.

pulse deficit—The difference between the rate of an apical pulse and the rate of a radial pulse.

pulse oximeter—A device that measures the oxygen level in arterial blood.

pulse pressure—The difference between systolic and diastolic blood pressure.

puncture—Injury caused by a pointed object such as a needle or nail.

pupil—Opening or hole in the center of the iris of the eye; allows light to enter the eye.

pustule—Small, elevated, pus- or lymph-filled area of the skin.

pyrexia—Fever.

pyuria—Pus in the urine.

Q

quadrants—Fourths of a specific area.

quality control technicians—Individuals who test materials and products before, during, and after production to make sure the characteristics of the material or product are correct and to ensure they conform to specifications.

R

race—Classification of people based on physical or biological characteristics.

radiation exposure—An environmental hazard that is a major concern in radiology departments and dental offices; risks of exposure are involved with use radiographs and radioactive iodine in procedures.

radiation therapy—The use of high-energy particles to decrease the size of tumors and treat cancer.

radiographs—X-rayss; an images produced by radiation.

radiologic technologists (RTs)—Individuals who use X-rays, radiation, nuclear medicine, ultrasound, and magnetic resonance to diagnose and treat disease.

radiolucent—Transparent to X-rays; permitting the passage of X-rays or other forms of radiation.

radiopaque—Not transparent to X-rays; not permitting the passage of X-rays or other forms of radiation.

radius—Long bone of the forearm, between the wrist and elbow.

rales (rawls)—Bubbling or noisy sounds caused by fluid or mucus in the air passages.

range of motion (ROM)—The full range of movement of a muscle or joint; exercises designed to move each joint and muscle through its full range of movement.

rate—Number per minute, as with pulse and respiration counts.

rationalization—Defense mechanism involving the use of a reasonable or acceptable excuse as explanation for behavior.

ratios—Comparison used to show relationships between numbers or like values; for example, how many of one number or value is present as compared with the other.

reagent strip—Special test strip containing chemical substances that react to the presence of certain substances in the urine or blood.

reality orientation (RO)—Activities to help promote awareness of time, place, and person.

recall—To call back; letter or notice that reminds a patient to return for periodic treatment or examination.

receipt—Written record that money or goods has been received.

reciprocal—The multiplicative inverse of a number or fraction; a fraction that has been inverted or turned upside down so the denominator becomes the numerator.

record—A collection of related information in a database; a document that contains all of a patient's information.

recreational therapists (TRs)—Individuals who use recreational and leisure activities as forms of treatment to minimize patients' symptoms and improve physical, emotional, and mental well-being; also called *therapeutic recreation specialists*.

recreational therapy assistants—Individuals who work under the supervision of recreational therapists or other health care professionals; also called *activity directors* or *therapeutic recreation assistants*.

rectal temperature—Temperature taken in the rectum; an internal measurement and the most accurate of all methods of taking temperatures.

rectum—The final 6–8 inches of the large intestine and is a storage area for indigestibles and wastes.

red marrow—Soft tissue in the epiphyses of long bones.

reference initials—Initials placed at the bottom of a letter to indicate the writer and/or preparer.

reference plane—A real or imaginary flat surface from which an angle is measured.

refractometer—An instrument used to measure the specific gravity of urine.

refracts—Bends light.

registered nurses (RNs)—Licensed individuals who work under the direction of physicians to provide total care to patients.

regression—A defense mechanism that involves retreating to a previous developmental level that provided more safety and security than the current level the individual is experiencing.

regular diet—A balanced diet usually used for the patient with no dietary restrictions.

rehabilitation facilities—Provide care to help patients who have physical or mental disabilities obtain the maximum self-care and function. Services may include physical, occupational, recreational, speech, and hearing therapy.

religion—Spiritual beliefs and practices of an individual.

renal pelvis—A funnel-shaped structure that is the first section of the ureter.

repression—Defense mechanism involving the transfer of painful or unacceptable ideas, feelings, or thoughts into the subconscious.

reproductive system—Body system that produces new life; consists of gonads, ducts to carry the sex cells and secretions, and accessory organs.

reservoir—An area where the infectious agent can live.

Resident's Bill of Rights—Rights guaranteed to residents of long-term care facilities; residents must be informed of these rights, and a copy must be posted in each facility.

resistant—Able to oppose; organisms that remain unaffected by harmful substances in the environment.

respiration—The process of taking in oxygen (inspiration) and expelling carbon dioxide (expiration) by way of the lungs and air passages.

respirations—Measurements that reflect the breathing rate of the patient; include respiration count, rhythm, and character of respirations; abnormal respirations usually indicate that a health problem or disease is present.

respiratory system—The body system that consists of the lungs and air passages; responsible for taking in oxygen and removing carbon dioxide.

respiratory therapists (RTs)—Individuals who, under physicians' orders, treat patients with heart and lung diseases by administering oxygen, gases, or medications; using exercise to improve breathing; monitoring ventilators; and performing diagnostic respiratory function tests.

respiratory therapy technicians (RTTs)—Individuals who work under the supervision of respiratory therapists and administer respiratory treatments, perform basic diagnostic tests, clean and maintain equipment, and note and inform therapists of patients' responses and progress.

responsibility—Being held accountable for actions or behaviors; willing to meet obligations.

restoration—Process of replacing a diseased portion of a tooth or a lost tooth by artificial means, including filling materials, crowns, bridges, or dentures.

restraints—Protective devices that limit or restrict movement.

résumé—A summary of a person's work history and experience, submitted when applying for a job.

retina—The sensory membrane that lines the eye and is the immediate instrument of vision.

retractors—Instruments used to hold or draw back the lips or sides of a wound or incision.

rheostats—Foot controls in dental units; used to operate handpieces.

rhythm—Referring to regularity; regular or irregular.

ribs—Also called *costae*; 12 pairs of narrow, curved bones that surround the thoracic cavity.

rickettsiae—Parasitic microorganisms that live on other living organisms.

right atrium—One of the four chambers of the heart; receives blood as it returns from the body cells.

right lymphatic duct—Part of the lymphatic system; the short tube that receives all of the purified lymph from the right side of the head and neck, the right chest, and the right arm.

right to die—A legal right under the Patient Self-Determination Act that allows an individual to determine whether or not to accept medical care to continue life.

right ventricle—One of the four chambers of the heart; receives blood from the right atrium and pumps the blood into the pulmonary artery, which carries the blood to the lungs for oxygen.

robotic surgery—Performing surgery with a mechanical device that is computer controlled.

Roman numerals—Symbols in the old Roman notation that represent numbers.

root—The anatomic portion of a tooth that is below the gingiva (gums); helps hold the tooth in the mouth.

rotation—Movement around a central axis; a turning.

rounding numbers—Changing numbers to the nearest ten, hundred, thousand, and so on.

S

safety—Needs that are important when physiological needs have been met; include the need to be free from anxiety and fear, and the need to feel secure in the environment.

Safety Data Sheet (SDS)—Information sheet that must be provided by the manufacturer for all hazardous products.

safety standards—Set of rules designed to protect both the patient and the health care worker.

sagittal plane—Imaginary line that divides the body into left and right sections.

saliva ejector—Handpiece in dental units that provides a constant, low-volume suction to remove saliva and fluids from the mouth.

salivary glands—Glands of the mouth that produce saliva, a digestive secretion.

salutation—A greeting; the greeting in a letter (for example, "Dear").

satisfaction—Fulfillment or gratification of a desire or need.

scalpels—Instruments with a knife blades used to incise (cut) skin and tissue.

scapula—Shoulder blade or bone.

school health services—Provide emergency care for victims of accidents and sudden illness; perform tests to check for health conditions such as speech, vision, and hearing problems; promote health education; and maintain a safe and sanitary school environment. Many school health services also provide counseling.

sclera—White outer coat of the eye.

scope of practice—The procedures, processes and actions that health care providers are legally permitted to perform in keeping with the terms of their professional license.

screen—To evaluate; to determine the purpose of telephone calls so they can be referred to the correct person.

scrotum—Double pouch containing the testes and epididymis in the male individual.

search engine—Computer program designed to locate specific information on the Internet.

sebaceous gland—Oil-secreting gland of the skin.

self-actualization—Achieving one's full potential.

self-motivation—Ability to begin or to follow through with a task without the assistance of others.

semicircular canals—Structures of the inner ear that are involved in maintaining balance and equilibrium.

seminal vesicle—One of two saclike structures behind the bladder and connected to the vas deferens in the male individual; secretes thick, viscous fluid for semen.

senile lentigines—Dark-yellow or brown spots that develop on the skin as aging occurs.

sensitive—Susceptible to a substance; organisms that are affected by an antibiotic in a culture and sensitivity study.

sensitivity—Ability to recognize and appreciate the personal characteristics of others.

septum—Membranous wall that divides two cavities.

sequential compression device (SCD)—A device that continually inflates and deflates compression hose on the legs to stimulate circulation in the legs.

sexuality—Sexual life and experience; people's feelings concerning their masculine/feminine natures, their ability to give and receive love and affection, and their roles in reproduction of the species.

shock—Clinical condition characterized by various symptoms and resulting in an inadequate supply of blood and oxygen to body organs, especially the brain and heart.

sigmoidoscope—Instrument used to examine the sigmoid, or S-shaped, section of the large intestine.

sign—Objective evidence of disease; something that is seen.

signature—A person's name written by that person.

silicone—An impression material, usually polysiloxane or polyvinylsiloxane, used to take impressions of the teeth and or dental arches.

Sims'—The patient lies on his or her left side with the right leg bent up near the abdomen.

sinus—Cavity or air space in a bone.

Sitz baths—Special baths given to apply moist heat to the genital or rectal area.

skeletal muscle—Type of muscle that is attached to bones and causes body movement.

skeletal system—Bodily system made up of bones.

skin puncture—A small puncture made in the skin to obtain capillary blood.

small intestine—That section of the intestine that is between the stomach and large intestine; site of most absorption of nutrients.

Snellen charts—Special charts that use letters or symbols in calibrated heights to check visual acuity.

social—Pertaining to relationships with others.

social workers (SWs)—Individuals who assist patients who have difficulty coping with various problems by helping them make adjustments in their lives and/or referring them to community resources for assistance.

sodium-restricted diets—Special diets containing low or limited amounts of sodium (salt).

soft diet—Special diet containing only foods that are soft in texture.

somatic nervous system—A main division of the nervous system; carries messages between the CNS and the body.

soft palate—Tissue at the back of the roof of the mouth; separates the mouth from the nasopharynx.

specific gravity—Weight or mass of a substance compared with an equal amount of another substance that is used as a standard.

speculum—Instrument used to dilate, or enlarge, an opening or passage in the body for examination purposes.

speech–language pathologists—Individuals who identify, evaluate, and treat patients with speech and language disorders; also *called speech therapists* or *speech scientists*.

sphygmomanometer—Instrument calibrated for measuring blood pressure in millimeters of mercury (mm Hg).

spinal cavity—Section of the dorsal cavity that contains the spinal cord.

spinal cord—A column of nervous tissue extending from the medulla oblongata of the brain to the second lumbar vertebra in the vertebral column.

spiritual—The beliefs and practices of an individual; spiritual needs are an important aspect of care.

spirituality—Individualized and personal set of beliefs and practices that evolve and change throughout an individual's life.

spleen—Ductless gland below the diaphragm and in the upper-left quadrant of the abdomen; serves to form, store, and filter blood.

splinter forceps—Instruments with sharp points used to remove splinters and foreign objects from the skin and/or tissues.

sprain—Injury to a joint accompanied by stretching or tearing of the ligaments.

spreadsheet—A computer document created by special software that is used to access a computer's ability to perform high-speed math functions.

standard precautions—Recommendations that must be followed to prevent transmission of pathogenic organisms by way of blood and body fluids.

statement–receipt—Financial form that shows charges, amounts paid, and balance due.

statistical data sheets—A form that contains patient demographics; usually completed on a patient's first visit to an office or health agency.

stem cells—Cells that are capable of becoming any of the specialized cells in the body; two main types include embryonic stem cells from a developing fetus and somatic or adult stem cells.

stereotyping—Process of assuming that everyone in a particular group is the same.

sterile—Free of all organisms, including spores and viruses.

sterile field—An area that is set up for certain procedures and is free from all organisms.

sterilization—Process that results in total destruction of all microorganisms; also, surgical procedure that prevents conception of a child.

sternum—Breastbone.

stethoscope—Instrument used for listening to internal body sounds.

stoma—The opening of an ostomy on the abdominal wall.

stomach—Enlarged section of the alimentary canal, between the esophagus and the small intestine; serves as an organ of digestion.

stone—A gypsum material used to form dental models.

stool specimen—Feces specimen examined by the laboratory, usually to check for ova and parasites or the presence of fats, microorganisms, and other abnormal substances.

strain—Injury caused by excessive stretching, overuse, or misuse of a muscle.

stress—Body's reaction to any stimulus that requires a person to adjust to a changing environment.

stress test—An electrocardiogram (ECG) that is obtained while the patient is exercising or after the patient has been given medication to create a heart response similar to active exercise.

stroke—*See* **cerebrovascular accident**.

subcutaneous—Beneath the skin.

subcutaneous fascia (hypodermis)—Layer of tissue that is under the skin and connects the skin to muscles and underlying tissues.

subject line—Part of letter referencing the reason for writing.

sudoriferous gland—Sweat-secreting gland of the skin.

suffix—An affix attached to the end of a word.

suicide—Killing oneself.

superficial—Term that relates to structures within the body; indicates that the structures are located near the body surface.

superior—Above, on top of, or higher than.

supination—Turning a body part upward; turning "palm up."

supine—The patient lies flat on the back, face upward.

suppression—Defense mechanism used by an individual who is aware of unacceptable feelings or thoughts but refuses to deal with them.

surgical (elastic) hose—Elastic or support hose used to support leg veins and increase circulation.

surgical scissors—Special scissors used to cut tissue.

surgical technologists technicians (STs)—Individuals who, working under the supervision of RNs or physicians, prepare patients for surgery; set up instruments, equipment, and sterile supplies in the operating room; and assist during surgery by passing instruments and supplies to the surgeon; also called *operating room technicians*.

susceptible host—A person likely to get an infection or disease, usually because body defenses are weak.

suture—Surgical stitch used to join the edges of an incision or wound; also, an area where bones join or fuse together.

suture-removal set—Set of instruments, including suture scissors and thumb forceps, used to remove stitches (sutures).

sympathetic—That division of the autonomic nervous system that allows the body to respond to emergencies and stress; also, to understand and attempt to solve the problems of another.

system—A group of organs and other parts that work together to perform a certain function.

systole—Period of work, or contraction, of the heart.

systolic—Measurement of blood pressure taken when the heart is contracting and forcing blood into the arteries.

T

tachycardia—Fast, or rapid, heartbeat (usually more than 100 beats per minute in an adult).

tachypnea—Respiratory rate above 25 respirations per minute.

tact—Having the ability to say or do the kindest or most fitting thing in a difficult situation.

tarsal—One of seven bones that forms the instep of the foot.

team player—A personal/professional characteristic required in health care careers; working well with others.

teamwork—Cooperative effort by the members of a group to achieve a common goal.

technology—Applying scientific knowledge for practical purposes to find answers and fix problems.

teeth—Structures in the mouth that physically break down food by chewing and grinding.

telemedicine—The use of video, audio, and computer systems to provide medical and/or health care services.

telepharmacies—The use of video, audio, and computer systems to manage and dispense medications.

temperature—The measurement of the balance between heat lost and heat produced by the body.

temporal scanning thermometers—Specialized electronic thermometers that use an infrared scanner to measure the temperature in the temporal artery of the forehead.

temporal temperature—Measurement of body temperature at the temporal artery on the forehead.

temporary—Dental material used for restorative purposes for a short period of time until permanent restoration can be done.

tendon—Fibrous connective tissue that connects muscles to bones.

tension—Uncomfortable inner sensation, discomfort, strain, or stress that affects the mind.

terminal illness—An illness that will result in death.

testes—Gonads or endocrine glands that are located in the scrotum of the male and that produce sperm and male hormones.

thalamus—That structure in the diencephalon of the brain that acts as a relay center to direct sensory impulses to the cerebrum.

The Joint Commission (TJC)—A nonprofit, U.S.-based organization that was created to ensure that patients receive the safest, highest quality care in any health care setting.

therapeutic diets—Diets used in the treatment of disease.

thermal blankets—Special blankets which contain coils that can be filled with air or fluid to warm or cool a patient's body.

thermotherapy—Use of heat applications for treatment.

thoracic cavity—Section of the ventral cavity located in the chest that contains the esophagus, trachea, bronchi, lungs, heart, and large blood vessels.

thoracic duct—Main lymph duct of the body; drains lymph from the lymphatic vessels into the left subclavian vein.

thrombocyte—Also called a *platelet*; blood cell required for clotting of the blood.

thrombus—A blood clot.

thymus—Organ in the upper part of the chest, lymphatic tissue and endocrine gland that atrophies at puberty.

thyroid gland—Endocrine gland that is located in the neck and regulates body metabolism.

time management—System of practical skills that allows an individual to use time in the most effective and productive way.

tissue—A group of similar cells that join together to perform a particular function.

tissue forceps—An instrument with one or more fine points (teeth) at the tips of blades; used to grasp tissue.

tongue—Muscular organ of the mouth; aids in speech, swallowing, and taste.

tongue blade/depressor—A wood or plastic stick used to depress the tongue so the throat can be examined.

tonsil—Mass of lymphatic tissue found in the pharynx (throat) and mouth.

tort—A wrongful or illegal act of civil law not involving a contract.

towel clamps—Instruments with pointed ends that lock together; used to attach surgical drapes to each other and/or clamp dissected tissue.

toxicologists—Individuals who design, plan, and conduct experiments and trials to study the safety and biological effects of chemical agents, drugs, and other substances on the body.

trachea—Windpipe; air tube from the larynx to the bronchi.

transcribe—Put a word and/or its meaning in written form.

transcultural health care—Health care based on the cultural beliefs, emotional needs, spiritual feelings, and physical needs of a person.

transfer (gait) belt—Band of fabric or leather that is placed around a patient's waist; grasped by the health care worker during transfer or ambulation to provide additional support for the patient.

transient ischemic attacks (TIAs)—A brief episode that disrupts the blood flow to the brain and causes the same symptoms as a cerebrovascular accident or stroke; frequently called a *ministroke*.

transmission-based precautions—Methods or techniques of caring for patients who have communicable diseases.

transport technicians—Individuals who transport patients by assisting them to move in and out of vehicles, ambulances, and helicopters.

transverse plane—Imaginary line drawn through the body to separate the body into a top half and a bottom half.

Trendelenburg—The patient lies on the back with the head lower than the feet, or with both the head and feet inclined downward.

triage—A method of prioritizing treatment.

TRICARE—The U.S. government health insurance plan for all military personnel.

tricuspid valve—Flap or cusp between the right atrium and right ventricle in the heart.

tri-flow (air-water) syringe—Handpiece in dental units that provides air, water, or a combination of air and water for various dental procedures.

trifurcated—Having three roots (as do some teeth).

tuning fork—An instrument that has two prongs and is used to test hearing acuity.

24-hour urine specimen—Special urine test in which all urine produced in a 24-hour period is collected in a special container.

tympanic membrane—The eardrum.

tympanic thermometers—Specialized electronic thermometers that use an infrared ray to record the aural temperature in the ear.

typing and crossmatch—A determination of blood types and antigens prior to a blood transfusion.

U

ulcer—An open lesion on the skin or mucous membrane.

ulna—Long bone in the forearm, between the wrist and elbow.

ultrasonic units—Pieces of equipment that clean using sound waves.

ultrasonography—Noninvasive, computerized scanning technique that uses high-frequency sound waves to create pictures of body parts.

underweight—A body weight that is 10–15 percent less than the desired weight, or a BMI less than 18.5.

unilateral—Affecting only one side.

uninterrupted power supply (UPS)—A device that provides battery backup when the electrical power fails or drops to an unacceptable voltage level.

Universal/National Numbering System—Abbreviated means of identifying the teeth.

ureter—Tube that carries urine from the kidney to the urinary bladder.

ureterostomy—Formation of an opening on the abdominal wall for drainage of urine from a ureter.

urethra—Tube that carries urine from the urinary bladder to outside the body.

urinalysis—Examination of urine by way of physical, chemical, or microscopic testing.

urinary-drainage unit—Special device used to collect urine and consisting of tubing and a collection container usually connected to a urinary catheter.

urinary meatus—External opening of the urethra.

urinary sediment—Solid material suspended in urine.

urinary system—Body system responsible for removing certain wastes and excess water from the body and for maintaining the body's acid–base or pH balance; *see also* **excretory system**

urinate—To expel urine from the bladder.

urine—The fluid excreted by the kidney.

urine specimen—Common specimen, used for a variety of laboratory tests such as urinalysis.

urinometer—Calibrated device used to measure the specific gravity of urine.

U.S. Department of Health and Human Services (USDHHS)—A national agency that deals with the health problems in the United States; its goal is to protect the health of all Americans, especially those people who are in need; provides more grant money than any other federal agency.

uterus—Muscular, hollow organ that serves as the organ of menstruation and the area for development of the fetus in the female body.

V

vacuoles—Pouchlike structures found throughout the cytoplasm that have a vacuolar membrane with the same structure as the cell membrane.

vagina—Tube from the uterus to outside the body in a female individual.

value-based compensation—A health payment plan in which doctors and providers are paid a certain amount for each diagnosis or disease regardless of the number of services provided.

variable expenses—In a budget, an expenses that can change or be adjusted (for example, expenses for clothing and entertainment).

vas (ductus) deferens—Also called the *ductus deferens*; the tube that carries sperm and semen from the epididymis to the ejaculatory duct in the male body.

vasoconstriction—Constriction (decrease in diameter) of the blood vessels.

vasodilation—Dilation (increase in diameter) of the blood vessels.

vein—Blood vessel that carries blood back to the heart.

venipuncture—Surgical puncture of a vein; inserting a needle into a vein.

ventilation—Process of breathing.

ventral cavities—Body cavities separated into two distinct cavities (thoracic and abdominal cavities) by the diaphragm.

ventricle—One of two lower chambers of the heart; also, a cavity in the brain.

vermiform appendix—A small projection of the cecum, part of the large intestine.

vertebrae—Bones of the spinal column.

vesicle—Blister; a sac full of water or tissue fluid.

vestibule—Small space or cavity at the beginning of a canal.

villi—Tiny projections from a surface; in the small intestine, projections that aid in the absorption of nutrients.

Veteran's Administration—A federal agency that provides health care for veterans and their families; also is America's largest integrated health care system, providing care at hospitals, medical centers and outpatient sites serving 9 million enrolled veterans each year.

veterinarians (DVMs or VMDs)—Individuals who work to prevent, diagnose, and treat diseases and injuries in animals.

veterinary assistants—Individuals who feed, bathe, and groom animals; exercise animals; prepare animals for treatment; assist with examinations; clean and sanitize cages, examination tables, and surgical areas; and maintain records; also called *animal caretakers*.

veterinary technologists/technicians (VTs)—Individuals who, working under the supervision of veterinarians, assist with the handling and care of animals, collect specimens, assist with surgery, perform laboratory tests, take and develop radiographs, administer prescribed treatments, and maintain records; also called *animal health technicians*.

virtual learning—An online teaching and learning environment that uses computers and the Internet to allow teachers to present information and activities and, at times, even engage and interact with students.

viruses—Programs that contain instructions to alter the operation of computer programs, erase or scramble data on the computer, and/or allow access to information on the computer.

visceral (smooth) muscle—Type of muscle that is found in the internal organs of the body; contracts to cause movement in these organs.

visual acuity—Ability to perceive and comprehend light rays; seeing.

vital signs—Determinations that provide information about body conditions; include temperature, pulse, respirations, and blood pressure.

vitamins—Organic substances necessary for body processes and life.

vitreous humor—Jelly-like mass that fills the cavity of the eyeball, behind the lens.

voice mail—A common feature of most ARU systems; if the individual is not available, the caller is instructed to leave a message and/or directed to contact another person.

void—To empty the bladder; urinate.

volume—The degree of strength of a pulse (for example, strong or weak).

voluntary—Under one's control; done by one's choice or desire.

voluntary agencies—Agencies supported by donations, membership fees, fundraisers, and federal or state grants. They provide health services at the national, state, and local levels; *see also* **nonprofit agencies**.

vulva—External female genitalia; includes the labia majora, labia minora, and clitoris.

W

walker—A device that has a metal framework and aids in walking.

warm-water bags—Rubber or plastic devices designed to hold warm water for dry-heat application.

wellness—State of being in good health; well.

wheals—Itchy, elevated areas with an irregular shape.

wheezing—Difficult breathing with a high-pitched whistling or sighing sound during expiration.

whole numbers—Numbers that are traditionally used to count (1, 2, 3, ...); they do not contain fractions.

willingness to learn—A personal/professional characteristic required in health care careers; adaptability to changes and preparedness to pursue additional education required to remain competent in a particular field.

withdrawal—Defense mechanism in which an individual either ceases to communicate or physically removes self from a situation.

word roots—Main words or parts of words to which prefixes and suffixes can be added.

workers' compensation—Payment and care provided to an individual who is injured on the job.

World Health Organization (WHO)—An international agency sponsored by the United Nations and concerned with compiling statistics and information on disease and addressing serious health problems throughout the world.

wound—An injury to tissues.

wound VAC—A medical device that applies negative pressure to a wound to promote healing and prevent infections.

Y

yellow marrow—Soft tissue in the diaphysis of long bones.

Pulse deficit, 489
Pulse oximeters, 341, 483
Pulse pressure, 491
Puncture, 520
Pupil, 188
Pyelonephritis, 225
Pyrexia, 470

Q

Quality control technicians, 77

R

Race, 293. *See also* Cultural diversity
Radiation exposure, 391
Radiation hazards, 391–392
Radiation therapists, 69
Radiation therapy, 339
Radiographers, 69
Radiologic technologists (RTs), 69
Radiolucent, 664
Radiopaque, 664
Rales, 485
Range-of-motion (ROM) exercises, 904–913
Rapamune, 38
Rapid identification test kits, 680
Rate, pulse, 468, 483
Rate, respirations, 485
Rationalization, 265
Ratios, 363
Reality orientation (RO), 284
Recall letter, 961
Receipt, record, 978, 982
Reciprocal fractions, 360
Record. *See* Medical record
Recreational therapists (TRs), 63
Recreational therapy assistants, 64
Rectal temperatures, 470, 477–478
Rectum, 217
Red blood cells (RBCs), 708, 711
  blood film or smear, 700
Red marrow, 168
Reflexology, 21
Refractometer, 721
Refracts, 188
Registered nurses (RNs), 58
Registration, 45
Regression, 266
Regular diet, 323
Rehabilitation clinics, 30
Rehabilitation facilities, 31
Reiki, 21
Religion, 299–304
Renal calculus, 225–226
Renal failure, 226
Renal pelvis, 224
Repression, 265–266
Reproductive system, 278–279
  female reproductive system, 237–241
  male reproductive system, 234–236
  sexually transmitted infections, 242–243
Reservoir, defined, 411
Resident's Bill of Rights, 118
Respirations, 209, 468, 485–486
Respiratory shock, 525
Respiratory system, 276

diseases and abnormal conditions, 210–213
process of breathing, 209
respiratory organs and structures, 207–209
stages of respiration, 209–210
Respiratory therapists (RTs), 64
Respiratory therapy technicians (RTTs), 64
Restoration, definition of, 660
Restraints, 876–882
Résumé, 571–577
  credentials, 573
  educational background, 572
  employment objective, job desired, or
    career goal, 571
  with information centered, 573
  with left margin highligts, 574
  other activities, 573
  personal identification, 571
  references, 574
  skills, 572–573
  work or employment experience, 572
Retina, 188
Retirement, 280
Retractors, 759
Reverse isolation, 454
Rheostats, 613
Rhinitis, 212
Rh negative, 704
RhoGAM injection, 705
Rh positive, 704
Rh system, 704
Rhythm, pulse, 468, 483
Rickettsiae, 408
Right lymphatic duct, 205
Robotic surgery, 338
Rod of Asclepius, 4–5
Roller gauze bandages, 557, 558
Roman Catholic, 303
Roman numerals, 366
Rongeur forceps, 623
Root, 593
Root canal, 594
Root (extraction) elevator, 622, 623
Root-tip pick, 622, 623
Rotation, 176
Rounding numbers, 363
Routine stool specimen, 868, 873–874
Routine urine specimen, 866–867, 869–870
Rubber-base, 632
Rule of nines, 532, 533
Ruptured disk, 173
Russian Orthodox, 303

S

Safety
  accidents, preventing, 382–397
  bloodborne pathogen standard, 391
  body mechanics, 380–382
  chemical hazards, 382–391
  environmental, 391–396
  equipment, 392–393
  fire, 397–400
  injuries, preventing, 382–397
  patient/resident, 393–395
  personal safety, 395–396
  physiological needs, 263

solutions, 392–393
  standards, 382
Safety Data Sheets (SDSs), 382–390
Saliva ejector, 613
Salivary glands, 215
SARS (severe acute respiratory syndrome), 408
Saturated fats, 311
Scalers, 619, 620
Scalpels, 759
Scope of practice, 45
Scrotum, 234
Search engines, 347
Sedation, 647–648
Sediment, 724
Sedimentation rate, 708
Sediplast Westergren method, 710
Sed rate, 708
Seizure, first aid, 553
Self-actualization, 264
Self-curing composite, 662
Semicircular canals, 192
Seminal vesicles, 234
Semi-solid medications, 776–777
Senile lentigines, 275
Sensitivity, personal, 293
Septic shock, 525
Sequential compression devices (SCDs), 885
Seventh Day Adventist, 303
Severe acute respiratory syndrome (SARS), 408, 450
Severe full-thickness burns, first aid, 533
Severe partial-thickness burns, first aid, 533
Sexual abuse, 111
Sexuality, physiological needs, 263
Sexually transmitted infections, 242–243
  chlamydia, 242
  gonorrhea, 242
  herpes, 242
  pubic lice, 242
  syphilis, 242
  trichomoniasis, 243
Shaving, 823, 832–834
Shingles, 187
Shock
  causes of, 524
  definition of, 524
  first aid, 524–527
  signs and symptoms, 524
  treatment for, 525
  types of, 525
Shower, 821, 840–842
Side or interproximal surface, of tooth, 628
Sigmoidoscope, 752
Silicone, 632–633
Sims' (Left Lateral), patient position, 741
Sinuses, 169, 208
Sinusitis, 212
Sitz baths, 926
Skeletal muscle, 175
Skeletal system
  bone of, 171
  defined, 167
  diseases and abnormal conditions, 171–172
  joints, 170
Skills-USA, 987–988
Skin, 193
SkinGun, for burns treatment, 563